Caring for Adolescent Patients

●●●●●● 2ND EDITION ●●●●●●

Section on Adolescent Health
American Academy of Pediatrics

Cynthia B. Aten, MD, FAAP
Edward M. Gotlieb, MD, FAAP, FSAM
Editors

American Academy of Pediatrics
141 Northwest Point Blvd
Elk Grove Village, IL 60007-1098

American Academy of Pediatrics Department of Marketing and Publications Staff

Maureen DeRosa, MPA
Director, Department of Marketing and Publications

Mark Grimes
Director, Division of Product Development

Diane E. Beausoleil
Senior Product Development Editor

Holly Kaminski
Coordinator, Product Development

Sandi King, MS
Director, Division of Publishing and Production Services

Kate Larson
Manager, Editorial Services

Jason Crase
Editorial Specialist

Theresa Wiener
Manager, Editorial Production

Leesa Levin-Doroba
Manager, Print Production Services

Linda Diamond
Manager, Graphic Design

Peg Mulcahy
Graphic Designer

Jill Ferguson
Director, Division of Marketing and Sales

Linda Smessaert
Manager, Publication and Program Marketing

2nd edition
1st edition, 1994 (published as *Practicing Adolescent Medicine: A Collection of Resources*)

Library of Congress Control Number: 2004101688
ISBN-10: 1-58110-135-X
ISBN-13: 978-1-58110-135-5
MA0279

The recommendations in this publication do not indicate an exclusive course of treatment or serve as a standard of medical care. Variations, taking into account individual circumstances, may be appropriate.

9-132/0905

1 2 3 4 5 6 7 8 9 10

SECTION ON ADOLESCENT HEALTH 2005–2006 EXECUTIVE COMMITTEE

Richard B. Heyman, MD, FAAP, Chairperson

Cynthia B. Aten, MD, FAAP

Margaret J. Blythe, MD, FAAP

Melanie A. Gold, DO, FAAP

Janice Dixon Key, MD, FAAP

Kathryn Love-Osborne, MD, FAAP

D. Paul Robinson, MD, FAAP

Lisa Kessler Tuchman, MD, MPH

Staff

Karen Smith

For information on joining the Section on Adolescent Health, visit www.aap.org/sections/adol.

Table of Contents

Introduction

The book you are holding is a collection of resources taken from publications of the American Academy of Pediatrics (AAP). It has been created at the urging of the Executive Committee of the Section on Adolescent Health (SOAH) of the AAP as a part of its ongoing efforts to increase its educational offerings to section members and all AAP members.

When this project was suggested at an Executive Committee meeting in the fall of 2002, one of us (Cynthia B. Aten, MD, FAAP) agreed to take on the task provided the other one of us (Edward M. Gotlieb, MD, FAAP, FSAM) would agree to join the effort. Dr Gotlieb edited the original manual produced by the SOAH Executive Committee, *Practicing Adolescent Medicine: A Collection of Resources* (1994), which remains a highly useful reference. Some of the articles in that book are timeless, with plenty of wisdom for today's practitioners. However, all of the articles are more than 10 years old, and it was deemed time to produce an updated collection of resources—enter your editors.

There has been a substantial change in focus in the current book from the earlier publication. *Practicing Adolescent Medicine* was primarily intended as a challenge to pediatricians to overcome perceived barriers to caring for adolescents. At that time, specialists in fields other than pediatrics provided the vast number of adolescent medical visits, and most AAP publications on adolescents came only from the Committee on Adolescence or SOAH. Today, the following 3 changes have occurred:

1. A major shift in the care of adolescents toward pediatricians and mid-level pediatric providers
2. The development of sub-boards in adolescent medicine and expanded training programs, which are producing a highly trained but small group of specialist pediatricians who cannot possibly provide all adolescents with care
3. A much more extensive collection of published materials about adolescent issues across many AAP committees, councils, sections, and task forces

This new publication, therefore, no longer needs to encourage pediatricians to provide care for adolescents; they are doing it. Rather, it needs to bring under one cover some of the many AAP adolescent resources for the busy practitioner to turn to in the heat of battle.

Our goal was to gather a practical compendium of AAP materials pertaining to adolescent health and medical care. We combed through *Adolescent Health Update, Pediatrics®, Pediatrics in Review®, AAP News,* and SOAH newsletters to gather resources and were delighted with the wealth we found. We have included references to other useful articles, particularly those in the SOAH journal, *Adolescent Medicine Clinics* (formerly known as *Adolescent Medicine: State of the Art Reviews,* before its purchase by Elsevier). Current policy statements from the Committee on Adolescence and Committee on Substance Abuse are included in the appropriate sections of the book. Policy statements from other AAP committees are referenced if they seemed especially useful for the care of adolescents.

Inevitably with the passage of time and the publication of new research, certain things in this manual will lose their timeliness. To keep the materials associated with this publication fresh, SOAH plans to post updates on these and new topics of interest on its Web site, www.aap.org/sections/adol. There, we also hope to include questionnaires, patient and parent handouts contributed by section members, and other materials that did not fit within the space limitations of this book.

Our thanks go to Diane Beausoleil in the AAP Department of Marketing and Publications for her many contributions and good-humored forbearance and guidance through the creation of this manual. Much assistance and support came from the AAP SOAH staff people, Tammy Hurley and Karen Smith; thanks, you capable and terrific women.

We also thank the members of the SOAH Executive Committee during the book's development— Melanie A. Gold, DO, FAAP; Margaret J. Blythe, MD, FAAP; Kathryn Love-Osborne, MD, FAAP; D. Paul Robinson, MD, FAAP; Janice Dixon Key, MD, FAAP; and Robert M. Cavanaugh, MD, FAAP.

They gave generously of their time and expertise in reviewing the contents, though the responsibility for the outcome rests entirely with your editors.

The chairs of the SOAH Executive Committee during the book's preparation, Jennifer Johnson, MD, FAAP, and her successor, Richard B. Heyman, MD, FAAP, provided enthusiastic support and when necessary, reality checks to our endeavors.

May you find these pages useful.

Cynthia B. Aten, MD, FAAP   cynthiaaten@earthlink.net

Edward M. Gotlieb, MD, FAAP, FSAM   edward.gotlieb@emory.edu

Advice for Treating Children With Antidepressants

Lynn Wegner, M.D., FAAP, chair of the AAP Section on Developmental and Behavioral Pediatrics, offers the following advice to clinicians treating pediatric patients who are considering or are currently taking antidepressants. The following suggestions are not approved AAP policy. The Academy is working with the American Psychiatric Association, American Academy of Child and Adolescent Psychiatry and the American Academy of Family Physicians to develop a joint advisory that will be issued to pediatricians and other physicians in the next several months.

Before You Prescribe

- Depression is characterized by both internalizing symptoms expressed by the child (e.g., mood, feeling of guilt, being criticized by others) and externalizing symptoms observed by parents and teachers (withdrawal, irritability, and changes in appetite and sleep). Once symptoms have been identified, physicians should verify the symptoms are sustained, neurovegetative and interfere with several domains of functioning (poor sleep, appetite).

- When providing a full suicide assessment, questions should be asked directly of the child, family members, friends and teachers, if possible. Questions should identify previous self-destructive thoughts and attempts. The child should be asked for all of the "reasons for living" he/she can articulate.

- Provide a complete physical exam to eliminate any confounding/co-morbid physical elements.

- Ask parents/caregivers to remove weapons from the home, particularly guns, and any medications that should not be accessible to the child.

- After discussing with the patient and guardian the risks and benefits of treatment, obtain informed consent for medication use. Physicians should keep a printed form or handwritten/dictated note of informed consent from the guardians and have it clearly documented in the child's medical records. The clinician also should have established a plan with the referral psychiatrist (if available) should self-destructive actions occur to assure timely intervention.

Children on Antidepressant Medications

- Tools such as the Beck Depression Inventory and Children's Depression Inventory-Revised may be used to monitor the child's response to treatment. While rating scales are not definitive for diagnosing depression, they can help guide questions during follow-up monitoring appointments. Suicide should be discussed at each visit. Although the greatest risk appears to be in the first 40 days after diagnosis and medical treatment initiation, the clinician must explore this topic regularly.

As the Academy and other groups formulate appropriate monitoring guidelines for primary care physicians, Dr. Wegner offers the following suggestions, based on her experience:

- *Newly diagnosed children:* Parents and child should have a telephone number where they can reach a clinician 24/7 if they have any concerns about the child appearing more despondent, irritable, etc. The child should be seen in the office approximately weekly for weeks 1–4, then biweekly for the next two months. After 12 weeks, office visits should be every three months or sooner if needed.

- *Children who require dosage changes:* Advise the parents to observe changes in mood/behavior and either have office appointments or telephone confirmation once weekly for one month, then office appointments once every three months.
- *Children on medication 12 weeks or longer:* Children who have been taking antidepressants for 12 weeks or longer and do not require dosage changes should be seen in the office every three months.

For more information on the FDA's decision to provide "black box" warnings on all antidepressant medications, visit www.aapnews.org/cgi/content/full/e2004145v1.

Language of FDA's "Black Box" Warning

SUICIDALITY IN CHILDREN AND ADOLESCENTS

Antidepressants increase the risk of suicidal thinking and behavior (suicidality) in children and adolescents with major depressive disorder (MDD) and other psychiatric disorders. Anyone considering the use of [Drug Name] or any other antidepressant in a child or adolescent must balance this risk with the clinical need. Patients who are started on therapy should be observed closely for clinical worsening, suicidality, or unusual changes in behavior. Families and caregivers should be advised of the need for close observation and communication with the prescriber. [Drug Name] is not approved for use in pediatric patients except for patients with [Any approved pediatric claims here]. (See Warnings and Precautions: Pediatric Use)

Pooled analysis of short-term (4 to 16 weeks) placebo-controlled trials of nine antidepressant drugs (SSRIs and others) in children and adolescents with MDD, obsessive compulsive disorder (OCD), or other psychiatric disorders (a total of 24 trials involving over 4400 patients) have revealed a greater risk of adverse events representing suicidal thinking or behavior (suicidality) during the first few months of treatment in those receiving antidepressants. The average risk of such events on drug was 4%, twice the placebo risk of 2%. No suicides occurred in these trials.

ANTIDEPRESSANTS DRUGS WITH BLACK BOX WARNING LABEL

Anafranil (clomipramine HCl)
Aventyl (nortriptyline HCl)
Celexa (citalopram HBr)
Cymbalta (duloxetine HCl)
Desyrel (trazodone HCl)
Effexor (venlafaxine HCl)
Elavil (amitriptyline HCl)
Lexapro (escitalopram oxalate)
Limbitrol (chlordiazepoxide/amitriptyline)
Ludiomil (Maprotiline HCl)
Luvox (fluvoxamine maleate)
Marplan (isocarboxazid)
Nardil (phenelzine sulfate)
Norpramin (desipramine HCl)
Pamelor (nortriptyline HCl)
Parnate (tranylcypromine sulfate)
Paxil (paroxetine HCl)
Pexeva (paroxetine mesylate)
Prozac (fluoxetine HCl)
Remeron (mirtazapine)
Sarafem (fluoxetine HCl)
Serzone (nefazodone HCl)
Sinequan (doxepin HCl)
Surmontil (trimipramine)
Symbyax (olanzapine/fluoxetine)
Tofranil (imipramine HCl)
Tofranil-PM (imipramine pamoate)
Triavil (Perphenaine/Amitriptyline)
Vivactil (protriptyline HCl)
Wellbutrin (bupropion HCl)
Zoloft (sertraline HCl)
Zyban (bupropion HCl)

www.fda.gov/cder/drug/antidepressants

FDA Calls for Black Box Warnings on Antidepressants

The Food and Drug Administration (FDA) approved recommendations from two advisory committees calling for "black box" warnings on antidepressants that will be used in children.

After a two-day public meeting in September, the committee called for black box warnings, a warning that is used only when the drug poses an extremely serious risk to patients.

Richard Gorman, M.D., FAAP, AAP Committee on Drugs chair, represented the Academy on one of the advisory committees. The Academy has been advocating for strong labeling changes after the FDA's revelation this past summer of a potential link to increased suicide or suicidal thoughts in children on the medication.

The committees voted 15–8 to urge black box warnings and also voted unanimously to extend any warning to all antidepressant medications, not just one. In reaching its decision, the committee heard evidence from FDA officials, researchers and parents. It also used the latest FDA analysis to make its decision, which showed 2% to 3% of children who used the medications experienced suicidal thoughts or behavior that potentially could be linked to their medications. The results are available because of the Best Pharmaceuticals for Children Act, a federal law that encourages pharmaceutical companies to conduct pediatric drug studies.

The committee's call received widespread media attention and has parents and pediatricians asking what next to do for children who experience depression. The committee discussed how the information potentially could impact children who have responded positively to a drug; however the majority of the committee believed that the black box warning was still the best solution. A number of committee members also called for wording in the black box label about both the drug's potential negative effects and lack of efficacy results.

"The committee saw very strong evidence of potential harm; because of that I wanted to see the warning strengthened," Dr. Gorman said. "The controlled clinical trial results as a result of Best Pharmaceuticals failed to show efficacy for any of the drugs except Prozac. This combination of potential adverse effects and no efficacy should give physicians pause when prescribing these medicines."

Although some pediatricians have claimed to stop prescribing these medications to their patients, the advisory committee did not contraindicate the drugs for pediatric use. The committee felt that recommendation could deprive children who have experienced positive results of access to much needed treatments.

The pharmaceutical industry has stated that it will comply with the FDA's call, but it still believes antidepressants for pediatric use can be helpful and supports careful and ongoing patient monitoring. The American Academy of Child and Adolescent Psychiatry (AACAP) spoke out against the FDA advisory committees' recommendation of a black box, saying that such a warning would have too much of a negative effect on children. However, AACAP still is supportive of strengthening warnings but nothing as severe as a black box.

The Academy is supportive of a call to strengthen the warnings and believes that physicians should have all of the relevant information about a drug available to them when making treatment decisions.

For more information, go to www.aap.org/moc, click on federal affairs, or contact Elaine Vining, AAP Department of Federal Affairs, (800) 336-5475, ext. 3005, or evining@aap.org.

Medical Care
for Adolescents

Age Limits of Pediatrics, American Academy of Pediatrics, Council on Child Health, *Pediatrics,* 1972;49:463

Comments by Iris F. Litt, MD

The purview of pediatrics includes the growth, development, and health of the child and therefore begins in the period before birth when conception is apparent. It continues through childhood and adolescence when the growth and developmental processes are generally completed. The responsibility of pediatrics therefore may begin during pregnancy and usually terminates by 21 years of age.[1]

Commentary

Short and concise, yet this Statement developed by the Council on Child Health of the American Academy of Pediatrics (AAP) and published in 1972 had a monumental impact on the health of teenagers, as well as on the practice of pediatrics.

An earlier position of the AAP (1938) had defined the upper limits of pediatric practice to extend "well into adolescence."[2] Although some pediatricians at the time were seeing early adolescents, many chose to discontinue care for patients who were approximately 12 years of age. The age cutoff for admission to hospital pediatric services was 14 years. It is noteworthy that in 1969, the Council on Child Health had been charged with updating this position. What transpired in the 3 years that intervened reflects perceptions about the respective practice domains of the other specialties, as well as changing views about the health of adolescents.

According to those close to the debates that took place, the Statement went forth only after reassurance from the leaders of those other fields that such an extension of the age limits of pediatrics would not be opposed. That views about adolescent health changed over a 30-year period reflects the results of research, as well as the realization that the developmental perspective of the pediatrician would best serve teenagers.

In relationship to this critical Statement, let us consider the five stages of evolution of the field of adolescent medicine over its 40-year history (dating from the time of the establishment of the first training program at the Children's Hospital in Boston, MA, by Dr J. Roswell Gallagher):

1. recognition of the biologic uniqueness of adolescents;
2. recognition of systematic differences among groups of adolescents (based on pubertal stage and timing, gender, ethnicity, chronic illness, etc);
3. recognition of the interaction of psychosocial and biologic factors in determining health of teenagers;
4. recognition that physicians require special skills and orientation to best care for adolescents; and
5. advocacy for special health care needs of adolescents.

Research by pediatricians, as well as our colleagues from other disciplines including psychiatry, psychology, and education, has been primarily responsible for the first three of these stages in evolution of the field. Many publications in *Pediatrics* over the years have advanced our knowledge of these special developmental aspects of teenagers. Among the earliest of these are reports establishing age-appropriate reference

From the Department of Pediatrics, Division of Adolescent Medicine, Stanford University School of Medicine, Stanford, California.

Received for publication Mar 19, 1998; accepted Mar 19, 1998.

Address correspondence to: Iris F. Litt, MD, Department of Pediatrics, Division of Adolescent Medicine, Stanford University School of Medicine, 750 Welch Rd, Suite 325, Palo Alto, CA 94304.

standards for growth[3-6]; and consideration of gender-based health problems more common in adolescents than in either children or adults.[7]

Attention of pediatricians to the psychosocial needs of this age group is to be found in publications in *Pediatrics* in the late 1950s. McClendon,[8] Deisher and O'Leary,[9] Milman,[10] and Salber,[11] for example, focused on delinquency, school phobia, and smoking, respectively.

It appears that the fourth of these stages—recognition of the special skills needed for care of teenagers—coincides with the time of publication of this Statement by the AAP. It legitimized care of adolescents by pediatricians, and to some, had the force of a mandate to pediatricians to do so. Not all pediatricians, however (especially those trained in more traditional programs focusing on infant care and infectious diseases), felt comfortable and knowledgeable in the care of teenagers. In response to the sense among many pediatricians that they were ill-equipped to meet the special needs of teenagers, the AAP undertook a major effort to provide continuing medical education to provide the needed skills. The resultant increase in interest and expertise in the care of adolescents by pediatricians is, perhaps, the most important legacy of this publication.

In recent discussions with some of my colleagues who were already working with teenagers, including Drs Deisher and Rauh, we recall that at the time we felt that this publication legitimized what we had been doing. Of great importance, it also led to increased resources and space within academic pediatric departments. This occurred at a time when federal monies available for hospital construction supported the building of inpatient units for adolescent patients.

The most valuable result of this redefinition of the age limits of pediatrics was, undoubtedly, the opportunity to teach a growing number of trainees interested in adolescents. The creation of the Section on Adolescence by the AAP also was an outgrowth of the recognition of the need for continuing medical education of pediatricians in practice. Because the Society for Adolescent Medicine had been formed in 1968, primarily by pediatricians and a few internists, and held its early national scientific meetings in concert with those of the AAP, there was synergy in the training effort.

The impact of publication of this Statement also can be felt in the increasing requirements by the Residency Review Committee for inclusion of formalized training in adolescent medicine in pediatric programs.

Most recently, the force of this statement was felt in the documentation for the need for subspecialty certification in adolescent medicine by the American Board of Pediatrics. The establishment of subspecialty certification ensures that there will be academicians capable of training generalist pediatricians to provide primary care to teenagers. It also is significant that this was a conjoint SubBoard with the American Board of Internal Medicine, paving the way for eventual improvement in management of the transition of health care from adolescent to adult settings as they mature.

The issue of interface with internal medicine was critical in the deliberations that led to the setting of the upper age limit of adolescence at 21 years. According to Sherrel Hammar, MD (personal communication), this reflected acknowledgment of the difficulty faced by teenagers with chronic illnesses in finding appropriate care providers when they reached adulthood. The improved longevity of many of these patients is, happily, leading to efforts to train internists and family practitioners in their care.

Despite the importance of this definitional Statement to the care of teenagers by pediatricians, it is sobering to find that only 7% of office visits to all physicians are by adolescents, despite the fact that they constitute almost 20% of the population. Moreover, more family practitioners than pediatricians are providing the care. The sad reality is that 25 years after this Statement was published, most teenagers still are not getting any care, let alone the care they deserve.

References

1. American Academy of Pediatrics, Council on Child Health. Age limits of pediatrics. *Pediatrics*. 1972;49:463
2. American Academy of Pediatrics. Age limits of pediatrics. *J Pediatr*. 1938;13:127, 266

3. Maresh MM. Growth of heart related to bodily growth during childhood and adolescence. *Pediatrics.* 1948;2:382–404

4. Ferris BG, Whittenberger JL, Gallagher JR. Maximum breathing and vital capacity of male children and adolescents. *Pediatrics.* 1952;9:659–670

5. Reed RB. Patterns of growth in height and weight from birth to eighteen years of age. *Pediatrics.* 1959;24:904–921

6. Burke BS. Caloric and protein intakes of children between one and eighteen years of age. *Pediatrics.* 1959;24:922–940

7. Heald F, Masland R, Sturgis SH, Gallagher JR. Dysmenorrhea in adolescence. *Pediatrics.* 1957;1:121–127

8. McClendon PA. Pediatric care and delinquency. *Pediatrics.* 1957;20:1–3

9. Deisher RW, O'Leary JF. Early medical care of delinquent children. *Pediatrics.* 1960;25:329–336

10. Milman DH. School phobia in older children and adolescents: diagnostic implications and prognosis. *Pediatrics.* 1961;28:462–471

11. Salber EJ. Smoking habits of high school students related to intelligence and achievement. *Pediatrics.* 1962;29:780–787

Improving the Delivery of Adolescent Clinical Preventive Services Through Skills-Based Training

Julie L. Lustig, PhD*; Elizabeth M. Ozer, PhD*; Sally H. Adams, PhD*; Charles J. Wibbelsman, MD‡;
C. Daniel Fuster, MD§; Robert W. Bonar, MD‡; and Charles E. Irwin, Jr, MD*

ABSTRACT. *Objective.* To examine the efficacy of skills-based training workshops on primary care providers' screening and counseling practices with adolescents during routine outpatient well visits.

Design. Sixty-three primary care providers in outpatient pediatric departments within a managed health care organization participated in two 4-hour workshops on clinical preventive services for adolescents. The workshops focused on adolescent health, confidentiality, screening, and anticipatory guidance/brief counseling for 5 risk behaviors including: helmet and seatbelt use, tobacco use, alcohol use, and sexual behavior. A pre/post-test design was used to assess clinicians' screening and counseling practices during the pretraining and post-training periods. Independent adolescent reports of clinicians' practices were obtained from 2 samples of 14- to 16-year-old adolescents immediately after their routine well visit in the outpatient clinics. One sample of adolescents reported during a pretraining period and a separate sample reported during a period after the training.

Results. Adolescent reports indicated that after the training workshops, the average percentage of adolescents screened by their primary care providers increased significantly for seatbelt use (from mean 38% to 56%), helmet use (from mean 27% to 45%), tobacco use (from mean 64% to 76%), alcohol use (from mean 59% to 76%), and sexual behavior (from mean 61% to 75%). Additionally, the average percentage of adolescents offered brief counseling by their clinicians increased significantly after training in the areas of seatbelt use (from mean 36% to 51%), helmet use (from mean 25% to 43%), and sexual behavior (from mean 42% to 58%). Improvement after the training in brief counseling for tobacco use was marginally significant (from mean 60% to 69%) and for alcohol use was not significant, although there was an increase. Clinicians also

significantly increased their discussion of the limits of confidentiality with their adolescent patients after the training workshops (from mean 32% to 45%).

Conclusions. This study offers strong support for the efficacy of skills-based training for primary care providers as a method for increasing screening and counseling practices with adolescents. The present findings suggest that with appropriate skills-based training, practicing clinicians can implement several of the national guidelines that direct them to provide preventive services for multiple behaviors in a routine outpatient visit. Screening and counseling in these visits are important in the early identification, detection, and prevention of behaviors associated with the primary adolescent morbidities and mortalities. Thus, enhancing the delivery of clinical preventive services is an important step in the prevention of untoward health outcomes for youth. *Pediatrics* 2001;107:1100–1107; *primary care, provider training, preventive services, adolescents, risk behavior.*

ABBREVIATIONS. HMO, health maintenance organization; SD, standard deviation; AROV, Adolescent Report of the Visit.

The majority of adolescent morbidity and mortality can be attributed to preventable risk factors.[1] These include unhealthy behaviors such as substance use and abuse, unsafe sexual behavior practices, and risky vehicle use.[2-4] Often, these risky behaviors remain unidentified until an adolescent develops health problems, such as a sexually transmitted disease, that require acute medical care.[1,5-7] Primary care providers for adolescents are in a unique position to screen for

From the *Division of Adolescent Medicine, Department of Pediatrics, School of Medicine, University of California, San Francisco, San Francisco, California; ‡Kaiser Permanente, Northern California, Department of Pediatrics; and §Kaiser Permanente, Southern California, Department of Pediatrics.

This work was presented in part in a plenary session at the annual meeting of the Society for Adolescent Medicine; March 23, 2000; Washington, DC, and at the annual meeting of the Society for Prevention Research; June 1, 2000; Montreal, Quebec.

Received for publication Jul 13, 2000; accepted Oct 4, 2000.

Address correspondence to Julie L. Lustig, PhD, University of California–San Francisco, School of Medicine, Department of Pediatrics, Division of Adolescent Medicine, 3333 California St, Suite 245, Box 0503, San Francisco, CA 94143-0503. E-mail: jlustig@itsa.ucsf.edu

risky behaviors and to provide anticipatory guidance and brief counseling.

To facilitate the provision of preventive services to adolescents, national recommendations have been developed and disseminated as a guide for physicians, including the American Medical Association's *Guidelines for Adolescent Preventive Services,*[8] the Maternal and Child Health Bureau's *Bright Futures,*[9] the American Academy of Pediatrics' *Health Supervision Guidelines,*[10] and the Department of Health and Human Services' *The Clinician's Handbook, Put Prevention Into Practice.*[11] In general, these guidelines recommend that all adolescents have an annual, confidential preventive services visit during which time primary care providers screen, educate, and counsel their adolescent patients on a range of issues that affect adolescent health. However, despite the dissemination of guidelines, evidence that adolescents trust health providers, and findings that adolescents are willing to talk with providers about topics outlined in the guidelines,[12-16] implementation of clinical preventive services remains far below recommended levels.[12,17-20]

Green and colleagues'[21,22] Precede-Proceed model provides a framework that organizes many factors likely to contribute to the low rates of implementation of clinical preventive services. The framework includes predisposing factors (eg, attitudes, knowledge), enabling factors (eg, perceived self-efficacy, skills), and reinforcing factors (eg, positive reinforcement and support) that influence providers' behavior.[21-23] Predisposing factors include the necessary attitudes and motivation to perform a behavior; enabling factors include the competence, skills, and resources necessary to perform the behavior; and reinforcing factors are those that support or reward the behavior.[22,23] Training clinicians in the delivery of preventive services for adolescents may address many of these factors through the provision of education, skills, and opportunities to increase their perceived competence.[24,25] Nevertheless, primary care providers who see adolescent patients have reported insufficient training as the most significant barrier to their delivery of preventive health care to adolescents.[26] Furthermore, there

is a paucity of studies to determine efficacious training intervention approaches, particularly with adolescents.

In a review of interventions to improve practices of health professionals, Oxman and colleagues[24] reported that comprehensive approaches to training that use intrasession practice and rehearsal are more effective than is distribution of materials or didactic sessions alone. However, training interventions often rely on lectures and distribution of materials.[25,27]

Few investigators have evaluated training interventions that use both didactic and interactive methods and focus on clinicians who serve pediatric patients. The limited studies that have been conducted focus on training medical students and residents and typically address only a single category of risky behavior. For example, Klein and colleagues[28] implemented a smoking cessation curriculum for pediatric residents that included didactic seminars and small group exercises. Both residents' self-reports and exit interviews with patients' parents revealed few significant differences in screening and counseling practices between residents who participated in the training and those who did not participate.

Kokotailo and colleagues demonstrated the efficacy of a training program focused on pediatric residents' screening and counseling of adolescent patients regarding alcohol and other drug use. The training included education and role-plays about assessment and interviewing skills. Analysis of videotapes of clinician interviews with confederate patients yielded significant improvement for the intervention group compared with the control group in use of screening techniques and interviewing skills.[29] This study suggests that a more comprehensive approach to training that includes skill enhancement may be an effective method for improving practices of clinicians seeing adolescents. However, this study included only pediatric residents, was limited to a focus on substance use, and relied on analyses of clinician interviews with confederate patients to evaluate clinicians' performance.

As illustrated by these examples, another important limitation to most studies on clinician training is that they focus on a single category of behavior. Given the high rates of covariation among risk behaviors,[5,30-33] and that guidelines recommend screening and counseling in multiple risk areas, it is important to train clinicians to discuss a range of risk behaviors. In addition, it has been shown that discussion of confidentiality and the limits of confidentiality increase disclosure to clinicians about risky behaviors in a medical visit.[34] However, discussion of confidentiality rarely is emphasized in training interventions nor evaluated as an outcome of training.

In 1 recent study, some of these limitations were addressed. Sanci and colleagues[35] evaluated the impact of a 12-hour training program for family physicians on delivery of health care to adolescent patients. Physician self-report and videotapes of simulated patients revealed that physicians improved in their discussion of confidentiality, comfort, and self-perceived knowledge and skill. An important next step is to evaluate the efficacy of training practicing clinicians to screen and counsel on multiple risky behaviors and to use reports from their actual adolescent patients as a measure of clinician behavior in a pediatric visit.

The present study is an evaluation of skills-based training workshops for primary care providers in outpatient pediatric clinics within a health maintenance organization (HMO). The training workshops were a central component of a larger model for implementing clinical preventive services with adolescents in the health care setting, drawing on the Precede-Proceed framework.[21,22,36] The goal of the training workshops was to enhance clinicians' screening and brief counseling of adolescents regarding a set of important risky behaviors and to improve their discussion of confidentiality. Bandura's Social Cognitive Theory[37,38] guided the development of the training workshops, which emphasized knowledge, self-efficacy, and skills. Our primary hypothesis was that clinician screening, counseling, and discussion of confidentiality with adolescents during routine well visits would increase after the provision of skills-based training.

Methods

DESIGN

The present study is a pre-post evaluation of the effectiveness of training workshops to increase clinician screening, counseling, and discussion of confidentiality practices with adolescent patients during routine physical examination visits. Independent adolescent reports of clinician screening and counseling practices were obtained from 2 separate groups of adolescents who attended well-visits with their clinicians: 1 group during a pretraining baseline period and the second after the training during the posttraining period. The independent reports completed by adolescents during each of the time periods served as the basis of the analyses of change in clinician practices from the pretraining to the posttraining period. All procedures were approved by the internal review boards at the University of California, San Francisco and the participating HMO.

CLINICIAN PARTICIPANTS

We conducted training workshops in 3 outpatient pediatric clinics within a large group model HMO. These clinics were selected based on their provision of care to large numbers of adolescents (eg, ≥3000 visits per year of 14-year-old patients) and their agreement to be part of a longitudinal study on clinical preventive services with adolescents. In addition, because of an interest in studying general pediatric care, we selected general pediatric clinics that did not have separate active teen clinics within them. Seventy-nine clinicians from the 3 outpatient pediatric clinics were invited to attend the training workshops. All 79 clinicians signed informed consent forms indicating their agreement to attend the training sessions and participate in the study. The chiefs of pediatrics for each clinic encouraged and facilitated clinician attendance. The clinicians were released from their regular clinic schedules, and the HMO was reimbursed for the clinicians' release time by study funds. The clinicians also received continuing medical education credits. Seventy-five (95%) clinicians participated in the workshops, and the remaining 4 had previous commitments (eg, vacations, maternity leave) and were trained at a later date.

The analyses presented here include clinicians who attended the scheduled training workshops and who saw at least 1 adolescent study patient before the training and 1 adolescent study patient after the training, resulting in a final N of 63 clinicians. Eighty-four percent of the 63 clinicians were pediatricians, and 16% were nurse practitioners. Sixty-two percent of all clinicians were female. The average number of years since training was 17 (standard deviation [SD] 6.2; range: 2-37) and none of the clinicians were board-certified in adolescent medicine.

ASSESSMENT OF CLINICIAN PRACTICES

Adolescent Reporters

Reports were obtained from 2 samples of adolescents regarding their clinician's behavior after their physical examinations. The first sample had seen their clinicians before the training workshops and the second sample had seen their clinicians after the workshops. Participants were recruited using lists obtained from the clinics of adolescents with scheduled physical examination or sports physical visits. Parents and adolescents were first sent a letter describing the study that was followed up by a telephone recruitment call. Approximately 92% of adolescents (and parents) contacted agreed to participate in the study. A total of ~71% of those who agreed to participate completed their study visits and the questionnaire. Informed consent was obtained from all adolescents and their parent or legal guardian.

The pretraining assessment period lasted an average of 3 months in the 3 sites. During the pretraining period, 267 14- to 16-year-old adolescents (mean age: 15.0; SD: 0.79) completed questionnaires, immediately after their routine prescheduled physical examination visit, that asked detailed questions about what had taken place during the well-visit (described below). The pretraining sample was comprised of 46% females. Forty-seven percent of the pretraining sample were white, 20% were Hispanic, 12% were black, 9% were Asian, 2% were Native American, and 10% were classified as other. The posttraining assessment period began immediately after the training and lasted an average of 2.8 months in the 3 sites. The posttraining sample consisted of 265 14- to 16-year-old adolescents (mean age: 14.75; SD: 0.80) who also completed questionnaires immediately after their routine physical examinations. The posttraining sample was comprised of 49% females. Fifty-nine percent of the sample were white, 14% were Hispanic, 14% were black, 7% were Asian, 1% were Native American, and 5% were classified as other.

Measure of Clinician Practices

The assessment measure of clinician screening and counseling practices is based on independent individual reports from adolescents. This type of measure yields a unique appraisal of clinician practices that is free of the confounding influences of clinician self-report and social desirability biases. Few studies have included independent adolescent reports of clinician practices. Klein and colleagues[39] found that adolescent reports were valid indicators of actual clinicians' behavior with their adolescent patients.

In the present study, we developed a questionnaire, the "Adolescent Report of the Visit" (AROV), that adolescents completed immediately after their routine physical examination and well visit (which are allotted an average of 24 minutes, range 20–30 minutes). Clinicians whose patients completed the questionnaire were not made aware which patients were participating in the study. The AROV is a 39-item self-report questionnaire that includes questions on whether clinicians screen or offer brief counseling messages for each of the 5 target risk areas (helmet, seatbelt, tobacco use, alcohol use, and sexual behavior) and whether confidentiality is explained.

Construct validity was obtained by correlating scores on the adolescents' reports of clinician screening with scores on a self-report questionnaire completed by clinicians. On the clinician measure, each clinician reported his/her frequency of screening adolescents over the past 30 days on each of the risk areas. Significant correlations were found for 4 of the 5 risk areas. An example of a screening question on the AROV is: "Did your doctor ask if you smoke or chew tobacco?"

The counseling items presented in this study varied depending on the risk area of focus. In the safety areas of seatbelt and helmet use, clinicians were trained to encourage all adolescents to use their seatbelts and helmets, regardless of the adolescent's reported behavior. In the areas of tobacco use, alcohol use, and sexual behavior, clinicians gave different counseling messages to adolescents depending on whether the adolescent reported engaging in the risky behaviors. In these 3 areas, the present analyses included the counseling messages given to nonengaging adolescents that reflect reinforcement and counseling to maintain their positive behaviors (preventive or anticipatory counseling). A sample item is: "Did your doctor encourage you to remain a nonsmoker or nontobacco user?" The response categories were dichotomous yes or no. Counseling messages given to adolescents who reported engaging in risky behaviors are not included in the present

analyses because the numbers of adolescents engaging in the risky behaviors were relatively low and resulted in each clinician having very few, if any, reports with which to conduct the analyses.

Evaluation of clinician discussion of confidentiality included 2 components: 1) whether or not clinicians explained that there were certain things the clinician would not disclose to the adolescent's parent (general confidentiality); and 2) whether or not clinicians discussed the limits of confidentiality.

In creating the adolescent report variable, each adolescent report was associated with the clinician who conducted the visit, and each specific item was summed and averaged across the questionnaires for that clinician. The resulting score for each item (eg, screening for tobacco use) represented the percentage of visits during which a clinician screened or counseled in each risk area, or discussed confidentiality with adolescents in the study. (For example, if a clinician saw 4 adolescents and 2 reported being asked if they used tobacco and 2 reported not being asked, that clinician's score for screening in tobacco use would be 0.50). Each clinician therefore had a mean score representing his/her practices across adolescent reports during the pretraining period for each risk area and a mean representing his/her practices during the posttraining period for each risk area. In addition, we created variables that reflected the aggregate or sum of the mean scores across all risk areas for both clinician's screening practices (aggregate screening) and counseling practices (aggregate counseling); 1 each for the pretraining and posttraining assessment periods.

The mean number of adolescent reports per clinician was the same during the pretraining period (mean: 4.2; SD: 2.7; range: 1–17) and the posttraining period (mean: 4.2; SD: 3.0; range: 1–17). Each clinician's score was a composite of adolescent reports obtained over the course of several months during either the pretraining or posttraining period. Therefore, the composite score reflects clinician behavior throughout the duration of the assessment periods. Although there was variability in the number of visits per clinician, the number of visits was not correlated significantly with the clinician scores on screening and counseling, thus indicating that number of visits did not influence whether clinicians screened or counseled during those visits.

TRAINING WORKSHOPS

The training workshops were developed using Bandura's Social Cognitive Theory[37,38] to address multiple factors that influence implementation of preventive services for adolescents. Social Cognitive Theory emphasizes the importance of knowledge, attitudes, self-efficacy, and skills in creating behavior change. The training workshops instructed primary care providers in a brief office-based intervention and addressed these variables as mediators of clinician behavior change.[22,40]

We assembled an advisory panel of adolescent medicine specialists from the study HMO to review our plan for the workshops. Workshops were conducted by a panel comprised of all authors on this study. In addition, we used educational theater actors from the HMO to portray adolescents, and to participate in demonstration and practice role-plays. Training manuals were developed to include information on each topic, lists of related resources in the clinic and local community, relevant empirical articles, and a bibliography.

The workshops were divided into two 4-hour sessions. Each workshop was repeated to facilitate the attendance of as many clinicians as possible. As suggested by the review of effective interventions for health care professionals,[24] the workshops contained 4 components: 1) didactic; 2) discussion; 3) demonstration role-plays; and 4) interactive role-plays. The first didactic component included presentations on statistics for adolescent risk behaviors and health in the United States, adolescent development, the role of primary care clinicians in reducing risky behaviors leading to adolescent morbidities and mortalities, a general framework for interviewing adolescents, confidentiality, useful screening questions and brief counseling messages both for adolescents engaging in risky behaviors and those not engaging, and prioritizing in the clinical visit. The second component was comprised of interactive question and answer sessions and discussion after the presentations. The third component involved demonstration role-plays with adolescent patients. Role-plays demonstrated a clinical visit with an adolescent patient and began with a discussion of confidentiality, then moved to brief screening, and counseling on the 5 target risk behaviors. The fourth component involved group practice wherein an actor used case scenarios to role-play an adolescent patient with a clinician, and 2 facilitators along with the other clinicians in the group offered immediate feedback. The training was videotaped for clinicians who were unable to attend.

ANALYSIS PLAN

We conducted paired t test analyses for each set of mean scores, comparing pretraining to posttraining changes in behavior. There were 3 sets of outcome variables: 1) screening for helmet and seatbelt use, tobacco use, alcohol use, and sexual behavior, and an aggregate screening score across target areas; 2) counseling on helmet and seatbelt use, tobacco use, alcohol use, and sexual behavior, and an aggregate counseling score across areas; and 3) general discussion of confidentiality and discussion of the limits of confidentiality.

Three sets of analyses were conducted. The first set includes paired t tests evaluating change in clinician screening from pretraining to posttraining, both for the specific risk areas and the aggregated screening score. The second set of analyses includes paired t tests evaluating change in clinician brief counseling from pretraining to posttraining, both for the specific risk areas and the aggregated counseling score. The third set includes paired t tests evaluating pretraining to posttraining changes in the 2 aspects of clinician discussion of confidentiality.

Results

SCREENING

Paired t tests indicated that, based on adolescent reports, clinician screening practices increased significantly from pretraining to posttraining in each of the 5 risk areas: helmet use (from mean 27% to 45%); seatbelt use (from mean 38% to 56%); tobacco use (from mean 64% to 76%); alcohol use (from mean 59% to 76%); and sexual behavior (from mean 61% to 75%) (Table 1). The paired t test also indicated that the aggregated screening score across all 5 risk areas increased significantly from pretraining to posttraining (mean pretraining 50%; SD 0.27 to mean posttraining 65%; SD 0.23; t = 4.59; P < .000).

Table 1. Average Percentage of Adolescents Screened Pretraining and Posttraining by Their Clinician

Screening Variable	Pretraining		Posttraining		Paired t Value
	Mean Percentage	SD	Mean Percentage	SD	
Helmet	27	32	45	36	3.95***
Seatbelt	38	36	56	38	3.67***
Tobacco	64	36	76	28	2.57*
Alcohol	59	37	76	28	3.22**
Sexual behavior	61	37	75	30	2.43*

N = 63.
* P <.05.
** P <.01.
*** P <.001.

BRIEF COUNSELING

Clinicians' brief counseling increased from the pretraining to posttraining period. Specifically, t tests of change in clinicians' counseling practices across all adolescents showed significant increases for clinicians' encouragement to wear a helmet (from mean 25% to 43%) and encouragement to use a seatbelt (from mean 36% to 51%). Counseling adolescents who were not sexually active to delay sexual activity increased significantly (from mean 42% to 58%) (Table 2). Counseling nontobacco users to continue not to use tobacco increased marginally (from mean 60% to 69%) and counseling nondrinkers to not begin drinking increased, but the difference from pretraining to posttraining was not significant (51% to 61%). The aggregate score for counseling across all 5 risk areas increased significantly from pretraining to posttraining (mean pretraining: 43%; SD: 0.26 to mean posttraining: 56%; SD: 0.26; t = 3.95; P < .000).

CONFIDENTIALITY

The 2 components of discussion of confidentiality were analyzed separately: discussion of general confidentiality (ie, information that would not be disclosed to parents) and discussion of the limits of confidentiality (ie, information that would be disclosed to parents if necessary). Pretraining to posttraining increase in clinician discussion of

Table 2. Average Percentage of Adolescents Who Received Brief Counseling Pretraining and Posttraining by Their Clinician

Brief Counseling Variable	n of Clinicians	Pretraining		Posttraining		Paired t Value
		Mean Percentage	SD	Mean Percentage	SD	
Helmet	63	25	32	43	35	3.98**
Seatbelt	62	36	35	51	37	3.39**
Tobacco	61	60	37	69	33	1.71*
Alcohol	62	51	35	61	34	1.63
Sexual behavior	60	42	34	58	36	3.47**

* $P < .10$.
** $P < .001$.

general confidentiality occurred in the expected direction, but was not significant (from 44% to 52%). However, clinician discussion of the limits of confidentiality increased significantly (mean pretraining: 32%; SD: 0.31 to mean posttraining: 45%; SD: 0.32; $t = 2.29$; $P < .03$).[a]

Discussion

In this study, we examined the efficacy of skills-based training workshops designed to enhance clinicians' delivery of preventive services to their adolescent patients in a group model HMO. These findings support the hypothesis that clinicians' screening, counseling, and discussion of confidentiality with their adolescent patients increase significantly after skills-based training workshops. These training workshops offer a promising approach to facilitate the implementation of national guidelines that recommend screening and counseling adolescents on a range of risky behaviors.

TRAINING PRACTICING CLINICIANS

The training workshops in the present study were provided to practicing clinicians in a busy health care environment. Studies of education and training for clinicians typically focus on medical students and residents,[27,28,41,42] despite the need for studies of training of clinicians already in

practice. In the present study, although clinicians had been trained an average of 17 years ago, they attended the trainings and modified their practices significantly after our trainings. Indeed, we trained 95% of eligible clinicians, and posttraining clinician evaluations revealed positive responses to the training and retention of the material covered (eg, clinician reports averaged 4.7 out of 5 on meeting objectives of the trainings). Clinicians therefore were exposed to the full "dose" of trainings and played an active role in the workshops.

This high rate of attendance and involvement may have been attributable, in part, to our efforts to collaborate with the clinicians, chiefs of the departments, and administrators in each of the clinics throughout the process of planning, scheduling, and implementing the trainings. In addition, clinicians seemed highly motivated to learn new skills to facilitate their work with their adolescent patients, perhaps because of the introduction of this HMO's preventive services guidelines, along with increased awareness of high rates of adolescent morbidity and mortality attributable to risky behavior. Thus, the present findings offer support for the integration of continuing education, such as skills-based trainings, for clinicians practicing within the health care system.

The trainings were conducted in a group model HMO where such trainings were feasible and the screening and counseling methods could be incorporated into clinicians' practices. In other health care environments, modifications may be necessary in the logistics of conducting the trainings and in the methods of incorporating prevention

---

[a]We also conducted analyses using adolescent reports across clinician visits, not associating visits with individual clinicians, to obtain the rates of screening and counseling practices across the 3 clinics. χ^2 analyses showed that the majority of results were the same as results using mean scores for each clinician, suggesting a similar pattern of findings.

into the clinical settings. It is noteworthy that national guidelines are recommending the integration of preventive services and it will be important to explore methods of effectively conducting trainings to implement these services in a wide range of practice settings.

MULTIPLE BEHAVIOR APPROACH

In this study, we targeted multiple behaviors rather than focusing solely on 1 target risk behavior. Studies of clinician trainings typically target a single risk area such as tobacco use,[28,43-45] alcohol and drug use,[29] or sexually transmitted diseases,[46] despite the literature suggesting that there is high covariation among various risk behaviors.[5,30-33] Given the challenges imposed by the national guidelines to screen and counsel on many behaviors in clinicians' visits with adolescents, we are encouraged by findings from the present study that clinicians increased their queries to teens in all risky behaviors during their brief office visits. In our trainings, we emphasized methods to efficiently address multiple areas of risk in a routine physical examination visit. These results suggest that the trainings facilitated clinicians' efficacy to incorporate preventive services into their actual visits with adolescents and to give attention to a range of risky behaviors, including sensitive topics such as sexual behavior and substance use.

VARIATION ACROSS RISKY BEHAVIORS

The workshops were associated with significant increases in overall clinician screening and counseling of adolescent patients for risky behaviors. When examined individually by target risk behaviors, clinicians' screening practices improved significantly from the pretraining to posttraining periods for all 5 behaviors. Brief counseling, however, increased significantly for safety and sexual behavior, but not for substance use. Independent adolescent reports of their clinician visits is considered a stringent measure of clinician provision of services to their adolescent patients in an actual patient encounter,[28] suggesting there is variation in clinicians' counseling practices.

The most marked improvement in clinicians' screening and brief counseling was in the target areas of helmet and seatbelt use. There is a paucity of research on clinician practices regarding safety, and the limited research suggests that it is difficult to alter clinicians' practices in the area of injury prevention.[47] However, relative to our other target areas, helmet and seatbelt use screening and counseling are fairly straightforward issues that do not require extensive assessment or clinical sensitivity.

We obtained significant improvement in clinicians' screening for tobacco and alcohol use; marginally significant changes in counseling for tobacco use, and an increase in counseling for alcohol use that was not statistically significant. The counseling variable reflected brief counseling for teens who were not currently smoking or drinking and emphasized encouragement to continue refraining from those behaviors. It is plausible that some clinicians did not introduce a discussion of the complex topic of substance use because of lack of time and resources. Although we provided lists of resources in the clinic and local community, additional tools and resources such as health risk screening questionnaires, counseling prompts, and support staff may be needed to increase clinicians' comfort initiating a discussion about substance use.[24,36,48] Thus, training alone was sufficient to improve screening for substance use, but additional system-level interventions may be needed for consistent, ongoing improvement in counseling.

In the target area of sexual behavior, clinicians' screening of all adolescents and brief counseling of nonsexually active adolescents to delay onset of sexual activity improved significantly after the training workshops. Little research has been conducted to improve clinicians' screening and counseling regarding adolescents' sexual behavior. The limited studies that address screening and counseling on sexual behavior typically focus on at-risk or high-risk patients.[46,49] The present study is unique in its primary prevention focus on adolescent patients, including those who had not begun to engage in risky sexual behavior. We recruited our study patients from prescheduled well-visits, and the majority were not sexually active. The workshops therefore emphasized training on preventive counseling, such as delaying onset of sexual activity for adolescents as a method to prevent sexually transmitted diseases, human immunodeficiency virus infection, and pregnancy, as well as counseling for sexually active adolescents that emphasized options to maximize their health and safety. Preventive and early interventions and health promotion are both important in reducing negative behavioral and health outcomes[41] and the present findings suggest that training is 1 useful method to improve such interventions.

Finally, discussion of the limits of confidentiality increased significantly after the trainings, whereas general discussion of confidentiality did not show a significant increase. Preventive guidelines recommend that clinicians discuss confidentiality in an adolescent visit,[8,9] yet clinicians generally are not instructed in how to discuss this topic with their adolescent patients. In the present study, clinicians increased their discussions about the particular circumstances under which they would need to disclose information to an adolescents' parent. Perceiving that a visit is confidential has been found to be a significant correlate of adolescents' willingness to disclose personal information.[34] Informing adolescents about the limited circumstances under which information would be disclosed is an important component of a confidentiality discussion. Ford and colleagues[34] demonstrated that discussion of the limits of confidentiality was not associated with reductions in adolescent patients' willingness to disclose information.

In the current study, although there was a positive increase in discussion about issues that would not be disclosed, it is interesting that the improvement was not significant, whereas, the increase in discussion of the limits of confidentiality was significant. This may in part have resulted because the pretraining rate of discussion of general confidentiality was substantially higher than the rate of discussion of the limits of confidentiality, thus creating a ceiling effect. Alternatively, our training workshops emphasized mandatory reporting and clarification of the limits of confidentiality. Future trainings should equally emphasize the importance of explaining to patients the type of information that will remain confidential, as well as the type of information that will be disclosed.

LIMITATIONS AND FUTURE DIRECTIONS

Although these findings are promising, it is important to note limitations to the methodology. Although we used an internal comparison, we did not use a randomized, controlled design to evaluate our training workshops. Also, the clinics we selected to participate in our study of the implementation of preventive services may not be representative of all clinics within the HMO, thus limiting generalizability. The chiefs of pediatrics and clinicians in the clinics were interested in improving their services for adolescents and had agreed to participate in the training workshops and longitudinal study.

Finally, because this study was part of a larger study in which additional system interventions were later added, the data are limited to immediate follow-up within 3 months posttraining. Future studies are needed to examine the longitudinal effects of the trainings, using ongoing feedback, reinforcement, and booster sessions that are important in maintaining effects of training.[24]

Conclusion

This study offers strong support for the efficacy of skills-based workshops for primary care clinicians to improve screening and counseling practices with adolescents in a health care setting. The enhancement of screening across all 5 target risk behaviors suggests that training workshops alone significantly improve screening across a broad array of behaviors. Screening for risky behaviors is a critical component of an outpatient pediatric visit for adolescents wherein clinicians may identify and detect risky behaviors early. Provision of counseling in complex areas such as substance use may require additional system-level interventions to address organizational/system factors that influence service delivery, such as a need for charting tools and additional staff resources. However, skills-based workshops alone are associated with improvement in screening and counseling practices and may represent an important component of a larger system intervention to enhance overall delivery of clinical preventive services. Ongoing research is being conducted to examine a larger system model, including adolescent screening questionnaires, clinician prompts, forms, and additional staff resources, to improve the delivery of preventive services. Improving such services is an essential step in the prevention of untoward behavioral and health outcomes for youth.

Acknowledgements

This research was supported primarily by Grant Number 96-42 from The California Wellness Foundation. Additional support was provided through grants from the Maternal and Child Health Bureau, Health Resources and Services Administration, Department of Health and Human Services, the Interdisciplinary Leadership Training in Adolescent Health (Project #MCJ-000978), the Policy Information and Analysis Center for Middle Childhood and Adolescence (Project #MC-00023), and the National Adolescent Health Information Center (Project #MCJ-06A80).

We thank Susan Millstein, PhD, for her contributions to the design of the study and of the training workshops, and Carol Bandura Cowley, MSN, CPNP, for her assistance in conceptualizing the training workshops, contributions to the development of materials, and her helpful insights. We also appreciate the technical assistance and consultation in developing the trainings of Art Elster, MD, Missy Fleming, PhD, Janet Gans-Epner, PhD, and Pat Levenberg, PhD, of the Department of Adolescent Health at the American Medical Association. We thank Anne Claiborne for her skillful assistance in developing the materials for the trainings, organizing the workshops, and preparing this manuscript. We also appreciate the assistance of Scott Burg in preparing materials for the trainings and Denise Mailloux in the final preparation of the manuscript. Finally, we are grateful to the clinicians in the 3 Kaiser Permanente Northern California Clinics who participated in the training workshops and demonstrated an interest in improving preventive health care for adolescents.

References

1. Ozer EM, Brindis CD, Millstein SG, Knopf DK, Irwin CE Jr. *America's Adolescents: Are They Healthy?* San Francisco, CA: University of California, San Francisco, National Adolescent Health Information Center; 1998

2. Centers for Disease Control and Prevention. *CDC Wonder Online Database, Mortality Data Set (Compressed).* Atlanta, GA: Centers for Disease Control and Prevention. Available at: http://wonder.cdc.gov/mortsql.shtml. Accessed July 2000

3. Kann L, Warren CW, Harris WA, et al. *Youth Risk Behavior Surveillance—United States, 1993.* Atlanta, GA: Surveillance and Evaluation Research Branch, Division of Adolescent and School Health, Centers for Disease Control and Prevention; 1996

4. *National Health Interview Survey. Research for the 1995-2004 Redesign. Series 2: Data Evaluation and Methods Research.* Publ. No. 126. Hyattsville, MD: US Department of Health and Human Services, Centers for Disease Control and Prevention, National Center for Health Statistics; 1999

5. Elliott DS. Health-enhancing and health-compromising lifestyles. In: Millstein SG, Petersen AC, Nightingale EO, eds. *Promoting the Health of Adolescents.* New York, NY: Oxford University Press; 1993:119–145

6. Jessor R, Donovan JE, Costa FM. *Beyond Adolescence: Problem Behavior and Young Adult Development.* Vol. 15. New York, NY: Cambridge University Press; 1991:312

7. Riley A, Leaf P, Horwitz S, Lustig J, Vaden-Kiernan M. Detection of psychosocial problems among children with significant medical problems. Presented at: Annual International Conference on Mental Disorders in the General Health Care Sector; October 20, 1994; McLean, VA

8. Elster AB, Kuznets NJ, American Medical Association. *AMA Guidelines for Adolescent Preventive Services (GAPS): Recommendations and Rationale.* Baltimore, MD: Williams & Wilkins; 1994:191

9. Green M, Palfrey JS. Bright futures: guidelines for health supervision of infants, children and adolescents. Arlington, VA: National Center for Education in Maternal and Child Health; 2000

10. Stein ME. *Health Supervision Guidelines.* 3rd ed. Elk Grove Village, IL: American Academy of Pediatrics; 1997

11. *The Challenge and Potential for Assuring Quality Health Care for the 21st Century.* Washington, DC: Domestic Policy Council (US), United States Department of Health and Human Services; 1999

12. Blum RW, Beuhring T, Wunderlich M, Resnick MD. Don't ask, they won't tell: the quality of adolescent health screening in five practice settings. *Am J Public Health.* 1996;86:1767–1772

13. Joffe A, Radius S, Gall M. Health counseling for adolescents: what they want, what they get, and who gives it. *Pediatrics.* 1988;82:481–485

14. Levenson PM, Morrow JR, Morgan WC, Pfefferbaum BJ. Health information sources and preferences as perceived by adolescents, pediatricians, teachers and school nurses. *J Early Adolesc.* 1986;6:183–195

15. Malus M, LaChance PA, Lamy L, Macaulay A, Vanasse M. Priorities in adolescent health care: the teenager's viewpoint. *J Fam Pract.* 1987;25:159–162

16. Steiner BD, Gest KL. Do adolescents want to hear preventive counseling messages in outpatient settings? *J Fam Pract.* 1996;43:375–381

17. Ellen JM, Franzgrote M, Irwin CE Jr, Millstein SG. Primary care physicians' screening of adolescent patients: a survey of California physicians. *J Adolesc Health.* 1998;22:433–438

18. Franzgrote M, Ellen JM, Millstein SG, Irwin CE Jr. Screening for adolescent smoking among primary care physicians in California. *Am J Public Health.* 1997;87:1341–1345

19. Igra V, Millstein S. Current status and approaches to improving preventive services for adolescents. *JAMA.* 1993;269:1408–1412

20. Halpern-Felsher BL, Ozer EM, Millstein SG, et al. Preventive services in a health maintenance organization: how well do pediatricians screen and educate adolescent patients? *Arch Pediatr Adolesc Med.* 2000;154:173–179

21. Green LW, Eriksen MP, Schor EL. Preventive practices by physicians: behavioral determinants and potential interventions. *Am J Prev Med.* 1988;4(suppl 4):101–110

22. Green LW, Kreuter MW. *Health Promotion Planning: An Educational and Ecological Approach.* 3rd ed. Mountain View, CA: Mayfield Publishing Co; 1999

23. Walsh JM, McPhee SJ. A systems model of clinical preventive care: an analysis of factors influencing patient and physician. *Health Educ Q.* 1992;19:157–175

24. Oxman AD, Thomson MA, Davis DA, Haynes RB. No magic bullets: a systematic review of 102 trials of interventions to improve professional practice. *CMAJ.* 1995;153:1423–1431

25. Davis DA, Taylor-Vaisey A. Translating guidelines into practice: a systematic review of theoretic concepts, practical experience and research evidence in the adoption of clinical practice guidelines. *Can Med Assoc J.* 1997;157:408–416

26. Blum RW, Bearinger LH. Knowledge and attitudes of health professionals toward adolescent health care. *J Adolesc Health.* 1990;11:289–294

27. Gemson DH, Ashford AR, Dickey LL, et al. Putting prevention into practice: impact of a multifaceted physician education program on preventive services in the inner city. *Arch Intern Med.* 1995;155:2210–2216

28. Klein JD, Portilla M, Goldstein A, Leininger L. Training pediatric residents to prevent tobacco use. *Pediatrics.* 1995;96:326–330

29. Kokotailo PK, Langhough R, Neary EJ, Matson SC, Fleming MF. Improving pediatric residents' alcohol and other drug use clinical skills: use of an experiential curriculum. *Pediatrics.* 1995;96:99–104

30. Irwin CE Jr, Igra V, Eyre S, Millstein S. Risk-taking behavior in adolescents: the paradigm. *Ann N Y Acad Sci.* 1997;817:1–35

31. Hawkins JD, Catalano RF, Miller JY. Risk and protective factors for alcohol and other drug problems in adolescence and early adulthood: implications for substance abuse prevention. *Psychol Bull.* 1992;112:64–105

32. Lindberg LD, Boggess S, Porter L, Williams S. *Teen Risk Taking: A Statistical Portrait.* Washington, DC: The Urban Institute; 2000

33. Millstein SG, Irwin CE Jr, Adler NE, Cohn LD, Kegeles SM, Dolcini MM. Health-risk behaviors and health concerns among young adolescents. *Pediatrics.* 1992;89:422–428

34. Ford CA, Millstein SG, Halpern-Felsher BL, Irwin CE Jr. Influence of physician confidentiality assurances on adolescents' willingness to disclose information and seek future health care: a randomized controlled trial. *JAMA.* 1997;278:1029–1034

35. Sanci LA, Coffey CM, Veit FC, et al. Evaluation of the effectiveness of an educational intervention for general practitioners in adolescent health care: randomised controlled trial. *BMJ.* 2000;320:224–230

36. Lustig JL, Ozer EM, Adams SH, et al. Addressing adolescent risk behaviors in health care settings: developing a clinic based preventive intervention. Presented at: Annual Conference of the Society for Prevention Research; June 22, 1999; New Orleans, LA

37. Bandura A. *Social Foundations of Thought and Action: A Social Cognitive Theory.* Englewood Cliffs, NJ: Prentice Hall; 1986

38. Bandura A. *Self-efficacy: The Exercise of Control.* New York, NY: WH Freeman; 1997

39. Klein JD, Graff CA, Santelli JS, Hedberg VA, Allan MJ, Elster AB. Developing quality measures for adolescent care: validity of adolescents' self-reported receipt of preventive services. *Health Serv Res.* 1999;34:391–404

40. Lawrence RS. Diffusion of the US preventive services task force recommendations into practice. *J Gen Intern Med.* 1990;5(suppl):S99–S103

41. Millstein SG, Petersen AC, Nightingale EO. *Promoting the Health of Adolescents: New Directions for the Twenty-first Century.* New York, NY: Oxford University Press; 1993

42. Cohen SJ, Halvorson HW, Gosselink CA. Changing physician behavior to improve disease prevention. *Prev Med.* 1994;23:284–291

43. Cummings SR, Coates TJ, Richard RJ, et al. Training physicians in counseling about smoking cessation: a randomized trial of the "Quit for Life" program. *Ann Intern Med.* 1989;110:640–647

44. Kottke TE, Solberg LI, Brekke ML, Conn SA, Maxwell P, Brekke MJ. A controlled trial to integrate smoking cessation advice into primary care practice: doctors helping smokers, Round III. *J Fam Pract.* 1992;34:701–708

45. Strecher VJ, O'Malley MS, Villagra VG, et al. Can residents be trained to counsel patients about quitting smoking? Results from a randomized trial. *J Gen Intern Med.* 1991;6:9–17

46. Rabin DL, Boekeloo BO, Marx ES, Bowman MA, Russell NK, Willis AG. Improving office-based physicians' prevention practices for sexually transmitted diseases. *Ann Intern Med.* 1994;21:513–519

47. Hansen K, Wong D, Young PC. Do the Framingham Safety Surveys improve injury prevention counseling during pediatric health supervision visits? *Pediatrics.* 1996;129:494–498

48. Cabana MD, Rand CS, Powe NR, et al. Why don't physicians follow clinical practice guidelines? A framework for improvement. *JAMA.* 1999;82:1458–1465

49. Ward J, Sanson-Fisher R. Does a 3-day workshop for family medicine trainees improve preventive care? A randomized control trial. *Prev Med.* 1996;25:741–747

Normal Adolescent Growth

The following summary is adapted from a lecture by Elizabeth Alderman, MD, FAAP, at the AM:PREP course in Montreal in September 2003. Details on racial differences in sexual maturation may be found in the following article: Sun SS, Schubert CM, Chumlea WC, et al. National estimates of the timing of sexual maturation and racial differences among US children. *Pediatrics.* 2002;110:911–919

Please note that some of the data may be outdated because of the lack of recent studies, and all the ages stated are approximations. We recommend considering consultation with a pediatric endocrinologist before undertaking an extensive workup.

(Thanks to Marcia E. Herman-Giddens, PA, DrPH, for her review of this paper.)

First evidence of onset of puberty
- Thelarche (breast development) in girls (for ~15%, adrenarche first—varies by race).
- Gonadarche (testicular development) in boys.
- Sequence of specific maturational events is almost uniform. However, there is tremendous variation in timing.

Breast development in girls
- Age range: 6 or 7 to 14 years, depending on race. Unilateral onset of breast development is normal—other breast will follow within 6 months.
- Mean age
  - ~ Non-Hispanic black: 9.5 years
  - ~ Mexican American: 9.8 years
  - ~ Non-Hispanic white: 10.4 years

Menarche about 2.5 years after thelarche
- By the time menarche has occurred, a girl has attained 90% to 95% of her adult height. Growth after menarche is limited to 2 to 4 inches.

Breast development (sexual maturity rating [SMR])
- SMR 1: Prepubertal breast
- SMR 2: Breast bud formation under areola
- SMR 3: Breast mound enlargement/ enlarged areola
- SMR 4: Secondary mound formation under areola (Menarche will typically occur during this brief stage if it has not occurred in SMR 3.)
- SMR 5: Mature adult breast

Gynecomastia
- May begin at SMR 2 in boys
- Is a common finding in boys SMR 2 to 4 (present in about 60%)
- Usually resolves spontaneously
- Lasts until SMR 5 in less than 10%
- Because of altered ratio of estrogens/ androgens—usually physiologic
- 75% bilateral

Gonadal development in boys
- Begins between 9 and 14 years (Mean has been previously reported as 11.5—it is not known what it is now.)
- Enlargement of testes first in 98% of boys, complete in 2 to 5 years
- SMR 1: Preadolescent
- SMR 2: Enlargement of testes/scrotum— scrotum skin reddens, no change in penis
- SMR 3: Enlargement of penis in length— further growth of testes/scrotum
- SMR 4: Enlargement of width of penis— darkening of scrotal skin/enlarging with testes
- SMR 5: Adult size/shape

Reproductive ability in boys
- Ejaculation 1 year after testes enlarge. Sperm as early as SMR 2 in first morning urine. Impregnation is possible at SMR 3. Definite fertility expected in SMR 4.

- At SMR 3, most boys masturbate and begin to ejaculate.
- Mature sperm in ejaculate prior to peak height velocity, coincident with acne and axillary hair.

Pubic hair development in boys and girls

- SMR 1: Vellus hair
- SMR 2: Sparse, long, downy, at base of penis/along labia
- SMR 3: Darker, coarser, curlier, extends laterally
- SMR 4: Adult-type hair (much coarser), greater extension
- SMR 5: Adult type extending to medial aspect of thighs

Adrenarche

- May precede thelarche and gonadarche. Timing of adrenarche may or may not be correlated to gonadarche.
- Adrenal androgens include dehydroepiandros-terone (DHEA), dehydroepiandrosterone sulfate (DHEAS), androstenedione.
- Pubic and axillary hair in girls.
- Pubic/axillary/facial hair in boys (chest hair is postpuberty).

Axillary hair/sweat glands

For boys

- At SMR 4, pubic and axillary hair appear.
- 1 year later, facial hair begins laterally above upper lip, moves medially, then to chin. Appearance of chin hair has been postulated to mark the end of puberty.
- Change of voice at SMR 3 to 4 pubic hair.

For girls

- Axillary hair appears 1 year after pubic hair.
- At SMR 2 pubic hair, sweat glands are func-tional, though girls can have body odor before axillary hair.

Menarche

- Physiologic leukorrhea, because of estrogen stimulation of the vaginal mucosa occurs 3 to 6 months prior to menarche.
- Onset of menarche SMR 3 to 4, related to peak in weight velocity.
- Average age 12.5 years in United States, but ethnic differences.

- 2 years after breast bud, 1 year after peak height velocity.
- Ovulatory cycles may not be established for 2 to 3 years.

Bottom line

Girls

- If no breast development by age 13.25 years, delayed puberty
- If onset of pubic hair occurs before age 7 years in white girls or before age 6 years in black girls, precocious puberty (see Kaplowitz PB, Oberfield SE. Reexamination of the age limit for defining when puberty is precocious in girls in the United States: implications for evaluation and treatment. *Pediatrics*. 1999; 104:936–941)

Boys

- If no testicular enlargement by age 14 years, delayed puberty
- If onset of pubertal changes occur before age 9 years, precocious puberty

Linear growth

- No growth spurt without influence of sex steroids (estrogen, progesterone, testosterone). Epiphyseal closure controlled by estradiol.
- Growth spurt related to bone age, not chronological age. Bone age will not go beyond 13.6 years without sex steroids, and there will be no change in body proportions. Potential growth if bone age is behind chrono-logical age. Abnormal if bone age is greater than 2 standard deviations above or below the mean for age.
- Accounts for 20% to 25% of adult height and lasts about 2 years in both sexes.
- Girls begin growth spurt at average age 10 years.
  - ~ Peak height velocity at average age 11.5 years, 8 to 9 cm/y.
  - ~ Peak weight velocity occurs after peak height velocity.
- Boys begin growth spurt at average age 11.5 years.
  - ~ Peak height velocity at average age 13.5 years, 9 to 10 cm/y.
  - ~ Peak height velocity and peak weight velocity occur together.

- External changes are the most striking, but similar dimensional increase occurs in every body system except brain and lymphatic system, where total tissue decreases.
- Mid-parental height is a good estimate of predicted final height at end of growth.
  - ~ Most adolescents achieve final adult height within 2 inches of male parental height.

Boys: $\dfrac{(\text{father's height} + 13 \text{ cm or } 5 \text{ in}) + \text{mother's height}}{2}$

Girls: $\dfrac{(\text{father's height} - 13 \text{ cm or } 5 \text{ in}) + \text{mother's height}}{2}$

Weight gain during puberty

- Girls gain most weight in adipose tissue, which increases to about 25% of body weight. Estrogen causes deposition of this fat in the pelvis, breasts, upper back, and arms. Lean body mass decreases from 80% of body weight in early puberty to 75% at maturity.
- Boys gain most weight in muscle tissue. Lean body mass increases from 80% of body weight in early puberty to 90% because of androgens. Adult male has 1.5 times the lean body mass of the adult female.
- 50% of adult weight is gained during puberty.

Body mass index—Centers for Disease Control and Prevention growth charts

- Weight (kg)/height (m^2) or weight (lb)/height (in^2) $\propto$ 703.
- Overweight is >95th percentile for age.
- At risk for obesity 85th to 94th percentile for age.
- No consensus guidelines for underweight, but many consider those who are <5th percentile to be underweight.

Office-Based Care of Adolescents: Part 1
Creating a Teen-Friendly Office

by David Y. Rainey, MD, MPH, FAAP

Adolescence is a unique and critically important developmental stage. Pediatricians who enjoy caring for adolescent patients recognize the need for creative and effective approaches to their care. While caring for teens and young adults in the office setting can be fun, professionally rewarding, and financially viable, maintaining an adolescent practice requires some extra effort. This article opens a 2-part series designed to help pediatricians provide appropriate, cost-effective, office-based care for adolescents. Part 2 of this series, which will appear in the February 2004 issue of *Adolescent Health Update,* will consider financial aspects of caring for adolescent patients.

Not a Kid Anymore

The transition from pediatric to adolescent care begins in late childhood. When children reach age 12, for example, they can be told that for their next checkup they will be seen as a teenager (or during "teen hours"). This is the time to explain to teens and their parents how future health supervision visits will differ from pediatric visits. First, younger adolescents will still be seen with parents, but as they grow older they should anticipate increasing time alone with their pediatrician, especially during a health supervision visit. (Assure parents that you are always willing to communicate with them in person or by telephone as necessary.) Second, the concept of confidentiality can be broached. Third, adolescents should be taught to begin taking more responsibility for their health (eg, they should know their health history and what medications they take).

By midadolescence, parents will be in the waiting room most of the time and the clinical interview topics will expand to include honest discussion about sensitive matters (eg, smoking, substance abuse, sexuality). Remind parents that pediatricians are trained to counsel teenagers regarding such issues, complementing the health education and guidance provided at home. Anticipatory guidance also should address peer pressure, progress in school, and emotional well being.

Patients in late adolescence may come to appointments by themselves. College students are encouraged to return during summer break and other holidays and to follow up during the school year by telephone. College students—and

Goals and Objectives

Goal: Pediatricians will learn concepts and skills that support appropriate, friendly, cost-effective, office-based care for adolescents.

Objectives: After reading this article, pediatricians will be better prepared to

- Describe how the physician/patient/ parent relationship changes as patients enter adolescence
- Practice developmentally appropriate anticipatory guidance
- Become familiar with techniques and tools to screen for health risk behaviors
- Discuss the nature and timing of laboratory or other screening procedures
- Describe the nature, extent, and limitations of confidentiality
- List the resources needed for a successful practice
- Discuss strategies for tailoring the office environment to the care of adolescents

David Y. Rainey, MD, MPH, FAAP, is medical director of Forsyth Adolescent Medicine affiliated with Novant Health and is a clinical assistant professor of pediatrics at the Wake Forest University School of Medicine in Winston-Salem, North Carolina.

parents—should be cautioned against the use of e-mail to communicate confidential concerns because it may not be possible to ensure complete security of electronic communications.

While the patient/physician/parent relationship changes in adolescence, the essential skills required to maintain an effective pediatrician/patient relationship remain constant. The pediatrician whose practice includes a thriving adolescent medicine component is likely to be one who enjoys adolescents and preventive health care, is comfortable talking about sensitive issues such as those related to drugs, smoking, and sexuality, and is skillful in treating common adolescent health problems (eg, sports-related injuries, acne, dysmenorrhea). In caring for adolescents, it is extremely important to ask questions and to keep asking them. Teens need to be prompted to communicate fears and concerns about personal health matters. They need to understand why their doctors raise these delicate topics. Pediatricians who work successfully with adolescents make use of every encounter to provide developmentally appropriate anticipatory guidance.

Confidentiality and Privacy Issues

Maintaining confidentiality is a critical element of patient trust. It is essential that adolescent patients and their parents know from the outset what will be kept confidential and what must be reported. If this conversation is conducted properly, the patient should feel assured that sensitive issues will be kept private except in specific cases, such as potential suicide and mandated reporting of abuse. A complete discussion of confidentiality and adolescent care is beyond the scope of this paper. Pediatricians should become familiar with state and federal laws pertaining to consent for and confidentiality of care related to sexually transmitted infections (STIs), pregnancy, abortion, substance abuse, and mental health issues.

OFFICE VISITS

Time alone with the pediatrician becomes a feature of the preventive care visit around age 12 or 13, depending upon the maturity level of

the child and the anxiety level of the parent. Almost invariably, the parent will agree to leave for a few minutes for the examination part of the visit, which can then accommodate further history-taking and preventive counseling. In fact, parental refusal to leave for part of an older teen's health maintenance visit may signal an unhealthy relationship, such as enmeshment or even abuse. Establishing a pattern of some private time during *all* office visits promotes maturity and autonomy and makes it easier to ask important questions. It can be difficult to ask necessary questions during a sick visit because the parent, appropriately concerned about the adolescent's illness, may not wish to leave the room. However if the pattern has been established, the parent will find it more natural and will expect to leave for part of the evaluation.

Sometimes it is simply impractical or not in the adolescent's best interest to keep an issue confidential. In these situations, talk to your patient about the pros and cons of telling his or her parents. Offer to help them tell their parents about the situation so they can receive the support and help that they need. When confidentiality must be breached, make sure the adolescent patient understands why. When possible, give the patient options regarding how his or her parents will be involved.

A parent will sometimes request or demand that a drug test be performed on their teenager. Except in extenuating circumstances, this should not be done without the patient's full understanding and consent. For a more detailed discussion of this topic, please refer to the Consultant's Corner column accompanying the most recent issue of *Adolescent Health Update* (*AAP News.* July 2003;23:19).

CHARTING/RECORD KEEPING

Specific considerations apply to documentation. When a confidential issue is charted, some practitioners stamp the page with a red "confidential" stamp. This accommodates easier retrieval and quick identification if copying the chart becomes necessary. Of course, records of any kind should not be left out on counters, and laboratory requests or results should not be openly displayed on examination room doors where they may be viewed by passers-by.

Adolescents can independently consent to receive certain services, most often those related to sexually transmitted diseases, reproductive health, and substance abuse. The right to consent has generally been considered to carry with it a right to confidentiality protection and the right to determine who has access to information about the confidential care. Under the federal medical privacy regulations adopted under the Health Information Portability and Accountability Act (often referred to as the HIPAA Privacy Rule), however, the link between consent and confidentiality is not as clear.

The HIPAA Privacy Rule recognizes that minors sometimes have the right to consent to their own health care and also acknowledges that parents sometimes support an agreement of confidentiality between an adolescent and a health care professional. However, the HIPAA rule defers to other laws—referred to as "state or other law"—to determine whether a parent will have access to information in these circumstances. When state laws are silent on this issue, discretion is vested in health care provider (or health plan) to decide whether to grant parents access to the information. It is therefore essential for health care professionals to understand the specific laws that apply in their state on this issue.

Often, parents request their child's records because they suspect that their teen is engaging in certain behaviors. If parents ask to see a chart that contains sensitive or confidential information, an adversarial relationship can almost always be avoided by meeting with the parents in the office for a sensitive and careful discussion exploring and addressing their concerns and fears. Thankfully, these situations are rare. They should be resolved based on state and federal laws, the specific facts and circumstances of the situation, and a good measure of common sense. There will be times when a parent may not agree and will persist in demands that are in conflict with efforts to preserve confidentiality. It may help to confer with an experienced colleague, or seek an opinion from a hospital risk management department.

REIMBURSEMENT FOR CONFIDENTIAL CARE

The time spent seeing an adolescent can almost always be reimbursed, as most adolescents have some medical reason to see the pediatrician. A teen who wants to discuss concerns about an STI, for example, will often make an appointment to address abdominal pain or dysuria. It is usually possible to assign an accurate and appropriate charge for an office visit based on less sensitive and less confidential (often symptom-based) *CPT* codes. There should always be sufficient support for the diagnosis in the office notes.

Reimbursement for confidential laboratory tests is more problematic. If adolescent patients are aware that a charge for a specific test (eg, an assay for chlamydia) might appear on a notice or bill sent to the parent, they may seek care elsewhere (fracturing continuity of care), or worse, forego care entirely. A number of strategies may be employed alone or in combination to obtain reimbursement without violating the patient's confidentiality:

● A third party payer covers the cost of laboratory tests in a way that does not compromise confidentiality. This is ideal.

● It is possible to facilitate family communication. Often, adolescent patients are willing to disclose a great deal to parents if they can be helped to frame the disclosure in a less "incriminating" context.

● A mechanism is established to allow patients to pay using confidential accounts. Charge the adolescent only what it costs the office for the test and set up a confidential account to which the adolescent can make payment of any amount at any time. Although the office may lose some revenue with this arrangement, the cost is low relative to the benefits. We have found that adolescents are willing to pay something for confidential services and appreciate the effort to maintain confidentiality.

● The adolescent agrees to pay for services rendered and prefers that the bill be sent to them directly, often at a non-home address.

● The laboratory conducting confidential tests agrees to bill the practice directly, rather than sending a bill to the patient's home.

Tools for Office-Based Health Promotion and Screening

Excellent screens and tips for anticipatory guidance are available to assist pediatricians caring for adolescents in a primary care office practice.

The **Guidelines for Adolescent Preventive Services** (GAPS) program was created in 1992 by the American Medical Association. This comprehensive package of recommendations is delivered in a series of preventive health visits between ages 11 and 21. GAPS makes 24 recommendations in 14 topic areas ranging from psychological adjustment to infectious diseases. The recommendations consider health care delivery, health guidance, screening, and immunizations. GAPS is designed to investigate any needs and concerns related to adolescent health and risk-taking behaviors. Age-appropriate screening questionnaires for adolescents and parents to be used at initial and periodic visits are available in English and Spanish. Reproducible GAPS forms also include a preventive services tracking chart, body mass index (BMI) charts, blood pressure graphs for males and females, and health guidance prompt sheets. Both the recommendations and rationale document (#OP947093ADS) and the GAPS implementation forms (#OPO22497ADS) can be ordered from the AMA at (800) 621-8335. Forms can also be downloaded from the AMA Web site (www.ama-assn.org/ama/pub/category/1980.html).

Bright Futures, a health promotion and disease prevention initiative for infants, children, adolescents, and their families, was launched by the federal Maternal and Child Health Bureau Health Resources and Services Administration more than a decade ago. The Academy was recently awarded grant monies to promote Bright Futures; over the next 5 years, the content will be updated and integrated with the AAP *Guidelines for Health Supervision III.* To learn more about how Bright Futures guidelines and materials can be employed in office-based health promotion and health risk prevention activities for adolescents, please check the new Web site at http://brightfutures.aap.org.

Screening in the Adolescent Office

Health screening, a core objective in adolescent care, should identify areas of concern and facilitate anticipatory guidance. The best instruments will reveal signs of risk-taking and symptoms of significant physical and emotional health concerns while also providing evidence of protective factors, strengths, and good health choices that can be identified and reinforced. Good screening instruments will encourage both adolescent and parent to raise topics that they might otherwise hesitate to broach. They will also make it easier to initiate dialogue about subjects such as sexuality, sexual orientation, mental health concerns, or substance abuse.

A number of screening instruments are included in the resource list on page 31. The *AMA Guidelines for Adolescent Preventive Services* (GAPS), available through the American Medical Association, features check lists by age group that can be downloaded from the Internet. *Bright Futures: Guidelines for Health Supervision of Infants, Children, and Adolescents,* and the *AAP Guidelines for Health Supervision III,* also excellent, are available through the American Academy of Pediatrics. These tools permit confidential screening of adolescents who present for health maintenance examinations and can also be used to survey parental concerns. (Preventive health services guidelines from *GAPS* and *Bright Futures* are compared in a 1998 review by Elster.)

Pediatricians can also screen for health risk behaviors during the clinical interview and physical examination. Helpful tools such as the HEADSS mnemonic described on the next page, and the CRAFFT screen for substance abuse described in the July 2003 issue of *Adolescent Health Update (AHU* 15:3), provide an efficient, consistent framework to address important topics. The results of health risk behavior screening can then be transcribed quickly to the medical record.

Keep in mind that screening for strengths and skills that can be recognized and reinforced is every bit as important as screening for vulnerabilities and health risk behaviors. Accelerated growth in cognitive skills, new awareness of personal qualities and limitations, and even

HEADSS A Psychological Review of Systems

The HEADSS mnemonic describes a systematic interview method developed by Eric Cohen, MD, at Los Angeles Children's Hospital. The HEADSS interview is designed to identify youth at highest risk for morbidity and mortality. Sample prompts that might come up in each category are suggested below.

H–Home
Who lives with the patient? Where? Does the patient have his or her own room? Any recent moves or new people in the home environment?

E–Education/employment
How is school performance? Ask about failed grades/classes, suspensions, dropping out, future education, and relations with teachers. What is employment history?

A–Activities
What does the patient do for fun with peers? Clubs, sports, church, hobbies, reading, TV, video games, music? Delinquency?

D–Drugs
Is there alcohol and tobacco use by peers, patient, and family? Ask about amount, frequency, source, patterns of use/abuse.

S–Sexuality
Inquire about sexual orientation, degree and types of sexual experience, number of partners, pregnancy, abortion history, contraception use, STIs, and sexual abuse.

S–Suicide/depression
Ask about sleep, appetite, boredom, withdrawal, hopelessness, history of suicide attempts, depression, family history, preoccupation with death, and drug and alcohol involvement.

Source: Cohen E, Mackenzie RG, Yates GL. HEADSS, a psychosocial risk assessment instrument: implications for designing effective intervention programs for runaway youth. *J Adolesc Health.* 1991;12:539–544

---

constructive risk-taking are important and normal features of adolescence. The clinical assessment should reinforce success, progress, and strengths, and assure that these positive developments are appreciated and noted in discussions with both teen and family.

SCREENING PROCEDURES

Adolescents are uniquely at risk for a number of health risks that deserve special attention. The AAP Recommendations for Preventive Pediatric Health Care, available at www.aappolicy.org, are a reliable means to that end. Considerations include the following:

- *Routine Annual Procedures:* A comprehensive assessment will incorporate a medical and psychosocial history and a physical examination, including a hypertension check, verification that immunizations are current (see next page), and evaluation as to the need for a tuberculin test.

- *Behavioral/developmental assessment:* This part of the interview can be structured as described in the HEADSS mnemonic (see box above). The CRAFFT test, a useful screen for substance abuse, was described in the July 2003 issue of *AHU* (15:3).

- *Nutrition and Exercise:* All adolescents should be counseled regarding diet and exercise and assessed for problematic eating behaviors. A body mass index (BMI) assessment (weight in kg/height in meters^2) should be calculated and plotted annually. Given the explosive rise in the prevalence of obesity, glucose intolerance, and diabetes, as well as eating disorders, consider screening when appropriate. American Diabetes Association recommendations on screening children and adolescents for type 2 diabetes were discussed in the July 2000 issue of *AHU* (12:3). If the family history reveals hypercholesterolemia or is unknown, a random or fasting cholesterol or fasting lipid profile should be considered in accordance with the AAP policy statement, Cholesterol in Childhood (www.aappolicy.org).

- *Depression:* When depressive symptoms are present, further investigation with screening tools such as the Beck Depression Inventory or Zung Self-Rating Depression Scale can assist with the evaluation. For further reading, see the July 2001 issue of *AHU* (13:3).

- *Gynecologic and STI screens:* Menstruating adolescents should have an annual hematocrit or hemoglobin. For those who are not sexually active and do not have specific gynecologic issues or problems, routine pelvic examinations and Pap smears should begin by age 21. All sexually active females should have an annual pelvic examination, and all sexually active adolescents should have an annual STI screen. Newer urine-based STI testing techniques (specifically, noninvasive non-culture procedures, such as nucleic acid amplification tests) permit rapid detection of common infections such as gonorrhea and chlamydia (October 2001 issue of *AHU:* 14:1). Of course, females can still be screened by other procedures (eg, DNA techniques using samples obtained from the cervix) as part of an annual gynecologic exam.

Immunizations

Immunization recommendations are continually updated by the AAP and the Advisory Committee on Immunization Practices. A second MMR and the hepatitis B series are now generally completed before adolescence; this should be verified. Varicella vaccine is indicated for any teenager without a history of clinical disease. Tetanus boosters (Td) are recommended at 10 to 12 years and every 10 years thereafter.

Meningococcal vaccine is strongly recommended for college freshmen or high school students who will be living on campus. This vaccine is now required in many states for incoming college freshmen, and while it still may not be reimbursed by insurance companies, it is recommended by the AAP, the CDC Advisory Committee on Immunization Practices, and the American College Health Association.

Office Resources

Providing healthcare for adolescents calls for clinical skills not involved in dealing with younger patients. The most important ingredient is an appreciation for teens' unique point of view and an interest in helping to guide them through adolescent development. Staff members who will interact with adolescents in your practice should genuinely enjoy teenagers. Nurses, receptionists, and other personnel should make your patients feel welcome, and demonstrate that they respect young adults and their growing independence. Certain skills and interests within a practice permit a more comprehensive approach to the care of adolescent patients.

Gynecology

Those pediatricians who feel comfortable with or choose to maintain their gynecologic skills can readily manage the majority of gynecologic concerns experienced by adolescents, caring for dysmenorrhea, dysfunctional uterine bleeding and contraceptive needs, screening for and diagnosing common STIs, performing routine pelvic examinations, and interpreting Pap smears. Ideally, the pediatrician will provide these services. Those who are not comfortable performing these procedures can provide many gynecologic services while referring patients to a gynecologist in the community for pelvic examinations and Pap smears.

Sports medicine

Many adolescents are involved with organized athletics and many more are recreational athletes. Your practice should be able to accommodate preparticipation sports exams, evaluation of acute injuries, and planning for rehabilitation and follow-up. This reduces the need for frequent orthopedic referral. When a pediatrician in the group also volunteers as a team physician, the practice as a whole will benefit. Close association with orthopedists and physical therapists in the area is helpful, as is ongoing participation in sports medicine CME.

Mental health

Diagnosing and treating mental health issues in adolescent care is crucial, particularly in view of increasingly limited access to these providers. It is important to remain current with new developments in psychiatric care and psychopharmacology. Some practices have addressed the mental health needs of patients by establishing a close affiliation with a therapist who can spend some time in the office (perhaps one day a week for a large practice or one half-day every other week for a smaller practice) seeing referrals. Adolescents appreciate the option of coming back to our office for counseling. A mental health colleague is also a great source for ongoing education and informal consultation. This arrangement can facilitate and expedite rapid referral for psychiatric care, as most therapists have professional relationships with psychiatrists.

Other clinical skills

Adolescents also frequently consult dermatologists, radiologists, and nutritionists. Only a very large adolescent medicine practice can support on-site experts in these fields. Providers should be comfortable offering basic nutrition advice and first-line management of issues in dermatology such as acne and eczema.

Designated teen nurse

Another valuable human resource is a nurse who has expertise in adolescent care and, more important, who likes teenagers. This individual can perform triage, provide telephone advice to patients and parents, and act as a ready and trusted contact. The right person can help with clinical work, follow up on Pap smear results, administer medroxyprogesterone acetate (DMPA) injections, provide contraceptive counseling, act as a chaperone when necessary, and serve as an on-site health educator. A nurse who can make teenagers feel connected and cared for can easily become the single most important reason your office runs smoothly.

Referral directory

A frequently updated personal directory of local experts and resources, from eating disorders support groups to inpatient drug treatment centers and Al-Anon chapters, is invaluable. Families also appreciate endorsements of teen-friendly providers when specialty consultation is required.

THE ENVIRONMENT AND SUPPLIES

A small section of the pediatric practice can be devoted to adolescents, even if it is just one or two rooms with appropriate decor. Pediatric patients who see that "big kids" are treated a little differently will eagerly anticipate graduating to the new arrangement. If this is impractical, another arrangement may be to set aside specific times for adolescents only, perhaps with slightly bigger appointment slots, when interruptions from crying infants will be at a minimum.

Continuity of care in adolescent medicine requires well-maintained follow-up systems. Adolescents are seen in the office less often than younger patients, which makes it doubly important to maintain a good reminder system for follow-up visits. Such systems can identify teens who have not appeared for annual or at least biannual health supervision appointments. They are especially important in tracking adolescents with abnormal Pap smear results and certain chronic conditions such as diabetes or asthma.

If possible, it is preferable to schedule most adolescent preventive care visits after school. A pediatrician who sees large numbers of adolescents might consider an early morning "urgent care clinic," when those who are not too sick can be seen and get to school. In our morning clinic, no appointment is necessary and perhaps 10 to 15 patients with mild illnesses or injuries can be accommodated in the first hour. Evening hours might be considered, although this may not be cost effective if the required staff are not well utilized. It may be effective to offer evening sports preparticipation examination sessions in July and August to accommodate the typically high demand for these physicals in anticipation of fall sport programs.

The nurse's work-up of the adolescent patient should be done in private, not in the hallway, as sometimes occurs in a busy pediatric practice. Adolescents may not want everyone knowing how tall they are and how much they weigh. One model would be a small private room for patient work-up; another would be to have scales and stadiometers in each adolescent examining room. It is especially important to have at least one room with a very accurate scale for patients with eating disorders, who typically should be weighed in a gown.

Rooms for adolescent care should be large enough to accommodate patient, parent, and physician. If possible, all adolescent rooms should have tables that permit pelvic examinations so that patients will not need to move to another room. Equipment should include appropriately sized examination tables and blood pressure cuffs, scoliometer, and supplies for gynecologic examination. It is essential to have a large adult blood pressure cuff and a thigh cuff on hand for obese patients. For a gynecologic examination, disposable plastic speculae with detachable light sources are useful, eliminating the need for sterilization. Most adolescent pelvic examinations are done with the slightly narrower Pederson speculum. A few standard (Graves), narrow (Huffman), and pediatric speculae should also be available.

In addition to the usual supplies, the office should consider keeping a treatment room stocked with equipment to administer IV fluids for dehydrated patients. Simple incision and drainage procedures, laceration repair, and partial excisions of toenails are common in adolescent practice. Ankle and wrist splints are frequently needed to manage acute injuries. It is helpful to keep a well-stocked sample closet for teenagers, particularly for medications that might be prescribed confidentially. Samples will help supply teenagers with oral contraceptive pills in a timely way for emergency use. Condoms should be available for demonstration and distribution.

Written health education materials are crucial. Adolescent examining rooms should be stocked with patient education pamphlets addressing topics such as alcohol and substance abuse, STI prevention, contraceptive options, and mental health issues. Brochures on good nutrition, common sports injuries, body piercing, tattoos, and eating disorders are also popular. At present, 30 teen brochures are published by the AAP (www.aap.org/bookstore).

Conclusion

Pediatricians are developmental specialists, and as such are well-suited to offer valuable medical care, health advice, and encouragement during the challenging and rewarding time of adolescence. Taking care of adolescents is different from treating younger pediatric patients. It is enormously gratifying and energizing to guide and assist youth as they traverse adolescence and enter adulthood. To be sure, office-based care of adolescents requires some preparation and flexibility, particularly in terms of scheduling, skills, and supplies. If done well, these arrangements will encourage teens to feel welcome, unique, and respected, and will contribute to continuity of care. The ultimate reward of adolescent care is to see adolescents successfully reach adulthood prepared and motivated to practice good health habits and enjoy a healthy, vibrant, and productive life.

Acknowledgment

The editors would like to acknowledge technical review by Jerald L. Zarin, MD, MBA, FAAP, for the AAP Section on Administration and Practice Management, and consultation with Abigail English, JD, director, Center for Adolescent Health & the Law, on confidentiality issues.

Further Reading

American Academy of Pediatrics, Committee on Infectious Diseases. Immunization of adolescents: recommendations of the Advisory Committee on Immunization Practices, the American Academy of Pediatrics, the American Academy of Family Physicians, and the American Medical Association. *Pediatrics.* 1997;99:479–488

American Academy of Pediatrics. Confidentiality in adolescent health care. *AAP News.* April 1989. (Policy statement adopted April 1989 and reaffirmed May 2000; available at http://www.aap.org/policy/104.html)

American Academy of Pediatrics, Committee on Infectious Diseases. Meningococcal disease prevention and control strategies for practice-based physicians (addendum: recommendations for college students). *Pediatrics.* 2000;106:1500–1504

Braverman PK, Strasburger VC. Office-based adolescent health care: issues and solutions. *Adolescent Medicine: State of the Art Reviews.* 1997;8

Centers for Disease Control and Prevention. Meningococcal disease and college students: recommendations of the advisory committee on immunization practices. *MMWR.* 2000;49(RR-7):11–20

Dailard C. New medical records privacy rule: the interface with teen access to confidential care. *The Guttmacher Report.* 2003;6 (Available at www.guttmacher.org/pubs/journals/gr060106.html)

Elster AB. Comparison of recommendations for adolescent clinical preventive services developed by national organizations. *Arch Pediatr Adolesc Med.* 1998;152:193–198

Rainey DY, Brandon DP, Krowchuk DP. Confidential billing accounts for adolescents in private practice. *J Adolesc Health.* 2000;26:389–391

Sigman G, Silber TJ, English A, Epner JE. Confidential health care for adolescents: position paper of the Society for Adolescent Medicine. *J Adolescent Health.* 1997;21:408–415. (Available at www.adolescenthealth.org/html/confidential.html)

RESOURCES FOR PHYSICIANS

On the Internet

AAP Section on Adolescent Health. *Adolescent Health Update* is one of many projects of the Academy's Section on Adolescent Health, which provides resources and links on care of adolescents. http://www.aap.org/sections/adol/

Alan Guttmacher Institute. A nonprofit organization focused on sexual and reproductive health research, policy analysis, and public education. http://www.agi-usa.org

Adolescent Health Working Group. Variety of materials; a synchronized presentation titled *Confidentiality, Minor Consent, and Practice Concerns When Treating Teen Patients* may be of particular interest. http://www.ahwg.net

National Adolescent Health Information Center. Specifically, a paper titled *Assuring the Health of Adolescents in Managed Care: A Quality Checklist for planning and evaluating components of adolescent care.* http://youth.ucsf.edu/nahic/img/4.pdf

National Center for Youth Law. Good general resource. A compilation of "Selected California Minor Consent Laws," for example, while not applicable to other states, gives a fine overview of the types of issues impacted by state consent laws. A comprehensive resource on state minor consent laws is under development. http://www.youthlaw.org

In Print

American Diabetes Association. Type 2 diabetes in children and adolescents. *Pediatrics.* 2000;105:671–680

American Academy of Pediatrics, Committee on Adolescence. Identifying and treating eating disorders. *Pediatrics.* 2003; 111:204–211

American Academy of Pediatrics, Committee on Infectious Diseases. Recommended childhood and adolescent immunization schedule—United States, 2003. *Pediatrics.* 2003;111:212–216. (Available online at www.cispimmunize.org)

American Academy of Pediatrics, Committee on Practice and Ambulatory Medicine. Recommendations for preventive pediatric health care. *Pediatrics.* 2000;105:645–646

Beck AT, Steer RA, Brown GK. *Beck Depression Inventory®-II.* San Antonio, TX: The Psychological Corporation. (1-800-872-1726 or www.psychorp.com)

Elster AB, Kuznets MJ, eds. *AMA Guidelines for Adolescent Preventive Services (GAPS): Recommendations and Rationale.* Baltimore, MD: Williams & Wilkins; 1994. (Downloadable forms and background on implementation available at http://www.ama-assn.org/ama/pub/category/1980.html)*

Green M, Palfrey J, eds. *Bright Futures: Guidelines for Health Supervision of Infants, Children, and Adolescents*—2nd ed, revised. Arlington, VA: National Center for Education in Maternal and Child Health; 2002. (Under revision; more information available at http://brightfutures.aap.org)**

American Academy of Pediatrics. *Guidelines for Health Supervision III.* Elk Grove Village, IL; 1997. (2002 edition available; under revision)**

---

*   *Available from the American Medical Association (www.ama-assn.org or 1-800/621-8335).*

** *Available from the American Academy of Pediatrics (www.aap.org or 1-888/227-1770 or www.aap.org/bookstore).*

Helpful and Informative Web Sites for Teenagers and Parents

Today's adolescent is typically very familiar with computers and with the Internet. While many parents worry appropriately about material available on the Web, the Internet also provides many helpful and accurate sources of information for parents and teens. A number of helpful sites are listed below. In general, these sites are not appropriate for younger children. Parents are well advised to explore these sites with their teens or screen them independently.

RESOURCES FOR TEENS AND PARENTS

http://www.aap.org
American Academy of Pediatrics. Brochures and books for teens and their parents.

http://www.adolescenthealth.org
Tips for teens and parents sponsored by the Society for Adolescent Medicine

http://www.highschoolhub.org
Learning portal for free online educational resources for high school students

http://www.teengrowth.com
Physician-directed interactive site where adolescents can find sound information on a variety of health issues.

http://www.teenhealthfx.com
Award-winning site where questions from teens are addressed by physicians, mental health clinicians, and other professionals

http://www.teenshealth.org
Health information site sponsored by The Nemours Center for Children's Health Media

http://www.youthsource.org
International flavor (from Australia). Anything from A–Z.

SEXUALITY

Content about teen sexual health, pregnancy and contraception, STIs, HIV/AIDS, gynecology questions, and making good choices

http://www.goaskalice.com
Columbia University's health question and answer Internet service

http://www.iwannaknow.org
American Social Health Association

http://www.siecus.com
Sexuality Information and Education Council of the US

http://www.sxetc.org
A web site for teens by teens—Network for Family Life Education—Rutgers University

http://www.teenwire.com
Planned Parenthood Web site

MENTAL HEALTH AND SUBSTANCE ABUSE

Content about substance abuse, ADHD, depression, and anxiety

http://www.add.org
National Attention Deficit Disorder Association

http://www.addictionresourceguide.com
Getting help, finding treatment

http://www.chadd.org
Children and Adolescents with ADHD (CHADD)

http://www.clubdrugs.org
Service of the National Institute on Drug Abuse

http://www.nimh.nih.gov
National Institute of Mental Health

http://nmha.org
National Mental Health Association

http://www.samhsa.gov/oas/oasftp.htm
US Department of Health and Human Services Substance Abuse and Mental Health Services Administration

http://theantidrug.com
Site for parents from the National Youth Anti-Drug Media Campaign

MEDIA AND INTERNET SAFETY

Savvy advice about media messages and surfing the Internet

http://www.aap.org/mediamatters
Academy project that highlights how the media influence children and adolescents

http://www.apa.org/pubinfo/violence.html
American Psychological Association material about how violence on television affects children and how its impact can be moderated through parental involvement

http://www.mediafamily.org
Safety tips for surfers from the National Institute on Media and the Family. Advice for parents on how to talk to their children about Internet use

> Resources are included as sources of general information only. Their content has not been reviewed or endorsed by the American Academy of Pediatrics.

This patient education sheet is distributed in conjunction with the October 2003 issue of Adolescent Health Update, *published by the American Academy of Pediatrics. The information in this publication should not be used as a substitute for the medical care and advice of your pediatrician.*

Pediatricians are encouraged to photocopy this page for distribution to patients and parents.

A Nutrition Scorecard

by Kathy Scalzo, MA, RD

Does your breakfast give you a smart start in the morning? Do you pay attention to how you feel when you eat right...and when you don't? Use this form to grade yourself!

Breakfast

How often do you eat a healthy breakfast? Breakfast eaters feel sharper. They have more energy, they're thinner, and they live longer. To take good care of yourself, don't run out the door on an empty stomach or go with a sweet treat instead of a solid start.

Give yourself 1 point for every day in the last week that you ate a healthy breakfast.

Breakfast points	

5-A-Day: Fruits and Vegetables

Fruits and vegetables are some of your body's best friends. Both are natural sources of vitamin A, vitamin C, fiber, and folate (also known as folic acid). Guys and girls should have at least 2 pieces of fruit and 3 servings of vegetables a day for a total of 5-A-Day.

Super fruits:	Power veggies:
Strawberries	Spinach
Kiwi	Okra
Pineapple	Asparagus

Give yourself 1 point for every serving of fruits or vegetables you had yesterday. Then give yourself an extra-credit point for each super fruit and power veggie.

5-A-Day points	

Nutrition Scorecard:

0–15 points:	Starting today, I'm planning to pay more attention to what I eat and drink
16–22 points:	I get the concept, now I need to put it into action all the time
23 points or better:	Right on track. Great job!

Liquid Assets

Do you drink enough to meet your needs? You are what you eat AND what you drink! Smart choices will make your body work better. Fill in the blanks below and then grade yourself. Add the number of healthy drinks, and then subtract the number of drinks that handled your thirst but did nothing for your body. For example, if you had 12 cups of healthy drinks and 3 cups of "empty" drinks, your score is 9.

For good health, you need at least 11 cups of healthy drinks, for example:	You Drank
8 cups water	_____ cups
2 cups 1% low-fat or skim milk	_____ cups
1 cup 100% juice	_____ cups
Total good choices (add)	_____ cups

For good health, you DON'T need these liquids...	You Drank
Alcohol, wine or beer*	_____ cups
Soda	_____ cups
Coffee or tea	_____ cups
Total drinks that DON'T help your health (subtract)	"empty" _____ cups

There are lots of good reasons for teens to avoid alcohol. Dehydration is one of them

Enter your liquid asset points (cups of good choices minus empty cups) below:

Liquid asset points	
Now total your score	

If you want to improve your score, why not sit down with your family and talk about it? Looking good and feeling sharp have a lot to do with eating right!

Kathy Scalzo, MA, RD, is the nutritionist for the Schneider Children's Hospital school-based health program in New Hyde Park, New York.

This patient education sheet is distributed in conjunction with the October 2003 issue of Adolescent Health Update, *published by the American Academy of Pediatrics. The information in this publication should not be used as a substitute for the medical care and advice of your pediatrician. Comments and suggestions on Nutrition Notes should be forwarded to Marc Jacobson, MD FAAP (jacobson@lij.edu).*

Pediatricians are encouraged to photocopy this page for distribution to patients and parents.

Supported by an unrestricted educational grant from the Nestle Nutrition Institute™

Office-Based Care of Adolescents: Part 2 Practice Strategies and Coding Procedures for Proper Payment

by Peter D. Rappo, MD, FAAP

In part 1 of this 2-part series on practice management considerations in office-based care of adolescents (AHU 2003;16:1), author David Y. Rainey, MD, MPH, FAAP, considered nonfinancial considerations in creating what he described as a "teen-friendly office." In this second installment, Peter D. Rappo, MD, FAAP, presents advice and information about billing, coding, and office procedure that is of interest to pediatricians who care for adolescents.

Introduction

The challenges of modern practice require that primary care physicians understand and adhere to sound fiscal and management strategies. Effective practice strategies to assure proper billing and coding require a commitment to systematic, precise documentation. This is particularly important for the pediatrician caring for adolescents and young adults, whose office visits are often longer and more complex due to medical, developmental, and psychosocial issues that emerge during this time. This article will provide an overview of essential elements that provide the pediatrician with the tools required to successfully obtain appropriate compensation for adolescent care.

Billing for office visits requires an understanding of two coding systems: *Current Procedural Terminology (CPT®)*, published by the American Medical Association,* and the *International Classification of Diseases, Clinical Modification, 9th edition (ICD-9-CM)*, published by the World Health Organization. The *CPT* code tells the insurer what was done during the office visit (ie, the procedure or type of visit) and the *ICD-9* code tells why it was done (ie, the diagnosis). Inaccurate coding may lead to improper data collection, misidentification of patient diagnosis, inappropriate payment, and potential charges of fraud and abuse.

While this article will describe requirements of *CPT* and *ICD-9-CM*, these descriptions are not a substitute for the far more detailed and precise information in the text of the *CPT* and *ICD-9* manuals. Our discussion is descriptive and skeletal; *CPT* and *ICD-9* are prescriptive and comprehensive. **For billing, always rely upon information in the current, original *CPT* and *ICD-9-CM* texts.**

Goals and Objectives

Goal: Pediatricians will better understand coding, payment, and office management issues related to the care of adolescents.

Objectives: After reading this article, the pediatrician will be better prepared to:
- Describe appropriate and correct coding procedures
- Explain the requirements for appropriate documentation of an office encounter and how documentation affects coding and reimbursement
- Discuss strategies to address the challenges related to insurance reimbursement for certain services, such as mental health care
- Discuss practical challenges relevant to coding and appropriate payment

---

* *American Medical Association* Current Procedural Terminology (CPT®). *Any 5-digit numeric* Physicians' Current Procedural Terminology, *fourth edition, CPT codes, service descriptions, instructions and/or guidelines are copyright 2003 American Medical Association. All Rights Reserved.*

Peter D. Rappo, MD, FAAP, is the former vice president for pediatrics at Beansprout Networks and a member of the National Nominating Committee of the American Academy of Pediatrics (AAP). Dr Rappo, a former chair of the AAP Committee on Practice and Ambulatory Medicine and a former member of the Adolescent Health Update *editorial advisory board, practices primary care pediatrics in the Boston area. He has a particular interest in the care of children with special health care needs.*

CPT Coding and Documentation

Pediatricians and office staff need to understand *CPT* so that appropriate data elements are submitted to payers and vendors. A quick guide to the fundamental principles of *CPT* coding is shown in Table 1. There are separate codes for new and established patients (See Tables 2–3). A few comments:

- Since the system assumes that a new patient encounter should be compensated at a greater relative value than an established patient visit, the clinician should strive, if appropriate, to utilize the new patient code. The <u>first encounter</u> of a new patient with a new physician should be coded as the new patient visit. If an <u>established</u> patient has not seen the clinician for 3 or more years, then that patient may be also viewed as new. When seeing a patient who is established with a colleague in the practice for the first time as an on-call or a covering physician, that patient encounter is not new to the coverage system or practice and there is no opportunity for enhanced payment.

- Traditionally, the <u>consultation codes</u> in *CPT* **(99241–99245)** are utilized by pediatric subspecialists when evaluating a patient at the request of the primary care physician. A consultation generally requires a formal (ideally written) request that identifies the reason for the referral and a written report detailing what was accomplished during the consultation. There are times when a generalist can use these consultation codes, specifically when the request for the evaluation comes from another source, such as a surgeon requesting preoperative clearance or a school system inquiring about a child's medical condition.

- In general, physicians will not use **99211,** which is employed to bill for services provided by nurses.

This article will focus on procedures done in the office setting, the site for most encounters involving adolescents. The rationale for codes must be documented in the patient's chart in compliance with documentation guidelines stipulated by the U.S. Centers for Medicare & Medicaid Services (CMS). These guidelines are required whenever federal funds are involved. Many private payers use them also.

Two versions of the documentation guidelines (1995 and 1997) are currently acceptable and either can be used for any visit. Both are published on the CMS Web site (http://cms.hhs.gov/physicians/) and are included in coding manuals (see resource list). In general, pediatricians will find that the 1995 guidelines are easier to follow. The 1997 guidelines, however, offer tailored alternatives when coding for medical care focused on a particular organ system.

Precision is essential in coding and documentation. Clinicians are well advised to create and use templates that identify the elements required to document the visit properly. Many physicians devise simple checklists for this purpose. Tables 2 and 3, reprinted from the Academy's excellent new resource, the *Quick Reference Guide to Pediatric Coding and Documentation for Adolescent Medicine: A Companion to Coding for Pediatrics,* may be helpful in this regard.

The critical documentation components which determine the level of evaluation and management (E&M) visits are (1) history, (2) physical exam, (3) medical decision making, (4) counseling, (5) coordination of care, (6) nature of the

Table 1. Principles of *CPT*

CPT is structured around ten basic principles:

1) Set fees independent of reimbursement. A pediatrician's fees are based on work performed, time, and effort. Even when contractual write-offs are averaging around 30%, the physician who accepts "what they pay" as payment in full guarantees a downward reimbursement spiral.

2) Design a superbill or routing slip for your practice that lists your commonly used codes.

3) Take responsibility for selecting procedure and diagnosis codes. This is not the responsibility of the office staff.

4) Document services to support the codes.

5) Use separate codes for different encounters.

6) Set a separate fee commensurate with the effort and time involved with each code.

7) Use a modifier when altering a standard fee.

8) Understand local variations in coding and reimbursement.

9) Review and update your codes and fees on at least an annual basis.

10) Inquire about lowered or changed or noncompensated charges.

presenting problem, and (7) time. The first three (history, examination and medical decision making) are key components in all instances except those where more than half the visit is devoted to counseling and coordination of care. In that case, <u>time</u> is the controlling factor to determine the level of service.

In general, medical decision making will serve as the basis for determining the level of complexity of an office visit for coding purposes. Medical decision making is understood to be a mixture of knowledge, mental effort, and iatrogenic risk necessary to confirm and act on a diagnosis. (See Tables 4, 4A)

If counseling or coordination of care drive 50% or more of any physician/patient and/or family encounter for a standard office visit, time recommendations in the *CPT* text descriptions can be used to determine the code for the visit. There are individual counseling codes, also time-based, for counseling to promote prevention of injuries, avoidance of substance abuse, proper diet and exercise, etc. The series **99401–99404** is for individual preventive counseling; codes change with every 15 minutes of counseling time (eg, **99401** equaling 15 minutes, **99402** equaling 30 minutes, etc.). Additional time for parent-only counseling, if required, is also coded as counseling time. Group counseling is billed with **99411–99412.**

It is important to remember that, <u>in the event of an audit, a procedure that is not specifically documented in the chart is a procedure that did not occur.</u> The medical record should always specify each of the systems or elements that were completed in order to meet the documentation standard. Failure to meet the documentation standard can make the physician vulnerable to charges of fraud.

WELL-ADOLESCENT CARE

Preventive medicine codes are used to bill for the annual well-patient visit. Codes **99384** (new) and **99394** (established) are employed for patients ages 12–17, and **99385** (new) and **99395** (established) are employed for patients ages 18–39. Federal documentation guidelines require, and the Academy's Recommendations

for Preventive Pediatric Health Care recommend, that well-patient examinations include a comprehensive history and physical along with appropriate counseling and anticipatory guidance. It is important to note that this documentation standard is at variance with the AMA *Guidelines for Adolescent Preventive Services* (GAPS) recommendations, which do not stipulate a comprehensive physical examination at each annual visit.

(continued on page 40)

Talking Point

Those Mysterious Modifiers
A modifier is a 2-digit add-on code that tells the insurer's computer, "This one's different." Modifiers signal that the encounter involved more or less work than it usually might, or perhaps that an additional procedure was required. The two digit modifier is appended to the five digit *CPT* code that it is linked to.

Modifiers that are particularly useful in primary care or adolescent practice include:
- **-21** Prolonged evaluation and management (E&M) service (eg, a visit that takes longer than the usual time allotment for a visit)
- **-25** Significant, separate E&M service (eg, dealing with a medical problem at the same time that one is doing a well adolescent exam)
- **-52** Reduced service
- **-53** Discontinued procedure (failed attempt to draw blood, for example)
- **-57** Decision for surgery (eg, removing a wart at the time of a physical exam)
- **-76** Repeat procedure by the same physician (eg, multiple nebulization treatments for an asthmatic)

A number of *CPT* code descriptors include <u>suggested time allotments</u>, but these are guidelines rather than absolute parameters. Although there are time suggestions for most office visit and consultative codes, the experienced and efficient clinician will find that he is often able to accomplish evaluation and management services in less than the suggested time. Codes that are explicitly time-determined are those for case management, review of records or documents without patient contact, and encounters where more than 50% of the visit time is used for purposes of counseling.

Coding for New and Established Patient Office Visits

These tables illustrate the reasoning that drives the selection process when coding for office-based evaluation and management services. The series **99201–99205** for new patients and **99211–99215** for established patients will "fit the bill" about 80% of the time. When coding, ensure that criteria for 2 of the 3 key components (history, physical examination, and medical decision making) are met or exceeded.

Table 2. Office or Other Outpatient Services (New Patient)

Document either **all 3 key components** (history, examination, and medical decision making) OR time spent counseling the patient.

	99201	99202	99203	99204	99205
History					
Level of history	Problem focused	Expanded problem focused	Detailed	Comprehensive	Comprehensive
CC	Required	Required	Required	Required	Required
HPI	1–3 elements	1–3 elements	4+ elements OR 3+ chronic or inactive conditions	4+ elements OR 3+ chronic or inactive conditions	4+ elements OR 3+ chronic or inactive conditions
ROS	Not required	1 system	2–9 systems	10–14 systems	10–14 systems
PFSH	Not required	Not required	1 of 3 elements	3 of 3 elements	3 of 3 elements
Physical Examination					
Level of examination	Problem focused	Expanded problem focused	Detailed	Comprehensive	Comprehensive
1995	1 system	2–4 systems	5–7 systems	8 or more systems	8 or more systems
1997	1–5 elements	6–11 elements	12 or more systems	Comp multisystem OR GU	Comp multisystem OR GU
Medical Decision Making					
Level of MDM	Straightforward	Straightforward	Low	Moderate	High
Face-to-Face Time					
Typical times	10 minutes	20 minutes	30 minutes	45 minutes	60 minutes
Relative Value Units/2005 Medicare Payment Conversion Factor=37.8975					
Total RVUs/$	0.97/$36.76	1.72/$65.18	2.56/$97.02	3.62/$137.19	4.58/$173.57

Table 3. Office or Other Outpatient Services (Established Patient)

Document either **2 or 3 key components** (history, examination, and medical decision making) OR time spent counseling the patient.

	99211	99212	99213	99214	99215
History					
Level of history	Not required	Problem focused	Expanded problem focused	Detailed	Comprehensive
CC	Not required	Required	Required	Required	Required
HPI	Not required	1–3 elements	1–3 elements	4+ elements OR 3+ chronic or inactive conditions	4+ elements OR 3+ chronic or inactive conditions
ROS	Not required	Not required	1 system	2–9 systems	10–14 systems
PFSH	Not required	Not required	Not required	Not required	Not required
Physical Examination					
Level of examination	Not required	Problem focused	Expanded problem focused	Detailed	Comprehensive
1995	Not required	1 system	2–4 systems	5–7 systems	8 or more systems
1997	Not required	1–5 elements	6–11 systems	12 or more elements	Comp multisystem OR GU
Medical Decision Making					
Level of MDM	Not required	Straightforward	Low	Moderate	High
Face-to-Face Time					
Typical times	5 minutes supervision*	10 minutes	15 minutes	25 minutes	40 minutes
Relative Value Units/2005 Medicare Payment Conversion Factor=37.8975					
Total RVUs/$	0.57/$21.60	1.02/$38.66	1.39/$52.68	2.18/$82.62	3.17/$120.14

Tables 2 and 3 are reprinted from Bradley J, Blythe M, eds. *Quick Reference Guide to Pediatric Coding and Documentation for Adolescent Medicine: A Companion to Coding for Pediatrics.* Elk Grove Village, IL: American Academy of Pediatrics; 2004:22, 24

Legend for Tables 2 and 3

Abbreviations in Tables 2 and 3 refer to items specified in the Centers for Medicare and Medicaid Services (CMS) 1995 and 1997 Documentation Guidelines for Evaluation and Management Services (DGs), which can be found at http://cms.hhs.gov/physicians/.

History

CC: chief complaint (symptom, problem, condition, diagnosis, physician-recommended return, or other reason for the encounter)

HPI: history of present illness (elements may include location, quality, severity, duration, timing, context, modifying factors, and associated signs/symptoms)

PFSH: past (experiences with illnesses, surgeries, injuries, and treatments), family (medical events in the family, including diseases that may be hereditary or place the patient at risk), and social (age-appropriate review of past and current activities) history

ROS: review of systems (systems to specify may include: constitutional, eyes, ears/nose/mouth/throat, cardiovascular, respiratory, gastrointestinal, genitourinary, musculoskeletal, integumentary, neurological, psychiatric, endocrine, hematologic/lymphatic, and allergic/immunologic)

Physical Examination

The 1995 and 1997 federal documentation guidelines differ from one another in several respects. These require a more detailed presentation than our space allows. Please see the online documentation guidelines (http://cms.hhs.gov/physicians/) for more information.

Table 4. Medical Decision Making

Two of the three elements in columns 2–4 below must be met or exceeded to justify the level of decision making indicated in column 1. For an explanation of risk assessment (column 4), please see Table 4A.

Type of decision making	Number of diagnoses or management options	Amount and/or complexity of data to be reviewed	Risk of complications and morbidity or mortality*
Straightforward	Minimal	Minimal or none	Minimal
Low complexity	Limited	Limited	Low
Moderate complexity	Multiple	Moderate	Moderate
High complexity	Extensive	Extensive	High

Reprinted from 1995 and 1997 federal documentation guidelines for evaluation and management services, Centers for Medicare and Medicaid Services (available at http://cms.hhs.gov/physicians/)

*See Table 4A below

Table 4A. Risk of Complications and Morbidity or Mortality

The risk of complications helps to determine the level of complexity in medical decision making.

Level of risk	Examples of presenting problem(s)	Examples of diagnostic procedure(s) ordered	Examples of management options selected
Minimal	Single, minor problem (eg, URI, insect bite)	Chest x-ray, UA, laboratory tests	Supportive care, superficial dressing
Low	Two or more minor acute problems or one stable chronic problem (eg, stable hypertension)	Pulmonary function tests, noncardiovascular imaging studies without contrast (eg, barium enema), clinical lab tests	Over-the-counter drugs, physical therapy, IV fluids
Moderate	Chronic illness with mild exacerbation, 2 or more stable chronic conditions, acute complicated illness or injury (eg, cystitis with fever, head trauma with loss of consciousness)	Diagnostic endoscopy with no identified risk factors, lumbar puncture, thoracentesis	Prescription drugs, minor surgery with identified risk factors
High	Chronic illness with severe exacerbation, acute or chronic illness that poses immediate threat to life or function	Cardiovascular imaging	Drug therapies that require close monitoring for toxicity, decision not to resuscitate

Derived and excerpted from the "Table of Risk" in the 1995 and 1997 federal documentation guidelines for evaluation and management services (http://cms.hhs.gov/physicians/)

If a separate problem requiring referral or further evaluation is identified during a routine well-patient examination and that problem requires significant time and attention, a standard office visit code (**99211–99215** for an established patient) can be employed with a **-25** modifier attached and appropriate documentation to show that two separate procedures were accomplished at that visit.

OTHER *CPT* CODES

A few special codes merit brief mention.

- **99361** (30 minutes) or **99362** (60 minutes): Team conference code employed when a clinician calls for a conference in the office, school setting, etc., with other interested parties
- **99374** (less than 30 minutes per month) or **99375** (more than 30 minutes per month): Oversight to assure that a care plan is properly followed by a home health agency is billed as ongoing coordination of care
- **99358** (60 minutes) and **99359** (each additional 30 minutes): Prolonged physician service without direct face-to-face patient contact (eg, review of information to evaluate for job disability or prolonged review of records for another reason).
- Certain "off-hours" codes may be added to the office visit code:
  - **99050:** services provided in office at times other than regularly scheduled hours, or days when office is normally closed
  - **99058:** services provided on an emergency basis in office

CONSULTATION VIA TELEPHONE AND THE INTERNET

CPT allows for billing of telephone consultations under codes **99371–99373.** Prolonged services codes can be used to bill for a telephone consultation that is longer than 30 minutes (**99358** for the first hour). Third party payers rarely pay for telephone consultation; this is a difficult issue and resolution is a work in progress.

When the payer considers telephone calls to be an uncovered service it is possible to bill a patient directly for this time if this is discussed with the parents in advance. It is not possible to bill Medicaid patients directly for this service.

CPT has not yet created virtual codes to allow for electronic consultation via secure messaging technology over the Internet. Ironically, some insurers that do not cover telephone consultation are reportedly considering virtual consultation as a limited, covered benefit. Such a move should help to refocus the issues involved in compensation for telephone consultation.

Diagnosis Coding

The *ICD-9-CM* is organized into three volumes, a tabular list of diseases and injuries, an alphabetical index of the same categories, and a list of procedures. Two supplementary classifications deserve additional mention. E codes are descriptions of injuries and poisonings, which are very useful in capturing and categorizing the causes of accidents. V codes are used to describe factors other than a disease, injury, or accident that prompt a need for care. Although V codes can be used as either primary or secondary reasons for the encounter, they are best used as secondary because many insurers' computers are programmed to accept only "diagnosis" codes and to reject V codes automatically.

Talking Point

Why submit bills with codes that are rarely reimbursed?

The rationale for submitting a code that accurately reflects the services provided despite the likelihood that it will not be reimbursed is an important "big picture" argument:

1. An unused *CPT* code will never be reimbursed.
2. Increased use of a code encourages insurers to create a profile and consider the need for payment.
3. Use of these codes demonstrates the range of services necessary for adolescent patients.

Those who write the budgets for third party payment need to appreciate the range of typical services in adolescent care so that they can calculate appropriate capitation rates.

MENTAL HEALTH SERVICES

The overlap between medical and mental health issues is complicated by insurance contracts with "carve out" arrangements under which only mental health professionals can be compensated for services billed under "mental health" diagnostic codes. Such provisions discourage pediatricians who endeavor to provide coordinated, comprehensive, complete, and compassionate care for adolescent patients.

Mental health issues that emerge or can exacerbate in adolescence include mood disorders, family conflict, oppositional defiant disorder, adjustment disorder of childhood, somatization disorders, substance use, attention deficit/hyperactivity disorder, and eating disorders such as anorexia nervosa, bulimia nervosa, and compulsive overeating. Mental health care is typically compensated under a diagnostic coding system published by the American Psychiatric Association, the *Diagnostic and Statistical Manual of Mental Disorders, Fourth Edition, Text Revision (DSM-IV-TR)*, and the American Academy of Pediatrics' companion primary care version, *The Classification of Child and Adolescent Mental Diagnoses in Primary Care: Diagnostic and Statistical Manual for Primary Care (DSM-PC Child and Adolescent Version)*. *DSM-IV* and *DSM-PC* provide algorithmic criteria to assist in identifying the appropriate *ICD-9* code for mental health diagnoses.

Some health insurers will not compensate pediatricians for treatment of mental health disorders. Others will compensate pediatricians for mental or behavioral health services only if medication management for the disorder is the primary reason for the visit, or medical comorbidities are addressed and documented as part of the visit. Compensation problems are often regional; there are ongoing tensions in this regard.

Clinicians may not be compensated if V codes are used as the primary diagnosis of mental health conditions; the issue relates to the linkage between what the physician codes for and what procedure code he or she uses. If regional practices allow reimbursement for a mental health *DSM-IV* or *DSM-PC* code, that would be the first choice.

In all cases, the 2 pages of psychiatric *CPT* codes in the *CPT* manual are restricted to use by mental health clinicians.

Compliance, Fraud, and Abuse

The first Medicare anti-fraud and abuse legislation was passed in 1972 as an outgrowth of the False Claims Act of 1860, legislation designed to punish vendors during the Civil War who billed the government inappropriately for goods and services. White-collar crime has become a top priority for the Justice Department, with an anticipated cost in 2003 of $240 million for enforcement.

Fraud is defined as submission of claims for services not provided. Abuse refers to the systematic submission of such claims whether advertent or inadvertent. Red flags for potential accusations of fraud and abuse include:

1) Coding for all evaluation and management services at one or two levels
2) Consultations without referrals
3) Billing for resident services without appropriate supervision or documentation by attendings.
4) Billing for nonallowed services
5) Excessive charges
6) Services not provided as claimed
7) Routine waiver of copays
8) Advertising for free services

Sanctions for fraud and abuse violations can include financial penalty, restriction of privileges, loss of medical licensure, and criminal proceedings including fines, recoupment and prison sentences. Systematic overcoding, upcoding, and inappropriate provision of services are illegal and unethical practices undertaken at the peril of the individual pediatrician.

Establishing Sound Office Policies

After coding, information is transmitted to the patient or insurer for payment. Charges need to be entered and submitted to the insurer on the day that the service was provided. It is important to see that statements returned by insurers to offices are promptly resolved; these are all too often put aside. Insurance companies use "explanation of benefits" forms (EOBs) to explain reasons for denials or rejection of services. Statements rejected because of lack of medical necessity can be rebilled with documentation to support the need for the service. Failing to follow up on payment rejections in a timely manner will often result in missed payment timelines. Each practice should look at repeated systematic rejections for the same services, claims that are denied for registration errors, and inappropriate procedures related to bundling or unbundling of services. [Bundling of services refers to the inappropriate combining of services (lab, immunization, procedures) as part of a patient visit.] Insurers expect that copayments will be collected at the time of service.

Office personnel must clearly understand the importance of administrative and billing procedures to prevent inadvertent disclosure of sensitive or confidential information, as when diagnosis codes on "explanation of benefits" forms sent by insurers to parents unexpectedly compromise confidentiality. Pediatricians should know state and federal laws pertaining to confidentiality and assure that their office procedures are compliant with those laws. (Please refer to part 1 of this series for a more thorough discussion of confidentiality in adolescent care.)

Summary

Many clinicians who routinely negotiate medical matters that are far more complicated than billing, coding, and collections find office management bewildering and hopelessly complex. Yet it is critical that clinicians understand the systems, rules of the road, and rationale for the payment structures within which their practices operate.

While there are many consulting firms available to assist those who are reluctant to master these concepts, these consultants come at a cost to the practice. Pediatricians who are able to deal with the complexities of adolescent health care and provide services to meet the medical, social, mental health, and behavioral needs of this group of patients are entirely capable of acquiring the skills required to manage their practices with skill and satisfaction.

References and Resources

American Academy of Pediatrics. *Coding for Pediatrics 2004.* 9th ed. Elk Grove Village, Illinois: American Academy of Pediatrics; 2003

American Academy of Pediatrics. *2004 Pediatric ICD-9-CM Coding Flip Chart.* Elk Grove Village, Illinois: American Academy of Pediatrics; 2003

American Academy of Pediatrics. *The Classification of Child and Adolescent Mental Diagnoses in Primary Care: Diagnostic and Statistical Manual for Primary Care (DSM-PC Child and Adolescent Version).* Elk Grove Village, Illinois: American Academy of Pediatrics; 1996

American Hospital Association. *ICD-9-CM Expert for Physicians, Volumes 1&2—2004.* West Valley City, Utah: Ingenix (St. Anthony/Medicode); 2003

American Medical Association. *CPT 2004—Current Procedural Terminology, Professional Edition.* Chicago, Illinois: American Medical Association; 2003

American Psychiatric Association. *Diagnostic and Statistical Manual of Mental Disorders, Fourth Edition, Text Revision. (DSM-IV-TR).* Washington DC: American Psychiatric Association; 2000

Bradley J, Blythe M, eds. *Quick Reference Guide to Pediatric Coding and Documentation for Adolescent Medicine: A Companion to Coding for Pediatrics.* Elk Grove Village, Illinois: American Academy of Pediatrics; 2003

Centers for Medicare & Medicaid Services. *1995 Documentation Guidelines for Evaluation and Management Services.* Available at http://cms.hhs.gov/physicians/. Accessed October 31, 2003

Centers for Medicare & Medicaid Services. *1997 Documentation Guidelines for Evaluation and Management Services.* Available at http://cms.hhs.gov/physicians/. Accessed October 31, 2003

Acknowledgment

The editors would like to acknowledge technical review by Margaret J. Blythe, MD, FAAP, for the AAP Section on Adolescent Health. Dr. Blythe and coeditor Joel F. Bradley, MD, FAAP, recently completed work on a new coding manual for adolescent care, *Quick Reference Guide to Pediatric Coding and Documentation for Adolescent Medicine,* published earlier this year by the American Academy of Pediatrics as a companion to the manual, *Coding for Pediatrics.* (The new coding manual is available from the Academy at www.aap.org/bookstore or 1-888/227-1770.)

Questions and Answers About Coding in Clinical Practice

Q. *One of my colleagues is code-phobic. I need to come up with a way to help him understand that there is a logic to CPT. Most of what we do falls into the established patient office visit codes (99211–99215). Can you come up with a simple way to describe what they mean?*

A. The best way to learn *CPT* is to use it, but to break through that coding anxiety syndrome, try this:

99211	Probably, but now always, a nursing visit (TB test, dressing change, weight check, blood pressure check)
99212	Straightforward, simple, single-system problem
99213	Usual, average clinical encounter
99214	Oh, no, this will take a while
99215	We just finished the marathon; who's next?

Q. *Let's say that an established 17-year-old patient reveals substance use in the course of an annual well-adolescent visit, and the visit extends to 40 minutes, including 25 minutes for counseling around sexuality and sexually transmitted infections (STIs). How do I code?*

A. Code for the well adolescent exam (*CPT* **99394**) linked to *ICD-9* code **V20.2.** One could add modifier **-21** to indicate a prolonged visit, but preferably one would use, in addition to the well-examination code, an office visit code **(99211–99215)** with a modifier **-25** attached and linked to code **V65.45** for counseling around STI issues to report the additional service. Since 25 minutes of the visit was for counseling, time would determine the selection of the *CPT* code for compensation, in this case **99214** for an established patient. In all cases, both the well exam and the STI counseling time should have clearly definable, separate documentation.

Q. *I do a lot of medication checks for patients with ADHD, depression, anxiety, etc. I am told that psychiatric CPT codes are unavailable to pediatricians. How do I code for medication management?*

A. The above assertion is correct; pediatricians should not employ codes designed for psychiatric professionals. However, since you are performing the service, use standard office visit evaluation and management codes linked to the *ICD-9* code for ADHD **(314.01).**

Q. *What coding strategies will allow me to be compensated without compromising patient confidentiality related to a reproductive health matter? For example, what codes would be used for care of a patient with a sexually transmitted infection?*

A. The only way to be sure that confidential information would not turn up at home on an EOB is to bill the patient directly, provided that she is not insured by Medicaid, which would be a federal violation of the Medicaid program. Some coding choices will minimize the risk of inadvertent disclosure. If the patient is a young woman, a diagnosis of vaginitis **(616.01)** would address STI symptoms. For a young man with painful urination caused by urethritis, possibly a sexually transmitted infection, the code would be **597.80.** In patients with an asymptomatic sexually transmitted infection, it would be **079.98.**

Q. *I have treated several patients who are obese but whose physical examinations reveal normal cholesterol, blood pressure, and glucose, etc. Their insurance carriers refuse to accept the condition of obesity as a primary diagnosis. Can you suggest an effective way to educate these payers?*

A. Although more exact coding is almost always preferred by insurers, obesity seems to be the exception. There seems to be a sentiment in the insurance world that obesity is not a reimbursable condition unless it is associated with specific comorbidities (eg, hypertension), which are less common in the adolescent patient. It is hoped that the new AAP Task Force on Obesity will be addressing this difficult issue.

Q. How do I code for ongoing care of adolescents with puberty-related medical issues (eg, growth concerns, precocious puberty, gynecomastia of puberty, menstrual problems not related to sexual behavior)?

A. Patients with established problems, such as puberty-related issues, would have evaluation and management codes utilized that reflect the service completed. If a patient came in for a visit because he was upset about delayed puberty and short stature, and counseling dominated 50% of the 20-minute encounter, then the clinician would employ a **99213**.

Q. I had a patient who reported increasing problems with irregular menses and dysmenorrhea on her annual well-adolescent check-up. Rather than ask her to come back, I extended the visit to do a gynecologic exam. How do I bill for the extra time required on that visit?

A. The gynecologic exam is included in the descriptor for the comprehensive well-adolescent examination **(99394)**. While it can be difficult for pediatric generalists to schedule sufficient time for both the comprehensive exam (measurements, history, physical, and appropriate anticipatory guidance) along with the gynecologic exam, that is the model. A return visit, if required, could be coded as an office visit **(99212–99215)** with an appropriate diagnosis code (eg, **626.4**, irregular menses). This scenario seems to punish the efficient physician and reward less efficient, separate encounters, but sometimes a single encounter is the best solution.

Section I Further Reading

Fisher M. Adolescent health assessments and promotion in office and school settings. *Adolesc Med.* 1999;10:71–86

Prazar GE. A private practitioner's approach to adolescent problems. *Adolesc Med.* 1998;9:229–241

Common Medical Problems

Back Pain in the Adolescent: A User-Friendly Guide

by Jordan D. Metzl, MD, FAAP

"Jodie," a 15-year-old female volleyball player, comes to the office complaining of steadily increasing low back pain of 4 weeks' duration. She cannot recall any specific injury, and instead describes an aching pain in her lumbar spine that has developed over the course of the season and has worsened every time she plays. "The past month has been terribly painful," she says.

When asked specifically, Jodie describes a "dull ache at the bottom of my spine," that hurts, "especially when I serve." She denies paresthesia or radiculopathy into the feet or toes as well as pain that awakens her in the night. The pain is clearly worse after volleyball, she says, and is worst when she serves the ball. "I can barely serve it hurts so much," she says.

When they arrive in the office for further evaluation, Jodie and her mom say that they want to figure out what's wrong and take care of it right away. "I love playing volleyball and I have to get back as soon as possible," she says.

The pediatrician in this fictional vignette must quickly sort out the many possible causes of Jodie's back pain. The most common sources of back pain in adolescence are bone-related, muscular, and discogenic, although other etiologies must be considered.

This article will discuss the most common types of back pain and briefly address less typical etiologies. The text will give clues for appropriate evaluation, treatment, and referral of adolescents who present to the medical office with back pain.

How Common Is It?

Studies suggest that between 70% and 80% of the general population will experience low back pain at some point in their lives.[1] In the majority of adult cases, pain is located in the lumbar spine and is termed "mechanical." This type of back pain is largely related to muscular weakness, inflexibility, cartilaginous disk abnormality, and arthritic degeneration of the lumbar spine.

Back pain is also common in adolescents. Retrospective school-based surveys of 1700 and 1400 adolescents found that 27% and 30%, respectively, had experienced low back pain at some time in the past.[1] Another study of 100 student athletes ages 12 to 18 who presented to the sports medicine clinic of a children's hospital for evaluation of back pain attributed the pain to spondylolysis in 47%, disk problems in

Goals and Objectives

After reading this article, pediatricians who care for patients with back pain will be better prepared to:
- List the types of back pain most commonly seen in adolescents
- Do a comprehensive assessment
- Perform an appropriate physical examination
- Complete a differential diagnosis
- Identify criteria for further diagnostic evaluation
- Discuss the role of imaging and other diagnostic tools
- Develop a management plan for treatment of the most common forms of back pain
- Delineate criteria for referral

Jordan D. Metzl, MD, FAAP, is the medical director of the Sports Medicine Institute for Young Athletes, Hospital for Special Surgery, New York City and Old Greenwich, CT. Dr. Metzl, who treats pediatric, adolescent, and adult athletes, is on the editorial boards of Pediatrics, Pediatric Emergency Care, *and* Pediatric Annals, *and is the author of* The Young Athlete, A Sports Doctor's Complete Guide for Parents *(Little, Brown and Company, 2002).*

11%, lumbosacral strain of muscle-tendon units in 6%, and lordotic or mechanical causes in 26%.[2]

Taking the History

In evaluating back pain in an adolescent, the history is a key part of the equation.

Listen closely to ascertain the mechanism of injury. Elicit information about types of movement and activities associated with pain. Ask about prior injuries or periods of back pain. Inquire as to the site of pain and whether or not it radiates. (See *Checklist for the Clinical Encounter*)

The Physical Examination

Physical examination of the patient with back pain includes observation of gait and posture followed by active motion, strength, and neurosensory tests.

To begin the physical examination of the spine, ask patients to let you watch them walk across the room. Ideally, they should be in a gown that is open in back, dressed in shorts, with no top and no brassiere. Look to see whether they have a normal gait. Are they comfortable? Are they tilted to one side? Next, look at the spine. Is the hip height equal on both sides? Are the shoulders equal on both sides? If there is a fold of skin above the hips, does one side look more creased than the other?

ACTIVE MOTION TESTS

Ask the patient to move as directed while you observe the lumbar spine.

- Instruct the patient to bend all the way forward. Pain bending forward is most often discogenic. Do the Adams test for scoliosis, asking the patient to extend her arms and put both palms together, then slowly bend forward from the waist. Stand behind the patient and position your field of gaze at the level of the spine. Look for asymmetry of the thoracic cage or lower back. Curvature in the spine suggests scoliosis, which may be further assessed by x-ray.

- Ask the patient to bend backward. Pain on bending backward often suggests spondylolysis or a stress fracture.

- Instruct the patient to put hands on hips and twist back to left and right, looking for any pain on either side of the spine. Pain with twisting would be consistent with muscle spasm or muscle pain.

- Ask the patient to sit on the examining table with legs dangling for a straight leg raise test. Straighten out one leg, then the other, and look for any pain associated with one side or the other. If there is pain bending forward and with a leg raise on a specific side, consider a disk problem on that side.

FURTHER EXAMINATION

After the active motion tests, examine the patient further via palpation, strength testing, and a neurosensory examination.

- Palpate the spine and look for areas of tenderness along spinal processes (bones).

- Palpate the iliac crest, specifically cartilaginous apophyses or growth plates.

- L5 disk herniation would cause weakness of the hallucis longus muscle. To test for that, ask the patient to extend the great toe upward against your resistance.

- Test quadriceps and hamstring muscles, asking the patient to push the leg out as if to kick, then pull it back, both times against your resistance.

- L4 weakness would be detected with inversion of the foot. To test for this, ask the patient to evert the foot against resistance.

- Check for L4 nerve root involvement by assessing dorsal and plantar flexion of the foot.

- Check reflexes in the patellar tendon, the L4 nerve root. A diminished reflex in the L4 nerve root suggests a possible disk herniation between the L3 and L4 vertebrae.

- Look for a diminished Achilles reflex, which would indicate disk herniation at the L5 level.

Findings from the physical examination will direct the clinician's next steps, which may include further diagnostic tests, physical therapy, and/or referral to a specialist. Weak or diminished

---

Checklist for the Clinical Encounter

The following questions can help structure history-taking for back-related problems:

1. What was the mechanism of injury (eg, acute traumatic injury, overuse injury, specifics that led to injury)?
2. (If not injury-related): When did this pain begin? How did it begin? Do you remember what you were doing the day before the onset of pain? Was the onset acute or insidious? Have you had pain like this before?
3. What activity makes the pain worse (eg, pressure, movement in a given direction, rest)? Do any sports activities make it worse (eg, serving a volleyball, bending backward in dance class, twisting in basketball)?
4. Does the pain awaken you at night?
5. What eases the pain?
6. Are there neurological or radicular symptoms?
7. What is the prior history of injuries or problems?
8. Where is the pain located (lumbar, upper/lower thoracic, midline, paraspinal)?
9. Are there any other symptoms on the review of systems (eg, bowel or bladder problems, abdominal pain, fever, weight loss)?
10. Are there symptoms not related to the back that suggest systemic infection, neoplasm, or a collagen vascular problem (eg, fever or painful joints)?
11. Is there a family history of back stiffness or spondyloarthropathy?

---

reflexes may suggest a nerve problem or a herniated disk. Consider referral to an orthopedic or sports medicine specialist if there is pain on bending forward or backward, pain on the straight leg test, diminished deep tendon reflexes, or apophyseal pain on palpation.

Most Common Types of Back Pain

Most adolescent back pain will fall into 3 general categories: muscular, bone-related, and discogenic. **(See Table 1)**

MUSCULAR BACK PAIN

Roughly 30% of all cases of back pain in adolescents is muscular in origin. When an adolescent comes to the office with a complaint of back pain, what clues would suggest muscular pain?

Muscular pain in the adolescent back tends to occur on one or both sides of either the thoracic or lumbar spine, most often during or after twisting or lifting. Sometimes there is a history of acute injury, as in the case of a teen who twists during a baseball game and develops an acute back spasm with a sharp pain along the side of the lumbar spine in the paraspinous muscles.

More often, however, the scenario for muscular back pain is an overuse injury, as in the adolescent who lugs a 60-pound backpack to school daily and then complains of an ache in the paraspinous muscle group.

The specific findings on physical examination of the adolescent with muscular back pain include tenderness to palpation along the paraspinous muscles and the feeling of a "knot" in the back.

Adolescents with muscular back pain generally will <u>not</u> have pain with forward flexion (bending forward) or extension (bending backward). Rather, muscular back pain tends to occur with spinal rotation. To best elicit this finding, the examiner should have the patient slowly twist from side to side while stabilizing the hips. The slow twist will cause the muscles to hurt because they are tight and in spasm.

A Word About Scoliosis

Although scoliosis does not directly produce back pain, muscular back pain is a common secondary finding in adolescents who have a scoliotic curve, which is why it is important to rule out scoliosis if a diagnosis of muscular back pain is entertained.

Table 1. Common Causes of Back Pain

Clues to Pathophysiology	Muscular	Bone-Related	Discogenic
Site of pain	Localized to paraspinous muscles	Localized to center of spine	
Pain during activity	X	X	X
Pain after activity	X	X	X
Pain bending forward			X
Pain bending backward		X	
Straight raised leg test elicits pain			X
Pain with twisting	X		
Radiating pain		May occur if there is spondylolisthesis and the degree of slip is sufficient to impinge on the nerve root	X
Strength testing			Strength tests involving the great toe, inverted foot, thigh, and hip flexor may show weakness
Neurosensory exam	Unremarkable	Reflex deficiencies may signal spondylolisthesis that has progressed to compress spinal nerve roots.	Reflex deficiencies may signal disk herniation; tingling toes may suggest spinal cord compression
Radiologic Tests	Consider x-ray only if pain persists more than 6 weeks, occult fracture is suspected, or scoliosis is also present	X-rays—1 AP, 1 lateral, and 2 oblique views. Consider MRI if concerned about fracture. If spondylolysis is suspected but not clear on x-ray, MRI will reveal edema	X-rays—1 AP and 1 lateral. MRI considered gold standard; rarely CT if MRI not clear.
Activity modification	Patients should be encouraged to return to play as soon as they can, using their judgment and taking nonsteroidal anti-inflammatory drugs as needed.	Sports hiatus for younger patients with spondylolysis that may heal with rest. Older patients can play with or without a brace once they are pain-free, but must postpone return to play until nerve-related symptoms resolve.	Bed rest is not recommended
Indications for referral	Associated scoliosis	Spondylolysis, spondylolisthesis, or pain that persists for more than a month despite physical therapy, regardless of x-ray findings	Always
Treatment plan	Physical therapy, which may include referral to a sports-oriented physical therapist	Referral to a sports-oriented physical therapist and either a sports medicine specialist or a sports-oriented pediatric orthopedist	Referral to a sports-oriented physical therapist and sports medicine specialist or sports-oriented pediatric orthopedist. Their options will include bracing or steroid injection and, if all else fails, microdiskectomy

Patients with both scoliosis and pain are candidates for referral because one cannot assume the pain is due to scoliosis and must therefore pursue other causes.

Evaluation for possible scoliosis is best done by performing the forward-flexion maneuver known as the Adams test, described previously. If physical findings suggest scoliosis, a Scoliometer can help to confirm the diagnosis. An inclination reading between 5 and 7 degrees indicates that further evaluation is required. Definitive diagnosis is made through a spine radiograph.

Diagnosis and Treatment of Muscular Back Pain

In general, the physical examination is sufficient for diagnosis and evaluation of muscular back pain. However, if there is scoliosis associated with the pain, spinal radiographs are recommended for measurement of the curve.

While anti-inflammatory agents are sometimes helpful for temporary pain management, steroids and muscle relaxants generally are not indicated. Treatment of muscular back pain involves muscular stretching and strengthening, which may include referral to a physical therapist. The referral should stipulate a diagnosis of muscular back pain and recommend a plan for evaluation and treatment including ultrasound, electrical stimulation, heat, and ice. With physical therapy, muscular back pain will usually resolve within 4 to 6 weeks. In our office, we encourage patients to remain active when being treated and schedule an interim check at 3 weeks. For student athletes, this includes return to sports as soon as they can. More activity does not typically cause increased problems with muscular back pain, so these patients can be encouraged to use their judgment.

BONE-RELATED BACK PAIN

Bone-related back pain accounts for roughly 25% to 50% of back pain in adolescents and is most often seen in more athletic teens. The most common scenario for this presentation is the adolescent athlete who comes in complaining of pain in the lumbar spine with extension. This is generally an athlete who uses the spine for repetitive extension maneuvers, such as the gymnast, figure skater, ballerina, or volleyball player.

Bone-related back pain is most often a result of overuse. In overuse or repetitive stress injury, edema in the bone signals stress that may progress to an overt stress fracture known as a *spondylolysis*, a crack in the pars interarticularis.

Micheli and Wood found that nearly half of young athletes who presented to a sports medicine clinic with back pain had spondylolysis.[2] However, spondylolysis is often asymptomatic. A study of 145 Indiana University football players screened for spondylolysis in the 1970s revealed that 47% of those with spondylolysis were asymptomatic when they started college and 40% remained pain-free at graduation.[3] Spondylolysis is not uncommon and patients with spondylolysis who are pain-free require no treatment.

Keys to Diagnosis and Treatment of Muscular Back Pain:

1. Location of pain is generally paraspinous, not midline
2. Radicular symptoms are absent
3. Scoliosis has been ruled out
4. Physical therapy should be started as soon as possible

Keys to Diagnosis and Treatment of Bone-Related Back Pain

1. What seems to make it worsen? Pain on bending backward (extension) should be considered bone-related pain until proven otherwise.
2. Back pain that awakens an adolescent from sleep and worsens at night but does not worsen with activity is suspicious for neoplasm, most commonly benign osteoid osteoma.
3. The treatment of bone-related back pain most commonly involves bracing, physical therapy, and rarely, surgery.
4. Patients are most often referred to a sports medicine specialist or sports-oriented pediatric orthopedist.
5. Physical therapy should be initiated promptly. The ideal physical therapy referral will be to someone who understands the patient's sport and can address the specific athletic maneuvers that may have precipitated or exacerbated the condition.
6. In most cases, patients can resume normal activities as soon as they are pain-free, with bracing as indicated.

The most common location for spondylolysis is in the fifth lumbar vertebrae at the base of the spine. Either through congenital causes or through bilateral spondylolysis, the affected vertebrae can slip. When this occurs, the patient has a condition known as *spondylolisthesis.*

Physical Examination, Work-up, and Treatment

The specific physical exam findings of an adolescent with suspected bone-related back pain include pain with extension maneuvers (bending backward). This is in contrast to muscular pain, which worsens with twisting. The neurological examination for patients with bone-related back pain is usually normal, although abnormalities are seen when the spondylolisthesis has slipped to where it is compressing the spinal nerve roots.

The work-up and treatment for bone-related back pain in the adolescent depends upon the type of pain. In the case presented at the beginning of this article, an adolescent volleyball player came in with a complaint of back pain with extension that had worsened over the past several months until she could no longer play volleyball without significant pain. The history of pain with extension that limits the adolescent's ability to participate in sports should immediately trigger the presumptive diagnosis of spondylolysis in the mind of the health practitioner.

The work-up for suspected spondylolysis includes four radiographs: AP, lateral, and two oblique views. The AP view is important to assess the curvature of the spine and the lateral view is important to investigate for spondylolisthesis,

---

Talking Point

Explaining the plan for diagnosis and treatment
To explain spondylolysis, tell patients that there has been too much pressure on the bones of their spine and those bones have started to crack. Emphasize that their condition is not uncommon and can be treated. Stress that complying with the regimen for physical therapy will strengthen core muscles so that these injuries do not remain symptomatic.

---

slip of the vertebrae. The oblique views, taken at 45 degree angles from the midline on either side of the lumbar spine, are used to investigate for a crack across the pars interarticularis (often described as the neck of the "Scotty dog"), the hallmark of long-standing spondylolysis.[4]

X-ray and physical examination are usually sufficient for diagnosis of spondylolysis, but if in doubt an MRI can show edema in the bone before it cracks. The quality of MRI magnets can vary, which is why SPECT (CT plus bone scan) is sometimes used to confirm the diagnosis.

Treatment is indicated when the patient has persistent pain bending backward. If this occurs, the patient should be referred to a sports medicine specialist or sports-oriented pediatric orthopedist. Patients with spondylolysis should also be referred for physical therapy with a sports-oriented physical therapist. Physical therapy will strengthen abdominal or core muscles, correct the mechanical problem of overloading the spine, and reduce discomfort. If the patient has back pain but not pain when bending backward and the x-ray indicates spondylolysis, many clinicians will allow a month of physical therapy before referring the patient for evaluation by a specialist.

Treatment for spondylolysis depends upon the age of the patient and age of the lesion. It may include a period of bracing, physical therapy, and the use of a bone stimulator to facilitate healing. In patients with spondylolysis who are younger than 10 or 11 years of age, it is possible to attain bone healing. These patients take a respite from sports for a few months while they continue with physical therapy and are followed with CT or MRI. Older adolescents can generally return to sports as soon as they are pain-free. Continued physical therapy, bracing, and judicious use of NSAIDs will usually be all that is needed to return to their sport.

The work-up for suspected spondylolisthesis is generally finished after the radiographs. MRI can be used to evaluate adolescents with discogenic symptoms that might accompany spondylolisthesis when spinal stenosis, a narrowing of the spinal canal, is present, or when the degree of slip is sufficient to cause nerve root compression.

Spondylolisthesis is a graded entity most often described in terms of H.W. Meyerding's 5-category classification system. To measure the degree of slippage, the examiner takes a lateral view of the lumbosacral junction, then measures the slip as a percentage of the length of the superior border of the sacrum. Meyerding's grade I is a 1% to 25% slip. Grade II is a 26% to 50% slip. Slips of 50% or more (grade III or more) are considered high-grade. Grade III is a 51% to 75% slip, grade IV is a 76% to 100% slip, and grade V, spondyloptosis, is a slip greater than 100%.[5]

The treatment for spondylolisthesis is rarely surgical. Symptoms generally improve with physical therapy. Occasionally, surgery is necessary if the symptoms persist and the degree of slippage is sufficiently severe.

DISCOGENIC (NERVE-RELATED) BACK PAIN

Discogenic back pain, which accounts for 50% of back pain in adults, accounts for roughly 10% of back pain in adolescents.[2] Discogenic pain is caused by the herniation of an intervertebral disk and subsequent impingement on either a central or peripheral nerve. These teens will often present to the office complaining of lumbar spine pain that worsens with bending forward, and may sometimes be accompanied by radiating pain into the hip or thigh.

Unlike muscular or bone-related back pain, which is acute, discogenic pain tends to wax and wane, and does not always follow a typical activity-pain correlation. For this reason, discogenic back pain can persist for months and even years without proper diagnosis or treatment.

The typical patient with adolescent variant discogenic back pain comes to the office complaining of pain with bending forward. Occasionally, nerve impingement symptoms are the cause for concern, as in the patient who presents with thigh weakness and may also be suffering from undiagnosed lumbar radiculopathy. Discogenic back pain can cause radicular pain into the feet as it does in adults, but in adolescents, radicular pain more commonly stops at the level of the thigh and upper leg.

Evaluation and Treatment

The evaluation and treatment of discogenic lumbar spine pain in the adolescent patient begins with a good history. The presence of nerve-related findings on the physical exam, classically a worsening of pain with forward flexion, will confirm clinical suspicions. Straight leg testing, raising the leg to an extended position while the patient is seated at the edge of the examination table, is the best way to identify discogenic pain because straightening the affected leg impinges the nerve root. The diminution of either the patellar or Achilles reflex on the affected side reinforces a preliminary determination that the pain is nerve-related.

Keys to Diagnosis and Treatment of Discogenic Back Pain

1. Have a proper index of suspicion if evaluation reveals pain with forward flexion and radicular pain.
2. Rule out underlying spondylolisthesis with x-rays.
3. Initial management is nonsurgical. Refer the patient for physical therapy and also to a sports-oriented pediatric orthopedist.

Radiographs are important. Generally, AP and lateral views of the lumbar spine are sufficient to show any underlying bone causes of discogenic back pain. The classic finding is spondylolisthesis, in which slippage of the vertebra weakens the disk, making it prone to herniation and nerve root impingement. In higher grades of spondylolisthesis, the spinal canal can become narrowed by the vertebrae themselves, causing unremitting radicular pain.

Physical findings are corroborated via MRI, the gold standard for diagnosis. Imaging will show bone, nerve, and disc. MRI is used in combination with physical exam and x-ray findings to chart the best course for treatment. In adolescents, the first step is generally physical therapy to strengthen the core abdominal musculature. Bed rest is no longer recommended. Occasionally, a temporary back brace is used to augment core stability during the strengthening phase. If this treatment fails, epidural spinal injection of steroids at the level of the disk herniation has been used with moderate success. If this fails, surgical microdiskectomy, in which the surgeon removes a little piece of the disk, is the surgical treatment of choice for most adolescents. It must be stressed, however, that the vast majority of adolescents will not require surgery.

Less Common Causes of Back Pain

NEOPLASM-RELATED BACK PAIN

Back pain can result from bone tumors. A significant aspect of bone pain caused by neoplasm is that it does not seem to worsen after activity. Instead, the pain is constant and worsens at night. When adolescents complain of back pain that awakens them from sleep, neoplasm should be strongly suspected. These patients should be evaluated with both radiographs and an MRI of the spine, as x-rays alone may miss a lesion. Only an MRI is fully diagnostic for neoplastic disease.

An extremely common neoplasm in the adolescent age group is osteoid osteoma, a small, benign tumor that appears in the second decade of life, hurts more at night than during the day, and most often occurs in the femur, tibia, extremities, and lumbar spine. The pain from osteoid osteoma initially responds well to nonsteroidal anti-inflammatory drugs (NSAIDs); a history of night pain that is successfully treated with NSAIDs should raise clinical suspicion for this entity.

Neoplastic disease should be considered when the history and symptomatology do not fit any of the classic patterns and the patient's condition does not improve over time. There are a number of uncommon tumors and cysts of the spinal canal and extraspinal area that may be present. Although MRI evidence is diagnostic, not all MRIs are equally reliable. When symptoms persist over 6 to 8 weeks, fit no pattern, and worsen at night, consider referral to a specialist.

SYSTEMIC CAUSES

Systemic causes, such as infectious or rheumatologic diseases should be suspected when the history is unclear, there is no trauma, the pain is not consistent with the physical examination, and systemic symptoms such as fever or fatigue are present. Pain can occur with all activities and may not be limited to the back. The intensity of the pain experience may seem to be out of proportion to the physical examination. Listen for reports of pain in multiple joints and the extremities; these patients are typically referred either to a pediatric rheumatologist or infectious disease specialist.

X-ray may reveal inflammation. Laboratory tests should include CBC with differential, erythrocyte sedimentation rate, HLA B27, and C-reactive protein. Consider screening patients who live in or travel to areas endemic for Lyme disease. Results may show elevated HLA B27, indicating possible spondyloarthropathy, which is the most common systemic cause of back pain. Spondyloarthropathy is signaled by sacroiliitis, or inflammation of the sacroiliac space, and peripheral arthritis, often in the lower extremity.

Conclusion

With a proper history, physical exam, and testing, diagnosis of adolescent patients with back pain can be accomplished efficiently. Successful treatment will be rewarding for both the patient and pediatrician.

Acknowledgment

The editors would like to acknowledge technical review by David M. Siegel, MD, MPH, FAAP, University of Rochester School of Medicine and Dentistry and Rochester General Hospital, Rochester, New York.

References and Resources

1. Olsen TL, Anderson RL, et al. The epidemiology of low back pain in an adolescent population. *Am J Public Health.* 1992;82:606–608
2. Micheli LJ, Wood R. Back pain in young athletes. Significant differences from adults in causes and patterns. *Arch Pediatr Adolesc Med.* 1995;149:15–18
3. McCarroll JR, Miller JM, Ritter MA. Lumbar spondylolysis and spondylolisthesis in college football players. A prospective study. *Am J Sports Med.* 1986;14:404–406
4. Smith JA, Hu SS. Management of spondylolysis and spondylolisthesis in the pediatric and adolescent population. *Orthop Clin North Am.* 1999;30:487–499, ix
5. Meyerding H. Low backache and sciatic pain associated with spondylolisthesis and protruded intervertebral disc: Incidence, significance and treatment. *J Bone Joint Surg.* 1947;23:461–470

Patient Resource Page

Balance Routines to Stay In the Game

Most people play sports, dance, or work out because they enjoy it. Regular exercise is a great way to stay fit. It is also a mental charge and an attitude booster.

Anyone who has spent time on the disabled list knows that it can be hard work to wait for your body to heal. Good planning can keep you in the game and off the bench.

Many injuries are caused by a sudden impact or a fall, but *overuse injuries* are more common. Overuse injuries are often the result of doing too much, too soon. They can also happen when somebody ignores warning signs and "plays with pain."

TOO MUCH

While it is fun to focus on what you do best, your body pays a price when you use the same muscles again and again. The gymnast who works on her back-bend every afternoon puts a lot of stress on the same bones and joints. The baseball pitcher who practices his fast ball hour after hour does the same.

It is possible to have too much of a good thing. Athletes need to vary their routines and rest their muscles. Daily exercise is great, but the key is variety. Visit the pool once a week. Play something different in the off-season. To stay on top of your game, make sure you aren't putting the same stresses on your body day after day.

If your sport or activity is important to you, protect your opportunity to stay with it! Successful athletes take care of their bones, attend to their joints, and remember to warm-up and cool-down.

TOO SOON

In adolescence, the growth plates of your long bones are still maturing. They need to be protected while they're growing. When coaches and teachers tell you to ease up and vary your routine,

that's what they're thinking about. It's wonderful fun to work hard at your sport, but give your body time to grow into the task.

The teen years are prime time for bone growth and development, so don't forget to give your body the nourishment it needs. Eat a balanced diet, and make sure you are getting enough calcium. (Low-fat dairy products and fortified breakfast cereals are a good place to start.)

A WORD TO THE WISE

Sports are a terrific way to stay healthy and sharp. And it's great to enjoy what you do best. But if you have pain, don't ignore it. If you're hurting, there's a reason. Find out why! See your doctor, and while you're there, talk to your pediatrician about ways to keep your whole body in mind when you work and play.

Stretch and Strengthen Tips

Regular warm-up and cool-down exercises improve muscle tone and prepare your body to compete. To learn some new stretches, check out *Exercises for Young Athletes* under "Sports/Exercise" on the American Academy of Orthopedic Surgeons' Web site (**http://orthoinfo.aaos.org**).

Strength training is another way to build bone and muscle. Strength training, which should not be confused with body building, often calls for free weights, exercise bands, and resistance balls. If you're interested, first get checked by your doctor, then ask him or her, your coach, or your trainer to suggest qualified people who can get you started and keep you on track.

Another good place to learn more about these topics is the Web site sponsored by the American College of Sports Medicine (**www.acsm.org**).

This patient education sheet is distributed in conjunction with the February 2005 issue of Adolescent Health Update, *published by the American Academy of Pediatrics.*

The information in this publication should not be used as a substitute for the medical care and advice of your pediatrician.

Pediatricians are encouraged to photocopy this page for distribution to patients and parents.

Caring for Adolescents With Somatic Concerns

by Sara B. Kinsman, MD, PhD

Adolescents frequently present with concerns related to physical function and pain. The majority of these concerns are age-specific and self limited. However, a minority of adolescents will have multiple somatic concerns or chronic concerns that are not related to a known medical condition.

Somatic concerns are physical symptoms that do not suggest a specific developmental or disease process. The pediatrician's approach to caring for these adolescents is critically important to their healing. By validating the adolescent's experience, understanding the family's concerns, encouraging effective coping strategies, and addressing comorbid conditions, the pediatrician can help these patients function to their fullest and assure that they do not undergo unnecessary medical examinations and treatments. A holistic approach to caring for these complex adolescents is wise, effective, and rewarding.

TALKING ABOUT SOMATIC CONCERNS

The term "somatization" refers to the experience of physical symptoms or changes in function that are not related to a known disease process. As medical knowledge in the field of somatic symptoms has advanced, we have begun to better understand how the development and activation of the neuroendocrine system relates physical and emotional experiences.[1-4] Terms such as "organic," "nonorganic," and "functional" are now considered outmoded.

Spectrum of Clinical Presentations

The clinical presentation of somatic concerns varies widely, from adolescents with developmental concerns to older adolescents with complex somatoform disorders.

THE ADOLESCENT WITH DEVELOPMENTAL CONCERNS

Young adolescents may be intensely concerned about normal developmental changes. For example, some girls experience pain with breast budding. Although this is not uncommon, it can be frightening if unexpected or unexplained. If an aunt, grandmother, or mother has suffered or died from breast cancer, the adolescent may have even more concern about this normal developmental event. In such a situation, the pediatrician can ask questions that explore the patient's fears, then provide reassurance that painful breast budding is normal and not related to breast cancer. The clinical interview may provide an opportunity to further discuss the adolescent's concerns about cancer or the loss of a family member.

Objectives

After reading this article, pediatricians who care for patients with somatic concerns will be better able to:
- Understand the development and physiological basis for somatic symptoms
- Formulate a differential diagnosis
- Validate the patient's experience with a thorough history and physical examination
- Develop a collaborative approach and comprehensive therapy plan aimed at improving function and relieving symptoms

Sara B. Kinsman, MD, PhD, is an assistant professor of pediatrics in the Division of Adolescent Medicine, The Children's Hospital of Philadelphia, and a fellow at the Psychoanalytic Center of Philadelphia.

SOMATOFORM DISORDERS: A BRIEF OVERVIEW

As described in the *Diagnostic and Statistical Manual of Mental Disorders, Fourth Edition, Text Revision (DSM-IV-TR)*, published by the American Psychiatric Association, *somatoform disorders* involve reports of physical symptoms that suggest a general medical condition but are not fully explained by that condition. Symptoms must cause distress, functional impairment, or medical help-seeking. Somatoform disorders are distinct from intentional reports of physical symptoms or pain, such as in factitious disorders or malingering, which are beyond the scope of this paper.

- *Somatization disorder* describes a specific somatoform disorder characterized by recurring, multiple, clinically significant complaints of pain in at least 4 different body sites, 2 symptoms of gastrointestinal distress, 1 sexual or reproductive symptom, and 1 pseudoneurologic symptom over the course of the disorder. This disorder is typically diagnosed in adults over 20 years of age.

- *Undifferentiated somatoform disorder* is diagnosed when 1 or more somatic complaints not limited to pain alone (eg, fatigue) persist for 6 months or longer

- Patients with *pain disorder* report pain in one or more sites that causes significant distress or functional impairment.

- *Conversion disorder* involves symptoms or deficits that suggest a neurological condition in the absence of another diagnosis. A psychological stressor may precede the symptom and psychological factors can be associated with the symptom or deficit, though the patient may not recognize this association.

- *Hypochondriasis* is a fear of having or a belief that one has a serious disease. The fear or belief is based on a misinterpretation of bodily symptoms.

- Patients with *body dysmorphic disorder* are concerned about a perceived defect in their appearance such as exaggerated perception of a minor physical difference. (Body dysmorphic disorder is distinct from the body image disturbance seen in anorexia nervosa.)

- *Somatoform disorder not otherwise specified (NOS)* is the diagnosis when the pattern of somatoform symptoms does not meet criteria for another specific somatoform disorder.

SOMATIC CONCERNS IN ADOLESCENCE

While the majority of adolescents in the pediatrician's office will not have a somatoform disorder, most adolescents will at some point have concerns related to pain and function. A combination of developmental and social changes during adolescence places these patients at greater risk for somatization.

- *Cognitive and emotional maturation is occurring.* Although adolescents may appreciate more complex information and see connections between emotional and situational experiences, they may not know how to organize or communicate about what they are starting to understand. Young adolescents are accustomed to expressing concerns in physical terms and expressing anxiety with symptoms. For example, a child who was being teased incessantly in the second grade may not have been able to verbalize the need for a "mental health" day, but his or her nausea before school in the morning may have justified staying home. As children mature through adolescence they will recognize the meaning of the queasiness and learn to manage environmental stress through a variety of strategies that encourage continued functionality. The pediatrician can be vital in helping the adolescent develop these effective coping strategies.

- *There may be a history of early or chronic trauma.* The loss of a parent when the adolescent was a toddler may be "remembered" in the same way the young child experienced the loss—physical discomfort. Research has shown that individuals exposed to chronic trauma without amelioration may develop lifelong alterations in baseline cortisol levels and exaggerations in cortisol responses to stress.[5] This "neurological vigilance" results in physical responses to environmental stressors that differ from those of individuals who do not share that history. Fortunately, researchers believe that neuroplasticity, which permits children to learn from fearful situations, also permits them to relearn adaptive strategies to manage situations that may be reminiscent of a past event.[6,7]

- *The physical concern is an entrée to seek help from a trusted adult.* Although most pediatricians expect to help their patients manage all the developmental tasks of adolescence, including the emotional challenge of developing autonomy, most adolescents feel that they must have a physical complaint to get help from their pediatrician.

- *The physical concern that brings them into the pediatrician's office is often the stressor.* Adolescents may not understand that their bodies respond to their environment. Sometimes it can be helpful to explain the physiological links between tension headaches and overworking, butterflies in the tummy and examinations, blushing and public speaking, sexual arousal and attraction. It is important to recognize that not all patients will understand and appreciate these examples, and will be mainly focused on the physical concern that brought them into the office.

Comprehensive Assessment

The first step in developing a therapeutic relationship is to validate the patient's experience. Showing respect for what the individual is feeling, even when the description is confusing and complex, is the first step toward helping the patient feel well. The assessment should include the history of the present illness, family history, psychosocial history, and an assessment of comorbid conditions.

HISTORY AND VALIDATION

Adolescents with somatic concerns will appreciate evidence of genuine interest in their condition. A detailed history affirms the pediatrician's concern and facilitates a thorough differential diagnosis. A confusing constellation of symptoms or an extraordinary level of anxiety about those symptoms in a patient who appears to be well might prompt questions about the accuracy of the patient's account. In this situation, try to

understand the meaning of his or her concern. For example, a careful history may reveal that the adolescent who reports having trouble seeing despite a completely normal ophthamological examination is afraid that she has developed a brain tumor, because that is what happened to her sister when she was the same age. With this insight, you can focus on the meaning of the concern to the patient and family.

To assess the impact of your patient's symptoms, inquire about activities of daily life and routine. It can be extremely helpful for an adolescent, and separately a parent, to keep a 3-day diary or log of these activities.

Family History

The family history should include evaluation of health concerns among family members, including depression, anxiety, alcohol misuse, illicit or prescription drug use, suicide attempts, undiagnosed medical conditions, early or unusual morbities (eg, death of a sibling from lupus in late adolescence), and any history of somatic concerns. For example, you might ask, "Do [patient's name]'s symptoms remind you of

---

Guide to the Clinical Interview

The history should include both physical sensations and underlying thoughts and feelings about the problems. Consider the questions below when interviewing a patient with multiple distressing symptoms.

What does the [symptom: pain/tightness/weakness] mean to you?

What does the [symptom: pain/tightness/weakness] mean to your family?

Are you frightened by the [symptom: pain/tightness/weakness]? Why or why not?

What part of your body do you think the problem comes from?

What is your best guess as to what's going on?

What scares you most about this problem?

What is the worst thing that you can imagine this problem might be?

anyone else in the family?" This question may prompt the parent to tell you about specific issues in the family or a history of somatic concerns among close family members.

Psychosocial History

It is essential to spend time alone with adolescent patients so that a confidential psychosocial history can be completed. The psychosocial history should include questions about the following:

- *School:* current school performance as compared to past school performance; future aspirations
- *Home:* household composition and function with special attention to early losses of care providers, conflicts and domestic violence, and marital discord
- *Activities:* current and past enjoyment of activities
- *Drug use:* those that exacerbate symptoms (eg, stimulants such as nicotine, which increase palpitations) and those used to treat symptoms (eg, alcohol)
- *Relationships:* current and past friendships, romantic relationships, and sexual orientation
- *Emotional, physical, or sexual abuse,* now or in the past
- *Mood:* depressive feelings, anxiety, and suicidality

Assessing Comorbid Conditions

Evaluating psychiatric comorbidities is an essential part of the work-up for adolescents with unexplained somatic concerns. A number of studies have supported the strong association between somatoform disorders and other psychiatric conditions, such as depression, anxiety, obsessive-compulsive disorder, panic disorder, and substance-related disorders.[8,9] Validated screening tests for both depression and anxiety are available; these sometimes help adolescents express feelings that they may not be aware of, or are reluctant to raise. (See resource list, page 63)

PHYSICAL EXAMINATION

A careful physical examination is needed to exclude medical conditions that are part of the differential diagnosis. It also validates the patient's report and helps assure both patient and family that "something life threatening" does not underlie the discomfort.

The history obtained from the patient will influence the emphasis of the physical examination. For example, in some circumstances the clinician may give particular attention to the abdominal, musculoskeletal, or neurological examinations. At other times, suspected fibromyalgia might prompt a check of trigger points for pain sensitivity. (See *AHU* 2003;15:2). It is also possible for physical findings (eg, a neurologic deficit that defies anatomic patterns) to support the diagnosis of somatization. While examining these patients, be especially gentle and ask the patient's permission before palpating sensitive areas.

DIFFERENTIAL DIAGNOSIS

When an adolescent presents with multiple, chronic, or nonspecific concerns, it is important to consider a thorough differential diagnosis. For example, diffuse abdominal pain without other gastrointestinal symptoms may be an indication of lactose intolerance or inflammatory bowel disease. Fatigue and poor appetite accompanied by possible depression or anxiety may be caused by an endocrine disorder such as hypo- or hyperthyroidism or Addison's disease. Body aches, fatigue, and fever may be presenting complaints in a rheumatologic illness such as rheumatoid arthritis. Headaches may have organic causes, such as an occult malignancy, especially if associated with weight loss, adenopathy, or fever. Sensory or motor changes, gait disturbances, or a change or loss in muscle strength or function may signal neurological disease such as multiple sclerosis. Some disorders, such as irritable bowel syndrome, meet criteria for somatoform disorder, but have specific treatment regimens. These patients may benefit from consultation with a specialist such as a gastroenterologist.

Rather than share your full differential diagnosis, discuss the specific medical concerns, including somatic diagnoses, with the patient and family and explain that you are thoroughly considering the possible etiologies of your patient's symptoms.

DIAGNOSTIC WORK-UP

Order only necessary diagnostic tests and explain your expectations regarding test results at the outset. For example, let's assume that you have ordered a complete blood count, erythrocyte sedimentation rate, and stool hemoccult for a patient with abdominal pain, despite a very low clinical suspicion of inflammatory bowel disease. In this instance, you might tell the adolescent and family, "I am almost certain that these tests will be normal. I'm ordering these things to be thorough. Now let's see how we can start to help you to feel better." Avoid ordering tests to "prove" that the patient is healthy, since this will not reassure an anxious family that you have not missed a rare medical condition.

Management

Pediatricians can explain to adolescents and their families that somatic concerns are recognized entities that appear to be more common among adolescents than other age groups.

Assure the family that somatic symptoms are not life threatening or progressively debilitating. For some patients and families, providing a symptom-based diagnosis that is consistent with the patient's concerns (eg, "abdominal pain") can avoid confusion and prevent mislabeling especially as treatment begins and a full work-up is in progress.

The pediatrician will want to avoid labeling the patient anxious or stressed if the patient's only experience is a somatic concern. For these patients, using a symptom-based label is most consistent with their experience, especially because the majority of adolescents will not meet full criteria for a somatoform disorder. As the treatment phase progresses, patients may be able to make associations between past, ongoing, or upcoming events and their somatic concerns. Anecdotal observations about the limitations of "test-based" medicine may also be helpful in your conversations with these patients. For example, you might say, "We have no specific medical tests for irritable bowel syndrome or migraines, but we now have effective approaches to manage these conditions." Likewise, for a nonspecific

somatic illness the pediatrician might say, "We do not have a specific test to explain why you are not moving your right foot, but your symptom is consistent with what we call a somatic concern or conversion disorder. We can treat this with physical therapy and talking therapy. The physical therapy coordinates the body and the talking therapy coordinates your feelings about this illness. Sometimes with talking, patients recognize a challenge in the past, present, or the future that is affecting them." Thus, even without specific testing, the pediatrician can prescribe treatment for the body and the mind.

A primer on how neurotransmitters operate in the brain and rest of the body can sometimes break down old notions about mind-body dualism.[1,10] The pediatrician might say, "The body has a few messengers called neurotransmitters that connect the brain, the heart, the stomach, and all the muscles. For example, if you burn your hand, the damaged skin sends a message to your brain and signals from your brain make the hand move and speed up your heart rate. You might yell 'ouch' and you might feel angry. We don't think about these actions; the brain and the body are so well connected it happens automatically. Well, sometimes this system gets worked up for other reasons. For example, when someone gets ready to go to college, the brain might get worried in advance about the upcoming change. With that worry, a young person may not get restful sleep, or may get tense muscles and an upset stomach. He or she may raise concerns related to being tired, achy, or nauseous. This is confusing when senior year of high school is going so well. Luckily, there are a lot of things we can do to help people whose neurotransmitters are 'gearing up for a challenge' or 'overdoing it.'"

For a few adolescents and their families, biases about psychological conditions are so strong that an environmental stressor theory is very difficult to accept. And while some families will be reassured that a comorbid condition such as anxiety is associated with the somatic concerns, other families will feel confused. In such situations, it is helpful for the pediatrician to acknowledge the mind-body connection and focus on the adolescent's physical concerns and improved overall functioning. With improved function, adolescents and their families are sometimes better able to understand and accept environmental theories or the diagnosis of comorbid conditions.

TREATMENT PLAN

Although patients and families may be frustrated by the lack of a specific treatment for their condition, if the pediatrician can be optimistic, help the adolescent regain function, and assure the family that symptom relief will follow, many adolescents will work diligently toward healing.

Advocate a "care versus cure" *rehabilitative approach,* which encourages a return to usual activities and responsibilities even if symptoms persist. A detailed, realistic, graded plan to manage symptoms and regain function should be developed in partnership with the adolescent through a collaborative process that empowers the patient to function to his or her fullest.

It is most helpful to establish and work with a "treatment team." Members will vary depending upon the adolescent's presentation. Typically, your team will include the adolescent, the family, the pediatrician, the school nurse or guidance counselor, a counselor (individual or family therapist)

Areas of Function to Ask About

Exercise

Diet

Sleep

School performance

Activities and interests

Family life

Peer relationships

Drug use

Depression, anxiety, and suicidality

Sexual behavior

Physical, emotional, or sexual abuse

Stressors: past, recent, or future

---

who is knowledgeable of somatic literature and skilled with adolescents, and other complementary providers. These may include, but are not limited to, a (1) physical therapist, (2) chiropractor, (3) massage therapist, (4) acupuncturist, (5) homeopathic therapist, or (6) yoga or tai chi teacher. The box below shows the areas of function that a pediatrician may want to ask about when developing a treatment plan.

RESUMING A ROUTINE

The adolescent with somatic symptoms may have fallen out of synchrony with daily activities. Ask your patient which aspects of function he or she can resume immediately and work together to reintroduce them. Ideally, the adolescent with somatic symptoms can quickly return to some routines, such as waking at school time, showering, getting dressed, joining family for breakfast and dinner, completing some household chores, and starting to catch up in 1 or 2 subjects.

Return to school can be more complex. For the adolescent with many absences who has not kept up with schoolwork, resuming the responsibilities and pace of school can be overwhelming and confusing. Talk to the adolescent and parents about coordinating a catch-up plan with the school guidance team and teachers. This can help overcome fears associated with school reentry. It is important to appreciate that many adolescents do not have sophisticated executive functioning skills that would enable them to multitask and "catch up" in several subjects simultaneously. Parents might ask the school to permit part-time attendance and a plan to complete makeup work. Tutoring programs may be wise, especially for students who have missed important educational material. In-school accommodations can also be helpful. For example, adolescents with severe irritable bowel symptoms may benefit from access to a private bathroom when necessary. Adolescents may feel reassured that they can "rest" in the nurse's office or other calm space if necessary. School nurses can become vital members of the treatment team by facilitating in-school accommodations.

PHYSICAL RECONDITIONING

For many patients with functional somatic complaints, physical reconditioning will be the first step in the recovery process.[11] Conditioning goals should be achievable and can be advanced every few days. If the adolescent has been "couch-bound," suggest walking out to get the mail every day and circling the dining-room table twice every 2 hours. What may seem like minimal progress will enable the adolescent to propose a healing regimen and take things at a pace that assures success. Some adolescents will ask if they might attend their teams' practices, but not participate; this can be a great motivator and will facilitate valuable peer contact. Others will make great strides by working with a physical therapist to stretch painful muscles, release trigger spots, and use deep breathing. Programs that support intense aerobic reconditioning have reported very successful short- and long-term wellness.

INDIVIDUAL AND FAMILY THERAPY

Most patients and families will benefit from working with an individual or family therapist who is experienced with somatic complaints and can help adolescents understand somatization and associated comorbid disorders. In making a referral, it is crucial to assure that the selected therapist is skilled in this area. He or she should be able to help the adolescent interpret and cope with physical sensations and discomfort, identify strengths and coping skills that can be used to manage symptoms, and address the inevitable disappointments, such as changes in peer relationships, that are associated with chronic illness. The therapist should also be able to help family members learn to respond appropriately as improvements occur and should know how to encourage positive parenting skills.

PAIN MANAGEMENT

Almost two-thirds of somatic complaints include an element of pain or discomfort. Pediatricians should be prepared to address the issue of pain management with both adolescents and their families.[12,13] Pain management may be needed while the adolescent works to increase overall functioning and even after full function has returned. A number of nonpharmacological and pharmacological approaches may be effective.

Nonpharmacological Pain Management

Alternative nonpharmacologic approaches are utilized effectively to manage pain and other somatic concerns. Massage, tender point release, acupuncture, and stretching exercises included in yoga, tai chi, or pilates may alleviate musculoskeletal pain. Hypnotherapy and visualization or meditation techniques have also proven helpful. Before referring a patient for alternative or complementary care, ask adolescents and families about their feelings regarding nontraditional methods. These approaches may also help teens deal with stress, which in turn affects their symptom experience and overall well being.

Pharmacological Pain Management

Medications can help patients with somatic complaints, but patients who take these drugs require careful supervision. For example, while intermittent use of nonsteroidal anti-inflammatory

---

Resources for the Clinician

Beck AT, Steer RA, Brown GK. *Beck Depression Inventory—Primary Care (BDI-PC)*. San Antonio, TX: Harcourt Assessment, Inc; 1996

Beck AT, Steer RA, Brown GK. *Beck Depression Inventory®—II*. San Antonio, TX: Harcourt Assessment, Inc; 1996

March JS. *Multidimensional Anxiety Scale for Children (MASC)*. San Antonio, TX: Harcourt Assessment, Inc; 1997

Campo JV, Fritz G. A management model for pediatric somatization. *Psychosomatics*. 2001;42:467–476

Kohli R, Li BU. Differential diagnosis of recurrent abdominal pain: new considerations. *Pediatr Ann*. 2004;33:113–122

The Beck Inventories and MASC screen can be ordered from Harcourt Assessment (1-800-211-8378 or www.psychcorp.com)

medications can ease some types of discomfort, supervision by the pediatrician is important to avoid overuse, gastrointestinal irritation, and rebound headaches. The most important message for adolescents with somatic concerns is that there is no "magic pill," and that many different modalities can be tried to increase function and manage symptoms.

Narcotic analgesics pose short-term and long-term challenges, and should be avoided. While a few adolescents will receive some benefit from low-dose, short-term use (eg, an ability to tolerate more aggressive physical therapy), others may report that even a high dose is ineffective. In these situations, the pediatrician may acknowledge that narcotics will not be beneficial and increasing dosages may even be harmful. After assuring that the adolescent is not addicted to illicitly obtained narcotics, these patients should be weaned from potentially addictive pharmaceuticals.

Low-dose tricylcic antidepressants (TCAs) can be extremely helpful in treating somatic conditions in adults with chronic pain. In prescribing TCAs for adolescents, make it clear that symptoms will not be alleviated immediately. In addition, because TCAs have been associated with potentially lethal overdose, assess for suicidal ideation and history of suicide attempts. This assessment should include not only the adolescent, but also anyone in the home who may have access to the medication. Some cardiologists recommend a baseline EKG to evaluate the adolescent's potential risk for a cardiac arrhythmia, particularly if high-dose TCA treatment may be required in the future.

Because of the risks associated with tricylcic antidepressant use, some have advocated selective serotonin reuptake inhibitors (SSRIs) as initial therapy for chronic pain disorders. Recent findings have linked increased use of SSRIs in adolescents with an increased risk of suicidal ideation and have brought the safety of this class of medications for adolescents into question. At this writing, there have been no clinical trials addressing the risk/benefit ratio of SSRIs in the treatment of chronic pain syndromes in adolescent populations.

Pediatricians using SSRIs should inform the patient and family of potential risks, monitor the patient for increased impulsivity and suicidality, and perhaps consult with a psychiatrist or pain specialist experienced with adolescents.

MANAGING FATIGUE

Fatigue is common among adolescents with somatic concerns, who often report irregular sleep patterns, too much sleep, and nonrestorative sleep. A differential diagnosis of fatigue should include iron-deficiency anemia, endocrine dysfunction, sleep disorders, and comorbid conditions such as depression or anxiety.

To help your patients develop a restorative sleep program, teach them about sleep hygiene. Explain that people who spend time online or watching television near bedtime often have trouble falling asleep. Encourage an evening routine (eg, a hot bath, tooth brushing, reading, deep breathing, and refraining from computer use or television watching for 30 minutes before bed). Strongly encourage a regular and specific sleep/wake schedule, which is also observed on the weekends (eg, wake up at 7:00 am daily and attempt to fall asleep at 11:00 pm daily). For some adolescents, particularly those who are highly scheduled, finding time to relax or meditate while listening to music can be very important. Recommend that patients engage in daily aerobic activity with mild to moderate aerobic exercise early in the day and avoid caffeine and alcohol.

While not FDA-approved for use in adolescents, medications such as zolpidem, zaleplon, or trazadone, which are sometimes used as sleep aids in adults, may be used in rare circumstances. Emphasize that this is a short-term solution. One downside of using a sleep-inducing medication is that the patient may not experience the benefits of adopting a healthy lifestyle and may instead feel that a medication is the answer for their somatic concerns. The pediatrician will also want to be aware of the possibility of a primary sleep dysfunction and consider pursuing further evaluation.

ONGOING TREATMENT PLAN

Once a plan and healing team are in place, the pediatrician will want to schedule frequent visits to assess symptoms, minimize symptom-based calls to the practice, and monitor progress. It may take several visits to establish the team and treatment plan. In addition to coordinating the care plan, the pediatrician is also the team member charged with communicating with the adolescent's high school, college, community team, or workplace. Together with the adolescent, the pediatrician can develop a plan that is practical and supports the broader goals of increased functionality.

Some adolescents will regain function and see their symptoms resolve very quickly. For these patients, continue to provide support and remain accessible. It is essential that the adolescent and family understand that they need not wait until there is a crisis to contact you. When the patient is feeling better, plan to talk about the somatic event and consider what elements of the treatment plan worked to heal symptoms. Once a stressor is over and somatic symptoms have passed, patients may assume that they will not recur. Suggest to the adolescent that there could well be future similar stressors (such as romantic "breakups"). Talk about ways to cope with the intense feelings associated with such a loss. These focused brief therapeutic discussions can set the groundwork for a supportive relationship between the adolescent and the pediatrician for years to come.

When the adolescent's symptoms take time to resolve, stay vigilant for potential diagnoses that were not initially obvious. Frequent contact with other team members is important and essential to assure that everyone is working together to address the evolving needs and concerns of the patient.

Conclusion

Adolescent patients with unexplained somatic symptoms provide some of the most complex, challenging, and rewarding encounters in pediatric practice. Resolution usually involves pediatrician and patient as well as other members of the treatment team working together.

Research exploring long-term outcomes of adolescents with unexplained somatic symptoms suggests that while some will continue to have concerns related to somatization and associated comorbidites, many are able to resume normal activities. Pediatricians who effectively address the health care needs of adolescents with unexplained somatic concerns will form useful therapeutic alliances and enable more adolescents with somatic concerns to manage symptoms and function to their fullest.

Acknowledgment

The editors would like to acknowledge technical review by John V. Campo, MD, FAAP, an associate professor of psychiatry and pediatrics at the Western Psychiatric Institute & Clinic, University of Pittsburgh, and Richard B. Heyman, MD, FAAP, chair, AAP Section on Adolescent Health.

Selective Bibliography

Cassidy JT. Progress in diagnosis and understanding chronic pain syndromes in children and adolescents. *Adolesc Med.*1998;9:101–114, vi

Chambliss CR, Heggen J, Copelan DN, Pettignano R. The assessment and management of chronic pain in children. *Pediatr Drugs.* 2002;4:737–746

Dierker LC, Albano AM, Clarke GN, et al. Screening for anxiety and depression in early adolescence. *J Am Acad Child Adolesc Psychiatry.* 2001;40:929–936

Goldenberg DL. Fibromyalgia syndrome a decade later: what have we learned? *Arch Intern Med.* 1999;159:777–785

Halligan PW, Athwal BS, Oakley DA, Frackowiak RS. Imaging hypnotic paralysis: implications for conversion hysteria. *Lancet.* 2000;355:986–987

Lindstrom J. Autoimmune diseases involving nicotinic receptors. *J Neurobiol.* 2002;53:656–665

Shapiro B. Building bridges between body and mind: the analysis of an adolescent with paralyzing chronic pain. *Int J Psychoanal.* 2003;84:547–561

Silber TJ, Pao M. Somatization disorders in children and adolescents. *Pediatr Rev.* 2003;24:255–264

Winter LB, Steer RA, Jones-Hicks L, Beck AT. Screening for major depression disorders in adolescent medical outpatients with the Beck Depression Inventory for Primary Care. *J Adolesc Health.* 1999;24:389–394

References

1. Ledoux JE. *The Emotional Brain: The Mysterious Underpinnings of Emotional Life.* New York, NY: Touchstone Books; 1998

2. Rogan MT, LeDoux JE. Emotion: systems, cells, synaptic plasticity. *Cell.* 1996;85:469–475

3. Hakala M, Karlsson H, Ruotsalainen U, et al. Severe somatization in women is associated with altered cerebral glucose metabolism. *Psychol Med.* 2002;32:1379–1385

4. Stam R, Akkermans LM, Wiegant VM. Trauma and the gut: interactions between stressful experience and intestinal function. *Gut.* 1997;40:704–709

5. Charney DS, Deutch AY, Krystal JH, Southwick SM, Davis M. Psychobiologic mechanisms of posttraumatic stress disorder. *Arch Gen Psychiatry.* 1993;50:295–305

6. Yehuda R. Post-traumatic stress disorder. *N Engl J Med.* 2002;346:108–114

7. Stiles J. Neural plasticity and cognitive development. *Dev Neuropsychol.* 2000;18:237–272

8. Campo JV, Fritsch SL. Somatization in children and adolescents. *J Am Acad Child Adolesc Psychiatry.* 1994; 33:1223–1235

9. Lieb R, Pfister H, Mastaler M, Wittchen HU. Somatoform syndromes and disorders in a representative population sample of adolescents and young adults: prevalence, comorbidity and impairments. *Acta Psychiatr Scand.* 2000;101:194–208

10. Shannon JR, Flattem NL, Jordan J, et al. Orthostatic intolerance and tachycardia associated with norepinephrine-transporter deficiency. *N Eng J Med.* 2000;342:541–549

11. Sherry DD, Wallace CA, Kelley C, Kidder M, Sap L. Short- and long-term outcomes of children with complex regional pain syndrome type I treated with exercise therapy. *Clin J Pain.* 1999;15:218–223

12. Shapiro BS. Treatment of chronic pain in children and adolescents. *Pediatr Ann.* 1995;24:148–150, 153–156

13. Eccleston C, Malleson PN, Clinch J, Connell H, Sourbut C. Chronic pain in adolescents: evaluation of a programme of interdisciplinary cognitive behaviour therapy. *Arch Dis Child.* 2003;88:881–885

Questions and Answers About Somatic Symptoms

Q. *What are somatic symptoms?*

A. Somatic symptoms fall into two categories. Some are changes in body function. Others relate to discomfort or pain. Somatic symptoms are common and are not life threatening.

Q. *What types of symptoms are common?*

A. Headaches, stomachaches, chest pains, backaches, joint pains, arm or leg swelling, changes in skin color, dizziness, tiredness, difficulty concentrating, and sometimes difficulty moving part of the body.

Q. *Are somatic symptoms real?*

A. Absolutely! Somatic symptoms are real in the same way that blushing is real, or perspiring is real, or headaches are real.

Q. *I've been told that these symptoms are all in my head. Is that true?*

A. No, your symptoms are real. Sometimes somatic symptoms are tied to stress. Physical or somatic feelings are one way that the thinking and acting parts of the human body are connected. For example, when we get nervous about an upcoming test or performance, sometimes our heart beats faster than usual. Doctors call this the mind-body connection. This connection allows our bodies to respond to what is going on in the world around us. Sometimes even stresses from early childhood, like the death of a parent or fighting in the home, can trigger pain in the body during the adolescent years.

Q. *Can puberty be associated with these symptoms?*

A. Yes! As adolescents mature they must learn to accept many changes in their bodies, including a lot of weight gain and growing to adult height. It is not surprising that young adolescents, in particular, notice and sometimes experience discomfort related to growing up.

Q. *My doctor wants me to talk about feelings, but I want to talk about my pain.*

A. This makes sense. Many adolescents are used to talking about how their body is feeling and not their emotions. For example, second graders who are being teased can't ask mom for a "mental health" day, but as they deal with the teasing day after day, they might feel nervous from the stress of being hassled by kids at school and develop tension in their abdomen, or a "tummyache." The second grader's parents might give him or her a break from the stressful school environment for a day. As young people go through adolescence they begin to recognize that the "tummyache" comes when they are nervous about dealing with a tough situation. Soon your body can teach you when you are stressed. Talking about it usually helps. Even if this doesn't feel comfortable or make sense, try talking to someone you trust.

Q. *Is there a medical explanation for somatic symptoms?*

A. Yes. Neurotransmitters are the body's messengers of pain, discomfort, temperature, energy, learning, breathing, digesting food, and many other things. Somatic disorders can throw them off-balance for a little while. Your system should come back into balance as you work with your treatment team and begin to follow a good sleep schedule with regular meals and lots of exercise.

Q. *Is there a medicine to make me feel better?*

A. No, but you will probably be working with a team of health care providers, including your pediatrician and perhaps a counselor, physical therapist, and others.

Q. *What can I do to feel better?*

A. Try a combination of the things that help most people. For example, set up a regular routine for each day. Do your best to catch up with your schoolwork. Eat regular, balanced meals. Follow a plan for regular physical therapy and/or work with someone who can help you become physically fit. Sleep on a regular schedule (wake up by 7:00 am, every day!), and try to get at least 8 hours of sleep each night. Consider talking to a counselor. Get treatment for any other conditions that may make your somatic symptoms worse, such as panic disorder, anxiety, or depression.

Q. *I'm doing everything I'm supposed to do, but I still don't feel better.*

A. In most cases, you probably won't start to feel better until *after* you have been doing everything you're supposed to do for a while. This can be very frustrating, but you'll get there! So keep working with your treatment team. Healing takes time.

Chest Pain in Children

Steven M. Selbst, MD*

Case Presentation

A 15-year-old boy presents to the emergency department with chest pain for 1 week. The pain began as mild left chest discomfort when he was hit over the ribs while playing football. Three days ago he reported a headache, neck stiffness, and worsening chest pain, especially when walking. He described the pain as aching, stabbing, and much worse with exertion. The patient has had no fever or symptoms of an upper respiratory tract infection, but he complains of mild dizziness with standing. He vomited twice yesterday and now complains of nausea. His past medical history is noncontributory.

The physical examination reveals an alert, talkative, obese male. Vital signs are: temperature, 38.3°C (oral); pulse, 72 beats/min; respirations, 24 breaths/min; and blood pressure, 128/84 mm Hg. The heart rate increases to 96 beats/min with standing and 116 beats/min with walking. Examination of the head, eyes, ears, nose, and throat is unremarkable. The neck is mildly tender, and there is pain with flexion. The chest examination reveals mild tenderness over the sternum and no pain over the ribs. The cardiac rhythm is regular, and no murmur is appreciated. The lungs are clear, and the abdomen is soft and nontender, with no mass or organomegaly. Findings on the remainder of the physical examination are normal.

The chest radiograph shows clear lung fields, but the heart is enlarged slightly. Electrocardiography shows left axis deviation, normal sinus rhythm, possible right ventricular hypertrophy, and ST elevation in the inferolateral leads.

About 3 hours after arrival at the emergency department, the boy becomes unresponsive, is found to have a ventricular arrhythmia, and develops cardiac arrest. He cannot be resuscitated. An autopsy reveals evidence of myocarditis.

Introduction

Chest pain is a frequent complaint among children; it occurs in 6 in 1,000 who present to an urban pediatric emergency department or walk-in clinic. Chest pain occurs equally in boys and girls and is found in children of all ages. The mean age of children who have this complaint is about 12 years. Young children are more likely to have a cardiorespiratory cause for their pain, such as cough, asthma, pneumonia, or heart disease; adolescents are more likely to have pain associated with a psychogenic disturbance.

Many patients and their families associate chest pain with heart disease, and they are understandably frightened by media reports of sudden death in young athletes. Often the symptom of chest pain disturbs the child's daily routine; about one third of children who have this complaint are awakened from sleep by the pain and one third miss school because of it. The case reported here is unusual; most studies have shown that pediatric chest pain rarely is due to serious organic pathology. However, the complaint should be taken seriously because underlying heart disease can be present. In general, a thorough history and careful physical examination can guide the pediatrician as to when to order laboratory studies and when to refer a child who has chest pain to a specialist for further evaluation.

Differential Diagnosis

CARDIAC DISEASE

Previously undiagnosed cardiac disease is a rare cause of chest pain in children (Table 1). Myocardial infarction can result from anomalous coronary arteries, and there may be no warning of this underlying condition. However, some children will have a pansystolic, continuous, or mitral regurgitation murmur or gallop rhythm that suggests myocardial dysfunction. Other children may have had a previous condition that results in a higher likelihood of angina or infarction, such as long-standing diabetes mellitus, Kawasaki disease, chronic anemias, or use of cocaine.

*Associate Professor of Pediatrics, University of Pennsylvania School of Medicine; Acting Division Chief, Division of Emergency Medicine, The Children's Hospital of Philadelphia, Philadelphia, PA.

TABLE 1. Cardiac Disorders Leading to Pediatric Chest Pain

Coronary artery disease—Ischemia/Infarction
- Anomalous coronary arteries
- Coronary arteritis (Kawasaki disease)
- Long-standing diabetes mellitus

Arrhythmia
- Supraventricular tachycardia
- Ventricular tachycardia

Structural abnormalities
- Hypertrophic cardiomyopathy
- Severe pulmonic stenosis
- Aortic valve stenosis
- Mitral valve prolapse

Infection
- Pericarditis
- Myocarditis

In many cases, exercise induces the chest pain with these disorders because coronary blood flow is limited. Therefore, pain with exertion should be given careful consideration. Syncope also may be associated.

Some children may have an arrhythmia that causes signs and symptoms such as palpitations or abnormalities on cardiac examination. Supraventricular tachycardia is the most common of these arrhythmias, but premature ventricular beats or tachycardia also can lead to brief, sharp chest pain.

One structural abnormality that deserves mention is hypertrophic obstructive cardiomyopathy. This disorder has an autosomal dominant pattern of inheritance, so there often is a family history of the condition. Children who have this disorder have a murmur that may be audible when standing or performing a Valsalva maneuver. The patients are at risk for ischemic chest pain, especially when exercising. Most other structural disorders of the heart rarely cause chest pain, although severe pulmonic stenosis with associated cyanosis and aortic valve stenosis can lead to ischemia. The pain in these conditions may be described as squeezing, choking, or a sensation of pressure in the sternal area. These maladies almost always are diagnosed before the child presents with pain, and the associated murmurs are found on physical examination. Finally, mitral valve prolapse (MVP) may cause chest pain by papillary muscle or left ventricular endocardial ischemia, and a midsystolic click and late systolic murmur are found in many cases. However, studies show that MVP is no more common in children who have chest pain than in the general population.

Cardiac infections should be considered as important, although uncommon, causes of pediatric chest pain. For instance, pericarditis presents with sharp, stabbing pain that improves when the patient sits up and leans forward. The child who has this infection usually is febrile; is in respiratory distress; and has a friction rub, distant heart sounds, neck vein distention, and pulsus paradoxus. Myocarditis is a more common infection and sometimes can present more subtly. The adolescent in the case report presented with many classic features of this disease. Such children have pain for several days that is mild and not disruptive. After a few days of fever and other systemic symptoms such as vomiting and lightheadedness, the patient may develop pain or shortness of breath on exertion. Examination may reveal muffled heart sounds, fever, a gallop rhythm, or tachycardia that is out of proportion to the degree of fever present. As noted in the case report, the patient also may have orthostatic changes in pulse or blood pressure (pulse increase 30 beats/min, blood pressure decrease by >20 mm Hg when moving from supine to standing position). This often is misinterpreted as volume depletion because the children who have this infection may not be taking oral fluids well and, indeed, may be mildly dehydrated. However, this finding will not always improve with fluid resuscitation; if not, cardiogenic causes such as myocarditis should be suspected. A chest radiograph usually will show cardiomegaly in both of these infections (Fig. 1), and the electrocardiogram will be abnormal, prompting a further evaluation, such as an echocardiogram.

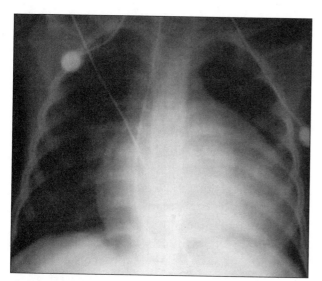

Figure 1. Radiograph of a child who has myocarditis. Note the markedly enlarged heart.

TABLE 2. Noncardiac Causes of Pediatric Chest Pain

Musculoskeletal disorders
- Chest wall strain
- Direct trauma/contusion
- Rib fracture
- Costochondritis

Respiratory disorders
- Severe cough
- Asthma
- Pneumonia
- Pneumothorax/pneumomediastinum
- Pulmonary embolism

Psychologic disorders
- Stress-related pain

Gastrointestinal disorders
- Reflux esophagitis
- Esophageal foreign body

Miscellaneous disorders
- Sickle cell crises
- Abdominal aortic aneurysm (Marfan syndrome)
- Pleural effusion (collagen vascular disease)
- Shingles
- Pleurodynia (coxsackievirus)
- Breast tenderness (pregnancy, physiologic)

Idiopathic

MUSCULOSKELETAL PAIN

This is one of the most common diagnoses in children who have chest discomfort (Table 2). Active children frequently strain chest wall muscles while wrestling, carrying heavy books, or exercising. Direct trauma to the chest may result in a mild contusion of the chest wall or, with more significant force, a rib fracture, hemothorax, or pneumothorax. In most cases there is a straightforward history of trauma, and the diagnosis is clear. Certainly, a careful physical examination will reveal chest tenderness or pain with movement of the torso or upper extremities.

Costochondritis is a related disorder that is common in children. The diagnosis is made by eliciting tenderness over the costochondral junctions with palpation. The pain may be bilateral, and it generally is sharp and exaggerated by physical activity or breathing. Such pain may persist for several months.

RESPIRATORY CONDITIONS

Children who have severe, persistent cough, asthma, or pneumonia may complain of chest pain due to overuse of chest wall muscles. The diagnosis is made by history or the findings of rales, wheezes, tachypnea, or decreased breath sounds. Some children may complain of chest pain with exercise due to exercise-induced asthma, which can be determined quite readily with a treadmill test. An occasional child will develop a spontaneous pneumothorax (Fig. 2) or pneumomediastinum and complain of pain with respiratory distress. Children at high risk for these conditions are those who have asthma, cystic fibrosis, and Marfan syndrome, but previously healthy children may rupture an unrecognized subpleural bleb with minimal precipitating factors. With this condition, the patient typically would be in respiratory distress, with decreased breath sounds on the affected side (if the pneumothorax is significant) and palpable subcutaneous air. Of course, adolescents who snort cocaine are at risk for similar barotrauma and may complain of severe, sudden chest pain with associated anxiety, hypertension, and tachycardia. Finally, pulmonary embolism is extremely rare in pediatric patients, but may be considered in the adolescent girl who has dyspnea, fever, pleuritic pain, cough, and hemoptysis. The likelihood of this diagnosis is increased if she is using oral

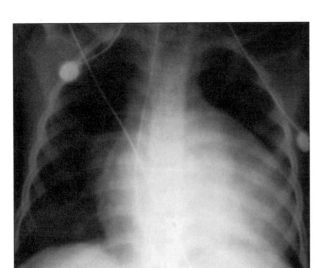

Figure 2. Radiograph of a child who has tension pneumothorax on the right. Note the shift of the mediastinum to the left.

contraceptives or recently has had an abortion. Young males who have recent leg trauma also are at some risk for pulmonary embolism.

PSYCHOGENIC DISTURBANCES

Such disturbances can precipitate chest pain in both boys and girls at equal rates. Often the anxiety and stress that results in somatic complaints is not easily apparent; not all of these children present with hyperventilation or an anxious appearance. However, if the child has had a recent major stressful event, such as separation from friends, divorce in the family, or school failure that correlates temporally with the onset of the chest pain, it is reasonable to conclude that the symptoms are related to the underlying stress. The perception of pain that is a result of emotional conflict also may have its roots in unresolved chronic issues in the child or within the family. A family history of depression or a somatization disorder predisposes a child to psychosomatic symptoms. A family member or friend who has experienced chest pain, especially as a result of cardiac disease, may trigger a heightened perception of mild pain in a child that is due to a common problem such as musculoskeletal trauma or costochondritis. Recent research in

neuropsychological mechanisms of apparent psychogenic pain suggests that many of these children experience or perceive mild pain in the form of an exaggerated response.

GASTROINTESTINAL DISORDERS

Such conditions as reflux esophagitis often cause chest pain in young children and adolescents. The pain is described classically as burning, substernal in location, and worsened by reclining or eating spicy foods. Many gastroenterologists believe that manometric studies are required for children who have persistent unexplained chest pain. However, this condition also can be diagnosed with a therapeutic trial of antacids. Likewise, some young children will complain of chest pain following the ingestion of a coin or other foreign body that lodges in the esophagus. In general, the child or parent may give a clear history of recent foreign body ingestion, and a simple radiograph can confirm the diagnosis. Infants and young children who have an esophageal foreign body are more likely to gag with food than complain of chest pain.

MISCELLANEOUS CAUSES

Some instances of chest pain are related to underlying diseases. For instance, sickle cell disease may lead to vaso-occlusive crises or acute chest syndrome. Marfan syndrome may result in chest pain and fatal dissection of an abdominal aortic aneurysm. Collagen vascular disorders may lead to pleural effusions, and shingles may result in severe chest pain that precedes or occurs simultaneously with the classic rash. Likewise, infection with coxsackievirus may lead to pleurodynia with paroxysms of sharp pain in the chest or abdomen. Children also may complain of chest pain when there is breast tenderness from physiologic changes of puberty or from early changes of pregnancy.

Unfortunately, in 20% to 45% of cases of pediatric chest pain, no diagnosis can be determined with certainty. The child's pain is labeled as idiopathic in many such cases.

Clinical Approach to Chest Pain

A complete history and careful physical examination will reveal the etiology of chest pain in most cases. The family history may be helpful because disorders such as hypertrophic obstructive cardiomyopathy are familial. The medical history may reveal asthma, which places the patient at risk for more serious causes of pain. Previous heart disease or conditions such as Kawasaki disease may increase the risk for cardiac pathology.

The physician should determine if the pain is frequent, severe, or interrupts the child's daily activity. Children who wake from sleep because of the pain are more likely to have an organic etiology, although it may not necessarily be serious. Asking the patient to locate and describe the pain is not always helpful because young children are vague in their descriptions. However, burning pain in the sternal area suggests esophagitis, and sharp stabbing pain that is relieved by sitting up and leaning forward suggests pericarditis in a febrile child. The onset of pain also should be determined because children who have an acute onset are more likely to have an organic etiology. Those who have chronic pain that has gone without a diagnosis are much more likely to have idiopathic or psychogenic etiologies.

Any precipitating factors should be elicited. A history of trauma, muscle strain, or choking on a foreign body may be quite relevant. Also, chest pain that occurs with exercise should be taken seriously; it may relate to cardiac disease or, more commonly, to exercise-induced asthma. Chest pain associated with syncope, fever, or palpitations is more significant. The physician may determine that the pain is part of an underlying systemic disorder such as a collagen vascular disease if joint pain, rash, or fever has been present. The physician should inquire about possible stressful conditions at home or school, and the diagnosis of psychogenic pain should not be a diagnosis of exclusion. Finally, in adolescents who have chest pain, it is appropriate to ask about substance abuse (cocaine, in particular) or use of oral contraceptives.

A careful physical examination is likely to point to the cause of pain. A general examination should identify the child in severe distress who needs immediate treatment for life-threatening conditions such as pneumothorax. Hyperventilation should be distinguished from respiratory distress by the absence of cyanosis or nasal flaring. Signs of chronic disease (pallor, poor growth) may suggest that the chest pain is one symptom of a more complex problem such as a tumor or collagen vascular disease. Rashes or bruises on parts distant from the chest may indicate unrecognized trauma to the torso. The abdomen deserves careful evaluation because it may be a source of pain that is referred to the chest.

A complete chest examination is essential. This is likely to reveal rales, wheezes, or decreased breath sounds if there is pulmonary pathology or murmurs, rubs, muffled heart sounds, or arrhythmias if there is cardiac pathology. The chest wall should be evaluated for signs of trauma, tenderness (suggesting musculoskeletal pain), or subcutaneous air (suggesting a pneumothorax or pneumomediastinum).

Laboratory Evaluation and Referral

The boy presented in the case report had worrisome findings of fever, shortness of breath, pain with exertion, abnormal vital signs, and an abnormal cardiac examination, which warranted laboratory evaluation and urgent treatment.

Laboratory studies usually confirm previously known disorders or abnormal findings that are suspected clinically. If the history is acute in onset (began in the past 2 or 3 days) or is indicative of pulmonary problems or cardiac disease, a chest radiograph or electrocardiogram is indicated. If there is pain on exertion, one should be particularly concerned about cardiac disease or asthma and consider referral for exercise stress tests or pulmonary function tests. If the pain is associated with syncope or palpitations, one should consider referral for Holtor monitoring to look for an arrhythmia or structural heart disease. Chest pain in patients who have a history of previous heart disease usually is not serious, but the examining physician may be more comfortable reviewing the child's chest film, obtaining an electrocardiogram, or referring the patient to the cardiologist. This group represents only a small percentage of children who have chest pain.

If the physical examination is abnormal, laboratory studies are justified. A chest radiograph can be quite helpful if the patient has fever, respiratory distress, or decreased or abnormal breath sounds. Fever with chest pain is highly correlated with pneumonia. As illustrated by the case report, pericarditis or myocarditis should be considered in the febrile child who has chest pain; radiographs may reveal cardiomegaly. Moreover, an abnormal cardiac examination, including unexplained tachycardia, arrhythmia, murmur, rub, or click, warrants an electrocardiogram.

Laboratory studies are not necessary in the child who has chronic pain, a normal physical examination, and no history suggestive of cardiac or pulmonary disease. The family should be reassured that the child is unlikely to have a serious etiology for the pain and that studies would be unhelpful. If this strategy is not successful, then noninvasive studies should be considered to alleviate the family's anxiety. Likewise, it is not necessary to obtain an echocardiogram to look for mitral valve prolapse in all children who have ill-defined chest pain.

Blood counts and sedimentation rates are of limited value unless collagen vascular disease, infection, or malignancy is suspected. A drug screen may be indicated in the older child who has acute pain that is associated with anxiety, tachycardia, hypertension, or shortness of breath.

The child should be referred to an emergency department if he or she is in severe distress or has a history of significant trauma. Referral to a specialist should be considered if an esophageal foreign body is noted or if the patient has a serious emotional problem that cannot be managed in the office. The child who has known or suspected heart disease, syncope, palpitations, or pain on exertion may be served best by referral to a cardiologist.

When a specific etiology for the pain is found, such as pneumonia, it can be treated. In most cases of musculoskeletal, psychogenic, or idiopathic pain, the child will respond to reassurance, analgesics, rest, and perhaps heat and relaxation techniques. If esophagitis is suspected, a trial of antacids may be beneficial.

Appropriate follow-up should be arranged because many children who have ill-defined pain have persistent symptoms for many months. Although serious organic pathology is unlikely to be found in the future, the physician must ascertain that the child is participating in his or her usual activities. Also, the physician should observe for significant psychoemotional problems or exercise-induced asthma that previously was unrecognized. Follow-up, with an emphasis on further exploration of the cause of pain if appropriate or an explanation for pathophysiologic pain, may prevent the development of cardiac or pulmonary "nondisease."

Summary

Chest pain is a common complaint among children of all ages. It rarely is due to cardiac disease, but deserves careful evaluation for this possibility, with laboratory tests performed in limited cases. The child who has pain of acute onset that interferes with sleep, is precipitated by exercise, or is associated with dizziness, palpitations, syncope, or shortness of breath should be evaluated with the aid of laboratory tests. This includes at least a chest radiograph and electrocardiogram. Also, pain in the child who has a history of coin ingestion, trauma, previous cardiac disease, or conditions that put him or her at risk for developing cardiac pathology deserve further study. Likewise, those who have a history of conditions such as asthma, Marfan syndrome, or sickle cell disease warrant special consideration. Finally, most of those who have an abnormal physical examination (fever, respiratory distress, abnormal breath sounds, cardiac murmur, abnormal rhythm or heart sounds, palpable subcutaneous air, or obvious trauma) also require a chest radiograph and an electrocardiogram. However, the child who has chronic chest pain but appears quite well and has a normal physical examination with no worrisome history needs reassurance and careful follow-up rather than extensive studies.

Suggested Reading

Hallagan LF, Dawson PA, Eljaiek LF. Pediatric chest pain: case report of a malignant cause. *Am J Emerg Med.* 1992;10:43–45

Selbst SM. Evaluation of chest pain in children. *Pediatrics in Review.* 1986;8:56–62

Selbst SM, Ruddy R, Clark BJ. Chest pain in children: followup of patients previously reported. *Clin Pediatr.* 1990;29:374–377

Selbst SM, Ruddy RM, Clark BJ, Henretig FM, Santulli T. Pediatric chest pain: a prospective study. *Pediatrics.* 1988; 82:319–323

Weins L, Sabath R, Ewing L, et al. Chest pain in otherwise healthy children and adolescents is frequently caused by exercise-induced asthma. *Pediatrics.* 1992;90:350–353

Zeltzer L, Arnoult S, Hamilton A, De Laura S. Visceral pain in children. In: Hyman P, DiLorenzo C, eds. *Pediatric Gastrointestinal Motility Disorders.* New York, NY: Academic Professional Information Services; 1994:155–176

Contemporary Management of Adolescents With Diabetes Mellitus
Part 1: Type 1 Diabetes

by Donald P. Orr, MD, FAAP

Diabetes mellitus is a group of metabolic disorders characterized by hyperglycemia resulting from defects in insulin secretion, insulin action, or both. The most common subtypes of diabetes mellitus include Type 1, Type 2, those associated with cystic fibrosis, and the rare maturity-onset diabetes of youth. Pediatricians are well positioned to care for adolescents with diabetes, especially those they have cared for over time. The clinician, however, must be up-to-date on the newest treatment modalities and possess the skills to manage individuals with diabetes.

The management of diabetes has changed dramatically in the past 10 years. Recent studies have demonstrated that better glycemic control reduces significantly the risk for eye, nerve, and renal complications. Application of state-of-the art methods in diabetes management to all individuals with diabetes would increase life span, decrease the years the individual must live with serious complications, increase the quality of life-added-years, and be cost effective. Newer insulin preparations, insulin delivery devices like insulin pens and pumps, less painful blood-letting devices, and a wide array of blood glucose testing devices, including some with memory capacity whose content can be downloaded to personal computers, make self-management and improved control feasible for most adolescents.

Pediatricians may believe that adolescents are incapable or unwilling to accept newer insulin regimens that require multiple insulin injections and more frequent blood glucose (BG) testing. Clearly, there is no "one size fits all" approach to adherence, and some adolescents will be unwilling or unable to accept these changes. However, with proper education and encouragement, most will be able to improve their control and many will be able to use the more complicated insulin routines recommended for adults, adolescents, and some pre-adolescents.

Although consultation with a diabetes specialist may be difficult in certain remote areas, it is often appropriate. When a specialist evaluation is medically indicated, it may be necessary to educate patients and payers regarding the necessity of such a referral.

This issue of *Adolescent Health Update* presents the first segment of a two-part series on diabetes management. Part 1 offers a brief overview and focused discussion of the care of adolescents with Type 1 diabetes. In July 2000, part 2 of this series will address Type 2 diabetes in adolescents.

Learning Objectives

After reading this article, pediatricians will be able to describe
- Prevalence and trends of Type 1 diabetes
- New diagnostic criteria
- Diagnostic evaluation
- Optimal management, including use of newer insulin preparations and blood glucose monitoring and insulin-delivery technologies
- Anticipatory guidance and monitoring for complications
- Indications for referral to subspecialists
- Psychosocial factors complicating self-management

Donald P. Orr, MD, FAAP, is professor and director, Section of Adolescent Medicine and Adolescent/Young Adult Diabetes Program, Department of Pediatrics, Indiana University Medical Center, Indianapolis. Dr. Orr is the immediate past editor of Adolescent Health Update. *He was a founding member of the original* Adolescent Health Update *editorial board.*

This issue will not address the management of patients in diabetic ketoacidosis. The text presumes that pediatricians have a working knowledge of BG testing devices, standard twice-daily split mixed-insulin regimens of short- and intermediate-acting insulins, and sick-day management.

A word about the value of a multidisciplinary team: Self-management of diabetes requires that patient and parents understand the relationships between insulin action, food intake, and exercise. Successful self-management requires that patients and parents are educated in all aspects of the disease. It is impossible to manage diabetes without a good understanding of the influence of food in determining BG levels.

A *diabetes team* consisting of a certified diabetes educator (usually a nurse) and a dietitian has an important role in essential patient and parent education in contemporary concepts regarding management of diabetes. These professionals teach, counsel, and reinforce patients' self-management. Patients will not achieve good self-management unless they can capably estimate their CHO intake.

The primary care pediatrician who cares for diabetic adolescents must have the ability to be reached 24 hours per day. Sick day management guidelines should be clearly spelled out. The physician should be prepared to teach regimens and algorithms for correction (both base algorithms and correction algorithms), and be available to adjust dosages daily if needed. Pediatricians who are not prepared to allow the time required to teach these skills and to make dosage adjustments when required must have certified diabetes educators (CDEs) working with them who are available and capable of making daily adjustments.

Incidence and Prevalence

The incidence of Type 1 diabetes (T1DM) varies by race/ethnicity and country, with the highest rates in areas most distant from the equator. It is estimated that there are over 500,000 individuals in the United States with Type 1 diabetes. The US prevalence of T1DM is approximately 1.7/1000 persons under age 19 years. For reasons that are unclear, the incidence is increasing worldwide. The ages of peak incidence in the United States are late childhood and early/mid adolescence.

Chronic hyperglycemia is associated with long-term microvascular (retinopathy, nephropathy and neuropathy) and macrovascular (coronary artery disease, stroke) complications. The direct and indirect costs of diabetes care were estimated at $98 billion in 1997. The medical conditions associated with diabetes among the elderly account for a significant share of these

Table 1. Glycemic Control Targets for Adolescents and Adults[1]

Biochemical Index	Normal	Goal	Action Indicated[2]
Average preprandial BG (mg/dl)[3]	< 110	80–120	< 80 or > 140
Average 2 hour postprandial BG (mg/dl)[3] (rapid-acting insulin users only)	< 120	150–180	> 180
Average bedtime BG (mg/dl)[3]	< 120	100–140	< 100 or > 160
Average 3:00 am BG (mg/dl)	< 110	80–100	< 80 or > 120
HbA$_{1c}$ (%)	< 6	< 7	> 8

1. These values are generally not indicated for preadolescents. The values shown in this table are by necessity generalized to the entire population of individuals with diabetes. Patients with comorbid diseases, the very young and older adults, and others with unusual conditions or circumstances may warrant different treatment goals. These values are for nonpregnant adults.

2. "Action indicated" depends on individual patient circumstances. Such actions may include enhanced diabetes self-management education, comanagement with a diabetes team, referral to an endocrinologist, change in pharmacological therapy, initiation of or increase in SMBG, or more frequent contact with the patient. HbA$_{1c}$ is referenced to a nondiabetic range of 4.0–6.0% (mean 5.0%, SD 0.5%).

3. Measurement of capillary blood glucose

Adapted with permission from: American Diabetes Association. Standards of medical care for patients with diabetes mellitus. *Diabetes Care.* 1999;22(suppl 1):S32–S41. (Table 1, S32). Copyright 1999, American Diabetes Association.

costs. Still, the costs attributable to Type 1 were estimated to be $20 billion in 1993.

Better glycemic control significantly reduces the risk of progressive microvascular complications. The 1994 Diabetes Control and Complications Trial (DCCT), a landmark randomized clinical study of 1,441 individuals with T1DM, demonstrated that better glycemic control significantly reduces the risk for long-term complications. A total of 195 adolescents were included in the DCCT. Normalization of BG levels was the goal in the experimental (intensive) group and required more intensive insulin regimens via multiple injections or continuous subcutaneous insulin injection pumps (CSII pumps), as well as frequent BG testing, extensive education about diet, and monthly visits. Among those in the intensive group (for whom the target HbA1c was < 6%), adults were able to achieve an average HbA1c of 7.2% and adolescents were able to achieve an average HbA1c of 8.0%. The DCCT found that risk reduction for microvascular complications among adults and adolescents with Type 1 and Type 2 diabetes varies from 30% to 76%, depending on the complication. As a result of this study, diabetes regimens that target normalization of BG are increasingly considered "standard of care." (See Table 1)

Compared with conventionally treated patients (typically those on only two insulin injections), the average intensively treated individual would gain 15.3 years of life free from any significant microvascular or neurologic complication and live 5.1 years longer. The challenge remains to translate the findings of the DCCT to the larger number of individuals with diabetes, especially adolescents.

Diagnosis

The American Diabetes Association (ADA) recently modified the diagnostic criteria for diabetes mellitus. The revised ADA diagnostic criteria are shown in Table 2. _Most important is the recommendation that the oral glucose tolerance test not be used routinely for diagnosis._ ADA diagnostic criteria will be discussed in depth in Part 2 of this series.

Unless detected very early in the course of the disease, individuals with T1DM are generally

Table 2. American Diabetes Association Criteria for Diagnosis of Diabetes Mellitus

1. Symptoms of diabetes plus casual plasma glucose concentration ≥ 200 mg/dl. (Casual is defined as any time or day without regard to time since last meal.)

   or

2. FPG ≥ 126 mg/dl. Fasting is defined as no caloric intake for at least 8 h.

   or

3. 2-h PG ≥ 200 mg/dl during an oral glucose tolerance test (OGTT). The test should be performed as described by WHO using a glucose load containing the equivalent of 75-g anhydrous glucose dissolved in water.

In the absence of acute metabolic decompensation, these criteria should be confirmed by repeat testing on a different day. The third measure (OGTT) is not recommended for routine clinical use.

Adapted with permission from: The Expert Committee on the Diagnosis and Classification of Diabetes Mellitus. Report of the expert committee on the diagnosis and classification of diabetes mellitus. *Diabetes Care.* 1999;22(suppl 1):S5–S19. (Table 3, S12). Copyright 1999, American Diabetes Association.

symptomatic (polyuria, polydipsia, polyphagia, weight loss), not overweight, and often at least mildly ketotic at the time of diagnosis. It is usually (but not always!) quite easy to distinguish Type 1 from Type 2. For example, a proportion of patients with T2DM may present in ketoacidosis when under severe metabolic stress and will require initial treatment with insulin. This finding has been particularly noted among African-American T2DM patients.

Measurement of autoantibodies [pancreatic islet β-cell, glutamic acid decarboxylase (GAD_{65}), IA-2 or IA-2β (tyrosine phosphatases), insulin] is generally not indicated unless the etiologic classification is unclear. Consultation with a diabetes specialist is suggested in these circumstances. More difficult diagnostic categories will be discussed in Part 2 of this series.

MONITORING

Diabetes treatment regimens are designed to lower BG (and resultant HbA1c). Treatment plans should take into account patient safety and individual ability to carry out the treatment regimen. Although normal levels of BG are the goal, most patients (adult and adolescent) are not able to achieve consistently normal levels of glycated hemoglobin. However, any consistent lowering of glycated hemoglobin will reduce the rates of complications. The preprandial BG target for adolescents is 80 to 120 mg/dl.

Glycated hemoglobin should be measured at each visit (generally quarterly) and the results discussed with the adolescent in relation to blood glucose test results. Glycated hemoglobin values reflect the average blood glucose over the previous 6 to 8 weeks; BG records must also be examined because the adolescent may have dramatic (even dangerous) swings in BG that would not be evident in the percent of glycated hemoglobin. Several different assays are available, each with its own normal (nondiabetic) range. It is preferable to use a single test and laboratory to avoid confusion. It has been suggested that all glycated hemoglobin assays be standardized and reported in values equivalent to HbA1c (which was used in the DCCT). A rapid (9 minute) sensitive and specific immunoassay method to determine HbA1c has become available. This makes it easier to discuss the results at the time of the office visit. Having the results of the glycated hemoglobin level available at the time of the visit has been shown to result in significantly improved control among adults. Therefore, it is preferable that the adolescent have the test performed before visiting the physician. Discussing the results at the next visit or by telephone is less satisfactory. Based upon the DCCT HbA1c values, the target A1c is 7%.

Blood glucose testing devices change rapidly and vary in their characteristics. Many contain memory to store the date, times, and test results, some can be downloaded to personal computers, and most (but not all) are calibrated to reflect plasma glucose (about 10 mg/dl to 15 mg/dl higher than blood glucose). The physician should become familiar with a few devices. Patients should be encouraged to test on a single brand of meter to assure that test results are comparable. (See resource list, page 12.)

INSULIN DELIVERY DEVICES

Insulin delivery devices have changed along with regimens. Syringes, pens, and external pumps are now in common use.

Insulin syringes: Insulin syringes are available in 0.3, 0.5, and 1.0 cc sizes with needles of varying gauges (28g to 30g) and lengths (5/16 and 1/2 inch). Adolescents usually prefer one type over another. Check with your local diabetes educator or one of the Web sites for additional information.

Insulin pens: The availability of insulin pens has facilitated the use of newer insulin regimens. Several devices are available that contain short-acting, rapid-acting, NPH, and 70/30 (70% NPH/30% short-acting) insulin, in a cartridge containing 150 units, or as a disposable device containing 150 or 300 units. These devices are about the size of a fountain pen and can be carried easily in purse or shirt pocket. The required dose is simply "dialed" and then injected. Disposable needles must be prescribed. Pens and insulin cartridges from different manufacturers are interchangeable.

CSII pumps: These permit ultimate flexibility in designing an insulin regimen, enabling the patient to compensate more easily for exercise as well as large and small variations in carbohydrate intake (including skipped meals and the tendency of BG to increase between 3:00 am and 6:00 am, known as the "dawn phenomenon"). Multiple basal insulin rates can be preprogrammed. The patient must determine the amount of insulin to be delivered for each mealtime or compensatory bolus and instruct the pump to deliver this amount at the correct time. Candidates for CSII pumps are very motivated patients who are willing to test at least four times daily (and often more frequently, including between 2:00 am and 3:00 am when required), actively monitor carbohydrate intake, adjust insulin doses with each meal or snack, and commit to frequent contact with the diabetes team. Individuals with markedly elevated HbA1c levels are generally poor candidates for pump therapy. Adolescents who wish to use CSII should be referred to a diabetes team experienced with CSII and adolescents.

INSULIN REGIMENS

Adjusting the dose of short- or rapid-acting insulin administered before meals takes into account the fact that BG levels vary considerably from day to day even for the most conscientious individual. The use of corrective sliding scales for rapid/short-acting insulins gives the adolescent more control and allows for more immediate compensation for hypo- and hyperglycemia. In making adjustments of intermediate-acting insulins, stress that the patient should monitor patterns for 2 to 3 days before increasing the dose.

Number of insulin injections: Inflexible traditional regimens of twice-daily injections of mixed insulin (short- and intermediate-acting) are being replaced by multiple daily injections (MDI) of short- or rapid-acting insulin. At least three injections are generally required. These permit greater flexibility in matching insulin dose to dietary carbohydrate (CHO) content and more frequent correction for variations in BG levels. Although MDI regimens necessitate insulin injection during the school day, this rarely presents a problem. Schools are increasingly accustomed to accommodating students with special health needs and the ADA Web site provides additional information in this regard.

Some adolescents (especially those using NPH insulin) will have already adopted a "split night-time dose" regimen of rapid/short-acting insulin with dinner and intermediate-acting insulin with the bedtime snack. This regimen facilitates management of fasting hyperglycemia associated with the long interval between dinner and breakfast compared to the duration of action of the intermediate insulin, large bedtime snack, and the dawn phenomenon. Institution of an MDI regimen would necessitate a fourth injection at lunchtime.

Insulin preparations: The pharmacological characteristics of human insulin preparations are shown in Table 3. Human insulin has replaced older animal preparations for most patients. Analogues of human insulin have been developed to control the absorption times and duration of action. Rapid-acting insulin analogues are absorbed more rapidly from subcutaneous tissues than human insulin preparations. This reduces the need for administration 30 to 60 minutes prior to eating (required with the use of Regular insulin) and results in less hyperglycemia and hypoglycemia 4 to 6 hours later. This is especially important at night when hypoglycemia is most dangerous. Insulin lispro (eg, Humalog) is a currently available rapid-acting analogue. Two additional insulin analogues are likely to be available in the near future: insulin aspart (eg, NovoRapid), a rapid-acting analogue

Table 3. Characteristics of Human Insulin Preparations

Informal description	Proprietary or other name	Onset (hours)	Peak (hours)	Effective duration (hours)	Maximum duration (hours)	Technical description
rapid-acting	lispro	.25	1 to 2	2 to 3	4	insulin analogue
rapid-acting	aspart*	.25	1 to 2	2 to 3	4	insulin analogue
short-acting	Regular	.5 to 1	2 to 3	3 to 6	4 to 6	insulin
intermediate-acting	NPH	2 to 4	4 to 10	10 to 16	14 to 18	insulin isophane [suspension]
intermediate-acting	Lente	3 to 4	4 to 12	12 to 18	16 to 20	insulin zinc [suspension]
long-acting	Ultralente	6 to 10	12 to 18	18 to 20	20 to 30	insulin zinc [suspension] extended

* new drug application on file with the FDA

Not yet available is insulin glargine, a long-acting insulin analogue providing basal insulin with once-daily injection; new drug application on file with FDA available in Europe, and insulin glargine, a long-acting, peakless insulin analogue that provides basal insulin when injected once daily.

MDI REGIMENS

Lunch-time insulin: The easiest multiple dose regimen consists of adding pre-lunch short- or rapid-acting insulin to a standard twice-daily schedule. This accommodates decreased insulin sensitivity, increased food intake, and variation in lunch foods occurring during adolescence. When these events occur, the dose of morning intermediate-acting insulin increases disproportionate to the amount of short- or rapid-acting insulin. Even with large doses of intermediate-acting insulin, pre-dinner BG levels tend to be elevated. This is due, in part, to the shorter duration of action of human NPH insulin, leading to hyperglycemia in two-shot regimens. Importantly, on twice-daily regimens, the risk for hypoglycemia in late afternoon increases when the adolescent fails to eat a planned late afternoon snack, exercises unexpectedly before dinner, or delays dinner.

Two options are available if predinner BG levels are elevated. One option is to add an amount of short- or rapid-acting insulin sufficient to reduce the predinner BG to target levels based on previous BG records (without reducing the dose of prebreakfast intermediate insulin). Alternatively, estimate the amount of short- or rapid-acting insulin required for the adolescent's lunch-time carbohydrate intake, and reduce the morning intermediate-acting insulin by the same amount. The results of a week's BG testing before each meal and before bedtime snack will guide the pediatrician and adolescent in making necessary adjustments. (See Table 4 for an example of a plan.) Remind the adolescent that regardless of the morning intermediate-acting dose, delaying lunch more than an hour presents a risk of hypoglycemia.

A word of caution to clinicians: Adolescents who object to the inconvenience of an injection at lunch or bedtime may agree to please the physician, begin with good intentions, then fail to adhere. An additional injection alone does not assure improved control, and not all adolescents are good candidates for an MDI regimen. Additional

Table 4. Adding Prelunch Insulin to Twice-Daily Regimen

Typical lunch: Big Mac,™ large fries, diet drink

CHO: 7 carbohydrate exchanges (105 g)

Estimate insulin bolus dose: One unit of regular insulin will cover 10 g CHO.

Action: Reduce the morning Lente dose by 10 units Administer 10 units of short-acting insulin before lunch. (The bolus dose may be adjusted up/down from 10 units using a corrective sliding scale to compensate for prelunch BG values.)

injections should be based on the overall mutual treatment goals. *Two injections of sufficient amounts and types of insulin are superior to surreptitious omission of the third or fourth injection.* If the level of control is acceptable and the adolescent does not desire greater flexibility, twice-daily injections are fine.

Basal Bolus Regimens: The principle of a basal bolus regimen is to provide 40% to 50% of the total daily dose of insulin (TDD) as intermediate/long-acting (referred to as basal dose) and the remainder as short- or rapid-acting. Short- or rapid-acting injections are to be taken before all meals (bolus). Basal bolus regimens are designed to more closely mimic physiologic secretion of insulin. Several regimens of short/rapid, intermediate, and long-acting insulin are commonly used, based on the timing of meals, lifestyle of the adolescent, and individual preference of the physician. Lunch-time short/rapid-acting insulin also permits easier compensation for after-school exercise by allowing reduction of the prelunch insulin dose on exercise days—an attractive alternative for adolescents who do not want to rely on additional pre-exercise carbohydrate and the associated calories. If the adolescent wishes a late afternoon snack, then he/she may need to use regular insulin as the prelunch insulin or inject presnack rapid-acting insulin. Two common basal bolus regimens are presented here. For additional regimens see the reading list.

First basal bolus regimen: For most individuals, the peak of human Ultralente insulin is sufficiently blunted at steady state to use as a peakless basal insulin. Dividing the Ultralente into two equal doses with the second dose given before dinner tends to work better because there is sufficient basal insulin available during the day to allow delay in lunch times with less likelihood of hyperglycemia. As with other MDI plans, the exact doses at each meal depend on the amount of CHO consumed, the time of day (generally slightly more is required at breakfast), the level of planned activity, and the overall sensitivity to insulin. For the first week of therapy, the patient should be asked to adhere as closely as possible to his/her meal plan, perform BG testing before each meal, and obtain several 3:00 am BG tests. The individual doses of short/rapid-acting insulin are then adjusted based on the BG test following that dose (eg, breakfast short/rapid-acting insulin dose is adjusted to achieve the desired BG before lunch). The second dose of Ultralente is adjusted based on the 3:00 am and breakfast BG values. Remember that Ultralente insulin has a long half-life and it will take 4 to 5 days to begin to achieve a steady state. BG levels may be elevated the first several days, but the doses of short/rapid-acting insulin can be adjusted accordingly when BG is > 300 mg/dl. Urinary ketones should be determined when BG is ≥ 350 mg/dl and the adolescent instructed to call for advice whenever ketones are ≥ moderate levels. Additional insulin is required at that time. (See Table 5 for an example)

In general, a safe starting point for the initial distribution of insulin with MDI is:

- 40% to 50% of the total daily insulin dose (TDD) as basal, divided into two equal doses
- 15% to 25% TDD prebreakfast as short/rapid-acting
- 15% TDD prelunch as short/rapid-acting
- 15% to 25% TDD predinner as short/rapid-acting
- 0% to 10% TDD bedtime snack as short/rapid-acting

The doses of short/rapid-acting insulin are adjusted after one week based upon the pattern of preprandial BG values for the meal following each insulin injection. Interpretation of these BG test results will be easiest if the CHO content at mealtimes remains relatively constant (eg, the adolescent consumes the same amount of CHO

Table 5. Changing to a Basal Bolus Regimen

70 kg male	Bedtime snack—15 g CHO	
Current:	Breakfast	13 R/29 L
	Dinner	14 R/14L
TDD:	70 units	
New regimen:		
Basal:	32 units	
	Breakfast	16 Ultralente
	Dinner	16 Ultralente
Rapid-acting:	38 units	
	Breakfast	13 rapid-acting
	Lunch	13 rapid-acting
	Dinner	13 rapid-acting

at each breakfast). For example, the dose of prelunch rapid/short-acting insulin is increased or decreased based on the subsequent predinner BG. Sufficient BG testing results must be available to determine patterns of BG values.

The next step after starting an MDI regimen is to develop a corrective sliding scale for short/rapid-acting insulin doses. This permits regular compensation for variations in premeal BG. After an additional 1 to 2 weeks of testing, the physician and patient can identify the times when premeal BG levels remained relatively level (ie, <50 mg/dl apart). This dose of insulin is then selected as the amount to be taken prior to the preceding meal when BG is 70 to 150 mg/dl. In general, it is safe to estimate that one unit of rapid- or short-acting insulin will lower the BG 50 mg, and adjust the sliding scale accordingly. For those occasions when BG testing does not take place, the adolescent should administer the dose of rapid/short-acting insulin that is usually taken at that meal. At this stage of self-management, the adolescent should be encouraged to maintain as consistent a CHO intake within each meal as is possible. (See Table 6 and the "dosage hints" chart on page 85.)

When the patient achieves prebedtime snack BG levels in the target range, and elevated 3:00 am BG levels (target 80 to 120 mg/dl), adding rapid-acting insulin at the bedtime snack or reducing the CHO content of the snack is indicated. The second dose of Ultralente may

Table 6. Example of a Corrective Sliding Scale for Rapid-Acting Insulin

Rapid-acting dose that usually maintains BG between 70 and 150

from breakfast to lunch:	11 units
from lunch to dinner:	8 units
from dinner to HS snack:	9 units

Examples of a corrective sliding scale for rapid-acting dosing

Preprandial BG expressed mg/dl	Rapid-acting dose units at breakfast	Rapid-acting dose units at lunch	Rapid-acting dose units at dinner
< 70	10	7	8
70 to 150	11	8	9
151 to 200	12	9	10
201 to 250	13	10	11
251 to 300	14	11	12
301 to 350	15	12	13
351 to 400	16	13	14
401 to 450	17	14	15
> 450	18	15	16

be adjusted after approximately 5 days based on 3:00 am and fasting BG levels. Adolescents with a large dawn phenomenon may have difficulty preventing fasting hyperglycemia with this regimen. Options include replacing the second injection of Ultralente with an intermediate insulin at the bedtime snack or *adding* a small amount of intermediate insulin at bedtime. *Replacing* bedtime Ultralente with intermediate insulin may reduce the flexibility of the timing of lunch. If overall HbA1c levels are in the desired range, some adolescents choose to simply compensate with increased amounts of rapid-acting insulin at breakfast. Adolescents requiring such complex MDI regimens should be referred to a diabetes specialist and may consider the use of CSII pump if sufficiently motivated.

Second basal bolus regimen: Patients who count carbohydrates often do best with an MDI regimen of basal long-acting insulin (as described previously) and a bolus (meal-time) rapid/short-acting dose based on the amount of CHO eaten and a corrective sliding scale to compensate for the pre-meal BG. This allows the greatest flexibility in eating. The adolescent counts the CHO to be consumed at a given meal, divides it by the CHO/insulin ratio to obtain the dose of short/rapid-acting insulin, and then adjusts this dose based on the premeal BG value, using a corrective sliding

scale as described above. It is then possible to re-evaluate the effectiveness of each meal's bolus dose by examining the average BG values of the subsequent meal over time. For example, if the 2-week average prelunch BG level is 200, this indicates that the breakfast bolus dose needs to be increased by approximately one unit. There are two ways to begin this regimen.

Example 1. It is easiest to transition an adolescent from the MDI plan just described. Examine the BG and CHO intake values for *each* meal over a several-week period. Find the days on which the BG remains reasonably level from one meal to the next; divide the gm/CHO by the units of insulin taken to identify the amount of CHO covered by each unit of short/rapid-acting insulin (CHO/insulin ratio). For example, 90 gm CHO consumed (6 carbs) at lunch and 8 units of insulin maintain the BG at about the same level from lunch to dinner. Therefore, each 11 gm CHO will require about 1 unit of insulin *at that meal time*. The CHO/insulin ratio should be estimated for each meal because they are likely to be different. Modifications can then be made based on several weeks of BG and CHO records.

Example 2. For adolescents who are being changed from a standard twice daily regimen, estimate the long-acting dose as described previously and estimate a "typical" CHO/insulin ratio of 15 gm CHO for each unit of short/rapid acting insulin. After several weeks, adjust the ratios *for each meal time* based on BG and CHO records.

Symptomatic and asymptomatic nocturnal hypoglycemia are potentially serious consequences of better control. The use of rapid-acting preparations at dinner-time results in less night-time hypoglycemia. These insulins are most effective when administered about 15 minutes before eating, but they also perform well when given immediately prior to the meal. They may also be given immediately after a meal at which large amounts of fat have been consumed. The shorter duration of action makes it safer to administer insulin when additional carbohydrate is consumed between meals, including bedtime, and affords greater dietary flexibility. The midmorning snack may be eliminated.

Dietary Management

Initial and continuing education are prerequisites of successful control. All newly diagnosed patients and their parents should be referred to an experienced certified diabetes educator (CDE) and a dietitian (assuming that the CDE is not also a dietitian). The American Association of Diabetes Educators maintains a Web site (www.aadenet.org) where clinicians will find information about how to locate local CDEs. Also, the American Diabetes Association has accredited diabetes programs throughout the United States (see www.diabetes.org), and most larger hospitals have diabetes education programs.

Dietary carbohydrate is the major determinant of blood glucose levels and therefore meal-related insulin requirements. It is crucial that adolescents are able to accurately estimate the amount of CHO consumed at each meal. The diabetes exchange system for meal planning has been refined to allow more accurate estimation of CHO. This simplifies meal planning and facilitates more precise estimation of premeal insulin doses. Two counting methods are available.

*Counting **carbs:*** Standard servings of starch/bread, fruit, and milk, are considered to be equal in CHO value (about 15 G per *carb*). Values are obtained from food lists and food product nutrition labels. If the adolescent

---

Dosage Hints

For average adolescent with total daily insulin dose of about 1 unit/kg

- 1 unit short/rapid-acting insulin will usually lower blood glucose by 50 to 100 mg/dl
- 8 to 15 gm carbohydrate will require about 1 unit of short/rapid-acting insulin
- 10 to 15 gm dietary carbohydrate will usually change blood glucose by about 40 to 60 mg

---

desires very tight control, vegetables or meat (~1/3 *carb* per serving) may be counted. The premeal insulin bolus is calculated as units of short-acting per *carb*. This method is easiest, less time consuming, but less accurate. See the reading list for additional information.

*Counting **grams** of CHO:* The specific CHO gram value for all foods eaten at a given meal is calculated. The premeal insulin bolus is calculated by dividing the total grams of CHO by insulin/CHO ratio. (The insulin/CHO ratio is defined as the number of grams of CHO covered by one unit of short-acting insulin). This is the most accurate method, but it is time consuming and requires math skills to add and divide two- and three-digit numbers.

SPECIAL CONSIDERATIONS

Improved glycemic control increases the risk of severe hypoglycemia. A mild hypoglycemic event can go unrecognized, increasing the risk for more dangerous future episodes. Among the adolescents in the intensive group of the DCCT, 80% experienced at least one episode of severe hypoglycemia requiring assistance during the 9-year study. Adolescents with limited cognitive ability, those who refuse to perform any BG testing, those who unpredictably skip meals, and those lacking awareness of hypoglycemia, are at high risk for severe hypoglycemia, and should have higher HbA$_{1c}$ as a goal. (See Table 1.)

Excessive weight gain is associated with improved control unless the meal plan is modified. In the DCCT, weight gain was a more significant problem for adolescents in the intensive group, 44% of whom became overweight (BMI > 27.8 kg/m^2 for males and > 27.3 kg/m^2 for females) compared to 28% in the control group. This can be particularly problematic for adolescent women, who may resort to administering less insulin or omitting doses altogether, thus increasing the risk of long-term sequelae. This practice is far less common among adolescent men. Most of these young women do not fulfill diagnostic criteria for eating disorders according to *DSM-IV*. Although eating disorders occur in patients with diabetes, current data suggest that eating disorders are not more common among adolescents with diabetes than among those without diabetes. Regular attention to the adolescent's weight is important. Improved control when achieved solely by increased insulin doses and frequent hypoglycemia with the resultant need for additional CHO will cause weight gain. Patients should work with the treatment team to decide whether hyperglycemia will be treated with increased insulin or decreased CHO intake. Chronic poor control (elevated HbA$_{1c}$) associated with unrealistically large reported insulin doses (>1.5 u/kg/day) should prompt consideration of intentional under-dosing or insulin omission in an attempt to prevent weight gain.

Alcohol use is common among older adolescents and young adults, including many with diabetes. Alcohol cannot be converted to glucose; it tends to inhibit gluconeogenesis and interfere with the counter-regulatory responses to insulin-induced hypoglycemia. It also impairs judgment. Severe hypoglycemia may result many hours after as little as two ounces of alcohol, especially when consumed on an empty stomach. Anticipatory guidance should stress that alcohol may be dangerous for adolescents with diabetes. Some patients may have the mistaken impression that they should compensate for alcohol by taking additional insulin. This is especially dangerous. Individuals who drink alcohol should eat additional CHO at the time of the alcohol consumption,

Table 7. Guidelines for Exercise

For most people, the safe pre-exercise blood glucose range is from 100 to 250 mg/dl. If your glucose is less than 100 mg/dl, or if it's dropping down to close to 100, have a snack to raise it before exercising, as shown below. When BG is between 100 and 150 mg/dl, many people do not require a snack unless the exercise is intense. However, test during exercise and be prepared to snack to keep your glucose up if necessary. For every hour of planned exercise, be ready to consume at least 10 to 15 grams of carbohydrate. A blood glucose between 151 and 250 is optimal for safe exercise.

Metabolic control before exercise
- Avoid exercise if fasting blood glucose (FBG) > 350 mg/dl
- Avoid exercise if FBG > 250 and ketones are present
- If blood glucose (BG) < 100 mg/dl eat carbohydrates (CHO) based on estimated intensity of exercise

Monitor BG before and after exercise
- Identify usual BG response to exercise to determine if insulin must be reduced or CHO consumed
- Be prepared to test in the middle of the night if the exercise is intense

Food intake
- Consume enough CHO to avoid hypoglycemia
- Have short-acting CHO foods available during and after exercise

Examples of regimens tailored to intensity of exercise are shown below:

Intensity of exercise	Examples	Suggested snack
mild/moderate (< 30 minutes)	walking, cycling	15 g CHO
moderate (1 hour)	tennis, swimming, jogging, golfing, or leisurely cycling	30 g CHO*
intense	football, hockey, racquetball, basketball, strenuous cycling, swimming, shoveling snow	45 g CHO*

* Some guidelines suggest adding a protein serving after moderate or intense exercise

Pediatricians are encouraged to photocopy Table 7 for distribution to patients.

inform others that they have diabetes, and not drive.

Driving: Neuroglycopenia is especially dangerous when driving. Adolescents should have a source of rapid-acting CHO (eg, glucose tablets, hard candy, regular soda) available whenever driving and should wear an ID bracelet. They should be encouraged to test BG before driving at times when they are likely to experience hypoglycemia (eg, after they have skipped a meal or exercised).

Pregnancy: Contraception education for all adolescent women with diabetes is essential. All commonly used hormonal contraceptives are compatible with diabetes and do not influence control. The pediatrician should consider early pregnancy in the differential diagnosis of unexplained hypoglycemia.

Exercise: Failure to compensate for exercise may result in hypoglycemia during, immediately after, or many hours after exercise. General guidelines for exercise are offered in Table 7.

Experience with intensified regimens (basal-bolus) using rapid-acting insulin has shown that it is no longer always necessary to add supplemental CHO based on the intensity and duration of the planned exercise. It is better to encourage adolescents to determine their responses to particular exercise when BG is > 100 mg/dl by checking BG levels before, during, and after activity. This enables the patient to know whether exercise lowers BG during or afterward. In general, short periods of moderate exercise (< 30 minutes) require no CHO supplementation. With sufficient planning, it is generally possible to reduce the dose of insulin acting during the exercise period by one to three units and reduce the risk for hypoglycemia. This is easiest for individuals on MDI, particularly those on rapid-acting insulins, who can reduce the amount of insulin injected that covers the period of the exercise. The amount of dose reduction depends on the intensity of the exercise. Adjusting intermediate-acting insulin is possible but more difficult, and requires planning, frequent BG testing, and knowledge of the adolescent's individual response to exercise. When reduction of insulin dose is not possible or is insufficient, anticipatory supplementation with CHO is required.

MONITORING FOR COMPLICATIONS

All microvascular complications are related to the duration of diabetes and level of BG. Macrovascular complications are also influenced by blood pressure. Elevated blood pressure significantly increases the risk and progression of all complications. Blood pressure should be measured at every visit. Sustained elevations of diastolic pressure above 85 or systolic pressure above 135 should be treated with an antihypertensive agent, preferably an angiotensin converting enzyme (ACE) inhibitor. The extent of the evaluation for an underlying cause of elevated blood pressure will depend on the exact circumstances of each patient. (See Table 8)

Early detection of progressive retinopathy and macular edema permits the use of vision-sparing laser photocoagulation. The risk of other autoimmune complications (primarily thyroiditis with resultant hypothyroidism) continues through

Table 8. Guidelines for Screening for Complications

Complication	Test	Frequency	Abnormality	Action
neuropathy	foot screen	quarterly	see text	see text
thyroiditis*	TSH	yearly	elevated	thyroid replacement therapy
retinopathy	dilated eye exam	yearly	see text	see text
nephropathy	microalbumin	yearly	> 30µ / mg creatinine or > 30 mg / 24 hours	ACE inhibitor
dyslipidemia	lipid profile	1 to 2 years	elevated	see text

*Antithyroid antibody levels determined at diagnosis may not predict risk for subsequent thyroid disease.

adolescence. Sustained microalbuminuria is an indication of nephropathy. Treatment with ACE inhibitors as indicated has been shown to reduce the progression of diabetic nephropathy. Such cases warrant referral to a diabetes specialist.

Dyslipidemia (elevated levels of LDL, total cholesterol and triglycerides, and reduced levels of HDL cholesterol) is common in poorly controlled diabetes and contributes to cardiovascular complications. If the dyslipidemia persists after improved glycemic control, or if better control is not possible, referral to a diabetes specialist is encouraged for consideration of treatment with lipid-lowering medication While diabetic neuropathy is rarely symptomatic during adolescence, examination of the feet for pulses, sensation, deep tendon reflexes, hygiene, calluses, and evidence of infection is indicated. The Semmes-Weinstein monofilament test for sensation is a rapid, sensitive screening test for distal sensory neuropathy. (See reading list, page 11.)

SELF-MANAGEMENT

Diabetes is a complex illness that requires many self-management skills, the ability to plan ahead and anticipate consequences of actions/inactions, and attention to detail. Younger adolescents generally lack the ability to plan for the distant future; thus the ultimate benefits (fewer complications and longer life) of better control are not strong motivators for behavioral change.

The pediatrician must negotiate with the adolescent patient, whose developmental level influences ability to appreciate the value of controlling the disease. The patient needs to understand that a pragmatic attitude toward necessary regimens will lead to improved blood glucose levels, which affect quality of life. Significant personal, family and diabetes team investments are required to achieve near normal blood glucose levels. Not all adolescents are able or willing to achieve excellent control, but almost all can be helped to improve their control and thus decrease their risks of sequelae.

Adolescents perform better in most areas of life when they have consistent parental support and involvement; diabetes is no different. Premature withdrawal of parental support, lack of involvement, and lack of supervision in diabetes management have been consistently associated with poorer control. Parents who expect their children and adolescents to remain in good control, who supervise and assist their efforts to maintain necessary regimens, and who gradually shift responsibility for self-maintenance, will find that their teens have better success.

Parents may assume that their adolescent can and should automatically take over all self-care responsibility at some arbitrary age—often 15 years. Even very motivated and skillful 15-year-old patients require some oversight from parents; many 17-year-olds still benefit from daily parental attention. The goal is to have parents transfer individual management responsibilities over time. A gradual transition from responsible parent to supportive observer, available to assist with insulin injections and blood glucose testing but no longer needed to complete the procedure, works best. Negotiating each responsibility may be necessary. At times, parents may temporarily reassume responsibility for a task previously transferred to their adolescent, including administering insulin in rare instances of recurrent diabetic ketoacidosis.

Concurrent psychopathology (depression, personality disorders, substance abuse disorder, eating disorder), low cognitive ability, and fear of hypoglycemia may also affect the adolescent's ability to adhere to the prescribed regimen.

IMPROVING CONTROL

The pediatrician's approach to the adolescent who has poor control has several facets.

- *Identify the reason for poor control and develop a strategy for remediation.* Serious psychopathology (including eating disorders) and recurrent DKA are indications for referral to mental health and diabetes specialists.
- *Identify one reasonable and measurable target behavior for action.* This might be the number of BG tests, remembering to record CHO at a specific meal each day, or making self-insulin adjustments based on BG or CHO intake.
- *Identify short-term reinforcers relevant to the adolescent.* Examples might include fewer symptoms of hypoglycemia or nocturia,

improved physical performance, more flexibility in timing and content of meals, rewards from parents, and greater independence.

● *Establish realistic time frame for accomplishment based on behavior and goal.* For example, encourage the teen to aim for a 20% reduction in average fasting BG over the next two weeks. (Remember that glycated hemoglobin levels reflect average blood sugar over a 6- to 8-week period. A 1% reduction [from 12% to 11%] over an 8-week period is significant.)

● *Provide frequent feedback.* This is a time to see the adolescent more frequently.

● *Encourage patients to participate in support groups and camps for teens.*

● *Consider referral to a diabetes specialist* if control has not improved within 6 months.

Conclusion

In summary, the well-informed pediatrician who has access to a CDE and experienced dietitian can help adolescent patients with diabetes improve their control and adopt more flexible insulin regimens. Improved glycemic control offers the adolescent significant reduction in the risk for long-term sequelae, longer duration of living without serious complications and with enhanced quality-of-life, and the likelihood of longer life. It is worth the investment.

Further Reading

Betschart J, Thom S. *In Control—A Guide for Teens with Diabetes.* Minneapolis MN: Chronimed; 1995

American Diabetes Association. Report of the Expert Committee on the Diagnosis and Classification of Diabetes Mellitus. *Diabetes Care.* 1999;22(suppl):S5–S19

American Diabetes Association. *Intensive Diabetes Management.* Clinical Education Series, 1995. Write to the ADA at 1660 Duke Street, Alexandria, VA 22314

American Diabetes Association. *Carbohydrate Counting. Getting Started (Level 1), Moving On (Level 2), Using Insulin Ratios (Level 3)* (#5606-04)

Franz, MJ. Alcohol and diabetes. Part II—its metabolism and guidelines for occasional use. *Diabetes Spectrum.* 1990; 3:210–216

Linder B. Improving diabetic control with a new insulin analog. *Contemp Pediatr.* 1997;14:5273

DCCT Research Group. Effect of intensive diabetes treatment on the development and progression of long-term complications in adolescents with insulin-dependent diabetes mellitus: Diabetes Control and Complications Trial. *J Pediatr.* 1994; 125:177–188

DCCT Research Group. Diabetes Control and Complications Trial (DCCT): the effect of intensive treatment of diabetes on the development and progression of long-term complications in insulin-dependent diabetes mellitus. *N Engl J Med.* 1994; 329:977–986

Mayfield JA, Reiber GE, Sanders LJ, Janisse D, Pogach LM. Preventive foot care in people with diabetes. *Diabetes Care.* 1998;21:2161–2177

Useful Internet Resources

American Diabetes Association: www.diabetes.org

Juvenile Diabetes Foundation: www.jdf.org

National Institute of Diabetes and Digestive and Kidney Diseases of the National Institutes of Health (NIDDK Diabetes): www.niddk.nih.gov/health/diabetes/dylb/ home.htmb (Diabetes information for parents and adolescents)

Children with Diabetes—www.childrenwithdiabetes.com (Site is designed for type 1 children and their parents, but may be of interest to adolescents. Features include reviews of different BG testing devices.)

National Heart, Lung, and Blood Institute (NHLBI National Diabetes Center)—www.diabetes-mellitus.org

American Association of Diabetes Educators— www.aadenet.org (This site includes geographically-sorted lists of certified diabetes educators)

American Association of Clinical Endocrinologists and The American College of Endocrinology—www.aace.com/clin/ guides/diabetes_ guide.html (AACE practice guidelines for diabetes—not specific to adolescents)

PlanetRx—This is an e-commerce site, but useful: www.diabetes.com

Nutrition in the Fast Lane: www.fastfoodfacts.com. (This nutrition guide for fast foods is also available by writing Franklin Publishing Incorporated, 310 N. Alabama Street, Indianapolis, In 46204, or calling 800-634-1993.)

Acknowledgment

The editors would like to acknowledge technical review by Robert P. Schwartz, MD, chair and Francine R. Kaufman, MD, from the AAP Section on Endocrinology.

Contemporary Management of Adolescents With Diabetes Mellitus
Part 2: Type 2 Diabetes

by Donald P. Orr, MD, FAAP

Type 2 diabetes mellitus (T2DM) is increasingly recognized among adolescents, particularly obese adolescents from certain ethnic/racial groups (African Americans, Native Americans, Hispanics and Asians/Pacific Islanders).

As with type 1 diabetes (T1DM), the chronic hyperglycemia associated with T2DM presents a risk for serious long-term sequelae, including the development of accelerated cardiovascular disease, end-stage renal disease, limb amputations, and visual impairment. Pediatricians are well positioned to recognize patients who are at risk for T2DM, counsel them and their parents about prevention, screen at-risk individuals, make early diagnosis, and provide optimal treatment. For further background on diabetes in adolescents, readers are referred to part 1 of this series (*AHU* 12:2).

Prevalence

There has been a steady increase in the prevalence of T2DM (formerly called noninsulin dependent diabetes) in the United States, which now affects 6.6% of those aged 20 to 74 years. T2DM now accounts for at least 10% of the diabetes diagnosed in children and adolescents in the United States, and the proportion is increasing.

There are important demographic variations in the prevalence of T2DM. Within the United States, African Americans have a 2-fold increase in risk, Hispanics a 2.5-fold increase, and Native Americans a 5-fold increase compared to whites. The risk is slightly higher for females and those living in poverty, probably secondary to the added risk of obesity. More than 40% of the children of those with T2DM have a lifetime risk for T2DM.

However, because individuals are usually asymptomatic for long periods of time, up to 50% of persons with T2DM are currently undiagnosed, yet at risk for long-term sequelae.

Pathophysiology and Etiology

Whereas T1DM is entirely a defect in insulin secretion, T2DM involves multiple defects in the ability of the body to maintain normal glucose homeostasis. T2DM involves: (1) insulin resistance and (2) a defect in insulin secretion or progressive beta cell failure.

Obesity increases insulin resistance and predisposes to diabetes. Children of diabetic parents become more insulin resistant with additional weight gain compared to those without a family history of diabetes, demonstrating the combined effects of genetics and environment.

Screening and Diagnosis

It has been estimated that the prevalence of T2DM would double if all those who met the criteria

---

Learning Objectives

After reading this article, pediatricians will be able to describe
● Prevalence and trends of type 2 diabetes mellitus (T2DM)
● Clinical presentation
● Diagnostic evaluation
● Stepped management, including the role of diet, exercise, the use of oral hypoglycemic medications, and insulin
● Indications for referral to subspecialists

Donald P. Orr, MD, FAAP, is professor and director, Section of Adolescent Medicine and Adolescent/Young Adult Diabetes Program, Department of Pediatrics, Indiana University Medical Center, Indianapolis. Dr. Orr is the immediate past editor of Adolescent Health Update, *and was a founding member of the* Adolescent Health Update *editorial board.*

were diagnosed. Among adults, T2DM usually goes undiagnosed for years until fasting hyperglycemia is present and symptoms appear. With increased rates of obesity in children and adolescents, it is likely that there is a substantial amount of undiagnosed T2DM in this age group; these adolescents are at risk for long-term sequelae.

The American Academy of Pediatrics and the American Diabetes Association (ADA) concurrently published a consensus statement, "Type 2 Diabetes in Children and Adolescents," in the March 2000 issues of *Pediatrics* and *Diabetes Care*. The statement was authored by a consensus panel of the ADA, with representation from the Academy, the Centers for Disease Control and Prevention, and the National Institutes of Health. Their recommendations for T2DM screening of children and adolescents are shown in Table 1. The expert panel recommends screening individuals at risk for T2DM every two years beginning at age 10, or beginning at puberty if puberty occurs at a younger age.

Annual screening may be considered for members of high risk groups, including youth who are obese, have a parent with T2DM, are African American, Hispanic, Asian/Pacific Islander, or Native American, *and* have evidence of insulin resistance (eg, hypertension, dyslipidemia, polycystic ovary syndrome, acanthosis nigricans).

The revised ADA criteria for diagnosis of diabetes were outlined in the previous issue of *Adolescent Health Update*. Fasting plasma glucose (FPG) > 110 and < 126 is considered impaired fasting glucose (IFG); 2-h PG ≥ 140 and < 200 mg/dl on an oral glucose tolerance test (OGTT) represents impaired glucose tolerance (IGT). *In the absence of pregnancy, neither IFG nor IGT is considered to be a clinical entity;* rather they represent risk factors for diabetes and cardiovascular disease. IFG or IGT prompt repeat OGTT in 3 months. Risk factors such as obesity and sedentary lifestyle should be addressed.

As the ADA consensus committee observed, FPG and 2-h PG are suitable screening tests for T2DM. The FPG is preferred because of convenience and cost. As with any screening test, abnormal results must be confirmed at another time. No data exist on the use of random levels of PG, BG, insulin, or C-peptide as screening tests; they are not acceptable substitutes for FPG or 2-h PG. If a capillary blood testing device is used to measure glucose in screening, the physician must confirm that the results are calibrated to PG and not whole BG. HbA$_{1c}$ is currently recommended for monitoring glycemia but not for diagnosis.

Table 1. Testing for Type 2 Diabetes in Children

● Criteria*
  Overweight (BMI>85th percentile for age and sex, weight for height >85th percentile, or weight >120% of ideal for height)

  Plus

  Any two of the following risk factors:
  —Family history of type 2 diabetes in first- or second-degree relative
  —Race/ethnicity (American Indian, African-American, Hispanic, Asian/Pacific Islander)
  —Signs of insulin resistance or conditions associated with insulin resistance (acanthosis nigricans, hypertension, dyslipidemia, polycystic ovary syndrome)
● Age of initiation: Age 10 years or at onset of puberty if puberty occurs at a younger age
● Frequency: Every 2 years
● Test: Fasting Plasma Glucose preferred

*Clinical judgment should be used to test for diabetes in high-risk patients who do not meet these criteria.

Reprinted with permission from: American Diabetes Association. Type 2 diabetes in children and adolescents. *Diabetes Care.* 2000; 23:381–389 (Table 4, 386). Copyright 2000, American Diabetes Association.

Classification and Clinical Presentation

Diabetes is classified depending on the natural history, degree of insulin resistance, and level of hyperglycemia. Table 2 presents an overview of the characteristics of the common types of diabetes. Figure 1 depicts clinical classification schemata based on whether the mode of presentation is acute with moderate/severe ketoacidosis, or insidious.

T2DM refers to individuals who have insulin resistance and relative (rather than absolute) insulin deficiency. At least initially, they do not require exogenous insulin to survive. The age of diagnosis corresponds to the time of pubertal development, when there is physiologic insulin resistance as an additional contributing factor.

Table 2. Characteristics of the Common Types of Diabetes

	Type 1	Type 2	Atypical	Maturity Onset Diabetes of Youth (MODY)
Age	childhood	pubertal (?)	pubertal	pubertal
Onset	acute; severe	mild-severe; often insidious	acute; severe	mild; insidious
Insulin secretion	very low	variable	moderately low	variable
Insulin sensitivity	normal	decreased	normal	normal
Insulin dependence	permanent	no until late	variable	no until late
Racial/ethnic groups at increased risk	all (low in Asians)	African Americans, Hispanics, Native Americans, Asian/Pacific Islanders	African Americans	all
Genetics	polygenic	polygenic	autosomal dominant	autosomal dominant
Proportion of those with diabetes	~80%	10%–20%	5%–10%	rare
Association: obesity	no	strong	variable	no
Acanthosis Nigricans	no	yes	no	no
Autoimmune etiology	yes	no	no	no

Reprinted with permission from: Rosenbloom et al. Emerging epidemic of type 2 diabetes in youth. *Diabetes Care.* 1999;22:345–354. (Table 2, 346). Copyright 1999, American Diabetes Association.

Although still primarily a diagnosis of adults, T2DM does occur among children, most commonly during adolescence.

Individuals with T2DM are usually obese, and if not obese may have an increased predominance of abdominal fat (central adiposity) which is causally implicated in insulin resistance. Acanthosis nigricans, hyperpigmentation with thickening of the skin into velvety, irregular folds in flexural or redundant skin areas (neck, axilla, beneath breasts, elbows), is common in youth with T2DM (86% in one series). Acanthosis nigricans is also found in about 7% of healthy school children and is most prevalent in Hispanic and African Americans. It is associated with obesity, hyperinsulinemia, and insulin resistance.

Obese individuals with insidious onset of hyperglycemia, and those who present with non-ketotic severe hyperglycemia (BG > 750 mg/dl), usually have T2DM, and additional testing for classification is generally not useful. If there is a family history of T2DM, ask about those family members: their age at diagnosis, whether they were overweight when the condition was identi-

fied, and how they were treated. Whether antibodies should be drawn on every patient suspected of having T2DM, or on selected patients as identified in Figures 1A/B, is a matter for consultation. Similarly, pediatricians who are familiar with insulin and C-peptide ratios may choose to order these tests prior to treatment, but interpretation of levels will usually require the advice of a diabetes specialist.

ATYPICAL T2DM OF AFRICAN AMERICANS

Winter and colleagues described a special form of T2DM found in African American youth: atypical diabetes mellitus. These patients may not be obese, do not have acanthosis nigricans, and may present acutely with ketoacidosis. There appears to be normal insulin sensitivity but moderately low insulin secretion. When acutely ill at presentation, they require insulin, thus leading to a misclassification as T1DM. Insulin can usually be withdrawn after recovery from the acute episode, and patients managed with traditional regimens for T2DM described as follows.

MATURITY ONSET DIABETES OF YOUTH (MODY)

Maturity onset diabetes of youth (an autosomal dominant condition) occurs rarely, and has been described among all racial/ethnic populations. MODY is an entity distinct from T2DM. It is characterized by impaired insulin secretion with minimal or no defects in insulin action (resistance) and insidious presentation before age 25. Patients usually can be managed initially with oral hypoglycemic agents. The clinical presentation appears to vary broadly from asymptomatic hyperglycemia to weight loss and dehydration.

Initial Management

Regardless of the ultimate classification, acutely ill adolescents and those who have significant hyperglycemia (≥ 300 mg/dl) require initial treatment with insulin and intravenous fluids if dehydrated or ketoacidotic. Insulin therapy may later be withdrawn and traditional T2DM treatment instituted. It is important to remember that the initial use of insulin does not commit the pediatrician to long term use when subsequent evidence (such

as family history, presence of insulin resistance, or failure to develop ketonemia in the absence of exogenous insulin) suggests that the diagnosis is not T1DM. Consultation with a diabetes expert is indicated when the diagnosis is unclear. For those who are not ill at diagnosis, management with medical nutrition therapy and exercise may be sufficient for a time. Most will eventually require drug therapy.

Monitoring

Blood glucose, lipid profile, blood pressure, and signs of complications are monitored in patients with T2DM. Monitoring for complications was discussed in Part 1 of this series. T2DM is not an autoimmune process and it is not necessary to screen for thyroiditis.

BLOOD GLUCOSE

Self-monitoring for blood glucose provides immediate feedback on BG control between visits, demonstrates the effect of a specific behavior such as alteration in carbohydrate (CHO) intake, and can empower the adolescent as part

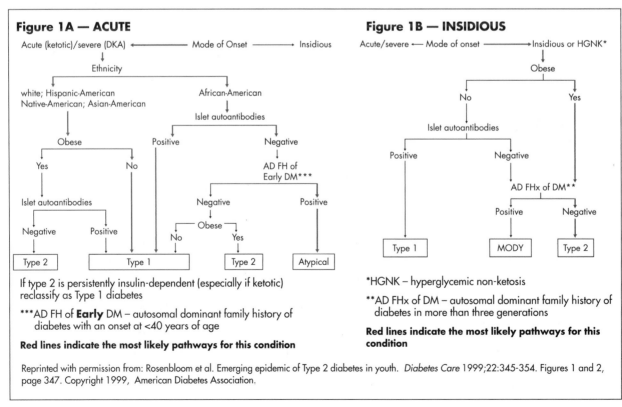

Figure 1. Clinical classifications of DM in children and adolescents

of the therapeutic team. Fasting BG is the major determinant of mean day-long BG level reflected in glycohemoglobin levels; postprandial BG contributes relatively less to glycohemoglobin levels. Devices that use capillary blood samples to measure glucose may be calibrated to reflect PG or whole BG. Either is acceptable for self-monitoring. Waiting until the next HbA$_{1c}$ after the clinic visit does not provide sufficient reinforcement for behavior change.

The recommendations for frequency of BG testing are less specific than for T1DM; in general, obtaining daily FBG and random pre-meal levels should be satisfactory in T2DM. Target levels of BG and HbA$_{1c}$ have been detailed in the first part of this two-part series, and remain the same regardless of the type of diabetes.

DYSLIPIDEMIAS

Dyslipidemias are common in T2DM; they increase the risk for cardiovascular disease two- to four-fold, and reflect various degrees of insulin resistance, obesity, diet, and poor glycemic control. The typical pattern is elevated triglyceride (TG) and decreased high density lipoprotein (HDL) cholesterol. Although all hypoglycemic agents improve glycemic control and tend to lower TG and LDL (see Table 3), if LDL levels of <130 mg/dl have not been attained with better glycemic control, weight loss (if appropriate), and reduced intake of saturated fat, then referral to a diabetes specialist is indicated. Yearly measurement of fasting lipid profiles is recommended among those with previously abnormal profiles or ongoing poor glycemic control. Measurement every other year is probably sufficient among the remainder of children and adolescents with T2DM.

Ongoing Management

Treatment of T2DM targets the known pathophysiological aspects of the disease: insulin resistance, hepatic overproduction of glucose, and relative insulin deficiency. Remember, T2DM is a progressive disease that appears to eventually require the use of exogenous insulin. This usually takes many years if the patient is able to successfully alter dietary and exercise habits.

Table 3. Comparison of Oral Hypoglycemic Agents Prescribed for Adolescents

Effect	Biguanides[1]	Sulfonylureas[2]	Glucosidase inhibitors[3]
Mechanism of action	Decrease hepatic glucose production; increase muscle insulin sensitivity	Increase insulin secretion	Decrease GI absorption
Duration of Action	> 3–4 weeks	12–24 hours	~ 4 hours (postprandial period)
Decrease in FPG (mg/dl)	60–70 mg/dl	60–70 mg/dl	20–30 mg/dl
Decrease in HbA$_{1c}$(%)	1.5–2.0	1.2–2.0	0.7–1.0
Triglyceride level	Decrease	No effect*	No effect*
HDL cholesterol level	Slight increase	No effect*	No effect*
LDL cholesterol level	Decrease	No effect*	No effect*
Body weight	No effect or decrease	Increase	No effect
Plasma insulin	Decrease	Increase	No effect
Adverse effects	GI disturbance; lactic acidosis[4] rare	Hypoglycemia	GI disturbance

1. Metformin is the only current agent in this class
2. Commonly prescribed second generation sulfonylurea drugs include glyburide, glipizide, and glimepiride. Closely related to these is repaglinide, similar to sulfonylurea drugs in most respects, but with a duration of action of 4 to 6 hours
3. This class includes acarbose and miglitol
4. Incidence of .03 cases per 1000 patient years (see text)

*Independent of effect due to lowered BG

The pediatrician should work with a certified diabetes educator and/or nutritionist as described in the previous issue. A stepped approach to management is used, adding components when needed to maintain glycemic control. Treatment goals are the same as for T1DM described in the previous issue. Plan to re-evaluate progress every 4 to 6 weeks, making necessary changes until the adolescent achieves the targeted level of control (ie, HbA$_{1c}$ as close to normal as possible). In addition to visits, phone contact is extremely important. When control is optimized, the frequency of visits may be reduced to quarterly.

Although it is not possible for all adolescents and their families to achieve normal BG levels, it is important that this remain a goal, because any reduction of HbA$_{1c}$ will translate to decreased risk of complications. Stressing the importance of good control at each visit will underscore the seriousness of diabetes to the adolescent and his/her family.

NUTRITION AND EXERCISE

Modifications in diet and exercise are the mainstay of treatment. There is no longer a standard "ADA" diet. Rather the distribution of CHO, protein and fat is individualized by patient needs. The goals are: (1) near normal BG levels, (2) normal serum lipid levels, (3) weight loss, when indicated, and (4) normal growth and development

The CHO intake should be distributed evenly throughout the day to include snacks. As discussed in Part 1, CHO intake is limited because of the abnormal insulin secretion patterns. Weight reduction is encouraged for the obese through participation in a program of regular aerobic exercise and reduced caloric intake. Very low calorie diets (eg, <1000 calories/day) have been used in obese adults. Such diets are not recommended for adolescents.

Referral to a dietitian experienced with T2DM and with adolescents is indicated and may prove beneficial in helping the obese adolescent implement a weight reduction program. For further guidance, refer to previous issues of *Adolescent Health Update* concentrating on obesity (10:2) and nutrition (9:2).

Exercise, independent of weight loss, is important because it increases glucose transport into skeletal muscle resulting in lower levels of BG. The goal should be at least 150 minutes per week of brisk walking. Depending on the level of conditioning and obesity, this may begin with as little as 10 to 15 minutes of brisk walking or low-impact aerobic activity several times per week with gradual increase to at least 150 minutes per week. Organized diet and exercise programs may prove beneficial for adolescents who prefer group support and activities. Recruiting the family to exercise may improve compliance, because of the high likelihood that other members of the family are obese and have undiagnosed T2DM.

The effect of CHO restriction (as a part of total caloric reduction) may be seen within 4 days with reduction of postprandial BG. The effects of weight loss may take months and will be reflected in lower FBG levels. Studies from obese adults with T2DM suggest that a FBG < 180 mg/dl after individuals have lost 2.3 kg has a 62% positive predictive value that diet therapy will be effective in achieving control; the positive predictive value is 79% after 4.5 kg have been lost. Failure to see improvement in FBG in the face of substantial weight loss suggests that diet/exercise alone will be insufficient to achieve satisfactory control.

ORAL HYPOGLYCEMIC AGENTS

If, despite dietary and activity modifications, significant improvement in BG control (manifest as levels of HbA$_{1c}$ dropping to 8% or less) has not been attained after 3 months, an oral hypoglycemic agent or insulin should be added. Although no data specific for adolescents are available on the long-term use of oral hypoglycemic agents, it is reasonable to include these as the next treatment options. An increasing array of oral hypoglycemic agents is available, with each group targeting different metabolic components—insulin secretory defect, elevated hepatic glucose output, and insulin resistance.

When using oral agents, remember that:
1. The response to oral agents follows a sigmoid curve with a rapid rise in therapeutic activity, leveling off and gradual tapering to maximal therapeutic effect

2. Half the maximal dosage yields more than half the maximal effect (60%–80%)
3. Side effects increase slowly at low dosages and then more rapidly at higher doses

About 25% of adults will achieve an HbA$_{1c}$ < 8% on monotherapy, 50% a partial response and 25% will fail to respond to a single oral agent. No oral agent should be used during pregnancy; insulin must be substituted and referral to a high-risk obstetrical program is indicated.

BIGUANIDES

Many pediatric endocrinologists use a biguanide as the first line oral hypoglycemic agent for obese adolescents. There is a nearly completed clinical trial of biguanides in children and adolescents. Biguanides lower FBG by reducing hepatic glucose output. (See Table 3) Because they are not associated with weight gain and modest weight loss is not uncommon, they are a good initial medication for use in obese patients. In addition, biguanides improve lipid profiles with reduction of total and LDL cholesterol and TG and increase of HDL. The major side effects are mild gastrointestinal symptoms that generally resolve; they may be minimized by slowly increasing the dose. Hypoglycemia is uncommon and lactic acidosis, a potentially serious condition associated with the predecessor biguanide (phenformin), is extremely rare with the only available agent in this class, *metformin.*

Metformin may be given once or twice daily. Begin with 500 mg daily, and increase 500 mg every 2 to 3 weeks to a maximum daily dose of 2200 mg. Although 2200 mg may sound like too much for an adolescent, some patients will require it. There are no data on the use of metformin in adolescents at present.

Eighty percent of the effect on BG is seen at 1500 mg, therefore if there is no response at this dose after 6 to 8 weeks, it is unlikely that metformin will be effective as a single agent. Because biguanides are metabolized by the kidney, they should be withheld in conditions such as dehydration and when radiographic contrast agents are used. They may be used in combination with insulin and sulfonylurea drugs as discussed next.

SULFONYLUREA DRUGS AND REPAGLINIDE

Sulfonylureas (SUs) enhance insulin release from the ß-cell and may also decrease insulin resistance. (See Table 3) The first generation agents (eg, tolbutamide, tolazamide, chlorpropamide) were associated with multiple drug interactions and hypoglycemia and are rarely used. The newer agents (eg, glipizide, glyburide, glimepiride) have fewer side effects, but potential interactions with sulfonamides, fluconazole and ciprofloxacin may result in hypoglycemia. These agents may be given as a single morning dose. Begin at the lowest dose and increase the dose every 14 to 21 days, based on levels of FBG, until target BG levels are reached, side effects occur, or the maximum dose is reached.

A related medication, *repaglinide,* also enhances insulin secretion but operates through a mechanism different from SUs; it must be administered before each meal.

These medications are less effective when BG levels are over 250 mg/dl, therefore, the pediatrician should consider initial use of insulin in this situation, replacing the insulin with an SU when FBG levels have been lowered. A disadvantage of SUs is weight gain, which tends to further increase insulin resistance. Therefore, some specialists do not select SUs as initial medications in obese patients.

GLUCOSIDASE INHIBITORS

Acarbose and *miglitol* are glucosidase inhibitors that delay the absorption of CHO from the intestine, thereby reducing the rise in BG levels following a meal. These are most useful when employed in conjunction with other hypoglycemic agents to assist in managing postprandial hyperglycemia. Gastrointestinal symptoms (eg, crampy abdominal pain, loose stools, flatus) are common and limit their use. Glucosidase inhibitors are not associated with weight gain or hypoglycemia. They must be given before each meal, not to exceed three times per day, starting at 25 mg and slowly increasing the dose to a maximum of 300 mg tid. Although there are no data on use with adolescents, experience is not expected to be different from that among adults.

THIAZOLIDINEDIONES

Thiazolidinediones increase insulin action in muscle, adipose tissue, and probably in the liver. Troglitazone, the first available agent in this class, was withdrawn by the FDA in March 2000 because of the drug's association with fatal liver toxicity. Newer thiazolidinediones, pioglitazone and rosiglitazone, are thought to be safer, but *their use is not recommended in children and adolescents until further information is available.*

COMBINATION REGIMENS

Consider consulting a diabetes specialist about combining oral agents or adding insulin when a single medication has not achieved the desired degree of control. The rationale for combining agents includes the additive effect because they operate through different physiologic mechanisms, fewer side effects, and lower cost (if dosages are lower).

When combining oral agents, increase the dose of the first drug until maximum dose has been reached or side effects limit further increases. Add the second medication at the lowest dose and increase slowly, watching for hypoglycemia. If target levels of BG control have not been achieved in 4 to 6 months, the addition of insulin is indicated. Some clinicians would choose to add insulin instead of a second oral agent. No data are available for adolescents.

Insulin may be used as a single night-time dose (to lower FBG) or in divided doses as with T1DM. Adding a single night-time dose to an oral regimen has the advantage that lower doses of insulin and the oral agent may be used. Begin with a single dose of intermediate-acting insulin at the bedtime snack or long-acting at dinner. An initial dose of 5–10 units is safe. Increase the dose until the desired level of FBG is achieved. Adolescents who have a large CHO intake at dinner may benefit from the addition of regular or rapid-acting insulin with this meal. This dose of short-acting insulin is adjusted based on bedtime BG levels.

Indications for Referral

In addition to those indications discussed previously, referral is appropriate when diagnosis is unclear, there is failure to achieve target BG levels after 6 months, or when the use of combination therapies is being considered.

Follow-up

Follow-up, described in the previous issue of *Adolescent Health Update,* is the same for T1DM and T2DM with the exception that there is no need to test for autoimmune complications in T2DM. Considerations include monitoring to assure proper control, the role of the multidisciplinary diabetes team in education and encouraging adherence, and scheduled screens for common complications.

Summary

The pediatrician who is interested in diabetes can play an integral role in the care of patients with T2DM. However, specialty consultation when indicated and collaboration with a multidisciplinary team are crucial. Early recognition, consistent follow-up, and aggressive treatment will increase the likelihood of achieving improved control and reducing the risk for long-term complications.

Further Reading

American Diabetes Association. Type 2 diabetes in children and adolescents. *Diabetes Care.* 2000;23:381–389. (Concurrently published in *Pediatrics.* 2000;105:671–680)

Fagot-Campagna A, Pettitt DJ, Engelgau MM, et al. Type 2 diabetes among North American children and adolescents: An epidemiologic review and a public health perspective. *J Pediatrics.* 2000;136:664–672

Rosenbloom AL, Joe JR, Young RS, Winter WE. Emerging epidemic of type 2 diabetes in youth. *Diabetes Care.* 1999; 22:345–354

Scott CR, Smith JM, Cradock MM, Pihoker C. Characteristics of youth-onset noninsulin-dependent diabetes mellitus and insulin-dependent diabetes mellitus at diagnosis. *Pediatrics.* 1997;100:84–91

Winter WE, Maclaren NK, Riley WJ, Clarke DW, Kappy MS, Spillar RP. Maturity-onset diabetes of youth in black Americans. *N Eng J Med.* 1987;316:285–291

Acknowledgment

The editors would like to acknowledge technical review by Arlan L. Rosenbloom, MD, FAAP, who chaired the American Diabetes Association consensus panel on T2DM in children and adolescents, and Francine R. Kaufman, MD, FAAP, executive committee member of the AAP Section on Endocrinology.

Diagnosis and Management of Headache in Children

Balbir V. Singh, MD* and E. S. Roach, MD*

Introduction

Headache is an age-old problem that affects both children and adults; it is mentioned as far back as 5000 BC in Babylonian and Sumarian writings and later is described by Hippocrates and Galen. In spite of more than 50 epidemiologic studies, there is no consensus on the prevalence of headache. The prevalence of chronic headache varies widely in different studies, probably due to differences in case definition, selection criteria, and demographics of the study populations. Most recent studies suggest rates close to 5% for migraine, 15% for tension-type headache, and about 30% for infrequent nonmigrainous headaches. Nevertheless, most children who suffer migraines never come to medical attention.

The International Headache Society's classification system has replaced the old and somewhat confusing terminology with more descriptive terms (Table 1). Migraine is divided into three types: migraine without aura (Table 2), migraine with aura (Table 3), and complicated migraine. Tension and muscle contraction headache have been replaced by tension-type headache, admitting our ignorance of the pathophysiology of the disorder (Tables 4 and 5). Operational diagnostic criteria are used to increase both the sensitivity and the specificity of diagnosis.

Migraine

Migraine is an episodic syndrome characterized by headaches of varying intensity, duration, and frequency. Before puberty, migraine is slightly more common in boys; after puberty, it is two to three times more common in girls. Eighty percent of all migrainous headaches are comprised of migraine without aura. The headache often is

Table 1. Etiology of Recurrent Headaches

Vascular Headaches
    Migraine
    Arteriovenous Malformations

Tension-type Headache

Headache Due to Increased Intracranial Pressure
    Space-occupying Lesions
    Idiopathic Intracranial Hypertension (Pseudotumor cerebri)

Other Causes
    Systemic Diseases
    Sinusitis
    Ocular Diseases
    Temporomandibular Joint Diseases

unilateral (35%) and throbbing (55%), but it may be diffuse and continuous in more than 50% of the children. Other common signs and symptoms include pallor, irritability, malaise, and fatigue. Nausea, vomiting, and abdominal pain occur in about 90% of cases. The pain may last from minutes to several hours. Photophobia and phonophobia are common.

Severity of symptoms ranges from episodes that force the child to seek relief in a quiet and dark place to detection only upon direct questioning. The most accurate way to assess the severity of a headache in young children is to determine its effect on the child's normal activities. Family history of migraine is present in about 70% of patients. Stress; anxiety; lack of sleep; oversleeping; menstruation; hunger; and ingestion of alcohol, caffeine, and some foods (eg, chocolate, cheese, and monosodium glutamate) may precipitate an attack. Sleep provides relief to 95% of children.

*Division of Pediatric Neurology, Department of Neurology, The University of Texas Southwestern Medical Center, Dallas, TX.
Pediatrics in Review, *Vol 19, No. 4, April 1998*

Table 2. International Headache Society Diagnostic Criteria for Migraine Without Aura

- Headache attack lasts 4 to 72 h
- Headache has at least two of the following characteristics:
  —Unilateral location
  —Pulsating quality
  —Moderate to severe intensity
  —Aggravation by routine physical activity
- During headache, at least one of the following occurs:
  —Nausea and/or vomiting
  —Photophobia and phonophobia
- At least five attacks occur that fulfill the above criteria
- Results of the history, physical examination, and neurologic examination do not suggest any underlying organic disease

Table 3. International Headache Society Diagnostic Criteria for Migraine With Aura

- At least three of these four characteristics are present:
  —One or more fully reversible aura symptoms indicate focal cerebral cortical and/or brain stem dysfunction
  —At least one aura symptom develops gradually over more than 4 min
  —No aura symptom lasts more than 60 min (duration proportionally increases if more than one aura symptom is present)
  —Headache follows the aura with a free interval of less than 60 min (may begin before or with the aura). It usually lasts 4 to 72 h, but may be completely absent
- At least two attacks occur that fulfill the criteria listed above
- Results of the history, physical examination, and neurologic examination do not suggest any underlying organic disease

Migraine with aura constitutes 15% to 20% of vascular headaches. An aura most often consists of visual symptoms (eg, scintillating scotomas, blurred vision, hemianopsia), but almost any neurologic deficit can result from migraine. The aura typically is followed by a pounding headache on the opposite side. Other symptoms are similar to those of migraine without aura.

The term complicated migraine is used when the signs of an aura last throughout the headache or persist afterwards. Depending on the area of cerebral cortex affected, a complicated migraine may cause hemiparesis, sensory loss, aphasia, ophthalmoplegia, blindness, macropsia, micropsia, vertigo, ataxia, quadriparesis, transient global amnesia, confusional state, or loss of consciousness.

Tension-type Headaches

Tension-type headaches typically are generalized or focused posteriorly and may be described as a band-like sensation. They can be either episodic or chronic and are more common in adolescent girls than in children younger than 10 years of age. Nausea is rare, but fatigue and dizziness are common. The description of the headache and accompanying symptoms are often vague and nonspecific.

The mechanism through which pain is caused is not clear. Prolonged muscle contraction with accompanying ischemia of the involved muscles and psychogenic factors may play a role. Although the headaches may persist for weeks or months, they may not disrupt the child's regular activities. In some children, symptoms of tension-type headache and migraine overlap, making the diagnostic distinction more difficult. There may be secondary gain in the form of prolonged school absences in spite of good academic performance. Underlying factors include stress, depression, conversion, and adjustment reactions. The relationship of depression to tension-type headache is not straightforward. Many patients who have chronic daily headaches become depressed, but in some patients headaches are caused by depression and resolve as soon as depression improves.

Headaches Secondary to Increased Intracranial Pressure

The classic brain tumor headache—progressive, worse in the morning, and associated with nausea and vomiting—occurs only in a minority of patients who have brain tumors. More than 50% of children who have brain tumor develop increasingly frequent and severe headaches. Between the headaches, a patient who has a tumor often exhibits other symptoms, such as personality changes, diplopia, ataxia, and gait problems. If unilateral, the headache more often is on the side of the tumor. Nocturnal awakening, although worrisome, is not specific. In addition to specific focal deficits caused by the lesion,

Table 4. International Headache Society Diagnostic Criteria for Episodic Tension-type Headache

- Headache lasts 30 min to 7 days
- Headache has at least two of the following characteristics:
  —Pressing/tightening quality
  —Mild or moderate intensity
  —Bilateral location
  —No aggravation by routine physical activity
- No nausea or vomiting with headache
- Photophobia and phonophobia are absent, or one but not the other is present
- At least 10 previous headache attacks fulfill criteria above. Number of headache days <180/year, <15/month
- Results of the history, physical examination, and neurologic examination do not suggest any underlying organic disease

Table 5. International Headache Society Diagnostic Criteria for Chronic Tension-type Headache

- Average headache frequency ≥15 days/month (180 days/year) for ≥6 months
- Headache has at least two of the following pain characteristics:
  —Pressing/tightening quality
  —Mild or moderate intensity
  —Bilateral location
  —No aggravation by routine physical activity
- Both of the following:
  —No vomiting
  —No more than one of the following: nausea, photophobia, or phonophobia
- Results of the history, physical examination, and neurologic examination do not suggest any underlying organic disease

one should look for nonlocalizing signs such as sixth nerve palsy and papilledema. Headaches due to increased intracranial pressure may worsen with coughing, micturition, and defecation. Idiopathic intracranial hypertension is a relatively common cause of increased intracranial pressure in adults; in children, it usually is caused by local cranial or systemic disease. Most children do not have any of the characteristic symptoms seen with brain tumors and, therefore, do not require routine imaging studies.

Headache Due to Systemic Disease

An acute headache as a single event can be the beginning of chronic or recurrent headaches, but it is more likely to be due to a systemic disease. Almost any febrile disease can cause headache, but some illnesses characteristically are associated with headaches, including upper respiratory tract infections, sinusitis, otitis media, infectious mononucleosis, and systemic lupus erythematosus. Rarely, a headache may be caused by dental disease, chronic lung disease with carbon dioxide retention, acute and severe hypertension, and temporomandibular joint disease. Conditions requiring urgent and specific management, such as meningitis, subarachnoid hemorrhage, and subdural hematoma, should be investigated.

History

As with most other conditions, the history is the most important part of the evaluation of a child who has headaches. Parents usually are the primary source of information, but discussion with the child and sometimes the teachers may provide useful clues. Noting disparity between the parent's and child's story and observation of the interaction between them sometimes can be helpful. A complete description of headaches should include information on length of history, aura, frequency, localization, quality of pain, duration, time of day or days of week, course over weeks or months, associated symptoms, precipitating or aggravating factors, other medical problems, and effect of pain medications on the headaches. In addition, a detailed social history is extremely important in patients who have long-standing headaches. Other neurologic symptoms, such as visual and auditory disturbances, ataxia, focal weakness, seizures, personality changes, and deterioration in school performance, must be investigated.

On the basis of history, headaches can be divided into four major types:
1. Acute (usually due to acute systemic illness)
2. Recurrent (most often due to migraine)
3. Chronic nonprogressive (most often due to tension-type headache)
4. Chronic and progressive (as with a tumor)

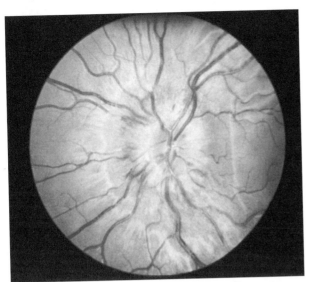

Figure 1. Papilledema in a 9-year-old girl who presented with a 2-month history of headaches due to a posterior fossa tumor with secondary hydrocephalus.

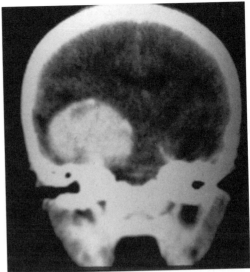

Figure 2. Coronal cranial CT scan of a 12-year-old girl who had focal seizures and a 1-month history of headaches shows a large, contrast-enhancing tumor. This ganglioglioma was removed completely and did not recur.

Physical Examination

The general physical examination should emphasize blood pressure measurements, auscultation of the head for a bruit (suggesting an arteriovenous malformation), and measurement of head size (for evidence of chronically elevated intracranial pressure). A detailed neurologic examination should be performed in all patients, including assessment of the mental status and examination of both discs for papilledema (Fig. 1) and, in advanced cases, for secondary optic atrophy. Cranial nerves, motor abilities, gait, deep tendon reflexes, and sensory systems should be evaluated.

Investigations

Most children who have brain tumors have abnormal results on physical examination within 6 months of the onset of headaches. Therefore, children who have chronic or recurrent nonprogressive headaches without any focal signs generally do not need laboratory or radiographic studies. In patients who have chronic headaches in whom results of neurologic examination are normal, the chances of a computed tomographic (CT) scan demonstrating an abnormality requiring neurosurgical intervention (Fig. 2) is low, and it is unlikely that magnetic resonance imaging (MRI) would have a much higher yield. CT or

MRI is indicated in patients who have symptoms of migraine if there is a change in the headache pattern or focal signs or symptoms or if there is a history of seizures, complicated migraines, persistent unilateral headaches, or symptoms of increased intracranial pressure. Patients who have signs and symptoms of increased intracranial pressure but normal findings on MRI should undergo a lumbar puncture to measure intracranial pressure.

Treatment

MIGRAINE

Treatment of migraine can be divided into three categories: 1) general measures, 2) symptomatic management, and 3) prophylactic therapy. In children who have frequent migraines, educating the child and the parents about changes in lifestyle that can lower stress and avoid provoking factors affect the frequency of headache significantly. A headache diary that includes a description of preheadache events can be very helpful in identifying provocative factors. In children who have mild or infrequent migraines, common analgesics such as acetaminophen or ibuprofen may be effective, particularly if taken early in the headache. Others may require naproxen, metoclopramide, ergotamine preparations, or combinations containing sympathomimetic drugs, sedatives, and analgesics.

Prophylactic treatment is reasonable in children who suffer more than two incapacitating headaches per month or in those who have recurrent complicated migraine. Commonly used prophylactic drugs include amitriptyline, propranolol, and cyproheptadine. They are started at a low dose that gradually is increased until symptoms are controlled or side effects develop. If the patient does not respond to these drugs, verapamil, naproxen, fluoxetine, or sodium valproate may be tried. To determine if the headaches have abated, the medicines can be tapered during a school break, restarting treatment only if headaches return.

Several studies have documented the efficacy of biofeedback and relaxation techniques in children. Finger temperature biofeedback and relaxation techniques can be used as a primary treatment or as an adjunct to medical management.

TENSION-TYPE HEADACHE

Potentially addictive drugs should be avoided for patients who have tension-type headaches. Symptomatic treatment should begin with acetaminophen, ibuprofen, or naproxen. Antidepressants such as amitriptyline, imipramine, or doxepin are particularly effective in patients who have accompanying symptoms of depression and in those who have overlapping symptoms of migraine and tension-type headaches. Psychological evaluation followed by psychotherapy, relaxation therapy, counseling, and biofeedback are helpful in some patients. Muscle activity biofeedback is particularly useful for some children who experience tension-type headaches.

Suggested Reading

Barlow CF. *Headaches and Migraine in Childhood.* Philadelphia, Penn: JB Lippincott Co; 1984

Barlow CF. Migraine in the infant and toddler. *J Child Neurol.* 1994;9:92–94

Brown JK. Migraine and migraine equivalents in children. *Develop Med Child Neurol.* 1977;19:683–692

Headache Classification Committee of the International Headache Society. Classification and diagnostic criteria for headache disorders, cranial neuralgias and facial pain. *Cephalgia.* 1988;8(suppl 7):1–98

Igarashi M, May WN, Golden GS. Pharmacologic treatment of childhood migraine. *J Pediatr.* 1992;120:653–657

Jay CJ, Tomase LG. Pediatric headaches: a one year retrospective analysis. *Headache.* 1981;21:5–9

Lai CW, Ziegler DK, Lansky LL, Torres F. Hemiplegic migraine in childhood: diagnostic and therapeutic aspects. *J Pediatr.* 1982;101:696–699

Rothner AD. The migraine syndrome in children and adolescents. *Pediatr Neurol.* 1986;2:121–126

Evaluating Adolescents With Fatigue: Ever Get Tired of It?

Robert M. Cavanaugh, Jr, MD*

Introduction

Unexplained fatigue in adolescents is a common and frustrating complaint that can pose a challenge for even the most experienced physicians. Although the cause usually is benign and self-limited, occasionally there is a serious underlying disorder. This symptom cannot be dismissed without performing a thorough medical history, detailed psychosocial profile, and careful physical examination. Selective use of laboratory and radiologic studies should be considered when specifically indicated. If the cause remains unclear, sequential visits often provide clues for the practitioner and reassurance for the family. The purpose of this article is to offer guidelines to the clinician caring for adolescents who have prolonged, unexplained fatigue and to stress the value of a thorough history and physical examination.

Definitions

For purposes of this discussion, fatigue will be defined as abnormal exhaustion after usual activities. An arbitrary cutoff of 1 month is used to distinguish acute from chronic fatigue. The term chronic fatigue syndrome is avoided because criteria for this condition are not clearly established in children or adolescents, and data must be extrapolated from studies in adults. The term neurally mediated hypotension is used to describe a fall in blood pressure in response to assuming the upright posture, physical events, and emotional stressors. Affected patients may be syncopal or presyncopal. Neurally mediated hypotension also is referred to in the literature as neurocardiogenic

Objectives

After completing this article, readers should be able to:
1. Describe the key elements of the history and physical examination in adolescents who are fatigued.
2. Develop a differential diagnosis for fatigue in adolescents.
3. Delineate appropriate laboratory and radiologic studies to evaluate adolescents who are fatigued.
4. Describe specific treatments and supportive therapy for adolescents who are fatigued.

syncope, vasovagal reflex, vasodepressor syncope, and autonomic dysfunction.

Approach to the Evaluation

The best way to approach a problem of this nature is to establish a good relationship with adolescents and their parents so they will trust your recommendations and not pressure you into unnecessary tests or referrals. The examination begins when the family enters the office by greeting the patient first to establish a direct relationship immediately. It is worthwhile to obtain the history while the patient is fully clothed because adolescents usually feel more relaxed under these circumstances. Initially, the patient and parents are interviewed together, assuring both parties that there will be adequate time later to speak

*Associate Professor, Director of Adolescent Medicine, Department of Pediatrics, SUNY Upstate Medical University, Syracuse, NY.

This paper is dedicated to the memory of Dr. David H.P. Streeten, whose pioneering research has benefitted countless numbers of adolescents who have unexplained fatigue and who has served as an inspiration to all of us who work so closely with these very special and challenging patients.

Pediatrics in Review, *Vol 23, No. 10, October 2002*

with the examiner alone. While taking the history, the clinician should demonstrate a willingness to listen and be particularly alert for any clues of a hidden agenda or an underlying illness.

More sensitive issues are discussed with the patient alone. Every effort must be made to assure privacy and confidentiality when obtaining personal information from adolescents. Credit must be give to Cohen, who has refined a method for organizing the psychosocial history that was developed by Berman in 1972. This system has been expanded and modified further at the SUNY Upstate Medical University Adolescent Medicine Center in Syracuse. The questions are structured in an easily remembered format that stresses the importance of connecting with adolescents **HEADS FIRST** (Table 1). This approach emphasizes that "getting into adolescent heads" is just as necessary as performing a physical examination. In many instances, the information obtained during the psychosocial interview is key to elucidating the cause of unexplained fatigue in teenagers.

The issues outlined in Table 1 can be addressed with the traditional verbal approach, using the suggested cue words, or by having the patient complete a self-administered personal questionnaire. With either method, the questions should be answered privately and reviewed confidentially with the examiner unless the patient specifically requests otherwise. Most parents respect their adolescents' need for privacy and appreciate the opportunity for them to receive one-on-one counseling with an experienced health professional.

There is considerable overlap in the signs and symptoms caused by the various underlying conditions associated with fatigue. Manifestations are often subtle and should be correlated closely with the overall clinical picture. Thus, clinicians must have a high index of awareness when interpreting historical data, physical findings, and other pertinent information in adolescents who have unexplained fatigue.

Key Elements of the History

The onset, severity, and duration of the fatigue as well as any aggravating or relieving factors are explored when taking the history. Particular attention should be paid to any significant changes in

Table 1. The "HEADS FIRST" Approach to Psychosocial-Medical Issues of Adolescence

Home: Separation, support, "space to grow"
Education: Expectations, study habits, achievement
Abuse: Emotional, verbal, physical, sexual
Drugs: Tobacco, alcohol, marijuana, cocaine, others
Safety: Hazardous activities, seatbelts, helmets

Friends: Confidant, peer pressure, interaction
Image: Self-esteem, looks, appearance
Recreation: Exercise, relaxation, TV, media games
Sexuality: Changes, feelings, experiences, identity
Threats: Depressed or upset easily, harm to self or
others

the patient's physical activity level, exercise tolerance, and ability to keep up with peers. Lack of sleep due to getting to bed later, difficulty falling asleep, frequent nighttime awakening, or getting up earlier in the morning should be considered. A careful review of systems is also essential, with close attention to any constitutional symptoms, such as unexplained fevers, chills, sweating, anorexia, weight loss, or lymphadenopathy, which may suggest the presence of an underlying infection, malignancy, or other inflammatory process. A history of an antecedent "mono-like" illness with negative diagnostic studies is relatively common and suggestive of an infectious cause. However, the significance of this association is unknown.

Recent weight gain as well as weight loss should alert the clinician to the possibility of a nutritional disorder, psychosocial problem, or underlying medical condition. Teenagers who have eating disorders often resort to desperate, even dangerous measures to improve their self-esteem or to enhance their image. Attempts at weight reduction often involve self-injurious behaviors, such as severe caloric deprivation, excessive exercise, self-induced vomiting, and the use of appetite suppressants, laxatives, diuretics, or emetics. Fatigue from rapid fluid shifts or hypokalemia is especially common among bulimics, whose weight may fluctuate dramatically as a result of the frequent episodes of binging and purging. In contrast, patients who have the purely restrictive form of anorexia nervosa usually seem to have boundless energy, even in a state of severe emaciation.

Adolescents who engage in competitive activities in which thinness or "making weight" are judged important to success are believed to be particularly susceptible to unhealthy weight control practices. Such activities include body building, cheerleading, dancing (especially ballet), distance running, diving, figure skating, gymnastics, horse racing, modeling, rowing, swimming, weight-class football, and wrestling. As the preoccupation with thinness supersedes the desire to be healthy, physically active young women are at risk for a group of signs and symptoms known as the female athlete triad. Lack of information and the strong desire to win contribute to this condition, which consists of abnormal eating patterns, amenorrhea, and osteoporosis. In many instances, these girls become less competitive as they begin to tire more easily and have less stamina.

Adolescents should be screened for stress, anxiety, and depression, which frequently are associated with fatigue in this age group. The three most common sources of conflict are problems at home, strained peer relationships, and school-related difficulties. Having a job or not having a job for those in financial need may be an added source of pressure. The practitioner also should look for feelings of sadness, changes in behavior, difficulty concentrating, declining school performance, and other symptoms of depression. Most teens respond openly when asked if they get upset or depressed easily and if they have ever felt like hurting themselves or someone else. Any positive responses can be pursued by asking the patient to "tell me about this." It must be stressed that adolescents who are actively suicidal or homicidal require immediate intervention by mental health experts, legal authorities, or both.

Recent exposure to the Epstein-Barr virus as well as to other contagious diseases such as hepatitis, human immunodeficiency virus, and tuberculosis should be determined. Asking about pets, tick bites, recent travel, and water supply sometimes is fruitful. A search also should be made for symptoms of cardiac disorders, pulmonary conditions, endocrinopathies, gastrointestinal problems, and renal abnormalities. The menstrual history should be obtained from adolescent girls, looking for amenorrhea, irregular periods, or excessive bleeding, which may suggest the possibility of an intrauterine or ectopic pregnancy, spontaneous miscarriage, recent termination, or threatened abortion. In addition, the patients should be asked about the use of any over-the-counter or prescribed medications that have a known sedative effect.

The clinician also should inquire about symptoms of neurally mediated hypotension, a condition that has been associated with unexplained fatigue in adolescents. Neurally mediated hypotension leads to symptoms after prolonged periods of upright posture, standing in place, standing in the shower, and even sitting. It is especially common when the patient is in a warm environment and after emotionally stressful events. In addition, it may be seen immediately after exercise or soon after eating in some patients as blood flow is shifted to the intestines during the process of digestion.

Common symptoms of neurally mediated hypotension include recurrent light-headedness and fainting, which often are associated with postexertional fatigue for 24 to 72 hours. Of particular note, persistent fatigue is a prominent feature of this condition in many adolescents, even if there is no history of fainting. In addition, headaches, myalgias, and mental confusion may occur. The latter frequently is described by patients as being in a "mental fog," with difficulty concentrating, trouble paying attention, having a hard time staying on task, and having problems finding the right words. Occasionally, shortness of breath with or without chest pain may occur.

Physical Examination

TEMPERATURE

Any history of recurrent or persistent fever should be documented in the clinician's office. Unexplained temperature elevation suggests the presence of an underlying infection, neoplasm, or other inflammatory process such as Crohn disease. Hypothermia occurs frequently in patients who have experienced rapid or excessive weight loss. This finding is especially common among adolescents who have eating disorders in whom the low body temperature helps to conserve energy to help compensate for losses from severe caloric deprivation or purging. In addition, hypothyroidism always should be suspected in teenagers who are fatigued, whose temperatures tend to run below normal, and who gain weight in spite of what appear to be appropriate restrictions in dietary intake.

PULSE

Anxiety and stress are the most common causes of tachycardia in the practitioner's office. They also are important sources of fatigue in adolescents, especially in patients who are not sleeping well. Marijuana is another frequent cause of tachycardia and should be considered in teenagers who appear to be excessively tired or poorly motivated. Stimulant drugs that have been prescribed, purchased over-the-counter, or taken illegally may cause an accelerated heart rate. Fatigue is relatively common when the effects of these drugs begin to wear off. Endocrine abnormalities, including Addison disease, diabetes mellitus, and hyperthyroidism, as well as a number of pulmonary and cardiovascular conditions may cause an elevated pulse rate in patients who are fatigued.

Significant weight loss from voluntary caloric restriction is characteristically accompanied by sinus bradycardia, especially in patients who are hypothermic. This is an important physical finding that may help to distinguish adolescents who have eating disorders or those who are simply getting in shape from those who have an underlying organic cause for their weight loss. On the other hand, unexplained weight gain in patients who have bradycardia and fatigue should raise the suspicion of hypothyroidism. A slow pulse rate also may be caused by various medications or street drugs that have a known sedative effect.

RESPIRATIONS

Abnormalities in the respiratory rate in association with fatigue may indicate a cardiac, pulmonary, or metabolic disorder. Variations in the breathing pattern also may be seen with the use, abuse, or withdrawal of many prescription drugs, over-the-counter medications, or street drugs.

BLOOD PRESSURE

As with tachycardia, anxiety and stress are the most common causes of hypertension identified in the examination room. However, the finding of elevated blood pressure in association with fatigue may be due to several important medical conditions, including connective tissue disorders, Cushing syndrome, hyperaldosteronism, hyperthyroidism, and renal abnormalities. Routine use, abuse, or withdrawal of over-the-counter drugs, prescription medications, or illicit psychoactive substances also may cause hypertension and fatigue.

Delayed orthostatic hypotension after prolonged standing also has been described in patients who have unexplained fatigue (discussed in greater detail later in this article). Hypotension also may be noted as an adverse effect of various medications or in relation to abuse of street drugs. Adolescents who have Addison disease are especially susceptible to dehydration with hypotension and cardiovascular collapse, particularly during periods of physical stress. Addison disease always should be suspected in adolescents who have unexplained fatigue, especially when there is associated weakness, anorexia, nausea, vomiting, or weight loss.

HEIGHT

It is very important to plot height routinely throughout the adolescent years. Failure of a patient to progress along the expected parameters should draw immediate attention to the possibility of an underlying systemic process affecting growth and causing unexplained fatigue. In contrast, a normal linear growth velocity all but excludes the presence of an underlying endocrinopathy, such as hypothyroidism or Cushing syndrome, which may cause fatigue in association with obesity. A normal linear growth velocity also lessens the possibility of chronic cardiac, pulmonary, gastrointestinal, or renal disorders in teenagers who are excessively tired.

WEIGHT

It is also very important to plot weight throughout adolescence. Patients who have excessive weight gain or loss should be evaluated carefully for the possibility of a nutritional disorder, psychosocial problem, or medical condition. Poor weight gain over time also may be a subtle manifestation of a serious underlying illness, such as inflammatory bowel disease, especially in adolescents who have an unexplained low energy level.

GENERAL APPEARANCE

The examiner's first impression about the patient's overall well-being can be very insightful. Does the patient look ill or well? Does the patient seem to be depressed, anxious, or stressed? Does the patient seem to be adequately nourished?

CUTANEOUS SIGNS

The skin may serve as a window to underlying systemic causes of fatigue in adolescents. Jaundice suggests the presence of hepatitis or hemolysis. A yellow cast to the skin due to hypercarotenemia may be seen in patients who have anorexia nervosa and ingest large amounts of yellow-orange fruits and vegetables. This is a benign physical finding that resembles icterus, but the sclera are not involved. It should prompt the clinician to consider the possibility of an eating disorder that may be otherwise unrecognized.

Cyanosis may indicate the presence of a significant abnormality in the cardiovascular or pulmonary system, especially when digital clubbing also is present. The findings may be extremely subtle and only detectable by meticulous examination. A patient of mine had a somewhat sallow appearance. He was tired all the time, but was otherwise totally asymptomatic. During the consultation, he had bounding pulses that eventually led to the diagnosis of a large pulmonary arteriovenous malformation as the cause of symptoms.

Pallor usually is associated with iron deficiency anemia resulting from inadequate dietary intake, rapid growth, or blood loss. The latter is especially common in adolescent girls who are having heavy menstrual periods. However, many other important causes of anemia must be considered in this age group, including chronic inflammation, hemolysis, malignancy, and vitamin B12 deficiency, the latter especially in those who are on a vegan diet. Fatigue is a relatively late manifestation of anemia and usually is noted only in moderate-to-severe anemia that has developed over time. Pallor also may be a sign of anxiety, abuse of psychoactive drugs, and the allergic tension fatigue syndrome.

Generalized hyperpigmentation may be seen in patients who have fatigue associated with Addison disease. A clue to this diagnosis is involvement of the unexposed areas of skin as well as accentuation of the hyperpigmentation over the axillae, nipples, umbilicus, genitalia, or extensor surfaces of the joints. The clinician also should look carefully at the dorsum of the hands for evidence of superficial ulcerations, calluses, or scars in patients who have bulimia. This is known as Russell sign and is caused by using the fingers to induce vomiting in an effort to control weight. Many patients who have bulimia suffer from fatigue because of fluid or electrolyte imbalance as well as associated depression. Other signs of self-mutilation, such as cuts, scars, scratches, burns, and carved-out tattoos, may be seen in patients suffering from anxiety, depression, and poor self-esteem.

A number of skin findings may provide insight into the presence of an underlying connective tissue disease, infectious process, or other inflammatory condition that could cause fatigue in adolescents. A butterfly or discoid rash and photosensitivity are associated with systemic lupus erythematosus. Flushed cheeks followed by the appearance of a lacy, reticulated rash over the trunk and extremities are found in Fifth disease, which may cause persistent fatigue in teenagers. An evanescent, salmon-colored rash that has irregular borders or serpiginous margins is seen in patients who have juvenile rheumatoid arthritis and frequently is accompanied by fever. Subcutaneous nodules also may occur with this condition and are located near the olecranon process, on the dorsal aspect of the hands or knees, near the ears, and over pressure areas such as the scapulae, sacrum, buttocks, and heels. These nodules are usually nontender.

In contrast, erythema nodosum is characterized by exquisitely tender, erythematous nodular lesions over the extensor surfaces of the extremities, especially on the pretibial surface of the legs. These lesions frequently recur and are associated with many inflammatory disorders that cause fatigue.

Raynaud phenomenon, with characteristic color changes of the fingers and toes, should raise suspicion of a connective tissue disease or other underlying cause. Nailbed capillary changes with dilation and tortuosity of the vessels may be a very subtle finding in patients who have collagen vascular diseases. Cutaneous sclerosis, especially of the digits and face, is associated with scleroderma. In addition, an erythematous, purplish discoloration of the eyelids, forehead, cheeks, temples, dorsal interphalangeal joints, and extensor surfaces of the extremities suggests dermatomyositis.

OCULAR AND ORAL SIGNS

The presence of "allergic shiners" or a bluish discoloration under the eyes often is seen with sinusitis as well as with the allergic tension fatigue syndrome. Injection of the bulbar conjunctivae is common among those who use marijuana. Sjögren syndrome is a chronic autoimmune disorder of unknown cause characterized by dry eyes, xerostomia, salivary gland enlargement, and a high incidence of connective tissue disease. Evidence of iritis or uveitis suggests the presence of a connective tissue disorder or other underlying inflammatory process, such as inflammatory bowel disease.

Several oral findings have been noted in patients who have eating disorders, including enamel erosion or caries, particularly over the inner aspect of the upper teeth. This finding probably is related to repeated exposure to gastric contents following self-induced vomiting. Swelling of the parotid and submandibular salivary glands also has been described in those who have bulimia. Enlargement of the submandibular glands may be especially difficult to distinguish from lymphadenopathy in the anterior cervical region. In most instances, the salivary tissue has a softer consistency than the enlarged nodes, but there may be considerable overlap. Infection or other causes of inflammation in the salivary glands also may be associated with fatigue.

Evidence of stomatitis, gingivitis, or glossitis in teenagers who are excessively tired may indicate an underlying systemic process. Recurrent mouth ulcers, especially if they are unusually severe or recalcitrant to therapy, are relatively common in Crohn disease or ulcerative colitis. Behçet syndrome is a rare multisystem vasculitis characterized by the triad of recurrent oral ulcers, iridocyclitis, and recurrent ulcers of the external genitalia as well as a variety of other findings that may be accompanied by fatigue. In addition, hyperpigmentation of the gums is seen with Addison disease.

MUSCULOSKELETAL SIGNS

The adolescent's strength should be assessed to differentiate conditions that are associated with muscular weakness from other causes of fatigue. Muscular dystrophy always must be considered. Patients who have myasthenia gravis often experience weakness only late in the day or after physical activity. The clinician should search for other signs of myasthenia gravis that sometimes are subtle, including evidence of ptosis, weakness of the extraocular muscles, and dysphagia. The diminished strength noted in dermatomyositis may be generalized, but it is predominantly proximal, with involvement of the limb girdles and anterior flexors.

Objective evidence of arthritis strongly supports an organic cause for the fatigue, such as connective tissue disease, inflammatory bowel disease, infection, or neoplasm. Localized bone pain or tenderness to direct palpation may be associated with anatomic lesions, both benign and malignant. Unexplained bone pain that awakens the patient at night is especially concerning for leukemia or similar invasive processes. Clubbing of the fingers or toes suggests the possibility of chronic pulmonary, cardiac, or liver disease.

NEUROLOGIC SIGNS

A careful neurologic examination should be performed to help exclude rare causes of fatigue in adolescents, such as multiple sclerosis. The Chiari malformation also may be associated with subtle neurologic signs in association with fatigue. I recently had a patient in whom the cerebellar tonsils protruded into the spinal canal and compressed the nerves innervating the palate. The floppy palatal tissue resulted in obstructive sleep apnea, and the patient awakened unrefreshed in the morning. The family sought medical attention after the teachers complained that the girl had been falling asleep in class. A decompression procedure was performed by neurosurgery, and the girl's fatigue resolved completely.

MISCELLANEOUS SIGNS

Facial tenderness suggests the presence of sinusitis, although this finding often is absent in this condition. Persistent lymphadenopathy may be seen with infection, malignancy, connective tissue disease, or other inflammatory processes. The thyroid gland should be palpated for any enlargement or nodules. Both hyperthyroidism and hypothyroidism may be associated with fatigue. The lungs, heart, and abdomen should be assessed carefully for any abnormalities that may provide a clue to the diagnosis. The costovertebral angles should be palpated for any tenderness that may suggest pyelonephritis, glomerulonephritis, or other renal abnormality. In addition, patients who have generalized ligamentous laxity frequently experience vague musculoskeletal pain and are tired, especially late in the day. Finally, the possibility of pregnancy should be considered in adolescent girls and a pelvic examination performed when indicated.

Differential Diagnosis

The differential diagnosis of fatigue is extensive and includes numerous organic disorders as well as many psychosocial-medical conditions (Table 2). Sometimes a combination of factors contributes to the fatigue, especially when it is unduly prolonged. It is relatively common for an initial medical illness to take on features of a psychiatric condition as the process evolves. Psychologic issues may emerge as the primary agenda or develop as a consequence of an organic illness. A psychiatric diagnosis should not be assigned solely by the process of exclusion; the appropriate diagnostic criteria must be met before such a diagnosis is made.

Symptoms of stress, anxiety, or depression may be especially difficult to sort out in adolescents who are fatigued. Failure to attend school may compound an already difficult situation by perpetuating progressive absenteeism. Clinicians should be alert to the possibility that masked school avoidance may be contributing to the fatigue. The hyperventilation syndrome may present with fatigue in association with difficulty breathing, chest pain, lightheadedness, headaches, abdominal pain, and numbness or tingling of the extremities. In addition, fatigue may be a sign of certain eating disorders, especially bulimia and obesity, which frequently are accompanied by poor self-esteem, feelings of guilt, and depression. Patients who have the purely restrictive form of anorexia nervosa typically do not tire easily unless they are moribund or the weight loss has been rapid.

Clinicians always should consider the possibility of Addison disease in adolescents who have unexplained fatigue, especially if there is associated weakness, anorexia, nausea, vomiting, or weight loss. There usually is generalized hyperpigmentation with involvement of unexposed surfaces as well as accentuation in areas of predilection, as described earlier. Hyperkalemia, hyponatremia, and hypoglycemia are useful diagnostic features, but are not always present. The most definitive diagnostic test is the ACTH stimulation test (described later). It is imperative to consider Addison disease in the differential diagnosis because if it is not recognized and treated, an adrenal crisis may supervene.

Many adolescents who have unexplained fatigue begin with a "mono-like" illness that never resolves completely, and all diagnostic testing results are negative. As with acute infectious mononucleosis, these patients often have a history of severe sore throat, fever, malaise, lymphadenopathy, headaches, nausea, myalgia, and arthralgia with or without evidence of

Table 2. Causes of Fatigue in Adolescents

Allergic tension fatigue syndrome

Cardiovascular disorders
  Arteriovenous fistula
  Cardiomyopathy
  Congenital heart disease
  Congestive heart failure
  Orthostatic hypotension
  Orthostatic tachycardia
  Subacute bacterial endocarditis

Chronic fatigue syndrome*

Connective tissue disease
  Dermatomyositis
  Fibromyalgia*
  Juvenile rheumatoid arthritis
  Mixed connective tissue disease
  Scleroderma
  Sjögren syndrome
  Systemic lupus erythematosus

Drugs
  Illicit
  Over-the-counter
  Prescribed

Endocrine diseases
  Addison disease
  Cushing syndrome
  Diabetes insipidus
  Diabetes mellitus
  Hyperaldosteronism
  Hyperthyroidism
  Hypothyroidism
  Others

Gastrointestinal diseases
  Chronic liver disease
  Inflammatory bowel disease

Genitourinary conditions
  Cystitis
  Glomerulonephritis
  Pregnancy
  Pyelonephritis

Granulomatous diseases
  Sarcoidosis
  Wegener granulomatosis

Hematologic/Oncologic diseases
  Anemia
  Leukemia
  Lymphoma
  Other malignancies

Infectious diseases
  Abscess (localized/occult)
  Bacterial (Lyme disease, tuberculosis)
  Fungal (coccidioidomycosis, histoplasmosis)
  Parasitic (toxoplasmosis)
  Viral (Epstein-Barr virus, hepatitis, human immunodeficiency virus)

Miscellaneous conditions
  Familial hypokalemic periodic paralysis
  Idiopathic
  Narcolepsy

Neurologic disorders
  Chiari malformation
  Muscular dystrophy
  Multiple sclerosis
  Myasthenia gravis

Otolaryngologic disorders
  Obstructive sleep apnea
  Sinusitis

Psychosocial-medical disorders
  Anorexia nervosa/bulimia
    Abuse of appetite suppressants, diuretics, emetics, or laxatives
    Dietary restriction
    Rapid and/or excessive weight loss ("voluntary")
    Self-induced vomiting
  Depression and grief
  Excessive physical activity
  Munchausen syndrome
  Munchausen syndrome by proxy
  Rapid or excessive weight gain
  Rapid or excessive weight loss (involuntary)
  Sleep disorders
    Inadequate sleep
    Insomnia
    Unrefreshing sleep
  Somatoform disorders
  Stress-related disorders
    Anxiety
    Hyperventilation syndrome
    Masked school avoidance or phobia
  Substance abuse
    Alcohol
    Depressants
    Marijuana
    Withdrawal of stimulants

Pulmonary diseases
  Asthma
  Cystic fibrosis

*Requires further validation in adolescents.

arthritis. Many of the symptoms recur or linger for months in association with the fatigue. In addition, whenever a diagnosis of infectious mononucleosis is being entertained, the clinician should consider the possibility of infection with *Toxoplasma gondii* or cytomegalovirus, which may cause similar symptoms.

The association between orthostatic blood pressure changes and prolonged fatigue was described by Streeten and Anderson in 1992, who studied seven patients who had lightheadedness, fatigue, "weakness," and sometimes syncope. Blood pressures were measured every minute with an automated oscillometer while the patients remained standing. There was no fall in blood pressure after standing for a few minutes, which is the endpoint in traditional testing. However, there was a severe fall in blood pressure in all patients after they stood for 13 to 30 minutes, often with syncope or presyncope. Rowe and associates later described four adolescents who had a history of fatigue and underwent tilt-table testing. This procedure induced significant hypotension in all after they were tilted upright for 12 to 23 minutes. Their fatigue improved dramatically after they were treated for orthostatic hypotension.

It is not known why patients who have prolonged fatigue develop these cardiovascular changes when they assume the upright posture. When normal individuals stand up, blood pools in the legs, catecholamines increase to compensate for the decreased venous return to the heart, and there is a compensatory increase in heart rate that involves more vigorous contractions. The reduced amount of bloodflow to the heart is pumped more efficiently to the vital organs, especially the brain. In contrast, when individuals who have neurally mediated hypotension stand up, there appears to be a "miscommunication" between the heart and the brain. The heart rate slows while the vessels in the arms and legs dilate. As a result, even more blood is taken from the brain, and the patients feel faint. Finally, an abnormal increase in heart rate after prolonged standing has been described in adolescents who have unexplained fatigue. This condition is known as delayed postural orthostatic tachycardia syndrome, and it may occur with or without hypotension.

Diagnostic Investigation

BASELINE SCREENING STUDIES

In many instances, no diagnostic studies are required after a thorough history and careful physical examination. The costs of investigative studies are high, and any unnecessary testing should be avoided unless specifically indicated. However, if the diagnosis remains uncertain, the

---

Table 3. Diagnostic Investigations for Unexplained Fatigue in Adolescents

Baseline Screening Studies
- Complete blood count with differential and platelet counts
- Erythrocyte sedimentation rate
- Serum electrolyte determination
- Liver enzymes, protein, and albumin
- Thyroxin, thyroid-stimulating hormone
- Morning cortisol versus ACTH stimulation test
- Serum human chorionic gonadotropin if pregnancy cannot be excluded
- Epstein-Barr virus viral capsid antigen immunoglobulin (Ig)M and IgG
- Human parvovirus B19 IgM titers
- Antinuclear antibody, rheumatoid factor, C3 and C4 complement, creatine phosphokinase
- Urinalysis, urine culture and sensitivity

Additional Diagnostic Studies
- Orthostatic blood pressure measurements
  - Indicated if fatigue persists, diagnosis remains uncertain, or symptoms of neurally mediated hypotension are present
  - Prolonged standing required rather than few minutes, as traditionally tested
  - Abnormal pooling of blood in lower extremities ("pale face, purple feet and legs")
  - Be prepared: drop in blood pressure may be precipitous! (Intravenous fluids should be available)
  - Automated oscillometer facilitates process
  - Tilt-table testing expensive, probably not necessary
- Sinus films
  - Plain radiographs versus computed tomography
- Additional studies (as indicated)
  - Human immunodeficiency virus testing, Lyme titers
  - Chest radiograph, purified protein derivative
  - Toxicology screen
  - Magnetic resonance imaging of brain for Chiari malformation
  - Cytomegalovirus and Toxoplasma titers

clinician should consider a screening evaluation that includes the baseline tests shown in Table 3.

The complete blood count, erythrocyte sedimentation rate, serum electrolytes, liver profile, and urinalysis allow rapid assessment of target organ status in response to a systemic illness. Rheumatologic studies help exclude systemic lupus erythematosus and other connective tissue diseases that may present with fatigue. Thyroid studies always should be performed because manifestations of thyroid conditions often are subtle early in the course of the illness. A high morning cortisol level goes against a diagnosis of Addison disease, but the ACTH stimulation test is the definitive test to exclude this condition. In normal individuals, the serum cortisol level increases two- to three-fold 1 hour after intravenous administration of a synthetic ACTH preparation. Patients who have Addison disease have a blunted response to this challenge.

It is important to test for infectious mononucleosis early in the course of the illness, whenever possible. The Epstein-Barr virus viral capsid antigen immunoglobulin (Ig)M (EBV-VCA IgM) rises rapidly, but the response is transient; it usually can be detected only for 4 weeks and occasionally up to 3 months. If the EBV-VCA IgM is negative and the Epstein-Barr virus viral capsid antigen IgG is positive, the patient has had infectious mononucleosis at an undetermined time in the past. This could be as recently as 1 month ago or as long as many years ago.

Erythema infectiosum or Fifth disease also may be associated with fatigue. The telltale rash frequently is subtle or sometimes not present. As with infectious mononucleosis, the best time to establish the diagnosis serologically is early during the course of the evaluation. Therefore, testing for this infection is recommended as part of the initial laboratory investigation. The acute IgM response to the causative agent, human parvovirus B19, may be detected for up to 4 months. A positive IgM response to this virus indicates a recent infection; a positive IgG response indicates a previous infection and immunity.

A urine culture is included in the baseline screening evaluation because chronic pyelonephritis occasionally presents with fatigue

without any other symptoms or physical findings. Finally, a serum pregnancy test should be ordered in adolescent girls if the possibility of pregnancy cannot be excluded.

ADDITIONAL DIAGNOSTIC STUDIES

Further investigation is warranted if the fatigue persists and the diagnosis remains uncertain. Orthostatic blood pressure testing is indicated at this point, especially if symptoms of neurally mediated hypotension are present. According to Streeten, prolonged standing for up to 40 minutes is required to test for delayed orthostatic hypotension. Use of an automated oscillometer facilitates this process by measuring the pulse and blood pressure automatically at preset intervals, usually 1 minute. In many instances, blood pools in the lower extremities, and venous return to the heart is decreased. The patients may develop presyncopal symptoms associated with a "pale face and purple feet" shortly before the blood pressure drops significantly. However, patients sometimes experience little or no warning that they are about to pass out, and the fall in blood pressure may be precipitous. Thus, this evaluation should be performed in a setting that is equipped adequately with intravenous fluids and similar supportive measures to manage such complications during the testing procedure. Finally, tilt-table testing is expensive, extremely uncomfortable, and not considered necessary in most cases.

Persistent sinusitis following an upper respiratory tract infection is relatively common among adolescents who have unexplained fatigue, particularly when headaches, nasal symptoms, and cough are present. Computed tomography of the sinuses is more sensitive than plain films and is considered by many to be the preferred radiologic study when sinusitis is suspected. If significant mucosal thickening or sinus opacification is found, we initiate treatment with appropriate antimicrobial therapy for presumed sinusitis. The duration of therapy is usually 2 to 3 weeks, and the patient then is reassessed. Although cause and effect have not been proven scientifically, many adolescents who are fatigued and have evidence of sinusitis show significant improvement after an adequate course of antibiotics.

Cytomegalovirus and *Toxoplasma* titers should be considered in patients who have a "mono-like" illness in whom the EBV-VCA IgM titers are negative. A purified protein derivative and chest radiograph are included in the evaluation if the symptoms persist or are unusually severe or if there has been potential exposure to an infectious respiratory agent. Magnetic resonance imaging of the brain should be considered whenever the history, physical findings, or clinical course suggest the presence of a neurologic condition, such as the Chiari malformation.

A urine toxicology screen is indicated in cases when the diagnosis remains unknown and the adolescent denies use of any drugs. The patient should be informed of the purpose of this test and give consent for it to be performed. Interpretation of the duration of detectability must take into account a number of variables, including the type of substance abused, the drug metabolism, and the half-life. The route of administration, frequency of ingestion, physical condition of the patient, and state of hydration also may affect the results.

Lyme disease is a very rare cause of fatigue in adolescents who have no objective evidence of infection, such as a history of erythema migrans, arthritis, facial nerve paralysis, carditis, meningitis, or encephalitis. The diagnosis can be difficult to make because of poor standardization and inappropriate use of serologic diagnostic tests. Currently, the Western immunoblot assay is the most useful diagnostic test for diagnosing Lyme disease. Human immunodeficiency virus testing should be considered, especially for patients who have a history of sexual activity, sexual abuse, transfusions, sharing of needles, and intravenous drug use. Any further diagnostic investigation should be dictated by the findings on history and physical examination and the clinical course.

Management

GENERAL PRINCIPLES

The treatment of prolonged, unexplained fatigue is supportive and should be tailored to meet individual patient needs. It is important to validate the symptoms and reassure adolescents and their parents as necessary. Although there is no known cure, the illness is not life-threatening, and it rarely is progressive. Most teenagers recover completely and do not have any residual disability or limitation in functioning. However, families should be forewarned that progress can be slow in an effort to minimize their frustration when rapid improvement does not occur. It is helpful to think of the time span for recovery in terms of weeks to months and occasionally 1 year or more. This may require a change of perspective for all parties involved, including patients, parents, and even practitioners.

NONPHARMACOLOGIC THERAPY

Affected adolescents require extra rest until they regain their strength and stamina. Whenever possible, exercise should be limited and paced carefully in an effort to avoid any setbacks. Activities should be increased progressively, as tolerated, to avoid deconditioning. Referral to a physical therapist who is skillful with teenagers can be very helpful. Patients should return to school as soon as possible to avoid the vicious cycle of fatigue, depression, social isolation, and school phobia. However, gradual school reentry is recommended because most teenage patients will not tolerate returning to a regular, full-day schedule all at once. Psychotherapy with supportive counseling and family therapy sessions frequently are beneficial.

PHARMACOLOGIC THERAPY

Pain management with acetaminophen or nonsteroidal anti-inflammatory medications such as ibuprofen should be prescribed as indicated for headache, arthralgia, myalgia, and other such discomfort. Symptoms of depression, with insomnia or nighttime restlessness, can be treated with sedating antidepressants such as amitriptyline at a low dose of 10 to 20 mg at bedtime. Symptoms of depression, with hypersomnia or psychomotor retardation, may respond to selective serotonin reuptake inhibitors such as fluoxetine, which tends to have a more stimulating effect in most individuals. The adverse effects of the medications should be reviewed with patients and their parents prior to initiation of therapy.

Patients who have documented orthostatic hypotension or orthostatic tachycardia may respond to measures that expand the intravascular volume and increase venous return to the heart. This includes *at least* 2 L/d of fluid in an otherwise normal adolescent who has no known contraindications. Larger volumes are needed to compensate for fluid losses during warmer weather or after vigorous exercise. Extra salt should be added to food to the point that it can be tasted readily. If this is not palatable, salt tablets can be taken as a supplement. The subculture of adolescents who have fatigue and normally restrict their salt intake for health reasons or those who consume limited amounts of fluids on a regular basis may be particularly susceptible to orthostatic changes unless they can follow these simple suggestions. Patients who do not respond to the previously noted measures should be considered for treatment with fludrocortisone acetate, a potent mineral corticoid that aids in fluid retention. Teenagers who are placed on this medication should be monitored closely for adverse effects, including hypertension, headaches, hypokalemia, and excessive weight gain with associated edema.

UNPROVEN THERAPIES

Many other medications have been used experimentally to treat adolescents who have prolonged, unexplained fatigue. However, none has been documented to be effective to date. Various dietary supplements, including vitamins, minerals, and coenzymes, also have been tried without proven benefit. The benefits of popular herbal energy supplements such as Ma Huang (a Chinese medicine term for ephedra) have not been established. Furthermore, many of these substances have potentially harmful adverse effects and may interact with medications or other remedies. For example, ephedrine (the stimulant derived from the ephedra plant) can cause vascular constriction, raise blood pressure, and produce sleeplessness, especially when combined with caffeine or other stimulants. Additional investigative studies are needed to validate the efficacy and safety of such agents before their use can be recommended.

Summary

Prolonged, unexplained fatigue is common in adolescents. Although the cause is unknown, the course is usually benign and self-limited. Clinicians must be aware of the extensive differential diagnosis because a serious underlying medical condition or psychiatric disorder occasionally occurs. A comprehensive, balanced approach is necessary, with particular emphasis on a careful medical history, detailed psychosocial profile, and thorough physical examination. Selected investigative studies should be ordered as indicated. Treatment is supportive because there is no known cure. Appropriate therapy should be initiated when a specific underlying condition is identified. Evaluation and treatment for orthostatic cardiovascular abnormalities should be considered when appropriate. Finally, when the diagnosis remains uncertain, close sequential follow-up sometimes is needed to allow the illness to "play out" or "burn out."

Suggested Reading

Fukuda K, Straus SE, Hickie I, Sharpe MC, Dobbins JG, Komaroff A. The International Chronic Fatigue Syndrome Study Group. The chronic fatigue syndrome: a comprehensive approach to its definition and study. *Ann Intern Med.* 1994;121:953–959

Goldenring JM, Cohen E. Getting into adolescent heads. *Contemp Pediatr.* 1988;5:75–90

Jordan KM, Landis DA, Downey MC, Osterman SL, Thurm AE, Jason LA. Chronic fatigue syndrome in children and adolescents: a review. *J Adolesc Health.* 1998;22:4–18

Krilov LR, Fisher M, Friedman SB, et al. Course and outcome of chronic fatigue in children and adolescents. *Pediatrics.* 1998;102:360–366

Rowe PC, Bou-Holaigah I, Kan JS, Calkins H. Is neurally mediated hypotension an unrecognized cause of chronic fatigue? *Lancet.* 1995;345:623–624

Stewart JM, Gewitz MH, Weldon A, Munoz J. Patterns of orthostatic intolerance: the orthostatic tachycardia syndrome and adolescent chronic fatigue. *J Pediatr.* 1999;135:218–225

Streeten DHP, Anderson GH. Delayed orthostatic intolerance. *Arch Intern Med.* 1992;152:1066–1072

Fibromyalgia Syndrome

by David M. Siegel, MD, MPH, FAAP

Fibromyalgia syndrome (FS) is a disorder characterized by widespread musculoskeletal pain, fatigue, and specific areas of soft tissue point tenderness on physical examination. It is a complex condition for which no specific cause or pathophysiologic mechanism has been identified. Given that complaints of pain and/or fatigue are not uncommon among adolescents, it is important to know how FS presents and to be familiar with the components of a judicious evaluation and differential diagnosis, as well as the principles of management, the expected natural history, and the circumstances that would prompt subspecialty consultation.

Epidemiology

Data regarding the prevalence of FS in a pediatric or adolescent population are limited. The overwhelming proportion (80%–90%) of those in the United States with FS are female and of white/European ethnic background, although no specific hereditary pattern has been observed. In the adult population, FS prevalence is estimated to be between 2% and 4% (as compared to 10% of the general population reporting chronic widespread pain, and 20% to 25% suffering from persistent regional pain). In our pediatric rheumatology clinic, FS is now the third most common new patient diagnosis, representing 7% of referrals. This is consistent with what has been found in a national pediatric rheumatology clinic registry.

Pathophysiology

The pathologic processes involved in FS are not well understood, but research offers some insights. A key element associated with FS is disturbed sleep. In a study of a small number of patients with FS, researchers found that when subjects attempted to enter deep sleep, higher-frequency alpha wave activity intruded, disrupting the normal (and necessary) periods of delta-wave sleep. Further, when subjects who did <u>not</u> have FS spent several consecutive nights in a controlled sleep environment where noise was generated to disrupt delta-wave sleep, the individuals developed symptoms of FS.

Recent research suggests that FS patients experience "central sensitization," a condition of amplified pain response mediated through the

> ## Learning Objectives
>
> After reading this article, pediatricians will be better able to identify, evaluate, and manage adolescents with fibromyalgia syndrome, and will be able to:
> - Recognize the symptoms and signs of fibromyalgia syndrome
> - List criteria for diagnosis
> - Discuss the differential diagnosis
> - Describe key aspects of the physical examination and elements of laboratory evaluation
> - Explain the principles of management, including the role of the pediatrician and when specialty consultation is required
> - Discuss the long-term prognosis of fibromyalgia syndrome

David M. Siegel, MD, MPH, FAAP, a professor of pediatrics and medicine, is chief of the Division of Pediatric Rheumatology and Immunology, and a member of the Division of Adolescent Medicine, in the Department of Pediatrics, Golisano Children's Hospital at Strong, University of Rochester School of Medicine and Dentistry. Dr Siegel is also the Edward H. Townsend Chief of Pediatrics, Rochester General Hospital, Rochester, New York.

midbrain by way of the dorsal horn of the spinal cord. This may explain the usually poor response of FS to peripherally acting analgesics and non-steroidal anti-inflammatory drugs (NSAIDs).

Diagnosis

The American College of Rheumatology (ACR) diagnostic criteria for FS are shown in **Table 1**. In this context, widespread pain is defined as significant discomfort in regions of the body both above and below the waist and on the right and left sides. With the exception of finding specific tender points, the physical examination should be completely normal.

In conducting a tender-point examination, the physician applies 4 kg of pressure (which is enough to indent a tennis ball) at 18 specific soft tissue sites using the thumb or other finger. While exerting 4 kg of pressure over the skin is generally uncomfortable, a positive tender-point examination is marked by visible "flinching" or withdrawal by the patient. FS tender points are symmetric with respect to the midline of the body. There are 9 locations reflected on the left and right sides. (See **Table 1** and **Figure 1**)

As part of the physical evaluation, the examiner presses on what should be nontender sites (or "control" points) such as the mid-deltoid or midquadriceps to confirm a sufficient range of patient response to vigorous soft tissue pressure. In adult patients, Wolfe, et al, reported that findings of widespread pain and at least 11 out of 18 tender points resulted in FS diagnostic sensitivity of 88.4% and specificity of 81.1%. In our study of 45 adolescents with FS (Siegel, et al), we found that 11 tender points were not mandatory for a working diagnosis. In a few cases there were only 2 or 3 tender points early in the course of the illness, although the mean cumulative tender point count over time was 9.7. We, therefore, recommend starting FS management early in teens with a consistent history, physical examination and laboratory evaluation (discussed next) even in the presence of fewer than 11 tender points at presentation. Subsequent response to therapy supports the diagnostic confirmation of FS. In

Table 1. The American College of Rheumatology 1990 Criteria for the Classification of Fibromyalgia*

1. History of widespread pain.

Definition. Pain is considered widespread when all of the following are present: pain in the left side of the body, pain in the right side of the body, pain above the waist, and pain below the waist. In addition, axial skeletal pain (cervical spine or anterior chest or thoracic spine or low back) must be present. In this definition, shoulder and buttock pain is considered as pain for each involved side. "Low back" pain is considered lower segment pain.

2. Pain in 11 of 18 tender point sites on digital palpation.

Definition. Pain, on digital palpation, must be present in at least 11 of the following 18 tender point sites:

  Occiput: bilateral, at the suboccipital muscle insertions.

  Low cervical: bilateral, at the anterior aspects of the intertransverse spaces at C5-C7.

  Trapezius: bilateral, at the midpoint of the upper border.

  Supraspinatus: bilateral, at origins, above the scapula spine near the medial border.

  Second rib: bilateral, at the second costochondral junctions, just lateral to the junctions on upper surfaces.

  Lateral epicondyle: bilateral, 2 cm distal to the epicondyles.

  Gluteal: bilateral, in upper quadrants of buttocks in anterior fold of muscle.

  Greater trochanter: bilateral, posterior to the trochanteric prominence.

  Knee: bilateral, at the medial fat pad proximal to the joint line.

Digital palpation should be performed with an approximate force of 4 kg. For a tender point to be considered "positive" the subject must state that the palpation was painful. "Tender" is not to be considered "painful."

*For classification purposes, patients will be said to have fibromyalgia if both criteria are satisfied. Widespread pain must have been present for at least 3 months. The presence of a second clinical disorder does not exclude the diagnosis of fibromyalgia.

Reprinted with permission from Wolfe F, Smythe HA, Yunus MB, et al. The American College of Rheumatology 1990 Criteria for the Classification of Fibromyalgia: Report of the Multicenter Criteria Committee. *Arthritis and Rheumatism.* 1990;33:160–172. Table 8, page 171. Copyright © 1990 American College of Rheumatology. Reprinted by permission of Wiley-Liss, Inc., a subsidiary of John Wiley & Sons, Inc.

addition to pain and tender points, adolescent patients with FS experience a wide array of other symptoms which accumulate over time as the natural history of the illness unfolds. (**Table 2**)

SPECIFIC SYMPTOMS OF NOTE

Sleep disturbance is virtually universal in these patients, and should be thoroughly explored in the history. Patients with FS typically fall asleep easily but experience nighttime awakening without obvious provocation.

These teens are restless sleepers, but they may not know it. If in doubt, ask others in the home who might be aware of their sleep movements, or ask patients where the bed covers are when they awaken. Patients with FS who have nonrestorative sleep report that they never feel rested in the morning. The adolescent who states that she feels much better (both with regard to fatigue and pain) when she allows herself a specific adequate amount of sleep (eg, 9 or 10 hours) is less likely to have FS and may only need guidance about appropriate sleep hygiene.

The *fatigue* of untreated FS is generally pervasive and only intermittently remitting. Patients are persistently tired whether they are trying to keep up with their usual physical, intellectual and recreational routines, or have withdrawn from most activity and are leading a sedentary life with minimal exertion and limited social

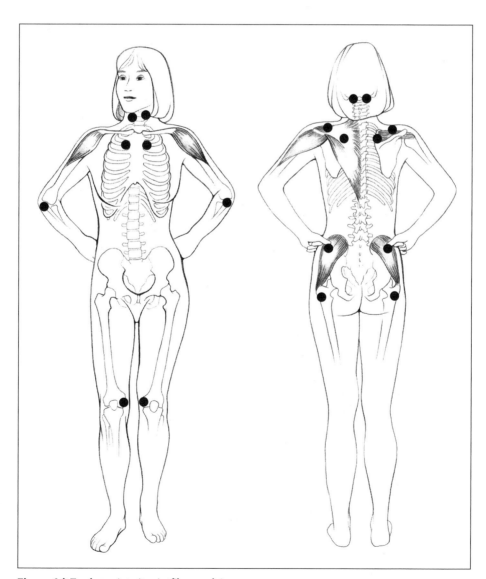

Figure 1.* Tender-point sites in fibromyalgia
*Bennett RM, Smythe HA, Wolfe F. Recognizing fibromyalgia. *Patient Care.* July 15, 1989:61.
Illustration by Marcia Hartsock, CMI. Reproduced with permission of the artist.

Table 2. Prevalence of Symptoms and Signs in Adolescents With FS

Symptom/Sign	Percent of Patients at Initial Presentation	Percent of Patients Over Time
Sleep disturbance	96	94
Diffuse pain	93	94
Headache	71	82
Fatigue	62	97
Morning stiffness	53	88
Morning fatigue	49	82
Depression	43	61
Subjective swelling*	40	59
Irritable bowel	38	46
Dysmenorrhea	36	42
Paresthesias	24	36
Anxiety	22	58
Raynaud's phenomenon	13	30

*Swelling reported by the patient (typically in the hands and fingers) but not confirmed by physician on physical examination (eg, "My rings are tighter than they used to be.")

contact. Most patients report the occasional "good day" during which they feel that their fatigue has abated and their pain has lessened, but attempts to resume previously abandoned activities invariably result in aggressive return of symptoms, often experienced as worse than before.

Adolescents with FS often struggle with concentration and memory as well as symptoms of *depression*. The clinical interview should determine whether the primary disorder is depression with associated somatization and fatigue, or if the mood disturbance is secondary to the pain and fatigue of FS. This distinction must be considered, and if suspicion of primary depression remains high, further psychological evaluation and assessment is warranted. Depression is quite common in FS, particularly among those with longstanding symptoms, and may require specific treatment.

It is important to ask about *light-headedness* (without vertigo), another common symptom in FS often associated with getting out of bed or otherwise arising quickly from a recumbent or seated position.

DIFFERENTIAL DIAGNOSIS

While the differential diagnosis in these patients can seem overwhelming at first, many illnesses that might appear to be suggested by a symptom or two are often quickly excluded as interview, physical, and laboratory data converge. Other symptoms seen in FS should be noted during the review of systems, but it is not practical to explore every nuance of each problem and clinicians should avoid embarking on extensive testing and subspecialty consultations unless other diagnoses are supported by the patient's presentation. Because of the prominence of musculoskeletal pain, rheumatologic disorders such as juvenile arthritis (JA) are often the initial consideration. An absence of inflammation as evidenced by the lack of joint (or soft tissue) warmth, erythema, swelling, or limitation of movement make JA unlikely. While patients with FS may complain of swelling of the hands, this is not the result of joint effusion. It may be subjective or due to soft tissue swelling probably resulting from autonomic dysfunction. ("My rings are too tight for my fingers in the morning.")

Patients with JA will also have longstanding signs of chronic illness, such as joint deformities or weight loss, and laboratory markers of inflammation that are not seen with FS. Other entities in the differential include Lyme disease, obstructive sleep apnea, viral infection, and chronic fatigue syndrome. **(Table 3)**

Indolent bacterial or mycobacterial infection might also enter into the differential diagnosis, but absence of documented fever, weight loss, infectious stigmata, or consistent serologies or other blood work serve to return the focus to FS.

LABORATORY

A prudent laboratory screen for patients in whom FS is supported by the history and physical examination should consist of a complete blood count with differential, erythrocyte sedimentation rate, Epstein-Barr viral titres, and, in the appropriate clinical context, Lyme titres and/or thyroid function studies. Lyme and EBV serologies must be interpreted carefully so as not to confuse evidence of past, resolved infection with acute illness.

Antinuclear antibody (ANA) is not a useful investigation unless there are signs or other tests that suggest autoimmune diseases. Low titre, positive ANA (eg, 1:40 or 1:80) often serves only to suggest misleading diagnostic pathways when the patient's presentation is not otherwise consistent with an inflammatory connective tissue disease. Rheumatoid factor is not helpful in evaluating a patient with suspected FS.

If there are signs suggestive of infectious, rheumatologic, or psychiatric illness, and the findings for FS are not present or convincing, consider subspecialty consultation. FS can be seen in patients who have another diagnosis as well, sometimes referred to as secondary FS (a finding more common in adults), and the clinician should be alert to this possibility.

Treatment

Management of FS centers around making a definitive diagnosis, implementing good sleep hygiene, initiating structured physical activity, prescribing medication, and considering mental health/behavioral interventions.

The diagnosis of FS is often delayed in adolescents. Initially, symptoms may be attributed to a viral syndrome or recent overexertion, and physician consultation is not sought. Often, by the time a diagnosis of FS is made and treatment is begun, the patient has not felt well for weeks or months.

Table 3. Features That Will Help to Exclude Other Diagnoses

Diagnosis	Clinical Features *not* seen in FS	Laboratory Results *not* seen in FS
Infectious mononucleosis	Fever Enlarged tonsils Adenopathy Hepatosplenomegaly	Epstein-Barr viral titres consistent with acute infection Elevated LFTs
Chronic Lyme disease	History of tick bite with typical cutaneous eruption (erythema migrans) Erythema migrans	+Lyme antibody with confirmatory test
Juvenile arthritis (systemic or polyarticular)	Fever Rash Swollen, red, warm joints Hepatosplenomegaly	Elevated ESR Elevated WBC Anemia
Systemic lupus erythematosus	Fever Rash Oral lesions Alopecia Serositis Renal disease	+ANA +Anti-dsDNA +Anti-Smith Leukopenia Anemia Thrombocytopenia
Obstructive sleep apnea	Snoring Apnea	Diagnostic sleep study

LFTs – Liver function tests
ESR – Erythrocyte sedimentation rate
WBC – White blood cell count
ANA – Antinuclear antibody
dsDNA – double-stranded DNA

During the period prior to diagnosis, a great deal of anxiety can mount as level of function and quality of life decline. At the time of presentation, many adolescents have already discontinued most physical activity, become disconnected from friends, and missed significant days of school. Treatment goals therefore include regular school attendance, resumption of normal physical exertion, and return to other daily activities. As transitioning from home tutoring back to school is often problematic, removal from school should be assiduously avoided.

The first step in management is to present and explain the diagnosis. Patient and family should be relieved to learn that FS definitively explains the symptoms and there is no evidence that infection, arthritis, or malignancy lurk in the background. They will be heartened to hear that the condition should improve with consistent treatment and a return to usual activities is a realistic expectation.

Once the diagnosis is clarified, the next step is to improve the quality of sleep. Cyclobenzaprine, a compound closely related to tricyclic antidepressants, is an appropriate starting intervention (10 mg every evening, 1½ to 2 hours before bedtime). Patients should be cautioned that they might experience side effects of dry mouth, blurry vision, drowsiness, or constipation, but for most adolescents these symptoms are mild and temporary. The initial sign of medication response is less nocturnal movement and awakening, followed by an increasingly refreshed feeling (restorative sleep) in the morning and less fatigue during the day. If there has been no change in the sleep disruption after 2 weeks, the dose should be increased to 20 mg nightly up to a maximum of 40 mg (this high a dose is not usually required). If the quality of sleep improves but the patient has great difficulty arising in the morning, either the dose is too high or the medication needs to be taken earlier in the evening, or both. Counsel patients to be careful about medication timing. If drug administration is confirmed to have been a full 2 hours before bedtime but morning drowsiness persists, the initial dose should be halved to 5 mg.

If cyclobenzaprine is ineffective or poorly tolerated, low doses of a tricyclic antidepressant (TCA) [eg, nortriptyline (10–50 mg), amitriptyline (10–50 mg), or doxepin (10–50 mg)] 1½ to 2 hours prior to bedtime may help to suppress alpha wave intrusion into delta wave sleep. A baseline ECG is prudent in these patients along with appropriate education regarding the consequences of TCA overdose. The benefit of TCAs in FS does not establish a diagnosis of depression, since the effective doses are much lower than those required to treat affective disorders. Some reports have also described the utility of selective serotonin reuptake inhibitors (SSRIs) in FS, but in adolescents, initial management with cyclobenzaprine is preferred. Although melatonin and antihistamines might aid in promoting sleep initiation, they do not enhance restorative (stage IV) sleep. We do not recommend benzodiazepines in FS.

In addition to medication, the sleep schedule must also be addressed. Bedtime and wake-up time should be appropriate for the patient's age and school expectations, and should be consistent each day. Initially, weekend schedules should not vary from weekday timing by greater than 1½ hours both morning and night. Patients with FS might find themselves napping in the afternoons due to fatigue. Sleeping during the day should be discouraged, but if the adolescent is unable to stay awake, napping should occur at the same time each day and for no more than 45–60 minutes. Other guidance around sleep includes discontinuation of caffeine and bedtime use of television, VCRs, videogames, or other sources of stimulation. Teens should be reminded, also, that FS is one more reason to avoid alcohol.

RETURN TO PHYSICAL ACTIVITY

Moderate (not high endurance or contact) physical activity is an essential element during treatment of FS; exercise is required for physical reconditioning. Although patients might insist that they are too tired and in too much pain, encourage a combination of regular stretching and aerobic activity in their weekly schedule. Working with a physical therapist to outline a daily stretching routine complemented by mild exercise such as brisk walking or swimming for 20 to 30 minutes, 3 times each week, can be helpful. This also establishes a relationship that serves to structure an appropriate regimen under direct supervision while providing encouragement and support. The pace of exercise increase will be determined by how long the patient has been relatively inactive, how quickly sleep becomes restorative, and what the premorbid level of physical activity had been. Early on, the adolescent and family may need frequent, if brief, contact with the physician and physical therapist to keep on track with the treatment program.

Case Vignette: Encouraging Compliance

Maggie is a 14-year-old student athlete who has been your patient for 6 years. She presents complaining of fatigue and pain of 6-weeks duration that seemed to begin with a case of the "flu." Maggie is uncharacteristically subdued; she admits that she hurts all over and feels tired all the time regardless of how much she sleeps. She recalls nocturnal awakening with her bed covers strewn about the bed in the morning. She has missed basketball practice and games for 2 weeks. "A few months ago I was wishing she would stay home on a weekend night once in a while," her mom says, "but this isn't what I had in mind. She just doesn't seem to have the energy for anything. Something is wrong."

Your initial interview with Maggie includes a history and physical examination (with FS tender points), and blood tests to rule out rival diagnoses. Major considerations are Epstein-Barr virus (EBV) infection, chronic inflammatory conditions (eg, bacterial infection, inflammatory bowel disease, juvenile arthritis), obstructive sleep apnea, and primary depression. As an initial screen, laboratory studies include complete blood count with differential, erythrocyte sedimentation rate, C-reactive protein, and EBV titres.

It is clear that Maggie is discouraged about her lack of energy and pain, but depression does not seem to be the primary problem. You talk about sleep hygiene, describe the significance of positive tender points in FS, explain that medication might be helpful, and schedule a longer appointment to discuss test results.

When Maggie returns, you can tell her that all of her laboratory tests are normal, supporting your clinical impression of FS. You explain the diagnosis and reassure her that the prognosis is good. Maggie is heartened at first, but still clearly frustrated; she had hoped that medication alone would quickly get her back on the basketball court and instead you explain that a gradual return to activity is the best way to steadily improve without a relapse.

Maggie is not enthused about the strict sleep-wake schedule and supervised stretching and exercise that are part of the FS regimen. She has become inconsistent about getting up and going to school each day, and she is not all that eager to resume a regular morning routine. Maggie resists the idea that she will have to begin getting up relatively early in the morning on weekends and going to sleep Friday and Saturday nights only a bit later than on school nights.

However, Maggie wants to return to sport and her social life. When you talk about the sleep regimen, you frame it in terms of an athlete's "retraining," describing the brain's sleep patterns and explaining that the sleep abnormality observed in FS is a "medical" or physiologic reason to adhere to good sleep hygiene and begin medication. You emphasize that the sleep protocol is not punitive and that she can anticipate greater flexibility in her schedule once sustained improvement has occurred.

Some teens, especially nonathletes whose FS has persisted for months, will resist the notion that exercise will be helpful. Fortunately, Maggie is receptive to your explanation that accumulated weeks of pain, fatigue, and inactivity have resulted in a physically deconditioned state that calls for a graduated exercise program. She is willing to work with the physical therapist who will get her started, and understands that if she does too much too soon symptoms may recur.

You prescribe cyclobenzaprine and instruct her to expect change in the quality of her sleep within about 2 weeks. In concluding the visit, you tell Maggie and her parents that with adherence to the sleep-wake schedule, exercise routine, and medication, both the pain and fatigue should steadily begin to abate within 2 to 3 weeks after the onset of more normal sleep.

LIGHT-HEADEDNESS

When light-headedness is present, FS management should include adequate fluid intake (1500–2000 ml/day) and supplementation of dietary sodium (1 g NaCl daily). Formal tilt-table testing is not necessary if a history of postural light-headedness and/or orthostatic pulse changes are noted.

DEPRESSION

Depression is often a problem for patients with FS. As with all adolescents who are depressed, the clinician's first obligation is to assess the risk for suicidality or self-injury. If neither is present and the affective disorder is not severe, primary care counseling to explore strategies for coping with the pain and fatigue of FS should ensue. If signs of depression persist or mood worsens, a mental health professional experienced in working with adolescents (and, ideally, adolescents with chronic pain syndromes) should join the multidisciplinary team working with the patient and family. Adjunctive medication should be added to the treatment regimen if needed. The best choice for someone who is already taking a low-dose tricyclic at night is addition of an SSRI such as fluoxetine or paroxetine. Although not FDA approved for the treatment of FS, SSRIs may be beneficial, even in the absence of overt depression.

INTRACTABLE PAIN

For some adolescents with FS, severe pain persists despite therapy. This can be a very disabling problem, one that may undermine regular physical activity, interfere with resolution of depression (when present), and delay return to full function. Alternative modalities to try might include application of heat or cold, massage, acupressure, and acupuncture.

Injection of a limited number of tender points with 1% lidocaine solution is sometimes effective; this should only be undertaken by a rheumatologist or one experienced in this technique. Clinical trials of NSAIDs in FS have not been encouraging, but some individuals experience benefit and when helpful, NSAIDs can be used long term. Narcotic analgesics are not appropriate in FS.

Short-term (2–4 weeks) therapy with non-narcotic analgesics has a limited role. Propoxyphene can be used but dose and duration should be restricted given the risk of dependency. Another option is tramadol, a centrally acting analgesic agent. This medication can be very helpful, but again, as an opioid agonist, it is not suitable for long-term management of FS. Carbamazepine has been used in chronic pain states and is another alternative.

Although many patients will eventually be pain-free, this can take several months. Pain reduction sufficient to allow return to full activity despite periods of residual discomfort may be a more realistic therapeutic goal for these patients.

Consultation

Most patients with FS will present first to their primary care provider. While the pediatrician is ideally suited to make the diagnosis and begin therapy, subspecialty consultation may be indicated at several junctures. If the presentation of FS is atypical and/or the patient and family remain unconvinced of the diagnosis, consider referral to a pediatric rheumatologist. Inadequate response to initial therapy is another indication for rheumatologic input. If a pediatric rheumatologist is not accessible, consider participation by an adult rheumatologist comfortable and experienced in caring for adolescents.

The difference in the course of FS in adolescents as compared to adults affects choices about participation in support groups. While a support group can be invaluable, it is important to investigate the constituency first. If all the other members are adults, the adolescent may not relate well to the life tasks and challenges that will dominate discussion. Worse, the prognostic expectations among adult patients may be more negative and discouraging than for adolescents.

Seek mental health consultation for patients with significant depression and/or anxiety related to coping with the discomfort and limitations imposed by a chronic illness. Consultation with a pain management team is sometimes helpful, but again, there must be expertise in working with adolescents and in the current thinking regarding FS and its treatment.

Long-term Outlook

The physician can and should be optimistic regarding prognosis (see Siegel, et al). The course of FS in adolescents should be one of gradual recovery and return to full function, although symptoms may recur, especially in times of increased psychologic and/or physiologic stress.

Summary

FS is an important entity to consider when adolescents complain of diffuse pain and fatigue. With a focused history and physical examination, the pediatrician can identify this condition and initiate treatment without resorting to excessive laboratory studies or unnecessary subspecialty consultation. With appropriate management, the prognosis for adolescents with FS is very good.

Further Reading

Ballinger SH, Bowyer SL. Fibromyalgia: the latest "great imitator." *Contemp Pediatr.* 1997;14:140–154

Cassidy JT. Progress in diagnosis and understanding chronic pain syndromes in children and adolescents. *Adolesc Med.* 1998;9:101–114

Moldofsky H, Scarisbrick P. Induction of neurasthenic musculoskeletal pain syndrome by selective sleep stage deprivation. *Psychosom Med.* 1976;38:35–44

Schikler KN. Is it juvenile rheumatoid arthritis or fibromyalgia? *Med Clin North Am.* 2000;84:967–982

Siegel DM, Janeway D, Baum J. Fibromyalgia syndrome in children and adolescents: clinical features at presentation and status at follow-up. *Pediatrics.* 1998;101:377–382

Smythe HA, Moldofsky H. Two contributions to understanding of the "fibrositis" syndrome. *Bull Rheum Dis.* 1977-78;28:928–931

Wolfe F, Smythe HA, Yunus MB, Bennett RM, Bombardier C, Goldenberg DL, et al. The American College of Rheumatology 1990 Criteria for the Classification of Fibromyalgia. Report of the Multicenter Criteria Committee. *Arthritis Rheum.* 1990;33:160–172

Acknowledgment

The editors would like to acknowledge technical review by Kenneth A. Schikler, MD, FAAP, for the AAP Section on Rheumatology.

NUTRITION NOTES

Iron-Clad Facts for Adolescents

by Laura E. Primak, RD, CSP and Nancy F. Krebs, MD, MS

Why is iron important?

Your body needs iron to work properly. When you don't have enough iron in your diet, you can become *anemic,* causing you to feel tired. Anemia is a common problem for teenagers.

Athletes with low iron levels may notice that they are not able to perform as well. Iron is also important for proper brain function.

Getting enough iron will help your body work its best.

How can you make sure your body is getting enough iron?

It is important to eat iron-rich foods every day. Adolescent girls need about 14 mg iron per day and boys need about 11 mg per day.

Good Sources of Iron

Animal Sources
   3-oz red meat (hamburger or steak) provides 3–7 mg iron
   3-oz chicken, fish, or pork provides 1–3 mg iron

Other Sources (each 1–3 mg iron/serving)
   Ready-to-eat breakfast cereals, 1 cup
   Canned baked beans or kidney beans, 1/2 cup
   Cooked spinach, 1/2 cup
   Cooked enriched pasta, 1 cup
   Whole wheat bread, 2 slices
   Frozen cooked peas, 1/2 cup
   Enriched rice, 1 cup

Your body can use iron from meat or fish more easily, but other food sources of iron are good too. If you are low in iron, your doctor may want you to take an iron supplement or a vitamin with iron.

What will help your body to use the iron in foods you eat?

● Eating foods rich in vitamin C (oranges, grapefruits, tomatoes, broccoli, strawberries) with an iron-rich food
● Cooking food in a cast-iron skillet or pot

What will make it harder for your body to use iron in foods you eat?

● Too much caffeine (coffee, tea, coffee drinks, or caffeinated soda) with a meal
● Too much fiber
● Taking calcium tablets with meals. (If you take a calcium tablet, don't take it with meals.)

Choosing iron-rich foods every day is part of healthy eating!

Laura E. Primak, RD, CSP, is a registered dietitian in the department of pediatrics, University of Colorado Health Sciences Center (UCHSC). Nancy F. Krebs, MD, MS, an associate professor of pediatrics at the UCHSC, chairs the AAP Committee on Nutrition.

This patient education sheet is distributed in conjunction with the February 2003 issue of Adolescent Health Update, *published by the American Academy of Pediatrics.*

The information in this publication should not be used as a substitute for the medical care and advice of your pediatrician. Comments and suggestions on Nutrition Notes should be forwarded to Marc Jacobson, MD FAAP (jacobson@lij.edu).

Pediatricians are encouraged to photocopy this page for distribution to patients and parents.

Take Care of Yourself to Get Over Fibromyalgia Syndrome (FS)

What is FS? FS is an illness that causes pain and tiredness. The cause of FS is not known, but it is not arthritis. It does not cause inflammation or damage to the body's joints, muscles, or organs. FS is not a new medical problem, but we are beginning to understand more about it.

When most people find out they have FS, they feel relieved and worried at the same time. It is a relief to know why you have been feeling so bad for such a long time, and it is a worry not to know how soon you will be feeling better. The good news is that there is a treatment plan that works, and your medical team is there to help.

How is FS treated? FS treatment involves taking medication, sticking with a healthy sleeping schedule, doing the right stretching and exercise, and (sometimes) getting counseling.

Most teens with FS begin to feel better after the first couple weeks of treatment. They continue to have less pain and more energy over the next 2 to 3 months. One day they realize that they are back to normal.

You will know that you are starting to get better when you begin to sleep without a lot of tossing and turning and waking up in the middle of the night. You will feel this change in sleep *before* you start to be less tired and have less pain. Sticking with the treatment, you will find that your energy will increase and your pain will decrease.

Many teens find that the hardest part of FS treatment is the need to get up early each morning and go to bed around the same time each night, even on weekends. If you are used to taking long daytime naps, sleeping in and staying up late on weekends, this will have to change. Along with medicine, regular sleep is really important to getting better. The right kinds of stretching and exercise (not too much and not too little) are also keys to help your body recover from FS.

Will I get better? You may have heard or read that adults with FS never really get better. FS patients often do get better, and this is <u>especially</u> true for teens. The vast majority of adolescents with FS who keep up with their treatment can expect to feel better and get back to usual activity.

After you have recovered from FS, you might have some times (especially if you are stressed or not sleeping regularly) when it seems to be coming back. If this happens, let your doctor know right away so you can stay on top of it. These flare-ups are usually not as bad as the first, and don't last as long.

It is hard to be patient when you have been feeling bad and missing out on fun for a while, but patience is important now. Stay with your sleep schedule and your exercise plan, take your

---

Useful Points to Remember

- Fibromyalgia syndrome (FS) causes significant pain and often feels like arthritis, but it is not.
- Blood tests for arthritis (or other inflammation-related problems) are normal in FS.
- People with FS do not get the deepest, most restful stage of sleep when they are in bed at night, which leads to pain and fatigue. One of the first steps in treatment is to correct this sleep problem.
- Regular physical activity is an important part of treating FS. However, adolescents who push themselves to participate in demanding or competitive athletics too soon will find that their symptoms persist and their recovery is delayed. In this situation, *too much* exercise is not a good thing.
- Remember, the outlook for most adolescents with FS is generally good. It's all about staying on top of your sleep, exercise, and medication regimens.

This patient education sheet is distributed in conjunction with the February 2003 issue of Adolescent Health Update, *published by the American Academy of Pediatrics. The information in this publication should not be used as a substitute for the medical care and advice of your pediatrician.*

Pediatricians are encouraged to photocopy this page for distribution to patients and parents.

medicine, and expect good things. Before you know it, a little bit at a time, you'll gradually be your old self again.

Tip for patients and parents: The Arthritis Foundation Web site (www.arthritis.org) contains extensive information on fibromyalgia syndrome for patients and professionals.

The Fourth Report on the Diagnosis, Evaluation, and Treatment of High Blood Pressure in Children and Adolescents

National High Blood Pressure Education Program Working Group on High Blood Pressure in Children and Adolescents

ABBREVIATIONS. BP, blood pressure; NHBPEP, National High Blood Pressure Education Program; SBP, systolic blood pressure; DBP, diastolic blood pressure; NHANES, National Health and Nutrition Examination Survey; JNC 7, Seventh Report of the Joint National Committee on the Prevention, Detection, Evaluation, and Treatment of High Blood Pressure; NHLBI, National Heart, Lung, and Blood Institute; ABPM, ambulatory blood pressure monitoring; CVD, cardiovascular disease; BMI, body mass index; PRA, plasma renin activity; DSA, digital-subtraction angiography; ACE, angiotensin-converting enzyme; MRA, magnetic resonance angiography; CT, computed tomography; LVH, left ventricular hypertrophy.

Introduction

Considerable advances have been made in detection, evaluation, and management of high blood pressure (BP), or hypertension, in children and adolescents. Because of the development of a large national database on normative BP levels throughout childhood, the ability to identify children who have abnormally elevated BP has improved. On the basis of developing evidence, it is now apparent that primary hypertension is detectable in the young and occurs commonly. The long-term health risks for hypertensive children and adolescents can be substantial; therefore, it is important that clinical measures be taken to reduce these risks and optimize health outcomes.

The purpose of this report is to update clinicians on the latest scientific evidence regarding BP in children and to provide recommendations for diagnosis, evaluation, and treatment of hypertension based on available evidence and consensus expert opinion of the working group when evidence was lacking. This publication is the fourth report from the National High Blood Pressure Education Program (NHBPEP) Working Group on Children and Adolescents and updates the previous 1996 publication, "Update on the 1987 Task Force Report on High Blood Pressure in Children and Adolescents."[1]

This report includes the following information:

● New data from the 1999–2000 National Health and Nutrition Examination Survey (NHANES) have been added to the childhood BP database, and the BP data have been reexamined. The revised BP tables now include the 50th, 90th, 95th, and 99th percentiles by gender, age, and height.

● Hypertension in children and adolescents continues to be defined as systolic BP (SBP) and/or diastolic BP (DBP), that is, on repeated measurement, ≥95th percentile. BP between the 90th and 95th percentile in childhood had been designated "high normal." To be consistent with the Seventh Report of the Joint National Committee on the Prevention, Detection, Evaluation, and Treatment of High Blood Pressure (JNC 7), this level of BP will now be termed "prehypertensive" and is an indication for lifestyle modifications.[2]

● The evidence of early target-organ damage in children and adolescents with hypertension is evaluated, and the rationale for early identification and treatment is provided.

Received for publication Apr 29, 2004; accepted May 12, 2004.

Reprint requests to Edward J. Roccella, National High Blood Pressure Education Program, National Heart, Lung, and Blood Institute, National Institutes of Health, Bldg 31, Room 4A10, Center Dr, MSC 2480, Bethesda, MD 20892. E-mail: roccelle@nhlbi.nih.gov

This supplement is a work of the US government, published in the public domain by the American Academy of Pediatrics.

Pediatrics, Vol 114, No. 2, August 2004

- Based on recent studies, revised recommendations for use of antihypertensive drug therapy are provided.
- Treatment recommendations include updated evaluation of nonpharmacologic therapies to reduce additional cardiovascular risk factors.
- Information is included on the identification of hypertensive children who need additional evaluation for sleep disorders.

Methods

In response to the request of the NHBPEP chair and director of the National Heart, Lung, and Blood Institute (NHLBI) regarding the need to update the JNC 7 report,[2] some NHBPEP Coordinating Committee members suggested that the NHBPEP working group report on hypertension in children and adolescents should be revisited. Thereafter, the NHLBI director directed the NHLBI staff to examine issues that might warrant a new report on children. Several prominent clinicians and scholars were asked to develop background manuscripts on selected issues related to hypertension in children and adolescents. Their manuscripts synthesized the available scientific evidence. During the spring and summer of 2002, NHLBI staff and the chair of the 1996 NHBPEP working group report on hypertension in children and adolescents reviewed the scientific issues addressed in the background manuscripts as well as contemporary policy issues. Subsequently, the staff noted that a critical mass of new information had been identified, thus warranting the appointment of a panel to update the earlier NHBPEP working group report. The NHLBI director appointed the authors of the background papers and other national experts to serve on the new panel. The chair and NHLBI staff developed a report outline and timeline to complete the work in 5 months.

The background papers served as focal points for review of the scientific evidence at the first meeting. The members of the working group were assembled into teams, and each team prepared specific sections of the report. In developing the focus of each section, the working group was asked to consider the peer-reviewed scientific literature published in English since 1997. The scientific evidence was classified by the system used in the JNC 7.[2] The chair assembled the sections submitted by each team into the first draft of the report. The draft report was distributed to the working group for review and comment. These comments were assembled and used to create the second draft. A subsequent on-site meeting of the working group was conducted to discuss additional revisions and the development of the third-draft document. Amended sections were reviewed, critiqued, and incorporated into the third draft. After editing by the chair for internal consistency, the fourth draft was created. The working group reviewed this draft, and conference calls were conducted to resolve any remaining issues that were identified. When the working group approved the final document, it was distributed to the Coordinating Committee for review.

Definition of Hypertension

- Hypertension is defined as average SBP and/or diastolic BP (DBP) that is ≥95th percentile for gender, age, and height on ≥3 occasions.

- Prehypertension in children is defined as average SBP or DBP levels that are ≥90th percentile but <95th percentile.
- As with adults, adolescents with BP levels ≥120/80 mm Hg should be considered prehypertensive.
- A patient with BP levels >95th percentile in a physician's office or clinic, who is normotensive outside a clinical setting, has "white-coat hypertension." Ambulatory BP monitoring (ABPM) is usually required to make this diagnosis.

The definition of hypertension in children and adolescents is based on the normative distribution of BP in healthy children. Normal BP is defined as SBP and DBP that are <90th percentile for gender, age, and height. Hypertension is defined as average SBP or DBP that is ≥95th percentile for gender, age, and height on at least 3 separate occasions. Average SBP or DBP levels that are ≥90th percentile but <95th percentile had been designated as "high normal" and were considered to be an indication of heightened risk for developing hypertension. This designation is consistent with the description of prehypertension in adults. The JNC 7 committee now defines prehypertension as a BP level that is ≥120/80 mm Hg and recommends the application of preventive health-related behaviors, or therapeutic lifestyle changes, for individuals having SBP levels that exceed 120 mm Hg.[2] It is now recommended that, as with adults, children and adolescents with BP levels ≥120/80 mm Hg but <95th percentile should be considered prehypertensive.

The term white-coat hypertension defines a clinical condition in which the patient has BP levels that are >95th percentile when measured in a physician's office or clinic, whereas the patient's average BP is <90th percentile outside of a clinical setting.

Measurement of BP in Children

- Children >3 years old who are seen in a medical setting should have their BP measured.
- The preferred method of BP measurement is auscultation.

- Correct measurement requires a cuff that is appropriate to the size of the child's upper arm.
- Elevated BP must be confirmed on repeated visits before characterizing a child as having hypertension.
- Measures obtained by oscillometric devices that exceed the 90th percentile should be repeated by auscultation.

Children >3 years old who are seen in medical care settings should have their BP measured at least once during every health care episode. Children <3 years old should have their BP measured in special circumstances (see Table 1).

The BP tables are based on auscultatory measurements; therefore, the preferred method of measurement is auscultation. As discussed below, oscillometric devices are convenient and minimize observer error, but they do not provide measures that are identical to auscultation. To confirm hypertension, the BP in children should be measured with a standard clinical sphygmomanometer, using a stethoscope placed over the brachial artery pulse, proximal and medial to the cubital fossa, and below the bottom edge of the cuff (ie, ~2 cm above the cubital fossa). The use of the bell of the stethoscope may allow softer Korotkoff sounds to be heard better.[3,4] The use of an appropriately sized cuff may preclude the placement of the stethoscope in this precise location, but there is little evidence that significant inaccuracy is introduced, either if the head of the stethoscope is slightly out of position or if there is contact between the cuff and the stethoscope. Preparation of the child for standard measurement can affect the BP level just as much as technique.[5] Ideally, the child whose BP is to be measured should have avoided stimulant drugs or foods, have been sitting quietly for 5 minutes, and seated with his or her back supported, feet on the floor and right arm supported, cubital fossa at heart level.[6,7] The right arm is preferred in repeated measures of BP for consistency and comparison with standard tables and because of the possibility of coarctation of the aorta, which might lead to false (low) readings in the left arm.[8]

Correct measurement of BP in children requires use of a cuff that is appropriate to

Table 1. Conditions Under Which Children <3 Years Old Should Have BP Measured

History of prematurity, very low birth weight, or other neonatal complication requiring intensive care

Congenital heart disease (repaired or nonrepaired)

Recurrent urinary tract infections, hematuria, or proteinuria

Known renal disease or urologic malformations

Family history of congenital renal disease

Solid-organ transplant

Malignancy or bone marrow transplant

Treatment with drugs known to raise BP

Other systemic illnesses associated with hypertension (neurofibromatosis, tuberous sclerosis, etc)

Evidence of elevated intracranial pressure

the size of the child's upper right arm. The equipment necessary to measure BP in children, ages 3 through adolescence, includes child cuffs of different sizes and must also include a standard adult cuff, a large adult cuff, and a thigh cuff. The latter 2 cuffs may be needed for use in adolescents.

By convention, an appropriate cuff size is a cuff with an inflatable bladder width that is at least 40% of the arm circumference at a point midway between the olecranon and the acromion (see www.americanheart.org/presenter.jhtml?identifier=576).[9,10] For such a cuff to be optimal for an arm, the cuff bladder length should cover 80% to 100% of the circumference of the arm.[1,11] Such a requirement demands that the bladder width-to-length ratio be at least 1:2. Not all commercially available cuffs are manufactured with this ratio. Additionally, cuffs labeled for certain age populations (eg, infant or child cuffs) are constructed with widely disparate dimensions. Accordingly, the working group recommends that standard cuff dimensions for children be adopted (see Table 2). BP measurements are overestimated to a greater degree with a cuff that is too small than they are underestimated by a cuff that is too large. If a cuff is too small, the next largest cuff should be used, even if it appears large. If the appropriate cuffs are used, the cuff-size effect is obviated.[12]

Table 2. Recommended Dimensions for BP Cuff Bladders

Age Range	Width, cm	Length, cm	Maximum Arm Circumference, cm*
Newborn	4	8	10
Infant	6	12	15
Child	9	18	22
Small adult	10	24	26
Adult	13	30	34
Large adult	16	38	44
Thigh	20	42	52

*Calculated so that the largest arm would still allow the bladder to encircle arm by at least 80%.

SBP is determined by the onset of the "tapping" Korotkoff sounds (K1). Population data in children[1] and risk-associated epidemiologic data in adults[13] have established the fifth Korotkoff sound (K5), or the disappearance of Korotkoff sounds, as the definition of DBP. In some children, Korotkoff sounds can be heard to 0 mm Hg. Under these circumstances, the BP measurement should be repeated with less pressure on the head of the stethoscope.[4] Only if the very low K5 persists should K4 (muffling of the sounds) be recorded as the DBP.

The standard device for BP measurements has been the mercury manometer.[14] Because of its environmental toxicity, mercury has been increasingly removed from health care settings. Aneroid manometers are quite accurate when calibrated on a semiannual basis[15] and are recommended when mercury-column devices cannot be obtained.

Auscultation remains the recommended method of BP measurement in children under most circumstances. Oscillometric devices measure mean arterial BP and then calculate systolic and diastolic values.[16] The algorithms used by companies are proprietary and differ from company to company and device to device. These devices can yield results that vary widely when one is compared with another,[17] and they do not always closely match BP values obtained by auscultation.[18] Oscillometric devices must be validated on a regular basis. Protocols for validation have been developed,[19,20] but the validation process is very difficult.

Two advantages of automatic devices are their ease of use and the minimization of observer bias or digit preference.[16] Use of the automated devices is preferred for BP measurement in newborns and young infants, in whom auscultation is difficult, and in the intensive care setting, in which frequent BP measurement is needed. An elevated BP reading obtained with an oscillometric device should be repeated by using auscultation.

Elevated BP must be confirmed on repeated visits before characterizing a child as having hypertension. Confirming an elevated BP measurement is important, because BP at high levels tends to fall on subsequent measurement as the result of 1) an accommodation effect (ie, reduction of anxiety by the patient from one visit to the next) and 2) regression to the mean. BP level is not static but varies even under standard resting conditions. Therefore, except in the presence of severe hypertension, a more precise characterization of a person's BP level is an average of multiple BP measurements taken over weeks to months.

ABPM

ABPM refers to a procedure in which a portable BP device, worn by the patient, records BP over a specified period, usually 24 hours. ABPM is very useful in the evaluation of hypertension in children.[21-23] By frequent measurement and recording of BP, ABPM enables computation of the mean BP during the day, night, and over 24 hours as well as various measures to determine the degree to which BP exceeds the upper limit of normal over a given time period, ie, the BP load. ABPM is especially helpful in the evaluation of white-coat hypertension as well as the risk for hypertensive organ injury, apparent drug resistance, and hypotensive symptoms with antihypertensive drugs. ABPM is also useful for evaluating patients for whom more information on BP patterns is needed, such as those with episodic hypertension, chronic kidney disease, diabetes, and autonomic dysfunction. Conducting ABPM requires specific equipment and trained staff. Therefore, ABPM in children and adolescents should be used by experts in the field of pediatric hypertension who are experienced in its use and interpretation.

BP Tables

- BP standards based on gender, age, and height provide a precise classification of BP according to body size.
- The revised BP tables now include the 50th, 90th, 95th, and 99th percentiles (with standard deviations) by gender, age, and height.

In children and adolescents, the normal range of BP is determined by body size and age. BP standards that are based on gender, age, and height provide a more precise classification of BP according to body size. This approach avoids misclassifying children who are very tall or very short.

The BP tables are revised to include the new height percentile data (www.cdc.gov/growthcharts)[24] as well as the addition of BP data from the NHANES 1999–2000. Demographic information on the source of the BP data is provided in Appendix A. The 50th, 90th, 95th, and 99th percentiles of SBP and DBP (using K5) for height by gender and age are given for boys and girls in Tables 3 and 4. Although new data have been added, the gender, age, and height BP levels for the 90th and 95th percentiles have changed minimally from the last report. The 50th percentile has been added to the tables to provide the clinician with the BP level at the midpoint of the normal range. Although the 95th percentile provides a BP level that defines hypertension, management decisions about children with hypertension should be determined by the degree or severity of hypertension. Therefore, the 99th percentile has been added to facilitate clinical decision-making in the plan for evaluation. Standards for SBP and DBP for infants <1 year old are available.[25] In children <1 year old, SBP has been used to define hypertension.

To use the tables in a clinical setting, the height percentile is determined by using the newly revised CDC growth charts (www.cdc.gov/growthcharts). The child's measured SBP and DBP are compared with the numbers provided in the table (boys or girls) according to the child's age and height percentile. The child is normotensive if the BP is <90th percentile. If the BP is ≥90th percentile, the BP measurement should be repeated at that visit to verify an elevated BP.

BP measurements between the 90th and 95th percentiles indicate prehypertension and warrant reassessment and consideration of other risk factors (see Table 5). In addition, if an adolescent's BP is >120/80 mm Hg, the patient should be considered to be prehypertensive even if this value is <90th percentile. This BP level typically occurs for SBP at 12 years old and for DBP at 16 years old.

If the child's BP (systolic or diastolic) is ≥95th percentile, the child may be hypertensive, and the measurement must be repeated on at least 2 additional occasions to confirm the diagnosis. Staging of BP, according to the extent to which a child's BP exceeds the 95th percentile, is helpful in developing a management plan for evaluation and treatment that is most appropriate for an individual patient. On repeated measurement, hypertensive children may have BP levels that are only a few mm Hg >95th percentile; these children would be managed differently from hypertensive children who have BP levels that are 15 to 20 mm Hg above the 95th percentile. An important clinical decision is to determine which hypertensive children require more immediate attention for elevated BP. The difference between the 95th and 99th percentiles is only 7 to 10 mm Hg and is not large enough, particularly in view of the variability in BP measurements, to adequately distinguish mild hypertension (where limited evaluation is most appropriate) from more severe hypertension (where more immediate and extensive intervention is indicated). Therefore, stage 1 hypertension is the designation for BP levels that range from the 95th percentile to 5 mm Hg above the 99th percentile. Stage 2 hypertension is the designation for BP levels that are >5 mm Hg above the 99th percentile. Once confirmed on repeated measures, stage 1 hypertension allows time for evaluation before initiating treatment unless the patient is symptomatic. Patients with stage 2 hypertension may need more prompt evaluation and pharmacologic therapy. Symptomatic patients with stage 2 hypertension require immediate treatment and consultation with experts in pediatric hypertension. These categories are parallel to the staging of hypertension in adults, as noted in the JNC 7.[2]

Table 3. BP Levels for Boys by Age and Height Percentile

Age, y	BP Percentile	SBP, mm Hg							DBP, mm Hg						
		Percentile of Height							Percentile of Height						
		5th	10th	25th	50th	75th	90th	95th	5th	10th	25th	50th	75th	90th	95th
1	50th	80	81	83	85	87	88	89	34	35	36	37	38	39	39
	90th	94	95	97	99	100	102	103	49	50	51	52	53	53	54
	95th	98	99	101	103	104	106	106	54	54	55	56	57	58	58
	99th	105	106	108	110	112	113	114	61	62	63	64	65	66	66
2	50th	84	85	87	88	90	92	92	39	40	41	42	43	44	44
	90th	97	99	100	102	104	105	106	54	55	56	57	58	58	59
	95th	101	102	104	106	108	109	110	59	59	60	61	62	63	63
	99th	109	110	111	113	115	117	117	66	67	68	69	70	71	71
3	50th	86	87	89	91	93	94	95	44	44	45	46	47	48	48
	90th	100	101	103	105	107	108	109	59	59	60	61	62	63	63
	95th	104	105	107	109	110	112	113	63	63	64	65	66	67	67
	99th	111	112	114	116	118	119	120	71	71	72	73	74	75	75
4	50th	88	89	91	93	95	96	97	47	48	49	50	51	51	52
	90th	102	103	105	107	109	110	111	62	63	64	65	66	66	67
	95th	106	107	109	111	112	114	115	66	67	68	69	70	71	71
	99th	113	114	116	118	120	121	122	74	75	76	77	78	78	79
5	50th	90	91	93	95	96	98	98	50	51	52	53	54	55	55
	90th	104	105	106	108	110	111	112	65	66	67	68	69	69	70
	95th	108	109	110	112	114	115	116	69	70	71	72	73	74	74
	99th	115	116	118	120	121	123	123	77	78	79	80	81	81	82
6	50th	91	92	94	96	98	99	100	53	53	54	55	56	57	57
	90th	105	106	108	110	111	113	113	68	68	69	70	71	72	72
	95th	109	110	112	114	115	117	117	72	72	73	74	75	76	76
	99th	116	117	119	121	123	124	125	80	80	81	82	83	84	84
7	50th	92	94	95	97	99	100	101	55	55	56	57	58	59	59
	90th	106	107	109	111	113	114	115	70	70	71	72	73	74	74
	95th	110	111	113	115	117	118	119	74	74	75	76	77	78	78
	99th	117	118	120	122	124	125	126	82	82	83	84	85	86	86
8	50th	94	95	97	99	100	102	102	56	57	58	59	60	60	61
	90th	107	109	110	112	114	115	116	71	72	72	73	74	75	76
	95th	111	112	114	116	118	119	120	75	76	77	78	79	79	80
	99th	119	120	122	123	125	127	127	83	84	85	86	87	87	88
9	50th	95	96	98	100	102	103	104	57	58	59	60	61	61	62
	90th	109	110	112	114	115	117	118	72	73	74	75	76	76	77
	95th	113	114	116	118	119	121	121	76	77	78	79	80	81	81
	99th	120	121	123	125	127	128	129	84	85	86	87	88	88	89
10	50th	97	98	100	102	103	105	106	58	59	60	61	61	62	63
	90th	111	112	114	115	117	119	119	73	73	74	75	76	77	78
	95th	115	116	117	119	121	122	123	77	78	79	80	81	81	82
	99th	122	123	125	127	128	130	130	85	86	86	88	88	89	90
11	50th	99	100	102	104	105	107	107	59	59	60	61	62	63	63
	90th	113	114	115	117	119	120	121	74	74	75	76	77	78	78
	95th	117	118	119	121	123	124	125	78	78	79	80	81	82	82
	99th	124	125	127	129	130	132	132	86	86	87	88	89	90	90
12	50th	101	102	104	106	108	109	110	59	60	61	62	63	63	64
	90th	115	116	118	120	121	123	123	74	75	75	76	77	78	79
	95th	119	120	122	123	125	127	127	78	79	80	81	82	82	83
	99th	126	127	129	131	133	134	135	86	87	88	89	90	90	91
13	50th	104	105	106	108	110	111	112	60	60	61	62	63	64	64
	90th	117	118	120	122	124	125	126	75	75	76	77	78	79	79
	95th	121	122	124	126	128	129	130	79	79	80	81	82	83	83
	99th	128	130	131	133	135	136	137	87	87	88	89	90	91	91
14	50th	106	107	109	111	113	114	115	60	61	62	63	64	65	65
	90th	120	121	123	125	126	128	128	75	76	77	78	79	79	80
	95th	124	125	127	128	130	132	132	80	80	81	82	83	84	84
	99th	131	132	134	136	138	139	140	87	88	89	90	91	92	92
15	50th	109	110	112	113	115	117	117	61	62	63	64	65	66	66
	90th	122	124	125	127	129	130	131	76	77	78	79	80	80	81
	95th	126	127	129	131	133	134	135	81	81	82	83	84	85	85
	99th	134	135	136	138	140	142	142	88	89	90	91	92	93	93
16	50th	111	112	114	116	118	119	120	63	63	64	65	66	67	67
	90th	125	126	128	130	131	133	134	78	78	79	80	81	82	82
	95th	129	130	132	134	135	137	137	82	83	83	84	85	86	87
	99th	136	137	139	141	143	144	145	90	90	91	92	93	94	94
17	50th	114	115	116	118	120	121	122	65	66	66	67	68	69	70
	90th	127	128	130	132	134	135	136	80	80	81	82	83	84	84
	95th	131	132	134	136	138	139	140	84	85	86	87	87	88	89
	99th	139	140	141	143	145	146	147	92	93	93	94	95	96	97

The 90th percentile is 1.28 SD, the 95th percentile is 1.645 SD, and the 99th percentile is 2.326 SD over the mean.

For research purposes, the SDs in Table B1 allow one to compute BP Z scores and percentiles for boys with height percentiles given in Table 3 (ie, the 5th, 10th, 25th, 50th, 75th, 90th, and 95th percentiles). These height percentiles must be converted to height Z scores given by: 5% = −1.645; 10% = −1.28; 25% = −0.68; 50% = 0; 75% = −0.68; 90% = −1.28; and 95% = −1.645, and then computed according to the methodology in steps 2 through 4 described in Appendix B. For children with height percentiles other than these, follow steps 1 through 4 as described in Appendix B.

Table 4. BP Levels for Girls by Age and Height Percentile

Age, y	BP Percentile	SBP, mm Hg							DBP, mm Hg						
		Percentile of Height							Percentile of Height						
		5th	10th	25th	50th	75th	90th	95th	5th	10th	25th	50th	75th	90th	95th
1	50th	83	84	85	86	88	89	90	38	39	39	40	41	41	42
	90th	97	97	98	100	101	102	103	52	53	53	54	55	55	56
	95th	100	101	102	104	105	106	107	56	57	57	58	59	59	60
	99th	108	108	109	111	112	113	114	64	64	65	65	66	67	67
2	50th	85	85	87	88	89	91	91	43	44	44	45	46	46	47
	90th	98	99	100	101	103	104	105	57	58	58	59	60	61	61
	95th	102	103	104	105	107	108	109	61	62	62	63	64	65	65
	99th	109	110	111	112	114	115	116	69	69	70	70	71	72	72
3	50th	86	87	88	89	91	92	93	47	48	48	49	50	50	51
	90th	100	100	102	103	104	106	106	61	62	62	63	64	64	65
	95th	104	104	105	107	108	109	110	65	66	66	67	68	68	69
	99th	111	111	113	114	115	116	117	73	73	74	74	75	76	76
4	50th	88	88	90	91	92	94	94	50	50	51	52	52	53	54
	90th	101	102	103	104	106	107	108	64	64	65	66	67	67	68
	95th	105	106	107	108	110	111	112	68	68	69	70	71	71	72
	99th	112	113	114	115	117	118	119	76	76	76	77	78	79	79
5	50th	89	90	91	93	94	95	96	52	53	53	54	55	55	56
	90th	103	103	105	106	107	109	109	66	67	67	68	69	69	70
	95th	107	107	108	110	111	112	113	70	71	71	72	73	73	74
	99th	114	114	116	117	118	120	120	78	78	79	79	80	81	81
6	50th	91	92	93	94	96	97	98	54	54	55	56	56	57	58
	90th	104	105	106	108	109	110	111	68	68	69	70	70	71	72
	95th	108	109	110	111	113	114	115	72	72	73	74	74	75	76
	99th	115	116	117	119	120	121	122	80	80	80	81	82	83	83
7	50th	93	93	95	96	97	99	99	55	56	56	57	58	58	59
	90th	106	107	108	109	111	112	113	69	70	70	71	72	72	73
	95th	110	111	112	113	115	116	116	73	74	74	75	76	76	77
	99th	117	118	119	120	122	123	124	81	81	82	82	83	84	84
8	50th	95	95	96	98	99	100	101	57	57	57	58	59	60	60
	90th	108	109	110	111	113	114	114	71	71	71	72	73	74	74
	95th	112	112	114	115	116	118	118	75	75	75	76	77	78	78
	99th	119	120	121	122	123	125	125	82	82	83	83	84	85	86
9	50th	96	97	98	100	101	102	103	58	58	58	59	60	61	61
	90th	110	110	112	113	114	116	116	72	72	72	73	74	75	75
	95th	114	114	115	117	118	119	120	76	76	76	77	78	79	79
	99th	121	121	123	124	125	127	127	83	83	84	84	85	86	87
10	50th	98	99	100	102	103	104	105	59	59	59	60	61	62	62
	90th	112	112	114	115	116	118	118	73	73	73	74	75	76	76
	95th	116	116	117	119	120	121	122	77	77	77	78	79	80	80
	99th	123	123	125	126	127	129	129	84	84	85	86	86	87	88
11	50th	100	101	102	103	105	106	107	60	60	60	61	62	63	63
	90th	114	114	116	117	118	119	120	74	74	74	75	76	77	77
	95th	118	118	119	121	122	123	124	78	78	78	79	80	81	81
	99th	125	125	126	128	129	130	131	85	85	86	87	87	88	89
12	50th	102	103	104	105	107	108	109	61	61	61	62	63	64	64
	90th	116	116	117	119	120	121	122	75	75	75	76	77	78	78
	95th	119	120	121	123	124	125	126	79	79	79	80	81	82	82
	99th	127	127	128	130	131	132	133	86	86	87	88	88	89	90
13	50th	104	105	106	107	109	110	110	62	62	62	63	64	65	65
	90th	117	118	119	121	122	123	124	76	76	76	77	78	79	79
	95th	121	122	123	124	126	127	128	80	80	80	81	82	83	83
	99th	128	129	130	132	133	134	135	87	87	88	89	89	90	91
14	50th	106	106	107	109	110	111	112	63	63	63	64	65	66	66
	90th	119	120	121	122	124	125	125	77	77	77	78	79	80	80
	95th	123	123	125	126	127	129	129	81	81	81	82	83	84	84
	99th	130	131	132	133	135	136	136	88	88	89	90	90	91	92
15	50th	107	108	109	110	111	113	113	64	64	64	65	66	67	67
	90th	120	121	122	123	125	126	127	78	78	78	79	80	81	81
	95th	124	125	126	127	129	130	131	82	82	82	83	84	85	85
	99th	131	132	133	134	136	137	138	89	89	90	91	91	92	93
16	50th	108	108	110	111	112	114	114	64	64	65	66	66	67	68
	90th	121	122	123	124	126	127	128	78	78	79	80	81	81	82
	95th	125	126	127	128	130	131	132	82	82	83	84	85	85	86
	99th	132	133	134	135	137	138	139	90	90	90	91	92	93	93
17	50th	108	109	110	111	113	114	115	64	65	65	66	67	67	68
	90th	122	122	123	125	126	127	128	78	79	79	80	81	81	82
	95th	125	126	127	129	130	131	132	82	83	83	84	85	85	86
	99th	133	133	134	136	137	138	139	90	90	91	91	92	93	93

The 90th percentile is 1.28 SD, the 95th percentile is 1.645 SD, and the 99th percentile is 2.326 SD over the mean.

For research purposes, the SDs in Table B1 allow one to compute BP Z scores and percentiles for girls with height percentiles given in Table 4 (ie, the 5th, 10th, 25th, 50th, 75th, 90th, and 95th percentiles). These height percentiles must be converted to height Z scores given by: 5% = −1.645; 10% = −1.28; 25% = −0.68; 50% = 0; 75% = −0.68; 90% = −1.28; and 95% = −1.645 and then computed according to the methodology in steps 2 through 4 described in Appendix B. For children with height percentiles other than these, follow steps 1 through 4 as described in Appendix B.

USING THE BP TABLES

1. Use the standard height charts to determine the height percentile.

2. Measure and record the child's SBP and DBP.

3. Use the correct gender table for SBP and DBP.

4. Find the child's age on the left side of the table. Follow the age row horizontally across the table to the intersection of the line for the height percentile (vertical column).

5. There, find the 50th, 90th, 95th, and 99th percentiles for SBP in the left columns and for DBP in the right columns.

   ● BP <90th percentile is normal.

   ● BP between the 90th and 95th percentile is prehypertension. In adolescents, BP ≥120/80 mm Hg is prehypertension, even if this figure is <90th percentile.

   ● BP >95th percentile may be hypertension.

6. If the BP is >90th percentile, the BP should be repeated twice at the same office visit, and an average SBP and DBP should be used.

7. If the BP is >95th percentile, BP should be staged. If stage 1 (95th percentile to the 99th percentile plus 5 mm Hg), BP measurements should be repeated on 2 more occasions. If hypertension is confirmed, evaluation should proceed as described in Table 7. If BP is stage 2 (>99th percentile plus 5 mm Hg), prompt referral should be made for evaluation and therapy. If the patient is symptomatic, immediate referral and treatment are indicated. Those patients with a compelling indication, as noted in Table 6, would be treated as the next higher category of hypertension.

Primary Hypertension and Evaluation for Comorbidities

● Primary hypertension is identifiable in children and adolescents.

● Both hypertension and prehypertension have become a significant health issue in the young because of the strong association of high BP with overweight and the marked increase in the prevalence of overweight children.

● The evaluation of hypertensive children should include assessment for additional risk factors.

Table 5. Classification of Hypertension in Children and Adolescents, With Measurement Frequency and Therapy Recommendations

	SBP or DBP Percentile*	Frequency of BP Measurement	Therapeutic Lifestyle Changes	Pharmacologic Therapy
Normal	<90th	Recheck at next scheduled physical examination	Encourage healthy diet, sleep, and physical activity	—
Prehypertension	90th to <95th or if BP exceeds 120/80 even if <90th percentile up to <95th percentile†	Recheck in 6 mo	Weight-management counseling if overweight; introduce physical activity and diet management‡	None unless compelling indications such as chronic kidney disease, diabetes mellitus, heart failure, or LVH exist
Stage 1 hypertension	95th–99th percentile plus 5 mm Hg	Recheck in 1–2 wk or sooner if the patient is symptomatic; if persistently elevated on 2 additional occasions, evaluate or refer to source of care within 1 mo	Weight-management counseling if overweight; introduce physical activity and diet management‡	Initiate therapy based on indications in Table 6 or if compelling indications (as shown above) exist
Stage 2 hypertension	>99th percentile plus 5 mm Hg	Evaluate or refer to source of care within 1 wk or immediately if the patient is symptomatic	Weight-management counseling if overweight; introduce physical activity and diet management‡	Initiate therapy§

*For gender, age, and height measured on at least 3 separate occasions; if systolic and diastolic categories are different, categorize by the higher value.

†This occurs typically at 12 years old for SBP and at 16 years old for DBP.

‡Parents and children trying to modify the eating plan to the Dietary Approaches to Stop Hypertension Study eating plan could benefit from consultation with a registered or licensed nutritionist to get them started.

§More than 1 drug may be required.

Table 6. Indications for Antihypertensive Drug Therapy in Children

Symptomatic hypertension
Secondary hypertension
Hypertensive target-organ damage
Diabetes (types 1 and 2)
Persistent hypertension despite nonpharmacologic measures

● Because of an association of sleep apnea with overweight and high BP, a sleep history should be obtained.

High BP in childhood had been considered a risk factor for hypertension in early adulthood. However, primary (essential) hypertension is now identifiable in children and adolescents. Primary hypertension in childhood is usually characterized by mild or stage 1 hypertension and is often associated with a positive family history of hypertension or cardiovascular disease (CVD). Children and adolescents with primary hypertension are frequently overweight. Data on healthy adolescents obtained in school health-screening programs demonstrate that the prevalence of hypertension increases progressively with increasing body mass index (BMI), and hypertension is detectable in ~30% of overweight children (BMI >95th percentile).[26] The strong association of high BP with obesity and the marked increase in the prevalence of childhood obesity[27] indicate that both hypertension and prehypertension are becoming a significant health issue in the young. Overweight children frequently have some degree of insulin resistance (a prediabetic condition). Overweight and high BP are also components of the insulin-resistance syndrome, or metabolic syndrome, a condition of multiple metabolic risk factors for CVD as well as for type 2 diabetes.[28,29] The clustering of other CVD risk factors that are included in the insulin-resistance syndrome (high triglycerides, low high-density lipoprotein cholesterol, truncal obesity, hyperinsulinemia) is significantly greater among children with high BP than in children with normal BP.[30] Recent reports from studies that examined childhood data estimate that the insulin-resistance syndrome is present in 30% of overweight children with BMI >95th percentile.[31] Historically, hypertension in childhood was considered a simple independent risk factor for CVD, but its link to the other risk factors in the insulin-resistance syndrome indicates that a broader approach is more appropriate in affected children.

Primary hypertension often clusters with other risk factors.[31,32] Therefore, the medical history, physical examination, and laboratory evaluation of hypertensive children and adolescents should include a comprehensive assessment for additional cardiovascular risk. These risk factors, in addition to high BP and overweight, include low plasma high-density lipoprotein cholesterol, elevated plasma triglyceride, and abnormal glucose tolerance. Fasting plasma insulin concentration is generally elevated, but an elevated insulin concentration may be reflective only of obesity and is not diagnostic of the insulin-resistance syndrome. To identify other cardiovascular risk factors, a fasting lipid panel and fasting glucose level should be obtained in children who are overweight and have BP between the 90th and 94th percentile and in all children with BP >95th percentile. If there is a strong family history of type 2 diabetes, a hemoglobin A1c or glucose tolerance test may also be considered. These metabolic risk factors should be repeated periodically to detect changes in the level of cardiovascular risk over time. Fewer data are available on the utility of other tests in children (eg, plasma uric acid or homocysteine and Lp[a] levels), and the use of these measures should depend on family history.

Sleep disorders including sleep apnea are associated with hypertension, coronary artery disease, heart failure, and stroke in adults.[33,34] Although limited data are available, they suggest an association of sleep-disordered breathing and higher BP in children.[35,36]

Approximately 15% of children snore, and at least 1% to 3% have sleep-disordered breathing.[35] Because of the associations with hypertension and the frequency of occurrence of sleep disorders, particularly among overweight children, a history of sleeping patterns should be obtained in a child with hypertension. One practical strategy for identifying children with a sleep problem or sleep disorder is to obtain a brief sleep history, using an instrument called BEARS.[37(table 1.1)] BEARS addresses 5 major sleep domains that provide a

Table 7. Clinical Evaluation of Confirmed Hypertension

Study or Procedure	Purpose	Target Population
Evaluation for identifiable causes		
History, including sleep history, family history, risk factors, diet, and habits such as smoking and drinking alcohol; physical examination	History and physical examination help focus subsequent evaluation	All children with persistent BP ≥95th percentile
BUN, creatinine, electrolytes, urinalysis, and urine culture	R/O renal disease and chronic pyelonephritis	All children with persistent BP ≥95th percentile
CBC	R/O anemia, consistent with chronic renal disease	All children with persistent BP ≥95th percentile
Renal U/S	R/O renal scar, congenital anomaly, or disparate renal size	All children with persistent BP ≥95th percentile
Evaluation for comorbidity		
Fasting lipid panel, fasting glucose	Identify hyperlipidemia, identify metabolic abnormalities	Overweight patients with BP at 90th–94th percentile; all patients with BP ≥95th percentile; family history of hypertension or CVD; child with chronic renal disease
Drug screen	Identify substances that might cause hypertension	History suggestive of possible contribution by substances or drugs.
Polysomnography	Identify sleep disorder in association with hypertension	History of loud, frequent snoring
Evaluation for target-organ damage		
Echocardiogram	Identify LVH and other indications of cardiac involvement	Patients with comorbid risk factors* and BP 90th–94th percentile; all patients with BP ≥95th percentile
Retinal exam	Identify retinal vascular changes	Patients with comorbid risk factors and BP 90th–94th percentile; all patients with BP ≥95th percentile
Additional evaluation as indicated		
ABPM	Identify white-coat hypertension, abnormal diurnal BP pattern, BP load	Patients in whom white-coat hypertension is suspected, and when other information on BP pattern is needed
Plasma renin determination	Identify low renin, suggesting mineralocorticoid-related disease	Young children with stage 1 hypertension and any child or adolescent with stage 2 hypertension
		Positive family history of severe hypertension
Renovascular imaging	Identify renovascular disease and any child or adolescent with stage 2 hypertension	Young children with stage 1 hypertension
Isotopic scintigraphy (renal scan) MRA Duplex Doppler flow studies 3-Dimensional CT Arteriography: DSA or classic		
Plasma and urine steroid levels	Identify steroid-mediated hypertension	Young children with stage 1 hypertension and any child or adolescent with stage 2 hypertension
Plasma and urine catecholamines	Identify catecholamine-mediated hypertension	Young children with stage 1 hypertension and any child or adolescent with stage 2 hypertension

BUN, blood urea nitrogen; CBC, complete blood count; R/O, rule out; U/S, ultrasound.

*Comorbid risk factors also include diabetes mellitus and kidney disease.

simple but comprehensive screen for the major sleep disorders affecting children 2 to 18 years old. The components of BEARS include: bedtime problems, excessive daytime sleepiness, awakenings during the night, regularity and duration of sleep, and sleep-disordered breathing (snoring). Each of these domains has an age-appropriate trigger question and includes responses of both parent and child as appropriate. This brief screening for sleep history can be completed in ~5 minutes.

In a child with primary hypertension, the presence of any comorbidity that is associated with hypertension carries the potential to increase the risk for CVD and can have an adverse effect on health outcome. Consideration of these associated risk factors and appropriate evaluation in those children in whom the hypertension is verified are important in planning and implementing therapies that reduce the comorbidity risk as well as control BP.

Evaluation for Secondary Hypertension

- Secondary hypertension is more common in children than in adults.
- Because overweight is strongly linked to hypertension, BMI should be calculated as part of the physical examination.
- Once hypertension is confirmed, BP should be measured in both arms and a leg.
- Very young children, children with stage 2 hypertension, and children or adolescents with clinical signs that suggest systemic conditions associated with hypertension should be evaluated more completely than in those with stage 1 hypertension.

Secondary hypertension is more common in children than in adults. The possibility that some underlying disorder may be the cause of the hypertension should be considered in every child or adolescent who has elevated BP. However, the extent of an evaluation for detection of a possible underlying cause should be individualized for each child. Very young children, children with stage 2 hypertension, and children or adolescents with clinical signs that suggest the presence of systemic conditions associated with hypertension should be evaluated more extensively, as compared with those with stage 1 hypertension.[38] Present technologies may facilitate less invasive evaluation than in the past, although experience in using newer modalities with children is still limited.

A thorough history and physical examination are the first steps in the evaluation of any child with persistently elevated BP. Elicited information should aim to identify not only signs and symptoms due to high BP but also clinical findings that might uncover an underlying systemic disorder. Thus, it is important to seek signs and symptoms suggesting renal disease (gross hematuria, edema, fatigue), heart disease (chest pain, exertional dyspnea, palpitations), and diseases of other organ systems (eg, endocrinologic, rheumatologic).

Past medical history should elicit information to focus the subsequent evaluation and to uncover definable causes of hypertension. Questions should be asked about prior hospitalizations, trauma, urinary tract infections, snoring and other sleep problems. Questions should address family history of hypertension, diabetes, obesity, sleep apnea, renal disease, other CVD (hyperlipidemia, stroke), and familial endocrinopathies. Many drugs can increase BP, so it is important to inquire directly about use of over-the-counter, prescription, and illicit drugs. Equally important are specific questions aimed at identifying the use of nutritional supplements, especially preparations aimed at enhancing athletic performance.

PHYSICAL EXAMINATION

The child's height, weight, and percentiles for age should be determined at the start of the physical examination. Because obesity is strongly linked to hypertension, BMI should be calculated from the height and weight, and the BMI percentile should be calculated. Poor growth may indicate an underlying chronic illness. When hypertension is confirmed, BP should be measured in both arms and in a leg. Normally, BP is 10 to 20 mm Hg higher in the legs than the arms. If the leg BP is lower than the arm BP or if femoral pulses are weak or absent, coarctation of the aorta may be present. Obesity alone is an insufficient explanation for diminished femoral pulses in the presence of high BP. The remainder of the physical examination should pursue clues found on history and should

Table 8. Examples of Physical Examination Findings Suggestive of Definable Hypertension

	Finding*	Possible Etiology
Vital signs	Tachycardia	Hyperthyroidism, pheochromocytoma, neuroblastoma, primary hypertension
	Decreased lower extremity pulses; drop in BP from upper to lower extremities	Coarctation of the aorta
Eyes	Retinal changes	Severe hypertension, more likely to be associated with secondary hypertension
Ear, nose, and throat	Adenotonsillar hypertrophy	Suggests association with sleep-disordered breathing (sleep apnea), snoring
Height/weight	Growth retardation	Chronic renal failure
	Obesity (high BMI)	Primary hypertension
	Truncal obesity	Cushing syndrome, insulin resistance syndrome
Head and neck	Moon facies	Cushing syndrome
	Elfin facies	Williams syndrome
	Webbed neck	Turner syndrome
	Thyromegaly	Hyperthyroidism
Skin	Pallor, flushing, diaphoresis	Pheochromocytoma
	Acne, hirsutism, striae	Cushing syndrome, anabolic steroid abuse
	Café-au-lait spots	Neurofibromatosis
	Adenoma sebaceum	Tuberous sclerosis
	Malar rash	Systemic lupus erythematosus
	Acanthrosis nigricans	Type 2 diabetes
Chest	Widely spaced nipples	Turner syndrome
	Heart murmur	Coarctation of the aorta
	Friction rub	Systemic lupus erythematosus (pericarditis), collagen-vascular disease, end stage renal disease with uremia
	Apical heave	LVH/chronic hypertension
Abdomen	Mass	Wilms tumor, neuroblastoma, pheochromocytoma
	Epigastric/flank bruit	Renal artery stenosis
	Palpable kidneys	Polycystic kidney disease, hydronephrosis, multicystic-dysplastic kidney, mass (see above)
Genitalia	Ambiguous/virilization	Adrenal hyperplasia
Extremities	Joint swelling	Systemic lupus erythematosus, collagen vascular disease
	Muscle weakness	Hyperaldosteronism, Liddle syndrome

Adapted from Flynn JT. *Prog Pediatr Cardiol.* 2001;12:177–188.

*Findings listed are examples of physical findings and do not represent all possible physical findings.

focus on findings that may indicate the cause and severity of hypertension. Table 8 lists important physical examination findings in hypertensive children.[39]

The physical examination in hypertensive children is frequently normal except for the BP elevation. The extent of the laboratory evaluation is based on the child's age, history, physical examination findings, and level of BP elevation. The majority of children with secondary hypertension will have renal or renovascular causes for the BP elevation. Therefore, screening tests are designed to have a high likelihood of detecting children and adolescents who are so affected. These tests are easily obtained in most primary care offices and community hospitals. Additional evaluation must be tailored to the specific child and situation. The risk factors, or comorbid conditions, associated with primary hypertension should be included in the evaluation of hypertension in all children, as well as efforts to determine any evidence of target-organ damage.

ADDITIONAL DIAGNOSTIC STUDIES FOR HYPERTENSION

Additional diagnostic studies may be appropriate in the evaluation of hypertension in a child or adolescent, particularly if there is a high degree of suspicion that an underlying disorder is present. Such procedures are listed in Table 7. ABPM, discussed previously, has application in evaluating both primary and secondary hypertension. ABPM is also used to detect white-coat hypertension.

RENIN PROFILING

Plasma renin level or plasma renin activity (PRA) is a useful screening test for mineralocorticoid-related diseases. With these disorders, the PRA is very low or unmeasurable by the laboratory and may be associated with relative hypokalemia. PRA levels are higher in patients who have renal artery stenosis. However, ~15% of children with arteriographically evident renal artery stenosis have normal PRA values.[40-42] Assays for direct measurement of renin, a different technique than PRA, are commonly used, although extensive normative data in children and adolescents are unavailable.

EVALUATION FOR POSSIBLE RENOVASCULAR HYPERTENSION

Renovascular hypertension is a consequence of an arterial lesion or lesions impeding blood flow to 1 or both kidneys or to ≥1 intrarenal segments.[43,44] Affected children usually, but not invariably, have markedly elevated BP.[40,44] Evaluation for renovascular disease also should be considered in infants or children with other known predisposing factors such as prior umbilical artery catheter placements or neurofibromatosis.[44,45] A number of newer diagnostic techniques are presently available for evaluation of renovascular disease, but experience in their use in pediatric patients is limited. Consequently, the recommended approaches generally use older techniques such as standard intraarterial angiography, digital-subtraction angiography (DSA), and scintigraphy (with or without angiotensin-converting enzyme [ACE] inhibition).[44] As technologies evolve, children should be referred for imaging studies to centers that have expertise in the radiologic evaluation of childhood hypertension.

INVASIVE STUDIES

Intraarterial DSA with contrast is used more frequently than standard angiography, but because of intraarterial injection, this method remains invasive. DSA can be accomplished also by using a rapid injection of contrast into a peripheral vein, but quality of views and the size of pediatric veins make this technique useful only for older children. DSA and formal arteriography are still considered the "gold standard," but these studies should be undertaken only when surgical or invasive interventional radiologic techniques are being contemplated for anatomic correction.[46]

Newer imaging techniques may be used in children with vascular lesions. Magnetic resonance angiography (MRA) is increasingly feasible for the evaluation of pediatric renovascular disease, but it is still best for detecting abnormalities in the main renal artery and its primary branches.[47-49] Imaging with magnetic resonance requires that the patient be relatively immobile for extended periods, which is a significant difficulty for small children. At present, studies are needed to assess the effectiveness of MRA in the diagnosis of children with renovascular disease. Newer methods, including 3-dimensional reconstructions of computed tomography (CT) images, or spiral CT with contrast, seem promising in evaluating children who may have renovascular disease.[50]

Target-Organ Abnormalities in Childhood Hypertension

- Target-organ abnormalities are commonly associated with hypertension in children and adolescents.
- Left ventricular hypertrophy (LVH) is the most prominent evidence of target-organ damage.
- Pediatric patients with established hypertension should have echocardiographic assessment of left ventricular mass at diagnosis and periodically thereafter.

● The presence of LVH is an indication to initiate or intensify antihypertensive therapy.

Hypertension is associated with increased risk of myocardial infarction, stroke, and cardiovascular mortality in adults,[2,51] and treatment of elevated BP results in a reduction in the risk for cardiovascular events.

Children and adolescents with severe elevation of BP are also at increased risk of adverse outcomes, including hypertensive encephalopathy, seizures, and even cerebrovascular accidents and congestive heart failure.[52,53] Even hypertension that is less severe contributes to target-organ damage when it occurs with other chronic conditions such as chronic kidney disease.[54-56] Two autopsy studies[57,58] that evaluated tissue from adolescents and young adults who had sudden deaths due to trauma demonstrated significant relationships between the level of BP, or hypertension, and the presence of atherosclerotic lesions in the aorta and coronary arteries. The exact level and duration of BP elevation that causes target-organ damage in the young has not been established.

One difficulty in the assessment of these relationships is that, until recently, few noninvasive methods could evaluate the effect of hypertension on the cardiovascular system. Noninvasive techniques that use ultrasound can demonstrate structural and functional changes in the vasculature related to BP. Recent clinical studies using these techniques demonstrate that childhood levels of BP are associated with carotid intimal-medial thickness[59] and large artery compliance[60] in young adults. Even healthy adolescents with clustering of cardiovascular risk factors demonstrate elevated carotid thickness,[61,62] and those with BP levels at the higher end of the normal distribution show decreased brachial artery flow-mediated vasodilatation. Overall, evidence is increasing that even mild BP elevation can have an adverse effect on vascular structure and function[63] in asymptomatic young persons.

LVH is the most prominent clinical evidence of target-organ damage caused by hypertension in children and adolescents. With the use of echocardiography to measure left ventricular mass, LVH has been reported in 34% to 38% of children and adolescents with mild, untreated BP elevation.[64-66] Daniels et al[67] evaluated 130 children and adolescents with persistent BP elevation. They reported that 55% of patients had a left ventricular mass index >90th percentile, and 14% had left ventricular mass index >51 g/m$^{2.7}$, a value in adults with hypertension that has been associated with a fourfold greater risk of adverse cardiovascular outcomes. When left ventricular geometry was examined in hypertensive children, 17% had concentric hypertrophy, a pattern that is associated with higher risk for cardiovascular outcomes in adults, and 30% had eccentric hypertrophy, which is associated with intermediate risk for cardiovascular outcomes.[67]

In addition, abnormalities of the retinal vasculature have been reported in adults with hypertension.[68] Few studies of retinal abnormalities have been conducted in children with hypertension. Skalina et al[69] evaluated newborns with hypertension and reported the presence of hypertensive retinal abnormalities in ~50% of their patients. On repeat examination, after the resolution of hypertension, these abnormalities had disappeared.

CLINICAL RECOMMENDATION

Echocardiography is recommended as a primary tool for evaluating patients for target-organ abnormalities by assessing the presence or absence of LVH. Left ventricular mass is determined from standard echocardiographic measurements of the left ventricular end-diastolic dimension, the intraventricular septal thickness, and the thickness of the left ventricular posterior wall and can be calculated as: left ventricle mass (g) = 0.80 [1.04(intraventricular septal thickness + left ventricular end-diastolic dimension + left ventricular posterior wall thickness)^3 − (left ventricular end-diastolic dimension)^3] + 0.6 (with echocardiographic measurements in centimeters). From these measures, the left ventricular mass can be calculated by using the equation of Devereux et al[70] when measurements are made according to the criteria of the American Society of Echocardiography.[71]

Heart size is closely associated with body size.[72] Left ventricular mass index is calculated to standardize measurements of left ventricular mass.

Several methods for indexing left ventricular mass have been reported, but it is recommended that height ($m^{2.7}$) be used to index left ventricular mass as described by de Simone et al.[73] This method accounts for close to the equivalent of the effect of lean body mass and excludes the effect of obesity and BP elevation on left ventricular mass. Some echo laboratories use height as the indexing variable. This calculation is also acceptable and is somewhat easier to use, because fewer calculations are needed.

Children and adolescents with established hypertension should have an echocardiogram to determine if LVH is present. A conservative cutpoint that determines the presence of LVH is 51 $g/m^{2.7}$. This cutpoint is >99th percentile for children and adolescents and is associated with increased morbidity in adults with hypertension.[73] Other references exist for normal children,[74] but unlike adults, outcome-based standards for left ventricular mass index are not available for children. In interpreting the left ventricular mass index, it should be remembered that some factors such as obesity and hypertension have pathologic effects on the heart, whereas others (such as physical activity, particularly in highly conditioned athletes) may be adaptive.

Ascertainment of left ventricular mass index is very helpful in clinical decision-making. The presence of LVH can be an indication for initiating or intensifying pharmacologic therapy to lower BP. For patients who have LVH, the echocardiographic determination of left ventricular mass index should be repeated periodically.

At the present time, additional testing for other target-organ abnormalities (such as determination of carotid intimal-medial thickness and evaluation of urine for microalbuminuria) is not recommended for routine clinical use. Additional research will be needed to evaluate the clinical utility of these tests.

Therapeutic Lifestyle Changes

- Weight reduction is the primary therapy for obesity-related hypertension. Prevention of excess or abnormal weight gain will limit future increases in BP.

- Regular physical activity and restriction of sedentary activity will improve efforts at weight management and may prevent an excess increase in BP over time.
- Dietary modification should be strongly encouraged in children and adolescents who have BP levels in the prehypertensive range as well as those with hypertension.
- Family-based intervention improves success.

Evidence that supports the efficacy of nonpharmacologic interventions for BP reduction in the treatment of hypertension in children and adolescents is limited. Data that demonstrate a relationship of lifestyle with BP can be used as the basis for recommendations. On the basis of large, randomized, controlled trials, the following lifestyle modifications are recommended in adults[2]: weight reduction in overweight or obese individuals[75]; increased intake of fresh vegetables, fruits, and low-fat dairy (the Dietary Approaches to Stop Hypertension Study eating plan)[76]; dietary sodium reduction[76,77]; increased physical activity[78]; and moderation of alcohol consumption.[79] Smoking cessation has significant cardiovascular benefits.[32] As information on chronic sleep problems evolves, interventions to improve sleep quality also may have a beneficial effect on BP.[80]

The potential for control of BP in children through weight reduction is supported by BP tracking and weight-reduction studies. BP levels track from childhood through adolescence and into adulthood[81-83] in association with weight.[84,85] Because of the strong correlation between weight and BP, excessive weight gain is likely to be associated with elevated BP over time. Therefore, maintenance of normal weight gain in childhood should lead to less hypertension in adulthood.

Weight loss in overweight adolescents is associated with a decrease in BP.[30,86-90] Weight control not only decreases BP, it also decreases BP sensitivity to salt[88] and decreases other cardiovascular risk factors such as dyslipidemia and insulin resistance.[32] In studies that achieve a reduction in BMI of ~10%, short-term reductions in BP were in the range of 8 to 12 mm Hg. Although difficult, weight loss, if successful, is extremely effective.[32,91-93] Identifying a complication of overweight such as hypertension can be a helpful motivator for patients and families to make changes. Weight control can render pharmacologic treatment unnecessary but should not delay drug use when indicated.

Emphasis on the management of complications rather than on overweight shifts the aim of weight management from an aesthetic to a health goal. In motivated families, education or simple behavior modification can be successful in achieving moderate weight loss or preventing additional weight gain. Steps can be implemented in the primary care setting even with limited staff and time resources.[32,91] The patient should be encouraged to self-monitor time spent in sedentary activities, including watching television and playing video or computer games, and set goals to progressively decrease these activities to <2 hours per day.[94] The family and patient should identify physical activities that the child enjoys, engage in them regularly, and self-monitor time spent in physical activities (30–60 minutes per day should be achieved).[94-96] Dietary changes can involve portion-size control, decrease in consumption of sugar-containing beverages and energy-dense snacks, increase in consumption of fresh fruits and vegetables, and regular meals including a healthy breakfast.[32,91,93,97,98] Consultation with a nutritionist can be useful and provide customized recommendations. During regular office visits, the primary care provider can supervise the child's progress in self-monitoring and accomplishing goals and provide support and positive feedback to the family. Some patients will benefit from a more intense and comprehensive approach to weight management from a multidisciplinary and specialized team if available.[91-93]

Despite the lack of firm evidence about dietary intervention in children, it is generally accepted that hypertensive individuals can benefit from a dietary increase in fresh vegetables, fresh fruits, fiber, and nonfat dairy as well as a reduction of sodium. Despite some suggestion that calcium supplements may decrease BP in children,[99,100] thus far the evidence is too limited to support a clinical recommendation.[101] Lower BP has been associated in children and adolescents with an increased intake of potassium,[100-103] magnesium,[100,101] folic acid,[101,104] unsaturated

fat,[100,105,106] and fiber[100,101,104] and lower dietary intake of total fat.[100,101] However, these associations are small and insufficient to support dietary recommendations for specific, individual nutrients.

Sodium reduction in children and adolescents has been associated with small reductions in BP in the range of 1 to 3 mm Hg.[100,103,107-110] Data from 1 randomized trial suggest that sodium intake in infancy may affect BP in adolescence.[111] Similarly, some evidence indicates that breast-feeding may be associated with lower BP in childhood.[112,113] The current recommendation for adequate daily sodium intake is only 1.2 g/day for 4- to 8-year-olds and 1.5 g/day for older children.[114] Because this amount of sodium is substantially lower than current dietary intakes, lowering dietary sodium from the current usual intake may have future benefit. Reduced sodium intake, with calorie restriction, may account for some of the BP improvement associated with weight loss.

Regular physical activity has cardiovascular benefits. A recent meta-analysis that combined 12 randomized trials, for a total of 1266 children and adolescents, concluded that physical activity leads to a small but not statistically significant decrease in BP.[115] However, both regular physical activity and decreasing sedentary activities (such as watching television and playing video or electronic games) are important components of pediatric obesity treatment and prevention.[32,91-93] Weight-reduction trials consistently report better results when physical activity and/or prevention of sedentary activity are included in the treatment protocol. Therefore, regular aerobic physical activity (30–60 minutes of moderate physical activity on most days) and limitation of sedentary activities to <2 hours per day are recommended for the prevention of obesity, hypertension, and other cardiovascular risk factors.[94-96] With the exception of power lifting, resistance training is also helpful. Competitive sports participation should be limited only in the presence of uncontrolled stage 2 hypertension.[116]

The scope of hypertension as a public health problem in adults is substantial. Poor health-related behaviors such as physical inactivity, unfavorable dietary patterns, and excessive weight gain raise the risk for future hypertension. The therapeutic lifestyle changes discussed previously may have benefit for all children in prevention of future disease, including primary hypertension. Accordingly, appropriate health recommendations for all children and adolescents are regular physical activity; a diet with limited sodium but rich in fresh fruits, fresh vegetables, fiber, and low-fat dairy; and avoiding excess weight gain.

Pharmacologic Therapy of Childhood Hypertension

- Indications for antihypertensive drug therapy in children include secondary hypertension and insufficient response to lifestyle modifications.
- Recent clinical trials have expanded the number of drugs that have pediatric dosing information. Dosing recommendations for many of the newer drugs are provided.
- Pharmacologic therapy, when indicated, should be initiated with a single drug. Acceptable drug classes for use in children include ACE inhibitors, angiotensin-receptor blockers, β-blockers, calcium channel blockers, and diuretics.
- The goal for antihypertensive treatment in children should be reduction of BP to <95th percentile unless concurrent conditions are present, in which case BP should be lowered to <90th percentile.
- Severe, symptomatic hypertension should be treated with intravenous antihypertensive drugs.

In adults, hypertension is typically a life-long condition. Most hypertensive patients will need to remain on medications for the rest of their lives. Usually, adults readily accept this fact, given the known long-term adverse consequences of untreated or undertreated hypertension.[117] In children, however, the long-term consequences of untreated hypertension are unknown. Additionally, no data are available on the long-term effects of antihypertensive drugs on growth and development. Therefore, a definite indication for initiating pharmacologic therapy should be ascertained before a drug is prescribed.

Table 6 summarizes the indications for use of antihypertensive drugs in children. These indications include symptomatic hypertension, secondary hypertension, established hypertensive target-organ damage, and failure of nonpharmacologic measures. Other indications for use of antihypertensive drugs can be considered depending on the clinical situation. For example, because the presence of multiple cardiovascular risk factors (elevated BP, dyslipidemia, tobacco use, etc) increases cardiovascular risk in an exponential rather than additive fashion,[118,119] antihypertensive therapy could be considered if the child or adolescent is known to have dyslipidemia.

The number of antihypertensive drugs has increased since the publication of the first task force report on BP control in children.[120] The number of drugs that have been studied systematically in children has increased also, largely because of incentives provided to the pharmaceutical industry under the auspices of the 1997 Food and Drug Administration Modernization Act (FDAMA) and the 2002 Best Pharmaceuticals for Children Act.[121-123] These developments have had both negative and positive consequences. Chief among the negative consequences is the lack of reliable pediatric data for older, commonly used compounds with expired patent protection. Currently, no incentives exist for industry-sponsored trials of such drugs, and alternative methods of stimulating pediatric studies such as those contained in the Best Pharmaceuticals for Children Act[123-125] have yet to come to fruition. On the other hand, publication of the results of industry-sponsored clinical trials and single-center case series will provide additional data that can be combined with prior recommendations based on expert opinion and collective clinical experience to guide the use of antihypertensive drugs in children and adolescents who require pharmacologic treatment.

Table 9 contains dosing recommendations for antihypertensive drugs in children 1–17 years old. It should be noted that many other drugs are available in addition to those listed in Table 9. Those drugs are not included in the table, however, because few or no pediatric data were available at the time this report was prepared.

Table 9. Antihypertensive Drugs for Outpatient Management of Hypertension in Children 1–17 Years Old*

Class	Drug	Dose†	Dosing Interval	Evidence‡	FDA Labeling§	Comments
ACE inhibitor	Benazepril	Initial: 0.2 mg/kg per d up to 10 mg/d Maximum: 0.6 mg/kg per d up to 40 mg/d	qd	RCT	Yes	1. All ACE inhibitors are contraindicated in pregnancy; females of childbearing age should use reliable contraception. 2. Check serum potassium and creatinine periodically to monitor for hyperkalemia and azotemia. 3. Cough and angioedema are reportedly less common with newer members of this class than with captopril. 4. Benazepril, enalapril, and lisinopril labels contain information on the preparation of a suspension; captopril may also be compounded into a suspension. 5. FDA approval for ACE inhibitors with pediatric labeling is limited to children ≥6 years of age and to children with creatinine clearance ≥30 ml/min per 1.73m².
	Captopril	Initial: 0.3–0.5 mg/kg/dose Maximum: 6 mg/kg per d	tid	RCT, CS	No	
	Enalapril	Initial: 0.08 mg/kg per d up to 5 mg/d Maximum: 0.6 mg/kg per d up to 40 mg/d	qd–bid	RCT	Yes	
	Fosinopril	Children >50 kg: Initial: 5–10 mg/d Maximum: 40 mg/d	qd	RCT	Yes	
	Lisinopril	Initial: 0.07 mg/kg per d up to 5 mg/d Maximum: 0.6 mg/kg per d up to 40 mg/d	qd	RCT	Yes	
	Quinapril	Initial: 5–10 mg/d Maximum: 80 mg/d	qd	RCT, EO	No	
Angiotensin-receptor blocker	Irbesartan	6–12 years: 75–150 mg/d ≥13 years: 150–300 mg/d	qd	CS	Yes	1. All ARBs are contraindicated in pregnancy; females of childbearing age should use reliable contraception. 2. Check serum potassium, creatinine periodically to monitor for hyperkalemia and azotemia. 3. Losartan label contains information on the preparation of a suspension. 4. FDA approval for ARBs is limited to children ≥6 years of age and to children with creatinine clearance ≥30 ml/min per 1.73m².
	Losartan	Initial: 0.7 mg/kg per d up to 50 mg/d Maximum: 1.4 mg/kg per d up to 100 mg/d	qd	RCT	Yes	
α- and β-Blocker	Labetalol	Initial: 1–3 mg/kg per d Maximum: 10–12 mg/kg per d up to 1200 mg/d	bid	CS, EO	No	1. Asthma and overt heart failure are contraindications. 2. Heart rate is dose-limiting. 3. May impair athletic performance. 4. Should not be used in insulin-dependent diabetics.
β-Blocker	Atenolol	Initial: 0.5–1 mg/kg per d Maximum: 2 mg/kg per d up to 100 mg/d	qd–bid	CS	No	1. Noncardioselective agents (propranolol) are contraindicated in asthma and heart failure. 2. Heart rate is dose-limiting. 3. May impair athletic performance. 4. Should not be used in insulin-dependent diabetics. 5. A sustained-release formulation of propranolol is available that is dosed once-daily.
	Bisoprolol/HCTZ	Initial: 2.5/6.25 mg/d Maximum: 10/6.25 mg/d	qd	RCT	No	
	Metoprolol	Initial: 1–2 mg/kg per d Maximum: 6 mg/kg per d up to 200 mg/d	bid	CS	No	
	Propranolol	Initial: 1–2 mg/kg per d Maximum: 4 mg/kg per d up to 640 mg/d	bid–tid	RCT, EO	Yes	
Calcium channel blocker	Amlodipine	Children 6–17 years: 2.5–5 mg once daily	qd	RCT	Yes	1. Amlodipine and isradipine can be compounded into stable extemporaneous suspensions. 2. Felodipine and extended-release nifedipine tablets must be swallowed whole. 3. Isradipine is available in both immediate-release and sustained-release formulations; sustained-release form is dosed qd or bid. 4. May cause tachycardia.
	Felodipine	Initial: 2.5 mg/d Maximum: 10 mg/d	qd	RCT, EO	No	
	Isradipine	Initial: 0.15–0.2 mg/kg per d Maximum: 0.8 mg/kg per d up to 20 mg/d	tid–qid	CS, EO	No	
	Extended-release nifedipine	Initial: 0.25–0.5 mg/kg per d Maximum: 3 mg/kg per d up to 120 mg/d	qd–bid	CS, EO	No	

Table 9. Antihypertensive Drugs for Outpatient Management of Hypertension in Children 1–17 Years Old*

Class	Drug	Dose†	Dosing Interval	Evidence‡	FDA Labeling§	Comments
Central α-agonist	Clonidine	Children ≥12 years: Initial: 0.2 mg/d Maximum: 2.4 mg/d	bid	EO	Yes	1. May cause dry mouth and/or sedation. 2. Transdermal preparation also available. 3. Sudden cessation of therapy can lead to severe rebound hypertension.
Diuretic	HCTZ	Initial: 1 mg/kg per d Maximum: 3 mg/kg per d up to 50 mg/d	qd	EO	Yes	1. All patients treated with diuretics should have electrolytes monitored shortly after initiating therapy and periodically thereafter. 2. Useful as add-on therapy in patients being treated with drugs from other drug classes. 3. Potassium-sparing diuretics (spironolactone, triamterene, amiloride) may cause severe hyperkalemia, especially if given with ACE inhibitor or ARB. 4. Furosemide is labeled only for treatment of edema but may be useful as add-on therapy in children with resistant hypertension, particularly in children with renal disease. 5. Chlorthalidone may precipitate azotemia in patients with renal diseases and should be used with caution in those with severe renal impairment.
	Chlorthalidone	Initial: 0.3 mg/kg per d Maximum: 2 mg/kg per d up to 50 mg/d	qd	EO	No	
	Furosemide	Initial: 0.5–2.0 mg/kg per dose Maximum: 6 mg/kg per d	qd-bid	EO	No	
	Spironolactone	Initial: 1 mg/kg per d Maximum: 3.3 mg/kg per d up to 100 mg/d	qd-bid	EO	No	
	Triamterene	Initial: 1–2 mg/kg per d Maximum: 3–4 mg/kg per d up to 300 mg/d	bid	EO	No	
	Amiloride	Initial: 0.4–0.625 mg/kg per d Maximum: 20 mg/d	qd	EO	No	
Peripheral α-antagonist	Doxazosin	Initial: 1 mg/d Maximum: 4 mg/d	qd	EO	No	May cause hypotension and syncope, especially after first dose.
	Prazosin	Initial: 0.05–0.1 mg/kg per d Maximum: 0.5 mg/kg per d	tid	EO	No	
	Terazosin	Initial: 1 mg/d Maximum: 20 mg/d	qd	EO	No	
Vasodilator	Hydralazine	Initial: 0.75 mg/kg per d Maximum: 7.5 mg/kg per d up to 200 mg/d	qid	EO	Yes	1. Tachycardia and fluid retention are common side effects. 2. Hydralazine can cause a lupus-like syndrome in slow acetylators. 3. Prolonged use of minoxidil can cause hypertrichosis. 4. Minoxidil is usually reserved for patients with hypertension resistant to multiple drugs.
	Minoxidil	Children <12 years: Initial: 0.2 mg/kg per d Maximum: 50 mg/d Children ≥12 years: Initial: 5 mg/d Maximum: 100 mg/d	qd-tid	CS, EO	Yes	

FDA indicates Federal Drug Administration; ARB indicates angiotensin-receptor blocker; bid, twice daily; HCTZ, hydrochlorothiazide; qd, once daily; qid, four times daily; tid, three times daily.

*Includes drugs with prior pediatric experience or recently completed clinical trials.

†The maximum recommended adult dose should not be exceeded in routine clinical practice.

‡Level of evidence upon which dosing recommendations are based. CS indicates case series; EO, expert opinion; RCT, randomized controlled trial.

§FDA-approved pediatric labeling information is available. Recommended doses for agents with FDA-approved pediatric labels are the doses contained in the approved labels. Even when pediatric labeling information is not available, the FDA-approved label should be consulted for additional safety information.

‖Comments apply to all members of each drug class except where otherwise stated.

Long-term clinical endpoint data from randomized trials such as the Antihypertensive and Lipid-Lowering Treatment to Prevent Heart Attack Trial support the preferential use of specific antihypertensive drugs in adults.[2,126] However, pediatric clinical trials of antihypertensive drugs have focused only on their ability to lower BP and have not compared the effects of these drugs on clinical endpoints. Therefore, because all classes of antihypertensive drugs have been shown to lower BP in children, the choice of drug for initial antihypertensive therapy resides in the preference of the responsible physician. Some diuretics and β-adrenergic blockers, which were recommended as initial therapy in the first and second task force reports,[25,120] have a long history of safety and efficacy based on clinical experience in hypertensive children, and these drugs remain appropriate for pediatric use. Similarly, some members of the newer classes of antihypertensive drugs, including ACE inhibitors, calcium channel blockers, and angiotensin-receptor blockers,[127-130] have been studied in children and, based on short-term use, shown to be safe and well-tolerated with satisfactory BP reductions in hypertensive children.

Specific classes of antihypertensive drugs should be used preferentially in certain hypertensive children with specific underlying or concurrent medical conditions. Examples include the use of ACE inhibitors or angiotensin-receptor blockers in children with diabetes and microalbuminuria or proteinuric renal diseases, and the use of β-adrenergic blockers or calcium channel blockers in hypertensive children with migraine headaches. This approach is similar to that outlined in the recent JNC 7 report, which recommends specific classes of antihypertensive drugs for use in adults in certain high-risk categories.[2]

All antihypertensive drugs should be prescribed in a similar fashion: The child is initially started on the lowest recommended dose listed in Table 9. The dose can be increased until the desired BP goal is achieved. Once the highest recommended dose is reached, or if the child experiences side effects from the drug, a second drug from a different class should be added. Consideration should be given to combining drugs with complementary mechanisms of action such as an ACE inhibitor with a diuretic or a vasodilator with a diuretic or β-adrenergic blocker. Because little pediatric experience is available in using fixed-dose combination products, except for bisoprolol/hydrochlorothiazide,[131] routine use of these products in children cannot be recommended at this time.

For children with uncomplicated primary hypertension and no hypertensive target-organ damage, the goal BP should be <95th percentile for gender, age, and height, whereas for children with chronic renal disease, diabetes, or hypertensive target-organ damage, the goal BP should be <90th percentile for gender, age, and height. Again, this approach is similar to the recommended treatment of hypertension in adults with additional cardiovascular risk factors or comorbid conditions.[2]

Important adjunctive aspects to the drug therapy of childhood hypertension include ongoing monitoring of target-organ damage as well as BP monitoring, surveillance for drug side effects, periodic monitoring of electrolytes in children treated with ACE inhibitors or diuretics, counseling regarding other cardiovascular risk factors, and continued emphasis on nonpharmacologic measures. It also may be appropriate to consider "step-down" therapy in selected patients. This approach attempts a gradual reduction in the drug after an extended course of good BP control, with the eventual goal of completely discontinuing drug therapy. Children with uncomplicated primary hypertension, especially overweight children who successfully lose weight, are the best candidates for the step-down approach. Such patients require ongoing BP monitoring after the cessation of drug therapy as well as continued nonpharmacologic treatment, because hypertension may recur.

Severe, symptomatic hypertension with BP well above the 99th percentile occurs in some children, usually those with underlying renal disease, and requires prompt treatment. Hypertensive emergencies in children are usually accompanied by signs of hypertensive encephalopathy, typically causing seizures. Hypertensive emergencies should be treated by an intravenous antihypertensive that can produce a controlled reduction in BP, aiming to decrease the pressure by ≤25% over the first 8 hours after presentation and then gradually normalizing the BP over 26 to 48 hours.[132,133] Hypertensive urgencies are accompanied by less serious symptoms such as severe headache or vomiting. Hypertensive urgencies can be treated by either intravenous or oral antihypertensives depending on the child's symptomatology. Table 10 provides dosing recommendations for treatment of severe hypertension in children when prompt reduction in BP is indicated.

Figure 1 is a management algorithm that presents guidelines for evaluation and treatment of stage 1 and stage 2 hypertension in children and adolescents. The algorithm summarizes monitoring and intervention recommendations for children and adolescents with prehypertension and hypertension. Included in the algorithm are points at which the presence of overweight is considered in clinical decision-making. The algorithm also emphasizes the inclusion of evaluation for target-organ damage in children with established stage 1 and stage 2 hypertension.

Table 10. Antihypertensive Drugs for Management of Severe Hypertension in Children 1–17 Years Old

Drug	Class	Dose*	Route	Comments
Most useful[†]				
Esmolol	β-Blocker	100–500 µg/kg per min	IV infusion	Very short-acting; constant infusion preferred. May cause profound bradycardia. Produced modest reductions in BP in a pediatric clinical trial.
Hydralazine	Vasodilator	0.2–0.6 mg/kg per dose	IV, IM	Should be given every 4 h when given IV bolus. Recommended dose is lower than FDA label.
Labetalol	α- and β-Blocker	Bolus: 0.2–1.0 mg/kg per dose up to 40 mg/dose Infusion: 0.25–3.0 mg/kg per h	IV bolus or infusion	Asthma and overt heart failure are relative contraindications.
Nicardipine	Calcium channel blocker	1–3 µg/kg per min	IV infusion	May cause reflex tachycardia.
Sodium nitroprusside	Vasodilator	0.53–10 µg/kg per min	IV infusion	Monitor cyanide levels with prolonged (>72 h) use or in renal failure; or coadminister with sodium thiosulfate.
Occasionally useful[‡]				
Clonidine	Central α-agonist	0.05–0.1 mg/dose, may be repeated up to 0.8 mg total dose	po	Side effects include dry mouth and sedation.
Enalaprilat	ACE inhibitor	0.05–0.1 mg/kg per dose up to 1.25 mg/dose	IV bolus	May cause prolonged hypotension and acute renal failure, especially in neonates.
Fenoldopam	Dopamine receptor agonist	0.2–0.8 µg/kg per min	IV infusion	Produced modest reductions in BP in a pediatric clinical trial in patients up to 12 years
Isradipine	Calcium channel blocker	0.05–0.1 mg/kg per dose	po	Stable suspension can be compounded.
Minoxidil	Vasodilator	0.1–0.2 mg/kg per dose	po	Most potent oral vasodilator, longacting.

FDA indicates Food and Drug Administration; IM, intramuscular; IV, intravenous; po, oral.

*All dosing recommendations are based on expert opinion or case series data except as otherwise noted.

[†]Useful for hypertensive emergencies and some hypertensive urgencies.

[‡]Useful for hypertensive urgencies and some hypertensive emergencies.

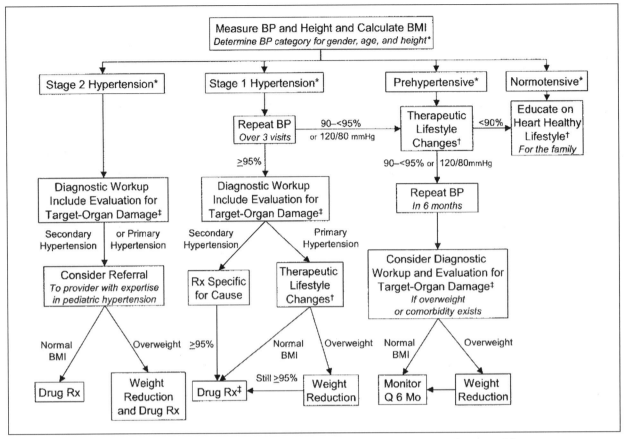

Figure 1. Management algorithm. Rx indicates prescription; Q, every. *, See Tables 3, 4, and 5; †, diet modification and physical activity; ‡, especially if younger, very high BP, little or no family history, diabetic, or other risk factors.

Appendix A. Demographic Data

See page 153.

Appendix B. Computation of Blood Pressure Percentiles for Arbitrary Gender, Age, and Height

To compute the SBP percentile of a boy who is age y years and height h inches with SBP = x mm Hg:

1. Refer to the most recent Centers for Disease Control and Prevention growth charts, which are available online, and convert the height of h inches to a height Z score relative to boys of the same age; this is denoted by Zht.

2. Compute the expected SBP (μ) for boys of age y years and height h inches given by

$$\mu = \alpha + \sum_{j=1}^{4} \beta_j(y-10)^j + \sum_{k=1}^{4} \gamma_k(Zht)^k$$

where α, $\beta_1...\beta_4$ and $\gamma_1... \gamma_4$ are given in the third column of Table B1.

3. Then convert the boy's observed SBP to a Z score (Zbp) given by $Zbp=(x-\mu)/\sigma$, where σ is given in the third column of Table B1.

4. To convert the BP Z score to a percentile (P), compute $P = \Phi(Zbp) \infty 100\%$, where $\Phi(Z)$ = area under a standard normal distribution to the left of Z. Thus, if Zbp = 1.28, then $\Phi(Zbp)$ = 0.90 and the BP percentile = 0.90 ∞ 100% = 90%.

5. To compute percentiles for SBP for girls, DBP (K5) for boys, and DBP (K5) for girls, use the regression coefficients from the fourth, fifth, and sixth columns of Table B1.

    For example, a 12-year-old boy, with height at the 90th percentile for his age-gender group, has a height Z score = 1.28, and his expected SBP (μ) is μ = 102.19768 + 1.82416(2) + 0.12776(2²) + 0.00249(2³) − 0.00135(2⁴) + 2.73157(1.28) − 0.19618(1.28)² − 0.04659(1.28)³ + 0.00947(1.28)⁴ = 109.46 mm Hg. Suppose his actual SBP is 120 mm Hg (x); his SBP Z score then equals

Appendix A. Demographic Data on Height/Blood Pressure Distribution Curves by Study Population

Source	Age, y	Gender		Ethnic Group							Persons Visits SBP Available		Persons Visits DBP.5 Available		Total No. of Persons Visits	
		Male	Female	Black	Hispanic	White	Asian	Native American	Other	Missing	Persons	Visits	Persons	Visits	Persons	Visits
National Institutes of Health	6–17	1896	1751	600	0	2963	0	0	84	0	3647	3647	3609	3609	3647	3647
Pittsburgh	1–5	148	137	108	0	176	0	0	0	1	285	893	0	0	285	893
Dallas	13–17	5916	5649	5266	1570	4729	0	0	0	0	11 565	21 860	11 565	21 852	11 565	21 860
Bogalusa	1–17	3751	3607	2480	0	4878	0	0	0	0	7358	15 882	0	0	7358	15 882
Houston	3–17	1457	1377	637	1341	748	23	0	0	85	2834	2834	0	0	2834	2834
South Carolina	4–17	3167	3263	3110	0	3320	0	0	0	0	6430	6430	6368	6368	6430	6430
Iowa	5–17	2099	1993	0	0	4092	0	0	0	0	4092	4092	0	0	4092	4092
Providence	1–3	230	231	24	4	431	0	0	2	0	461	898	371	560	461	898
Minnesota	9–17	9991	9418	3422	555	11 311	1677	644	1800	0	19 409	19 409	19 207	19 207	19 409	19 409
NHANES III	5–17	2465	2577	1770	1830	1324	64	10	12	32	5042	5042	4304	4304	5042	5042
NHANES 1999–2000	8–17	1041	1063	605	988	437	0	0	74	0	2104	2104	2076	2076	2104	2104
Total (percent of total)	1–17	32 161 (51)	31 066 (49)	18 022 (29)	6288 (10)	34 409 (54)	1764 (3)	654 (1)	1972 (3)	118 (0)	63 227	83 091	47 500	57 976	63 227	83 091

DBP .5, DBP (Korotkoff 5).

Table differs from the 1997 report: updated height percentile used; subjects whose height Z score was less than –6 or greater than 6 were excluded.

Table B1. Regression Coefficients From Blood Pressure Regression Models

Variable Name	Symbol	Systolic BP		Diastolic BP5	
		Male	Female	Male	Female
Intercept	α	102.19768	102.01027	61.01217	60.50510
Age					
Age–10	β_1	1.82416	1.94397	0.68314	1.01301
$(Age–10)^2$	β_2	0.12776	0.00598	0.09835	0.01157
$(Age–10)^3$	β_3	0.00249	0.00789	0.01711	0.00424
$(Age–10)^4$	β_4	0.00135	0.00059	0.00045	0.00137
Normalized height					
Zht	y_1	2.73157	2.03526	1.46993	1.16641
Zht^2	y_2	0.19618	0.02534	0.07849	0.12795
Zht^3	y_3	0.04659	0.01884	0.03144	0.03869
Zht^4	y_4	0.00947	0.00121	0.00967	0.00079
Standard deviation	σ	10.7128	10.4855	11.6032	10.9573
p^*		0.4100	0.3824	0.2436	0.2598
n (persons)		32 161	31 066	24 057	23 443
n (visits)		42 074	41 017	29 182	28 794

The coefficients were obtained from mixed-effects linear regression models. Diastolic BP5 indicates diastolic measurement at Korotkoff 5.

* The value of p represents the correlation between BP measurements at different ages for the same child after correcting for age and Zht. This computation was necessary because some studies contributing to the childhood BP database provided BP at more than 1 age.

$$(x-\mu)/\sigma = (120 - 109.46)/10.7128 = 0.984.$$
The corresponding SBP percentile = $\Phi(0.984)$
∞ 100% = 83.7th percentile.

References

CLASSIFICATION OF EVIDENCE

The scheme used for classification of the evidence is as follows: M indicates meta-analysis (use of statistical methods to combine the results from clinical trials); RA, randomized, controlled trials (also known as experimental studies); RE, retrospective analyses (also known as case-control studies); F, prospective study (also known as cohort studies, including historical or prospective follow-up studies); X, cross-sectional survey (also known as prevalence studies); PR, previous review or position statements; and C, clinical interventions (non-randomized). These symbols are appended to the citations in the reference list in parentheses. The studies that provided evidence supporting the recommendations of this report were classified and reviewed by the staff and the executive committee. The classification scheme is from the JNC 7 report and other NHBPEP working group reports (www.nhlbi.nih.gov/about/nhbpep/index.htm).[2,134-138]

1. National High Blood Pressure Education Program Working Group on Hypertension Control in Children and Adolescents. Update on the 1987 Task Force Report on High Blood Pressure in Children and Adolescents: a working group report from the National High Blood Pressure Education Program. *Pediatrics*. 1996;98: 649–658(PR)

2. Chobanian AV, Bakris GL, Black HR, et al. The seventh report of the joint national committee on prevention, detection, evaluation, and treatment of high blood pressure: the JNC 7 report. *JAMA*. 2003;289:2560–2572(PR)

3. Prineas RJ, Jacobs D. Quality of Korotkoff sounds: bell vs diaphragm, cubital fossa vs brachial artery. *Prev Med*. 1983;12:715–719

4. Londe S, Klitzner TS. Auscultatory blood pressure measurement—effect of pressure on the head of the stethoscope. *West J Med*. 1984;141:193–195

5. Prineas RJ. Blood pressure in children and adolescents. In: Bulpitt CJ, ed. *Epidemiology of Hypertension*. New York, NY: Elsevier; 2000:86–105. Birkenhager WH and Reid JL, eds. *Handbook of Hypertension*, Vol. 20.

6. Mourad A, Carney S, Gillies A, Jones B, Nanra R, Trevillian P. Arm position and blood pressure: a risk factor for hypertension? *J Hum Hypertens*. 2003;17:389–395

7. Netea RT, Lenders JW, Smits P, Thien T. Both body and arm position significantly influence blood pressure measurement. *J Hum Hypertens*. 2003;17:459–462

8. Rocchini AP. Coarctation of the aorta and interrupted aortic arch. In: Moller JH, Hoffmann U, eds. *Pediatric Cardiovascular Medicine*. New York, NY: Churchill Livingstone; 2000:570

9. Gomez-Marin O, Prineas RJ, Rastam L. Cuff bladder width and blood pressure measurement in children and adolescents. *J Hypertens*. 1992;10:1235–1241

10. American Heart Association. Home monitoring of high blood pressure. Available at: www.americanheart.org/presenter.jhtml?identifier=576. Accessed March 18, 2004

11. Prineas RJ. Measurement of blood pressure in the obese. *Ann Epidemiol*. 1991;1:321–336(PR)

12. Ostchega Y, Prineas RJ, Paulose-Ram R, Grim CM, Willard G, Collins D. National Health and Nutrition Examination Survey 1999–2000: effect of observer training and protocol standardization on reducing blood pressure measurement error. *J Clin Epidemiol.* 2003;56:768–774

13. Lewington S, Clarke R, Qizilbash N, Peto R, Collins R. Age-specific relevance of usual blood pressure to vascular mortality: a metaanalysis of individual data for one million adults in 61 prospective studies. *Lancet.* 2002;360:1903–1913(M)

14. Jones DW, Appel LJ, Sheps SG, Roccella EJ, Lenfant C. Measuring blood pressure accurately: new and persistent challenges. *JAMA.* 2003;289:1027–1030(PR)

15. Canzanello VJ, Jensen PL, Schwartz GL. Are aneroid sphygmomanometers accurate in hospital and clinic settings? *Arch Intern Med.* 2001;161:729–731(PR)

16. Butani L, Morgenstern BZ. Are pitfalls of oxcillometric blood pressure measurements preventable in children? *Pediatr Nephrol.* 2003;18:313–318(PR)

17. Kaufmann MA, Pargger H, Drop LJ. Oscillometric blood pressure measurements by different devices are not interchangeable. *Anesth Analg.* 1996;82:377–381

18. Park MK, Menard SW, Yuan C. Comparison of auscultatory and oscillometric blood pressures. *Arch Pediatr Adolesc Med.* 2001;155:50–53(RA)

19. O'Brien E, Pickering T, Asmar R, et al. Working Group on Blood Pressure Monitoring of the European Society of Hypertension International Protocol for validation of blood pressure measuring devices in adults. *Blood Press Monit.* 2002;7:3–17(PR)

20. O'Brien E, Coats A, Owens P, et al. Use and interpretation of ambulatory blood pressure monitoring: recommendations of the British hypertension society. *BMJ.* 2000;320:1128–1134(PR)

21. Sorof JM, Portman RJ. Ambulatory blood pressure measurements. *Curr Opin Pediatr.* 2001;13:133–137

22. Simckes AM, Srivastava T, Alon US. Ambulatory blood pressure monitoring in children and adolescents. *Clin Pediatr (Phila).* 2002;41:549–564(PR)

23. Lurbe E, Sorof JM, Daniels SR. Clinical and research aspects of ambulatory blood pressure monitoring in children. *J Pediatr.* 2004;144:7–16(PR)

24. Centers for Disease Control and Prevention, National Center for Health Statistics. 2000 CDC growth charts: United States. Available at: www.cdc.gov/growthcharts. Accessed March 18, 2004

25. Task Force on Blood Pressure Control in Children. Report of the Second Task Force on Blood Pressure Control in Children—1987. National Heart, Lung, and Blood Institute, Bethesda, Maryland. *Pediatrics.* 1987;79:1–25(PR)

26. Sorof J, Daniels S. Obesity hypertension in children: a problem of epidemic proportions. *Hypertension.* 2002;40:441–447(PR)

27. Ogden CL, Flegal KM, Carroll MD, Johnson CL. Prevalence and trends in overweight among US children and adolescents, 1999–2000. *JAMA.* 2002;288:1728–1732(X)

28. Reaven GM. Insulin resistance/compensatory hyperinsulinemia, essential hypertension, and cardiovascular disease. *J Clin Endocrinol Metab.* 2003;88:2399–2403

29. National Cholesterol Education Program. Third report of the Expert Panel on Detection, Evaluation, and Treatment of High Blood Cholesterol in Adults (Adult Treatment Panel III) final report. NIH Publication 02-5215. Bethesda, MD: National Heart, Lung, and Blood Institute, National Cholesterol Education Program; 2002(PR)

30. Sinaiko AR, Steinberger J, Moran A, Prineas RJ, Jacobs DR Jr. Relation of insulin resistance to blood pressure in childhood. *J Hypertens.* 2002;20:509–517(RA)

31. Cook S, Weitzman M, Auinger P, Nguyen M, Dietz WH. Prevalence of a metabolic syndrome phenotype in adolescents: findings from the Third National Health and Nutrition Examination Survey, 1988–1994. *Arch Pediatr Adolesc Med.* 2003;157:1–827(X)

32. Williams CL, Hayman LL, Daniels SR, et al. Cardiovascular health in childhood: a statement for health professionals from the Committee on Atherosclerosis, Hypertension, and Obesity in the Young (AHOY) of the Council on Cardiovascular Disease in the Young, American Heart Association. *Circulation.* 2002;106:143–160(PR)

33. Quan SF, Gersh BJ. Cardiovascular consequences of sleep-disordered breathing: past, present and future: report of a workshop from the National Center on Sleep Disorders Research and the National Heart, Lung, and Blood Institute. *Circulation.* 2004;109:951–957

34. Strohl KP. Invited commentary: to sleep, perchance to discover. *Am J Epidemiol.* 2002;155:394–395

35. Marcus CL, Greene MG, Carroll JL. Blood pressure in children with obstructive sleep apnea. *Am J Respir Crit Care Med.* 1998;157:1098–1103(X)

36. Enright PL, Goodwin JL, Sherrill DL, Quan JR, Quan SF. Blood pressure elevation associated with sleep-related breathing disorder in a community sample of white and Hispanic children: the Tucson Children's Assessment of Sleep Apnea study. *Arch Pediatr Adolesc Med.* 2003;157:901–904(F)

37. Mindell JA, Owens JA. *A Clinical Guide to Pediatric Sleep: Diagnosis and Management of Sleep Problems.* Philadelphia, PA: Lippincott, Williams & Wilkins; 2003:10

38. Sinaiko AR. Hypertension in children. *N Engl J Med.* 1996;335:1968–1973(PR)

39. Flynn JT. Evaluation and management of hypertension in childhood. *Prog Pediatr Cardiol.* 2001;12:177–188(PR)

40. Hiner LB, Falkner B. Renovascular hypertension in children. *Pediatr Clin North Am.* 1993;40:123–140(PR)

41. Dillon MJ, Ryness JM. Plasma renin activity and aldosterone concentration in children. *Br Med J.* 1975;4(5992):316–319(X)

42. Guzzetta PC, Potter BM, Ruley EJ, Majd M, Bock GH. Renovascular hypertension in children: current concepts in evaluation and treatment. *J Pediatr Surg.* 1989;24:1236–1240(C)

43. Watson AR, Balfe JW, Hardy BE. Renovascular hypertension in childhood: a changing perspective in management. *J Pediatr.* 1985;106:366–372

44. Dillon MJ. The diagnosis of renovascular disease. *Pediatr Nephrol.* 1997;11:366–372(PR)

45. Mena E, Bookstein JJ, Holt JF, Fry WJ. Neurofibromatosis and renovascular hypertension in children. *Am J Roentgenol Radium Ther Nucl Med.* 1973;118:39–45(RE)

46. Shahdadpuri J, Frank R, Gauthier BG, Siegel DN, Trachtman H. Yield of renal arteriography in the evaluation of pediatric hypertension. *Pediatr Nephrol.* 2000;14:816–819(RE)

47. Binkert CA, Debatin JF, Schneider E, et al. Can MR measurement of renal artery flow and renal volume predict the outcome of percutaneous transluminal renal angioplasty? *Cardiovasc Intervent Radiol.* 2001;24:233–239(F)

48. Marcos HB, Choyke PL. Magnetic resonance angiography of the kidney. *Semin Nephrol.* 2000;20:450–455(PR)

49. Debatin JF, Spritzer CE, Grist TM, et al. Imaging of the renal arteries: value of MR angiography. *AJR Am J Roentgenol.* 1991;157:981–990(F)

50. Vade A, Agrawal R, Lim-Dunham J, Hartoin D. Utility of computed tomographic renal angiogram in the management of childhood hypertension. *Pediatr Nephrol.* 2002;17:741–747(RE)

51. MacMahon S, Peto R, Cutler J, et al. Blood pressure, stroke, and coronary heart disease. Part 1, prolonged differences in blood pressure: prospective observational studies corrected for the regression dilution bias. *Lancet.* 1990;335:765–774(F)

52. Still JL, Cottom D. Severe hypertension in childhood. *Arch Dis Child.* 1967;42:34–39(PR)

53. Gill DG, Mendes dC, Cameron JS, Joseph MC, Ogg CS, Chantler C. Analysis of 100 children with severe and persistent hypertension. *Arch Dis Child.* 1976;51:951–956(F)

54. Johnstone LM, Jones CL, Grigg LE, Wilkinson JL, Walker RG, Powell HR. Left ventricular abnormalities in children, adolescents and young adults with renal disease. *Kidney Int.* 1996;50:998–1006(X)

55. Mitsnefes MM, Daniels SR, Schwartz SM, Khoury P, Strife CF. Changes in left ventricular mass in children and adolescents during chronic dialysis. *Pediatr Nephrol.* 2001;16:318–323(F)

56. Mitsnefes MM, Kimball TR, Witt SA, Glascock BJ, Khoury PR, Daniels SR. Left ventricular mass and systolic performance in pediatric patients with chronic renal failure. *Circulation.* 2003;107:864–868(X)

57. Berenson GS, Srinivasan SR, Bao W, Newman WP III, Tracy RE, Wattigney WA. Association between multiple cardiovascular risk factors and atherosclerosis in children and young adults. The Bogalusa Heart Study. *N Engl J Med.* 1998;338:1650–1656(F)

58. McGill HC Jr, McMahan CA, Zieske AW, Malcom GT, Tracy RE, Strong JP. Effects of nonlipid risk factors on atherosclerosis in youth with a favorable lipoprotein profile. *Circulation.* 2001;103:1546–1550

59. Davis PH, Dawson JD, Riley WA, Lauer RM. Carotid intimal-medial thickness is related to cardiovascular risk factors measured from childhood through middle age: the Muscatine Study. *Circulation.* 2001;104:2815–2819(F)

60. Arnett DK, Glasser SP, McVeigh G, et al. Blood pressure and arterial compliance in young adults: the Minnesota Children's Blood Pressure Study. *Am J Hypertens.* 2001;14:200–205(F)

61. Knoflach M, Kiechl S, Kind M, et al. Cardiovascular risk factors and atherosclerosis in young males: ARMY study (Atherosclerosis Risk-Factors in Male Youngsters). *Circulation.* 2003;108:1064–1069(X)

62. Sanchez A, Barth JD, Zhang L. The carotid artery wall thickness in teenagers is related to their diet and the typical risk factors of heart disease among adults. *Atherosclerosis.* 2000;152:265–266

63. Barnes VA, Treiber FA, Davis H. Impact of transcendental meditation on cardiovascular function at rest and during acute stress in adolescents with high normal blood pressure. *J Psychosom Res.* 2001;51:597–605(RA)

64. Belsha CW, Wells TG, McNiece KL, Seib PM, Plummer JK, Berry PL. Influence of diurnal blood pressure variations on target organ abnormalities in adolescents with mild essential hypertension. *Am J Hypertens.* 1998;11:410–417(F)

65. Sorof JM, Alexandrov AV, Cardwell G, Portman RJ. Carotid artery intimal-medial thickness and left ventricular hypertrophy in children with elevated blood pressure. *Pediatrics.* 2003;111:61–66

66. Hanevold C, Waller J, Daniels S, Portman R, Sorof J. The effects of obesity, gender, and ethnic group on left ventricular hypertrophy and geometry in hypertensive children: a collaborative study of the International Pediatric Hypertension Association. *Pediatrics.* 2004;113:328–333(X)

67. Daniels SR, Loggie JM, Khoury P, Kimball TR. Left ventricular geometry and severe left ventricular hypertrophy in children and adolescents with essential hypertension. *Circulation.* 1998;97:1907–1911(X)

68. Svardsudd K, Wedel H, Aurell E, Tibblin G. Hypertensive eye ground changes. Prevalence, relation to blood pressure and prognostic importance. The study of men born in 1913. *Acta Med Scand.* 1978;204:159–167(F)

69. Skalina ME, Annable WL, Kliegman RM, Fanaroff AA. Hypertensive retinopathy in the newborn infant. *J Pediatr.* 1983;103:781–786(X)

70. Devereux RB, Alonso DR, Lutas EM, et al. Echocardiographic assessment of left ventricular hypertrophy: comparison to necropsy findings. *Am J Cardiol.* 1986; 57:450–458(RE)

71. Sahn DJ, DeMaria A, Kisslo J, Weyman A. Recommendations regarding quantitation in M-mode echocardiography: results of a survey of echocardiographic measurements. *Circulation.* 1978;58:1072–1083

72. Daniels SR, Kimball TR, Morrison JA, Khoury P, Witt S, Meyer RA. Effect of lean body mass, fat mass, blood pressure, and sexual maturation on left ventricular mass in children and adolescents. Statistical, biological, and clinical significance. *Circulation.* 1995;92:3249–3254(X)

73. de Simone G, Daniels SR, Devereux RB, et al. Left ventricular mass and body size in normotensive children and adults: assessment of allometric relations and impact of overweight. *J Am Coll Cardiol.* 1992;20:1251–1260(F)

74. Daniels SR, Kimball TR, Morrison JA, Khoury P, Meyer RA. Indexing left ventricular mass to account for differences in body size in children and adolescents without cardiovascular disease. *Am J Cardiol.* 1995; 76:699–701(X)

75. He J, Whelton PK, Appel LJ, Charleston J, Klag MJ. Long-term effects of weight loss and dietary sodium reduction on incidence of hypertension. *Hypertension.* 2000;35:544–549(F)

76. Sacks FM, Svetkey LP, Vollmer WM, et al. Effects on blood pressure of reduced dietary sodium and the Dietary Approaches to Stop Hypertension (DASH) diet. DASH-Sodium Collaborative Research Group. *N Engl J Med.* 2001;344:3–10(RA)

77. Vollmer WM, Sacks FM, Ard J, et al. Effects of diet and sodium intake on blood pressure: subgroup analysis of the DASH-sodium trial. *Ann Intern Med.* 2001;135: 1019–1028(RA)

78. Whelton SP, Chin A, Xin X, He J. Effect of aerobic exercise on blood pressure: a meta-analysis of randomized, controlled trials. *Ann Intern Med.* 2002;136:493–503(M)

79. Xin X, He J, Frontini MG, Ogden LG, Motsamai OI, Whelton PK. Effects of alcohol reduction on blood pressure: a meta-analysis of randomized controlled trials. *Hypertension.* 2001;38:1112–1117(M)

80. Ayas NT, White DP, Manson JE, et al. A prospective study of sleep duration and coronary heart disease in women. *Arch Intern Med.* 2003;163:205–209(X)

81. Cook NR, Gillman MW, Rosner BA, Taylor JO, Hennekens CH. Combining annual blood pressure measurements in childhood to improve prediction of young adult blood pressure. *Stat Med.* 2000;19:2625–2640(F)

82. Lauer RM, Mahoney LT, Clarke WR. Tracking of blood pressure during childhood: the Muscatine Study. *Clin Exp Hypertens A.* 1986;8:515–537(F)

83. Lauer RM, Clarke WR. Childhood risk factors for high adult blood pressure: the Muscatine Study. *Pediatrics.* 1989;84:633–641(F)

84. Clarke WR, Woolson RF, Lauer RM. Changes in ponderosity and blood pressure in childhood: the Muscatine Study. *Am J Epidemiol.* 1986;124:195–206(F)

85. Burke V, Beilin LJ, Dunbar D. Tracking of blood pressure in Australian children. *J Hypertens.* 2001;19: 1185–1192(F)

86. Figueroa-Colon R, Franklin FA, Lee JY, von Almen TK, Suskind RM. Feasibility of a clinic-based hypocaloric dietary intervention implemented in a school setting for obese children. *Obes Res.* 1996;4:419–429(RA)

87. Wabitsch M, Hauner H, Heinze E, et al. Body-fat distribution and changes in the atherogenic risk-factor profile in obese adolescent girls during weight reduction. *Am J Clin Nutr.* 1994;60:54–60(C)

88. Rocchini AP, Key J, Bondie D, et al. The effect of weight loss on the sensitivity of blood pressure to sodium in obese adolescents. *N Engl J Med.* 1989;321:580–585(C)

89. Rocchini AP, Katch V, Anderson J, et al. Blood pressure in obese adolescents: effect of weight loss. *Pediatrics.* 1988;82:16–23(RA)

90. Sinaiko AR, Gomez-Marin O, Prineas RJ. Relation of fasting insulin to blood pressure and lipids in adolescents and parents. *Hypertension.* 1997;30:1554–1559(X)

91. Robinson TN. Behavioural treatment of childhood and adolescent obesity. *Int J Obes Relat Metab Disord.* 1999; 23(suppl 2):S52–S57(PR)

92. Epstein LH, Myers MD, Raynor HA, Saelens BE. Treatment of pediatric obesity. *Pediatrics.* 1998;101: 554–570(PR)

93. Barlow SE, Dietz WH. Obesity evaluation and treatment: expert committee recommendations. The Maternal and Child Health Bureau, Health Resources and Services Administration and the Department of Health and Human Services. *Pediatrics.* 1998;102(3). Available at: www.pediatrics.org/cgi/content/full/102/3/e29(PR)

94. Krebs NF, Jacobson MS. Prevention of pediatric overweight and obesity. *Pediatrics.* 2003;112:424–430(PR)

95. U.S. Department of Health and Human Services. *The Surgeon General's Call to Action to Prevent and Decrease Overweight and Obesity.* Rockville, MD: U.S. Department of Health and Human Services, Public Health Service, Office of the Surgeon General; 2001(PR)

96. Gutin B, Owens S. Role of exercise intervention in improving body fat distribution and risk profile in children. *Am J Human Biol.* 1999;11:237–247(RA)

97. Siega-Riz AM, Popkin BM, Carson T. Trends in breakfast consumption for children in the United States from 1965–1991. *Am J Clin Nutr.* 1998;67:748S–756S

98. Warren JM, Henry CJ, Simonite V. Low glycemic index breakfasts and reduced food intake in preadolescent children. *Pediatrics.* 2003;112(5). Available at: www.pediatrics.org/cgi/content/full/112/5/e414(RA)

99. Gillman MW, Hood MY, Moore LL, Nguyen US, Singer MR, Andon MB. Effect of calcium supplementation on blood pressure in children. *J Pediatr.* 1995;127: 186–192(RA)

100. Simons-Morton DG, Hunsberger SA, Van Horn L, et al. Nutrient intake and blood pressure in the Dietary Intervention Study in Children. *Hypertension.* 1997;29: 930–936(RA)

101. Simons-Morton DG, Obarzanek E. Diet and blood pressure in children and adolescents. *Pediatr Nephrol.* 1997; 11:244–249(PR)

102. Miller JZ, Weinberger MH, Christian JC. Blood pressure response to potassium supplementation in normotensive adults and children. *Hypertension.* 1987;10:437–442(C)

103. Sinaiko AR, Gomez-Marin O, Prineas RJ. Effect of low sodium diet or potassium supplementation on adolescent blood pressure. *Hypertension.* 1993;21:989–994(RA)

104. Falkner B, Sherif K, Michel S, Kushner H. Dietary nutrients and blood pressure in urban minority adolescents at risk for hypertension. *Arch Pediatr Adolesc Med.* 2000; 154:918–922(X)

105. Stern B, Heyden S, Miller D, Latham G, Klimas A, Pilkington K. Intervention study in high school students with elevated blood pressures. Dietary experiment with polyunsaturated fatty acids. *Nutr Metab.* 1980;24: 137–147(C)

106. Goldberg RJ, Ellison RC, Hosmer DW Jr, et al. Effects of alterations in fatty acid intake on the blood pressure of adolescents: the Exeter-Andover Project. *Am J Clin Nutr.* 1992;56:71–76(F)

107. Cooper R, Van Horn L, Liu K, et al. A randomized trial on the effect of decreased dietary sodium intake on blood pressure in adolescents. *J Hypertens.* 1984;2: 361–366(RA)

108. Falkner B, Michel S. Blood pressure response to sodium in children and adolescents. *Am J Clin Nutr.* 1997;65: 618S–621S(PR)

109. Gillum RF, Elmer PJ, Prineas RJ. Changing sodium intake in children. The Minneapolis Children's Blood Pressure Study. *Hypertension.* 1981;3:698–703(RA)

110. Howe PR, Cobiac L, Smith RM. Lack of effect of short-term changes in sodium intake on blood pressure in adolescent schoolchildren. *J Hypertens.* 1991;9:181–186(RA)

111. Geleijnse JM, Hofman A, Witteman JC, Hazebroek AA, Valkenburg HA, Grobbee DE. Long-term effects of neonatal sodium restriction on blood pressure. *Hypertension.* 1997;29:913–917(RA)

112. Martin RM, Ness AR, Gunnell D, Emmett P, Smith GD. Does breastfeeding in infancy lower blood pressure in childhood? The Avon Longitudinal Study of Parents and Children (ALSPAC). *Circulation.* 2004;109:1259–1266(F)

113. Wilson AC, Forsyth JS, Greene SA, Irvine L, Hau C, Howie PW. Relation of infant diet to childhood health: seven year follow up of cohort of children in Dundee infant feeding study. *BMJ.* 1998;316:21–25(F)

114. Panel of Dietary Intakes for Electrolytes and Water, Standing Committee on the Scientific Evaluation of Dietary Reference Intakes, Food and Nutrition Board, Institute of Medicine. *Dietary Reference Intakes for Water, Potassium, Sodium, Chloride, and Sulfate.* Washington, DC: National Academies Press; 2004. Available at: www.nap.edu/books/0309091691/html. Accessed March 18, 2004(PR)

115. Kelley GA, Kelley KS, Tran ZV. The effects of exercise on resting blood pressure in children and adolescents: a meta-analysis of randomized controlled trials. *Prev Cardiol.* 2003;6:8–16(M)

116. American Academy of Pediatrics, Committee on Sports Medicine and Fitness. Athletic participation by children and adolescents who have systemic hypertension. *Pediatrics.* 1997;99:637–638(PR)

117. Klag MJ, Whelton PK, Randall BL, et al. Blood pressure and end-stage renal disease in men. *N Engl J Med.* 1996; 334:13–18(F)

118. Yusuf HR, Giles WH, Croft JB, Anda RF, Casper ML. Impact of multiple risk factor profiles on determining cardiovascular disease risk. *Prev Med.* 1998;27:1–9(X)

119. Kavey RE, Daniels SR, Lauer RM, Atkins DL, Hayman LL, Taubert K. American Heart Association guidelines for primary prevention of atherosclerotic cardiovascular disease beginning in childhood. *Circulation.* 2003;107: 1562–1566(PR)

120. Blumenthal S, Epps RP, Heavenrich R, et al. Report of the task force on blood pressure control in children. *Pediatrics.* 1977;59:797–820(PR)

121. The Food and Drug Administration Modernization Act of 1997. Pub L 105–115

122. Wells TG. Trials of antihypertensive therapies in children. *Blood Press Monit.* 1999;4:189–192(PR)

123. Flynn JT. Successes and shortcomings of the Food and Drug Modernization Act. *Am J Hypertens.* 2003;16: 889–891(PR)

124. Best Pharmaceuticals for Children Act of 2002. Pub L 107–109

125. U.S. Department of Health and Human Services, National Institutes of Health. List of drugs for which pediatric studies are needed. *Fed Regist.* 2003;68: 2789–2790

126. ALLHAT Officers and Coordinators for the ALLHAT Collaborative Research Group. Major outcomes in high-risk hypertensive patients randomized to angiotensin-converting enzyme inhibitor or calcium channel blocker vs diuretic: The Antihypertensive and Lipid-Lowering Treatment to Prevent Heart Attack Trial (ALLHAT). *JAMA.* 2002;288:2981–2997(RA)

127. Wells T, Frame V, Soffer B, et al. A double-blind, placebo-controlled, dose-response study of the effectiveness and safety of enalapril for children with hypertension. *J Clin Pharmacol.* 2002;42:870–880(F)

128. Soffer B, Zhang Z, Miller K, Vogt BA, Shahinfar S. A double-blind, placebo-controlled, dose-response study of the effectiveness and safety of lisinopril for children with hypertension. *Am J Hypertens.* 2003;16:795–800(RA)

129. Sakarcan A, Tenney F, Wilson JT, et al. The pharmacokinetics of irbesartan in hypertensive children and adolescents. *J Clin Pharmacol.* 2001;41:742–749

130. Trachtman H, Frank R, Mahan JD, et al. Clinical trial of extended-release felodipine in pediatric essential hypertension. *Pediatr Nephrol.* 2003;18:548–553(RA)

131. Sorof JM, Cargo P, Graepel J, et al. Beta-blocker/thiazide combination for treatment of hypertensive children: a randomized double-blind, placebo-controlled trial. *Pediatr Nephrol.* 2002;17:345–350(RA)

132. Adelman RD, Coppo R, Dillon MJ. The emergency management of severe hypertension. *Pediatr Nephrol.* 2000; 14:422–427(PR)

133. Vaughan CJ, Delanty N. Hypertensive emergencies. *Lancet.* 2000;356:411–417(PR)

134. Sheps SG, Roccella EJ. Reflections on the sixth report of the Joint National Committee on Prevention, Detection, Evaluation, and Treatment of High Blood Pressure. *Curr Hypertens Rep.* 1999;1:342–345(PR)

135. Ingelfinger JR. Renovascular disease in children. *Kidney Int.* 1993;43:493–505(PR)

136. World Health Organization. World health report 2002: reducing risks, promoting healthy life. Geneva, Switzerland: 2002. Available at: www.who.int/whr/2002. Accessed March 11, 2004

137. U.S. Department of Health and Human Services, National Heart, Lung, and Blood Institute. National High Blood Pressure Education Program. Available at: www.nhlbi.nih.gov/about/nhbpep/index.htm. Accessed March 18, 2004

138. JNC 6. National High Blood Pressure Education Program. The sixth report of the Joint National Committee on prevention, detection, evaluation, and treatment of high blood pressure. *Arch Intern Med.* 1997;157:2413–2446(PR)

Hypertension

Victoria F. Norwood, MD*

Objectives

After completing this article, readers should be able to:

1. Describe the criteria for determining normal blood pressure versus hypertension.
2. Recognize, evaluate, and treat essential hypertension.
3. Delineate the staged evaluation of patients who have probable secondary hypertension.
4. Know the differential diagnoses of hypertension across pediatric age groups.
5. Recognize and treat hypertensive emergencies.
6. Describe the different mechanisms of action of the classes of antihypertensive drugs.

Introduction

Hypertension is a major public health issue in industrialized nations, affecting approximately 20% of adults. The close associations of hypertension with atherosclerosis, coronary and cerebrovascular disease, diabetes, and end-stage renal disease make it a major contributor to the most common causes of morbidity and mortality in adult populations. Although the prevalence of hypertension in the pediatric age group is significantly less (1% to 3%), and many of these patients are affected only mildly, pediatricians are appropriately situated to diagnose and manage many of these disorders. Education, anticipatory guidance, early detection, accurate diagnosis, and effective therapy may help to improve the long-term outcomes of children and adolescents affected by this "silent killer."

Definitions and Measurements

A definition of hypertension ideally is based on a threshold level of blood pressure that divides those at risk for adverse outcomes from those who have no increased risk. Unfortunately, an identifiable cutoff does not exist; arbitrary thresholds have been established based on epidemiologic data compiled from large numbers of children in the United States. The current normative values, as detailed most recently in the "Update on the 1987 Task Force Report on High Blood Pressure in Children and Adolescents" published in *Pediatrics* in 1996, includes more than 60,000 healthy children (approximately 50:50, male:female) of whom 56% are white, 29% black, 9% Hispanic, 3% Asian, and 4% other. Because blood pressure is regulated by a variety of genetic, demographic, and environmental factors, it is important to recognize that these standards, which are the best available, may not reflect accurately the norms or the risks for children outside the United States or those who have medical illnesses.

By current definitions, blood pressure is normal if the average systolic and diastolic readings on repeated measurements are below the 90th percentile for age, gender, and height. Patients who have readings between the 90th and 95th percentile are considered borderline. Significant hypertension exists if either systolic or diastolic averages are greater than the 95th percentile for age, gender, and height (Table 1). "Severe" hypertension is defined as systolic or diastolic values greater than the 99th percentile. Therefore, all children and adolescents whose blood pressures are greater than the 95th percentile should be evaluated thoroughly and some form of treatment initiated. Patients whose blood pressures are between the 90th and 95th percentile

*Chief, Pediatric Nephrology, University of Virginia, Children's Medical Center, Charlottesville, VA.

Pediatrics in Review, Vol 23, No. 6, June 2002

Table 1. 95th Percentile Blood Pressure Readings for Children by Age and Height Percentiles (mm Hg)

Age (y)	Girls			Boys		
	5th Percentile	50th Percentile	95th Percentile	5th Percentile	50th Percentile	95th Percentile
1	101/57	104/58	107/60	98/55	102/53	106/59
6	108/71	111/73	114/75	109/72	114/74	117/76
12	120/79	123/80	126/82	119/79	123/81	127/83
17	126/83	129/84	132/86	132/85	136/87	140/89

Adapted from Update on the 1987 Task Force on High Blood Pressure in Children and Adolescents. *Pediatrics.* 1996;98:4.

should be observed carefully and evaluated if risk factors are present; tracking data suggest that this subgroup is more likely to develop overt hypertension over time than more normotensive children.

Accurate measurement of blood pressure requires the proper equipment, practice, and patience. Blood pressure is measured most conveniently and inexpensively in the office by using a standard mercury sphygmomanometer and a stethoscope and employing commercially available cuffs. A large adult cuff or thigh cuff is necessary for the unusually large or obese teen. Automated oscillometric devices are useful but expensive and require significantly more maintenance and calibration. However, these automated devices can be very helpful in evaluating infants and small children in whom resting, quiet, auscultatory readings often are difficult to obtain. As shown in the Figure, an appropriate cuff size is one in which the cuff *bladder* width is equal to approximately 70% of the acromion-olecranon distance (or 40% of the midarm circumference); the bladder length should encircle the arm completely. Inappropriately small cuffs will give aberrantly high readings; inappropriately large cuffs will underestimate the true reading. Measurements should be taken after 3 to 5 minutes of resting. Children should have measurements taken while sitting with the arm at the level of the heart, and infants should have measurements taken while supine. Current recommendations suggest the use of the first (onset of tapping) and fifth (loss of tapping) Korotkoff sounds for auscultatory readings in children and adolescents.

Although performed most commonly in the clinic, monitoring of blood pressure in the home by appropriately trained family members can be helpful, especially when there are concerns of possible "white coat" hypertension. Readings can be taken more frequently during the day and records kept for comparison with the values obtained in the office. Patients or their families should be trained in accurate measurement of blood pressure if pharmacologic therapy is likely. The use of 24-hour ambulatory blood pressure monitoring systems is gaining in popularity, especially for adults, in whom continuous ambulatory measurements have been shown to correlate with effectiveness of therapy and changes in end-organ damage more so than random office or home measurements. Unfortunately, there are few normative data for these readings in children

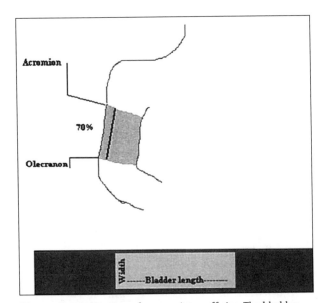

Figure. Determination of appropriate cuff size. The bladder width should cover approximately 70% of the acromion-olecranon distance, and the bladder length should encircle the arm completely.

or adolescents. Controversy abounds regarding the appropriate statistical analysis and setpoints needed to diagnose hypertension accurately in the pediatric age group, but these techniques are likely to become standardized and used more widely in the near future.

Hypertension is usually described as primary (or "essential") or secondary, resulting from a definable cause. Therefore, by definition, essential hypertension is a diagnosis of exclusion. Although by far the most common cause of hypertension in the adult population, essential hypertension is a significant pediatric diagnosis only within the adolescent age group. The younger the patient and the more severe the hypertension, the more likely that a secondary cause will be found. The astute pediatrician should tailor his or her evaluation appropriately.

Causes

When considering the potential causes and planning the evaluation of hypertension in the pediatric population, it can be helpful to determine whether the patient is experiencing acute

Table 2. Causes of Acute and Chronic Hypertension in the Pediatric Population

Acute	Chronic
Renal	**Renal**
Acute poststreptococcal glomerulonephritis	Chronic renal insufficiency or failure, any cause
Hemolytic uremic syndrome	Chronic glomerulopathies
Acute nephritis, any cause	Obstructive uropathy
Acute renal failure, any cause	Polycystic kidney disease (dominant or recessive)
Renal or urinary tract surgery	Reflux nephropathy
	Postrenal transplantation
Vascular	**Vascular**
Renal artery thrombosis/embolus	Renal artery stenosis (intrinsic or extrinsic)
Patent ductus arteriosus	Coarctation of the aorta
	Systemis vasculitis
	Williams syndrome
Medications	**Medications**
Steroids	Steroids
Decongestants/cold preparations	Erythropoietin
Oral contraceptives	Cyclosporine/tacrolimus
Amphetamines/cocaine/phencyclidine	Oral contraceptives
Rebound on discontinuation of antihypertensives	
Beta-adrenergic agonists/theophylline	
Caffeine/nicotine	
Trauma	**Endocrine**
Burns	Pheochromocytoma
Traction (especially femoral)	Cushing syndrome
Perirenal hematoma	Congenital adrenal hyperplasia
Increased intracranial pressure	Hypo/hyperthyroidism
Spinal cord injury	Neuroblastoma
	Hyperparathyroidism
	Primary hyperaldosteronism
	Genetic hypertensive endocrinopathies
Miscellaneous	**Miscellaneous**
Volume overload	Essential hypertension
Hypercalcemia	Obesity
Autonomic dysfunction (Guillian-Barré)	Bronchopulmonary dysplasia
Anxiety/pain	Sleep apnea
Seizures	Increased intracranial pressure
	Pregnancy

(and potentially transient) or chronic elevations in blood pressure. Table 2 lists the major categories of processes that cause acute and chronic hypertension. Patients may experience more than one cause of elevated blood pressure; mixed mechanisms are common in the chronically ill infant and child.

It is also important to note that the causes of hypertension vary with age; an infant or young child almost inevitably has a secondary cause such as congenital renal or cardiovascular disease. Older children may present late with congenital diseases or develop acquired disease such as reflux nephropathy or chronic glomerulonephritis. Most pediatricians are hesitant to confer a diagnosis of essential hypertension on a prepubertal child prior to a comprehensive evaluation. However, essential hypertension, with or without obesity, is by far the most common cause by adolescence.

Transient hypertension very commonly results from anxiety, medications, or acute reversible renal disease. "White coat" hypertension refers to the finding of elevated blood pressure readings in the clinical setting that is not confirmed in more relaxed environments or with continuous ambulatory monitoring. It is important to recognize that many types of stress exacerbate the hypertensive response. Importantly, sympathetic nervous system activity is enhanced and stress-induced blood pressure responses are augmented in children who have a family history of essential hypertension. Therefore, the findings of intermittent or "white coat" hypertension in a child or adolescent who has a family history of hypertension warrant close follow-up for the possible development of sustained hypertension.

Of the causes of hypertension listed in Table 2, acute and chronic renal parenchymal disease are the most common in preadolescents. Many glomerulonephritides and congenital anomalies are found easily during early screening phases, but reflux nephropathy frequently is missed and always should be considered. Recurrent urinary tract infections commonly are missed or considered of minimal importance; unfortunately, the renal parenchymal scarring often is silent until late childhood when significant, even malignant, hypertension develops in approximately 10% of

affected patients. Congenital obstructions of the urinary tract are associated frequently with hypertension, even in the absence of renal insufficiency. Unilateral ureteropelvic junction obstructions are not uncommonly diagnosed as the cause of severe hypertension in the absence of urinary or serum evidence of renal disease. In the intensive care nursery, renal ischemic events are not unusual because of the frequent use of umbilical artery catheters; renal artery thrombus always should be considered in this population, especially when the hypertension is severe. Congenital renal cystic disease (autosomal dominant and autosomal recessive polycystic diseases, cystic dysplasia, or large simple cysts) commonly is associated with hypertension in childhood.

Coarctation of the aorta accounts for up to one third of the cases of hypertension in infancy and occasionally presents in older populations. Fibromuscular dysplasia resulting in proximal or distal renal artery stenosis occurs in as many as 8% to 10% of children who have severe hypertension in referral centers. When renal vascular lesions are diagnosed, other vascular anomalies, such as midaortic hypoplasia and intracranial lesions, also should be considered. Williams syndrome often is associated with multiple vascular stenoses, and the autoimmune vasculitides may present with severe hypertension from large vessel involvement. Not all renovascular lesions are intrinsic to the kidney vasculature. Compression of the renal artery from malignant tumor or neurofibroma can cause significant hypertension. In the nursery setting, transient hypertension may be seen following ligation of a ductus arteriosus or repair of an aortic coarctation. Although the elevated blood pressures in these infants usually require only temporary treatment, long-term follow-up is warranted because recurrent hypertension may indicate the development of restenosis.

Pharmacologic agents, both legal and illicit, commonly produce elevations in blood pressure. Corticosteroids, oral contraceptives, antidepressants, sympathomimetic eye and nose drops, decongestants, beta-agonist bronchodilators, theophylline, nonsteroidal antiinflammatory drugs, recombinant erythropoietin, cyclosporine, and nicotine have been implicated as causative or contributory to hypertension. Cocaine, amphetamines, and phencyclidine may be the cause, especially in teens, of transient or severe hypertension. Rebound hypertension from rapid withdrawal of antihypertensive drugs should be considered when blood pressure worsens in a previously well-controlled patient.

Trauma can result indirectly in hypertension from pain and fluid resuscitation. Undetected elevations of intracranial pressure should be considered as a possibility in the critically injured child. Femoral traction commonly results in increased blood pressure due to reflex-mediated alterations in central nervous system function, and spinal cord trauma may cause frustrating swings between reflex-mediated hypertension and hypotension. Renal trauma can cause ischemia, infarction, compression, and scarring of the renal parenchyma, with long-term hypertension as a consequence.

The endocrine system abnormalities causing hypertension are numerous, but individually infrequent. Catecholamine-secreting tumors are concerning because of the potential for episodic hypertensive crisis. Although classically paroxysmal, the presentation of pheochromocytoma is rarely straightforward in childhood; many children fail to complain of flushing, tachycardia, or sweating. Approximately 88% of children who have pheochromocytomas experience sustained, rather than intermittent, hypertension. Children who have neuroblastoma often have associated hypertension, but blood pressure abnormalities rarely are the initial finding. Abnormalities of the adrenal axis also result in hypertension due to excessive glucocorticoid or mineralocorticoid effects. Cushing syndrome in children may be caused by primary pituitary oversecretion of adrenocorticotropic hormone (ACTH) or from adrenal tumors. Primary hyperaldosteronism is an uncommon cause of hypertension in the pediatric age group, but it should be considered in the presence of hypokalemia. Congenital adrenal hyperplasias (11-beta hydroxylase deficiency or 17-alpha hydroxylase deficiency) result in hypertension due to mineralocorticoid effects of elevated steroid metabolites. Hyper- and

hypothyroidism can cause hypertension from increased cardiac output and fluid retention, respectively. In patients who have end-stage renal disease, secondary or tertiary hyperparathyroidism often exacerbates preexisting hypertension. A number of genetically determined hypertensive states have benefited from advances in molecular biology. Liddle syndrome results from a constitutively activated sodium channel in the distal tubule. Glucocorticoid-remediable aldosteronism results from a chimeric gene in which aldosterone production is controlled aberrantly by ACTH. The syndrome of "apparent mineralocorticoid excess" results from an inability to inactivate cortisol activity effectively at the mineralocorticoid receptor.

Essential hypertension is the most common cause of elevated blood pressure in adolescents and young adults. As mentioned previously, it is a "diagnosis of exclusion" that should not be attributed to a patient merely because of age. A number of theories have been proposed to explain the existence of essential hypertension, and it is likely that many of them are partially responsible in some populations. Abnormal renal ability to maintain appropriate balance between body sodium content and blood pressure, clinically undetectable reduction in glomerular filtration, increased sympathetic nervous system activity, primary dysfunction of the renin-angiotensin system, insulin resistance, and mental stress all may contribute to a constant state of relatively high blood pressure. The normal circadian decline of blood pressure at night often is lost prior to the onset of overt hypertension, suggesting that a number of homeostatic mechanisms are likely participants.

Essential hypertension clearly tracks with a family history of hypertension, and children whose blood pressures are measured in the higher percentiles tend to remain in those higher percentiles in adulthood. Racial influences are strong; the incidence of hypertension in African-American adolescents and adults is twice that of Caucasians. Approximately 50% of patients who have essential hypertension are salt-sensitive, which should be considered when discussing therapies. Obesity is a common cofactor in the development of essential hypertension, with approximately 50% of hypertensive teens qualifying as obese. Although poorly understood, obesity probably contributes to blood pressure control through high sodium intake and insulin resistance among other factors. The so-called "syndrome X" of hypertension, obesity, hyperlipidemia, and diabetes mellitus is clearly a major cause of long-term cardiovascular morbidity and mortality.

Clinical Presentation

It is unusual for pediatric hypertension to be diagnosed as a result of patient complaint or symptom; most hypertension is clinically silent. For this reason, it is appropriate to measure blood pressure as a part of all routine medical examinations. Patients who have severe hypertension may complain of headache, vision changes, nosebleeds, or nausea and should be treated immediately. Hypertensive emergencies are defined as the presence of severe hypertension associated with life-threatening or organ-threatening complications, including encephalopathy (seizures, stroke, focal deficits), acute heart failure or myocardial infarction, pulmonary edema, dissecting aortic aneurysm, acute renal failure, or eclampsia. The term "malignant hypertension" implies hypertension-induced vascular damage that includes myointimal proliferation and fibrinoid necrosis. This pathology of the microvasculature frequently is responsible for the symptoms of a hypertensive crisis. Severe hypertension always should be considered in the differential diagnosis of congestive heart failure in childhood, even in the absence of other symptoms or diseases suggestive of high blood pressure.

Evaluation

Questions often arise regarding who to evaluate for hypertension and how far the evaluation should proceed. Documentation of sustained hypertension is warranted prior to additional evaluation in children and adolescents who exhibit only minimal elevations in blood pressure. Current recommendations suggest that all patients who have persistent blood pressures greater than the 95th percentile be evaluated more thoroughly. Because tracking data suggest that patients whose blood pressures are between the 90th and 95th percentile develop overt hypertension at a higher frequency than more normotensive patients, they should be followed carefully. Many clinicians begin evaluations for patients who have other risk factors, including a history of umbilical lines, recurrent urinary tract infections, diabetes, other cardiovascular disease, or a significant family history. Clearly, any person who has severe hypertension should be evaluated immediately and thoroughly. (A more extensive evaluation algorithm is available in the electronic version of this article.)

The extent of the evaluation depends on the age of the child, the severity of the hypertension, the extent of end-organ damage, and the long-term risk factors for the individual patient. A thorough personal and family history should include specific questions regarding neonatal course, urinary tract infections, other significant medical illnesses or traumas, medication use, and family history of hypertension, early cardiovascular or cerebrovascular events, or end-stage renal disease. The physical examination includes evaluation for four extremity pulses and blood pressure, bruits, and skin lesions in addition to the standard components.

The initial phases of evaluation should characterize the severity of the hypertension and identify common causes that require additional evaluation. Most physicians obtain routine chemistries and blood counts to document renal function, electrolyte levels (usually normal, but helpful in cases of unsuspected renal disease, endocrinopathies, or high-renin states), and overall health. A lipid profile may be appropriate based on the history and if the patient is obese. Urinalysis and spot or timed urine collections for hematuria, proteinuria, and creatinine clearance are important screens for underlying renal disease. Renal ultrasonography is helpful in searching for underlying renal pathology. Doppler ultrasonography of the renal vessels may be reassuring, although results are operator-dependent, the technology is insensitive for mild or distal lesions, and there are no age-dependent norms. This technology is expected to become more available and sensitive in the future. Cardiac evaluation is important in the search for causes (eg, coarctation of the aorta) and for defining the extent of end-organ damage. The presence of left ventricular hypertrophy is considered "damage" that warrants both therapy and follow-up. Electrocardiography and chest radiography have been standard studies for cardiac evaluations in the past, but they are insensitive. Most clinicians use echocardiography for more definitive and quantifiable information. Ophthalmologic evaluation is helpful in determining the long-term effects of hypertension, although children do not suffer from retinal changes as frequently as do hypertensive adults.

Faced with an obese adolescent who has a negative medical history, normal laboratory screening results, negative findings on ultrasonography, and a positive family history, most clinicians would halt the evaluation, make an initial diagnosis of essential hypertension, and begin considering therapy. Additional evaluation can be undertaken later if the clinical course suggests a secondary cause.

More intensive evaluation is warranted when the initial screening evaluation detects a possible secondary cause, when the age of the patient rules out essential hypertension, or when the hypertension is severe. Measurement of plasma renin, aldosterone, cortisol and cortisol precursors, and thyroid functions as well as urine drug screens may be considered, depending on the possible diagnoses. Renin and aldosterone are elevated in renal parenchymal disease and renovascular disease, although salt intake, antihypertensive medications, and laboratory capabilities can cloud the usefulness of these tests. They should be obtained when electrolyte abnormalities (usually hypokalemic alkalosis) suggest the possibility of endocrine causes of hypertension. In the presence of congenital urinary tract anomalies, nuclear imaging with ^{99}Technetium-MAG3 or DTPA can evaluate bilateral function and possible obstruction; DMSA or glucoheptonate can identify areas of renal ischemia and scarring with more accuracy and less radiation than standard intravenous pyelography.

The appropriate evaluation for renovascular disease remains controversial and changes frequently as newer technologies progress. Although invasive, the gold standard remains angiography with selective renal vein renin sampling. Importantly, in skilled hands, arteriography can be followed immediately by balloon angioplasty, thereby providing the necessary therapeutic intervention during the same procedure. Nuclear imaging with MAG3 or DTPA pre- and postdosing with captopril or another angiotensin-converting enzyme inhibitor (ACEI) has been used to detect a hypoperfused kidney or renal segment. So-called "captopril scans" are more sensitive and specific than standard intravenous pyelography, but are not well standardized for children and still miss a number of renal vascular lesions. Significant functional deterioration in one kidney following ACEI administration is highly suggestive of an ipsilateral renal artery stenosis. Unfortunately, studies that have abnormal baseline findings or no change following ACEI administration are indeterminate, and bilateral stenosis remains very difficult to detect by using this methodology. Magnetic resonance imaging (MRI) provides another option for renal vascular imaging. There are few data on its use in pediatric renovascular disease, but it should be useful for main renal artery lesions and likely will become more standardized and sensitive in the future. Similarly, computed tomography (CT) angiography with venous injections can be useful in the hands of skilled practitioners. Choosing the appropriate vascular imaging study for an individual patient requires consideration of the available radiologic capabilities and expertise.

The evaluation for possible pheochromocytoma requires measurement of timed urinary catecholamines. In these tumors, epinephrine, norepinephrine, and their metabolites (vanillylmandelic acid and homovanillic acid) are elevated. Ultrasonography and CT results can be negative because many of the tumors are small. However, nuclear imaging with MIBG (a radioiodinated compound that localizes to storage granules in neural crest cells) is very sensitive and helpful when the tumor is located elsewhere than the traditional adrenal or paraganglionic positions. Localization with MRI is improving. Due to the high morbidity of sympathetic storm, the prudent clinician should rule out pheochromocytoma in any severely hypertensive patient prior to undertaking any invasive procedure.

The detailed evaluation of the endocrinologic causes of hypertension is beyond the focus of this review. However, genetic and biochemical tools are developing rapidly, and many of these previously mysterious diseases now have defined molecular mechanisms.

Treatment

Although the decision to treat a child who has severe hypertension and end-organ damage is relatively straightforward, the management of a child or adolescent who has relatively mild hypertension and no end-organ damage remains controversial. In these situations, many clinicians begin with conservative measures, progressing to pharmacologic therapy only when conservative measures fail or the hypertension worsens.

NONPHARMACOLOGIC

The goal of treatment for pediatric hypertension is to decrease the short-and long-term risks of cardiovascular diseases and end-organ disease that result from high blood pressure. However, reducing the blood pressure alone is insufficient for this objective; the issues of obesity, hyperlipidemia, smoking, and glucose intolerance also must be addressed. Treatments include both nonpharmacologic and pharmacologic options. The most commonly used nonpharmacologic treatments are salt restriction, weight loss, exercise, and cessation of smoking. Restriction of sodium chloride intake from the astounding 8 to 10 g/d of the usual North American diet to a more modest but still sufficient level of 4 to 5 g/d has been shown in a number of studies to lower blood pressure readings by approximately 8 mm Hg. Although reduced salt intake is not always apparently beneficial to an individual patient, instruction in reducing salt intake (initially to the level of a "no added salt diet") should be a part of the lifestyle changes suggested to anyone who has borderline or documented hypertension. There are no current recommendations for the use of supplemental potassium, calcium, or magnesium in the treatment of pediatric hypertension. The associations between obesity and hypertension are strong; in some studies, obesity accounts for as much as 45% of hypertension in adolescents. Therefore, nutritional counseling for weight loss should be a part of the therapeutic strategy for managing hypertension in the overweight child. Diets low in fat and rich in fruits and vegetables generally reduce sodium intake and may provide additional advantages beyond weight loss. When undertaking weight loss programs for obese children, it is crucial to enlist the full support of the family to achieve success. Unfortunately, this frequently is not achieved, and significant weight loss is both uncommon and often transient.

The addition of exercise to a hypertensive child's lifestyle has beneficial effects on both blood pressure and overall health. The American College of Sports Medicine recommends aerobic exercise three to four times per week at a level that achieves 60% to 85% of maximal heart rate. Static exercise also can improve long-term blood pressure, although many clinicians are hesitant to recommend it and often discourage it. The largest theoretical risk is to patients who have uncontrolled hypertension and choose to participate in static sports. Pressures greater than 400/300 mm Hg and 290/230 mm Hg have been recorded in normotensive athletes performing weightlifting maneuvers without adverse effects. However, many clinicians are reluctant to allow these types of exercise in hypertensive patients until their resting blood pressures are brought into the normal range. Combinations of aerobic and static exercise can be allowed for appropriately monitored patients, and patients who want to undertake static training should start with lower weight and more repetitions, followed by staged increases in the weight and decreases in the repetitions. Forcing children and adolescents to participate in activities they do not enjoy will not encourage long-term lifestyle changes that encourage exercise. Rather, working with them to achieve their athletic goals will more likely keep them exercising.

No episodes of sudden death in children or adolescents have been attributed to hypertension alone. In the absence of cardiovascular abnormalities or end-organ dysfunction, sports participation should not be limited on the basis of hypertension alone. Prior to the initiation of an exercise program for a hypertensive child, the clinician should explore the history for cardiovascular complaints with exercise, thoroughly examine the patient, and review the echocardiogram. Standardized exercise stress testing is used by many centers to determine clearance for organized sports, although no effects on patient outcome have been reported. The current recommendations from the American Academy of Pediatrics limits competitive sports and highly static exercise in patients who have severe hypertension only until their hypertension is under adequate control and there is no evidence of end-organ damage (such as arrhythmia or ST-segment depression). Dynamic exercise and participation in organized sports is encouraged for all other patients whose hypertension is less severe or is well-controlled.

PHARMACOLOGIC

Although conservative measures clearly can reduce blood pressure, these options are often insufficient for the treatment of hypertension because of patient and family compliance problems. In the presence of end-organ involvement or when nonpharmacologic methods fail, drug therapy should be initiated. When comparing and choosing from the available pharmacologic therapies, the clinician must consider efficacy, dosing availability and frequency, adverse effects, and cost. The most effective treatment is usually the one that the patient will take. Only in the very recent past have clinical trials been performed to document dosing and efficacy for antihypertensives in the pediatric age group. Current United States Food and Drug Administration guidelines now mandate such studies prior to the release of new agents, which decreases the "trial-and-error" approach that has been used in this arena in the past. Many of the newer agents (Table 3) are being studied in the pediatric population.

ANGIOTENSIN CONVERTING ENZYME INHIBITORS (ACEIs). These agents block the conversion of angiotensin I to angiotensin II, thereby preventing the vasoconstrictive and salt-retaining effects of the renin-angiotensin system. Additional actions include blocking the action of kininase II, which leads to increases in vasodilatory kinins. Although also used in low-renin hypertension, these drugs are most efficacious in the settings of renin-mediated hypertension, such as reflux nephropathy, chronic glomerulonephritis, and renovascular disease. They have additional renal protective effects in states of prevalent glomerulosclerosis (especially diabetic nephropathy) and may slow the progression of renal insufficiency from a number of acquired and inherited renal diseases. Captopril, the initial drug in this class, largely has been supplanted by longer-acting forms (enalapril, lisinopril, fosinopril, quinapril, benazepril, ramipril). Dosing for small children continues to be difficult; tablets usually must be divided and ground and possibly compounded into short-acting liquid forms.

Adverse effects of ACEIs are generally few, but include impairment of renal functional when the glomerular filtration rate (GFR) is less than 30 mL/min, in the presence of bilateral renal artery disease or renal artery disease in a single kidney, or following kidney transplantation. This effect is due to the loss of angiotensin II-mediated efferent arteriolar tone that maintains GFR in these situations; the effect is transient following discontinuation of the medication, but it can be temporarily severe. Other adverse effects include hyperkalemia (uncommon if GFR is normal), neutropenia, anemia, dry cough (1% to 5%), and angioedema. These medications do not affect cardiovascular performance and, therefore, are good options for the hypertensive athlete. ACEIs should be used with caution and education in females of childbearing potential because they are contraindicated in the second and third trimesters of pregnancy due to fetal anuria, calvarial defects, failure of renal developmental, and fetal death.

ANGIOTENSIN RECEPTOR BLOCKERS (ARBs). Although experience with these new agents in the pediatric population is minimal, ARBs (losartan, candesartan) directly prevent the action of angiotensin II on cell membrane receptors. Accordingly, these drugs are most useful in states of renin-mediated hypertension and appear to

Table 3. Commonly Used Pharmacologic Agents for Pediatric Hypertension*

Emergency Use

Drug	Dose	Route	Major Adverse Effects/Comments
Nifedipine	0.2 to 0.5 mg/kg (max, 10 mg/dose)	PO or SL	Hypotension, flushing, tachycardia, use with care in the presence of coronary or aortic disease
Nicardipine	5 to 10 mcg/kg per minute	Continuous IV	Similar to nifedipine
Sodium nitroprusside	0.3 to 8 mcg/kg per minute	Continuous IV	Hypotension, metabolized to cyanide/thiocyanate, titrate carefully
Labetalol	0.3 to 1.0 mg/kg q 10 min (max, 20 mg)	IV bolus	Hypotension, bradycardia, bronchospasm. Do not use in asthma, heart block, obstructive lung disease, or pulmonary edema
	or		
	0.4 to 3 mg/kg per hour	Continuous IV	

Chronic Use

Drug	Dose	Adverse Effects/Comments
Angiotensin Converting Enzyme Inhibitors		
Captopril	0.5 to 2.0 mg/kg q 8 h or 0.05 to 0.5 mg/kg q 6 to 8 h in neonates	May cause rash, neutropenia, hyperkalemia, cough. Use with caution in renal insufficiency. Contraindicated in pregnancy. May be compounded to 1 mg/mL suspension with a 14-day shelf limit
Enalapril	0.1 to 0.5 mg/kg per day divided qd or bid	As with captopril
Lisinopril	2.5 to 20 mg/d	As with captopril
Angiotensin Receptor Blockers		
Losartan	25 to 100 mg/d divided qd or bid	Little pediatric experience. Use with caution in renal insufficiency or hyperkalemia. Contraindicated in pregnancy
Candesartan	2 to 32 mg qd	As with losartan
Calcium Channel Blockers		
Nifedipine (extended release)	20 to 60 mg qd	May cause peripheral edema, flushing, tachycardia, headache. Cannot be suspended
Amlodipine	2.5 to 10 mg qd	May be compounded into suspension. Adverse effects as with nifedipine
Isradipine	2.5 to 10 mg divided qd or bid	As with amlodipine
Beta-adrenergic Antagonists		
Propranolol	0.5 to 4.0 mg/kg per day divided q 6 to 8 h	May cause bradycardia, bronchospasm. Do not use in asthma, heart block, obstructive lung disease, or pulmonary edema
Atenolol	1 to 2 mg/kg qd	As with propranolol
Labetalol	4 to 40 mg qd divided bid or tid	Mixed alpha/beta blocker. May be compounded into 10 mg/mL suspension. Adverse effects as with propranolol
Diuretics		
Furosemide	0.5 to 2.0 mg/kg per dose bid or qid	May cause hypokalemia, hypercalciuria, dehydration
Bumetanide	0.05 to 0.1 mg/kg per dose qd or bid	As with furosemide
Hydrochlorothiazide	2 to 3 mg/kg per day divided bid	May cause hypokalemia, hyperlipidemia, dehydration
Metolazone	2.5 to 10 mg qd	As with hydrochlorothiazide
Central Alpha-adrenergic Blockers		
Clonidine	2.5 to 10 mcg/kg per day divided qd or tid	May cause drowsiness, bradycardia, dry mouth. *Do not withdraw rapidly.* Available as transdermal patch and may be compounded as 0.1 mg/mL suspension
Alpha methyldopa	10 to 65 mg/kg per day divided bid or qid	Proven safety profile in pregnancy
Peripheral Alpha-adrenergic Blockers		
Prazosin	1 to 20 mg/d divided bid or tid	May cause syncope, orthostatic hypotension, salt retention. Titrate slowly
Direct Vasodilators		
Hydralazine	0.5 to 7.5 mg/kg per day divided bid or qid	May cause orthostatic hypotension, headache, and salt retention. Use with caution in renal or liver disease
Minoxidil	0.1 to 1 mg/kg divided bid or qd	Adverse effects as for hydralazine, plus significant hirsutism

*Pediatric dosing guidelines have not been officially established for the majority of these agents. These recommendations are based on common practice.

have fewer adverse effects than ACEIs, although the effects on renal function and potassium balance are similar. Importantly, the effects on fetal development are identical to those of ACEIs, making ARBs contraindicated in pregnancy.

CALCIUM CHANNEL BLOCKERS. These agents inhibit calcium movement into vascular smooth muscle, thereby inhibiting vasoconstriction. Because the dihydropyridines (nifedipine, nicardipine, amlodipine, isradipine, felodipine) are most selective for arteriolar smooth muscle, they are used most commonly to treat hypertension. They are effective for treatment of hypertensive emergencies and for chronic therapy because of their good safety and efficacy profiles and few adverse effects. Short-acting nifedipine no longer is used in adults who have hypertensive crises because of hypotensive morbidity and mortality among patients who have underlying coronary artery or cerebrovascular disease. No similar problems have been encountered in children, and oral or sublingual nifedipine continues to be used commonly in pediatric patients who have hypertensive emergencies. Convenient and appropriate dosing of calcium channel blockers is difficult in the young child because long-acting tablets are available only in larger doses. Isradipine and amlodipine can be compounded into liquid forms if necessary. Nicardipine is gaining use as an emergency and intensive care drug. It is administered as a continuous, titratable, intravenous infusion as an alternative to nitroprusside or labetalol. Adverse effects of the calcium channel blockers are usually minimal, but they include peripheral edema, flushing, tachycardia, nausea, headache, and postural hypotension; their frequency is decreased with the use of the sustained-release preparations.

BETA-ADRENERGIC ANTAGONISTS. These agents decrease cardiac output, peripheral vascular resistance, renin secretion, and central nervous system sympathetic activity by blocking the beta receptors. The most extensively used beta blocker in pediatric experience is the prototype, propranolol. However, its adverse effect profile is substantial, and its lack of selectivity for cardiovascular receptors results in problems with bronchoconstriction, insulin resistance, and altered lipid profiles. Many pediatricians now use labetalol, which also has significant alpha-adrenergic blockade properties and, therefore, significant synergistic vasodilation. Adverse effects of all drugs in this class include bradycardia, syncope, central nervous system depression, and rarely, hematologic problems. In the adolescent population these drugs also carry the significant adverse effects of decreased sexual potency and decreased exercise capacity, with subsequent compliance problems.

DIURETICS. Diuretics exert their antihypertensive effects by promoting salt and water excretion. Although long a mainstay in the treatment of adult hypertension, their use has decreased as newer options have been developed. However, they frequently are used as second- or third-line medications and are especially helpful in states characterized by fluid retention. In fact, diuretics should be considered the first line of treatment for hypertension due to acute poststreptococcal glomerulonephritis.

The so-called "loop diuretics" (furosemide, bumetanide) act on the ascending loop of Henle by blocking the Na-K-2Cl cotransporter. These agents are extremely helpful when rapid diuresis is necessary, and they are effective in patients who have renal insufficiency. Adverse effects include hypokalemic alkalosis, hypercalciuria and nephrocalcinosis, and ototoxicity, especially when used concomitantly with other ototoxic drugs. They are protein-bound and are less effective in hypoalbuminemic states, such as nephrotic syndrome and liver disease. Thiazides and metolazone prevent sodium transport in the distal tubule by blocking the Na-Cl cotransporter. They provide a more sustained but less vigorous diuresis than do loop diuretics. Adverse effects include hypokalemic alkalosis, glucose intolerance, and adverse effects on lipid profiles. They do not work well when GFR is low, but nephrocalcinosis and stone formation are not complications.

Potassium-sparing diuretics (spironolactone, amiloride, triamterene) block sodium reabsorption in the collecting duct by preventing the effects of aldosterone. As a class, they are weak diuretics, but they can help prevent potassium loss and are very effective for treatment of hypertension resulting from hyperaldosteronism or similar endocrinopathies.

When considering the use of diuretics for athletes, it is important to recognize that they are prohibited in many sports and carry the additional risks of electrolyte abnormalities that may be exacerbated in dehydrating conditions.

CENTRAL ALPHA2-ADRENERGIC BLOCKERS. These agents act via stimulation of alpha$_2$-adrenergic receptors in the central nervous system. Clonidine and methyldopa are used most commonly. Importantly, they have minimal cardiac or renal adverse effects, but dry mouth, depression, sedation, sleep disturbances, and impotence limit their use. Rarely, patients can experience autoimmune hemolytic anemia or hepatitis. Also of concern is severe rebound hypertension that can occur when the drug is discontinued rapidly. The transdermal delivery system for clonidine is a good alternative because it is associated with fewer sedation effects and compliance is better. The current primary use of methyldopa is in the treatment of hypertension in pregnancy, where its safety profile is unparalleled.

PERIPHERAL ALPHA$_1$-ADRENERGIC BLOCKERS. These agents cause peripheral vasodilatation by antagonizing vascular alpha$_1$ sympathetic receptors. Prazosin is used most commonly. Adverse effects include orthostatic hypotension and salt and fluid retention. Phenoxybenzamine and phentolamine also are members of this class of drugs, but their use generally is limited to the treatment of pheochromocytoma.

DIRECT VASODILATORS. These agents act through a number of mechanisms to cause direct vascular smooth muscle relaxation. Due to a high incidence of adverse effects (hypotension, salt and water retention, headache, tachycardia, flushing), they are not used routinely as first-line antihypertensives. In the past, hydralazine was favored because it was available in intravenous, liquid, and tablet forms and, therefore, could be used for all age groups and medical situations. Its use has been supplanted largely by minoxidil. Although a very effective antihypertensive, the well-known effects of severe hirsutism limit the use of minoxidil in pediatrics to patients who

have recalcitrant hypertension. Sodium nitroprusside acts as a vasodilator via nitric oxide donation. It remains the gold standard for hypertensive emergencies in the intensive care unit because it can be titrated minute to minute by continuous infusion. Metabolic byproducts (thiocyanate and cyanide) are a concern, especially among patients who have renal or hepatic disease, and the levels of these byproducts must be monitored after 24 hours of use. Diazoxide, once used commonly for hypertensive emergencies, has been replaced with oral nifedipine and intravenous labetalol or nicardipine.

SURGERY

Although not commonly considered a therapeutic option for hypertension, there are a few instances when surgery is an appropriate alternative to lifelong medication. Correction of a renal artery stenosis by balloon angioplasty or operative bypass procedures is needed to correct hypertension and preserve the function of the affected kidney. Similarly, in cases of segmental renal infarct, unilateral renal hypoplasia with diminished function, or chronic obstruction, partial or complete nephrectomy can be considered. To maximize the potential for complete resolution of hypertension, the affected and contralateral kidney should be evaluated carefully, including assessment of renal vein renin prior to surgical intervention. Removal of viable kidney tissue is not advised in the presence of global decreased kidney function. The other major role for surgical intervention for pediatric hypertension is in cases of pheochromocytoma. Although the urge to remove the tumor is strong, surgery should not be performed until the tumor has been blocked completely with appropriate medications. Knowledgeable pediatric anesthesia and surgical personnel must perform the surgery.

LENGTH OF THERAPY

The appropriate duration of treatment for a child or adolescent is unknown. Some patients require lifelong therapy; others may experience improvement or even resolution of their hypertension. For these reasons, if blood pressure is under excellent control and no organ system damage is present, medications can be tapered and discontinued under careful observation. When patients have been weaned from medication, they still should have their blood pressure monitored routinely because a significant number will become hypertensive again in the future.

Special Treatment Issues

ESSENTIAL HYPERTENSION

The decision to treat a patient who has essential hypertension often is controversial. Many affected teens will be only minimally hypertensive, and they and their families may be reluctant to begin therapy. Clearly, an initially conservative approach of dietary and exercise programs is appropriate as long as there is no evidence of end-organ damage. However, should medication be needed, it is important to maximize compliance and minimize adverse metabolic side effects. The agents used most commonly in these circumstance are long-acting calcium channel blockers and ACEIs. When considering ACEIs in adolescent girls of childbearing potential, it is imperative to educate them well about the fetotoxic effects of these medications.

HYPERTENSIVE ATHLETES

For the pediatric athlete for whom competition and performance are issues, ACEIs and calcium channel blockers are often excellent pharmacologic options because they do not suppress cardiovascular function. Diuretics are banned by many sports organizations and should be avoided because of the additional adverse effects of enhanced volume contraction.

NEONATAL HYPERTENSION

In the neonatal population, the most common causes of hypertension include congenital renal diseases, renal ischemic events, and a combination of cardiopulmonary disease and multiple drug regimens. Although nearly every medication discussed previously has been used in very young and preterm infants, there are very few data regarding long-term use and safety, and the majority of options do not facilitate appropriate dosing for very small patients. ACEIs work well

in renin-mediated hypertension due to renal ischemia or congenital obstructions. However, the clinician should be aware of the potential for abnormal renal development in the very preterm infant in whom nephrogenesis is incomplete. Each infant's special problems should be considered thoroughly prior to choosing an antihypertensive.

HYPERTENSIVE EMERGENCIES

Close monitoring is mandatory when treating the patient who has symptomatic hypertension to reduce blood pressure without producing potentially threatening hypotension. The goal of treatment of hypertensive urgencies is to reduce the blood pressure over a 24-hour period; it can be attempted with any of the previously listed oral medications. In many instances, dose increases in the patient's current medications may be sufficient. Oral or sublingual nifedipine is effective but short-lived, and additional, longer-acting medications should be added or increased. The addition of intravenous medications should be considered if oral options do not produce the desired results quickly. In the rare instance of a true hypertensive emergency that involves acute, life-threatening cardiovascular or cerebrovascular complications, intravenous medications and intra-arterial monitoring are mandatory. Oral or sublingual nifedipine are helpful in the initial stages of treatment, during establishment of access and delivery of other medications, but continuous intravenous infusions with sodium nitroprusside, nicardipine, or labetalol should be initiated as rapidly as possible.

Suggested Reading

American Academy of Pediatrics Committee on Sports Medicine and Fitness. Athletic participation by children and adolescents who have systemic hypertension. *Pediatrics.* 1997;99:637–638

Bao W, Threefoot SA, Srinivasan SR, Berenson GS. Essential hypertension predicted by tracking of elevated blood pressure from childhood to adulthood: the Bogalusa Heart Study. *Am J Hyperten.* 1995;8:657–665

Bartosh SM, Aronson AJ. Childhood hypertension: an update on etiology, diagnosis, and treatment. *Pediatr Clin North Am.* 1999;46:235–252

Feld LG, Waz WR. Treatment of hypertension. In: Barratt TM, Avner ED, Harmon WE, eds. *Pediatric Nephrology*. 4th ed. Baltimore, Md: Lippincott Williams & Wilkins; 1999: 1031–1049

Fivush B, Neu A, Furth S. Acute hypertensive crises in children: emergenices and urgencies. *Curr Opin Pediatr*. 1997;9:233–236

Miller K. Pharmacological management of hypertension in pediatric patients: a comprehensive review of the efficacy, safety and dosage guidelines of the available agents. *Drugs*. 1994;48:868–887

Sorof JM, Portman RJ. Ambulatory blood pressure monitoring in the pediatric patient. *J Pediatr*. 2000;136:578–586

Temple ME, Nahata MC. Treatment of pediatric hypertension. *Pharmacotherapy*. 2000;20:140–150

Update on the 1987 Task Force Report on High Blood Pressure in Children and Adolescents: A Working Group Report from the National High Blood Pressure Education Program. *Pediatrics*. 1996;98:649–658

Infectious Mononucleosis

John Peter, MD* and C. George Ray, MD†

Important Points

1. The etiologic agent for infectious mononucleosis is Epstein-Barr virus, although a mononucleosis-like syndrome can be caused by other viral agents, most notably cytomegalovirus.
2. The classic physical findings of infectious mononucleosis include fever, lymphadenopathy, pharyngitis, and splenomegaly.
3. Although the presence of heterophil antibodies is considered diagnostic of infectious mononucleosis, children younger than 4 years of age develop an antibody response less than 20% of the time.
4. The primary route of transmission for infectious mononucleosis is saliva; it rarely is spread via aerosol or fomites.
5. Treatment for infectious mononucleosis is generally supportive, with glucocorticoids indicated only for patients exhibiting evidence of airway obstruction.

History

Infectious mononucleosis (IM) was first described in the Russian medical literature in 1885. Epstein-Barr virus (EBV), the viral agent responsible for IM, is a ubiquitous herpesvirus first described by Epstein, Achong, and Barr in continuous cell lines derived from African Burkitt lymphoma tissues. The Henles first observed development of antibodies to EBV in a patient who had acute IM. Subsequent serologic surveys in 1967 confirmed EBV as the major cause of IM.

Epidemiology

EBV preferentially infects B lymphocytes and is transmitted primarily in saliva or, less commonly, by blood transfusion. It is not likely to be transmitted by aerosol or fomites. After an incubation period of 2 to 7 weeks following exposure, as many as 20% of the circulating B lymphocytes of adolescents or young adults developing IM are infected, although the number usually is closer to 1%. There is a subsequent increase in suppressor T lymphocytes during the acute phase of the infection, which produces a low or "inverted" T4/T8 (helper/suppressor) lymphocytic ratio. EBV is shed from the oropharynx for up to 18 months following the primary infection and is shed intermittently in 15% to 25% of healthy EBV-seropositive individuals for years. Immuno-suppressed individuals shed the virus more frequently. Most adults throughout the world (>80%) are EBV-seropositive.

The age of initial infection varies in different cultural and socioeconomic settings. In some poor urban settings or in developing countries, 80% to 100% of children are seropositive by 3 to 6 years of age. The majority of primary infections in such groups are subclinical or only mildly symptomatic. In economically privileged communities and developed countries, primary infection occurs later in life, often between the ages of 10 and 30 years. These cases are associated more often with clinical symptoms, usually a mononucleosis syndrome.

---

*Assistant Professor, Department of Pediatrics, Division of Emergency Medicine.

†Professor, Department of Pediatrics, Division of Infectious Disease, St. Louis University School of Medicine and Cardinal Glennon Children's Hospital, St. Louis, MO.

Given the widespread rate of infection in the general population, it may be assumed that EBV spreads relatively efficiently. However, in one family study, only 35% of nonimmune siblings developed EBV antibodies over 5.6 contact months after identification of the index case. Mononucleosis-like infections may occur more than once in immunocompetent individuals, but a confirmed case of symptomatic, acute reactivation of EBV disease never has been reported.

Clinical Aspects

Primary EBV infection in young children usually is asymptomatic or presents with such mild, nonspecific symptoms as upper respiratory tract infection, tonsillopharyngitis, or prolonged febrile illness with or without lymphadenopathy. Older children are more likely to develop the typical signs and symptoms of IM. After an incubation period of 2 to 7 weeks, prodromal symptoms of malaise, anorexia, and chills frequently precede the onset of the classic signs and symptoms of IM: fever, sore throat, malaise, and fatigue accompanied by tonsillopharyngitis and lymphadenopathy. Most patients also complain of headache. Periorbital edema may be seen. Fever may reach 39° to 40°C (102.2° to 104°F) and last 1 to 2 weeks. Adenopathy typically is nontender and involves both the anterior and posterior cervical lymph nodes, but diffuse adenopathy may be present. The pharyngitis is usually diffuse, and often there is a thick tonsillar exudate. Palatal petechiae also may be present. Splenomegaly develops in the first 3 weeks of illness in at least 50% of cases and hepatomegaly in about 30% to 50%. Mild hepatic tenderness may be present. In 5% of patients, a macular, petechial, scarlatiniform, urticarial, or erythema multiforme-like rash may appear. Administration of ampicillin- or amoxicillin-containing antibiotics can result in a pruritic, maculopapular eruption in 90% to 100% of patients, usually commencing 7 to 10 days after the first dose.

Mononucleosis due to cytomegalovirus (CMV) is the illness confused most frequently with EBV-induced IM. Patients who have CMV mononucleosis are, on average, older than those who have EBV-induced disease and exhibit fever and malaise as the major manifestations; pharyngitis and lymphadenopathy are less common than with EBV-induced IM.

Pharyngitis may be caused by a variety of other viral or bacterial organisms. Group A beta-hemolytic streptococci can be isolated from the throats of up to 30% of patients who have symptomatic IM and in nearly the same percentage of asymptomatic individuals. Therefore, isolation of this organism does not rule out IM. Malignancies or infection with adenoviruses, *Toxoplasma gondii*, rubella virus, human immunodeficiency virus (HIV), and hepatitis A virus also may produce a mononucleosis-like syndrome (Table 1).

EBV initially was believed to be the etiologic agent of chronic fatigue syndrome, an illness characterized by recurrent malaise, difficulty with concentration, headache, weakness, myalgias, arthralgias, pharyngitis, lymphadenitis, and low-grade fever. However, subsequent studies have not supported such an association. Although fewer than 5% of patients experience malaise and fever for as long as 3 to 4 months, some patients have been reported in whom signs and symptoms persisting for more than 6 months are associated with evidence of ongoing EBV replication. Some have labeled this disorder "chronic mono," but this is an extremely rare condition, and the etiology of the ongoing viral replication is uncertain.

Laboratory Evaluation

Although the classic tube heterophil titer is still performed in some laboratories, the "monospot" slide test is sensitive, specific, easily performed, and used more commonly. The sensitivity and specificity are 85% and 97%, respectively, in children older than 4 years of age. Symptomatic

---

TABLE 1. Conditions and Infections Producing a Mononucleosis-like Syndrome

- Malignancies
- Adenoviruses
- Toxoplasma
- Rubella
- Human immunodeficiency virus
- Hepatitis A
- Diphtheria

children younger than 4 years most often do not develop a heterophil antibody response to EBV, and the sensitivity in this age group is less than 20%. Up to 15% of patients who have IM may be heterophil-negative initially, then become positive on retesting during the second or third week of illness. Antibody concentrations decline after the acute illness has resolved but may be detectable for up to 9 months after the onset of illness. Therefore, a positive monospot test is not diagnostic of active disease.

Viral-specific serology should be used to diagnose EBV IM in children younger than 4 years of age who exhibit typical presentations and in patients who have atypical clinical presentations or severe, prolonged illnesses with negative heterophil tests (Table 2). Immunoglobulin M antibodies to the EBV capsid antigen (IgM anti-VCA) are produced at the time of the acute infection, persist for weeks to months, and do not reappear (Figure). Comparison of acute and convalescent sera shows a rise, a subsequent fall, and a lifelong persistence of IgG anti-VCA. Antibodies to EBV nuclear antigen (anti-EBNA) usually do not appear until 2 to 4 weeks after the onset of symptoms, so their absence in a previously well person who develops acute illness and is otherwise seropositive suggests an acute, primary EBV infection. Antibodies to EBV early antigens (EA) appear early in the infection, usually persist for several months, and can reappear at any time, either spontaneously or as a nonspecific response to a wide range of stressful stimuli.

Immunofluorescence is the most commonly used method for EBV serology, but it is labor-intensive and time-consuming. Several currently available commercial enzyme-linked immunosorbent assays (ELISAs) have varying degrees of sensitivity and specificity. Careful evaluation of

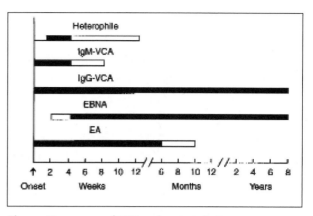

Figure. Time course of EBV serology in infectious mononucleosis. Open portions represent periods when detection is possible; dark portions represent periods when detection commonly occurs.

the performance of these kits is essential before any are adopted for routine use, but when used correctly, all are equally clinically effective.

Approximately 75% of patients who have IM demonstrate an absolute lymphocytosis (>50% lymphocytes, with total leukocytes >5,000/mm^3), often with more than 10% atypical lymphocytes, most of which are activated T cells. This lymphocytosis is the most reliable indicator of IM when the monospot slide test is negative and serology is not readily available. Transient neutropenia and thrombocytopenia are noted frequently, as are mild increases in serum IgA, IgG, and IgM and hepatocellular enzymes. The thrombocytopenia appears to be due to various mechanisms, including increased destruction by an enlarged spleen and the presence of antiplatelet antibodies. Frequently, patients develop antibodies to human erythrocyte antigens (anti-i), but significant hemolytic anemia is uncommon. In fewer than 1% of cases is the neutropenia, thrombocytopenia, and increased levels of hepatocellular enzymes and human erythrocyte antigens of any clinical significance.

Table 2. Interpretation of EBV Serology*

	IgG-VCA	IgM-VCA	EBV Nuclear Antigen	EBV Early Antigens
No evidence of infection	<10	<10	<2	<10
Acute infection	>10	≥10	<2	≥20
Convalescent infection	>10	Variable	>2	Variable
Remote past infection	≥10	<10	>2	≤20

*Values are expressed in reciprocal titers as measured by standard immunofluorescence methods.

Management

Treatment of IM is supportive. Adequate rest is advocated, but there is no evidence that bed rest hastens recovery. Fluids and a soft diet along with acetaminophen or ibuprofen will help ease the symptoms of pharyngitis and fever. Patients who have concurrent streptococcal pharyngitis should receive penicillin or erythromycin for 10 days to prevent poststreptococcal sequelae.

Patients who have splenomegaly should be advised to avoid contact sports to prevent the rare possibility of splenic rupture (estimated to be 0.1% to 0.2%). Interestingly, the majority of documented cases of splenic rupture are not accompanied by significant trauma. Although there is a wide range of recommendations for the timing of a return to contact sports, most experts agree that vigorous sports should be restricted until the spleen has returned to its normal size and protected location within the rib cage.

Recovery from IM is often gradual; in some individuals, malaise or fatigue lasts for 3 to 4 months. Glucocorticoids generally are indicated only for those who exhibit symptoms of upper airway obstruction, although some clinicians prescribe them to hasten the resolution of symptoms. Some limited studies suggest that corticosteroids hasten the resolution of fever and tonsillopharyngeal symptoms, but they do not provide significant or reproducible benefit for lymphadenopathy or hepatosplenic involvement. Some investigators have cautioned against the use of corticosteroids because of sporadic reports of an association between encephalitis or myocarditis in patients who have IM and are treated with steroids. Questions also have been raised about the possible adverse influence steroids might have on the development of long-term immunity to EBV. Most authorities advise against the routine use of corticosteroids in patients who have uncomplicated acute IM.

Several antiviral agents have been shown to inhibit the replication of EBV. The efficacy of acyclovir has been assessed in controlled studies of uncomplicated acute IM. Parenteral or high-dose oral acyclovir reduced oropharyngeal shedding of EBV. Despite this reduction in shedding, though, little or no clinical benefit was demonstrated in treating uncomplicated acute IM. The question has been raised about the possible beneficial effects of acyclovir for patients being treated with steroids in an attempt to restrict the potentially enhanced opportunity for the virus to replicate in the setting of steroid-induced immunosuppression. In one study, acyclovir suppressed oropharyngeal shedding of EBV even when steroids were administered. Although the combined regimen appeared to be clinically beneficial, the individual contribution of acyclovir to this effect was not delineated.

Prognosis

The majority of individuals who have IM experience an uneventful course and recover without residual problems, although complications do occur infrequently and may be dramatic. Hematologic complications include a self-limiting anti-i-mediated autoimmune hemolytic anemia, which resolves over a 1- to 2-month period in greater than 95% of affected individuals who are not treated. A mild thrombocytopenia may occur in up to 50% of patients; profound thrombocytopenia is rare. Similarly, mild granulocytopenia is common, but severe pancytopenia associated with infection and death has been reported. Both the thrombocytopenia and granulocytopenia usually resolve spontaneously in 3 to 6 weeks.

Neurologic complications of IM occur in about 1% of patients who have IM and may appear prior to the classic signs, symptoms, and laboratory findings. The most common neurologic complications are cranial nerve palsies and encephalitis. Cerebrospinal fluid findings generally are not helpful, and the clinical presentation in some patients resembles herpes simplex encephalitis. At least 85% of patients who have neurologic symptoms, even when severe, recover spontaneously. An "Alice-in-Wonderland" syndrome, characterized by metamorphopsia (distortion of sizes, shapes, and spatial relations of objects) has been reported.

Subclinical hepatitis is common in IM, with mildly to moderately elevated aminotransferases reported in 70% to 90% of patients. Chronic liver disease and liver failure are rare complications.

Fatal IM occurs in 1 in 3,000 cases, with the usual cause of death being fulminant hepatic failure. Children who have X-linked lympho-proliferative disease (Duncan syndrome) have no obvious manifestation of immunodeficiency until they become infected with EBV and develop hepatic failure. Up to 40% of affected males may die during their primary infection. The mechanism of liver injury appears to be due to abnormal T and natural-killer cell activity rather than to direct EBV infection of hepatocytes.

Despite the development of a significant neutropenia, serious bacterial superinfections are unusual. However, peritonsillar abscess has been observed, probably because up to 30% of patients have throat cultures positive for group A streptococci.

Infection with EBV has been associated with the development of nasopharyngeal carcinoma, a variety of lymphoproliferative disorders, and Burkitt lymphoma. However, IM usually runs a similar course in both immunocompetent and immunocompromised patients, and most EBV infections are clinically silent.

Summary

EBV-induced IM is a generally self-limited infection characterized by fever, pharyngitis, and adenopathy. Management consists of basic supportive measures and treatment of strepto-coccal pharyngitis when present. Corticosteroids may be considered for individuals who exhibit evidence of significant upper airway obstruction. To date there is little evidence to support the use of antiviral agents in immunocompetent patients. Complications of IM may arise, which can be life-threatening, but these are relatively rare.

Suggested Reading

Alpert G, Fleisher GR. Complications of infection with Epstein-Barr virus during childhood: a study of children admitted to the hospital. *Pediatr Infect Dis.* 1984;3:304–307

Domachowske JB, Cunningham CK, Cummings DL, Crosley CJ, Hannan WP, Weiner LB. Acute manifestations and neurologic sequelae of Epstein-Barr virus encephalitis in children. *Pediatr Infect Dis J.* 1996;15:871–875

Eshel GM, Eyov A, Lahat E, Brauman A. Alice in Wonderland syndrome, a manifestation of acute Epstein-Barr virus infection. *Pediatr Infect Dis J.* 1987;6:68

Straus SE, Cohen JI, Tosato G, Meier J. Epstein-Barr virus infections: biology, pathogenesis, and management. *Ann Intern Med.* 1993;118:45–58

Sumaya CV, Ench Y. Epstein-Barr virus infectious mononucle-osis in children. I. Clinical and general laboratory findings. *Pediatrics.* 1985;75:1003–1010

Sumaya CV, Ench Y. Epstein-Barr virus infectious mono-nucleosis in children. II. Heterophil antibody and viral-specific responses. *Pediatrics.* 1985;75:1011–1019

Svahn A, Magnusson M, Jagdahl L, Schloss L, Kahlmeter G, Linde A. Evaluation of three commercial enzyme-linked immunosorbent assays and two latex agglutination assays for diagnosis of primary Epstein-Barr virus infection. *J Clin Microbiol.* 1997;35:2728–2732

Tynell E, Aurelius E, Brandell A, et al. Acyclovir and pred-nisolone treatment of acute infectious mononucleosis: a multicenter, double-blind, placebo-controlled study. *J Infect Dis.* 1996;174:324–331

Inflammatory Bowel Disease

Jeffrey S. Hyams, MD*

Objectives

After completing this article, readers should be able to:

1. Describe the primary clinical difference between Crohn disease and ulcerative colitis.
2. List the greatest single risk factor for developing inflammatory bowel disease.
3. Delineate the primary presentation of children and adolescents who have Crohn disease.
4. Explain the effects of prolonged daily use of high-dose corticosteroids.
5. Describe the primary risk factor for intestinal cancer associated with both ulcerative colitis and Crohn disease.

Introduction

Inflammatory bowel disease (IBD) is a generic term used to describe two idiopathic disorders that are associated with gastrointestinal inflammation: Crohn disease (CD) and ulcerative colitis (UC). These disorders need to be distinguished from other conditions that may display similar clinical and laboratory findings, such as infection, allergy, and neoplasm. Because IBD also may be associated with a large array of extraintestinal manifestations, a knowledge of the clinical spectrum of these disorders is important to the clinician who may encounter associated pediatric problems such as growth delay, arthritis, hepatitis, and anemia. Once IBD is diagnosed, newer medical and surgical treatment modalities allow most affected children to lead relatively normal lives.

Definitions

The ultimate definition of UC and CD rests with the location and characteristics of inflammation within the gastrointestinal tract. In UC, a relatively homogeneous inflammatory process is confined to the mucosa, which starts in the rectum and involves a variable extent of colon proximally. Crypt abscesses are common. Contrary to historical belief, patients may have discontinuous inflammation at diagnosis or even rectal sparing, but over the course of the illness the inflammation becomes more confluent. Inflammation limited to the rectum, observed in 10% of patients, is termed ulcerative proctitis. In about 30% of cases, the disease is limited to the left side of the colon; in 40% to 50%, there is pancolitis.

The inflammation associated with CD may involve any portion of the alimentary tract, from mouth to anus. The earliest abnormality seen commonly is a superficial ulcer overlying a lymphoid follicle (aphthous lesion). Mucosal inflammation may become more generalized or remain patchy and may extend gradually into the submucosa, muscularis, and serosa. Transmural inflammation can result in fistula formation. Granuloma, believed to be pathognomonic for CD, is found only in a minority of patients. Inflammation is grossly limited to the terminal ileum in about 30% of cases, involves the ileum and colon in 60%, and is limited to the colon in 10% to 20%. Gastroduodenal inflammation is evident in about 30% to 40% of all patients. The advent of fiberoptic endoscopy has shown that microscopic disease frequently is present throughout the gastrointestinal system in many patients despite limited disease noted radiographically.

*Head, Division of Digestive Diseases and Nutrition, Connecticut Children's Medical Center; Professor of Pediatrics, University of Connecticut School of Medicine, Hartford, CT. Dr Hyams is a Consultant, National Treatment Registry for Remicade for Centocor, Inc.

Epidemiology and Genetics

IBD affects males and females equally; it is more common in whites than nonwhites, in northern than southern areas, in urban than rural areas, and in Jews than non-Jews. CD occurs with a higher frequency among patients who have Turner syndrome, Hermansky-Pudlak syndrome, and glycogen storage disease type IB.

The single greatest risk factor for the development of IBD is having a first-degree relative who has the disease. At the time CD is diagnosed, the likelihood of finding IBD in a first-degree relative of the proband is 10% to 25%. For a first-degree relative of a proband who has CD, the age-adjusted risk for developing CD during a lifetime is about 4%. The risk for relatives of probands who have UC is somewhat less than 4%. It has been suggested that the susceptibility loci for CD may exist on chromosomes 6 and 16. Within close distance to the chromosome 16 locus are genes involved in complement receptors, mycobacterial cell adhesion, B lymphocyte function, leukocyte adhesion, and the interleukin-4 (IL4) receptor. A perinuclear antineutrophil antibody (pANCA) is found in about 70% of individuals who have UC compared with 6% of those who have CD and is believed to represent a marker of a genetically controlled immunoregulatory disturbance. The presence of pANCA is concordant within families.

Pathogenesis

The cause(s) of IBD are not known. It also is not known whether UC and CD are two distinct diseases that have similar clinical manifestations or diseases that have different histopathologic and geographic localization and are causally linked. Genetic susceptibility has been suggested by the predisposition to IBD in certain ethnic groups and familial occurrence.

Most investigations have focused on possible infectious etiologies as well as immunologic disturbances. To date no specific infectious agent has been reproducibly associated with IBD. Several bacterial species, including *Salmonella*, *Shigella*, *Campylobacter*, and *Yersinia*, can cause acute intestinal inflammation, but the course of infection is self-limited, and histopathologic examination of affected tissue usually can differentiate infection from chronic IBD. No convincing data prove that *Mycobacterium paratuberculosis* has a role in the pathogenesis of CD despite suggestions to the contrary a number of years ago. It has been suggested that measles virus infection can result in a granulomatous vasculitis of mesenteric vessels that causes microvascular thrombosis and tissue ischemia and may be of importance in the pathogenesis of CD. Interestingly, IBD occurs less frequently among persons who have inherited disorders of coagulation such as hemophilia and von Willebrand disease.

Abnormalities in gastrointestinal immunoregulation appear to be important contributors to the etiology. The gut is under constant immunologic stimulation from microbial agents and dietary antigens. It is also rich in immunologically active cells, which work with the barrier function provided by epithelial cells to keep the noxious external world at bay. Accordingly, the gut is in a state of constant "physiologic inflammation," with a modest number of immune cells (lymphocytes, macrophages, plasma cells) present in the lamina propria. It is believed that this "physiologic" inflammation becomes uncontrolled in CD, resulting in pathologic inflammation, increased numbers of immune cells, and eventual tissue damage. Activated immune cells secrete a variety of soluble mediators of inflammation, including cytokines, arachidonic acid metabolites, reactive oxygen intermediates, and growth factors. Cytokines such as IL-1, IL-6, and IL-8 promote inflammation by increasing expression of vascular adhesion molecules, which attract inflammatory cells, increase eicosanoid production, induce nitric oxide synthase, and increase collagen production. This cascade leads to tissue destruction and remodeling with consequent fibrosis. Electrolyte secretion is stimulated by these mediators, which contributes further to diarrhea. Other causes of diarrhea in CD include malabsorption in the small intestine; loss of bile salts from the terminal ileus into the colon, affecting colonic electrolyte absorption; and bacterial overgrowth in the small bowel with bile salt deconjugation. Diffuse mucosal disease leads to exudation of serum proteins and bleeding.

Clinical Aspects

GASTROINTESTINAL

Virtually all patients who have UC present with bloody diarrhea, except those who have proctitis, in whom the stools may be formed. Abdominal pain in patients who have UC usually is limited to the peridefecatory period. Abdominal pain is a more prominent problem among those who have CD. The pain is usually more severe, occurs at any time of the day, and may awaken the child from sleep. It is most common in the right lower quadrant in those who have ileal or ileocecal disease and is periumbilical in those who have colonic or generalized small bowel disease. Epigastric pain, simulating ulcer, is observed in those who have gastroduodenal involvement. Diarrhea, occasionally bloody, is seen in about 50% of patients who have CD. Nausea and vomiting may be present with either UC or CD, particularly when the disease is severe. Perirectal inflammation with fissures and fistula occurs in about 25% of CD patients. Oral canker sores are noted in many patients who have CD. Fever occurs in UC only in the presence of fulminant disease. Fever may be insidious in CD, occur in the absence of severe gastrointestinal symptoms, and be diagnosed initially as a fever of unknown origin.

EXTRAINTESTINAL

The more common extraintestinal manifestations of IBD are shown in Table 1. Extraintestinal manifestations are noted in about 25% to 35% of patients and can be classified into several groups: 1) those directly related to disease activity, which usually respond to therapy directed against bowel disease (eg, fever, anemia); 2) those whose course is unrelated to bowel disease activity (eg, sclerosing cholangitis); 3) those that result from the presence of diseased bowel (eg, ureteral obstruction); and 4) those that arise from therapy (eg, drug-induced pancreatitis).

Growth failure occurs in up to 20% to 30% of children who have CD and in up to 10% of those who have UC. In the latter group, growth failure almost always is due to the prolonged use of high doses of corticosteroids. In CD, the pathogenesis of growth impairment is multifactorial and includes chronic undernutrition, corticosteroid administration, and possibly the effect of proinflammatory cytokines released from diseased bowel, which circulate and affect bone metabolism. Growth failure and delayed pubertal development may constitute the primary presentation in some children who have CD.

Two forms of arthritis are noted in patients who have IBD. The peripheral form (10% of patients) commonly affects the larger joints (knees, ankles, wrists, elbows) and usually is related to active colonic disease. The axial form, ankylosing spondylitis/sacro-iliitis, is rare in children. Although abnormal concentrations of serum aminotransferases are found in up to 15% of patients during their disease course, serious liver disease such as sclerosing cholangitis (3% of UC patients) and chronic active hepatitis (<1% of patients) is uncommon.

DIAGNOSIS

There is no substitute for a detailed clinical history and physical examination in the diagnosis of IBD. Not only can the diagnosis usually be suspected, but there are good clues suggesting whether the patient has UC or CD. Laboratory studies are used to confirm the diagnosis.

Table 1. Extraintestinal Manifestations of Inflammatory Bowel Disease

Site	Manifestation
Skin	Erythema nodosum, pyoderma gangrenosum
Liver	Fatty infiltration, sclerosing cholangitis, chronic hepatitis, cholelithiasis, Budd-Chiari syndrome
Bone	Osteopenia, aseptic necrosis
Joints	Arthralgias, arthritis, ankylosing spondylitis, sacro-iliitis
Eye	Uveitis, episcleritis, keratitis
Renal/urologic	Nephrolithiasis, obstructive hydronephrosis, enterovesical fistula, immune complex glomerulonephritis
Hematologic	Anemia (iron, folate, vitamin B12 deficiency), thrombocytosis, thrombocytopenia
Vascular	Thrombophlebitis, vasculitis, portal vein thrombosis
Pancreas	Pancreatitis
Other	Growth delay, pubertal delay, ? lymphoma, ? acute myelocytic leukemia

Enteric pathogens must be excluded by appropriate stool culture and parasite examination. *Salmonella, Shigella, Campylobacter, Escherichia coli* 0157:H7, *Yersinia, Aeromonas,* and *Clostridium difficile* infections may present with bloody diarrhea; *Giardia* and *Cryptosporidium* infection may present with watery diarrhea. Anemia is common and usually due to iron deficiency. Thrombocytosis reflects both the inflammatory state (IL-6 stimulates thrombopoiesis) and gastrointestinal bleeding. The erythrocyte sedimentation rate is elevated in 80% of patients who have CD and about 40% of those who have UC. Albumin levels are low, reflecting enteric protein loss and poor nutrition. Serum aminotransferases and gamma-glutamyltransferase should be measured to evaluate possible hepatic involvement. Commercial testing for pANCA is now available and occasionally used in the diagnosis of UC. Another antibody, anti-*Saccharomyces* (ASCA), is believed to indicate CD in some patients. In my experience, it is rarely necessary to test for these immune markers.

Colonic inflammation is diagnosed via endoscopic visualization (Fig. 1) and confirmed on histologic examination of biopsied tissue. There is virtually no role for barium enema in the diagnosis of colonic inflammation. Radiographic evaluation of the small bowel, with particular interest in the terminal ileum, is mandatory when looking for evidence of CD (Fig. 2). In more than 90% of patients, the clinician can reliably differentiate UC from CD with these examinations.

Management

The goals of therapy are to decrease bowel inflammation, address complications, and prevent recurrent or worsening disease.

PHARMACOLOGICAL THERAPY

Medications used to treat IBD can be divided into four categories: aminosalicylates, corticosteroids, immunomodulators, and antibiotics (Table 2). Patients who have severe colitis (more than five bloody stools per day, fever, hypoalbuminemia, anemia) require hospitalization, bowel rest with parenteral nutritional support, intravenous corticosteroids, and very careful monitoring. The past several years have

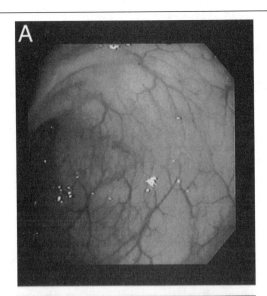
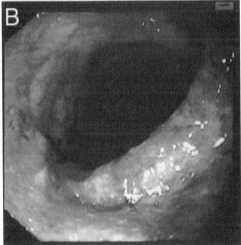
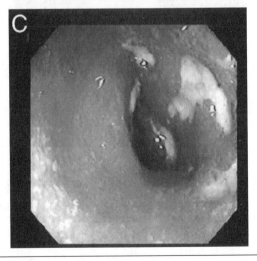

Figure 1. Endoscopic findings in inflammatory bowel disease. A. Normal-appearing colonic mucosa. Note the distinct vascular pattern and shiny appearance. B. Colonic mucosa in severe ulcerative colitis. Note the marked erythema, granularity, spontaneous bleeding, and loss of vascular pattern. C. Colonic mucosa in Crohn colitis. Note the multiple deep ulcers in the presence of erythematous mucosa.

seen increasing use of immunomodulators such as 6-mercaptopurine to decrease the amount of corticosteroids used to treat severe disease. Newer agents such as infliximab, an antitumor necrosis factor antibody, are being used to target the inflammatory response more selectively.

NUTRITION THERAPY

This type of therapy may be either primary or adjunctive in CD and is only adjunctive in UC. Elemental or polymeric formulas given as the sole source of nutrition may effect remission in up to 80% of those who have CD, but rapid relapse is common. Oral supplements and even nasogastric/gastrostomy feedings may be of critical importance in addressing chronic undernutrition and growth failure.

SURGICAL THERAPY

The goals of surgical therapy differ for UC and CD, although the indications often are similar. Uncontrolled gastrointestinal bleeding, bowel perforation, obstruction, unacceptable medication toxicity, and intractability can prompt surgery in either disorder. At times, surgical resection is used to treat growth failure, especially if it allows the discontinuation of corticosteroids. Perirectal disease may necessitate surgery in some who have CD. Carcinoma may occur in either condition and require operative intervention.

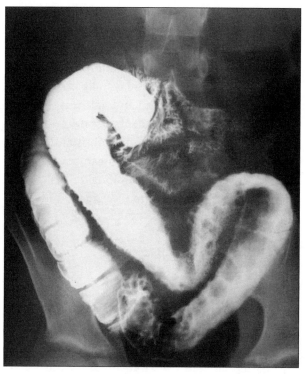

Figure 2. Radiographic findings in Crohn disease, with marked bowel wall thickening and nodularity in the distal ileum.

The surgical procedure of choice in UC is the ileal pouch anal anastomosis. This curative procedure can be performed either as a primary operation or in a staged approach, depending on the condition of the patient. Excellent long-term results have been demonstrated, although inflammation of the surgically created pouch

Table 2. Pharmacologic Therapy of Inflammatory Bowel Disease

Medication Class	Indications	Complications
Aminosalicylates ● Mesalamine ● Sulfasalazine	Mild-to-moderate UC, mild CD colitis, distal small bowel disease	Rash, bloody stools, headache, nausea, pancreatitis
Corticosteroids ● Prednisone	Moderate-to-severe small or large bowel disease	Cushingoid facies, growth suppression, osteopenia, cataracts, hypertension, acne
Immunomodulators ● Azathioprine ● 6-mercaptopurine ● Methotrexate ● Cyclosporine ● Infliximab	Severe small or large bowel disease, steroid dependency, severe fistulas, growth failure	Pancreatitis, bone marrow suppression, infection, renal damage, hypersensitivity
Antibiotics ● Metronidazole ● Ciprofloxacin	Perirectal fistula, abscess	Neuropathy, dysgeusia, nausea, fungal overgrowth

reservoir (pouchitis) develops in up to 40% of children. In CD, surgery is not curative because recurrent disease at the surgical site is very common. Segmental bowel resection is the most common procedure and usually involves the diseased terminal ileum and adjacent inflamed colon. Short segments of bowel that have been narrowed from fibrosis and do not have active inflammation can be treated with strictureplasty in which a longitudinal incision is made in the fibrotic segment and closed transversely.

PSYCHOLOGICAL THERAPY

The need for family education and reassurance cannot be overemphasized. Adolescents who have IBD may have a particularly difficult time because of issues of growth and pubertal delay, body image (cushingoid features, acne from corticosteroids), and social invalidism from abdominal pain and diarrhea. Counseling and peer support groups are very helpful.

Prognosis

IBD typically is marked by periods of exacerbation and remission. Most children (70%) who have UC will enter remission within 3 months following initial therapy, and approximately 50% will remain in remission over the next year. Colectomy within 5 years is required in up to 26% of children presenting with severe disease compared with 10% of those who have mild disease. Children who present with proctitis have up to a 70% likelihood of developing more extensive disease over time.

Only 1% of patients who have well-documented CD do not have at least one relapse after diagnosis and initial therapy. Those who have ileocolitis tend to have a poorer response to medical therapy and a greater need for surgery than do those who have only small bowel disease. Approximately 70% of children who have CD require surgery within 10 to 20 years of the original diagnosis.

The risk of cancer development in diseased bowel is significant, and patients who have long-standing colonic CD appear to be at similar risk to those who have UC. The two most critical risk factors for adenocarcinoma development in diseased colon are duration of colitis (especially >10 y) and extent of colitis (pancolitis>left-sided colitis>proctitis). The presence of sclerosing cholangitis in UC patients is also a major risk factor. Patients who have colonic disease of more than 8 to 10 years' duration should undergo annual to biannual screening colonoscopy to look for evidence of dysplasia. The finding of dysplasia prompts colectomy. Multifocal or synchronous tumors are present in 10% to 20% of patients who have UC.

Suggested Reading

Griffiths AM, Nguyen P, Smith C, et al. Growth and clinical course of children with Crohn's disease. *Gut.* 1993;34:939–944

Hyams JS. Crohn's disease. *Pediatr Clin North Am.* 1996; 43:255–277

Hyams JS. Extraintestinal manifestations of inflammatory bowel disease in children. *J Pediatr Gastroenterol Nutr.* 1994;19:7–21

Kirschner BS. Ulcerative colitis. *Pediatr Clin North Am.* 1996; 43:235–254

Is Chronic Fatigue Syndrome a Connective Tissue Disorder? A Cross-Sectional Study in Adolescents

E.M. van de Putte, MD*; C.S.P.M. Uiterwaal, PhD, MD‡; M.L. Bots, PhD, MD‡; W. Kuis, PhD, MD*; J.L.L. Kimpen, PhD, MD*; and R.H.H. Engelbert, PhD§

ABSTRACT. *Objectives.* To investigate whether constitutional laxity of the connective tissues is more frequently present in adolescents with chronic fatigue syndrome (CFS) than in healthy controls. Increased joint hypermobility in patients with CFS has been previously described, as has lower blood pressure in fatigued individuals, which raises the question of whether constitutional laxity is a possible biological predisposing factor for CFS.

Design. Cross-sectional study.

Participants. Thirty-two adolescents with CFS (according to the criteria of the Centers for Disease Control and Prevention) referred to a tertiary hospital and 167 healthy controls.

Methods. The 32 adolescents with CFS were examined extensively regarding collagen-related parameters: joint mobility, blood pressure, arterial stiffness and arterial wall thickness, skin extensibility, and degradation products of collagen metabolism. Possible confounding factors (age, gender, height, weight, physical activity, muscle strength, diet, alcohol consumption, and cigarette smoking) were also measured. The results were compared with findings in 167 healthy adolescents who underwent the same examinations.

Results. Joint mobility, Beighton score, and collagen biochemistry, all indicators of connective tissue abnormality, were equal for both groups. Systolic blood pressure, however, was remarkably lower in patients with CFS (117.3 vs 129.7 mm Hg; adjusted difference: −13.5 mm Hg; 95% confidence interval [CI]: −19.1, −7.0). Skin extensibility was higher in adolescents with CFS (mean z score: 0.5 vs 0.1 SD; adjusted difference: 0.3 SD; 95% CI: 0.1, 0.5). Arterial stiffness, expressed as common carotid distension, was lower in adolescents with CFS, indicating stiffer arteries (670 vs 820 μm; adjusted difference: −110 μm; 95% CI: −220, −10). All analyses were adjusted for age, gender, body mass index, and physical activity. Additionally, arterial stiffness was adjusted for lumen diameter and pulse pressure.

Conclusions. These findings do not consistently point in the same direction of an abnormality in connective tissue. Patients with CFS did have lower blood pressure and more extensible skin but lacked the most important parameter indicating constitutional laxity, ie, joint hypermobility. Moreover, the collagen metabolism measured by crosslinks and hydroxyproline in urine, mainly reflecting bone resorption, was not different. The unexpected finding of stiffer arteries in patients with CFS warrants additional investigation. *Pediatrics* 2005; 115:e415–e422. URL: www.pediatrics.org/cgi/doi/10.1542/peds.2004-1515; *chronic fatigue syndrome, connective tissue disease, cardiovascular factors, autonomic nervous system.*

ABBREVIATIONS. CFS, chronic fatigue syndrome; EDS, Ehlers-Danlos syndrome; HP, hydroxylysylpyridinoline; LP, lysylpyridinoline; CDC, Centers for Disease Control and Prevention; CIMT, carotid intimal-medial thickness; Hyp, hydroxyproline; CIS-20, Checklist Individual Strength-20; CI, confidence interval.

Chronic fatigue syndrome (CFS) is a frequently disabling illness of unknown etiology and variable prognosis. Scientific interest in the pathogenesis of this illness parallels the apparent increase in incidence.[1,2] However, despite all scientific efforts, a plausible cause for CFS has not been established yet. Until now, there is insufficient support for either a purely somatic or psychic chain of causation. CFS is viewed as a multifactorial illness, and

*From the Departments of *Pediatrics and §Pediatric Physical Therapy and Pediatric Exercise Physiology, Wilhelmina Children's Hospital, and ‡Julius Center for Health Sciences and Primary Care, University Medical Center Utrecht, Utrecht, Netherlands.*

Accepted for publication Nov 9, 2004.

doi:10.1542/peds.2004-1515

No conflict of interest declared.

Reprint requests to (E.M.v.d.P.) Department of Pediatric, Wilhelmina Children's Hospital, University Medical Center Utrecht, KE04.133.1, PO Box 85090, 3508 AB Utrecht, Netherlands. E-mail: e.vandeputte@wkz.azu.nl

a distinction is made between constitutional, initiating, and perpetuating factors on both the biological and psychosocial levels.[3]

The prognosis for adolescents with CFS seems to be better than for adults, although as many as 44% of adolescents remain ill with significant symptoms, as observed in an 8-year follow-up study.[4]

This study focuses on a constitutional biological factor, which may partly explain the symptoms of fatigue and pain. The main question is whether constitutional laxity of the connective tissues is present more frequently in adolescents with CFS than in healthy controls. One of the reasons to perform this study was the previous finding of increased joint hypermobility in adolescents with CFS.[5] Moreover, a former study in adolescents established the coexistence of CFS and Ehlers-Danlos syndrome (EDS) in a substantial part of the study population.[6] Fatigue is not a diagnostic criterion in EDS and not often emphasized in the medical literature, likely because of the highly unspecific nature of the symptom fatigue.[7] Also, in the more frequently diagnosed benign joint-hypermobility syndrome in childhood, fatigue is 1 of the clinical symptoms.[8-10]

Additional motivation for the hypothesis that constitutional laxity may play a role in CFS comes from the finding that just like in EDS, the clinical symptoms in benign joint-hypermobility syndrome are not restricted to the musculoskeletal system. Other organs are possibly involved, such as blood vessels (with lower systolic and diastolic blood pressure), skin (with higher skin extensibility), and bone (with a lower quantitative ultrasound measurement).[11] In addition, the patients with symptomatic generalized joint hypermobility have significantly lower excretion of urinary hydroxylysylpyridinoline (HP) crosslinks and lysylpyridinoline (LP) crosslinks.[11]

A relation between stiffness of joints and skin and blood pressure is not restricted to patients with a known collagen abnormality. Also, in healthy children we recently described a relation between stiffness of joints and laxity of skin and blood pressure.[12] Stiffness of joints seems to reflect other systemic changes in connective

tissue, and this putative multiple-organ involvement, together with the clinical finding of fatigue in collagen disorders, led to the main research question: Is constitutional laxity of the connective tissues a possible biological factor in CFS?

Methods

POPULATION

A group of 32 patients with CFS ranging in age from 12 to 18 years were included. These patients were referred to a specific CFS clinic of the University Medical Center Utrecht between January 2001 and May 2002. All patients were white and fulfilled the Centers for Disease Control and Prevention (CDC) criteria[13] for CFS at the time of inclusion. Supplementary to the CDC exclusion criteria, patients with an established diagnosis of a connective tissue disease were excluded ($n = 2$), as were patients with a known bone, skin, or joint disease ($n = 0$). Examination of the 32 patients took place in May 2002 during 2 special sessions at the hospital.

As a reference group, 363 adolescents aged 12 to 18 years from a secondary school were invited to participate; 167 adolescents (46%) agreed to participate and were examined during sessions at school over a total period of 3 weeks in April 2002. Adolescents with known diseases or disorders involving skin, joints, bone density, or vessels were not included.

MEASUREMENTS

A team of 4 examiners (physiotherapists) and the principal investigator (E.M.v.d.P.) conducted all measurements. The 4 physiotherapists were unaware of the study hypothesis. The same examiner conducted each specific measurement for all participants. No examiner was informed of the results of measurements taken by other examiners. All measurement procedures described below were similarly and in the same sequence applied to the patients and healthy controls (Table 1 summarizes the measurements in the applied sequence). Every 20 minutes the next participant started.

Body height and weight were measured, without shoes and heavy clothing, to the nearest 1 cm and 100 g, respectively. Body mass index

Table 1. Order of Measurements

Time, min	Measurement	Examiner
0	Rest	1
5	Blood pressure	1
7	Body height and body weight	2
8	Bone density	2
10	Skin extensibility (2 locations bilaterally)	2
13	Pain (2 locations bilaterally)	2
15	Joint mobility (34 joint motions in 9 joints bilaterally)	3
30	Myometry (4 locations bilaterally)	4
40	Ultrasonography carotid artery	5
60	Blood pressure	1
62	Questionnaires	1
80	Measurements completed	

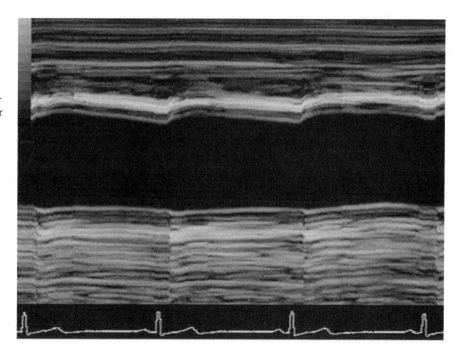

Figure 1. M-mode from the common carotid artery from which arterial stiffness was assessed. The upper white line reflects the near (closest to the skin) wall of the common carotid artery, which shows movement during the cardiac cycle. The black area reflects the lumen diameter, and the next white line reflects the far wall of the common carotid artery. The electrocardiogram tracing, indicating the phase of the cardiac cycle, is at the bottom of the image.

(BMI) was calculated as body weight in kilograms divided by the square of body height in meters.[14] Systolic and diastolic blood pressure and pulse rate were measured with participants in an upright sitting position at the right brachial artery with an automated device (Dynamap 1846 SX, Kritikon Inc, Tampa, FL) at the start and end of the examinations, each after a rest period of 5 minutes.

As an indicator of arterial stiffness, the distal part of the right common carotid artery was assessed by using B-mode carotid ultrasonography with a 7.5-MHz linear array transducer (SonoSite 180 Plus; SonoSite Ltd, Biggleswade, United Kingdom). The difference between systolic and diastolic lumen diameter was determined from an M-mode image and averaged over 3 cardiac cycles to provide an estimate of distension (ie, change in lumen diameter during the cardiac cycle/stroke change in diameter) (Fig 1). Other parameters of arterial stiffness were calculated as described recently by our group.[15] The arterial wall thickness was assessed on a longitudinal 2-dimensional ultrasound image of the carotid artery by measuring common carotid intimal-medial thickness (CIMT) over a 10-mm segment of the distal common carotid artery. The average of the intimal-medial thickness of 4 predefined angles was used for each subject as a measure for current wall thickness of the common carotid artery.[16] The actual measurements were performed offline. The sonographer and the reader were unaware of other participants' measurement data.

As a measure of stiffness of capsules and ligaments, the range of joint motion of 9 joints was assessed bilaterally to the nearest 5° with a standard 2-legged 360° goniometer, using the "anatomic-landmark" method.[17] Shoulder (anteflexion), elbow (flexion and extension), wrist (palmar and dorsal flexion), metacarpophalangeal, proximal interphalangeal, and distal interphalangeal joints of the second ray (flexion, extension), hip (flexion and extension), knee (flexion and extension), and ankle (plantar and dorsal extension) were examined. Children were asked to actively stretch or bend the joint maximally without interference by the investigator and without help of the ipsilateral muscles by use of contralateral limbs. Range of joint motion of all the participants was measured by the same physical therapist. The intrarater reliability, assessed in 25 joints of 8 subjects, was high (intraclass correlation: 0.97; $P < .001$). The mean difference between 2 measurements was 2.4 degrees (SD: 4.6). Based on 9 measurements, the Beighton score

was calculated as an indicator of the possible presence of generalized joint hypermobility (normal if <4; range: 0–9).[18]

As an index of skin extensibility, a vacuum-suction device was placed bilaterally at the ventral part of the forearm and at the medial part of the upper leg. Skin displacement as a result of a negative pressure of 10 kPa on the skin was indicated in millimeters. The reliability of this instrument has been shown to be high.[19]

Muscle strength was measured as a possible confounder, because it might partly explain maximal joint motion. The strength of the proximal and distal muscles in lower and upper extremities was measured with a hand-held myometer in Newtons. Measurements were performed sequentially 3 times, and the highest value was used for analysis. Shoulder abductors, grip strength, hip flexors, and dorsal extensors of the foot were measured bilaterally.

Quantitative ultrasound measurement of bone was performed in the right os calcis with a Sahara ultrasound device (Hologic QDR 4500; Hologic Inc, Waltham, MA) measuring broadband ultrasound attenuation (dB/MHz) and speed of sound (m/second) as indicators of bone quantity and stiffness, respectively.[20,21] Acoustic phantoms provided by the manufacturer were scanned daily without deviation over the duration of the study.

Degradation products of collagen (hydroxyproline [Hyp], crosslinks) were measured in overnight urine specimens. HP is the major collagen crosslink in articular cartilage, and another crosslink is LP, which is a bone-specific degradation marker, as is Hyp. Hyp and crosslink analysis was conducted as described previously.[22] Especially the amount of crosslink products correlates with joint mobility, with a lower amount of crosslinks in joint hypermobility and a higher amount of crosslinks in joint hypomobility.[11,23]

Pain is a nonspecific feature of CFS and of joint hypermobility. An algometer was used to measure pain threshold at 4 sites: 2 bony sites (right femur lateral condyle and right elbow lateral condyle) and 2 muscle sites (musculus deltoideus right upper arm and musculus vastus medialis right leg). With the algometer, an increasing pressure is applied to the reference points, and the subject is asked to react verbally when the level of pressure is perceived as pain; this level is subsequently designated as the pain threshold (scores: 0–11). Algometry has an excellent test-retest reliability.[24]

The total examination time for each participant was 60 minutes. After the physical examinations, the subjects had to complete questionnaires regarding fatigue (Checklist Individual Strength-20 [CIS-20]), physical activity (cycling, leisure sport, and gym), school attendance, and lifestyle behavior (sleep, smoking, drinking, diet). The CIS-20 asks about fatigue in the 2 weeks preceding the assessment. There are 4 respective subscales (fatigue with 8 items, concentration with 5 items, motivation with 4 items, and physical activity with 3 items), and each item is scored on a 7-point Likert scale. A high score indicates a high level of subjective fatigue and concentration problems and a low level of motivation and physical activity. The questionnaire has good reliability and discriminative validity.[25] The average time to complete these questionnaires was 20 minutes.

The medical ethics committee of the University Medical Center Utrecht approved this study. Written informed consent was obtained from the adolescents and their parents.

DATA ANALYSIS

Of all relevant variables, group-specific means and SDs or proportions were calculated for descriptive purposes. Joint motion, skin extensibility, and muscle force were determined at various locations. Because the absolute levels and the distributions differed considerably between locations, we calculated individual normal scores, the so-called z scores (z score = $[x_{index} - x_{mean}]$/SD or the number of SDs below or above the mean) for values at each location instead of simply averaging all measurement results. Subsequently, mean individual z scores were calculated by averaging z scores of all measured locations. These mean z scores, indicating individuals' ranks in the distribution of joint mobility, skin extensibility, or muscle strength, were used for additional analysis.

The data were analyzed with linear regression using a group indicator (patient = 1, control = 0) as an independent variable and the investigated parameter as a dependent (outcome) variable. Results are presented as linear-regression coefficients representing mean group differences for the investigated parameter with their corresponding 95% confidence intervals (95% CIs). The same models were used to adjust for possible confounding factors such as age, gender, BMI, and physical activity. For evaluations of arterial stiffness, we constructed several parameters of stiffness to enable comparison with other studies. All these stiffness parameters are constructed as ratios in different formulas as we have described.[15] However, in studies looking into etiology, analyses using ratios are difficult to interpret, because an observed relationship may be caused by the relation with the nominator, the denominator, or both. Therefore, a better approach in etiologic studies may be to use either the nominator or the denominator and adjust for the other factor in a regression model. Thus, we present the distension value (change in lumen diameter during the cardiac cycle), which is adjusted for pulse pressure and diastolic lumen diameter and additionally adjusted for age, gender, BMI, and physical activity, as the most appropriate measurement for stiff arteries in this etiologic study. A lower distension value inversely relates to a stiffer vessel, as do the cross-sectional compliance coefficient and the distensibility coefficient. The Peterson's modulus is closely related to the inverse of the distensibility coefficient. Young's elastic modulus provides direct information about the elastic properties of the wall material independent of the vessel geometry.[15]

Statistical significance was considered to be reached when 95% CIs did not include the null value, corresponding with a P value < .05.

Results

A summary of relevant characteristics of the adolescents with CFS is provided in Table 2. The majority of patients were females. There was considerable school absence and a high use of medication, and many patients were on a diet. Additionally, Table 2 shows a substantial use of health care services since the start of the symptoms, including psychotherapy and alternative treatment. Table 3 describes general characteristics of the adolescents with CFS and the controls. Both groups were comparable except for gender, BMI, and physical activity. Physical activity, computed in hours of physical activity per week, was 5.7 hours less in patients with CFS. Because gender, age, BMI, and physical activity may affect the studied collagen-related measurements, we considered them to be possible confounding factors. The patients with CFS showed a higher score on all the subscales of the CIS-20.

Table 4 shows the joint mobility in 5 bilateral joints in both groups and the mean (adjusted) difference in joint mobility between the adolescents with CFS and the healthy adolescents. There were no group differences in joint mobility in these 5 joints. The median Beighton score in the healthy adolescents was 2, similar to the median Beighton score in the CFS group. Comparison of the Beighton scores between the 2 groups in a linear-regression model (adjusted for age, gender, and BMI) showed no difference as well (regression coefficient: –0.35; 95% CI: –1.0, 0.3). Generalized joint hypermobility (Beighton score ≥4) was present in 29 of 167 (17%) healthy adolescents, whereas in the CFS group, 3 of the 32 adolescents with CFS (9%) showed hypermobility.

Mean differences in indicators of organ stiffness between patients with CFS and controls are presented in Table 5. Joint mobility of all the 34 examined joints did not differ between patients and controls. A separate analysis of small and large joints did not change this result. The skin of patients with CFS was more extensible, and adjustment for age, gender, and BMI did not materially change this finding.

There was a significant difference in muscle strength between the adolescents with CFS and

Table 2. Clinical Characteristics of Patients With CFS

Characteristics	CFS Cases (*n* = 32)
Gender, % females	88
Mean symptoms duration, months (range)	33 (6–192)
Start of symptoms, % of cases	
Acute	6
Insidious	50
After a minor illness	44
Side symptoms (CDC criteria),[13] % of cases	
Sleep disturbance	94
Prolonged generalized fatigue after levels of exercise	88
Generalized headache	84
Migratory arthralgia without joint swelling or redness	81
Forgetfulness, inability to concentrate	78
Myalgia	72
Sore throat	66
Painful lymph nodes (cervical or axillary)	56
School absence, % of cases	
Minimal (<5%)	12
Considerable (5–50%)	60
Almost complete non-school attendance (50–100%)	28
Overall use of diet, % of cases	50
Sugar-free diet	38
Other diet	28
Overall use of medication, % of cases	75
(Multi)vitamin supplements	66
Homeopathic medication	22
Ferro supplements	19
Melatonin	6
Antidepressive treatment	6
Pain medication	6
Use of health care services since start of symptoms, % visited (% active treatment)	
General practitioner	100 (37.5)
General pediatrician	93.8 (18.7)
Physiotherapist	65.6 (31)
Psychotherapist	37 (25)
Rehabilitation center	68.8 (40.6)
Alternative treatment	90.6 (6.3)

the healthy adolescents (mean difference in *z* score: –0.7; 95% CI: –1.0, –0.4), even when adjusted for age, gender, and BMI (mean difference in *z* score: –0.6; 95% CI: –0.9, –0.4).

There was a significant difference in systolic and diastolic blood pressure and pulse pressure between the groups at the start of the examination. Blood pressure levels were lower in patients with CFS (–13.5 adjusted difference in systolic blood pressure, –6.7 mm Hg adjusted difference in diastolic blood pressure), without any effect on the heart rate, which was similar for both groups at the start. At the end of the examination, the blood pressure was comparable for both groups, but the heart rate was faster for the CFS group (mean difference: 4.9; 95% CI: –0.1, 9.8). Arterial stiffness expressed as common carotid distension and adjusted for lumen diameter and pulse pressure showed that patients with CFS have a lower value of distension than controls, reflecting stiffer arteries. The analyses of the various arterial stiffness parameters point toward arterial stiffness in the patients with CFS compared with controls. Although some of the associations do not reach statistical significance, the consistency of the findings enhances the validity of the finding.

Table 3. Characteristics of Adolescents With CFS and Healthy Controls

	CFS Cases (n = 32)	Controls (n = 167)	Mean Difference (95% CI)	Adjusted Mean Difference (Adjusted for Age/Gender)
Age, y (SD)	16.0 (1.7)	15.5 (1.6)	0.5 (–0.1, 1.2)	
Gender, % girls	88	60	28 (9, 45)*	
Postmenarche, % girls	86	88		
White race, %	100	96		
Body height, cm (SD)	169.0 (8.8)	172.8 (9.8)	–3.7 (–7, –0)*	–2.7 (–5.7, 0.3)
Body weight, kg (SD)	63.8 (21.7)	60.7 (11.8)	3.1 (–2.2, 8.3)	2.4 (–2.3, 7.1)
BMI, kg/m² (SD)	22.0 (6.1)	20.2 (2.9)	1.8 (0.4, 3.2)*	1.3 (–0.9, 2.6)
Hours of physical activity per wk (SD)	2.3 (3.3)	8.0 (3.9)	–5.7 (–7.1, –4.3)*	–4.9 (–6.4, –3.5)*
Self-reported alcohol consumption, glasses per wk	0.4	2.7	–2.2 (–4.4, –0.1)*	–2.0 (–4.2, 0.2)
Self-reported cigarette smoking, number per day	1	1	0	0
Fatigue assessment: CIS-20 (20 items, 7-point Likert scale)				
Total mean score (20 items)	4.7	2.7	2.0 (1.6, 2.4)*	1.8 (1.4, 2.2)*
Subjective fatigue subscale (8 items), mean score	5.6	2.9	2.8 (2.3, 3.2)*	2.5 (2.0, 2.9)*
Concentration subscale (5 items), mean score	4.3	3.0	1.3 (0.7, 1.8)*	1.1 (0.5, 1.6)*
Motivation subscale (4 items), mean score	3.3	2.3	(0.7, 1.5)*	1.1 (0.7, 1.5)*
Physical-activity subscale (3 items), mean score	4.8	2.5	2.4 (1.9, 2.9)*	2.3 (1.8, 2.8)*

* Statistically significant associations (95% CI does not include the null value, corresponding with P <.05).

Table 4. Results and Mean Differences in Joint Mobility Between Patients With CFS and Healthy Controls

Joint Mobility	Patients With CFS, Mean (SD) (n = 32)	Controls, Mean (SD) (n = 167)	Difference (95% CI)	Adjusted Difference* (95% CI)
Right wrist palmar flexion	76.9 (7.6)	75.2 (8.3)	1.7 (–1.4, 4.8)	0.8 (–2.4, 3.9)
Left wrist palmar flexion	77.9 (7.3)	76.0 (8.3)	1.9 (–1.2, 5.0)	1.2 (–1.9, 4.4)
Right second-finger metacarpal extension	22.8 (11.5)	23.5 (10.4)	–0.7 (–4.7, 3.3)	–2.2 (–6.4, 1.8)
Left second-finger metacarpal extension	26.6 (12.0)	26.2 (12.0)	0.4 (–4.2, 4.9)	–1.3 (–5.9, 3.3)
Right elbow extension	3.4 (5.1)	3.5 (5.6)	0 (–2.2, 2.0)	–0.7 (–2.8, 1.4)
Left elbow extension	4.4 (4.4)	4.2 (5.9)	0.2 (–2.0, 2.3)	–0.5 (–2.7, 1.7)
Right hip flexion	111.3 (8.1)	112.4 (6.9)	–1.1 (–3.8, 1.6)	–0.4 (–2.8, 2.1)
Left hip flexion	111.9 (8.1)	113.5 (6.7)	–1.6 (–4.2, 1.1)	–1.0 (–3.4, 1.4)
Right knee extension	2.8 (3.8)	2.5 (4.0)	0.3 (–1.2, 1.8)	–0.3 (–1.8, 1.3)
Left knee extension	2.8 (3.8)	2.4 (3.9)	0.4 (–1.0, 1.9)	–0.2 (–1.7, 1.3)

* Adjusted for age, gender, and BMI.

Arterial wall thickness, as determined by the common CIMT, was equal for both groups. The bone parameters showed that there was less stiffness of bones in patients with CFS. Adjusting for confounding factors, including physical inactivity, attenuated this difference.

There were no clear differences between the groups with regard to collagen biochemistry (Table 5).

The mean pain threshold differed considerably between patients with CFS and controls. After adjusting for age, gender, and BMI, this lower pain threshold for patients with CFS remained.

Discussion

The results of our study do not consistently point toward an abnormality in connective tissue and therefore do not support the hypothesis that

Table 5. Results and Mean Differences in Indicators of Organ Stiffness Between Patients With CFS and Healthy Controls

	Patients With CFS, Mean (SD) (n = 32)	Controls, Mean (SD) (n = 167)	Difference (95% CI)	Adjusted Difference (95% CI)
Cardiovascular parameters				
Systolic blood pressure start, mm Hg	117.3 (14.2)*	129.7 (14.2)*	−12.6 (−18.0, −7.2)*	−13.5 (−19.1, −7.0)*†
Systolic blood pressure end, mm Hg	120.2 (12.8)	121.6 (13.5)	−1.4 (−6.5, 3.7)	
Diastolic blood pressure start, mm Hg	65.7 (7.2)*	70.5 (9.1)*	−4.8 (−8.2, −1.5)*	−6.7 (−10.5, −3.0)*†
Diastolic blood pressure end, mm Hg	67.7 (6.6)	67.6 (7.6)	0.1 (−2.7, 2.9)	
Pulse pressure start, mm Hg	51.6 (10.3)*	59.5 (12.1)*	−7.8 (−12.4, −3.2)*	−6.8 (−11.8, −1.8)*†
Pulse pressure end, mm Hg	52.5 (10.7)	54.0 (12.1)	−1.5 (−6.0, 3.0)	
Heart rate start, beats/min	83.5 (14.8)	83.0 (17.6)	0.5 (−6.0, 7.1)	
Heart rate end, beats/min	80.6 (12.2)	75.7 (13.1)	4.9 (−0.1, 9.8)	
Carotid artery stiffness				
Diastolic lumen diameter, m/10^3 (D)	5.37 (0.35)	5.48 (0.5)	−0.11 (−0.29, 0.08)	−0.12 (−0.31, 0.07)
Stroke change in diameter, m/10^3 (ΔD)	0.67 (0.22)*	0.82 (0.26)*	−0.15 (−0.24, −0.05)*	−0.11 (−0.22, −0.01)*‡
Cross-sectional compliance, mm^2/kPa (compliance coefficient)	0.84 (0.30)*	1.03 (0.42)*	−0.19 (−0.35, −0.04)*	−0.18 (−0.36, −0.01)*†
Distensibility coefficient, kPa^{-1} x 10^{-3} (distensibility coefficient)	37.8 (13.9)	43.6 (16.8)	−5.8 (−12.2, 0.5)	−6.1 (−13.4, 1.1)†
Peterson's modulus, kPa ∞ 10^3	0.06 (0.04)*	0.05 (0.03)*	0.01 (0.00, 0.02)*	0.01 (0.0, 0.02)*†
Young's elastic modulus, kPa ∞ 10^{-3}	0.37 (0.25)*	0.31 (0.14)*	0.06 (0.00, 0.13)*	0.04 (−0.03, 0.12)
Common CIMT, mm	0.48 (0.007)	0.48 (0.003)	0 (−0.02, 0.01)	
Joint mobility and skin extensibility				
Mean z score joint mobility (34 joints)	0.05 (0.43)	−0.01 (0.45)	0.06 (−0.11, 0.23)	0.02 (−0.17, 0.14)§
Mean z score skin extensibility (4 locations)	0.5 (0.73)*	−0.1 (0.77)*	0.6 (0.3, 0.9)*	0.3 (0.1, 0.6)*§
Bone parameters and collagen biochemistry				
Broadband ultrasound attenuation, dB/MHz	68.3 (12.2)	68.9 (15.0)	0.6 (−6.3, 5.0)	
Speed of sound, m/s	1547.8 (19.5)*	1559.6 (29.6)*	−11.8 (−22.7, −0.9)*	−5.6 (−17.3, 6.1)†
HP/LP	4.2 (0.5)*	3.9 (0.7)*	0.3 (0.1, 0.6)*	0.13 (−0.2, 0.4)†
HP/creatinine, μmol/mmol	130.4 (82.4)	138.1 (89.2)	−7.7 (−41.8, 26.4)	
Hyp/creatinine, μmol/mmol	60.4 (40.4)	68.1 (43.4)	−7.8 (−24.4, 8.8)	
LP/creatinine, μmol/mmol	31.5 (21.3)	36.5 (27.1)	−5.0 (−15.2, 5.1)	
Mean pain threshold, score	7.5*	9.8*	−2.3 (−2.9, −1.7)*	−2.0 (−2.7, −1.5)*§

* Statistically significant associations (95% CI does not include the null value, corresponding with P < .05).

† Adjusted for age, gender, BMI, and physical activity.

‡ Adjusted for age, gender, BMI, physical activity, and lumen diameter and pulse pressure.

§ Adjusted for age, gender, BMI, and muscle strength.

connective tissue laxity is a risk factor for the development of CFS in adolescents. Patients with CFS did have lower blood pressure during rest, more extensible skin, and less muscle strength but lacked the most important parameter indicating constitutional laxity: joint hypermobility. Another argument against constitutional laxity is the finding of an increased arterial stiffness in the patients with CFS. Moreover, the collagen metabolism measured by crosslinks and Hyp in urine, mainly reflecting bone resorption, did not differ between the 2 groups.

Before additional discussion about these results, some aspects of our study design need to be addressed. The cross-sectional design of our study limits causal interpretations. Furthermore, we attempted to measure all conceivable confounders of relations between stiffness parameters and disease status. However, we cannot exclude the possibility that there is residual confounding or unknown confounders. We do believe that we have sufficiently tackled problems with information bias, because examiners were blinded for other patient characteristics during measurement protocols.

Our results are incongruent with former studies with respect to joint mobility in adolescents with CFS. Whereas former studies established joint hypermobility in adolescents with CFS,[5,6] we found a remarkably similar joint motion in adolescents with CFS and controls and a congruent Beighton score. The question is whether the CFS population under study is a representative sample of the CFS adolescent population in the Netherlands, which is estimated to consist of 2000 cases (the prevalence rate in the 5- to 15-year age group according to CDC criteria is 0.2 in Great Britain).[26] Exact prevalence rates for the adolescent age group in the Netherlands are lacking. The Wilhelmina Children's Hospital is a tertiary referral center for CFS (50 new patients with fatigue each year) and for children with joint hypermobility. A child with joint hypermobility initially referred to the department of pediatric physiotherapy for hypermobility, and with possible CFS, is subsequently referred to the CFS clinic, and vice versa. Thus, the coincidence of being a tertiary clinic for both conditions and the internal referring for both conditions makes it unlikely that we missed the patient with CFS with joint hypermobility. We excluded from our initial sample of potential CFS cases 2 patients with a known collagen disorder (EDS, hypermobility type).

Because we were interested in generalized joint hypermobility, we applied the Beighton score for the assessment of hypermobility and in addition goniometry for the continuous measurement of joint mobility of 26 different joint movements.

The differences in systolic and diastolic blood pressure, which were evident only at the start of the examinations, are intriguing. The low blood pressure did not correlate with illness severity (CIS-20 score) or duration (Pearson correlation coefficients: 0.1 [$P = .6$] and –0.2 [$P = .2$], respectively), which makes a causal relationship between CFS and blood pressure not very likely. An association between systolic blood pressure and fatigue was established in a population study consisting of adult men and women with a linear trend showing more tiredness with lower systolic blood pressure.[27] In a subsequently published cross-sectional study in civil servants, this strong association between tiredness and systolic blood pressure was reestablished but seemed confounded by minor psychological dysfunction.[28] In this study we are not informed about minor psychological disturbances, and thus it is possible that the association between fatigue and blood pressure could be explained by unknown psychological factors.

Our study was explicitly not designed to study autonomic nervous dysfunction, which would have required appropriate measurements for the detection of orthostatic intolerance (eg, tilt-table testing). However, the lower blood pressure in sitting position in patients with CFS may be explained by alterations in the autonomic nervous system.[29]

Opposite to the finding of this lower blood pressure is the unexpected finding that patients with CFS do seem to have stiffer arteries than controls, established with different parameters of arterial wall stiffness and adjusted for possible confounding factors (age, gender, BMI, and physical activity). Residual confounding for lifestyle (smoking, alcohol consumption, and diet) and age of menarche was considered and investigated by determining for each factor the effect on the distension value. None of these factors influenced the distension value, and thus these lifestyle factors were not incorporated into the regression model. An explanation for stiffer arteries in patients with CFS is not available yet. It has not been reported in the literature, nor has increased cardiovascular disease among patients with CFS. It is credible that a stiffer carotid artery is the result of an increased BMI[30,31] and the decreased physical activity, but we adjusted for these possible confounding factors, as we did for lifestyle factors. There might be residual confounding in psychological factors, for example, the stress for patients with CFS to live with a disabling, unexplained condition.

The difference in arterial stiffness is not explained by arterial wall thickness, which was remarkably similar for both groups. Additional research is necessary to give more insight into this intriguing finding.

The difference in bone stiffness disappeared when we adjusted additionally for inactivity.

Bone-resorption parameters in an overnight urine sample were the same for both groups. We could have expected a less active process of formation and resorption of bone in the patients with CFS, because of the inactivity, but this was not reflected in the data, possibly because of the large variation in these measurements in both groups.

The pain perception differed considerably between patients and controls. Although this was to be expected, because pain is a frequent complaint of patients with CFS, this is the first study to confirm this difference. Little is known about nociception, processing, cortical perception, and reporting of pain.[32] It is surprising that the patients with CFS not only complain of more pain sensation on different locations but are also hypersensitive to visual,[33] acoustic,[34] and sensory signals. The processes underlying this increased sensory symptom perception in patients with CFS are not understood yet.

Conclusions

The findings of lower blood pressure, more extensible skin, arterial stiffening, and lower pain threshold in patients with CFS seem to be genuine but do not consistently point at a generalized abnormality in connective tissue. A more likely explanation is that these findings are caused by different mechanisms, such as complex disturbance of the autonomic nervous system in combination with a possible change in sensory symptom perception. More research is necessary to assess the pathogenicity of these findings and the reversibility after successful treatment of the adolescent with CFS.

Acknowledgments

The Royal Dutch Society for Physical Therapy provided a grant for biochemical analysis.

We thank the patients with chronic fatigue syndrome, the children of the secondary school De Breul in Zeist, and their parents for their willingness to participate in this study. Physiotherapists L. Hokke, A.A. Nijenhuis, M.J. Vis, and P.J. Wetselaar provided support in the conduct of the study. R. Meijer is gratefully acknowledged for his contribution to the collection of the ultrasound data. SonoSite Ltd (Biggleswade, United Kingdom) provided the ultrasound equipment (SonoSite 180 Plus) free of charge. The vascular measurements were performed under the supervision and guidance of the Vascular Imaging Center staff of the Julius Center for Health Sciences and Primary Care.

References

1. Bazelmans E, Vercoulen JH, Swanink CM, et al. Chronic fatigue syndrome and primary fibromyalgia syndrome as recognized by GPs. *Fam Pract.* 1999;16:602–604

2. Jason LA, Richman JA, Friedberg F, Wagner L, Taylor R, Jordan KM. Politics, science, and the emergence of a new disease. The case of chronic fatigue syndrome. *Am Psychol.* 1997;52:973–983

3. Wessely S, Hotopf M, Sharpe M. *Chronic Fatigue and its Syndromes.* New York, NY: Oxford University Press; 1999: 363–369

4. Gill AC, Dosen A, Ziegler JB. Chronic fatigue syndrome in adolescents: a follow-up study. *Arch Pediatr Adolesc Med.* 2004;158:225–229

5. Barron DF, Cohen BA, Geraghty MT, Violand R, Rowe PC. Joint hypermobility is more common in children with chronic fatigue syndrome than in healthy controls. *J Pediatr.* 2002;141:421–425

6. Rowe PC, Barron DF, Calkins H, Maumenee IH, Tong PY, Geraghty MT. Orthostatic intolerance and chronic fatigue syndrome associated with Ehlers-Danlos syndrome. *J Pediatr.* 1999;135:494–499

7. Beighton P, De Paepe A, Steinmann B, Tsipouras P, Wenstrup RJ. Ehlers-Danlos syndromes: revised nosology, Villefranche, 1997. Ehlers-Danlos National Foundation (USA) and Ehlers-Danlos Support Group (UK). *Am J Med Genet.* 1998;77:31–37

8. Murray KJ, Woo P. Benign joint hypermobility in childhood. *Rheumatology.* 2001;40:489–491

9. Grahame R, Bird HA, Child A. The revised (Brighton 1998) criteria for the diagnosis of benign joint hypermobility syndrome (BJHS). *J Rheumatol.* 2000;27: 1777–1779

10. Grahame R. Pain, distress and joint hyperlaxity. *Joint Bone Spine.* 2000;67:157–163

11. Engelbert RH, Bank RA, Sakkers RJ, Helders PJ, Beemer FA, Uiterwaal CS. Pediatric generalized joint hypermobility with and without musculoskeletal complaints: a localized or systemic disorder? *Pediatrics.* 2003;111:e248–e254

12. Uiterwaal CS, Grobbee DE, Sakkers RJ, Helders PJ, Bank RA, Engelbert RH. A relation between blood pressure and stiffness of joints and skin. *Epidemiology.* 2003;14: 223–227

13. Fukuda K, Straus SE, Hickie I, Sharpe MC, Dobbins JG, Komaroff A. The chronic fatigue syndrome: a comprehensive approach to its definition and study. International Chronic Fatigue Syndrome Study Group. *Ann Intern Med.* 1994;121:953–959

14. Gerver WJM, De Bruin R. *Paediatric Morphometrics: A Reference Manual.* Utrecht, Netherlands: Bunge; 1996

15. Stork S, van den Beld AW, von Schacky C, et al. Carotid artery plaque burden, stiffness, and mortality risk in elderly men: a prospective, population-based cohort study. *Circulation.* 2004;110:344–348

16. Liang Q, Wendelhag I, Wikstrand J, Gustavsson T. A multiscale dynamic programming procedure for boundary detection in ultrasonic artery images. *IEEE Trans Med Imaging.* 2000;19:127–142

17. Hogeweg JA, Langereis MJ, Bernards ATM, Faber JAJ, Helders PJM. Goniometry: variability in the clinical practice of a conventional goniometer in healthy subjects. *Eur J Phys Med Rehabil.* 1994;4:2–7

18. Beighton P, Solomon L, Soskolne CL. Articular mobility in an African population. *Ann Rheum Dis.* 1973;32:413–418

19. Hogeweg JA, Lemmers D, Temmink P. Skin compliance: measuring skin consistency in the spinal region of healthy children and adults. *Physiother Theory Pract.* 1993;205–214

20. Njeh CF, Boivin CM, Langton CM. The role of ultrasound in the assessment of osteoporosis: a review. *Osteoporos Int.* 1997;7:7–22

21. Gluer CC, Wu CY, Jergas M, Goldstein SA, Genant HK. Three quantitative ultrasound parameters reflect bone structure. *Calcif Tissue Int.* 1994;55:46–52

22. Bank RA, Bayliss MT, Lafeber FP, Maroudas A, Tekoppele JM. Ageing and zonal variation in post-translational modification of collagen in normal human articular cartilage. The age-related increase in nonenzymatic glycation affects biomechanical properties of cartilage. *Biochem J.* 1998;330:345–351

23. Engelbert RH, Uiterwaal CS, van de Putte E, et al. Pediatric generalized joint hypomobility and musculoskeletal complaints: a new entity? Clinical, biochemical, and osseal characteristics. *Pediatrics.* 2004;113:714–719

24. Hogeweg JA, Langereis MJ, Bernards AT, Faber JA, Helders PJ. Algometry. Measuring pain threshold, method and characteristics in healthy subjects. *Scand J Rehabil Med.* 1992;24:99–103

25. Vercoulen JH, Swanink CM, Fennis JF, Galama JM, van der Meer JW, Bleijenberg G. Dimensional assessment of chronic fatigue syndrome. *J Psychosom Res.* 1994;38:383–392

26. Chalder T, Goodman R, Wessely S, Hotopf M, Meltzer H. Epidemiology of chronic fatigue syndrome and self reported myalgic encephalomyelitis in 5–15 year olds: cross sectional study. BMJ. 2003;327:654–655

27. Wessely S, Nickson J, Cox B. Symptoms of low blood pressure: a population study. *BMJ.* 1990;301:362–365

28. Pilgrim JA, Stansfeld S, Marmot M. Low blood pressure, low mood? *BMJ.* 1992;304:75–78

29. Gerrity TR, Bates J, Bell DS, et al. Chronic fatigue syndrome: what role does the autonomic nervous system play in the pathophysiology of this complex illness? *Neuroimmunomodulation.* 2002;10:134–141

30. Sorof JM, Lai D, Turner J, Poffenbarger T, Portman RJ. Overweight, ethnicity, and the prevalence of hypertension in school-aged children. *Pediatrics.* 2004;113:475–482

31. Sorof JM, Alexandrov AV, Garami Z, et al. Carotid ultrasonography for detection of vascular abnormalities in hypertensive children. *Pediatr Nephrol.* 2003;18:1020–1024

32. Kuis W, Heijnen CJ, Sinnema G, Kavelaars A, van der Net J, Helders PJ. Pain in childhood rheumatic arthritis. *Baillieres Clin Rheumatol.* 1998;12:229–244

33. Potaznick W, Kozol N. Ocular manifestations of chronic fatigue and immune dysfunction syndrome. *Optom Vis Sci.* 1992;69:811–814

34. Beh HC. Effect of noise stress on chronic fatigue syndrome patients. *J Nerv Ment Dis.* 1997;185:55–58

Jaundice in Older Children and Adolescents

Dinesh Pashankar, MD, and Richard A. Schreiber, MD†*

Objectives

After completing this article, readers should be able to:

1. Describe the basic physiology of bilirubin metabolism, the two standard laboratory methods for its fractionation, and the classification of jaundice.
2. Characterize the features of Gilbert disease.
3. Identify the leading infectious cause of acute jaundice in older children and adolescents.
4. Delineate the clinical and biochemical features of Wilson disease and autoimmune hepatitis.
5. Compare and contrast liver function tests and tests of liver function.
6. Describe the "worrisome" clinical and laboratory signs of hepatic synthetic dysfunction in jaundiced patients that should prompt an immediate referral to a center where liver transplantation is available.

Abbreviations

ALP: alkaline phosphatase
ALT: alanine aminotransferase
ANA: antinuclear antibody
ASMA: anti-smooth muscle antibody
AST: aspartate aminotransferase
CNS: central nervous system
EBV: Epstein-Barr virus
GGT: gamma glutamyltransferase

HAV: hepatitis A virus
HBV: hepatitis B virus
HCV: hepatitis C virus
KF: Kayser-Fleischer
PT: prothrombin time
RE: reticuloendothelial

Introduction

Jaundice is defined as the presence of a yellow or yellow-greenish hue to the skin, sclera, and mucous membranes due to an elevation of serum bilirubin. In healthy individuals, the total serum bilirubin is less than 1 mg/dL (17 mcmol/L). Jaundice can be readily detected clinically when the total serum bilirubin is greater than 5 mg/dL (85 mcmol/L). Clinical jaundice occurs much less frequently in older children and adolescents than in neonates. Moreover, the differential diagnosis in this older age group differs markedly from that in newborns and young infants. This review provides a practical approach to the clinical evaluation of jaundice in the older child or adolescent. Because jaundice may be the presenting feature of life-threatening conditions such as fulminant liver failure, a prompt and logical evaluation is necessary to identify the more serious disorders that require urgent management.

Bilirubin Metabolism

Bilirubin is a product of heme metabolism. Heme is converted in the reticuloendothelial (RE) system to biliverdin and then to bilirubin by heme oxygenase and biliverdin reductase, respectively. Bilirubin is lipophylic and is bound to serum

Clinical Assistant Professor of Pediatrics, Division of Gastroenterology, Children's Hospital of Iowa, Iowa City, IA.

†Clinical Associate Professor of Pediatrics, University of British Columbia, Division of Gastroenterology, British Columbia's Children's Hospital, Vancouver, BC, Canada.

Additional media illustrating features of the disease processes discussed are available in the online version of this article at www.pedsinreview.org.

Pediatrics in Review, Vol 22, No. 7, July 2001

albumin in circulation from the RE system to the liver. The liver takes up the bilirubin-albumin complex through an albumin receptor. Bilirubin, but not albumin, is transferred across the hepatocyte membrane and transported through the cytoplasm to the smooth endoplasmic reticulum bound primarily to ligandin or Y protein, a member of the glutathione S-transferase gene family of proteins. There, the water-insoluble bilirubin is conjugated to water-soluble bilirubin monoglucuronide and diglucuronide by UDP-glucuronosyl transferase. The bilirubin conjugates are excreted through the canalicular membrane into the bile duct system by an energy-dependent process. Conjugated bilirubin flows in the bile to the intestine, where it is broken down by gut flora to urobilinogen and stercobilin.

Total serum bilirubin consists of an unconjugated fraction and conjugated fraction of bilirubin and a fraction of bilirubin glucuronide that is bound covalently to albumin known as delta-bilirubin. The newer Ektachem® slide method for bilirubin fractionation accurately measures the levels of unconjugated, conjugated, and total serum bilirubin. Delta-bilirubin concentration can be calculated from these figures (Table 1). With the traditional Diazo® method for bilirubin fractionation, indirect and direct bilirubin are measured and the total bilirubin is calculated. Unconjugated or indirect hyperbilirubinemia is defined biochemically by an increased total serum bilirubin level with less than 15% of the bilirubin in the direct or conjugated form. Conjugated or direct hyperbilirubinemia is characterized by the conjugated or direct fraction being greater than 20% of the total serum bilirubin.

Differential Diagnosis

The differential diagnosis of jaundice in an older child is extensive, encompassing some common conditions and many rare disorders (Table 2). A key practical first step is to classify the jaundice as unconjugated (indirect) or conjugated (direct) hyperbilirubinemia by using the previously noted Diazo or Ektachem method.

Table 1. Fractionation of Bilirubin

Diazo® Method

Total bilirubin = Direct bilirubin$_m$ + Indirect bilirubin^m

Ektachem® Slide Method

Total bilirubin$_m$ = Conjugated bilirubin^m + Unconjugated bilirubin^m + Delta bilirubin

The Diazo method measures the direct and indirect bilirubin and calculates the total. In the Ektachem slide method, the total, conjugated, and unconjugated bilirubin fractions are measured and the delta bilirubin is calculated. m = measured.

UNCONJUGATED HYPERBILIRUBINEMIA

Older children and adolescents who present with jaundice due to unconjugated hyperbilirubinemia are most likely to have a disorder associated with excessive hemolysis, such as hereditary spherocytosis, a red blood cell enzyme defect of pyruvate kinase or glucose-6-phosphate dehydrogenase, or a hemoglobinopathy (eg, sickle cell anemia and thalassemia). In these conditions, significant hemolysis leads to excess heme production and consequent increased circulating unconjugated bilirubin load.

Gilbert syndrome, an autosomal recessive disorder seen in 5% of the population, is another important cause of unconjugated hyperbilirubinemia in this age group. This inherited disorder of bilirubin metabolism is characterized by a mild unconjugated hyperbilirubinemia (usually 5 mg/dL [<85 mcmol/L]) due to a UGT1 gene mutation that impairs the function of the UDP glucuronosyl transferase enzyme. In affected adolescents or young adults, jaundice appears most often in association with an intercurrent mild infectious illness, fasting, or physical stress. Other than the modest elevation in unconjugated bilirubin, patients who have Gilbert syndrome are healthy and have no clinical or laboratory evidence of liver disease or hemolysis. An associated family history, although not always present, is diagnostic for the condition. There are no specific diagnostic laboratory tests. The prognosis is excellent, with no long-term sequelae.

The Crigler-Najjar syndromes types 1 and 2 are extremely rare autosomal recessive diseases that result from a complete absence (type 1) or

Table 2. Causes of Hyperbilirubinemia in Older Children

Unconjugated Hyperbilirubinemia
>   Hemolytic anemias
>   Gilbert syndrome
>   Crigler-Najjar syndrome

Conjugated Hyperbilirubinemia
Viral Infections
>   Hepatitis viruses A, B, C, D, E
>   Epstein-Barr virus
>   Cytomegalovirus
>   Herpes simplex

Metabolic Liver Disease
>   Wilson disease
>   Alpha-1-antitrypsin deficiency
>   Cystic fibrosis

Biliary Tract Disorders
>   Cholelithiasis
>   Cholecystitis
>   Choledochal cyst
>   Sclerosing cholangitis

Autoimmune Liver Disease
>   Type 1 (anti-smoooth muscle antibody)
>   Type 2 (anti-liver-kidney-microsomal antibody)

Hepatotoxins
>   Drugs: Acetaminophen
>   Anticonvulsants
>   Anesthetics
>   Antituberculous agents
>   Chemotherapeutic agents
>   Antibiotics
>   Oral contraceptives
>   Other: Alcohol, insecticides, organophosphates

Vascular Causes
>   Budd-Chiari syndrome
>   Veno-occlusive disease

limited activity (type 2) of the UDP-glucuronosyl transferase enzyme. Both conditions typically manifest as an unconjugated hyperbilirubinemia in the first few days of life, although exceptional cases of Crigler-Najjar type 2 presenting at an older age have been reported. Without the ability to conjugate and excrete bilirubin, patients who have type 1 disease exhibit markedly elevated serum bilirubin levels (25 to 35 mg/dL) [425 to 600 mcmol/L]), are at high risk to develop kernicterus, and require aggressive phototherapy. In contrast, patients who have type 2 disease usually have total serum bilirubin levels below

20 mg/dL (350 mcmol/L) because of the partially functioning UDP-glucuronosyl transferase enzyme, whose activity can be induced by phenobarbital. Indeed, the two types of Crigler-Najjar syndrome may be distinguished by treatment with phenobarbital. Patients who have type 1 disease show no response; those who have type 2 disease exhibit a dramatic decrease in serum bilirubin levels following the administration of phenobarbital.

Conjugated Hyperbilirubinemia

INFECTIONS

Infection with any of the hepatotropic viruses (A, B, C, D, or E) may cause jaundice in older children and adolescents. In these instances, the jaundice is due to conjugated hyperbilirubinemia resulting from intrahepatic cholestasis. Hepatitis A virus (HAV) infection, a self-limited illness induced by an RNA virus, is the most common infectious cause of acute jaundice in this age group. Young infants rarely develop jaundice when infected with HAV. Infants and young children who have HAV infection are usually asymptomatic or simply manifest signs and symptoms of viral gastroenteritis without icterus. In contrast, older children and adolescents have a prodrome of fever, headache, and general malaise followed by the onset of jaundice, abdominal pain, nausea, vomiting, and anorexia. There is biochemical evidence of a profound hepatitis characterized by significant elevations in aspartate aminotransferase (AST) and alanine aminotransferase (ALT) as well as a conjugated hyperbilirubinemia. Clinical symptoms and biochemical abnormalities completely resolve within 4 weeks in most patients. In rare cases, HAV can cause relapsing or persistent jaundice for months. However, HAV infection never leads to a chronic hepatitis, defined as hepatitis lasting for more than 6 months. Fulminant HAV infection, heralded by encephalopathy and significant hepatic dysfunction (ie, coagulopathy), is distinctly unusual, occurring in fewer than 1% of cases. Indeed, although viral or presumed viral hepatitis accounts for 75% to 80% of all cases of fulminant liver failure in children, most of these are the result of non-A through G hepatitis viruses.

The majority of pediatric patients who have hepatitis B virus (HBV) infection are asymptomatic. However, jaundice may occur in acutely infected older children. The most important routes for acquiring acute HBV infection in adolescence are horizontal—from highly infectious family members, from improperly sterilized syringes, or when adolescents practice high-risk sexual behavior with multiple partners and infrequent use of condoms. Many older children and adolescents chronically infected with HBV are foreign immigrants from endemic regions who had acquired infection through perinatal transmission. Older children who have chronic HBV infection are often asymptomatic carriers or they may have a limited, subclinical, biochemical hepatitis, evidenced by increased hepatic transaminase levels. Jaundice is an unusual manifestation in children who have chronic HBV infection, except in the rare instance of fulminant liver failure or end-stage liver disease and cirrhosis developing at a young age.

Most children who have hepatitis C virus (HCV) infection are older than 8 years of age and have contracted the infection through contaminated blood and blood products prior to 1992. With improved processing of blood and blood products, the chance of contracting HCV through these sources is now low, estimated at 1 per 100,000 units transfused. The more important source for pediatric HCV infection is through maternal-infant transmission. This indolent disease takes many decades to progress to end-stage liver disease. Thus, the vast majority of older children infected with this virus are asymptomatic. However, as with chronic HBV infection, jaundice may manifest in those very rare patients who have HCV infection and develop cirrhosis at an early age. Hepatitis D virus infection is uncommon in the United States, occurring only in patients already infected with HBV. Hepatitis E virus is prevalent in developing countries and typically presents acutely with jaundice, in a manner similar to HAV infection.

Epstein-Barr virus (EBV) infection can cause acute hepatitis and jaundice in older children and adolescents as a part of the infectious mononucleosis syndrome. Any child or adolescent who presents acutely with jaundice, especially in association with lymphadenopathy, sore throat, and mild splenomegaly, should be evaluated for EBV infection. In immunocompromised hosts, infection with herpes simplex virus, cytomegalovirus, or rare opportunistic agents can cause hepatobiliary disease with clinical jaundice, but a discussion of these is beyond the scope of this article. Jaundice with hepatic dysfunction as a result of gram-negative bacterial infections and sepsis is much more common in infants and young children than in older children and adolescents.

METABOLIC LIVER DISEASE

A variety of metabolic diseases of the liver may present with jaundice in older children. Wilson disease is an autosomal recessive disorder of copper metabolism, characterized by excess accumulation of copper in the liver, central nervous system (CNS), kidney, cornea, and other organs. The hepatic manifestations are protean, ranging from an acute hepatitis to fulminant hepatic failure with coagulopathy, ascites, and hepatic encephalopathy or a more indolent course with chronic hepatitis and cirrhosis. Wilson disease must be considered in the differential diagnosis of every older child or adolescent who presents with conjugated hyperbilirubinemia. Neuropsychiatric features may be dramatic, including motor system disturbances such as tremor, incoordination, and dysarthria, along with poor school performance, depression, neurosis, or psychosis. The CNS manifestations may present in concert with or independent of the hepatic symptoms. Kayser-Fleischer (KF) rings, a golden brown discoloration in the zone of the Descemet membrane of the cornea, is virtually always present when neurologic or psychiatric symptoms develop. However, KF rings may be absent in patients who have Wilson disease without neurologic involvement but who present with hepatic symptoms. Renal involvement is characterized by proximal tubular dysfunction, decreased glomerular filtration rate, and decreased renal plasma flow. Patients may manifest proteinuria, glucosuria, phosphaturia, uricosuria, aminoaciduria, renal tubular acidosis, and microscopic hematuria. Severe renal insufficiency may occur in patients who have fulminant or end-stage liver disease. Intravascular hemolysis with a Coombs-negative hemolytic anemia may develop because of the oxidative injury to red blood cell membranes induced by excess copper. Cardiac involvement, including ventricular hypertrophy and arrhythmias, has been reported in Wilson disease. Skeletal manifestations resulting from bone demineralization are not uncommon.

Alpha-1-antitrypsin deficiency, an autosomal codominantly inherited disease, can present with a conjugated hyperbilirubinemia at any age. Approximately 20% of patients who have the ZZ protease inhibitor phenotype will have liver disease. Although neonatal cholestasis is a more common presentation for this disorder, older children may have new-onset jaundice in association with alpha-1-antitrypsin deficiency, chronic hepatitis, or cirrhosis.

Hepatobiliary disease may occur in up to two thirds of patients who have cystic fibrosis. Pancreatic insufficiency and pulmonary disease used to be the dominant features of cystic fibrosis, which was associated with high morbidity and mortality at a young age. With improved treatments and longer life expectancy, liver disease has assumed greater importance, especially for older children and adolescents. The spectrum of hepatobiliary disorders in cystic fibrosis includes steatohepatitis, focal biliary and multilobular cirrhosis, cholelithiasis and cholecystitis, sclerosing cholangitis, and common bile duct stenosis. Any of these complications may be heralded by a conjugated hyperbilirubinemia.

BILIARY TRACT DISORDERS

Extrahepatic biliary tract disorders may cause an obstructive type of jaundice that is manifested by icterus, dark urine, acholic stools, and pruritus in association with a conjugated hyperbilirubinemia. Cholelithiasis can occur in older children, albeit infrequently. Gallstones in this age group may be idiopathic or may develop due to hemolytic disorders, cystic fibrosis, obesity, ileal resection, or long-term use of total parenteral nutrition. Although many children who have gallstones are asymptomatic, jaundice, periumbilical or right upper quadrant abdominal pain, vomiting, and fever may develop in cases of acute cholecystitis, choledocholithiasis, or pancreatitis. Ultrasonography is the safest, most sensitive, and most specific method of identifying gallstones.

Choledochal cysts are congenital cystic dilatations of the intrahepatic or extrahepatic biliary ducts. At least five subtypes have been described based on the anatomic site of cystic dilation along the biliary tree. Patients may present at any age with epigastric pain, fever, and jaundice. The most useful diagnostic study is abdominal ultrasonography. In older children, acute jaundice may develop in cases of intrahepatic cystic duct lesions that are associated with congenital hepatic fibrosis and autosomal recessive polycystic kidney disease.

Primary sclerosing cholangitis is a chronic fibro-obliterative disease of unknown etiology that involves the extrahepatic and intrahepatic bile ducts. In older children, this condition occurs most often in association with inflammatory bowel disease, although it may present rarely in otherwise healthy teenagers or in patients who have congenital or acquired immunodeficiency. Clinical features include jaundice, anorexia, fatigue, abdominal pain, and pruritus. The diagnosis is confirmed by cholangiography that shows a characteristic beading and stenosis of the common or intrahepatic bile ducts in the absence of choledocholithiasis.

AUTOIMMUNE HEPATITIS

Autoimmune hepatitis is a chronic progressive inflammatory liver disease of unknown etiology. Two major subtypes have been identified based on circulating autoantibodies. Type 1 disease, defined by the presence of anti-smooth muscle antibodies (ASMAs) and antinuclear antibodies (ANAs), typically presents in adolescent females as an acute hepatitis with symptoms of malaise, nausea, anorexia, fatigue, abdominal pain, and jaundice. Type 2 autoimmune liver disease, associated with the liver-kidney microsomal antibody, is a more rapidly progressive form that usually presents with similar symptoms in younger children and infants.

HEPATOTOXINS

A variety of drugs or environmental agents may be hepatotoxic and cause jaundice in older children and adolescents. Acetaminophen overdose is a leading cause of fulminant hepatic failure in these age groups. Hepatotoxicity develops in the face of glutathione depletion, after which any excess acetaminophen is metabolized by the hepatic P450 pathway to produce the hepatotoxic product NAPQI (N-acetyl-p-benzoquinoneimine). A distinct clinical course ensues, with initial nausea and vomiting, followed progressively by a quiescent period and acute liver dysfunction with jaundice and coagulopathy. Hepatic failure may develop with progressive encephalopathy and coma. Other hepatotoxic agents that can cause jaundice include erythromycin, sulfonamides, halothane, methotrexate, chemotherapy, anticonvulsants such as valproate and phenytoin, the antituberculous drug isoniazid, and oral contraceptives.

VASCULAR DISEASES

Vascular diseases of the liver may present with jaundice in older children. Veno-occlusive disease causing hepatic congestion and jaundice may be seen in children in the first few weeks following bone marrow transplantation.

Clinical Evaluation

Distinguishing between conjugated and unconjugated hyperbilirubinemia is a most important first step in diagnosis. Whereas the presence of dark urine, pale stools, or pruritus in a jaundiced patient suggests hepatobiliary disease with a conjugated hyperbilirubinemia, the absence of these symptoms does not specify the underlying type of jaundice, and laboratory studies are required. If the jaundice is associated with abdominal pain, it is important to document the nature, site, and severity of the pain. Cholecystitis or choledocholithiasis due to gallstone disease usually presents with severe epigastric or right upper quadrant pain, often accompanied by vomiting. For acute viral hepatitis, the abdominal pain characteristically is a dull ache in the right upper quadrant. Personality changes, inappropriate behavior, and disturbed sleep-wake cycle or worsening school performance in a child who has jaundice may indicate hepatic encephalopathy, suggesting fulminant hepatitis, or may represent features of the CNS complications of Wilson disease.

In reviewing the past history, it is important to inquire about risk factors for viral hepatitis, such as maternal-infant transmission, transfusion of contaminated blood products, intravenous drug abuse, high-risk sexual activity, travel history, or a history of infectious contacts. A detailed review of all medications is essential to search for potential hepatotoxic agents, especially acetaminophen abuse or misuse. Consanguinity or a family history for jaundice may suggest inherited metabolic conditions such as Wilson disease, alpha-1-antitrypsin deficiency, cystic fibrosis, or Gilbert syndrome.

The physical examination should focus on signs of chronic liver disease; the acute onset of jaundice in any child may be an initial clinical manifestation of previously unrecognized chronic liver disease. Pallor may suggest an acute hemolytic anemia or chronic liver disease. Malnutrition, palmar erythema, and spider nevi on the chest or upper extremities suggest chronic liver disease. Generalized lymphadenopathy and pharyngitis point to an EBV infection. The finding of KF rings on opthalmologic slitlamp examination suggests Wilson disease. The liver must be carefully palpated and percussed to assess its texture and measure its size and span. The normal liver span is approximately 9 to 12 cm in early adolescence. A nodular hard surface or a shrunken liver suggests cirrhosis. Sharp-edged, tender hepatomegaly typifies acute hepatitis. Splenomegaly may be present because of a hemolytic disease or acute EBV infection or it may be the singular sign for chronic liver disease with cirrhosis and portal hypertension. Abdominal distension or shifting dullness on percussion in the flanks may indicate ascites formation. Neurologic abnormalities, including confusion and delirium, asterixis, hyperreflexia, or decorticate or decerebrate posturing, are all features of hepatic encephalopathy. Early onset of encephalopathy in a patient who has newly diagnosed liver disease defines fulminant liver failure and portends a poor prognosis.

Table 3. Laboratory Evaluation of Hyperbilirubinemia in Older Children

Unconjugated Hyperbilirubinemia
- Complete blood count
- Reticulocyte count
- Blood smear
- Serum haptoglobins
- Direct and indirect Coombs test
- Hemoglobin electrophoresis
- Red cell enzyme assay
- Test for spherocytosis

Conjugated Hyperbilirubinemia
- Liver function tests (AST, ALT, ALP, and GGT)
- Synthetic liver function (prothrombin time, total protein, albumin, glucose, cholesterol, ammonia)
- Abdominal ultrasonography
- HAV IgM, HBsAg, IgM-antiHBcore, antiHCV, Monospot®/EBV titers
- Serum ceruloplasmin, 24-hour urinary copper excretion
- Serum IgG, autoantibodies (ANA, ASMA, anti-liver-kidney-microsomal antibody)
- Serum alpha-1-antitrypsin level and phenotype
- Liver biopsy

Laboratory Evaluation and Diagnosis

Bilirubin fractionation by the Ektachem or Diazo method is a necessary first step in the laboratory evaluation of any older child or adolescent who has jaundice (Table 3). Unconjugated hyperbilirubinemia in this age group is due most often to hemolytic disease. A complete blood count, reticulocyte count, direct and indirect Coombs tests, measurement of serum haptoglobins, and hemoglobin electrophoresis should be requested. Exceptionally, a Coombs-negative hemolytic anemia may be the sole presenting feature of Wilson disease. In the absence of hemolysis or elevated liver enzyme levels, Gilbert syndrome should be considered in the adolescent who has mild unconjugated hyperbilirubinemia.

Conjugated hyperbilirubinemia suggests hepatobiliary disease. The initial laboratory investigations should include a complete blood count, liver function tests (AST, ALT, alkaline phosphatase [ALP], gammaglutamyltransferase [GGT]), total protein, serum albumin, and a prothrombin time (PT). Although there is considerable overlap, predominant elevation of the AST and ALT suggests hepatocellular injury, and a prevailing elevation in the ALP and GGT suggests biliary tract disease. It is important to remember that the so-called "liver function tests" are a misnomer; they do not reveal anything about the synthetic function of the liver. Tests for liver function include a coagulation screen and measurements of serum glucose, cholesterol, ammonia, and albumin. Of these, the most sensitive test for synthetic liver function is the PT. Prolongation of the PT despite administration of vitamin K suggests significant hepatic dysfunction. Patients who have acute hepatitis and a marked coagulopathy that is not responsive to vitamin K or who manifest other "worrisome signs" (Table 4) should be referred promptly to a center that has expertise in the management of children who have advanced liver disease and where liver transplantation is readily available. For these more urgent cases, intensive supportive care and liver transplantation hold the greatest potential for survival.

Further laboratory investigations are directed toward establishing a diagnosis. Every patient who presents with conjugated hyperbilirubinemia should undergo abdominal ultrasonography to examine the hepatic architecture and to exclude biliary tract disease. Screening for the viral hepatitides should include serology for hepatitis A immunoglobulin M (IgM), hepatitis B surface antigen, IgM antibody to hepatitis B core antigen, and anti-HCV. A Monospot® test or serology for EBV is also highly recommended for the

Table 4. "Worrisome" Signs and Symptoms in the Jaundiced Older Child or Adolescent Who Has Acute Hepatitis

- Onset of hepatic encephalopathy
- Vitamin K-resistant prolongation of the prothrombin time
- Cerebral edema
- Serum bilirubin 18 mg/dL (>300 mcmol/L)
- Rising serum bilirubin with decreasing ALT/AST
- Rising serum creatinine
- Hypoglycemia
- Sepsis
- Ascites
- pH<7.3 in acetaminophen overdose

adolescent who presents with conjugated hyper-bilirubinemia. Measurement of serum alpha-1-antitrypsin levels and protease inhibitor phenotyping should be requested to exclude alpha-1-antitrypsin deficiency. Patients who have autoimmune hepatitis, jaundice, and an elevated ALT usually exhibit a high serum total protein relative to the albumin, reflecting an increased globulin fraction. This is a result of the significant hypergammaglobulinemia often found in association with autoimmune hepatitis. Aside from measuring the serum IgG, other tests for autoimmune hepatitis should include an ANA, ASMA, and anti-liver-kidney-microsomal anti-body. A liver biopsy is recommended to confirm the diagnosis.

Serum ceruloplasmin is a valuable screening test for Wilson disease. A decreased serum ceruloplasmin level is found in up to 80% of affected patients. Another useful diagnostic test is the 24-hour urinary copper excretion. In Wilson disease, the urinary copper excretion is typically greater than 100 mcg/24 h. Serum copper levels are not helpful in diagnosing Wilson disease except for those rare patients presenting with fulminant liver failure, in whom serum copper levels are significantly elevated. Other laboratory abnormalities often seen in Wilson disease include a low serum ALP, particularly when fulminant hepatic failure is present, and low serum phosphate and uric acid due to the associated Fanconi syndrome. Quantification of hepatic copper concentration in a liver biopsy tissue specimen (>250 mcg/g of dry weight liver) remains the gold standard for diagnosing Wilson disease.

Treatment

Specific treatment of the hyperbilirubinemia depends on the precise etiology. A detailed discussion of therapy for each individual disease state is beyond the scope of this article. In general, acute hemolytic crises require hyper-hydration and close monitoring of renal function. Immunosuppressive agents, such as prednisone, azathioprine, or cyclosporine, are used to treat autoimmune hepatitis. Penicillamine is the drug of choice for Wilson disease, although zinc

replacement and trientine also have been prescribed. N-acetyl-cysteine is recommended for the treatment of acetaminophen overdose. Patients who have acute viral hepatitis, especially hepatitis A, are prone to dehydration and require adequate fluid support. Passive immunoprophylaxis should be administered to all close family contacts of patients who have acute hepatitis A.

Any child who has conjugated hyperbilirubinemia and encephalopathy or biochemical features of hepatic synthetic dysfunction, best evidenced by a prolonged PT, is at high risk to develop a more fulminant course that has a fatal outcome. Close supervision and intensive supportive care are required, preferably by physicians who have expertise in the management of advanced pediatric liver disease.

Summary

The spectrum of diseases causing jaundice in older children and adolescents differs from that in the neonate and young infant. A sound knowledge of the differential diagnosis of unconjugated and conjugated hyperbilirubinemia in this age group provides the framework for a sensible approach to the clinical evaluation and laboratory investigation of these children. For patients who have acute hepatitis, a careful assessment of liver function is of critical importance. Signs and symptoms of liver dysfunction in a jaundiced patient should prompt an immediate referral to a tertiary center where expertise in the management of pediatric liver disease and hepatic transplantation is readily available.

Suggested Reading

D'Agata ID, Balistreri WF. Evaluation of liver disease in the pediatric patient. *Pediatr Rev.* 1999;20:376–389

Gourley GR. Disorders of bilirubin metabolism. In: Suchy F, ed. *Liver Disease in Children.* St. Louis, Mo: Mosby; 1994:401–413

Jonas M. Viral hepatitis. In: Walker WA, Durie PR, Hamilton JR, Walker-Smith JA, Watkins JB, eds. *Pediatric Gastrointestinal Disease.* St. Louis, Mo: Mosby; 1996:1028–1051

Mews C, Sinatra F. Chronic liver disease in children. *Pediatr Rev.* 1993;14:436–443

Roberts EA, Cox DW. Wilson disease. *Baillieres Clin Gastroenterol.* 1998:12:237–256

Metabolic Syndrome: Comments for the Newsletter

Elizabeth Goodman, MD, Professor of Child and Adolescent Health, Heller School for Social Policy and Management, Brandeis University, Waltham, MA

As noted in the Summer 2004 newsletter, Metabolic Syndrome was a hot topic at the 2004 PAS meetings. Metabolic Syndrome also figured prominently at the 2004 AAP National Conference. Pediatricians want more information about this syndrome, especially because there is little doubt that the rising rates of obesity, sedentary lifestyle, and Type 2 diabetes will likely lead to increasing risk among young people. Adolescents are in particular jeopardy in this regard, as rates of overweight, obesity, and Type 2 diabetes have soared in the past decade in this age group.[1] In addition, puberty is known to cause insulin resistance.[2] Despite these alarming trends and documented risks, little research has assessed metabolic syndrome among adolescents and no adolescent-specific definition exists.[3] However, clustering of cardiovascular risks among teens does occur, and increases risk of asymptomatic arteriosclerosis, even at this young age.[4] This article will review the current definitions of Metabolic Syndrome, and discuss assessment and treatment recommendations.

The clustering of cardiovascular risk factors now commonly referred to as the Metabolic Syndrome has been recognized for well over a decade. First described in 1988, this syndrome was initially known as the Insulin Resistance Syndrome, because insulin resistance was felt to be a key pathogenic component.[5] Since its description, this clustering has been variously described as insulin resistance syndrome, Syndrome X, the dysmetabolic syndrome, and more recently metabolic syndrome. Metabolic Syndrome is independently associated with both diabetes and cardiovascular disease.[6,7] A wide array of factors have been associated with Metabolic Syndrome including general obesity, central obesity, dyslipidemia, primarily in relation to triglyceride and high density lipoprotein (HDL-C) concentrations, hypertension, hyperinsulinemia, impaired glucose metabolism, microalbuminuria, abnormalities in fibrinolysis, and inflammation.[5,6] Insulin resistance, obesity, aging, a pro-inflammatory state, hormonal factors, sedentary lifestyle, and genetics have all been implicated in its pathogenesis.[5,6,8-10]

There are at least three health organizations that have created clinical criteria for defining this syndrome among adults. These include the World Health Organization (WHO),[11] the National Cholesterol Education Panel's Adult Treatment Panel III (NCEP)[12] and the American Association of Clinical Endocrinologists (AACE).[13] These definitions differ significantly. The AACE lists clinical criteria for diagnosis of Insulin Resistance Syndrome (IRS), including cut points for overweight; elevated blood pressure, triglycerides, fasting glucose, decreased HDL cholesterol, and other risks (family history of diabetes, hypertension or cardiovascular disease, sedentary lifestyle, polycystic ovary disease, increased age, ethnic group with high risk for type 2 diabetes of cardiovascular disease). However, no required number of these risks is specified for diagnosis of IRS. The diagnosis is left to clinical judgment, and with the development of diabetes, the diagnosis of IRS becomes inapplicable. In contrast, both the WHO and NCEP specify a minimum number of risk factors required for the diagnosis of Metabolic Syndrome and do not exclude those with Type 2 diabetes. The WHO explicitly includes and, in fact, requires insulin resistance for diagnosis of Metabolic Syndrome. Insulin resistance is defined either by presence of Type 2 diabetes, impaired fasting glucose, impaired glucose tolerance, or glucose uptake lower than the bottom quartile for the background population of interest using hyperinsulinemic, euglycemic clamp conditions.[10,11] Other risks include hypertriglyceridemia, hypertension, low HDL-C, obesity, and microalbuminuria.♦ The NCEP definition does not include hyperinsulinemia, focusing, instead, on associated metabolic parameters. These include hyperglycemia, hypertriglyceridemia, hypertension, low HDL-C, and abdominal obesity. Both the WHO and NCEP definitions require 3 risks for diagnosis of MS. For WHO-defined Metabolic Syndrome, these three risks include insulin resistance plus two out of three other risk parameters: 1) hypertension, 2) dyslipidemia (hypertriglyceridemia or low high-HDL-C), or 3) central obesity (high waist:hip ratio, or body mass index of at least 30). For NCEP-defined MS, any three risk factors will suffice. Although there are shared risk factors between the WHO and NCEP definitions (hyperglycemia,ℜ♦♦hypertriglyceridemia, hypertension, low HDL-C, and obesity), the cut points for hypertension, low HDL-C, and obesity differ between definitions. The WHO definition condenses some risks into parameters. Each risk is independent in the NCEP criteria.

The differences in these definitions have important implications for case identification. For example, a person with hyperglycemia, hypertriglyceridemia, and low HDL-C would have MS per the NCEP and potentially the AACE, but not the WHO, because both hypertriglyceridemia and low HDL-C are in the dyslipidemia component. An additional component, either hypertension or central obesity, would be required for WHO-defined MS. In contrast, a person with hyperinsulinemia, low HDL-C, and obesity would have MS per the WHO criteria, but not per the NCEP guidelines because hyperinsulinemia is not a risk factor used by the NCEP. An additional risk factor would be required for NCEP-defined MS, either hypertension, hypertriglyceridemia, or hyperglycemia, and the obesity would need to be abdominal obesity (high waist circumference).

Adult studies have contrasted the WHO and NCEP definitions among adults and found important differences in their prognostic ability and case identification.[8,15]

There is little published research on Metabolic Syndrome among teens. Almost all of the studies addressing Metabolic Syndrome in adolescence use a definition based on the NCEP criteria. Most use an age and gender specific percentile based definition for the various cut points of the NCEP risks. However, these cut points range from 75%–97.5% (5–25% for high density lipoprotein cholesterol (HDL-C)), depending on the study and the risk factor of interest.[3,16-19] One of the first such studies used data from NHANES III to describe prevalence of MS among 12–19 year olds.[3] Nearly 30% of overweight adolescents met their criteria for MS, which were developed to reflect the 90th percentile distribution of risks. How these cut points related to those identified by the NCEP for adults was not discussed. This is problematic, as the older adolescents in this sample could be categorized as adults and the adult criteria do not reflect percentiles of distribution. For example, among men in NHANES III, the 102 cm cut point for waist circumference, which is used in the NCEP definition, reflects the 70th percentile. The cut point among adult women—88cm—was the mean waist circumference among women.[20] The HDL-C cut point of 40 mg/dl was identical to the adult NCEP criteria for men, but more stringent than the NCEP's 50 mg/dl cut point for adult women. Such differences in criteria between adolescents and adults also create difficulties for understanding the developmental trajectory of cardiovascular risk clustering in this age group and can complicate clinical management as adolescents age into the adult years.

A conservative approach to this problem is to extend the adult guidelines for defining Metabolic Syndrome downward to adolescents. A recent study used this approach and compared

---

♦Of note, the European Group for the Study of Insulin Resistance subsequently (1999) modified the WHO definition for use in epidemiological studies, not clinical care, to obviate the need for euglycemic clamp studies. The EGIR definition defined insulin resistance as the top quartile of fasting insulin within the study population, changed the measurement of obesity (BMI and waist:hip ratio) to abdominal girth measured by waist circumference, and increased the cut point for triglycerides. (Balkau B, Charles MA. Diabet Med. 1999;16:442-443).

♦♦The American Diabetes Association recently recommended lowering the cutpoint for hyperglycemia from 110 mg/dl to 100mg/dl. (Genuth S, Alberti KG, Bennett P, et al. Diabetes Care. 2003;26:3160-3167).

and contrasted the NCEP and WHO definitions among youth.[21] This study demonstrated significant demographic differences depending on the definition used. Risk was about two-thirds lower among non-Hispanic white as opposed to non-Hispanic black youth when the WHO-based definition was used, but there were no black-white differences, nor were there any significant gender differences when the NCEP-based definition was applied. However, if the WHO-based definition was used, girls were at 26% greater risk than boys. There was poor agreement between definitions. Together, these findings and the adult studies suggest that the NCEP and WHO guidelines identify distinct yet overlapping populations with clustered CV risks.

Given the complexity of defining Metabolic Syndrome in adolescence, the evolving understanding of Metabolic Syndrome, and the lack of consensus regarding definition, it is not surprising that there is not universal agreement nor even general consensus regarding clinical assessment and treatment for Metabolic Syndrome in childhood and adolescence. However, there is consensus among the American Diabetes Association and American Heart Association that obesity prevention and treatment in childhood should be the first line approach to this problem.[22] There is also agreement that insulin resistance is associated with development of Type 2 diabetes, and that children and adolescence at risk for development of Type 2 diabetes, either by being overweight, belonging to a racial/ethnic group with a predisposition for developing Type 2 diabetes, having a family history of Type 2 diabetes, or having other signs of insulin resistance, such as acanthosis nigricans, polycystic ovary syndrome, dyslipidemia, or hypertension, should be assessed through use of a fasting glucose of oral glucose tolerance test.[22] There is insufficient data to support use of HgbA1c at the present time, and although measurement of insulin resistance through assessment of fasting insulin and glucose has been suggested as an alternative to the euglycemic clamp method, which is currently used for research purposes only, there is no current agreement as to how these should be applied.[22] Thus, continued efforts to prevent and

treat obesity among children and adolescents, and vigilant attention to the early diagnosis of diabetes provide the pediatrician with the most evidence-based methods for addressing metabolic syndrome in adolescence.

References

1. Ogden CL, Flegal KM, Carroll MD, Johnson CL. Prevalence and Trends in Overweight Among US Children and Adolescents, 1999-2000. *JAMA.* 2002; 288:1728-1732.

2. Potau N, Ibanez L, Rique S, Carrascosa A. Pubertal changes in insulin secretion and peripheral insulin sensitivity. *Horm Res.* 1997; 48:219-226.

3. Cook S, Weitzman M, Auinger P, Nguyen M, Dietz WH. Prevalence of a Metabolic Syndrome Phenotype in Adolescents: Findings From the Third National Health and Nutrition Examination Survey, 1988-1994. *Arch Pediatr Adolesc Med.* 2003;157:821-827.

4. Berenson GS, Srinivasan SR, Bao W, Newman WP 3rd, Tracy RE, Wattigney WA. Association between multiple cardiovascular risk factors and atherosclerosis in children and young adults. The Bogalusa Heart Study. *N Engl J Med.* 1998;338:1650-1656.

5. Reaven GM. Role of insulin resistance in human disease. *Diabetes.* 1988;37:1595-1607.

6. Meigs JB. Invited Commentary: Insulin Resistance Syndrome? Syndrome X? Multiple Metabolic Syndrome? A Syndrome At All? Factor Analysis Reveals Patterns in the Fabric of Correlated Metabolic Risk Factors. *Am J Epidemiol.* 2000;152:908-911.

7. Meigs JB, D'Agostino RB Sr, Wilson PW, Cupples LA, Nathan DM, Singer DE. Risk variable clustering in the insulin resistance syndrome. The Framingham Offspring Study. *Diabetes.* 1997;46:1594-1600.

8. Laaksonen DE, Lakka HM, Niskanen LK, Kaplan GA, Salonen JT, Lakka TA. Metabolic syndrome and development of diabetes mellitus: application and validation of recently suggested definitions of the metabolic syndrome in a prospective cohort study. *Am J Epidemiol.* 2002;156:1070-1077.

9. Yip J, Facchini FS, Reaven GM. Resistance to insulin-mediated glucose disposal as a predictor of cardiovascular disease. *J Clin Endocrinol Metab.* 1998;83:2773-2776.

10. Grundy SM, Brewer HB Jr, Cleeman JI, Smith SC Jr, Lenfant C, for the Conference Participants. Definition of Metabolic Syndrome: Report of the National Heart, Lung, and Blood Institute/American Heart Association Conference on Scientific Issues Related to Definition. *Circulation.* 2004;109:433-438.

11. Alberti KG, Zimmet PZ. Definition, diagnosis and classification of diabetes mellitus and its complications. Part 1: diagnosis and classification of diabetes mellitus provisional report of a WHO consultation. *Diabet Med.* 1998;15:539-553.

12. Expert Panel on Detection E, and Treatment of High Blood Cholesterol in Adults. Executive Summary of the Third Report of the National Cholesterol Education Program (NCEP) Expert Panel on Detection, Evaluation, and Treatment of High Blood Cholesterol in Adults (Adult Treatment Panel III). *JAMA.* 2001;285:2486–2497.

13. Einhorn D, Reaven GM, Cobin RH, et al. American College of Endocrinology position statement on the insulin resistance syndrome. *Endocr Pract.* 2003;9:237–252.

14. Balkau B, Charles MA. Comment on the provisional report from the WHO consultation. European Group for the Study of Insulin Resistance (EGIR). *Diabet Med.* 1999;16:442–443.

15. Ford ES, Giles WH. A comparison of the prevalence of the metabolic syndrome using two proposed definitions. *Diabetes Care.* 2003;26:575–581.

16. Raikkonen K, Matthews KA, Salomon K. Hostility predicts metabolic syndrome risk factors in children and adolescents. *Health Psychol.* 2003;22:279–286.

17. Weiss R, Dziura J, Burgert TS, et al. Obesity and the Metabolic Syndrome in Children and Adolescents. *N Engl J Med.* 2004;350:2362–2374.

18. Cruz ML, Weigensberg MJ, Huang TT, Ball G, Shaibi GQ, Goran MI. The metabolic syndrome in overweight Hispanic youth and the role of insulin sensitivity. *J Clin Endocrinol Metab.* 2004;89:108–113.

19. Frontini MG, Srinivasan SR, Berenson GS. Longitudinal changes in risk variables underlying metabolic Syndrome X from childhood to young adulthood in female subjects with a history of early menarche: the Bogalusa Heart Study. *Int J Obes Relat Metab Disord.* 2003;27:1398–1404.

20. Zhu S, Wang Z, Heshka S, Heo M, Faith MS, Heymsfield SB. Waist circumference and obesity-associated risk factors among whites in the third National Health and Nutrition Examination Survey: clinical action thresholds. *Am J Clin Nutr.* 2002;76:743–.

21. Goodman E, Daniels S, Morrison J, Huang B, Dolan L. Metabolic Syndrome in Adolescents: A Comparison of the WHO and NCEP Definitions. *J Pediatr.* 2004;145: 445–451.

22. Steinberger J, Daniels SR. Obesity, Insulin Resistance, Diabetes, and Cardiovascular Risk in Children: An American Heart Association Scientific Statement From the Atherosclerosis, Hypertension, and Obesity in the Young Committee (Council on Cardiovascular Disease in the Young) and the Diabetes Committee (Council on Nutrition, Physical Activity, and Metabolism). *Circulation.* 2003;107:1448–1453.

New Treatments for Asthma

Mary V. Lasley, MD*

Objectives

After completing this article, readers should be able to:

1. Define asthma.
2. List conditions that mimic asthma.
3. Delineate the factors that predict the persistence of asthma.
4. Describe the objective measurements of pulmonary function required for evaluation and treatment of asthma.
5. Explain the role of anti-inflammatory medications in the management of persistent asthma.
6. Determine when a child should be referred to an asthma specialist.

Epidemiology

Over the past 15 years, the number of people affected by asthma has more than doubled. Asthma is the most common pediatric chronic disease, afflicting nearly 5 million children younger than age 18 years in the United States. Asthma affects 1 of every 13 schoolchildren. Every year, asthma accounts for more than 3 million physician visits and 200,000 pediatric hospitalizations, with rates highest among African-American children. Asthma mortality nearly doubled between 1980 and 1993 (17 and 32 asthma deaths per 1 million population, respectively). More than 5,500 people die from asthma every year. Asthma is a major cause of school absenteeism, with an estimated 10 million missed schooldays each year. The economic impact of asthma is enormous, approaching $3 billion annually. This encompasses direct costs such as medical expenses and indirect costs of parents and caregivers taking time away from work to care for their ill children, which has been estimated at $1 billion annually.

Asthma severity is greater in urban minority populations, both African-American and Hispanic. Children living in inner cities often do not receive appropriate treatment to reduce their asthma severity and live in situations where it is difficult to control environmental exposures.

Pathogenesis

Inflammation is present even in the airways of young patients who have mild asthma. A complex orchestration of inflammatory cells (eg, mast cells, eosinophils, T lymphocytes, and neutrophils), chemical mediators (eg, histamine, leukotrienes, platelet-activating factor, bradykinin), and chemotactic factors (eg, cytokines, eotaxin) results in the underlying inflammation found in asthmatic airways (Fig. 1). Inflammation of the airways contributes to airway hyperresponsiveness, which is characterized as the tendency for the airways to constrict in response to allergens, irritants, viral infections, and exercise. It also results in edema, increased mucus production in the lungs, an influx of inflammatory cells into the airway, and epithelial cell denudation. Chronic inflammation can lead to airway remodeling, which results from a proliferation of extracellular matrix proteins and vascular hyperplasia (Fig. 1). Chronic remodeling may lead to irreversible structural changes and a progressive loss of pulmonary function. Exactly when the child is most susceptible to remodeling and whether therapeutic intervention can prevent this is still unknown.

---

*Clinical Assistant Professor of Pediatrics, University of Washington School of Medicine, Northwest Asthma & Allergy Center, Seattle, WA.

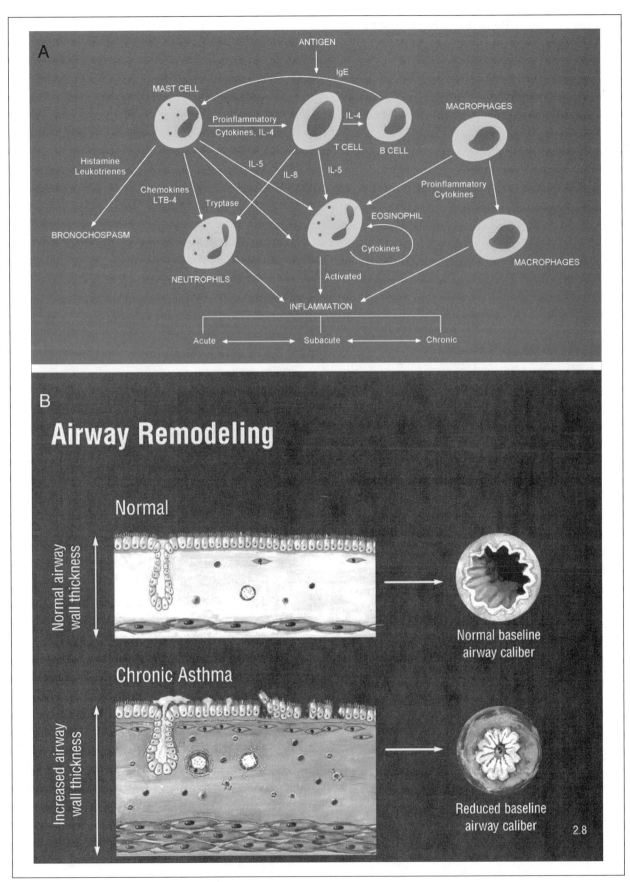

Figure 1. Airway inflammation in asthma. A. Cellular mechanisms involved in airway inflammation.
B. Airway remodeling due to chronic airway inflammation. Ig=immunoglobulin, IL=interleukin.

Airflow limitation due to the effects of airway inflammation leads to the respiratory symptoms of coughing, wheezing, shortness of breath, and chest tightness that are observed in children who suffer from asthma.

Diagnosis

It can be difficult to diagnose asthma in children; asthma often is underdiagnosed among infants and young children who wheeze during respiratory infections. It also is important to recognize that cough and wheeze do not always reflect asthma. Care is needed to avoid prescribing inappropriate prolonged asthma medications. Other conditions that mimic asthma are shown in Table 1. For some children, symptoms of wheezing accompanying respiratory infections subside in the preschool years; other children develop persistent symptoms. However, the strongest predictor for wheezing developing into asthma is atopy. Approximately 70% to 90% of children who have asthma and are older than 5 years of age have positive allergy skin tests. Other predictive factors include parental history of asthma, peripheral blood eosinophilia, wheezing episodes apart from upper respiratory tract infections, and presence of atopic dermatitis or allergic rhinitis.

Three steps for diagnosing asthma are to obtain a careful history, perform a thorough physical examination, and objectively measure pulmonary function. The history should elicit the child's symptoms of coughing, wheezing, shortness of breath or rapid breathing, or chest tightness and the frequency and severity of such symptoms. Symptoms tend to occur or worsen at night, waking the child or parent. Asthma symptoms frequently are exacerbated by viral infections, exposure to allergens and irritants (smoke, strong odors and fumes), exercise, emotions, and changes in weather/humidity. A family history of allergy and asthma is a useful finding; allergic diseases tend to occur in families. On examination, physical findings may be subtle. Wheezing may not be present. Evidence of other atopic diseases such as eczema or allergic rhinitis can help guide the clinician to the correct diagnosis.

If possible to obtain, objective measurements of pulmonary function (spirometry) are essential to establish the diagnosis and treatment of asthma. Spirometry should be undertaken at the initial visit as well as at return visits to document attainment of "normal" pulmonary functions. Spirometry testing can help monitor the patient's response to the treatment plan, assess the degree of reversibility with optimal asthma management, and measure the severity of an asthma exacerbation. Spirometry should be obtained at least annually to ensure preservation of airway function,

Table 1. Differential Diagnosis of Cough and Wheeze in Infants and Children

Upper Respiratory Tract	Middle Respiratory Tract	Lower Respiratory Tract
Allergic rhinitis	Bronchial stenosis	Asthma
Adenoid/tonsillar hypertrophy	Enlarged lymph nodes	Bronchiectasis
Foreign body	Epiglottitis	Bronchopulmonary dysplasia
Infectious rhinitis	Foreign body	Chlamydia trachomatis
Sinusitis	Laryngeal webs	Chronic aspiration
	Laryngomalacia	Cystic fibrosis
	Laryngotracheobronchitis	Foreign body
	Pertussis	Gastroesophageal reflux
	Toxic inhalation	Hyperventilation syndrome
	Tracheoesophageal fistula	Obliterative bronchiolitis
	Tracheal stenosis	Pulmonary hemosiderosis
	Tracheomalacia	Toxic inhalation
	Tumor	Tumor
	Vascular rings	Viral bronchiolitis
	Vocal cord dysfunction	

Adapted from Lemanske RF Jr, Green CG. Asthma in infancy and childhood. In: Middleton E Jr, Reed CE, Ellis EF, et al, eds. *Allergy: Principles & Practice.* 5th ed. St. Louis, Mo: Mosby-Year Book, Inc; 1998:878.

at visits where there are reports of pulmonary instability, and if there have been changes in the medication regimen. Children older than 5 years usually can perform spirometry maneuvers. Several practice sessions may be necessary for the younger child to master spirometry techniques.

Because atopy plays an important role in asthma persistence, allergy skin testing should be considered. A board-certified allergist offers the special skill of administering and interpreting skin tests to determine immediate hypersensitivity to aeroallergens. Studies have demonstrated that positive skin test results correlate strongly with bronchial allergen provocative challenges. In vitro tests, such as radioallergosorbent test and enzyme-linked immunosorbent assay, are other options to measure levels of antigen-specific immunoglobulin E. However, compared with skin testing, in vitro testing generally is not as sensitive in defining clinically pertinent allergens, is more expensive, and requires several days for results (compared with several minutes for skin tests).

Environmental Control

Optimal medical treatment of asthma is based on three key components: environmental control, pharmacologic therapy, and patient education, including acquisition of self-management skills.

Because children have a high incidence of allergy related to asthma, steps should be taken to minimize allergen exposure (Table 2). For all children who have asthma, common sense dictates that exposures to tobacco and wood smoke as well as viral infections be minimized.

Table 2. Controlling Factors Contributing to Asthma Severity

Major Indoor Triggers for Asthma	Suggestions for Reducing Exposure
Viral upper respiratory tract infections Influenza	● Limit exposure to viral infections (ie, smaller size child care) ● Administer annual influenza shots to children who have persistent asthma (who are not allergic to eggs)
Tobacco smoke, wood smoke	● Do not smoke around the child or in child's home ● Help parents and caregivers quit smoking ● Eliminate use of wood stoves and fireplaces
Dust mites	Essential actions: ● Encase pillow, mattress, and box spring in allergen-impermeable encasement ● Wash bedding in hot water weekly Desirable actions: ● Avoid sleeping or lying on upholstered furniture ● Minimize number of stuffed toys in child's bedroom ● Reduce indoor humidity to <50% ● If possible, remove carpets from bedroom and play areas; if not possible, vacuum frequently

Animal dander	● Remove the pet from the home or keep outdoors
	● If removal is not acceptable:
	   —Keep pet out of bedroom
	   —Use filters on air ducts in child's room
	   —Wash pet weekly (although evidence to support the benefit of this action has not been firmly established)

Cockroach allergens	● Do not leave food or garbage exposed ● Use boric acid traps ● Reduce indoor humidity to <50% ● Fix leaky faucets, pipes
Indoor mold	● Fix leaky faucets, pipes ● Avoid vaporizers ● Reduce indoor humidity to <50%

Adapted from American Academy of Allergy, Asthma & Immunology, Inc. *Pediatric Asthma: Promoting Best Practice*. Milwaukee, Wisc: American Academy of Allergy, Asthma, and Immunology, Inc; 1999:50.

Pharmacologic Therapy

Current therapy is based on the concept that chronic inflammation is a fundamental feature of the disease. The National Asthma Education and Prevention Program recently published an update on classification and treatment based on asthma severity. The stepwise approach for management of infants and young children is shown in Figure 2 and for children 5 years of age and older is shown in Figure 3. A short-acting bronchodilator should be available for all children who have asthma. Intermittent asthma is defined as the presence of asthma symptoms less frequently than twice weekly. To determine if a child is having more persistent asthma, the "rule of twos" can be helpful. The presence of daytime symptoms two or more times per week or nighttime awakening two or more times per month may indicate a need for daily controller medication that has anti-inflammatory activity. For infants and young children who have had three episodes of wheezing in the previous year as well as risk factors for the development of asthma (ie, parental asthma, peripheral blood eosinophilia, wheezing between upper respiratory tract infections, personal atopy) or who have severe exacerbations fewer than 6 weeks apart, long-term controller medications may be desirable.

The preferred first-line controller medication for children of all ages who have persistent asthma is inhaled corticosteroids. In clinical trials comparing inhaled corticosteroids with cromolyn, nedocromil, leukotriene modifiers, or theophylline, inhaled corticosteroids were the most effective medications in improving long-term asthma control. Low-dose inhaled corticosteroids are recommended for children who have mild persistent asthma. For children older than 5 years of age who have moderate persistent asthma, combining long-acting bronchodilators with low to medium doses of inhaled corticosteroids improves lung function and reduces rescue medication usage. The evidence for adding a leukotriene modifier or theophylline or for doubling the dose of corticosteroid is not as well supported by clinical studies. For children younger than 5 years of age who have moderate persistent asthma, medication combinations have not been as well studied. The preferred therapy is either a combination of low-dose inhaled corticosteroids and long-acting bronchodilators or medium doses of inhaled corticosteroids. High-dose inhaled corticosteroids and long-acting bronchodilators are the preferred therapies for children who have severe persistent asthma. The guidelines also recommend that patients be assessed every 1 to 6 months to determine whether medications should be reduced (step-down) or increased (step-up), depending on disease control.

Long-term controller medications are taken daily to achieve and maintain control of persistent asthma. Some controller medications, such as cromolyn, nedocromil, and theophylline, have been available for many years and will not be reviewed in this article. Discussion of the newer medications, including inhaled corticosteroids, leukotriene modifiers, and long-acting bronchodilators, follows.

INHALED CORTICOSTEROIDS

Inhaled corticosteroids are the most effective anti-inflammatory medications for the treatment of chronic persistent asthma. Inhaled corticosteroids are available as metered-dose inhalers (MDI), dry powder inhalers (DPI), and nebulizer solutions. The inhaled corticosteroids available in the United States include beclomethasone, budesonide, flunisolide, fluticasone, and triamcinolone, with mometasone forthcoming. Clinical trials with the next generation of inhaled corticosteroids are proceeding.

The greatest concern of parents and physicians about these medications is the risk of systemic corticosteroid activity. In general, if the medications are used in doses of less than 400 mcg/day (beclomethasone equivalent), there is little risk of systemic effects.

Information about the effects of corticosteroids on linear growth is conflicting in the literature. Short-term studies suggest growth delay of about 1 cm/y. The reliability of this growth delay is tempered by the apparent similarity of heights compared with normal peers demonstrated in long-term studies. The

Stepwise Approach for Managing Infants and Young Children (5 Years of Age and Younger) With Acute or Chronic Asthma

Classify Severity: Clinical Features Before Treatment or Adequate Control		Medications Required To Maintain Long-Term Control
	Symptoms/Day / Symptoms/Night	Daily Medications
Step 4 Severe Persistent	Continual / Frequent	■ **Preferred treatment:** – **High-dose inhaled corticosteroids** **AND** – **Long-acting inhaled beta$_2$-agonists** **AND**, if needed, – Corticosteroid tablets or syrup long term (2 mg/kg/day, generally do not exceed 60 mg per day). (Make repeat attempts to reduce systemic corticosteroids and maintain control with high-dose inhaled corticosteroids.)
Step 3 Moderate Persistent	Daily / > 1 night/week	■ **Preferred treatments:** – **Low-dose inhaled corticosteroids and long-acting inhaled beta$_2$-agonists** **OR** – **Medium-dose inhaled corticosteroids.** ■ Alternative treatment: – Low-dose inhaled corticosteroids and either leukotriene receptor antagonist or theophylline. .... If needed (particularly in patients with recurring severe exacerbations): ■ **Preferred treatment:** – **Medium-dose inhaled corticosteroids and long-acting beta$_2$-agonists.** ■ Alternative treatment: – Medium-dose inhaled corticosteroids and either leukotriene receptor antagonist or theophylline.
Step 2 Mild Persistent	> 2/week but < 1x/day / > 2 nights/month	■ **Preferred treatment:** – **Low-dose inhaled corticosteroid (with nebulizer or MDI with holding chamber with or without face mask or DPI).** ■ Alternative treatment (listed alphabetically): Cromolyn (nebulizer is preferred or MDI with holding chamber) OR leukotriene receptor antagonist.
Step 1 Mild Intermittent	≤ 2 days/week / ≤ 2 nights/month	■ No daily medication needed.

Goals of Therapy: Asthma Control
- ■ Minimal or no chronic symptoms day or night
- ■ Minimal or no exacerbations
- ■ Minimal use of short-acting inhaled beta$_2$-agonist (<1x per day, <1 canister/month)
- ■ No limitations on activities; no school/parent's work missed
- ■ Minimal or no adverse effects from medications

Step down
Review treatment every 1 to 6 months; a gradual stepwise reduction in treatment may be possible.

Step up
If control is not maintained, consider step up. First, review patient medication technique, adherence, and environmental control.

Quick Relief All Patients
- ■ Bronchodilator as needed for symptoms ≤ 2 times a week. Intensity of treatment will depend upon severity of exacerbation.
  - –Preferred treatment: Short-acting inhaled beta$_2$-agonists by nebulizer or face mask and space/holding chamber
  - –Alternative treatment: Oral beta$_2$-agonist
- ■ With viral respiratory infection
  - – Bronchodilator q 4 –6 hours up to 24 hours (longer with physician consult); in general no more than once every 6 weeks
  - – Consider systemic corticosteroid if exacerbation is severe or patient has history of previous severe exacerbations
- ■ Use of short-acting inhaled beta$_2$-agonists > 2 times a week in intermittent asthma (daily, or increasing use in persistent asthma) may indicate the need to initiate (increase) long-term control therapy.

Note
- The stepwise approach is meant to assist, not replace, the clinical decisionmaking required to meet individual patient needs.
- Classify severity: assign patient to most severe step in which any feature occurs.
- Gain control as quickly as possible (a short course of systemic corticosteroids may be required); then step down to the least medication necessary to maintain control.
- Provide parent education on asthma management and controlling environmental factors that make asthma worse (e.g., allergies and irritants).
- Consultation with an asthma specialist is recommended for patients with moderate or severe persistent asthma. Consider consultation for patients with mild persistent asthma.

Executive Summary of the NAEPP Expert Panel Report: Guidelines for the Diagnosis and Management of Asthma–Update on Selected Topics 2002. Bethesda, Maryland: National Heart, Lung, and Blood Institute. National Institutes of Health.
NIH Publication No. 02-5075 June 2002 http://www.nhlbi.nih.gov/guidelines/asthma/asthsumm.htm

Figure 2. Stepwise approach for managing infants and young children ≤5 y who have acute or chronic asthma. From NHLBI, National Asthma Education and Prevention Program. *Expert Panel Report: Guidelines for the Diagnosis and Management of Asthma— Update on Selected Topics.* 2002.

Stepwise Approach for Managing Asthma in Adults and Children Older Than 5 Years of Age: Treatment

Classify Severity: Clinical Features Before Treatment or Adequate Control			Medications Required To Maintain Long-Term Control
	Symptoms/Day Symptoms/Night	PEF or FEV₁ PEF Variability	Daily Medications

Step 4
Severe
Persistent
	Continual
	Frequent
		≤ 60%
		> 30%
			■ **Preferred treatment:**
			– **High-dose inhaled corticosteroids**
			  AND
			– **Long-acting inhaled beta₂-agonists**
			  AND, if needed,
			– Corticosteroid tablets or syrup long term (2 mg/kg/day, generally do not exceed 60 mg per day). (Make repeat attempts to reduce systemic corticosteroids and maintain control with high-dose inhaled corticosteroids.)

Step 3 Moderate Persistent	Daily > 1 night/week	> 60% – < 80% > 30%	■ **Preferred treatment:** – **Low-to-medium dose inhaled corticosteroids and long-acting inhaled beta₂-agonists.** ■ Alternative treatment (listed alphabetically): – Increase inhaled corticosteroids within medium-dose range OR – Low-to-medium dose inhaled corticosteroids and either leukotriene modifier or theophylline. If needed (particularly in patients with recurring severe exacerbations): ■ Preferred treatment: – Increase inhaled corticosteroids within medium-dose range, and add long-acting inhaled beta₂-agonists. ■ Alternative treatment (listed alphabetically): – Increase inhaled corticosteroids within medium-dose range and add either leukotriene modifier or theophylline.
Step 2 Mild Persistent	> 2/week but < 1x/day > 2 nights/month	≥ 80% 20–30%	■ **Preferred treatment:** – **Low-dose inhaled corticosteroids.** ■ Alternative treatment (listed alphabetically): cromolyn, leukotriene modifier, nedocromil, OR sustained release theophylline to serum concentration of 5–15 mcg/mL.
Step 1 Mild Intermittent	≤ 2 days/week ≤ 2 nights/month	≥ 80% < 20%	■ No daily medication needed. ■ Severe exacerbations may occur, separated by long periods of normal lung function and no symptoms. A course of systemic corticosteroids is recommended.

Goals of Therapy: Asthma Control
- Minimal or no chronic symptoms day or night
- Maintain (near) normal pulmonary function
- Minimal or no exacerbations
- Minimal use of short-acting inhaled beta₂-agonist (<1x per day, <1 canister/month)
- No limitations on activities; no school/work missed
- Minimal or no adverse effects from medications

 Step down
Review treatment every 1 to 6 months; a gradual stepwise reduction in treatment may be possible.

 Step up
If control is not maintained, consider step up. First, review patient medication technique, adherence, and environmental control.

Quick Relief All Patients
- Short-acting bronchodilator: 2 – 4 puffs short-acting inhaled beta₂-agonists as needed for symptoms.
- Intensity of treatment will depend on severity of exacerbation; up to 3 treatments at 20-minute intervals or a single nebulizer treatment as needed. Course of systemic corticosteroids may be needed.
- Use of short-acting inhaled beta₂-agonists > 2 times a week in intermittent asthma (daily, or increasing use in persistent asthma) may indicate the need to initiate (increase) long-term control therapy.

Note
- The stepwise approach is meant to assist, not replace, the clinical decisionmaking required to meet individual patient needs.
- Classify severity: assign patient to most severe step in which any feature occurs (PEF is % of personal best; FEV₁ is % predicted)
- Gain control as quickly as possible (consider a short course of systemic corticosteroids); then step down to the least medication necessary to maintain control.
- Provide education on self-management and controlling environmental factors that make asthma worse (e.g., allergens and irritants).
- Refer to an asthma specialist if there are difficulties controlling asthma or if step 4 care is required. Referral may be considered if step 3 care is required.

Executive Summary of the NAEPP Expert Panel Report: Guidelines for the Diagnosis and Management of Asthma—Update on Selected Topics 2002. Bethesda, Maryland: National Heart, Lung, and Blood Institute. National Institutes of Health. NIH Publication No. 02-5075 June 2002 http://www.nhlbi.nih.gov/guidelines/asthma/asthsumm.htm

Figure 3. Stepwise approach for managing asthma in adults and children >5 y. From NHLBI, National Asthma Education and Prevention Program. *Expert Panel Report: Guidelines for the Diagnosis and Management of Asthma—Update on Selected Topics. 2002.*

GREEN ZONE: Doing Well

- No cough, wheeze, chest tightness, or shortness of breath during the day or night
- Can do usual activities

And, if a peak flow meter is used,
Peak flow: more than _____
(80% or more of my best peak flow)

My best peak flow is: _____

Take These Long-Term-Control Medicines Each Day (include an anti-inflammatory)

Medicine	How much to take	When to take it

| Before exercise | ❏ | ❏ 2 or ❏ 4 puffs | 5 to 60 minutes before exercise |

YELLOW ZONE: Asthma Is Getting Worse

- Cough, wheeze, chest tightness, or shortness of breath, or
- Waking at night due to asthma, or
- Can do some, but not all, usual activities

-Or-

Peak flow: _____ to _____
(50% - 80% of my best peak flow)

FIRST → **Add: Quick-Relief Medicine – and keep taking your GREEN ZONE medicine**

_____ ❏ 2 or ❏ 4 puffs, every 20 minutes for up to 1 hour
(short-acting beta$_2$-agonist) ❏ Nebulizer, once

SECOND → If your symptoms (and peak flow, if used) *return to GREEN ZONE* after 1 hour of above treatment:
❏ Take the quick-relief medicine every 4 hours for 1 to 2 days.
❏ Double the dose of your inhaled steroid for _____ (7-10) days.
-Or-
If your symptoms (and peak flow, if used) *do not return to GREEN ZONE* after 1 hour of above treatment:
❏ Take: _____ ❏ 2 or ❏ 4 puffs or ❏ Nebulizer
(short-acting beta$_2$-agonist)
❏ Add: _____ _____ mg. per day For _____ (3-10) days
(oral steroid)
❏ Call the doctor ❏ before/ ❏ within _____ hours after taking the oral steroid.

RED ZONE: Medical Alert!

- Very short of breath, or
- Quick-relief medicines have not helped, or
- Cannot do usual activities, or
- Symptoms are same or get worse after 24 hours in Yellow Zone

-Or-

Peak flow: less than _____
(50% of my best peak flow)

Take this medicine:

❏ _____ ❏ 4 or ❏ 6 puffs or ❏ Nebulizer
(short-acting beta$_2$-agonist)

❏ _____ _____ mg.
(oral steroid)

Then call your doctor *NOW*. Go to the hospital or call for an ambulance if:
- You are still in the red zone after 15 minutes AND
- You have not reached your doctor.

DANGER SIGNS

- Trouble walking and talking due to shortness of breath
- Lips or fingernails are blue

- Take ❏ 4 or ❏ 6 puffs of your quick-relief medicine *AND*
- Go to the hospital or call for an ambulance (_____) *NOW!*

Figure 4. Sample asthma management plan for long-term control and for treating asthma exacerbations. Reprinted with permission from American Academy of Allergy, Asthma & Immunology, Inc. *Pediatric Asthma: Promoting Best Practice,* Milwaukee, Wisc: American Academy of Allergy, Asthma & Immunology, Inc; 1999.

Childhood Asthma Management Program (CAMP) trial provides the largest and longest double-blind, randomized trial of inhaled corticosteroid treatment compared with placebo in children as well as a cohort of children treated with nonsteroidal anti-inflammatory therapy (nedocromil). There was a 1.1-cm difference in growth between the children assigned to budesonide and those assigned to placebo that occurred as a result of a decrease in growth velocity. This reduction in growth velocity took place within the first year of steroid therapy and was not progressive thereafter. The CAMP Continuation Study is ongoing, and more information will be forthcoming about the growth of these children as they reach their adult heights. The practitioner must monitor for potential growth suppression in individual patients by regularly scheduled height measurements, preferably with a stadiometer.

Rinsing the mouth after inhalation of corticosteroids and using spacers help to lessen local adverse effects of dysphonia and candidiasis as well as to decrease systemic absorption from the gastrointestinal tract. To minimize adverse effects, the goal is to use the lowest effective dose that controls the child's asthma.

LEUKOTRIENE MODIFIERS

Leukotriene modifiers are a new class of oral daily-use asthma medication. Leukotrienes, synthesized via the arachidonic acid metabolism cascade, are potent mediators of inflammation and smooth muscle bronchoconstriction. Leukotriene modifiers have been designed to inhibit edema, mucus secretion, smooth muscle contraction, and eosinophil migration into the airways. There are two classes of leukotriene modifiers based on their site of action: leukotriene synthesis inhibitors (eg, zileuton) and cysteinyl leukotriene receptor antagonists (eg, zafirlukast and montelukast). Zileuton is approved for use in children older than 12 years of age. It is used less commonly than other leukotriene modifiers because of a need to monitor liver enzymes regularly, the possibility of drug interactions, and an initial dosing regimen of four times per day. The leukotriene receptor antagonists have much wider appeal. Zafirlukast has been approved for children older than 7 years of age and is administered twice daily. Montelukast is dosed once daily at night as 4-mg or 5-mg chewable tablets for ages 2 to 5 years and 6 to 14 years, respectively. A 10-mg tablet is available for adolescents older than 15 years. Pediatric studies demonstrate the usefulness of leukotriene modifiers in mild asthma and the attenuation of exercise-induced bronchoconstriction. These agents also are useful as steroid-sparing agents for patients whose asthma is more difficult to control.

Although leukotriene modifiers are considered "alternative therapy" for long-term control in children who have mild persistent asthma, they are appealing because of their easy administration and excellent safety profile. In addition, these medications do not provoke "steroid phobia" in families or physicians, which can be a reason for the undertreatment of asthma with inhaled corticosteroids.

LONG-ACTING BETA-2 AGONISTS

Newly available long-acting beta-2 agonists include formoterol and salmeterol. These medications are administered twice daily and exhibit bronchodilatory effects for up to 12 hours. It is important to recognize that these agents do not have any significant anti-inflammatory effects. Studies have demonstrated that adding a long-acting bronchodilator to inhaled corticosteroid therapy is more beneficial than doubling the dose of inhaled corticosteroids. Formoterol, available in the DPI form, is approved for use in children older than 5 years for maintenance asthma therapy and for prevention of exercise-induced asthma among children older than 12 years. Formoterol has a rapid onset of action that is similar to albuterol (15 min) compared

with a 30-minute onset of action for salmeterol. Salmeterol is available in the MDI form for children 12 years of age and older; the DPI form is approved for children 4 years of age and older.

In spring 2001, a fluticasone/salmeterol combination product, Advair® (GlaxoSmithKline), received United States Food and Drug Administration approval for children older than 12 years for maintenance treatment of asthma. It is available as a DPI in three doses, based on the amount of corticosteroid available (100 mcg, 250 mcg, or 500 mcg). Each of the strengths contains 50 mcg of salmeterol. Its advantages include possible improved compliance because it is administered as one puff twice daily and the combination of two potent asthma medications. Study trials for combination therapy for younger children are ongoing.

NOVEL THERAPIES

With an improved understanding of the basic mechanisms of airway inflammation, future asthma treatment will target the components of the inflammatory cascade. Possibilities include anti-immunoglobulin E and anticytokine therapies. Research is preliminary, and time will tell whether these therapies will be a helpful addition to the physician's armamentarium.

OTHER THERAPIES

The management of children in respiratory failure from status asthmaticus is beyond the scope of this article. Generally, medical therapy involves the use of frequent or continuous beta-2 agonist nebulization therapy and oral or intravenous corticosteroids. Chest physiotherapy can help move secretions to central airways, where cough can expel the secretions, and can be helpful in asthmatic patients who have coexisting chronic obstructive pulmonary disease or emphysema. Typically, these are not pediatric patients. Mucolytic agents, such as N-acetylcysteine, may induce bronchoconstriction and should be used with caution. Only when adequate mechanical ventilation is in progress should sedative, narcotic, or anxiolytic drugs be administered to the patient in status asthmaticus.

Patient Education

Education plays an important role in helping asthmatic patients and their families adhere to the prescribed therapy and needs to begin at the time of diagnosis. Key educational messages include basic asthma facts, the role of medications, environmental control measures, monitoring skills to recognize the symptoms of asthma that indicate adequate or inadequate asthma control, and an asthma management plan for exacerbations as well as daily control. Absorbing such information can be overwhelming in a 15-minute appointment, but other health care team members and office staff can help reinforce the educational messages. Education is an ongoing process, and information needs to be adjusted appropriately for the child as he or she ages and for the family as they become more educated. Many outside resources can provide additional educational services to families. The Asthma and Allergy Foundation of America (www.aafa.org), the American Lung Association (www2.lungusa.org), the Allergy and Asthma Network Mothers of Asthmatics (www.aanma.org), American Acadmey of Allergy, Asthma, and Immunology (www.aaaai.org), and American College of Allergy, Asthma, and Immunology (www.acaii.org) are excellent sources of information.

A key message for families is that children who have asthma should be seen not only when they are ill, but also when they are healthy. Regular office visits allow the health care team to review adherence to medication and control measures and to determine if medication doses need adjustment.

Families need to have an asthma management plan (Fig. 4) for daily care and for exacerbations. Peak flow monitoring is a self-assessment tool that encourages asthma management. Reliable measurements often can be obtained in children older than 5 years. Use of the peak flow meter is advisable for children who are "poor perceivers" of airway obstruction, who have moderate-to-severe asthma, or who have a history of severe exacerbations. Peak flow monitoring also can be useful for children recently diagnosed with asthma who are still learning to recognize asthma symptoms.

To use a peak flow meter, a child should be standing with the indicator placed at the bottom of the scale. The child must inhale deeply, place the device in the mouth, bite down on the mouthpiece, seal his or her lips around the mouthpiece, and blow out forcefully and rapidly. The indicator moves up the numeric scale. The peak expiratory flow rate (PEFR) is the highest number achieved. The test is repeated three times to obtain the best possible effort. Peak flow meters are available as low-range (measurement up to 300 L/s) and high-range (measurement up to 700 L/s). It is important to provide the appropriate range meter to obtain accurate measurements and to avoid discouraging the child whose blows barely move the indicator.

A child's personal best is the highest PEFR achieved over a 2-week period when stable. A written plan is based on the child's personal best. There are three PEFR zones, similar to a stoplight (Fig. 4). The green zone indicates a PEFR of 80% to 100% of the child's personal best value. In this zone, the child is likely asymptomatic and should continue with medications as usual. The yellow zone indicates a PEFR of 50% to 80% of the child's personal best value and generally coincides with the child having more asthma symptoms. Rescue medications such as albuterol are added to the therapy, and a phone call to the physician may be warranted if the peak flows do not return to the green zone within the next 24 to 48 hours or if asthma symptoms are increasing. The red zone indicates a PEFR below 50% and is a medical emergency. The rescue medication should be taken immediately. If the PEFR remains in the red zone or the child is experiencing significant airway compromise, a phone call to the physician or emergency care is needed.

When to Refer

Guidelines for when a child should be referred to an asthma specialist are shown in Table 3. To optimize care of the child who has asthma, the specialist must work closely with the primary care physician.

Suggested Reading

Agertoft L, Pedersen S. Effect of long-term treatment with inhaled budesonide on adult height in children with asthma. *N Engl J Med.* 2000;343:1064–1069

American Academy of Allergy, Asthma & Immunology, Inc. *Pediatric Asthma: Promoting Best Practice.* Milwaukee, Wisc: American Academy of Allergy, Asthma, and Immunology, Inc; 1999

Lemanske RF Jr, Green CG. Asthma in infancy and childhood. In: Middleton E Jr, Reed CE, Ellis EF, et al, eds. *Allergy: Principles & Practice.* 5th ed. St. Louis, Mo: Mosby-Year Book, Inc; 1998:877–900

NHLBI, National Asthma Education and Prevention Program. *Expert Panel Report: Guidelines for the Diagnosis and Management of Asthma—Update on Selected Topics.* NIH Publication No. 02-5075. Bethesda, Md: US Department of Health and Human Services; 2002. Downloadable version of the executive summary available at: http://www.nhlbi.nih.gov/guidelines/asthma/index.htm

NHLBI, National Asthma Education and Prevention Program. *Expert Panel Report II: Guidelines for the Diagnosis and Management of Asthma.* NIH Publication No. 97-4051. Bethesda, Md: US Department of Health and Human Services; 1997

The Childhood Asthma Management Program Research Group. Long-term effects of budesonide or nedocromil in children with asthma. *N Engl J Med.* 2000;343:1054–1063

Table 3. Referral to an Asthma Specialist

- Child has had a life-threatening asthma exacerbation.
- Goals of asthma therapy are not being met after 3 to 6 months of treatment; earlier if child appears unresponsive to treatment.
- Signs and symptoms are atypical. Consider other diagnoses.
- Other conditions complicate asthma or its diagnosis (eg, rhinitis, sinusitis, gastroesophageal reflux).
- Additional diagnostic testing is indicated (eg, pulmonary function testing, allergy skin testing).
- Child or family needs additional education and guidance on complications of therapy, problems with adherence, or avoidance of triggers.
- Child is being considered for immunotherapy.
- Child has severe persistent asthma.
- Child is younger than 3 years and has moderate or severe persistent asthma.
- Child has used prolonged courses of oral corticosteroids, high doses of inhaled corticosteroids, or more than two bursts of oral corticosteroids in 12 months.

Adapted from American Academy of Allergy, Asthma & Immunology, Inc. *Pediatric Asthma: Promoting Best Practice.* Milwaukee, Wisc: American Academy of Allergy, Asthma, and Immunology, Inc; 1999:80.

Palpitations, Syncope, and Sudden Cardiac Death in Children: Who's at Risk?

Anjan S. Batra, MD,* Arno R. Hohn, MD†

Objectives

After completing this article, readers should be able to:

1. Clarify the definition and terminology of palpitations, syncope, and sudden cardiac death (SCD).
2. Differentiate the relatively benign forms of palpitations and syncope from those that are associated with an increased risk of SCD.
3. Characterize the evaluation for palpitations of cardiac origin.
4. Describe the management of neurally mediated syncope.
5. Discuss the structural heart diseases predisposing to sudden death.
6. Define the guidelines for participation in competitive athletics for children who have common cardiac problems.

Case Reports

PATIENT 1

A 12-year-old female, who has a history of palpitations and exertional syncope, fainted while swimming. Her brother was near her and pulled her out of the water. The girl immediately regained consciousness and was found to have normal perfusion. The family history was significant for unexplained sudden death of the girl's older brother. Findings on physical examination of the patient were normal. Results of chest radiography were normal, but electrocardiography (ECG) revealed a sinus rhythm, with a corrected Q-T interval of 0.52 seconds.

PATIENT 2

A 16-year-old cross country runner had experienced several episodes of syncope. Each time she was caught prior to falling and was able to resume activities after some rest. Findings on her past medical history and family history were not significant. Physical examination results were normal. Chest radiography and ECG findings were normal, but a tilt table test showed onset of near-syncope accompanied by a significant decrease in the heart rate and blood pressure. The patient was started on a regimen of increased fluid intake and salt tablets prior to exercise. She has had no recurrences of syncope.

Overview

Palpitations and syncope are frequent presenting complaints to the pediatrician. Although mostly benign, these worrisome symptoms may be the prodrome of significant cardiac events. The devastating result could be brain damage or SCD. It is important to differentiate the relatively benign forms of palpitations and syncope from those that are associated with an increased risk of SCD.

PALPITATIONS

Palpitations are a subjective sensation of unduly strong, rapid, or irregular heart beats that may be related to cardiac arrhythmias. They also can be due to physiologic causes such as sinus tachycardia associated with anxiety or exercise or pathologic causes such as atrial fibrillation associated with hyperthyroidism and ventricular tachycardia in the long Q-T syndrome. Patients who have had palpitations should be evaluated carefully to rule out any significant arrhythmia before being allowed to participate in any competitive sports.

---

*Division of Cardiology, Riley Children's Hospital, Indiana University School of Medicine, Indianapolis, IN.
†Division of Cardiology, Children's Hospital of Los Angeles, University of Southern California, Los Angeles, CA.

A complete history is necessary to understand the nature of the palpitations. Inquiry should be made into the timing and circumstances that led to the palpitations; other associations with the onset of palpitations (eg, behavioral change); and a family history of syncope, palpitations, or SCD. A physical examination can rule out structural heart disease and systemic disorders. Although laboratory test results usually are normal, chest radiography is advised to rule out congenital heart disease and lung disease. ECG is needed to evaluate P waves, the presence of premature atrial beats or premature ventricular beats, and the Q-T interval. Commonly, these tests indicate a benign nature of the palpitations, leading to the great relief of those involved.

Asymptomatic patients who have premature atrial contractions or premature ventricular contractions, even if frequent, or short runs of unifocal ventricular tachycardia need not be referred to a cardiologist. Only reassurance is needed for the patient and family. If a cardiac origin of the palpitations is suspected, an extended evaluation usually is undertaken in collaboration with a pediatric cardiologist (Table 1).

SYNCOPE

Syncope is a temporary loss of consciousness due to generalized cerebral ischemia that usually is followed by rapid and complete recovery. In rare instances, anoxic seizures may result. Syncope may be preceded by palpitations, lightheadedness, dizziness, weakness, pallor, nausea, cold sweat, blurred vision, or hearing loss. Prompt relief from all symptoms usually occurs after lying down. Syncope may result from impaired response of the autonomic nervous system or from cardiac structural defects, especially those obstructing blood flow or from cardiac arrhythmias. The relatively uncommon long Q-T syndrome is an especially worrisome cause of syncope. Noncardiac mechanisms, such as metabolic, neurologic, and psychologic disorders, also may cause syncope.

Neurally mediated syncope, also referred to as vasovagal or neurocardiogenic syncope, is the most common form of syncope in children. It often is associated with orthostatic intolerance. It also has been reported that chronic fatigue

Table 1. Evaluation for Palpitations of Cardiac Origin

Initial Evaluation
- History and physical examination
- Chest radiography
- Electrocardiography

Advanced Evaluation (in association with a pediatric cardiologist)
- Echocardiography
- Holter monitoring
- Exercise stress test
- Electrophysiologic testing

syndrome in adolescents may be related to orthostatic intolerance. In such cases, the mechanism of syncope is reflex-mediated and originates from a decreased systemic venous return that leads to decreased left ventricular end diastolic volume. Increased mechanical contractility results in stimulation of cardiac vagal fibers and ultimately a paradoxic response of marked bradycardia, vasodilation, and hypotension. This chain of events is referred to as the Bezold-Jarisch reflex. Reflex syncope also may result from a hypersensitive autonomic response caused by different afferent input, such as micturition, swallowing, deglutition, coughing, sneezing, or defecation. Neurally mediated syncope may present in one of the three clinically recognized forms: cardioinhibitory (low blood pressure, bradycardia/asystole), vasodepressor (low blood pressure, no bradycardia), or mixed (low blood pressure, bradycardia).

Physical exhaustion, prolonged recumbency, conditions predisposing to peripheral vasodilation (exercise, hot weather), and pregnancy enhance the chance of having neurally mediated syncope, as do a variety of noxious stimuli, such as blood drawing or emotional stress. Affected patients have a decrease in blood pressure and heart rate with tilt table testing similar to that observed in vasodepressor syncope. Neurally mediated syncope rarely is associated with sudden death.

Because certain causes of syncope may be related to life-threatening conditions, a detailed evaluation should be undertaken whenever patients present with syncope. Those who have a family history of syncope, sudden death, myocardial disease, or arrhythmias and those who have exercise-associated syncope are at particularly high risk of SCD. Electrocardiography should be a part of the initial evaluation for all patients who present with syncope. A cardiology consultation is indicated when the cause of recurrent syncope cannot be identified, cardiac or arrhythmogenic syncope is identified, or a pacemaker is indicated for severe and recurrent syncope unresponsive to medical management. Further evaluation by the pediatric cardiologist often includes event monitoring, exercise stress testing, and tilt table testing.

Tilt table testing may be indicated under certain situations in which the cause of syncope is not clear. The American College of Cardiology published guidelines in 1996 on the indications for tilt table testing. It is generally agreed that tilt table testing should be reserved for patients who have recurrent syncope or for high-risk patients after a single syncopal episode. However, adolescents who describe prodromes of lightheadedness, nausea, and sweating before syncope most likely have neurally mediated syncope. These prodromes strongly suggest that tilt table testing is not necessary. The tilt table test consists of placing the patient in a head-up tilted position after a short period of lying prone. The tilt angle is between 60 and 80 degrees on a table that has a footplate and safety straps. The appropriate end point is induction of syncope or presyncope associated with intolerable hypotension and resulting in an inability to maintain postural tone.

Fluid therapy (Table 2) often is effective for neurally mediated syncope, especially of the vasodepressor type, and should be the primary mode of intervention in such patients. Other therapies that have been described include beta-blockers, volume expansion (with salt tablets or fludrocortisone), pseudoephedrine, disopyramide, and newer medications such as midodrine. These can be used individually or in combination. For patients in whom the neurally mediated syncope is frequent or sufficiently severe to cause anoxic seizures and unresponsive to conventional medical treatment, implantation of a pacemaker may be warranted.

Table 2. Management of Neurally Mediated Syncope

Evaluation

History and physical examination: negative for other causes of syncope

Electrocardiography: Normal, including QTc

Therapy

Trial of fluid therapy: 1 8-oz glass of any type of fluid on arising, at meals, and between meals (approximately q2 to 4 h) until the evening meal. Two 8-oz glasses of fluid such as "Gatorade™" prior to athletic participation, including practice.

Outcome

Approximately 90% will respond and need no referral

Referral

Refer nonresponders to a pediatric cardiologist

Sudden Cardiac Death

SCD is any natural death that occurs due to cardiac causes within minutes to 24 hours after the onset of symptoms. Cardiac deaths have been classified as arrhythmic deaths or due to circulatory collapse. SCD in children is relatively rare. There are about 600 SCDs in children annually compared with 7,000 to 10,000 deaths from sudden infant death syndrome and 300,000 to 400,000 SCD deaths in adults. The prevalence of SCD increases with age, accounting for 19% of sudden deaths in children between 1 and 13 years of age and 30% between 14 and 21 years.

The risk of SCD may be slightly higher in athletes involved in strenuous training. In a population of high school athletes in Minnesota, Maron and associates reported the risk of SCD to be approximately 1 in 200,000 per year and higher in male athletes. This low occurrence of SCD in competitive sports makes structuring of cost-effective broad-based participation screening guidelines for high school and college athletes difficult. In addition, the range of causes of sudden death on the athletic field may include causes for which it is impossible to screen. In rare instances, an athlete who has a structurally normal heart and no underlying pathology may suffer blunt trauma to the chest that causes a ventricular dysrhythmia and SCD. Labeled as commutio cordis, it is believed to be induced by the abrupt, blunt blow to an electrically vulnerable phase of electrical excitability within the myocardium. Athletes who have syncope or near-syncope warrant a more thorough evaluation to determine the cause. Current recommendations for disqualification from competitive athletics are based on the guidelines from the 26th Bethesda Conference (Table 3).

Structural Heart Diseases Predisposing to Sudden Death

The incidence of SCD in patients who have congenital heart disease is particularly high after repair of certain lesions. Following tetralogy of Fallot repair, patients have a 2% to 5% incidence of SCD, with ventricular arrhythmias being the most likely cause. Other surgically repaired lesions associated with a high incidence of arrhythmias and SCD include the Mustard or Senning operation for transposition of the great arteries and the Fontan operation for a single ventricle physiology. The latter lesions include hypoplastic left ventricles in which prior Norwood operations have been undertaken. Patients in these categories usually are limited to low-intensity competitive sports such as golf, billiards, and bowling, although certain individuals who have excellent surgical results and normal exercise test results may be allowed to participate in more dynamic sports. Atrial arrhythmias tend to dominate in these lesions. About 40% of SCDs in pediatric patients occur in those who have unoperated congenital or acquired heart disease. Several subgroups of such heart disease have been identified.

Table 3. Guidelines for Participation in Competitive Athletics for Common Cardiac Problems

Type of Cardiac Defect	Athletic Limitation
Tetralogy of Fallot	
Excellent result	No restrictions
Suboptimal result	Low-intensity competitive sports
Transposition of the Great Arteries	
Postoperative Mustard or Senning	Low and moderate static, low-dynamic sports
Arterial switch operation	No restrictions
Postoperative Fontan Operation	Low-intensity competitive sports
Hypertrophic Cardiomyopathy	Low-intensity competitive sports
Myocarditis	No competitive sports for 6 mo
Congenital Coronary Anomalies	No competitive sports until repaired
Kawasaki disease	
No coronary involvement	No restrictions
Minor residual abnormalities	Low static, low/moderate dynamic sports
Persistent coronary artery aneurysm or stenosis	Low-intensity competitive sports
Intermittent myocardial ischemia	No competitive sports
Aortic Stenosis	
Mild	No restrictions
Moderate	Low-intensity competitive sports
Severe	No competitive sports
Wolff-Parkinson-White Syndrome	No restrictions
Long QT Syndrome	No competitive sports
Pulmonary Hypertension	
Mild (<40 mm Hg peak pressure)	No restrictions
Moderate/severe (>40 mm Hg peak pressure)	No competitive sports
Marfan syndrome	
No aortic root dilation or mitral regurgitation	Low and moderate static, low-dynamic sports
Aortic root dilation	Low-intensity competitive sports

CARDIOMYOPATHIES AND MYOCARDITIS

Restrictive, hypertrophic, or dilated cardiomyopathies may predispose the patient to SCD. Of these, hypertrophic cardiomyopathy is the most common cause of SCD in adolescents in the United States. Patients may present with symptoms of chest pain, syncope, and palpitations associated with exercise or sudden death during exercise. Factors associated with an increased risk of SCD in patients who have hypertrophic cardiomyopathy include a strong family history of sudden death, clinical symptoms, a young age, presence of ventricular arrhythmia, and a thickened intraventricular septum. ECG may show left ventricular hypertrophy, ST-T wave changes, and deep and wide Q waves in the left precordial leads. Echocardiography is the principal diagnostic modality to judge the severity and progression of cardiomyopathy. Even though hypertrophic cardiomyopathy is a common cause of SCD in athletes in the United States, it is a rare cause of SCD in athletes in Italy. This may be related to the much more aggressive screening, including echocardiography, and disqualification from sports by Italian law of patients who have hypertrophic cardiomyopathy.

Arrhythmogenic right ventricular dysplasia and right ventricular cardiomyopathy have been reported as leading causes of SCD in athletes in studies performed in Italy, but they apparently are less common in other geographic regions, including the United States. These lesions are associated with a high frequency of cardiovascular symptoms and complications. Patients may present with ventricular arrhythmias (45%), congestive heart failure (25%), heart murmur (10%), complete heart block (5%), or sudden death (5%). First-degree relatives of 30% of the patients are affected. ECG usually shows a left bundle-branch pattern. Because limited data are available regarding the risks of athletic participation for such patients, they are best advised to refrain from participation in any competitive sports.

SCD has been reported in 14% to 42% of patients who had acute and chronic myocarditis and died either at rest or during exercise. These patients may present with a wide range of symptoms from subtle findings such as persistently increased heart rate or low-grade ventricular ectopy to severe congestive heart failure with cardiomegaly and poor exercise tolerance. Viruses have been identified as the most common causes of acute or chronic myocarditis.

CORONARY ARTERY DISEASE

Patients who have congenital or acquired coronary artery disease may present with SCD, with the disease being diagnosed at autopsy. The most common coronary artery anomaly leading to SCD is the left main coronary artery arising from the right sinus of valsalva. It may be difficult to recognize these patients prospectively because they usually are asymptomatic until the initiating event that is related to exercise. Routine 12-lead ECG and exercise stress testing are not much help in the diagnosis. A history of syncope, palpitations, or chest pain related to exercise is associated with an increased risk of anomalous origin of the coronary artery and warrants an echocardiogram to define the coronary arteries. It is reasoned that compression of the left coronary artery, which runs between the aorta and the pulmonary artery, causes coronary insufficiency and acute ischemia. This, in turn, predisposes the patient to fatal arrhythmias. Occasionally, patients who have an anomalous origin of the left coronary artery from the pulmonary artery may present in infancy with congestive heart failure. They also may die suddenly, presumably of an ischemic arrhythmia or cardiogenic shock.

Acquired coronary artery disease usually is the result of Kawasaki disease. Kawasaki disease may present with SCD in up to 2% of untreated patients. Such deaths may be related to rupture of a large coronary artery aneurysm, acute myocarditis, or a large coronary artery thrombosis. Familial hyperbetalipoproteinemia is an atherosclerotic heart disease inherited in an autosomal-dominant pattern that may cause SCD in homozygotic adolescents.

VALVULAR HEART DISEASE

Patients who have aortic valve disease, including aortic stenosis and chronic aortic regurgitation, may be asymptomatic or present with symptoms such as syncope, dyspnea, or chest pain. If palpitations are present, the patient may be suffering from arrhythmias associated with myocardial ischemia. Symptomatic patients usually have severe left ventricular obstruction and left ventricular hypertrophy. A high estimated valve gradient (>75 torr) measured by echocardiography indicates a risk for SCD. Recommendations for athletic participation are based on the severity of the aortic stenosis.

Mitral valve prolapse (MVP) is a relatively common and benign finding in the pediatric population that is associated with an excellent prognosis. However, patients who have MVP and ventricular arrhythmias, mitral regurgitation, prolonged Q-T interval, history of syncope or presyncope, and family history of sudden death should be considered at high risk to develop SCD. MVP also is seen frequently in association with Marfan syndrome and other connective tissue diseases. Isolated MVP or MVP in association with premature ventricular contractions does not require treatment. However, patients who have MVP and a history of syncope or complex ventricular arrhythmias, significant mitral regurgitation, or a family history of sudden death should restrict their activities to leisurely, noncompetitive sports.

ARRTHYTHMIAS AND LONG Q-T SYNDROME

Primary arrhythmias not associated with congenital cardiac malformation occasionally are encountered in the pediatric population and rarely may lead to SCD. These include Wolf-Parkinson-White (WPW) syndrome, isolated sick sinus syndrome, congenital complete atrioventricular block, and ventricular and supraventricular tachycardias. Syncope and palpitations are common presenting complaints in patients who have supraventricular tachycardias from WPW syndrome. SCD is rare in these patients and may occur from rapid conduction via the accessory pathway, leading to ventricular fibrillation. Because digoxin may potentiate this conduction via the accessory pathway, its use in treating WPW syndrome is controversial.

Complete heart block usually presents in infancy; in such patients, SCD generally is related to extreme bradycardia and a tendency to develop

ventricular arrhythmias. Sick sinus syndrome may manifest as marked sinus bradycardia, sinus arrest with slow junctional escape, tachycardia-bradycardia syndrome, or atrial fibrillation.

Patients who have long Q-T interval syndrome are at an increased risk for ventricular arrhythmias and SCD. They usually present with episodes of syncope and a family history of syncope and sudden death. The long Q-T syndrome is inherited in an autosomal-dominant pattern, with female predominance. The risk of cardiac events is higher in males until puberty and higher in females during adulthood. Affected patients exhibit a prolonged Q-T interval and at times profound bradycardia and ST-T wave changes on ECG. Medical therapy is initiated with betablocking drugs such as propranolol or atenolol. Beta blockers are associated with a significant reduction in cardiac events among patients who have the long Q-T syndrome. However, syncope, aborted cardiac arrest, and long Q-T syndrome-related death continue to occur among patients receiving beta blockers, particularly those who were symptomatic before starting the therapy.

PULMONARY HYPERTENSION

Pulmonary hypertension is another significant risk factor for SCD. Among patients who die of SCD, 11% to 17% have pulmonary hypertension associated with heart disease. Another 4% have primary pulmonary hypertension. Syncopal episodes and arrhythmias in patients who have pulmonary hypertension usually suggest a poor prognosis. Affected patients are at a high risk for SCD during pregnancy and delivery and during strenuous physical activities.

MARFAN SYNDROME

Marfan syndrome is associated with a decreased life expectancy, with 30% to 60% of patients having cardiovascular anomalies. Rupture of the dilated aortic root is the most common cause of SCD in these patients. Mitral valve prolapse with insufficiency is also common. Beta-blocker therapy is recommended for patients who have valve disease.

Conclusion

It is important for the pediatrician to understand the various cardiac and noncardiac causes of syncope. SCD in the young is rare. Often, judicious evaluation of the patient who has syncope can determine if he or she is predisposed to a higher risk of SCD. This, in turn, may reduce the risk of SCD substantially and obviate unnecessary restrictions for those in whom the symptoms are due to a benign or easily treatable cause.

Suggested Reading

Basso C, Maron BJ, Corrado D, Thiene G. Clinical profile of congenital coronary artery anomalies with origin from the wrong aortic sinus leading to sudden death in young competitive athletes. *J Am Coll Cardiol.* 2000;35:1493–1501

Corrado D, Basso C, Schiavon M, Thiene G. Screening for hypertrophic cardiomyopathy in young athletes. *N Engl J Med.* 1998;339:364–369

Futterman LG, Lemberg L. Sudden death in athletes. *Am J Crit Care.* 1995;4:239–243

Garson A Jr. Sudden death in a pediatric cardiology population, 1958–1983. In: Morganroth J, Horowitz LN, eds. *Sudden Cardiac Death.* New York, NY: Grune & Stratton; 1985:47–56

Kligfield P, Levy D, Devereux RB, Savage D. Arrhythmia and sudden death in mitral valve prolapse. *Am Heart J.* 1987; 113:1298–1307

Kullo IJ, Edwards WD, Seward JB. Right ventricular dysplasia: the Mayo Clinic experience. *Mayo Clin Proc.* 1995;70:541–548

Locati EH, Zareba W, Moss AJ, et al. Age and sex related differences in clinical manifestations in patients with congenital long Q-T syndrome: findings from the international LQTS Registry. *Circulation.* 1998;97:2237–2244

Maron BJ, Gohman TE, Aeppli D. Prevalence of sudden cardiac death during competitive sports activities in Minnesota high school athletes. *J Am Coll Cardiol.* 1998;32:1881–1884

Neuspiel DR, Kuller LH. Sudden and unexpected natural death in childhood and adolescence. *JAMA.* 1984;254:1321–1325

26th Bethesda Conference. Recommendations for determining eligibility for competition in athletes with cardiovascular abnormalities. *J Am Coll Cardiol.* 1994;24:867–892

Pancreatitis in Childhood

Michelle M. Pietzak, MD, and Dan W. Thomas, MD†

Objectives

After completing this article, readers should be able to:

1. Describe the challenge involved in diagnosing both acute and chronic pancreatitis.
2. Identify the radiologic study of choice in acute pancreatitis.
3. Identify the most common inherited disease involving the exocrine pancreas.
4. Delineate the pancreatic condition that is an absolute surgical indication, requiring necrosectomy (surgical debridement).
5. List the most common etiologies of pancreatitis in the child.

Definitions

Pancreatitis in children is a disease characterized by inflammation of the pancreas in the clinical setting of epigastric abdominal pain and usually is accompanied by elevated levels of pancreatic enzymes, amylase, and lipase. Pancreatitis can be categorized as acute, chronic, necrotic, hemorrhagic, and hereditary. The types are distinguished most frequently according to clinical and radiologic criteria; material obtained from the organ rarely is analyzed histologically.

Acute pancreatitis is a self-limited disorder causing nausea, vomiting, anorexia, abdominal pain, and marked elevations in enzymes. Bouts of acute pancreatitis may recur, but normal pancreatic function and morphology usually are restored between attacks. If the inflammatory process is progressive, morphologic changes may occur in the gland, leading to chronic pancreatitis, often with debilitating pain and possible irreversible loss of both exocrine and endocrine function. Protein ductal plugs may calcify in the gland, leading to chronic calcific pancreatitis, which indicates advanced disease. Relatively high mortality occurs in necrotizing hemorrhagic pancreatitis, where the inflamed gland can become infected secondarily with bacteria and sepsis can occur, often in association with subsequent multiorgan failure. Hereditary pancreatitis is an autosomal dominant condition that is characterized by recurrent attacks of pancreatitis, usually presenting during childhood within affected families.

Epidemiology

It is difficult to estimate the true incidence and prevalence of pancreatitis in children because most of the literature reports individual cases or small clusters of patients. Although pancreatitis is not seen as commonly in children as in adults, it most likely is underdiagnosed and requires a high index of suspicion on the part of the clinician. Acute pancreatitis is believed to be the most common pancreatic disorder in children, with cystic fibrosis second in prevalence.

Pathogenesis

Although the majority of adult cases of acute pancreatitis can be attributed to either alcohol or gallstone disease, the causes of acute pancreatitis in childhood are more numerous and include trauma, infection, medications, anatomic variants, and systemic and metabolic disorders. Gallstone pancreatitis is relatively common in adolescent females. Despite the varied causes,

*Assistant Professor of Clinical Pediatrics.

†Associate Professor of Pediatrics, Division of Gastroenterology and Nutrition, Childrens Hospital Los Angeles and Keck School of Medicine at the University of Southern California, Los Angeles, CA.

the clinical characteristics of acute pancreatitis follow a similar pattern. The severity of the disease and long-term complications may differ, depending on the cause. The primary initiating event, whether traumatic, infectious, or metabolic, is damage to the pancreatic acinar cell by the premature activation of digestive enzymes within the cell. The damaged acinar cell then attracts inflammatory cells and activates platelets and the complement system, which leads to the release of cytokines (such as tumor necrosis factor-alpha, interleukin-1, nitric oxide, and platelet activating factor), free radicals, and other vasoactive substances. These substances damage the gland directly, causing pancreatic edema, ischemia, necrosis, and eventual loss of glandular tissue. Systemically, often within hours of the initial insult, fever, hypotension, tachycardia, hypoxia, and capillary leak syndrome may occur in severe cases. The direct links between these chains of events are not well understood, but current research is targeting this inflammatory cascade for therapy that may be beneficial in all types of pancreatitis, regardless of the inciting event.

The various etiologies of pancreatitis are too numerous to be discussed in detail for this review (Table 1), which is limited to some of the more common causes and those in which recent advances in research have been made. Numerous drugs have been reported to be associated with pancreatitis. However, most of them have a proposed and unproved pathophysiology and do not have an established causal relationship (Table 2).

Infections from a variety of organisms, including bacteria, viruses, and parasites, account for a significant number of cases of pancreatitis worldwide. The *Escherichia coli* strain that produces verotoxin and is associated with hemolyticuremic syndrome, as well as varicella and influenza B that have been associated with Reye syndrome in the past, all have been implicated in causing acute pancreatitis in children. In developing areas, parasites such as *Ascaris* and *Clonorchis* may migrate into the biliary tree, causing obstructive jaundice, pancreatitis, and portal hypertension, and ultimately can lead to liver failure. In patients who have viral infections, such as human immunodeficiency virus, an elevated serum amylase level may be associated with parotid inflammation rather than pancreatitis. With such infections, determining serum amylase isoenzymes may be clinically useful.

Trauma is a significant and possibly the most common cause of acute pancreatitis in children in the United States. Blunt traumatic pancreatitis often results from motor vehicle and bicycle handlebar accidents. Findings on a physical examination that are consistent with trauma in the absence of a reliable history should raise the suspicion for child abuse. There usually are other associated intra-abdominal injuries in cases of significant blunt abdominal trauma. Duodenal hematoma or bowel rupture is not uncommon. In the absence of complete duct transection, nonoperative management is believed to be safe, and there usually are no long-term complications.

Congenital defects in the formation of the pancreas are rare, but can lead to chronic pancreatitis if not corrected. The most common anatomic variant, pancreatic divisum, occurs when the dorsal and ventral pancreatic ducts fail to fuse during a critical time in fetal development. As a result of this failure, pancreatic flow is directed primarily to the dorsal duct. This is believed to lead to relapsing pancreatitis, which eventually may require endoscopic or surgical treatment. However, some believe that pancreatic divisum is a normal anatomic variant and a rare cause of pancreatitis.

Cystic fibrosis, an autosomal recessive disease caused by mutations in the cystic fibrosis transmembrane conductance regulator (CFTR) gene, is thought to be the most common inherited disease involving the exocrine pancreas. CFTR is located on the apical membrane of the epithelial cells that line the pancreatic ducts, and it promotes dilution and alkalinization of the "juice" as it flows through the ducts. Up to 2% of individuals who have cystic fibrosis experience pancreatitis as a result of pancreatic ductal plugging due to mutant CFTR. There appears to be a strong correlation between specific CFTR mutations and idiopathic chronic pancreatitis, even in the absence of lung disease. Ongoing research is seeking to define the role of CFTR further in pancreatitis and other diseases of the pancreas.

Table 1. Conditions Associated With Acute and Chronic Pancreatitis in Childhood

Infections
- *Ascaris lumbricoides* (duct obstruction)
- *Campylobacter fetus*
- *Clonorchis sinensis* (duct obstruction)
- Coxsackie B virus
- Cytomegalovirus
- Echovirus
- Enterovirus
- Epstein-Barr virus
- *Escherichia coli*-verotoxin-producing
- Hepatitis A and B
- Human immunodeficiency virus
- Influenza A and B
- Legionnaire disease
- Leptospirosis
- Malaria
- Measles
- Mumps
- *Mycoplasma*
- Rubella
- Rubeola
- Typhoid fever
- Varicella
- *Yersinia*

Trauma
- Abdominal radiotherapy
- Accidental blunt injury
- Burns
- Child abuse
- Endoscopic retrograde cholangio-pancreatography or other ductal imaging using contrast
- Surgical trauma
- Total body cast

Anatomic
- Absence or anomalous insertion of the common bile duct or pancreatic duct
- Ampullary disease: diverticulum, stenosis
- Annular pancreas
- Anomalous choledochopancreaticoductal junction
- Aplasia of the pancreas
- Biliary tract malformations
- Choledochal cyst
- Choledochocele
- Cholelithiasis
- Duodenal obstruction (diverticulum, hematoma, tumor, stricture)
- Duodenal ulcer-perforated
- Duplication cyst (duodenum, gastro-pancreatic, common bile duct)
- Dysplasia of the pancreas
- Gastric trichobezoar
- Heterotopic pancreas
- Hypoplasia of the pancreas
- Pancreas divisum
- Pancreatic pseudocyst
- Sclerosing cholangitis
- Sphincter of Oddi dysfunction
- Tumors of the pancreas

Idiopathic
- Up to 25% of cases

Systemic/Metabolic/Hereditary
- Alpha-1-antitrypsin deficiency
- Anorexia nervosa
- Autoimmune diseases
- Brain tumor
- Bulimia
- Collagen vascular diseases
- Congenital partial lipodystrophy
- Crohn disease
- Cystic fibrosis
- Dermatomyositis
- Diabetes mellitus (ketoacidosis)
- Glycogen storage disease types Ia, Ib
- Head trauma
- Hemochromatosis
- Hemolytic-uremic syndrome
- Henoch-Schönlein purpura
- Hereditary pancreatitis
- Hyperalimentation
- Hypercalcemia
- Hyperlipidemia types I, IV, and V
- Hyperparathyroidism
- Hypertriglyceridemia
- Hypothermia
- Inborn errors of metabolism (organic acidemias, cytochrome c oxidase deficiency)
- Juvenile tropical pancreatitis
- Kawasaki disease
- Malnutrition with or without refeeding
- Periarteritis nodosa
- Peritonitis
- Renal failure with uremia
- Reye syndrome
- Sarcoidosis
- Septic shock
- Systemic lupus erythematosus
- Transplantation (bone marrow, heart, kidney, liver, pancreas)
- Ulcerative colitis
- Wilson disease

In the United States, the most common cause of chronic relapsing pancreatitis in childhood is believed to be hereditary pancreatitis. The gene defects in the two types of hereditary pancreatitis, which were reported in 1996, may shed some light on the pathophysiology of the nonhereditary forms of acute and chronic pancreatitis. Clinically similar, both types are autosomal dominant, with 80% penetrance. The majority of affected patients report symptoms before the age of 15 years, many before the age of 5 years. Type I hereditary pancreatitis involves a mutation in the gene that codes for cationic trypsinogen on chromosome 7q35; type II hereditary pancreatitis involves a different mutation in the same gene. Both mutations are believed to allow trypsinogen to become activated to trypsin within the pancreas instead of within the duodenum. This, in turn, may lead to

Table 2. Medications and Toxins Associated With Pancreatitis

Acetaminophen overdose	Diphenoxylate	Organophosphates
Alcohol	Didanosine	Penicillin
Amphetamines	Enalapril	Pentamidine
Anticoagulants	Erythromycin	Phenformin
L-Asparaginase	Estrogen	Piroxicam
Azathioprine	Ethacrynic acid	Procainamide
Boric acid	Furadantin	Propoxyphene
Calcium	Furosemide	Propylthiouracil
Carbamazepine	Heroin	Ranitidine
Cimetidine	Histamine	Rifampin
Chlorthalidone	Indomethacin	Salicylates
Cholestyramine	Isoniazid	Sulfasalazine
Cisplatin	Meprobamate	Sulfonamides
Clonidine	6-Mercaptopurine	Sulindac
Cytarabine	Mesalamine	Tetracycline
Corticosteroids	Methotrexate	Thiazides
Cyclophosphamide	Methyldopa	Trimethoprim-sulfamethoxazole
Cyproheptadine	Metronidazole	Valproic acid
Cytosine arabinoside	Nonsteroidal anti-inflammatory drugs	Vincristine
Diazoxide	Nitrofurantoin	Venom (scorpion, spider)
Dideoxycytidine	Opiates	Vitamin D
	Oxyphenbutazone	

uncontrolled activation of the other pancreatic enzymes within the gland's acinar cells, leading to autodigestion, inflammation, and resultant pancreatitis. Attacks of acute pancreatitis are only intermittent, perhaps because this uncontrolled activation only occurs when trypsinogen exceeds the inhibitory capacity of the "secondary brake" of the pancreas, pancreatic secretory trypsin inhibitor. Affected patients are at increased risk for pancreatic pseudocysts, exocrine and endocrine failure, and pancreatic adenocarcinoma.

Pancreatitis has been a reported complication in children who have received heart, kidney, liver, pancreas, and bone marrow transplants. It can be life-threatening following liver transplantation and is associated with retransplantation, emergency transplantation, and infectious peritonitis. As with autoimmune and collagen-vascular diseases, it is difficult to distinguish the contribution that medications play in this scenario versus the transplant or primary disease process.

Signs and Symptoms

The classic symptoms of pancreatitis in children are abdominal pain, nausea, vomiting, and anorexia. The quality of the pain may be sharp and sudden or constant. It may be located in the epigastrium or right upper quadrant or even in the periumbilical area, back, or lower chest. Eating usually triggers a worsening of the pain and vomiting. The emesis may be bilious. A family history of pancreatitis should prompt the clinician to ask about symptoms of hereditary and systemic/metabolic disorders, such as diarrhea, vasculitis, joint pain, rashes, and pulmonary disease.

A careful physical examination may provide more clues for differentiating pancreatitis from other, more common causes of acute abdominal pain in the child. Fever, if present, is usually low grade, but tachycardia and hypotension may be present early in the course of the illness. The child may be icteric, with a distended abdomen, decreased bowel sounds, and diffuse or localized tenderness and guarding on palpation. He or she may experience some pain relief when the knees are drawn up to a flexed trunk. In the case of severe hemorrhagic or necrotizing disease, Grey Turner sign (blue discoloration of the flanks) or Cullen sign (blue discoloration around the umbilicus) may be noted. In advanced disease, ascites, a mass (pseudocyst), or pulmonary findings may be appreciated. The physician always should be alert to additional physical evidence of child abuse.

Laboratory Tests

A complete blood count with differential count, chemistry panel, amylase, and lipase usually differentiate pancreatitis from other, more common causes of abdominal pain. Leukocytosis with bandemia, hemoconcentration, hyperglycemia, hypocalcemia, and elevated alkaline phosphatase, aspartate aminotransferase, alanine aminotransferase, and total bilirubin are frequent findings. Hypoxemia with hypoalbuminemia, hypocalcemia, and azotemia with elevated glucose and lactate dehydrogenase levels reflect more progressive disease and hemorrhagic pancreatic damage.

Although it has a relatively low sensitivity and specificity (75% to 92% and 20% to 60%, respectively), the serum amylase level remains the test used most frequently to confirm acute pancreatitis. By making the cut-off three to six times the upper limit of normal, specificity increases for pancreatitis, but at the expense of sensitivity. In addition, as shown in Table 3, hyperamylasemia may result from many diseases of nonpancreatic origin, and normal amylase levels may be seen in cases of pancreatitis. Measurement of the isoamylase levels to differentiate between enzymes of pancreatic and salivary origins is more discriminatory. Serum activity of amylase begins to increase 2 to 12 hours after the pancreatic insult and peaks at 12 to 72 hours after the onset of symptoms.

Serum lipase levels have a reported clinical sensitivity of 86% to 100% and clinical specificity of 50% to 99%. By increasing the cutoff level to greater than three times the upper limit of normal, sensitivity can by increased to 100% and specificity to 99%. Lipase levels remain elevated for a longer period of time in the plasma than do amylase levels, beginning to increase within 4 to 8 hours after symptoms, peaking at 24 hours, and decreasing over 8 to 14 days. It should be noted, however, that the degree of elevation of amylase and lipase in the plasma does not reflect the severity of the pancreatic disease. By using serum amylase and lipase determinations together, clinical sensitivity for the diagnosis of pancreatitis increases to 94%.

Plasma immunoreactive cationic trypsin, pancreatic elastase I, and phospholipase A_2 are serum enzymes that show higher sensitivities than amylase and lipase and correlate with disease severity. Unfortunately, they are not readily available in most centers.

The diagnosis of chronic pancreatitis depends on the assessment of pancreatic function and clinical and radiographic findings. Noninvasive tests of pancreatic function reflect decreased enzymes in the blood or stool or increased amounts

Table 3. Conditions Associated With Elevated Serum Amylase

Pancreatic	Salivary	Both (or Unknown)
● Aortic aneurysm–abdominal	● Anorexia nervosa	● Alcoholism
● Appendicitis	● Bulimia	● Burns
● Biliary duct obstruction	● Infection (mumps)	● Cardiopulmonary bypass
● Biliary tract disease	● Lung cancer	● Cirrhosis
● Choledocholithiasis	● Ovarian tumor/cyst	● Cystic fibrosis
● Endoscopic retrograde cholangiopancreatography	● Parotitis	● Diabetic ketoacidosis
● Intestinal infarction, obstruction, or perforation	● Pneumonia	● Drugs
● Pancreatic duct obstruction	● Prostate tumors	● Head trauma
● Pancreatic tumors	● Salivary duct obstruction	● Hepatitis
● Pancreatitis–acute, chronic	● Salpingitis	● Heroin addiction
● Perforated peptic ulcer	● Trauma	● Macroamylasemia
● Peritonitis		● Opiates
● Pseudocyst		● Renal insufficiency
		● Renal transplantation
		● Ruptured ectopic pregnancy

of malabsorbed food products. These tests include measuring serum pancreatic enzymes (amylase, lipase, isoamylase, and immunoreactive trypsinogen) and fecal assays for fat and pancreatic enzymes. However, due to the poor negative predictive value of these tests, chronic pancreatitis cannot be excluded confidently. These tests also may be falsely positive in the presence of intestinal bacterial overgrowth or other mucosal diseases of the small bowel. A recent study examining the usefulness of measuring fecal pancreatic elastase I versus the secretin-pancreozymin test in children who had cystic fibrosis and healthy controls reported a sensitivity of 100% and a specificity of 96% and may offer a valid noninvasive test to detect pancreatic insufficiency.

The "gold standard" for establishing pancreatic insufficiency involves direct testing of pancreatic function by administering intravenous cholecystokinin or secretin and measuring output of bicarbonate and pancreatic enzymes in pancreatic ductal secretions. If performed correctly, the sensitivity and specificity for this procedure range from 90% to 100% in the diagnosis of chronic pancreatitis. However, these tests require oroduodenal or endoscopic intubation, accurate placement of a duodenal catheter, and complete recovery of all duodenal secretions. Because these studies are difficult to perform and interpret, they usually are available only at tertiary centers.

Diagnosis

Although ultrasonography is the radiologic study of choice in pancreatitis, a simple radiograph of the kidneys, ureters, and bladder (KUB) may suggest the diagnosis. Findings of ileus, with colonic dilatation, a sentinel loop of dilated small bowel, obscured psoas margins, or a radiolucent "halo" around the left kidney, are suggestive of the disease. In chronic pancreatitis, calcifications may be seen in the area of the pancreatic parenchyma or ductal system. Changes in pancreatic size, contour, and echotexture are appreciated best with ultrasonography, as is the presence of dilated ducts, pseudocysts, abscesses, ascites, and associated gallstone disease. Computed tomography often is used to help manage the complications of pancreatitis, such as providing guidance in the

aspiration and drainage of an abscess, phlegmon, or pseudocyst or prior to surgical intervention.

Recurrent attacks of acute pancreatitis and chronic pancreatitis of unknown etiology require a detailed delineation of the pancreatic and biliary anatomy to rule out anatomic malformations, biliary strictures, and cholelithiasis. Cholangiopancreatography may be accomplished by endoscopic retrograde cholangiopancreatography (ERCP) or magnetic resonance cholangiopancreatography (MRCP) intraoperatively or via a percutaneous cholangiogram. ERCP is considered the study of choice to diagnose pancreas divisum and anomalous pancreaticobiliary duct junction. It has the added benefit of being a therapeutic modality, allowing sphincterotomy, stent placement, and stone removal, which can be performed at the time of diagnostic evaluation. These procedures should be undertaken at centers that have significant experience both in performing the studies and in managing childhood pancreatitis.

If an anatomic variant is suspected and ERCP is not possible, the next appropriate step is transduodenal exploration with intraoperative pancreatography. Surgical sphincteroplasty can be performed if minor or major papillae stenosis is found. MRCP has proven useful in determining the presence of pancreaticobiliary disease, the level of biliary obstruction, and the presence of malignancy and bile duct calculi. This procedure may prove useful in the patient who is unable to tolerate general anesthesia for ERCP or for an open laparotomy. Percutaneous cholangiography requires a skilled interventional radiologist and may be used when dilated bile ducts are present or through a biliary drain placed postoperatively (such as with postpancreatic debridement or postorthotopic liver transplant).

Management

The treatment of pancreatitis is primarily supportive, providing adequate hydration, pain relief, and "pancreatic rest" by decreasing the cephalic, gastric, and intestinal phases of pancreatic secretion. In the case of severe pancreatitis, the child is made *nil per os,* and nasogastric suction may be necessary to manage persistent vomiting or ileus. Parenteral nutrition should be initiated if the patient is expected to be without enteral feedings for more than 3 days to prevent protein catabolism. Antibiotics are indicated when there are clinical signs of sepsis, necrotic pancreatitis, or multiorgan system failure. Histamine$_2$ receptor antagonists may help prevent stress ulceration by reducing duodenal acidification.

It may be difficult to relieve pain completely, and opiates have been reported to worsen symptoms by increasing spasm of the sphincter of Oddi. Of all the pure opiate agonists, meperidine is the analgesic of choice by most clinicians for acute pancreatitis because it produces the least increase in enterobiliary pressure. We have used hydromorphone hydrochloride in many children who had severe acute pancreatitis, as well as in chronic pancreatitis, with excellent pain control. Chronic pancreatitis that leads to exocrine or endocrine insufficiency may require pancreatic enzyme replacement, insulin, or an elemental or low-fat diet to optimize nutritional status once enteral feedings are reinitiated.

The major cause of mortality in patients who have acute pancreatitis is septic complications, believed to arise from bacteria that have translocated from the small or large intestine via the mesenteric lymph nodes and lymphatics. This can lead to pancreatic abscess, infected pseudocyst, or pancreatic necrosis. These infections necessitate surgical intervention, but whether sterile necrosis requires operative management is still controversial. Evidence of infection within an area of necrosis can be obtained via fine-needle aspiration, with either ultrasonographic or CT guidance, for Gram stain and culture. The most common organisms recovered are *Escherichia coli*, *Klebsiella* sp, and other gram-negative enteric rods.

Antibiotics and intensive care unit management usually provide adequate support for the patient who has sterile necrosis, but persistent ileus, bowel perforation, portal vein thrombosis, and multisystem organ failure are indications for urgent surgical intervention. Infected pancreatic necrosis is an absolute surgical indication, requiring necrosectomy (surgical debridement). Debridement of the pancreatic and peripancreatic parenchyma is thought to stop the progression of the necrotizing process and resultant multiorgan

failure. Debridement, rather than partial or total pancreatic resection, is preferred because it preserves the exocrine and endocrine function of the gland. Multiple reoperations or continuous lavage with catheters left in the retroperitoneum may be necessary. Complications after necrosectomy include sepsis, hemorrhage, wound infection, and fistulas of the intestine, pancreas, and biliary system.

Prognosis

The chances of surviving an acute attack of severe pancreatitis are related to associated complications, which may affect virtually all organ systems, including pulmonary, cardiovascular, hematologic, gastrointestinal, renal, metabolic, and central nervous system (Table 4). Most cases of acute pancreatitis in children, which are uncomplicated and rarely progress to chronic pancreatitis, persist for only 5 to 7 days. The primary morbidity and mortality arise from septic shock, adult respiratory distress syndrome and respiratory failure, renal failure, and inflammatory masses of the pancreas. Criteria to predict the outcome from acute pancreatitis have been developed for adults (APACHE-II, Ranson), but they may not be as reliable in young children. Studies have shown a mortality rate of 5% to 17.5% from an initially mild presentation of acute pancreatitis and 80% to 100% from hemorrhagic pancreatitis or severe multisystem disorders. Exocrine and endocrine insufficiency are common after necrotizing pancreatitis, and the degree of dysfunction correlates with the extent of parenchymal necrosis.

Conclusion

The general clinician needs to have a high index of suspicion for pancreatitis when a child presents with the nonspecific symptoms of nausea, vomiting, and localized upper abdominal pain. A thorough history and physical examination that emphasizes recent infections, medications used, recent trauma, and underlying medical conditions may make the diagnosis clearer. Using serum enzyme testing alone (amylase and lipase) to diagnose both acute and chronic pancreatitis remains a challenge because although clinical

Table 4. Complications of Pancreatitis

Pancreatic	Gastrointestinal/Metabolic	Systemic
● Ascites	● Biliary obstruction	● Atelectasis
● Diabetes mellitus	● Bowel infarction	● Adult respiratory distress syndrome
● Exocrine insufficiency	● Gastritis	● Disseminated intravascular coagulation
● Necrotizing pancreatitis	● Gastrointestinal fistula	● Electrocardiographic changes
● Pancreatic abscess	● Hemorrhage	● Encephalopathy
● Pancreatic carcinoma	● Hepatic vein thrombosis	● Fat emboli
● Pancreatic duct strictures	● Hepatorenal syndrome	● Fat necrosis
● Pancreatic calculi	● Hyperglycemia	● Hypotension
● Pancreatic fibrosis	● Hyperkalemia	● Mediastinal abscess
● Pancreatic fistula	● Hypertriglyceridemia	● Pericardial effusion
● Pancreatic phlegmon	● Hypoalbuminemia	● Pleural effusion
● Pancreatic pseudocyst	● Hypocalcemia	● Pneumonitis
	● Ileus	● Psychosis
	● Jaundice	● Renal failure
	● Metabolic acidosis	● Renal vessel thrombosis
	● Peptic ulcer disease	● Respiratory failure
	● Portal vein thrombosis	● Sepsis
	● Varices-splenic vein	● Sudden death
		● Thrombosis

sensitivity has improved, clinical specificity remains suboptimal. Ultrasonography is the first radiographic study of choice in the child who has pancreatitis to look for evidence of congenital anomalies, biliary ductal dilatation, cholelithiasis, and infection. More detailed imaging of the pancreatic and biliary system should be performed in recurrent acute pancreatitis and chronic pancreatitis. Unlike the adult disease, in which the majority of cases are due to alcoholism or gallstone disease, pancreatitis in the child may be due to infection, trauma, abnormal anatomy, or hereditary or systemic diseases and the medications used to treat them. Nearly 25% of cases of childhood pancreatitis may remain idiopathic. Gallstone pancreatitis is not infrequent in teenagers. A family history of the disease should prompt the clinician to look for evidence of inherited biochemical or anatomic abnormalities.

Treatment is basically supportive in an effort to decrease the cephalic, gastric, and intestinal phases of pancreatic stimulation. Despite the varied etiologies, the course of acute pancreatitis in the child usually is limited, with complications being rare. However, the complications of this disease can involve virtually every organ system, and major morbidity and mortality can result despite aggressive supportive care. For severe cases or when complications occur, ERCP and pancreatic surgical and nonoperative radiologic intervention should be undertaken at a center that has significant expertise in caring for children who have pancreatic disorders.

Suggested Reading

Banks PA. Practice guidelines in acute pancreatitis. *Am J Gastroenterol.* 1997;92:377–385

Clain JE, Pearson RK. Diagnosis of chronic pancreatitis. *Surg Clin North Am.* 1999;79:829–845

Dodge JA. Paediatric and hereditary aspects of chronic pancreatitis. *Digestion.* 1998;suppl 4:49–59

Gates LK Jr, Ulrich CD II, Whitcomb DC. Hereditary pancreatitis. *Surg Clin North Am.* 1999;79:711–722

Guelrud M. Endoscopic therapy of pancreatic disease in children. *Gastrointest Endoscop Clin North Am.* 1998;3:195–219

Holland AJ, Davey RB, Sparnon AL, Chapman M, LeQuesne GW. Traumatic pancreatitis: long-term overview of initial nonoperative management in children. *J Paediatr Child Health.* 1999;35:78–81

Karne S, Gorelick FS. Etiopathogenesis of acute pancreatitis. *Surg Clin North Am.* 1999;79:699–710

Lerner A. Acute pancreatitis in children and adolescents. In: Lebenthal E, ed. *Gastroenterology and Nutrition in Infancy.* 2nd ed. New York, NY: Raven Press; 1989:897–906

Lerner A, Branski D, Lebenthal E. Pancreatic diseases in children. *Pediatr Clin North Am.* 1996;43:125–156

Oberlander TF, Rappaport LA. Recurrent abdominal pain during childhood. *Pediatr Rev.* 1993;14:313–319

Pieper-Bigelow C, Strocchi A, Levitt MD. Where does serum amylase come from and where does it go? *Gastroenterol Clin North Am.* 1990;19:793–810

Robertson MA, Durie PR. Pancreatitis. In: Walker WA, Durie PR, Hamilton JR, Walker-Smith JA, Watkins JB, eds. *Pediatric Gastrointestinal Disease.* 2nd ed. St. Louis, Mo: Mosby; 1996:1436–1465

Roy CC, Silverman A, Alagille D. Pancreatitis and pancreatic tumors. In: Roy CC, Silverman A, Alagille D, eds. *Pediatric Clinical Gastroenterology.* 4th ed. St. Louis, Mo: Mosby; 1995:986–1004

Stevenson RJ, Ziegler MM. Abdominal pain unrelated to trauma. *Pediatr Rev.* 1993;14:302–311

Tagge EP, Tarnasky PR, Chandler J, et al. Multidisciplinary approach to the treatment of pediatric pancreaticobiliary disorders. *J Pediatr Surg.* 1997;32:158–164

Tietz NW. Support of the diagnosis of pancreatitis by enzyme tests—old problems, new techniques. *Clin Chim Acta.* 1997; 257:85–98

Weizman Z. Acute pancreatitis. In: Wyllie R, Hyams JS, eds. *Pediatric Gastrointestinal Disease.* Philadelphia, Pa: WB Saunders Co; 1993:873–879

Prevention and Treatment of Type 2 Diabetes Mellitus in Children, With Special Emphasis on American Indian and Alaska Native Children

Sheila Gahagan, MD; Janet Silverstein, MD; and the Committee on Native American Child Health and Section on Endocrinology

ABSTRACT. The emergence of type 2 diabetes mellitus in the American Indian/Alaska Native pediatric population presents a new challenge for pediatricians and other health care professionals. This chronic disease requires preventive efforts, early diagnosis, and collaborative care of the patient and family within the context of a medical home. *Pediatrics* 2003;112:e328–e347. URL: http://www.pediatrics.org/cgi/content/full/112/4/e328; *type 2 diabetes mellitus, children, American Indian, Alaska Native, Native American, pediatric population.*

ABBREVIATIONS. AI/AN, American Indian/Alaska Native; AAP, American Academy of Pediatrics; IHS, Indian Health Service; CDC, Centers for Disease Control and Prevention; ADA, American Diabetes Association; PCOS, polycystic ovarian syndrome; BMI, body mass index; HbA$_{1c}$, glycosylated hemoglobin; OGTT, oral glucose tolerance test; FBG, fasting blood glucose; FPG, fasting plasma glucose; SMBG, self-monitoring of blood glucose; ACE, angiotensin-converting enzyme; LDL, low-density lipoprotein; HDL, high-density lipoprotein; NDEP, National Diabetes Education Program; NPH, neutral protamine Hagedorn; TZD, thiazolidinedione.

Statement of the Problem

Type 2 diabetes mellitus* is a new morbidity in children and adolescents.[1-4] For pediatric patients, it heralds earlier onset of cardiovascular disease, retinopathy, nephropathy, and neuropathy, with risk of impaired quality of life and premature death. The emergence of type 2 diabetes mellitus in young people is believed to be associated with changes in physical activity and nutrition that are ubiquitous in modern society. Not all populations are equally affected. American Indian/Alaska Native (AI/AN) children in the United States and Canada have a higher rate of this disease than do children of other ethnicities. Mexican American and black children are at increased risk. Vulnerable populations that exhibit new disease trends may be seen as the "canary in the coal mine," warning of hazards present for the entire population. In US children, the prevalence of type 2 diabetes mellitus is expected to exceed that of type 1 diabetes mellitus within 10 years. There is a compelling need for additional research, primary and secondary prevention efforts, and evidence-based treatment for youth with type 2 diabetes mellitus.

Purpose

These guidelines have been developed to assist in clinical decision making by primary health care professionals and are not intended to replace existing management protocols for the medical treatment of diabetes.[5] It is assumed that clinical care will be individualized for each child and adolescent. In keeping with the spirit of community pediatrics and the *Healthy People 2010* objectives, the American Academy of Pediatrics (AAP) believes that medical care for AI/AN children, like that of all other children, should be provided within a medical home, which "ideally should be accessible, continuous, comprehensive, family centered, coordinated, compassionate, and culturally effective. It should be delivered or directed by well-trained physicians who provide primary care and manage and facilitate essentially all aspects of pediatric care. The physician should be known

---

PEDIATRICS (ISSN 0031 4005). Copyright © 2003 by the American Academy of Pediatrics.

Type 1 diabetes mellitus is characterized by a lack of insulin production. Type 2 diabetes mellitus is a metabolic disorder secondary to an inability to appropriately use or make adequate insulin.

to the child and family and should be able to develop a partnership of mutual responsibility and trust with them."[6]

Methods

The AAP Committee on Native American Child Health, in collaboration with the Indian Health Service (IHS) Diabetes Program, the Centers for Disease Control and Prevention (CDC), and the AAP Section on Endocrinology, developed these guidelines to improve the medical care for AI/AN children with type 2 diabetes mellitus and those at risk of type 2 diabetes mellitus. This effort was greatly assisted by the 2000 American Diabetes Association (ADA) consensus statement on type 2 diabetes mellitus in children and adolescents.[2,3]

These guidelines were developed after a review of published data on type 2 diabetes mellitus in American Indian and First Nations[†] children[7-23] and are adapted from the medical literature on adults with type 2 diabetes mellitus.[5,24-29]

These guidelines were developed to support the role of the general pediatrician or other primary health care professional as the front line for care. The treatment of most AI/AN children with type 2 diabetes mellitus will be managed by primary health care professionals with specialty consultation. It is hoped that these guidelines will serve as a framework for the development of diabetes care programs and strategies aimed at decreasing the devastating impact of type 2 diabetes mellitus on AI/AN children and their families and communities. A section on primary prevention of type 2 diabetes mellitus is included and is based on existing data.

Primary and Secondary Prevention

Prevention must take highest priority and should focus on decreasing the risk, incidence, and consequences of type 2 diabetes mellitus among AI/AN children. Primary prevention efforts by primary health care professionals are recommended in 2 arenas: 1) general community health promotion and health education and 2) clinically based activities. Clinically based health promotion activities should not duplicate community-wide health promotion but instead should offer additive benefits. For example, if significant health education is offered at the community level, then motivational interviewing and collaborative problem solving can be offered in the clinical setting. When type 2 diabetes mellitus is the established diagnosis, secondary prevention efforts by primary health care professionals are important for the prevention of complications (eg, vascular, neural, renal, retinal). Early diagnosis and optimal medical care are the keys to effective secondary prevention.

To be effective, prevention efforts need a strong community base and acceptance. Current evidence suggests that modifiable risks for type 2 diabetes mellitus include obesity and lack of breastfeeding.[30] Primary prevention efforts can focus on the prevention of obesity in children and the promotion of breastfeeding. Preventing obesity in women of childbearing age is another primary prevention goal, because exposure to the environment of a diabetic pregnancy places the fetus at increased risk of future onset of diabetes.[30]

COMMUNITY ACTIVITIES

Community prevention activities are being developed in AI/AN communities on the basis of each tribe's unique needs and resources. Development and implementation of these activities should have the endorsement of appropriate tribal authorities. Ideally, these activities are multidisciplinary (eg, medical, nutrition, public health, nursing, health education) and include local businesses, community recreational programs, Head Start programs, and schools.[31,32] Tribal food and nutrition programs (eg, Special Supplemental Nutrition Program for Women, Infants, and Children; US Department of Agriculture's Food Distribution and Food Stamp program) have a prominent role in promoting foods that minimize the risk of obesity. Community programs and services should develop consistent messages and supply foods that assist in decreasing the prevalence of obesity. Studies to evaluate the effectiveness of community-based obesity and diabetes risk reduction efforts are in progress.[33,34]

Health care professionals can play a crucial role in their communities by raising community awareness about the importance of programs and facilities for physical activity and resources for healthy nutrition.[35] The powerful influence of physicians extends outside the clinic when they thoughtfully advocate for healthy lifestyles and good nutrition practices within the community.

Pediatricians and other health care professionals should advocate for school policy that requires daily physical activity for every child and for

---

[†]First Nations is the term used in Canada to identify Native or Aboriginal people. In this article, this term is used when citing research done in Canada.

physical fitness programs in the school and community. They should urge stores, restaurants, and schools to offer low-caloric density foods of high nutritional value in appropriate portions. Lack of physical activity is associated with the development of obesity, type 2 diabetes mellitus, and cardiovascular morbidity and mortality. Despite information on the importance of exercise, a low proportion of high school students participate in daily physical education classes.[36,37] Increasing physical activity should include participating in at least 30 minutes of physical activity daily, limiting sedentary activity (eg, watching television, playing video games, using a computer) to no more than 1 to 2 hours per day, and participating in sports. Community recreation programs and schools should encourage youth to participate in events that require physical activity. The community leadership should receive information on and understand the importance of physical activity and the value of having programs and facilities available for youth. Recommendations and programs should respect family, culture, and community values.

Health care professionals can use their expertise to provide prevention messages to the community on healthful lifestyles and good nutrition via local media (eg, radio, television, newspapers, posters). Prevention messages need to be thoughtfully developed to resonate with community and tribal culture and beliefs. Youth involvement in community prevention efforts can be highly effective.

Community involvement in the promotion and support of healthful lifestyles reinforces recommendations made in the health care setting. The engagement and empowerment of communities is critical for overall success in decreasing the disease burden of type 2 diabetes mellitus for the AI/AN population. Schools are integral in the successful management of type 2 diabetes mellitus (and other chronic illnesses) and potentially are important resources for promoting children's diabetes self-care, including blood glucose monitoring, appropriate recognition and treatment of hypoglycemia, and treatment of acute hyperglycemia.

CLINICALLY BASED PRIMARY AND SECONDARY PREVENTION ACTIVITIES

Health care professionals have influential roles in preventing type 2 diabetes mellitus among at-risk youth via direct patient care contacts. Children with 1 or more risk factors (see "Case Finding") identified by the ADA consensus panel on type 2 diabetes mellitus in children should be monitored closely.[2,3] Identification of disorders associated with insulin resistance, such as acanthosis nigricans, polycystic ovarian syndrome (PCOS), and family history of diabetes, should trigger education and the initiation of prevention activities.

Children whose body mass index‡ (BMI; see also "Physical Assessment") is greater than the 85th percentile for their age§ should receive appropriate counseling on nutrition, weight control, and physical activity. This is especially important because there is evidence that type 2 diabetes mellitus can be delayed or prevented by lifestyle interventions. These children may require treatment for hypertension and hyperlipidemia and should return for follow-up evaluation and additional lifestyle intervention within 3 months.

Until results of current prevention trials with oral hypoglycemic agents in youth are available, intervention using glucose-lowering drugs for prevention of diabetes is not recommended. (These medications are, however, recommended for treatment of children with diagnosed type 2 diabetes mellitus.)

Knowledgeable health care professionals (eg, nutritionists, health educators, physicians, nurses, community outreach workers) should guide nutrition interventions in AI/AN children and their families. Any intervention needs to consider growth and development in children. The most effective approach is appropriate reduction of calories along with increased energy expenditure. Specific recommendations need to

---

‡BMI is a measure based on weight and stature (kg/m²). A simple calculation can be made as follows: weight in pounds divided by height in inches, divided by height in inches again, and multiplied by 703.

§Growth charts developed by the CDC; see "Physical Assessment" for Web site address.

be individualized, and continued evaluation is crucial for long-term success. Individualized plans are based on collaboration with the child and the family to assess food preferences, timing and location of meals and snacks, food preparation, and desire to change behaviors. Family resources and the availability of low-calorie nutritious foods in the community must be considered. Pharmacologic therapy to decrease weight is not recommended for children until more safety and efficacy data are available. Very low-calorie diets and high-protein diets are contraindicated, except in a well-controlled research setting. Quick-fix weight loss programs are unsafe for children and rarely result in long-term weight control; furthermore, they do not promote lasting, healthful eating behaviors. Weight loss programs with the best results combine exercise and dietary components with behavior modification.[38] Accomplishing changes in the child's eating behavior and activity relies on changes made by the entire family.

Identification

The prevalence of type 2 diabetes mellitus in AI/AN children as well as AI/AN adults is higher than among other ethnic groups.[2,3,18] Among Pima Indian adolescents 15 to 19 years of age, the prevalence of type 2 diabetes mellitus estimated through screening increased significantly during the past 2 decades and reached 5% in the 1992–1996 time period.[19] (Although population-based prevalence estimates are not available for children and adolescents in the United States, a retrospective review estimated an incidence of 7.2 per 100 000 for black and white children and adolescents in southwestern Ohio in 1994.[20]) In Manitoba, Canada, the prevalence of type 2 diabetes mellitus diagnosed through screening was 3.6% for First Nations girls (0% for boys) 10 to 19 years of age in 1996–1997.[15] The prevalence of diagnosed diabetes (all types) among youth 15 to 19 years of age receiving services from the IHS was 0.45% in 1996, reflecting a 54% increase since 1988.[21] In Montana and Wyoming IHS clinics, the prevalence of diagnosed diabetes (all types) was 0.23% among American Indian youth 0 to 19 years of age in the period 1997–1999.[22,23] Therefore, the high burden of diabetes on AI/AN communities and their youth deserves specific research efforts directed toward better case identification.

POPULATION-BASED SCREENING

Many AI/AN communities are interested in population-based screening for type 2 diabetes mellitus. The evidence that microvascular complications of diabetes are strongly associated with previous hyperglycemia raises interest in earlier diagnosis during the asymptomatic period.[39] However, population-based screening for type 2 diabetes mellitus in high-risk children is not recommended, except as part of research efforts to advance knowledge about optimal prevention, diagnosis, and treatment.[40-43] Population-based screening remains controversial, because there are no data from controlled trials showing that earlier diagnosis improves long-term outcome. It is essential that studies be performed to determine the specificity, sensitivity, and cost-benefit of screening for type 2 diabetes mellitus in high-risk populations of children and adolescents.

The World Health Organization has recommended that before embarking on population-based screening, the following criteria be met[44]:
1. The condition should be an important health problem.
2. There should be an accepted treatment for patients with recognized disease.
3. Facilities for diagnosis and treatment should be available.
4. There should be a recognizable latent or early symptomatic stage.
5. There should be a suitable test or examination.
6. The test should be acceptable to the population.
7. The natural history of the condition, including development from latent to declared disease, should be understood adequately.
8. There should be an agreed policy on whom to treat as patients.
9. The cost of case finding should be economically balanced in relation to possible expenditure on medical care as a whole.
10. Case finding should be a continuing process and not a once-and-for-all project.

Although some of these criteria can be met, a key aspect to the second criterion is that there must be evidence that earlier identification improves clinical outcomes before the costs of this endeavor can be justified under nonresearch protocol.[44] The first results from the Diabetes Prevention Program show that diet and exercise delay the onset of diabetes and normalize blood glucose in adults.[45] Therefore, it is important to identify children and adolescents who are at risk of developing diabetes, such as those with obesity and signs of insulin resistance, to begin lifestyle management programs that could prevent and delay the development of diabetes. Many of these children will have impaired glucose tolerance.

Before beginning screening programs, health care systems and institutions must identify resources for intervention for people who will be identified with type 2 diabetes mellitus or altered glucose metabolism by the screening program. Screening programs can cause harm if effective treatment is not available.

If universal screening were performed in the United States on the basis of the ADA risk criteria for type 2 diabetes mellitus in youth, then 10% of US adolescents (2.5 million) 12 to 19 years of age would be tested.[43] This screening would not yield a large number of new diagnoses because of the low prevalence of type 2 diabetes mellitus in the general adolescent population.[46]

Screening efforts have been implemented as part of research initiatives for some high-risk populations. Among the Pima Indians, screening has been performed by the National Institutes of Health since 1965 as part of a longitudinal epidemiologic study. Because of the high prevalence of type 2 diabetes mellitus among Pima Indian children identified by the epidemiologic study, current efforts focus on measuring glycosylated hemoglobin (HbA_{1c}) concentration in children who are at risk and referring them for a 2-hour oral glucose tolerance test (OGTT) if the HbA_{1c} concentration is more than 5.5%.[18] Another survey conducted in 1996–1997 in 717 First Nations school youth 4 to 19 years of age from Manitoba identified 6 new cases and 2 previously identified cases by using the fasting blood glucose (FBG) concentration.[15] A survey of 276 Navajo students 13 to 20 years of age at 2 high schools found 1 case of diabetes and 8 cases of impaired glucose tolerance or impaired FBG concentration.[8] Future studies may identify specific criteria for screening children for type 2 diabetes mellitus in AI/AN populations.

Earlier diagnosis of diabetes may prevent or slow the development of complications if active treatment is implemented early and proves efficacious. In a world of limited resources, the benefits of screening efforts need to be assessed and balanced with those of other programs that may benefit the same population.

Some IHS areas and Indian tribes are developing screening and intervention programs for obesity and hypertension in youth. These efforts will result in identifying youth who are at increased risk of type 2 diabetes mellitus and have the potential to benefit from primary prevention interventions.

CASE FINDING

Although population-based screening is not recommended, early case finding and early initiation of treatment may prevent some sequelae of type 2 diabetes mellitus. Overweight children who have entered puberty (or who are older than 10 years) are considered at risk by the ADA if they meet 2 of the following criteria[2,3]:

- Family history of type 2 diabetes mellitus in first-or second-degree relative
- Race or ethnicity is American Indian, Alaska Native, black, Hispanic, or Asian/ Pacific Islander
- Presence of a condition associated with insulin resistance (acanthosis nigricans, hypertension, dyslipidemia, PCOS)

The following are definitions for being at risk for overweight[47]:

- BMI between the 85th and 95th percentiles for age and sex
- Weight-for-height ratio between the 85th and 95th percentiles

The following are definitions for being overweight:

- BMI greater than the 95th percentile for age and sex

- Weight-for-height ratio greater than the 95th percentile
- Weight greater than 20% of the ideal weight for height

The term "obese" is not defined for children by the CDC. Health care professionals should be knowledgeable about risk factors and make appropriate decisions to test individual patients.

DIAGNOSIS (CLINIC BASED)

The diagnosis of type 2 diabetes mellitus in a child or an adolescent usually will be made by an astute health care professional in a clinical setting rather than as a result of a screening program. Knowledge of the aforementioned risk factors will assist the health care professional in considering and making the diagnosis when the patient is asymptomatic. Symptomatic and asymptomatic disease manifestations are described in "Pharmacologic Management on the Basis of Clinical Manifestations."

Specialists should be consulted for children and adolescents in whom diabetic ketoacidosis is detected. Furthermore, subspecialty consultation is indicated for children with hyperglycemia (FBG >250 mg/dL [>13.9 mmol/L]) but without the clinical features, family history, or physical characteristics commonly associated with type 2 diabetes mellitus. In such cases, diagnostic differentiation between type 1 and type 2 diabetes mellitus may require additional studies, such as autoimmune markers (islet cell antibodies, glutamic acid decarboxylase antibodies), challenge tests with high-calorie nutritional supplements (eg, Sustacal and Boost Nutritional Energy Drink [Mead Johnson Nutritionals, Evansville, IN]) or glucagon, or assays of insulin or C peptide. Children with type 2 diabetes mellitus may have normal or high C peptide and fasting insulin concentrations. However, children with type 2 diabetes mellitus with toxic effects of glucose attributable to prolonged hyperglycemia before diagnosis may have transient low insulin concentrations and may benefit from a short course of subcutaneous insulin therapy. Specialty consultation also should be sought when youth are unable to achieve treatment goals in a reasonable time frame or when complications occur. Specialty consultation is helpful for youth with hyperlipidemia and hypertension.

The subspecialist often is a pediatric endocrinologist. However, the primary health care professional (eg, pediatrician, family physician, internist) who is responsible for the diabetes clinic in an AI/AN health care facility may be a clinically competent expert in the management of type 2 diabetes mellitus. In geographically isolated locations, telemedicine may facilitate specialty consultation.

Ongoing Evaluation and Monitoring for Type 2 Diabetes Mellitus in Children

HISTORY AND PSYCHOSOCIAL ASSESSMENT

A complete medical history, including a review of systems, is essential at diagnosis and at regular intervals (Table 1), with special attention to emotional disorders; eating disorders; alcohol, tobacco, and drug use; and family support. Emotional and behavioral disorders, particularly depression, have been associated with diabetes.[48-57] Psychosocial assessment is recommended at diagnosis and informally at every visit. Assessment may be performed on the basis of patient history or by using a standardized screening tool.[58,59] A social worker

Table 1. Ongoing Evaluation and Monitoring After Diagnosis: History

History Component	Frequency*	Recommendations
Interval history	Initially every 3 months	Include ROS
Psychosocial assessment		May use standardized questionnaire[78,79]
Eating disorder		Binge eating, bulimia
Substance abuse		Alcohol, tobacco, drugs
Family assessment		Strengths, needs

ROS indicates review of systems.

* Frequency of detailed history may decrease in case of metabolic control and low-risk social circumstances to every 6 to 12 months.

or a psychologist on the diabetes team can assist with this evaluation. If depression or another emotional disorder is identified, then treatment and referral should be initiated promptly.

Health care professionals and dietitians should screen for eating disorders as part of the standard nutrition evaluation for all children with type 2 diabetes mellitus.[60] Binge eating and bulimia are significant concerns. Psychiatrically defined eating disorders are differentiated from culturally normal behaviors, some of which may be unhealthful.

The use of alcohol, tobacco, and drugs should be evaluated in all children and adolescents in whom diabetes is newly diagnosed, and it should be reevaluated, at least informally, at every visit. The family's attitudes toward the use of these and other substances should be evaluated as well. Alcohol use may aggravate hypoglycemia caused by sulfonylureas or insulin and increase the risk of lactic acidosis in patients who use metformin.

Family support is essential to the child or adolescent with type 2 diabetes mellitus. The family's strengths and needs should be assessed so that necessary assistance can be offered. This assessment should include positive and negative role models in the home, availability of healthful foods (eg, fresh fruits and vegetables), financial resources, parental literacy, cultural beliefs about health and illness, and the family's understanding of diabetes. The involvement of the whole family in dietary and activity changes will promote successful management of the child's diabetes. A family history of diabetes and cardiovascular disease will influence the meaning of this illness within the family. Support services for the family may include health education, financial services, social services, mental health counseling, transportation, and home visiting. Socially disorganized families need early psychologic and social work intervention.

PHYSICAL ASSESSMENT

Although a complete physical examination is recommended for all children at diagnosis, special attention should be given to the following elements (Table 2).

Weight and height should be plotted on a growth chart. The weight goal should be based on BMI (weight [kg]/height^2 [m^2]). (The Web site for growth charts[61] is: www.cdc.gov/nchs/about/major/nhanes/growthcharts/charts.htm.) Weight should be measured at each visit, but height may be measured twice a year.

The blood pressure goal is less than the 90th percentile on the basis of height and weight standards. Blood pressure is assessed at each visit. Blood pressure control is discussed in "Decreasing Cardiovascular Risk"[62,63] (Table 3).

The skin, especially the back of the neck, the underarms, and the groin, should be evaluated for acanthosis nigricans, a thickened, hyperpigmented skin condition (Fig 1). Acanthosis nigricans often correlates with high BMI and insulin resistance. The resolution of acanthosis nigricans may be a useful marker for decreasing insulin resistance.[64] Insulin resistance may improve as weight decreases. The improvement of the skin condition as a result of better metabolic control is highly desirable to adolescents. Therefore, identification of this condition is especially useful as a motivator for adolescents. Other treatable skin conditions may occur in association with insulin

Table 2. Ongoing Evaluation and Monitoring After Diagnosis: Physical Examination

Physical Examination Component	Frequency	Recommendations
Weight	Initially every 3 mo*	
Height, BMI	Initially every 3 mo*	
Blood pressure	Initially every 3 mo*	
Skin	Every 12 mo	Acanthosis nigricans, hirsutism, tinea, acne
Foot	Every 12 mo but visual foot check every 3 mo	Pedal pulses, neurologic examination, nails

* May decrease to every 6 months if linear growth is complete and glucose is well controlled.

Table 3. Classification of Hypertension

Age (Years)	High Normal (mm Hg)*	Significant Hypertension (mm Hg)†	Severe Hypertension (mm Hg)‡
6–9	Systolic: 111–121	Systolic: 122–129	Systolic: >129 (129)§
	Diastolic: 70–77	Diastolic: 70–85	Diastolic: >85 (84)
10–12	Systolic: 117–122	Systolic: 126–133	Systolic: >133 (134)
	Diastolic: 75–81	Diastolic: 82–89	Diastolic: >89 (89)
13–15	Systolic: 124–135	Systolic: 136–143	Systolic: >143 (149)
	Diastolic: 77–85	Diastolic: 86–91	Diastolic: >91 (94)
16–18	Systolic: 127–141	Systolic: 142–149	Systolic: >149 (159)
	Diastolic: 80–91	Diastolic: 92–97	Diastolic: >97 (99)
>18	Not given	Systolic: [140–179]‖	Systolic: >(179)
	Not given	Diastolic: [90–109]	Diastolic: >(109)

* 90th to 94th percentile for age, boys and girls combined.

† 95th to 98th percentile for age, boys and girls combined.

‡ 99th percentile for age, boys and girls combined.

§ The values in parentheses are those used for the classification of severe hypertension by the 26th Bethesda Conference on cardiovascular disease and athletic participation.

‖ Because the Second Task Force did not discuss youth older than 18 years, the values in brackets are those for mild and moderate hypertension given by the 26th Bethesda Conference.

Adapted from American Academy of Pediatrics, Committee on Sports Medicine and Fitness. Athletic participation by children and adolescents who have systemic hypertension. *Pediatrics.* 1997;99:637–638

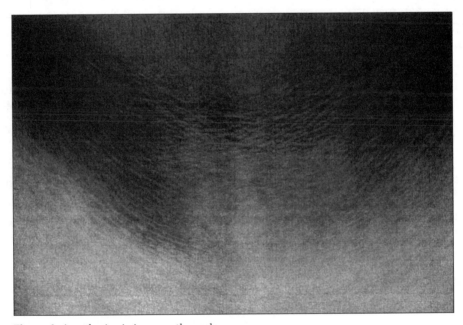

Figure 1. Acanthosis nigricans on the neck.

resistance, including tinea capitis, tinea corporis, and tinea pedis. Hirsutism or significant acne may be markers of hyperandrogenism in girls. Hirsutism is related to hyperinsulinism and is another potential motivating factor for adolescents to accomplish nutritional and physical activity goals.[65–67]

A thorough visual inspection of the feet, including pedal pulses (posterior tibial and dorsalis pedis) and a neurologic examination are recommended shortly after diagnosis and then annually (Fig 2). The monofilament examination for foot sensation is included to assess protective sensation.[68] This examination is performed using the 5.07 (10-g) Semmes-Weinstein nylon monofilament mounted on a holder that has been standardized to deliver a 10-g force when applied properly. Because the sensory deficits appear first in the most distal portions of the foot and progress proximally in a "stocking" distribution, the toes are the first areas to lose protective sensation. The examination should include assessment for treatable nail conditions, such as paronychia and ingrown toenails. The main purpose of the foot examination in children is to teach that foot care is an important health habit.

Nail care___________

Shoes: adequate length and width __________

Diagram

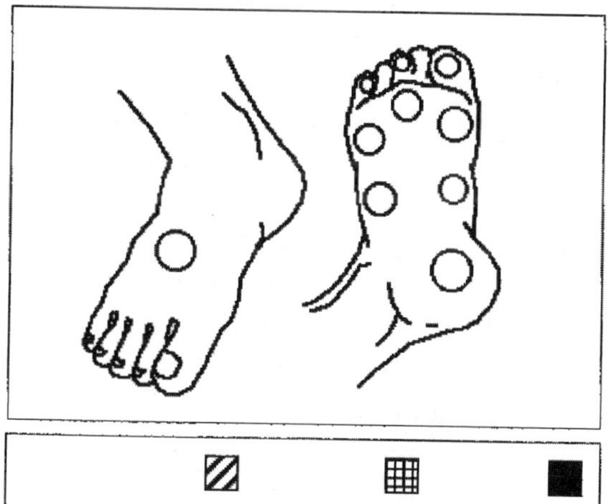

Pre-Ulcer

Label: Skin condition with R – Redness, S – Swelling, W – Warmth, D – Dryness, M – Maceration

	R	L
DP* pulse	________	________
Sensory Examination (5.07 monofilament, 10 g pressure)	________	________
Skin	________	________

*DP indicates dorsalis pedis.

Figure 2. Foot screening for youth with diabetes.

A funduscopic examination with dilation to detect signs of diabetic retinopathy is recommended shortly after diagnosis and then annually by an experienced eye care professional.[69,70]

Yeast vaginitis and balanitis are commonly seen in children and adolescents with type 2 diabetes mellitus.[71] Inspection of the vulva and penis should be included in the physical examination to screen for these disorders. Tanner staging of children and adolescents with type 2 diabetes mellitus should be performed every 3 to 6 months until puberty is complete, because early onset of puberty is noted in overnourished children.[72,73] A gynecologic examination for girls and a genital examination for boys may provide an opportunity to obtain additional sexual history and to offer abstinence and contraceptive counseling. Menstrual irregularities may be symptoms of PCOS in postpubertal girls.

LABORATORY EVALUATION

The fasting plasma glucose (FPG) concentration is the standard test for diagnosis. Monitoring is based on the FPG concentration and additional blood glucose measurements throughout the day. Fasting is defined as no consumption of food or any beverage other than water for at least 8 hours before testing. Most monitoring is performed by self-monitoring of blood glucose (SMBG) concentrations. Tables 4 and 5 include diagnostic and self-monitoring values.

The 2-hour postprandial glucose test provides information about glucose metabolism that is not provided by FPG measurement. It can be used for diagnosis together with FPG testing and must be used for monitoring.

Table 4. Impaired Glucose Metabolism

Test	Impaired	Diagnostic for Diabetes
Fasting glucose	≥110 mg/dL and <126 mg/dL	≥126 mg/dL
Impaired 2-h OGTT	≥140 mg/dL and <200 mg/dL	≥200 mg/dL

Measurement of HbA_{1c} concentration should be performed quarterly. The results should be available at the time of the patient visit and discussed with the patient. Technology is available to perform rapid HbA_{1c} testing. Many diabetes clinics have standing orders for the performance of HbA_{1c} testing before the health care professional's consultation and discussion with the patient. The HbA_{1c} result can verify SMBG data and is useful for identifying the need to adjust insulin dosage when SMBG data are unavailable. Setting realistic short-and long-term goals in consultation with a pediatric endocrinologist or other health care professional knowledgeable about childhood type 2 diabetes mellitus is recommended whenever possible. The HbA_{1c} concentration goal is less than 7.0% (or <1% above the laboratory reference range). This may not be achievable for all patients. Realistic goals should be individualized for each patient. HbA_{1c} concentration greater than 8.0% is associated with a substantial increase in complications.[74] Any sustained decrease is beneficial.

It is important to screen for proteinuria at diagnosis and annually. Testing for microalbuminuria is indicated if proteinuria is absent. Microalbuminuria is a high urinary albumin concentration that is not detected on routine dipstick testing. Microalbuminuria is defined as a urinary albumin excretion of 20 to 200 µg per minute (30–300 mg per day). Annual screening for microalbuminuria permits early identification and treatment of patients who are at risk of nephropathy. The recommended method of detection is the measurement of the albumin-creatinine ratio in a spot urine collection. An alternative method uses reagent tablets or dipsticks that detect microalbuminuria. When positive, the results of rapid tests should be confirmed by the urinary albumin-creatinine ratio in a timed urine collection. A patient is not designated as having microalbuminuria unless 2 of 3 collections performed within a 3- to 6-month period show increased concentrations. This test is not valid if the patient has a urinary tract infection or during menses. Although microalbuminuria may be encountered in patients in whom type 2 diabetes mellitus is newly diagnosed, proteinuria is the hallmark of diabetic nephropathy (Fig 3).[19,75,76]

The serum creatinine concentration should be determined at diagnosis and when indicated for drug therapy. Annual serum creatinine screening is indicated for patients with hypertension or microalbuminuria and for people taking angiotensin-converting enzyme (ACE) inhibitors.

Table 5. Ongoing Evaluation and Monitoring After Diagnosis: Laboratory Evaluation*

Test	Frequency	Recommendations
SMBG	Fasting and 2-h postprandial glucose daily	Individualized
FPG test	Initially and ongoing	
2-h postprandial glucose test	At diagnosis and as needed	
HbA_{1c}	Every 3 mo	
Urinalysis	Every 12 mo	
Microalbuminuria	Every 12 mo	
Creatinine	At diagnosis	And per protocol if there is hypertension, microalbuminuria, or ACE inhibitor treatment
Lipid profile	At diagnosis and every 12 mo	
LFTs	At diagnosis	Before initiating oral hypoglycemic agents

LFT indicates liver function test.

*More frequent monitoring at diagnosis, during initiation of new treatment, and during metabolic changes (illness, stress, increased activity, and growth).

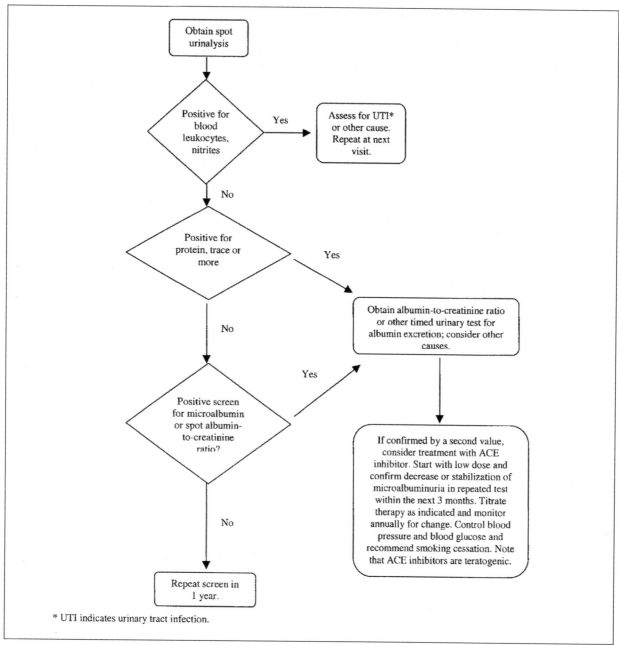

Figure 3. Annual evaluation and treatment for microalbuminuria.

A fasting lipid profile, including total cholesterol, low-density lipoprotein (LDL), high-density lipoprotein (HDL), and triglyceride concentrations, should be performed after diagnosis. The fasting lipid profile is best obtained after initial metabolic stabilization (1–3 months after diagnosis). The primary goal of therapy is to lower the LDL concentration,[77] which is discussed further in "Decreasing Cardiovascular Risk."

Liver function tests, including aspartate transaminase and alanine transaminase, should be performed before initiation of oral hypoglycemic therapy. Additional monitoring may be required depending on the person's drug regimen.

The concentrations of C peptide and insulin should not be measured routinely.[2,3] When differentiation between type 1 and type 2 diabetes mellitus is difficult, consultation with a subspecialist with expertise in type 2 diabetes mellitus in children and adolescents is recommended. There currently is no definitive diagnostic tool to differentiate between type 1 and type 2 diabetes mellitus. The differentiation typically is made clinically on the basis of obesity, family history, ethnicity, age, pubertal status, and evidence of insulin resistance (eg, acanthosis nigricans, PCOS).

Treatment

GOALS OF TREATMENT

The goals of treatment are adequate metabolic control (HbA$_{1c}$ concentration <7%) and prevention of microvascular and macrovascular complications. More specific treatment objectives include the following:

- Eliminating symptoms of hyperglycemia
- Assisting the patient in maintaining a reasonable body weight (weight stabilization)
- Decreasing cardiovascular risk factors: hypertension, hyperlipidemia, hyperglycemia, microalbuminuria, sedentary lifestyle, and use of tobacco products
- Achieving overall improvement in the child's physical and emotional well-being

Recommended treatment modalities include dietary modification, increased physical activity, decreased sedentary behaviors, and pharmacologic intervention (primarily metformin and insulin). Therapy to achieve these goals should be individualized on the basis of the child's age, other illnesses, lifestyle, self-management skills, and level of motivation. Education and other interventions that enhance self-care behaviors are essential for the successful management of type 2 diabetes mellitus. In general, weight loss is not recommended for prepubertal children. Children with morbid obesity and resultant health consequences, such as sleep apnea, may be referred to a subspecialist for weight reduction or a multidisciplinary child obesity clinic. Weight stabilization is the goal until girls are menstruating and boys have reached Tanner stage 5. After pubertal growth is complete, weight loss may be appropriate.

BARRIERS TO CARE

A functional and supportive environment is key in the treatment of children and adolescents with type 2 diabetes mellitus. One of the most serious barriers to achieving the goals of management is a dysfunctional family situation. The medical model of focusing only on the identified patient instead of treating the entire family further decreases the effectiveness of care.

Additional barriers exist for AI/AN youth. Environmental obstacles (eg, harsh climate, lack of transportation, limited access to healthy foods) create difficulties. Specific tribal or cultural issues, including beliefs and feelings about diabetes, may interfere with optimal self-care. For example, many families have a fatalistic attitude about diabetes: "My parents died of diabetes. I have it, and my children are going to get it." Eating and mood disorders, life stresses, and low self-esteem are common obstacles. Lack of appropriate role models, particularly healthy individuals living with diabetes, creates significant hardship for AI/AN children with diabetes. A low level of reading comprehension and proficiency in English may add additional barriers for some families. Furthermore, substance abuse is particularly problematic for many AI/AN children and their families. The health care system's frequent lack of understanding and respect for cultural beliefs may be a barrier to achieving optimal self-care. Many strategies have been shown to help overcome such barriers, including the use of trained professional interpreters, cultural competence and humility training for health care professionals and staff, and inclusion of members of the community in the design of clinical services.

TEAM MANAGEMENT

Multidisciplinary team management is strongly recommended for youth with type 2 diabetes mellitus. A primary health care professional alone usually cannot provide focused diabetes education, nutrition management, and psychosocial support. The team usually is composed of a physician, a registered dietitian, a nurse clinician, a social worker, and the patient and the family. The patient and the family are integral members of the team, and participation of the child or adolescent with the diabetes team should be frequent and ongoing. The diabetes team monitors the patient's knowledge about diabetes and its acute and chronic complications. The team also assesses and monitors the patient's knowledge and attitudes toward nutrition and physical activity. In addition, the team promotes the use of medications, SMBG, and problem-solving skills. Screening for barriers to self-care is recommended at each visit. The team assists in identification of achievable self-care goals that are appropriate for age and development level.

Many AI/AN health care facilities have existing diabetes clinics with multidisciplinary teams. It is highly recommended that these clinics organize a pediatric component so that youth receive developmentally appropriate care.

LIFESTYLE MODIFICATIONS

The cornerstones of initial treatment of type 2 diabetes mellitus are acquiring and integrating healthful behaviors in nutrition, exercise, and weight management. Frequent contact with the health care team is required to accomplish these goals. The approach to healthful living must be emphasized throughout diabetes treatment. Initially, type 2 diabetes mellitus in asymptomatic youth may be managed by lifestyle modification without adjunctive medication. Basic diabetes education, counseling, and SMBG should be included. The natural history of type 2 diabetes mellitus is one of progressive insulin insufficiency and deterioration of metabolic control.[78-84] Therefore, close monitoring and follow-up are important. Eventually, most people with type 2 diabetes mellitus require medication to achieve adequate metabolic control (Tables 4 and 5).

RESOURCES

Many resources are available for health care professionals and their patients to help achieve therapeutic goals. However, there is a great need for more culturally sensitive educational materials. Information prepared for adults often is confusing to children and adolescents. Furthermore, resources for children and families with type 1 diabetes mellitus do not apply easily to families affected by type 2 diabetes mellitus.

The National Diabetes Education Program (NDEP) is a federally sponsored initiative of the National Institute of Diabetes and Digestive and Kidney Diseases of the National Institutes of Health, the CDC, and more than 200 public and private partners to improve treatment and outcomes for people with diabetes, promote early diagnosis, and, ultimately, prevent the onset of diabetes. The objectives of the NDEP are to:

● Increase public awareness of the seriousness of diabetes and its risk factors and strategies for preventing diabetes and its complications
● Improve understanding about diabetes and its control and promote better self-management behaviors among people with diabetes
● Improve health care professionals' understanding of diabetes and its control and promote an integrated approach to care
● Promote health care policies that improve the quality of and access to diabetes care

Target audiences include people with diabetes and their families (with special attention to Hispanic, black, and Asian Americans; Pacific Islanders; and the AI/AN population); the general public; health care professionals; and health care payers, purchasers, and policy makers.

The NDEP has convened a Diabetes in Children and Adolescents Work Group to address awareness and education issues related to children with diabetes, including the growing emergence of type 2 diabetes mellitus in youth. Furthermore, the NDEP American Indian/Alaska Native Work Group is focusing on youth with diabetes. The NDEP aims to assist health care professionals in increasing their knowledge about type 2 diabetes mellitus in children and adolescents; diabetes education materials for patients and health care professionals can be obtained from NDEP. For more information about the NDEP, see its Internet site at http://www.ndep.nih.gov or call 800-438-5383. Materials for educators about the management of diabetes in school settings are available.

The ADA has a useful diabetes education program called WIZDOM, which includes specific patient education material in English and Spanish for youth with type 2 diabetes mellitus. Information can be found at the following Internet site: http://www.diabetes.org/wizdom/pod.asp.

Management Tools

SELF-MONITORING OF BLOOD GLUCOSE

The frequency of SMBG should be individualized. Daily fasting and 2-hour postprandial (after-dinner) glucose measurements are recommended.[5] More frequent monitoring is recommended during initiation of treatment. Furthermore, monitoring frequency should be increased during the following situations: insulin treatment, medication dosage adjustments, initiation of new therapies, increased activity, rapid growth, illness, and emotional stress. The frequency of SMBG may be negotiated with the patient and the family. For people who take insulin, the recommended frequency is before every meal and at bedtime. The recommended method is a blood glucose meter with memory. It can be instructive for patients to record their blood glucose results in a log to determine patterns. Reviewing these results with the patient at each visit is recommended. Many patients on medication will learn to make their own dosage adjustments on the basis of blood glucose patterns.

- Ideal targets: more than 50% of SMBG concentrations within target range:
  - Fasting: 80 to 120 mg/dL (4.4–6.7 mmol/L)
  - Postprandial (2 hours after start of meal): 100 to 160 mg/dL (5.6–8.9 mmol/L)
  - Bedtime: 100 to 160 mg/dL (5.6–8.9 mmol/L)

MEDICAL NUTRITION THERAPY

Meal planning, nutrition education, and exercise are primary treatment strategies for type 2 diabetes mellitus. All people with diabetes should receive regular nutrition counseling and consult with a registered dietitian or nutritionist or a diabetes educator at least every 6 to 12 months. Some children may require more frequent evaluation and counseling. The success of the child in adopting healthful eating habits is much more likely when the entire family follows the dietary recommendations. Other family members may be able to serve as role models. Assisting the family and the patient in change related to eating behavior is recommended.[85] For example, some families will choose to purchase more fruits and vegetables and make them more readily available to all family members. Families may choose to discourage eating outside of mealtimes and make rules about limiting eating while watching television. Weight management must be individualized for the patient initially and in follow-up visits. Each encounter is an opportunity for nutritional education.

DIABETES EDUCATION

Patients and their families require diabetes self-care information that is culturally relevant. It is important to recognize that there are many different tribal cultures. The National Standards for Diabetes Care and Patient Education provide guidelines for education program development with criteria specific for Native American health care facilities.[86] In addition, adolescents have distinct needs related to the culture of youth.

Education alone is not enough to motivate people to adopt more healthful behaviors. Children and adolescents, in particular, are not easily motivated by long-term health consequences, which seem irrelevant to them. They are more likely to be influenced by immediate concerns, such as physical attractiveness, feelings of well-being and acceptance, and their desire to be able to do more in school or sports. The use of motivational interviewing or collaborative problem solving may be useful in helping children and adolescents make and maintain necessary behavior changes.

PHYSICAL ACTIVITY EDUCATION

Physical activity is a cornerstone of the management of type 2 diabetes mellitus. Physical goals should be stated concretely. Exercise is associated with improvement in short- and long-term metabolic control,[87,88] and physical activity improves insulin sensitivity. All patients should be assessed for level of fitness and current exercise routines. Recommendations should be based on the patient's needs and current condition. It is important to assess the opportunities available within the family and the community. Adaptive physical education classes may be helpful for children who are overweight. Youth with obesity and type 2 diabetes mellitus are not likely to participate in organized sports, so other physical activity strategies are needed. Activities of daily living can be adapted to increase physical fitness.[88-91]

Sedentary activities should be limited, and positive alternatives should be emphasized. When making behavioral changes, simple, achievable goals promote efficacy. Children and adolescents are more likely to accept fitness goals when they are framed in terms of feeling better, looking better, or doing more.[31]

PRECONCEPTION COUNSELING AND MANAGEMENT

A sexual activity history should be obtained at diagnosis in postpubertal youth. Counseling about the necessity of metabolic control for healthful pregnancy outcomes should start at puberty. Abstinence counseling should be provided, if appropriate. Family planning options should be discussed with adolescents who are or may become sexually active. Pregnancy should be deferred until optimal glycemic control has been achieved to decrease first-trimester risks to the fetus, including congenital heart disease, caudal regression, and neural tube defects, and third-trimester risks of macrosomia, neonatal hypoglycemia, and hypocalcemia, all of which are common in preexisting type 2 diabetes mellitus and gestational diabetes. All oral hypoglycemic agents are contraindicated during pregnancy. Furthermore, treatment of diabetes may increase fertility and the likelihood of pregnancy in young women. Metformin, in particular, may improve ovarian function and ovulation.

IMMUNIZATIONS

Usual childhood immunizations (including hepatitis B, influenza, and pneumococcal immunizations) are recommended. Tuberculosis screening by purified protein derivative should be documented once after the diagnosis of diabetes and performed at appropriate intervals, as indicated by community-specific tuberculosis prevalence.

DENTAL EXAMINATIONS

Dental examinations are recommended every 6 months. Periodontal disease is more common in people with diabetes than in those without and has been called the sixth complication of diabetes

(the other 5 complications involve the heart, kidney, eyes, skin, and feet).[92-94]

Decreasing Cardiovascular Risk

IDENTIFICATION AND TREATMENT OF HYPERLIPIDEMIA

Children with type 2 diabetes mellitus are at risk of hyperlipidemia, which compounds their risk of premature cardiovascular disease. Although the American Heart Association recommends that children's total cholesterol concentration be less than 170 mg/dL (<4.40 mmol/L) and the LDL concentration be less than 110 mg/dL (<2.84 mmol/L), the ADA recommends a lower target concentration for LDL in adults with diabetes[28,87,95]: less than 100 mg/dL (<2.59 mmol/L). Because of the higher risk of cardiovascular disease in children with diabetes, the lower acceptable value recommended by the ADA is preferred. A lipoprotein analysis after a 12-hour fast is recommended to obtain triglyceride concentrations for computation of accurate LDL concentrations,[95] although recent evidence indicates non-HDL cholesterol is a better predictor of atherogenesis than LDL cholesterol. If a fasting measurement is not possible, then a measurement of the HDL concentration, along with the total cholesterol concentration, will provide an alternative. Other reliable analyses of the lipid profile may become available in the future. Children with an LDL concentration more than 100 mg/dL (>2.59 mmol/L) or a total cholesterol concentration more than 170 mg/dL (>4.40 mmol/L) should receive advice about other risk factors for cardiovascular disease, such as smoking and sedentary lifestyle. High triglyceride concentrations are increasingly recognized as an additional cardiovascular risk factor for people with diabetes. In addition to studies showing the benefit of decreasing the cholesterol concentration in adults, the Bogalusa Heart Study provides evidence that risk factors, such as a low HDL concentration, high triglyceride and LDL concentrations, and smoking, have clinical significance for development of cardiovascular disease beginning in childhood.[96-98]

The American Heart Association Step-One diet should be initiated for children with high total cholesterol or LDL concentrations. The Step-One diet includes fewer than 30% of total calories from fat, fewer than 10% of total calories from saturated fat, 10% or fewer calories from polyunsaturated fat, and cholesterol of no more than 100 mg/1000 cal. If cholesterol concentrations do not normalize despite a history of adherence to the Step-One diet, then the Step-Two diet is used. The Step-Two diet is lower in total cholesterol (67 mg/1000 cal) and saturated fat (<7% of total cal). People who follow these diets should be reevaluated every 6–12 months. More information about the Step-One and the Step-Two diets can be found on the American Heart Association's Internet site at http://www.americanheart.org. The assistance of a registered dietitian or other qualified nutrition professional is necessary to ensure adequacy of nutrients, vitamins, and minerals. Glycemic control, as well as therapy with metformin, can help to lower triglyceride and LDL concentrations. Cholesterol-lowering drug therapy should be considered for children older than 10 years if an adequate trial of diet therapy is unsuccessful after 6 to 12 months. An LDL concentration of 100 mg/dL or more (≥2.59 mmol/L) and 1 of the following risk factors or physical inactivity indicate a need for cholesterol lowering medication: family history of premature cardiovascular disease (55 years or younger), cigarette smoking, high blood pressure, low HDL concentration (<35 mg/dL [<0.91 mmol/L]), and obesity (≥95th percentile weight for height).

The recommended cholesterol-lowering medications for children include cholestyramine and colestipol hydrochloride. These medications are difficult to take because of the frequency of dosing and adverse gastrointestinal effects. Although the efficacy and safety of these medications have been documented in children, long-term data on improved morbidity and mortality are lacking.[77] The 3-hydroxy-3-methylglutaryl coenzyme A reductase inhibitors (statins) are now approved for use in children who have familial hyperlipidemia and are 10 years of age and older. They are being used and tested in pediatric populations for other indications. Rhabdomyolysis is a known adverse effect, and safety during pregnancy has not been proved. Specialty consultation may be helpful for treating youth with hyperlipidemia.

BLOOD PRESSURE CONTROL

In adults, tight blood pressure control has been shown to have a greater impact on cardiovascular disease risk reduction than blood glucose control.[99-102] Systemic hypertension is defined as systolic or diastolic pressure greater than or equal to the 95th percentile for age.[103] However, for children with type 2 diabetes mellitus, the blood pressure goal is less than the 90th percentile. Accurate blood pressure measurement is critical to the evaluation of suspected hypertension. The patient should be resting and comfortable. Cuff size, the position of the arm, the person's position (sitting or supine), and the speed of inflation and deflation of the cuff can affect the measurement. The cuff bladder width should be approximately 40% of the arm circumference midway between the olecranon and the acromion. The arm should be supported, and the cubital fossa should be at the level of the heart. The bell of the stethoscope should be placed over the brachial artery pulse. The cuff should be inflated to 20 mm Hg above the point at which the radial pulse disappears. The cuff is then deflated at a rate of 2 to 3 mm Hg per second. Automated devices are not as accurate for determining diastolic pressure. The diagnosis of hypertension should be confirmed in 3 separate consecutive examinations. For mild hypertension (slightly above the 95th percentile), the initial assessment should evaluate the possibility of renal disease. The evaluation of severe hypertension (≥99th percentile for age) should include an echocardiogram.

Conservative management (eg, lifestyle changes, such as weight decrease in postpubertal patients, nutrition, and exercise) is recommended as initial therapy. Sodium restriction may be difficult for adolescents. Significant reduction in blood pressure may be noted with weight loss and exercise programs. If blood pressure reduction is not achieved by lifestyle changes, then drug therapy will be necessary. ACE inhibitors are the usual first-line agents because of cardiovascular and renal benefits.[104,105] Because ACE inhibitors are teratogenic, another agent might be preferable for girls of childbearing age. Beta-blockers are an alternative unless the child is taking insulin, as symptoms of hypoglycemia may be masked.

SMOKING AND ALCOHOL CESSATION AND PREVENTION AND INCREASING PHYSICAL ACTIVITY

Smoking cessation and prevention of smoking initiation are essential for decreasing the risk of cardiovascular problems. Smoking is associated with an increased incidence of diabetes in adults.[106] It is important to screen for tobacco use and advise or refer for tobacco cessation if use is confirmed. Tobacco use information should be updated at each visit. Because of the greatly increased risk of macrovascular and microvascular disease in people who have diabetes and smoke,[107] children and adolescents who do not smoke or use other tobacco products should receive positive reinforcement and information about the importance of continued abstinence.

Alcohol affects insulin production and increases insulin resistance, which also increases the risk of cardiovascular complications. The independent risk of cardiovascular complications associated with alcohol consumption by people with diabetes is a long-term hazard for youth with diabetes. A more immediate risk is hypoglycemia caused by alcohol consumption.

Alcohol use may aggravate the hypoglycemia caused by sulfonylureas or insulin treatment, and it may increase the risk of lactic acidosis for patients who use metformin. Alcohol and drug use should be assessed at every visit. Adolescents are at risk of substance abuse, which may interfere with the achievement of treatment goals. Anticipatory guidance regarding alcohol avoidance is recommended, including for children and adolescents who do not use alcohol or other drugs. The benefits of not drinking should be emphasized. The effectiveness of creative strategies should be evaluated.

Increasing physical activity is a positive way to decrease risk of cardiovascular complications.

TREATMENT OF MICROALBUMINURIA

Microalbuminuria is a sign of incipient diabetic nephropathy and is a risk factor for cardiovascular complications. Microalbuminuria may be encountered in people who have a new diagnosis of type 2 diabetes mellitus. Proteinuria, conversely, is the hallmark of diabetic nephropathy. ACE inhibitors are indicated for proteinuria or microalbuminuria and have been shown to slow the rate of progression of nephropathy in adults. Improved glycemic and blood pressure control slows the progression of nephropathy. ACE inhibitors are an additional important treatment modality, as shown in the evaluation and treatment algorithm (Fig 3).

Pharmacologic Management on the Basis of Clinical Manifestations

The options for pharmacologic treatment include insulin; oral hypoglycemic agents, especially metformin; and any combination thereof. Intensive blood glucose control with insulin or sulfonylureas has been shown to decrease microvascular but not macrovascular complications.[79] The choice of medications is discussed in relation to the patient's status at diagnosis. The following sections are given in order of increasing severity and decreasing incidence.

IMPAIRED GLUCOSE METABOLISM

Patients with impaired glucose tolerance and impaired fasting glucose have glucose concentrations too high to be considered normal but do not meet the diagnostic criteria for diabetes. They are considered to have prediabetes. Patients with impaired fasting glucose have FPG$^{\parallel}$ concentrations of 110 mg/dL or more (≥6.1 mmol/L) but less than 126 mg/dL (<7.0 mmol/L). Patients with prediabetes have 2-hour OGTT results between 140 and 200 mg/dL (7.8 and 11.1 mmol/L [Table 5]). Compared with the FPG, the 2-hour OGTT will identify more people as having impaired glucose tolerance. Although the 2-hour OGTT is more sensitive than the FPG, it is not as reproducible. It is, therefore, important to identify which test was used for diagnosis. An increase in

---

$^{\parallel}$When glucose concentration is measured in a laboratory, plasma glucose concentration is measured. When a self-monitoring system is used, blood glucose concentration is measured; in most cases, these values are similar.

the postprandial glucose concentration precedes an increase in the FPG concentration in adults. The natural history of impaired glucose tolerance in children and adolescents has not been studied. The US Diabetes Prevention Program has shown that lifestyle interventions are more effective than metformin and both approaches are more promising than conventional treatment in reducing progression to diabetes in adults with impaired glucose tolerance.[108] Similarly, a study of Finnish adults was interrupted because of the success of the lifestyle intervention arm.[109] Patients with prediabetes and their families should receive nutrition and physical activity intervention and support. Their risk of diabetes should be discussed. Monitoring of weight, nutrition, physical activity, and FPG should be performed regularly (at least every 3 months). Some diabetes centers recommend SMBG for high-risk patients with impaired glucose metabolism.

ASYMPTOMATIC DIABETES

People with diabetes may be identified as part of community-based case-finding efforts or by primary health care professionals who test asymptomatic children and youth who are at risk of type 2 diabetes mellitus. Patients with an FPG concentration of 126 mg/dL or more ($\geq$7.0 mmol/L) or a 2-hour plasma glucose concentration of 200 mg/dL or more ($\geq$11.1 mmol/L), using a glucose load of 75 g of anhydrous glucose dissolved in water, but who do not have polyuria, polydipsia, or weight loss are considered to have asymptomatic type 2 diabetes mellitus. When diabetes is identified early, treatment with lifestyle modifications and SMBG (fasting and postprandial) may be instituted. If plasma glucose or HbA$_{1c}$ concentrations remain increased for 3 months, then treatment with oral agents or insulin should be started. Patients who attain euglycemia through lifestyle modification should be monitored every 3 months.

People with an FPG concentration greater than 250 mg/dL (>13.9 mmol/L) should be treated as if they have symptoms, even if they report none.

SYMPTOMATIC DIABETES WITHOUT KETOACIDOSIS

Symptoms include polyuria and polydipsia, nocturia, sleep apnea, vaginitis, dysuria, and even weight loss. Many families do not recognize polyuria and polydipsia in adolescents. Educational approaches to raise adolescent awareness about the potential significance of the symptoms of increased thirst and urination could encourage teenagers to alert their families and primary health care professionals.

Insulin

Initial treatment with subcutaneous insulin is suggested for children with FPG concentrations greater than 250 mg/dL (>13.9 mmol/L) and for children who are symptomatic. First Nations children with type 2 diabetes mellitus have been treated with subcutaneous insulin for 2 to 6 weeks followed by abrupt discontinuation of treatment with acceptable metabolic control.[110]

The use of insulin in children and adolescents with type 2 diabetes mellitus is safe.[2,3,111-113] Preliminary data suggest that early insulin therapy may preserve beta cell function in type 1 diabetes mellitus. This may be true in type 2 diabetes mellitus as well.[114,115] Symptomatic youth often have evidence of the toxic effects of glucose or a transient deterioration of beta cell function brought on by prolonged hyperglycemia. Thus, insulin often is needed for initial metabolic control. When C peptide or insulin concentrations are obtained at diagnosis, they may be uncharacteristically low. Therefore, if C peptide concentrations are measured to determine whether a patient has type 1 or type 2 diabetes mellitus, then it is best to wait until adequate metabolic control is obtained.

The recommended starting dose of insulin is individualized from 0.5 to 1.0 U/kg body weight per day. Additional insulin may be given if blood glucose concentrations do not fall below 150 mg/dL (8.3 mmol/L) before meals. Insulin dosage must be adjusted to achieve target blood glucose concentrations. Children and adolescents with type 2 diabetes mellitus often require much higher doses of insulin because of insulin resistance.

Insulin regimens must be individualized. Some patients may require only intermediate-acting insulin (isophane [neutral protamine Hagedorn (NPH)] or lente) given once or twice daily. Others may require short- or rapid-acting insulin (regular or lispro/aspart) and intermediate-acting insulin (NPH or lente) with a distribution of two thirds of the total dose before breakfast and one third of the total dose before dinner.[116] As with type 1 diabetes mellitus, an initial regimen might be to give the morning dose as one third regular or lispro/aspart and two thirds NPH or lente and the evening dose as one half regular or lispro/aspart and one half NPH or lente.[117] It may be more physiologically appropriate to give the evening intermediate-acting insulin at bedtime.[118] Lispro and aspart have certain advantages over regular insulin—its action profile provides insulin coverage for meals, and the dose can be adjusted according to the amount of food to be eaten. Other regimens that have proved successful are the use of the long-acting insulin glargine in conjunction with an oral hypoglycemic agent that increases endogenous insulin secretion to cover meals.

These dosage recommendations are to be considered a starting point, because insulin dosing must be adjusted on the basis of the blood glucose concentration. As metabolic control is achieved, insulin dosages start to decrease. It is not necessary to initiate insulin treatment with frequent dosing of rapid-acting insulin before meals. Using intermediate- and rapid-acting insulin early in treatment permits more rapid stabilization of glucose concentrations. When the health care professional judges that insulin will be required over the long-term, the person may be taught to give bolus insulin doses before meals, depending on the amount of carbohydrate to be consumed. Oral agents may be started once the glucose concentration is stabilized, and the insulin dosage gradually can be weaned. The glucose concentration usually is stable between 3 and 4 weeks after the initiation of therapy.[29]

Oral Agents

The recently completed United Kingdom Prospective Diabetes Study demonstrated that type 2 diabetes mellitus is a progressive disorder that can be treated initially with oral agent monotherapy.[79,80] Current recommendations for adults suggest beginning oral monotherapy if target glycemic goals are not achieved within 1 to 3 months of initial intervention of lifestyle modification. This period may not be practical for many AI/AN youth because of greater barriers to achieving activity and nutritional goals. A longer period may be warranted only if there is slow and steady improvement in achieving target glycemic goals.

Metformin is the only oral hypoglycemic agent approved for use in children. Data are not yet available regarding the safety, efficacy, or dosing of the other oral agents used to treat type 2 diabetes mellitus in children, although such data are available for adults. The biguanides (eg, metformin) and the sulfonylureas (eg, glyburide) have been part of the clinical experience in the treatment of type 2 diabetes mellitus in children. Sulfonylureas have been used for several years in the treatment of maturity-onset diabetes of youth, a set of rare, genetically determined diabetes. Use of metformin has increased in recent years, and clinical trials are in progress.

Metformin

The ADA consensus statement recommends that "if treatment goals with nutrition education and exercise are not met, pharmacologic therapy is indicated. The first oral agent should be metformin."[2,3,118] Metformin works by decreasing hepatic glucose production and enhancing insulin sensitivity. It is contraindicated for people with renal or hepatic disease, conditions that lead to hypoxia (eg, unstable asthma), or severe infection or those who abuse alcohol. It should be withheld before radiographic studies requiring the administration of radiocontrast dye. Metformin improves ovarian function, especially in women with PCOS, making family planning and contraception (when indicated) important. Lactic acidosis rarely has been reported.[119] Gastrointestinal adverse effects, such as abdominal discomfort and diarrhea, occur in approximately 20% to 30% of people who take metformin. These effects can be minimized by slowly titrating the dose and beginning with 250 mg each day, increasing to 250 mg twice daily, and finally increasing to 500 mg twice daily, if necessary. In adults, 80% to 85% of the maximal glucose-lowering effect is observed with a daily dose of 1500 mg. Most children who require treatment are at or above normal adult weight. Therefore, beginning at a dose of 500 mg per day would be considered safe. In adults, a clinically significant response at a dosage of less than 1500 mg per day is unusual. Metformin is supplied as 500- and 850-mg tablets and extended-release tablets. The maximum recommended daily dosage of metformin is 2550 mg. The current cost of metformin is approximately twice that of a second-generation sulfonylurea. However, less costly generic medications should soon be available. Advantages of metformin include decreased weight gain, possible weight loss, lower insulin concentrations, and improved lipid profile.[29,120]

Sulfonylureas

The primary mechanism of action of the sulfonylureas is enhancement of insulin secretion. In adults in whom type 2 diabetes mellitus has recently been diagnosed, good results have been achieved with mild to moderate fasting hyperglycemia (220–240 mg/dL [12.2–13.3 mmol/L]), good beta cell function as reflected by a high fasting C peptide concentration, and the absence of islet-cell or glutamic acid decarboxylase antibodies. No sulfonylureas are currently approved for use in children, although studies in the pediatric population with second-generation agents are ongoing. In most studies in adults, sulfonylureas have had neutral or slightly beneficial effects on plasma lipid concentrations. Weight gain is common with use, a negative effect in patients in whom weight loss is a major goal. Most pediatric endocrinologists use sulfonylureas with other agents when monotherapy with metformin or insulin sensitizers has failed. First-generation sulfonylureas (chlorpropamide, tolazamide, acetohexamide, and tolbutamide) must be given in higher doses than second-generation sulfonylureas (glyburide,

glipizide, and glimepiride). The second-generation sulfonylureas are largely free of drug interactions. The major adverse effect associated with sulfonylureas is hypoglycemia. Most of the hypoglycemic action of the sulfonylurea is observed with a daily dose that represents half of the maximally effective dose. Sulfonylureas may potentiate the hypoglycemia associated with alcohol use. Therefore, alcohol consumption is contraindicated when a person is taking a sulfonylurea. Other adverse effects are uncommon but include nausea; vomiting; and skin reactions, including rashes, purpura, and pruritus. Leukopenia, thrombocytopenia, hemolytic anemia, and cholestasis have been reported. Although a 1970 study[121] suggested that sulfonylureas may exacerbate coronary artery disease in people with type 2 diabetes mellitus, the ADA issued a statement in 1979 opposing any formal restrictions on use of the sulfonylurea agents on the basis of interpretation of that study. In addition, the United Kingdom Prospective Diabetes Study found no increased incidence of coronary artery disease for patients with type 2 diabetes mellitus who were assigned to intensive therapy with sulfonylureas, compared with patients who received dietary therapy without medications. The sulfonylureas have an additional advantage of low cost. Table 6 outlines the characteristics of select sulfonylureas.[122,123]

Repaglinide

Repaglinide is a new agent. Like the sulfonylureas, it enhances the release of insulin, but the response is quicker and of shorter duration than that of sulfonylureas. Repaglinide's glucose-lowering effect is additive to the glucose-lowering effect of metformin. Furthermore, repaglinide has no significant effect on plasma lipid concentrations. Repaglinide must be taken before each meal because of its short duration of action. Thus, its primary effect is on the postprandial blood glucose concentration.

Thiazolidinediones

Thiazolidinediones (TZDs) work primarily by increasing insulin sensitivity in muscle and adipose tissue with a lesser effect on hepatic glucose uptake. The first TZD to be marketed

Table 6. Pharmacologic Characteristics of Sulfonylureas[123]

Characteristics	Tolbutamide	Tolazamide	Chlorpropamide	Glipizide	Glyburide
Relative potency	1	5	6	100	150
Duration of action (h)	6–10	16–24	24–72	16–24	18–24
Dose (mg)					
Range	500–3000	100–1000	100–500	2.5–40*	1.25–20
Average	1500	250	250	10	7.5†
Doses per day (n)	2–3	1–2	1	1–2	1–2
Dosage forms available (mg)	250, 500	100, 250, 500	100, 250	5, 10	1.25, 2.5, 5
Diuretic	Yes	Yes	No	No	Yes
Frequency of severe hypoglycemia (%)	1	1	4–6	2–4	4–6
Overall frequency of side effects (%)	3	4	9	6	7

* Studies have shown that the maximum effective dose of glipizide is 10 mg/dL. Doses above this may cause decreased efficacy.

† Glyburide is available worldwide as better-absorbed micronized preparations. These preparations are available in 1.5-, 1.75-, 3-, 3.7-, and 6-mg tablets.

in the United States, troglitazone, was taken off the market because of hepatotoxic effects. However, the newer agents in this class seem to have an improved safety profile. Although not approved for children, clinical trials in the pediatric population are in progress. Because TZDs increase insulin sensitivity, they have a favorable effect on HDL and triglyceride concentrations. Studies in adults indicate that TZDs result in a 1% to 2% decrease in HbA$_{1c}$ values when used as monotherapy, although monotherapy is not recommended. Adverse effects include weight gain and fluid retention. TZDs may decrease the effectiveness of oral contraceptives. Another disadvantage is the high cost of this class of drugs. Dosing with pioglitazone hydrochloride is initiated at 15 mg daily with or without food. The dose can be increased after 8 to 12 weeks if the decrease in HbA$_{1c}$ is inadequate. The maximum daily dosage is 45 mg for monotherapy and 30 mg for combined therapy. The dosage does not need to be adjusted for patients with renal disease. Pioglitazone is available as 15-, 30-, and 45-mg tablets. Rosiglitazone maleate initially is given as a single 4-mg dose. The dose may be increased to 4 mg twice daily or 8 mg daily if the response is inadequate after 8 to 12 weeks; however, the maximum dosage is 8 mg daily. Like pioglitazone, rosiglitazone can be given with or without meals and does not need dosage adjustment for patients with renal failure. It is available in 4-and 8-mg tablets.

Acarbose

The α-glucosidase inhibitor acarbose was introduced in the United States in the late 1990s. It primarily affects postprandial glucose concentrations by delaying carbohydrate digestion.[124-126] Its major adverse effect, flatulence, has limited its acceptance in the pediatric population.

Combining Oral Agents

A maximal dose of a single oral agent (metformin or a sulfonylurea) may not maintain long-term acceptable glycemic control, according to ADA guidelines (FPG concentration <140 mg/dL [<7.8 mmol/L] or HbA$_{1c}$ value <8.0%).¶ Because type 2 diabetes mellitus is a progressive disease with decreasing beta cell function, most people with an initial acceptable response to monotherapy will require additional agents as their disease progresses.[127-129] Randomized, placebo-controlled studies of combination therapy support the effectiveness of this strategy for decreasing FPG and HbA$_{1c}$ concentrations.[130-132] When beta cells fail, insulin will need to be added to the therapeutic regimen.

Because metformin promotes weight loss and decreases lipid concentrations, it is preferred for use by overweight people with type 2 diabetes

---

¶The ADA currently recommends intensifying treatment on the basis of HbA$_{1c}$ concentration <8%. However, the recommended target goal for HbA$_{1c}$ concentration is <7%.

mellitus and dyslipidemia. The dose of metformin or sulfonylureas can be increased over a 4- to 8-week period until acceptable glucose control is achieved or the maximum dose is reached. If monotherapy fails with metformin, then a sulfonylurea should be added. It is prudent to assess whether the person is taking the medication as directed before initiating combination therapy. Patients may not take their medication for a variety of reasons, including denial of illness; fear of being labeled diabetic; fear of adverse effects, such as hypoglycemia; actual adverse symptoms; and lack of knowledge about the need for long-term treatment. If combination therapy with 2 oral agents does not achieve the desired therapeutic goal, then bedtime insulin or a third oral agent may be considered. Referral to a specialist in type 2 diabetes mellitus for children and adolescents is recommended when combination therapy has failed.

SYMPTOMATIC DIABETES WITH KETOACIDOSIS

Diabetic ketoacidosis is defined by a bicarbonate concentration less than 15 mmol/L (<15 mEq/L) and/or pH less than 7.25. Type 2 diabetes mellitus may manifest with ketosis and, uncommonly, with ketoacidosis. Therefore, clinical presentation with ketoacidosis does not preclude the diagnosis of type 2 diabetes mellitus.

Insulin

Children with diabetic ketoacidosis require initial treatment with intravenous insulin followed by subcutaneous insulin. High doses may be required because of the insulin resistance characteristic of type 2 diabetes mellitus.[133] Health care professionals, nurses, and laboratory professionals who care for a large number of patients with diabetic ketoacidosis are more likely to have the necessary clinical competence to provide this high-acuity care. When care by such personnel is not possible, consultation with a subspecialist is recommended. Excellent treatment protocols and guidelines are available for the treatment of ketoacidosis.[134-137] Once the patient's condition is stable, the important lifestyle modifications discussed previously can be addressed. As people often are willing to

consider major lifestyle changes during a crisis, this may be an optimal teachable moment.[137]

Conclusion

Type 2 diabetes mellitus in AI/AN youth is an alarming new morbidity that, without intervention, will lead to significant increased morbidity and mortality during adulthood. Health care professionals must address multiple medical and psychosocial concerns within the context of a medical home with the goal of coordinating comprehensive services from health care professionals and the community. Health care professionals who care for families affected by type 2 diabetes mellitus face the challenge of motivating people to adopt significant behavioral changes.

Several interventions have proved effective in preventing diabetes complications among adults, and evaluation of these interventions in children with type 2 diabetes mellitus is urgently needed. It is expected that clinical trials using behavioral and treatment interventions for children with diabetes will be developed. More knowledge about current care, gaps in care, and the natural history of the disease is forthcoming. Finally, results of research efforts in primary prevention of type 2 diabetes mellitus for adults and youth soon will be available. The increasing evidence base will challenge current treatment guidelines and ultimately improve the health of children with type 2 diabetes mellitus over their lifetimes.

TYPE 2 DIABETES SUBCOMMITTEE
Sheila Gahagan, MD, Chairperson
Indu Agarwal, MD
    AAP Committee on Native American
    Child Health
George Brenneman, MD
    AAP Committee on Native American
    Child Health
Anne Fagot-Campagna, MD, PhD
    Centers for Disease Control and Prevention
Kelly Moore, MD
    Indian Health Service
Terry Raymer, MD, CDE
    United Indian Health Services Inc
Janet Silverstein, MD
    AAP Section on Endocrinology

COMMITTEE ON NATIVE AMERICAN CHILD HEALTH
2002–2003
David C. Grossman, MD, MPH, Chairperson
Indu Agarwal, MD
Vincent M. Biggs, MD
George Brenneman, MD
Sheila Gahagan, MD
James N. Jarvis, MD
Harold Margolis, MD

LIAISONS
Joseph T. Bell, MD
    Association of American Indian Physicians
J. Chris Carey, MD
    American College of Obstetricians
    and Gynecologists
James Carson, MD
    Canadian Paediatric Society
Kelly R. Moore, MD
    Indian Health Service
Michael Storck, MD
    American Academy of Child and
    Adolescent Psychiatry

STAFF
Thomas Tonniges, MD

SECTION ON ENDOCRINOLOGY, 2002–2003
Janet Silverstein, MD, Chairperson
Kenneth Copeland, MD
Inger L. Hansen, MD
Francine R. Kaufman, MD
Susan R. Rose, MD
Robert P. Schwartz, MD
Surendra K. Varma, MD

LIAISONS
Judy Hartman, RN, BSN, MHS
    Pediatric Endocrinology Nursing Society

STAFF
Laura Laskosz, MPH

Acknowledgments

We thank Jill Ackermann, Ana Garcia, and Lindsay Sweet.

References

1. Rosenbloom AL, Joe JR, Young RS, Winter WE. Emerging epidemic of type 2 diabetes in youth. *Diabetes Care.* 1999;22:345–354
2. American Diabetes Association. Type 2 diabetes in children and adolescents. *Pediatrics.* 2000;105:671–680
3. American Diabetes Association. Type 2 diabetes in children and adolescents. *Diabetes Care.* 2000;23:381–389
4. Ludwig DS, Ebbeling CB. Type 2 diabetes mellitus in children—primary care and public health considerations. *JAMA.* 2001;286:1427–1430
5. American Diabetes Association. Clinical practice recommendations 1999. *Diabetes Care.* 1999;22 (suppl 1):S1–S114
6. American Academy of Pediatrics, Medical Home Initiatives for Children With Special Needs Project Advisory Committee. The medical home. *Pediatrics.* 2002;110:184–186
7. Fagot-Campagna A, Burrows NR, Williamson DF. The public health epidemiology of type 2 diabetes in children and adolescents: a case study of American Indian adolescents in the southwestern United States. *Clin Chim Acta.* 1999;286:81–95
8. Kim C, McHugh C, Kwok Y, Smith A. Type 2 diabetes mellitus in Navajo adolescents. *West J Med.* 1999;170:210–213
9. Dean HJ, Mundy RL, Moffatt M. Non–insulin-dependent diabetes mellitus in Indian children in Manitoba. *CMAJ.* 1992;147:52–57
10. Dabelea D, Pettitt DJ, Jones KL, Arslanian SA. Type 2 diabetes mellitus in minority children and adolescents. An emerging problem. *Endocrinol Metab Clin North Am.* 1999;28:709–729
11. Harris SB, Perkins BA, Whalen-Brough E. Non–insulin-dependent diabetes mellitus among First Nations children. New entity among First Nations people of north western Ontario. *Can Fam Physician.* 1996;42: 869–876
12. Young TK, McIntyre LL, Dooley J, Rodriguez J. Epidemiologic features of diabetes mellitus among Indians in northwestern Ontario and northeastern Manitoba. *Can Med Assoc J.* 1985;132:793–797
13. Dean H, Moffatt ME. Prevalence of diabetes mellitus among Indian children in Manitoba. *Arctic Med Res.* 1988;47:532–534
14. Dean H. NIDDM-Y in First Nation children in Canada. *Clin Pediatr (Phila).* 1998;37:89–96
15. Dean HJ, Young TK, Flett B, Wood-Steinman P. Screening for type-2 diabetes in aboriginal children in northern Canada. *Lancet.* 1998;352:1523–1524
16. Fox C, Harris S, Whalen-Brough E. Diabetes among Native Canadians in northwestern Ontario: 10 years later. *Chron Dis Can.* 1994;15:92–96

17. Harris SB, Gittelsohn J, Hanley A, et al. The prevalence of NIDDM and associated risk factors in native Canadians. *Diabetes Care.* 1997;20:185–187

18. Dabelea D, Hanson RL, Bennett PH, Roumain J, Knowler WC, Pettitt DJ. Increasing prevalence of type II diabetes in American Indian children. *Diabetologia.* 1998;41:904–910

19. Fagot-Campagna A, Knowler WC, Pettitt DJ. Type 2 diabetes in Pima Indian children: cardiovascular risk factors at diagnosis and 10 years later [abstract]. *Diabetes.* 1998;47:605

20. Pinhas-Hamiel O, Dolan LM, Daniels SR, Standiford D, Khoury PR, Zeitler P. Increased incidence of non-insulin-dependent diabetes mellitus among adolescents. *J Pediatr.* 1996;128:608–615

21. Ríos Burrows N, Acton K, Geiss L, Engelgau M. Trends in diabetes prevalence among American Indian and Alaska Native children, adolescents, and young adults, 1991–1997. Paper presented at the 11th Annual Indian Health Service Research Conference; April 26–28, 1999; Albuquerque, NM

22. Fagot-Campagna A, Pettitt DJ, Engelgau MM, et al. Type 2 diabetes among North American children and adolescents: an epidemiological review and a public health perspective. *J Pediatr.* 2000;136:664–672

23. Harwell TS, McDowall JM, Moore K, Fagot-Campagna A, Helgerson SD, Gohdes D. Establishing surveillance of diabetes in American Indian youth. *Diabetes Care.* 2001;24:1029–1032

24. Expert Committee on the Diagnosis and Classification of Diabetes Mellitus. Report of the Expert Committee on the diagnosis and classification of diabetes mellitus. *Diabetes Care.* 1999;22(suppl 1):S5–S19

25. American Diabetes Association. *Medical Management of Type 1 Diabetes.* 3rd ed. Alexandria, VA: American Diabetes Association; 1998

26. Libman I, Songer T, LaPorte R. How many people in the US have IDDM? *Diabetes Care.* 1993;16:841–842

27. Kahn CR. Banting Lecture: insulin action, diabetogenes, and the cause of type II Diabetes. *Diabetes.* 1994;43:1066–1084

28. American Diabetes Association. Standards of medical care for patients with diabetes mellitus. *Diabetes Care.* 1999;22(suppl 1):S32–S41

29. DeFronzo RA. Pharmacologic therapy for type 2 diabetes mellitus. *Ann Intern Med.* 1999;131:281–303

30. Pettitt DJ, Knowler WC. Long-term effects of the intrauterine environment, birth weight, and breast-feeding in Pima Indians. *Diabetes Care.* 1998;21 (suppl 2):B138–B141

31. Teufel NI, Ritenbaugh CK. Development of a primary prevention program: insight gained in the Zuni Diabetes Prevention Program. *Clin Pediatr (Phila).* 1998;37:131–141

32. Hood VL, Kelly B, Martinez C, Shuman S, Secker-Walker R. A Native American community initiative to prevent diabetes. *Ethn Health.* 1997;2:277–285

33. Caballero B, Davis S, Davis CE, et al. PATHWAYS: a school-based program for the primary prevention of obesity in American Indian children. *J Nutr Biochem.* 1998;9:535–543

34. Cook VV, Hurley JS. Prevention of type 2 diabetes in childhood. *Clin Pediatr (Phila).* 1998;37:123–129

35. American Academy of Pediatrics, Committee on Community Health Services. The pediatrician's role in community pediatrics. *Pediatrics.* 1999;103:1304–1307

36. American Academy of Pediatrics, Committee on Sports Medicine and Fitness and Committee on School Health. Physical fitness and activity in schools. *Pediatrics.* 2000;105:1156–1157

37. US Department of Health and Human Services. *Physical Activity and Health: A Report of the Surgeon General.* Atlanta, GA: US Department of Health and Human Services, Centers for Disease Control and Prevention, National Center for Chronic Disease Prevention and Health Promotion; 1996. Available at: http://profiles.nlm.nih.gov/NN/B/B/H/B/. Accessed June 6, 2003

38. Broussard BA, Sugarman JR, Bachman-Carter K, et al. Toward comprehensive obesity prevention programs in Native American communities. *Obes Res.* 1995;3 (suppl 2):289S–297S

39. Stratton IM, Adler AI, Neil HA, et al. Association of glycaemia with macrovascular and microvascular complications of type 2 diabetes (UKPDS 35): prospective observational study. *BMJ.* 2000;321:405–412

40. American Diabetes Association. Screening for diabetes. *Diabetes Care.* 2001;24(suppl 1):S21–S24

41. Centers for Disease Control, Diabetes Cost-Effectiveness Study Group. The cost-effectiveness of screening for type 2 diabetes. *JAMA.* 1998;280:1757–1763

42. Fagot-Campagna A, Saaddine JB, Flegal KM, Beckles GL. Diabetes, impaired fasting glucose, and elevated HbA$_{1c}$ in US adolescents: the Third National Health and Nutrition Examination Survey. *Diabetes Care.* 2001;24:834–837

43. Fagot-Campagna A, Saaddine JB, Engelgau MM. Is testing children for type 2 diabetes a lost battle? *Diabetes Care.* 2000;23:1442–1443

44. Wilson JMG, Jungner O. Principles. In: *Principles and Practice of Screening for Disease.* Geneva, Switzerland: World Health Organization; 1968:14–39

45. Diabetes Prevention Program Research Group. Reduction in the incidence of type 2 diabetes with lifestyle intervention or metformin. *N Engl J Med.* 2002;346:393–403

46. Rosenbloom AL. Is testing children for type 2 diabetes a lost battle? [letter]. *Diabetes Care.* 2000;23:1443

47. Himes JH, Dietz WH. Guidelines for overweight in adolescent preventive services: recommendations from an expert committee. *Am J Clin Nutr.* 1994;59:307–316

48. Lloyd CE, Dyer PH, Barnett AH. Prevalence of symptoms of depression and anxiety in a diabetes clinic population. *Diabet Med.* 2000;17:198–202

49. Peyrot M, Rubin RR. Persistence of depressive symptoms in diabetic adults. *Diabetes Care.* 1999;22:448–452

50. Warnock JK, Mutzig EM. Diabetes mellitus and major depression: considerations for treatment of Native Americans. *J Okla State Med Assoc.* 1998;91:488–493

51. Grandinetti A, Kaholokula JK, Crabbe KM, Kenui CK, Chen R, Chang HK. Relationship between depressive symptoms and diabetes among native Hawaiians. *Psychoneuroendocrinology.* 2000;25:239–246

52. Hanninen JA, Takala JK, Keinanen-Kiukaanniemi SM. Depression in subjects with type 2 diabetes. Predictive factors and relation to quality of life. *Diabetes Care.* 1999;22:997–998

53. Okamura F, Tashiro A, Utsumi A, Imai T, Suchi T, Hongo M. Insulin resistance in patients with depression and its changes in the clinical course of depression: a report on three cases using the minimal model analysis. *Intern Med.* 1999;38:257–260

54. Testa MA, Simonson DC. Health economic benefits and quality of life during improved glycemic control in patients with type 2 diabetes mellitus: a randomized, controlled, double-blind trial. *JAMA.* 1998;280:1490–1496

55. Eaton WW, Armenian H, Gallo J, Pratt L, Ford DE. Depression and risk for onset of type II diabetes. A prospective population-based study. *Diabetes Care.* 1996;19:1097–1102

56. Peyrot M, Rubin RR. Levels and risks of depression and anxiety symptomatology among diabetic adults. *Diabetes Care.* 1997;20:585–590

57. Kovacs M, Obrosky DS, Goldston D, Drash A. Major depressive disorder in youths with IDDM. A controlled prospective study of course and outcome. *Diabetes Care.* 1997;20:45–51

58. Talbot F, Nouwen A, Gingras J, Gosselin M, Audet J. The assessment of diabetes-related cognitive and social factors: the Multidimensional Diabetes Questionnaire. *J Behav Med.* 1997;20:291–312

59. Lustman PJ, Clouse RE, Griffith LS, Carney RM, Freedland KE. Screening for depression in diabetes using the Beck Depression Inventory. *Psychosom Med.* 1997;59:24–31

60. Herpertz S, Albus C, Wagener R, et al. Comorbidity of diabetes and eating disorders. Does diabetes control reflect disturbed eating behavior? *Diabetes Care.* 1998;21:1110–1116

61. Kuczmarski RJ, Ogden CL, Grummer-Strawn LM, et al. CDC growth charts: United States. *Adv Data.* 2000;314:1–27

62. American Academy of Pediatrics, Committee on Sports Medicine and Fitness. Athletic participation by children and adolescents who have systemic hypertension. *Pediatrics.* 1997;99:637–638

63. Kaplan NM, Devereaux RB, Miller HS Jr. 26th Bethesda conference: recommendations for determining eligibility for competition in athletes with cardiovascular abnormalities. Task Force 4: systemic hypertension. *J Am Coll Cardiol.* 1994;24:885–888

64. Burke JP, Hale DE, Hazuda HP, Stern MP. A quantitative scale of acanthosis nigricans. *Diabetes Care.* 1999;22:1655–1659

65. Barbieri RL. Hyperandrogenic disorders. *Clin Obstet Gynecol.* 1990;33:640–654

66. Hrnciar J, Hrnciarova M, Jakubikova K, Okapcova J. Hyperinsulinism as a major etiopathogenic link with arterial hypertension, hyperlipoproteinemia and hirsutism, II [in Slovak]. *Vnitr Lek.* 1992;38:438–447

67. Corenblum B, Baylis BW. Medical therapy for the syndrome of familiar virilization, insulin resistance, and acanthosis nigricans. *Fertil Steril.* 1990;53:421–425

68. Mayfield JA, Sugarman JR. The use of the Semmes-Weinstein monofilament and other threshold tests for preventing foot ulceration and amputation in persons with diabetes. *J Fam Pract.* 2000;49(11 suppl):S17–S29

69. Diabetes Quality Improvement Project Initial Measure Set (Final Version). Washington, DC: National Committee on Quality Assurance. Available at: http://www.ncqa.org/dprp/dqip2.htm. Accessed September 4, 2003

70. National Committee on Quality Assurance. Health Plan Employer Data and Information Set (HEDIS 1999). Available at: http://www.ncqa.org/Programs/hedis/newhedis.htm. Accessed June 6, 2003

71. Braverman IM. Cutaneous manifestations of diabetes mellitus. *Med Clin North Am.* 1971;55:1019–1029

72. Slyper AH. Childhood obesity, adipose tissue distribution, and the pediatric practitioner. *Pediatrics.* 1998;102(1). Available at: http://www.pediatrics.org/cgi/content/full/102/1/e4

73. Van Gaal LF, Wauters MA, Mertens IL, Considine RV, De Leeuw IH. Clinical endocrinology of human leptin. *Int J Obes Relat Metab Disord.* 1999;23(suppl 1):29–36

74. Eastman RC, Garfield SA. Prevention and treatment of microvascular and neuropathic complications of diabetes. *Prim Care.* 1999;26:791–807

75. American Diabetes Association and National Kidney Foundation. Consensus development conference on the diagnosis and management of nephropathy in patients with diabetes mellitus. *Diabetes Care.* 1994;17:1357–1361

76. Ritz E, Orth SR. Nephropathy in patients with type 2 diabetes mellitus. *N Engl J Med.* 1999;341:1127–1133

77. American Academy of Pediatrics, Committee on Nutrition. Cholesterol in childhood. *Pediatrics.* 1998; 101:141–147

78. Kahn SE. The importance of the beta-cell in the pathogenesis of type 2 diabetes mellitus. *Am J Med.* 2000;108(suppl 6A):2S–8S

79. UK Prospective Diabetes Study Group. Intensive blood-glucose control with sulphonylureas or insulin compared with conventional treatment and risk of complications in patients with type 2 diabetes (UKPDS 33). *Lancet.* 1998;352:837–853

80. UK Prospective Diabetes Study Group. Effect of intensive blood-glucose control with metformin on complications in overweight patients with type 2 diabetes (UKPDS 34). *Lancet.* 1998;352:854–865

81. Schneider SH, Morgado A. Effects of fitness and physical training on carbohydrate metabolism and associated cardiovascular risk factors in patients with diabetes. *Diabetes Rev.* 1995;3:378–407

82. Klimt CR, Knatterud GL, Meinert CL, Prout TE. A study of the effects of hypoglycemic agents on vascular complications in patients with adult-onset diabetes: design, methods and baseline results. *Diabetes.* 1970;19(suppl 2):747–783

83. United Kingdom Prospective Diabetes Study Group. United Kingdom Prospective Diabetes Study 24: a 6-year, randomized, controlled trial comparing sulfonylurea, insulin, and metformin therapy in patients with newly diagnosed type 2 diabetes that could not be controlled with diet therapy. *Ann Intern Med.* 1998;128:165–175

84. UK Prospective Diabetes Study Group. UKPDS 28: a randomized trial of efficacy of early addition of metformin in sulfonylurea-treated type 2 diabetes. *Diabetes Care.* 1998;21:87–92

85. Bielamowicz MK, Miller WC, Elkins E, Ladewig HW. Monitoring behavioral changes in diabetes care with the diabetes self-management record. *Diabetes Educ.* 1995;21:426–431

86. American Diabetes Association. National Standards for diabetes self-management education programs and American Diabetes Association review criteria. *Diabetes Care.* 1995;18:737–741

87. Bloomgarden ZT. American Diabetes Association Annual Meeting, 1998: insulin resistance, exercise, and obesity. *Diabetes Care.* 1999;22:517–522

88. Stolarczyk LM, Gilliland SS, Lium DJ, et al. Knowledge, attitudes and behaviors related to physical activity among Native Americans with diabetes. *Ethn Dis.* 1999;9:59–69

89. Myers L, Strikmiller PK, Webber LS, Berenson GS. Physical and sedentary activity in school children grades 5–8: the Bogalusa Heart Study. *Med Sci Sports Exerc.* 1996;28:852–859

90. Freund A, Johnson SB, Silverstein J, Thomas J. Assessing daily management of childhood diabetes using 24-hour recall interviews: reliability and stability. *Health Psychol.* 1991;10:200–208

91. Perusse L, Tremblay A, Leblanc C, Bouchard C. Genetic and environmental influences on level of habitual physical activity and exercise participation. *Am J Epidemiol.* 1989;129:1012–1022

92. Grossi SG, Genco RJ. Periodontal disease and diabetes mellitus: a two-way relationship. *Ann Periodontol.* 1998;3:51–61

93. Cherry-Peppers G, Ship JA. Oral health in patients with type II diabetes and impaired glucose tolerance. *Diabetes Care.* 1993;16:638–641

94. Loe H. Periodontal disease. The sixth complication of diabetes mellitus. *Diabetes Care.* 1993;16:329–334

95. American Academy of Pediatrics. National Cholesterol Education Program: report of the Expert Panel on Blood Cholesterol Levels in Children and Adolescents. *Pediatrics.* 1992;89:525–584

96. Berenson GS, Srinivasan SR, Nicklas TA. Atherosclerosis: a nutritional disease of childhood. *Am J Cardiol.* 1998; 82(10B):22T–29T

97. Bao W, Srinivasan SR, Valdez R, Greenlund KJ, Wattigney WA, Berenson GS. Longitudinal changes in cardiovascular risk from childhood to young adulthood in offspring of parents with coronary artery disease: the Bogalusa Heart Study. *JAMA.* 1997;278:1749–1754

98. Berenson GS, Srinivasan SR, Bao W, Newman WP III, Tracy RE, Wattigney WA. Association between multiple cardiovascular risk factors and atherosclerosis in children and young adults: the Bogalusa Heart Study. *N Engl J Med.* 1998;338:1650–1656

99. Estacio RO, Jeffers BW, Gifford N, Schrier RW. Effect of blood pressure control on diabetic microvascular complications in patients with hypertension and type 2 diabetes. *Diabetes Care.* 2000;23(suppl 2):B54–B64

100. Adler AI, Stratton IM, Neil HA, et al. Association of systolic blood pressure with macrovascular and microvascular complications of type 2 diabetes (UKPDS 36): prospective observational study. *BMJ.* 2000;321:412–419

101. UK Prospective Diabetes Study Group. Tight blood pressure control and risk of macrovascular and microvascular complications in type 2 diabetes: UKPDS 38. *BMJ.* 1998;317:703–713

102. Bakris GL, Williams M, Dworkin L, et al. Preserving renal function in adults with hypertension and diabetes: a consensus approach. *Am J Kidney Dis.* 2000;36: 646–661

103. Task Force on Blood Pressure Control in Children. Report of the Second Task Force on Blood Pressure Control in Children: 1987. *Pediatrics.* 1987;79:1–25

104. Miller K. Pharmacological management of hypertension in paediatric patients. A comprehensive review of the efficacy, safety and dosage guidelines of the available agents. *Drugs.* 1994;48:868–887

105. Sinaiko AR. Pharmacologic management of childhood hypertension. *Pediatr Clin North Am.* 1993;40:195–212

106. Godsland IF, Leyva F, Walton C, Worthington M, Stevenson JC. Associations of smoking, alcohol and physical activity with increased risk factors for coronary heart disease and diabetes in the first follow up cohort of the Heart Disease and Diabetes Risk Indicators in a Screened Cohort Study (HDDRISC-1). *J Intern Med.* 1998;244:33–41

107. Haire-Joshu D, Glasgow RE, Tibbs TL. Smoking and diabetes. *Diabetes Care.* 1999;22:1887–1898

108. Fujimoto WY. Background and recruitment data for the US Diabetes Prevention Program. *Diabetes Care.* 2000;23(suppl 2):B11–B13

109. Eriksson J, Lindstrom J, Valle T, et al. Prevention of type II diabetes in subjects with impaired fasting glucose tolerance: the Diabetes Prevention Study (DPS) in Finland. Study design and 1-year interim report on the feasibility of lifestyle intervention programme. *Diabetologia.* 1999;42:793–801

110. Dean H. Treatment of type 2 diabetes in youth: an argument for randomized controlled studies. *Paediatr Child Health.* 1999;4:265–270

111. Evans A, Krentz AJ. Benefits and risks of transfer from oral agents to insulin in type 2 diabetes mellitus. *Drug Saf.* 1999;21:7–22

112. Berger M, Jorgens V, Muhlhauser I. Rationale for the use of insulin therapy alone as the pharmacological treatment of type 2 diabetes. *Diabetes Care.* 1999;22(suppl 3):C71–C75

113. Hayward RA, Manning WG, Kaplan SH, Wagner EH, Greenfield S. Starting insulin therapy in patients with type 2 diabetes: effectiveness, complications, and resource utilization. *JAMA.* 1997;278:1663–1669

114. Muhammad BJ, Swift PG, Raymond NT, Botha JL. Partial remission phase of diabetes in children younger than age 10 years. *Arch Dis Child.* 1999;80:367–369

115. Greco AV, Caputo S, Bertoli A, Ghirlanda G. The beta cell function in NIDDM patients with secondary failure: a three year follow-up of combined oral hypoglycemic and insulin therapy. *Horm Metab Res.* 1992;24:280–283

116. Holleman F, Hoekstra JB. Insulin lispro. *N Engl J Med.* 1997;337:176–183

117. Gale EA. A randomized, controlled trial comparing insulin lispro with a human soluble insulin in patients with type I diabetes on intensified insulin therapy. The UK Trial Group. *Diabet Med.* 2000;17:209–214

118. Jones K, Arslanian S, McVie R, Tomlinson M, Park J. Metformin improves glycemic control in children with type 2 diabetes [abstract]. *Diabetes.* 2000;49:306

119. Dunn CJ, Peters DH. Metformin. A review of its pharmacological properties and therapeutic use in non-insulin dependent diabetes mellitus. *Drugs.* 1995;49:721–749

120. Bailey CJ. Biguanides and NIDDM. *Diabetes Care.* 1992;15:755–772

121. Meinert CL, Knatterud GL, Prout TE, Klimt CR. A study of the effects of hypoglycemic agents on vascular complications in patients with adult-onset diabetes, II. Mortality results. *Diabetes.* 1970;19(suppl):789–830

122. Bressler R, Johnson DG. Pharmacological regulation of blood glucose levels in non–insulin-dependent diabetes mellitus. *Arch Intern Med.* 1997;157:836–848

123. Gerich JE. Oral hypoglycemic agents. *N Engl J Med.* 1989;321:1231–1245

124. Rodger NW, Chaisson JL, Josse RG, et al. Clinical experience with acarbose: results of a Canadian multi-centre study. *Clin Invest Med.* 1995;18:318–324

125. Coniff RF, Shapiro JA, Seaton TB, Bray GA. Multicenter, placebo controlled trial comparing acarbose (BAY g 5421) with placebo, tolbutamide, and tolbutamide-plus-acarbose in non–insulin-dependent diabetes mellitus. *Am J Med.* 1995;98:443–451

126. Rosenstock J, Brown A, Fischer J, et al. Efficacy and safety of acarbose in metformin-treated patients with type 2 diabetes. *Diabetes Care.* 1998;21:2050–2055

127. DeFronzo RA, Goodman AM. Efficacy of metformin in patients with non–insulin dependent diabetes mellitus. *N Engl J Med.* 1995;333:541–549

128. Simonson DC, Kourides IA, Feinglos M, Shamoon H, Fischette CT. Efficacy, safety and dose-response characteristics of glipizide gastrointestinal therapeutic system on glycemic control and insulin secretion in NIDDM. Results of two multicenter, randomized, placebo-controlled clinical trials. *Diabetes Care.* 1997;20:597–606

129. Rosenstock J, Samols E, Muchmore DB, Schneider J. Glimepiride, a new once-daily sulfonylurea. A double-blind placebo-controlled study of NIDDM patients. *Diabetes Care.* 1996;19:1194–1199

130. Krentz AJ, Ferner RE, Bailey CJ. Comparative tolerability profiles of oral antidiabetic agents. *Drug Saf.* 1994;11:223–241

131. Hillebrand I, Boehme K, Frank G, Fink H, Berchtold P. The effects of the μ-glucosidase inhibitor BAY g 5421 (Acarbose) on meal-stimulated elevations of circulating glucose, insulin, and triglyceride levels in man. *Res Exp Med (Berl).* 1979;175:81–86

132. Haupt E, Knick B, Koschinsky T, Liebermeister H, Schneider J, Hirche H. Oral antidiabetic combination therapy with sulphonylureas and metformin. *Diabetes Metab.* 1991;17:224–231

133. Foster DW, McGarry JD. The metabolic derangements and treatment of diabetic ketoacidosis. *N Engl J Med.* 1983;309:159–169

134. Kaufman FR, Halvorson M. The treatment and prevention of diabetic ketoacidosis in children and adolescents with type I diabetes mellitus. *Pediatr Ann.* 1999;28: 576–582

135. Rosenbloom AL, Hanas R. Diabetic ketoacidosis (DKA): treatment guidelines. *Clin Pediatr (Phila).* 1996;35: 261–266

136. Harris GD, Fiordalisi I, Finberg L. Safe management of diabetic keto-acidemia. *J Pediatr.* 1988;113:65–68

137. Funnell MM. *A Core Curriculum for Diabetes Education.* Chicago, IL: American Association of Diabetes Educators; 1998

All clinical reports from the American Academy of Pediatrics automatically expire 5 years after publication unless reaffirmed, revised, or retired at or before that time.

Sinusitis

David Nash, MD,* and Ellen Wald, MD†

Objectives

After completing this article, readers should be able to:
1. Describe the clinical presentation of acute and chronic sinusitis.
2. Delineate the limited role for imaging studies in patients who have sinusitis.
3. Recognize if abnormal images of the paranasal sinuses imply bacterial infection.
4. Describe the microbiology of acute bacterial sinusitis.
5. Delineate appropriate antimicrobial therapy based on knowledge of the microbiology of acute bacterial sinusitis.

Definition

The term "sinusitis" describes an inflammation of the paranasal sinuses that can have a viral, allergic, or bacterial origin. The duration of respiratory symptoms can be used to categorize patients who have sinusitis. Acute bacterial sinusitis (ABS) is defined by nasal and sinus symptoms that have been present at least 10 (in most cases) days and fewer than 30 days. Subacute sinusitis is defined by nasal and sinus symptoms lasting longer than 4 weeks and fewer than 12 weeks. There is very little information comparing acute and subacute sinusitis, and this may ultimately prove to be an arbitrary distinction that does not affect etiology, diagnosis, or treatment. Chronic sinusitis is defined by symptoms of at least 12 weeks' duration. Because the etiology of chronic sinusitis is often unknown, treatment of this condition is controversial.

Epidemiology

Symptoms affecting the upper respiratory tract (nasal congestion, rhinorrhea, and cough) are the most common complaint in the pediatric office. One of the greatest challenges facing pediatricians is to distinguish between viral upper respiratory tract infections, allergic rhinitis, and sinusitis. A complicating factor is that both allergic rhinitis and viral upper respiratory tract infections predispose patients to acute or chronic sinusitis. Young children experience six to eight viral upper respiratory tract infections per year, of which 5% to 10% are estimated to be complicated by ABS. Allergic rhinitis also is extremely common, with a prevalence approaching 20% by adolescence. It is essential that pediatricians recognize that both allergic rhinitis and viral upper respiratory tract infections are many times more common than ABS.

Pathogenesis

The maxillary and ethmoid sinuses form during the third to fourth gestational month and, although very small, are present at birth. The maxillary sinuses are unique because the outflow tract sits high on the medial wall of the sinus cavity, thereby negating gravitational effects on drainage. The ethmoid sinus is comprised of multiple air cells, with each cell draining through a small, independent ostium into the middle meatus. The narrow caliber of these draining ostia predisposes to obstruction. The frontal sinus develops from an anterior ethmoid cell and moves to a position above the orbital ridge by the fifth or sixth birthday. The sphenoid sinuses are immediately

*Assistant Professor of Pediatrics, Division of Allergy, Immunology & Infectious Diseases, Children's Hospital of Pittsburgh.

†Professor of Pediatrics and Otolaryngology, University of Pittsburgh School of Medicine; Chief, Division of Allergy, Immunology & Infectious Diseases, Children's Hospital of Pittsburgh, Pittsburgh, PA.

anterior to the pituitary fossa and just behind the posterior ethmoids. Isolated involvement of the sphenoid sinuses is rare; they usually are infected as part of a pansinusitis. The ostiomeatal complex (OMC) is the area between the middle and inferior turbinates that represents the confluence of the drainage areas of the frontal, ethmoid, and maxillary sinuses (Figure). Within the OMC are several sites in which two mucosal layers make contact. Because the cilia move in opposite directions, secretions may be retained at these sites, creating the potential for infection even without physical obstruction of the ostia.

Physiology

Three key elements are important to the normal physiology of the paranasal sinuses: the patency of the ostia, the function of the ciliary apparatus, and the quality of secretions. Retention of secretions in the paranasal sinuses is usually due to one or more of the following: obstruction of the ostia, reduction in the number or function of the cilia, and overproduction or change in the viscosity of secretions.

The factors predisposing to ostial obstruction can be divided into those that cause mucosal swelling and those that are due to mechanical obstruction (Table 1). Although many conditions may lead to ostial closure, viral rhinosinusitis and allergic inflammation are the most frequent and most important. When the sinus ostium is obstructed completely, there is a transient increase in intrasinus pressure followed by the development of a negative intrasinal pressure. When the ostium opens again, the negative pressure within the sinus cavity relative to atmospheric pressure may allow the introduction of bacteria from the nasopharynx (which is heavily colonized with respiratory flora) into the usually sterile sinus cavity. Alternatively, sneezing, sniffing, and nose blowing associated with altered intranasal pressure may facilitate the entry of bacteria from the posterior nasal chamber into the sinuses.

The normal motility of the cilia and the adhesive properties of the mucous layer usually protect respiratory epithelium from bacterial invasion. The mucociliary apparatus may function abnormally because of either a direct cytotoxic effect on

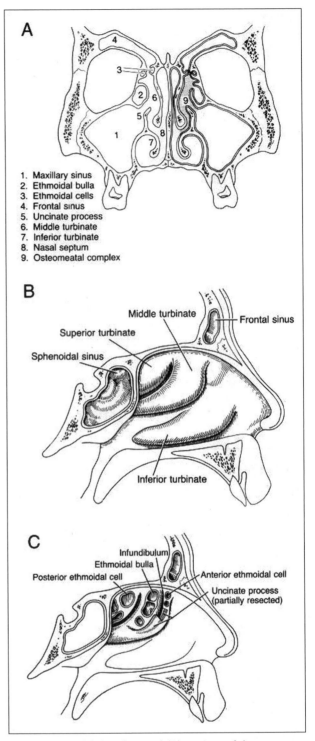

1. Maxillary sinus
2. Ethmoidal bulla
3. Ethmoidal cells
4. Frontal sinus
5. Uncinate process
6. Middle turbinate
7. Inferior turbinate
8. Nasal septum
9. Osteomeatal complex

Middle turbinate — Frontal sinus
Superior turbinate
Sphenoidal sinus
Inferior turbinate

Infundibulum
Ethmoidal bulla
Posterior ethmoidal cell — Anterior ethmoidal cell
Uncinate process (partially resected)

Figure. Coronal (A) and sagittal (B) sections of the nose and paranasal sinuses. The stippled areas represent the ostiomeatal complex. C. A view through the middle and superior turbinates, displaying the ethmoid air cells.

the cilia by respiratory viruses or a genetic defect in the microtubule structure of the cilia. The alteration of cilia number, morphology, and function may facilitate secondary bacterial invasion

Table 1. Factors Predisposing to Sinus Ostial Obstruction

Mucosal Swelling

Systemic disorder:
- Viral upper respiratory tract infection
- Allergic inflammation
- Cystic fibrosis
- Immune disorders
- Immotile cilia
- Second-hand smoke

Local insult:
- Facial trauma
- Swimming, diving
- Rhinitis medicamentosa

Mechanical Obstruction
- Choanal atresia
- Deviated septum
- Nasal polyps
- Foreign body
- Tumor
- Ethmoid bullae
- Encephalocele

of the nose and the sinuses. Cilia can beat only in a fluid medium. Alterations in the mucus, as in cystic fibrosis or asthma, may impair ciliary activity. The presence of purulent material in the acutely infected sinus also may impair ciliary movement, further compounding the effects of ostial closure.

Symptoms and Signs

ABS has two common clinical presentations that distinguish it from an uncomplicated episode of viral rhinosinusitis. The most common presentation involves persistent respiratory symptoms, including either nasal discharge of any quality (thin or thick; clear, mucoid, or purulent) or a cough that is present in the daytime, although it often worsens at night. Malodorous breath frequently is reported by parents of preschoolers. Complaints of facial pain and headache are rare, although the parent may note occasional painless morning eye swelling. The child may not appear very ill, and if fever is present, it usually is low grade. The persistence rather than the severity of symptoms in this presentation is of note. In the context of ABS, persistent symptoms are those that last from 10 to 30 days without improvement.

The 10-day mark separates simple viral rhinosinusitis from ABS. Most uncomplicated episodes of viral rhinosinusitis last 5 to 7 days. Although patients may not be asymptomatic by the tenth day, they are virtually always improved. Upper respiratory tract symptoms in children are common, but symptoms persisting for longer than 10 days are seen in a minority (<10%) of patients.

The second, less common presentation of ABS is a "cold" that seems more severe than usual. The severity is defined by a combination of high fever (at least 39.0°C [102.2°F]) and purulent nasal discharge. The quality of nasal discharge changes frequently during the course of an uncomplicated viral upper respiratory tract infection. It begins as a watery discharge and becomes thicker, colored, and opaque after a few days. Most often it remains purulent for several days, then clears again to a mucoid or watery consistency before resolving. If fever is present during the course of an episode of viral rhinosinusitis, it is at the outset and in association with other constitutional symptoms such as headache and myalgias. Usually the fever disappears and the respiratory symptoms begin. Accordingly, the combination of high fever and purulent nasal discharge for at least 3 to 4 consecutive days may signal a secondary bacterial infection of the paranasal sinuses. Affected patients may suffer from headaches behind or above the eye and occasionally experience periorbital swelling.

Patients who have subacute or chronic sinusitis present with a history of protracted (more than 30 days and not improving) respiratory symptoms. Nasal congestion (obstruction) and cough (day and night) are most common. Sore throat results from mouth breathing due to nasal obstruction. Nasal discharge (of any quality) and headache are less common; fever is rare. It is important to distinguish between protracted symptoms and recurrent symptoms because of implications for both etiology and treatment.

In general, physical examination of children who have either acute or chronic upper respiratory tract symptoms is most helpful in identifying conditions that may predispose to sinusitis. Unfortunately, the examination cannot distinguish between viral upper respiratory tract infections and ABS. Patients who have nasal polyps, poor growth, clubbing of the fingers, barrel chest, and respiratory findings may have cystic fibrosis. The immotile cilia syndrome almost always is associated with middle ear disease, and 50% of patients have situs inversus. The presence of atopic dermatitis, intermittent wheezing, Morgan-Dennie lines (skin folds under the lower eyelid), or a nasal crease suggests an allergic diathesis. Adenoidal hypertrophy either can predispose to ABS or, when the adenoids are infected, masquerade as sinusitis. The adenoids cannot be assessed by routine examination, requiring instead either radiographic imaging or flexible endoscopy of the nasopharynx. Patients who have immunodeficiency may lack tonsillar tissue and other lymph nodes and exhibit poor growth, clubbing of the fingers, and other signs of infection. However, normal findings on the physical examination do not rule out the possibility of immunodeficiency, and if the clinical history is compelling, additional laboratory evaluation is appropriate.

Diagnostic Methods

The need, if any, for radiographic imaging (plain film versus computed tomography [CT]) for children who have symptoms of sinusitis is controversial. Recent national guidelines on the treatment of sinusitis have emphasized the role of the clinical diagnosis, moving away from the use of radiographic imaging in patients who have uncomplicated ABS. Plain films are appropriate in older children who have recurrent acute sinusitis, vague symptoms, a poor response to antibiotic therapy, or a history of antibiotic hypersensitivity that makes therapy risky. Radiographic findings in patients who have ABS include diffuse opacification, mucosal thickening of at least 4 mm, or an air-fluid level. When these radiographic criteria were used in the clinical setting of either "persistent" or "severe" ABS, maxillary sinus aspirates contained a high density of bacteria in 75% of children.

CT should be reserved for patients who have either complicated ABS or who are being considered as surgical candidates (for either recurrent or chronic sinusitis). When CT imaging is obtained in these circumstances, a complete CT is indicated.

Any patient who has proptosis, impaired vision, limited extraocular movements, severe facial pain, notable swelling of the forehead or face, deep-seated headaches, or toxic appearance should receive a CT scan. The CT scan should not be used in patients who have simple upper respiratory tract symptoms because it does not distinguish between mucosal abnormalities due to viral infection and those due to ABS. CT scans of the paranasal sinuses in adults who had acute "colds" showed substantial mucosal abnormalities that resolved spontaneously, underscoring the fact that mucosal abnormalities within the paranasal sinuses are common in patients who have upper respiratory tract symptoms. In the setting of chronic sinusitis, the CT scan should be used as a guide for surgical intervention for patients who do not improve after completing maximal medical therapy. CT scans appear normal in up to one third of patients who have symptoms of chronic sinusitis.

Sinus Aspiration

Although maxillary sinus aspiration is not a routine procedure, it can be performed safely by a skilled otolaryngologist in the ambulatory setting using a transnasal approach. Current indications for maxillary sinus aspiration include: 1) failure to respond to multiple courses of antibiotics, 2) severe facial pain, 3) orbital or intracranial complications, and 4) evaluation of an immunocompromised host. Material aspirated from the maxillary sinus should be sent for quantitative aerobic and anaerobic cultures (if possible), fungal cultures, and Gram stain. The recovery of bacteria in a density of at least 10^4 cfu/mL is considered to represent true infection. The finding of at least one organism per high-power field on Gram stain of sinus secretions correlates with the recovery of bacteria in a density of 10^5 cfu/mL.

Microbiology of Sinusitis

Data on the microbiology of patients who have acute (10 to 30 days) and subacute (30 to 120 days) illnesses have highlighted the important bacterial pathogens as *Streptococcus pneumoniae*, *Haemophilus influenzae*, and *Moraxella catarrhalis*.

S pneumoniae is most common in all age groups, accounting for 30% to 40% of isolates. *H influenzae* and *M catarrhalis* are similar in prevalence, each accounting for approximately 20% of cases. Both *H influenzae* and *M catarrhalis* may be beta-lactamase-producing and, therefore, resistant to amoxicillin. Neither staphylococci nor respiratory anaerobes are common in ABS. Respiratory viral isolates include adenovirus, parainfluenza, influenza, and rhinovirus in approximately 10% of patients. For children who have chronic sinusitis, the role of bacterial agents is less clear. The results of cultures from children who have chronic sinusitis have been extremely variable; a high percentage of patients have had either sterile cultures or known contaminants, and the presence of anaerobes has ranged from almost 0 to more than 90%. The persistence of symptoms despite multiple courses of antimicrobials is counter to the hypothesis that bacterial pathogens play an important role in the etiology of chronic sinusitis.

Medical Treatment

Antimicrobial therapy is the backbone of the medical management of ABS. Recent guidelines published jointly by the Centers for Disease Control and Prevention and the American Academy of Pediatrics promoting the "Judicious Use of Antimicrobial Agents" suggest amoxicillin as a reasonable first choice for most cases of ABS in children. This is especially true if the episode of ABS is uncomplicated and mild to moderate in severity and if the patient has not recently (<1 mo) been treated with antimicrobial agents. The problem that has emerged during the past 5 years in the management of ABS is infection caused by *S pneumoniae* strains that are resistant to penicillin. The frequency of penicillin-resistant pneumococci varies geographically, and many isolates of pneumococci are resistant to other commonly used antimicrobials, such as cephalosporins, sulfamethoxazole-trimethoprim, and macrolides. Clinical situations in which alternative regimens are appropriate include: 1) failure to improve with conventional doses of amoxicillin, 2) recent treatment with amoxicillin (<1 mo), 3) attendance at child care, 4) occurrence of frontal

or sphenoidal sinusitis, and 5) presentation with protracted (>30 d) symptoms. Therapeutic options include high-dose amoxicillin (80 to 90 mg/kg per day), amoxicillin (45 mg/kg per day) plus amoxicillin with clavulanate (45 mg/kg per day), cefuroxime axetil, and cefpodoxime. Antibiotic selection should be guided by susceptibility results when available.

Patients who have orbital or central nervous system complications of sinusitis should be hospitalized and receive a parenteral antibiotic, subspecialty consultation, and surgical drainage when appropriate. If penicillin-resistant pneumococci are suspected, cefotaxime (300 mg/kg per day in four doses) with or without vancomycin (60 mg/kg per day in four doses) should be administered intravenously. The sinus should be aspirated to identify the infecting organism and aid in the selection of appropriate antimicrobial therapy.

Clinical improvement is prompt in nearly all children treated with an appropriate antimicrobial agent for uncomplicated ABS. Patients who are febrile at the initial encounter will become afebrile, and there is a remarkable reduction of nasal discharge and cough within 48 to 72 hours. If the patient does not improve or worsens in 48 hours, clinical re-evaluation is appropriate. If the diagnosis is unchanged, sinus aspiration may be considered to obtain precise bacteriologic information. Alternatively, an antimicrobial agent effective against beta-lactamase-producing bacterial species and penicillin-resistant pneumococci should be prescribed.

The appropriate duration of antimicrobial therapy for patients who have ABS has not been investigated systematically. Most can be treated with 10 to 14 days of therapy. Longer treatment courses have been used in those who have chronic sinusitis to avoid surgery. However, the use of antibiotic therapy for more than a few weeks is not supported by clinical studies, exposes patients to developing allergic hypersensitivity, and may increase the development of resistant organisms. Although antimicrobial prophylaxis has not been studied in patients who have recurrent ABS, it has proved useful to reduce symptomatic episodes of acute otitis media in patients who experience recurrent ear disease. A trial of antimicrobial prophylaxis may be appropriate for patients in whom there is no treatable underlying disorder and who have a history of responding to antibiotic therapy. Patients selected for a trial of antibiotic prophylaxis should have had at least three episodes of ABS in 6 months or four episodes in 12 months.

Adjuvant therapies such as antihistamines, decongestants, and anti-inflammatory agents have received little evaluation. Because antihistamines and decongestants have not been studied in patients who have sinusitis and have as much potential for harm as for benefit, they should not be used for treatment of ABS. The potential role of topical intranasal steroids as an adjunct to antibiotics has been evaluated recently in children and adults. The availability of agents that have a rapid onset of activity prompts their consideration for the management of acute symptoms, but the very modest beneficial effect of treatment does not justify their use. Nasal irrigation using either hypertonic or isotonic solutions has been shown to have a positive effect in some patients. Saline nasal irrigation is inexpensive, readily available, and devoid of side effects other than mild discomfort from hypertonic solutions. Further prospective studies are necessary to evaluate the role of these agents fully in sinusitis.

Complications

The major complications of ABS are rare and involve contiguous spread of infection to the orbit, bone, or central nervous system (Table 2). Subperiosteal abscess of the orbit and intracranial abscesses are the most common. Orbital infection is signaled by eye swelling, proptosis, and impaired extraocular eye movements; intracranial infection is suggested by signs of increased intracranial pressure, meningeal irritation, and focal neurologic deficits.

Table 2. Major Complications of Sinusitis

Orbital
- Inflammatory edema (preseptal or periorbital cellulitis)
- Subperiosteal abscess
- Orbital abscess
- Orbital cellulitis
- Optic neuritis

Osteomyelitis
- Frontal (Pott puffy tumor)
- Maxillary

Intracranial
- Epidural abscess
- Subdural empyema or abscess
- Cavernous or sagittal sinus thrombosis
- Meningitis
- Brain abscess

Surgical Therapy

Patients who have ABS seldom require surgical intervention unless they present with orbital or central nervous system complications. Rarely, sinus aspiration may be required in those who do not respond to aggressive antimicrobial management both to ventilate the sinuses and to obtain material for culture. When patients who have chronic sinusitis fail to improve with maximal medical therapy, sinus surgery might be considered. One academic otolaryngology center has reported that comprehensive evaluations for conditions that predispose children to chronic sinusitis combined with appropriate therapy directed toward these conditions dramatically reduced the number of surgical procedures. At present, the focus of surgical therapy is the ostiomeatal complex. Using an endoscope, most current surgical efforts attempt to enlarge the natural meatus of the maxillary outflow tract (by excising the uncinate process and the ethmoid bullae) and perform an anterior ethmoidectomy. The outcome of endoscopic sinus surgery is difficult to assess; all studies, including one meta-analysis, have been limited by retrospective designs and an absence of control groups. The precise population of children most likely to benefit from this surgery has not been delineated.

Suggested Reading

Gwaltney JM, Phillips CD, Miller RD, Riker DK. Computed tomographic study of the common cold. *N Engl J Med.* 1994; 330:25–30

McAlister WH, Kronemer K. Imaging of sinusitis in children. *Pediatr Infect Dis J.* 1999;18:1019–1020

Parsons DS. Chronic sinusitis: a medical or surgical disease? *Otolaryngol Clin North Am.* 1996;29:1–9

Wald ER, Milmoe GJ, Bowne A, Ledesma-Medina J, Salamon N, Bluestone CD. Acute maxillary sinusitis in children. *N Engl J Med.* 1981;304:749–754

Wald ER, Reilly JS, Casselbrant M, et al. Treatment of acute maxillary sinusitis in childhood: a comparative study of amoxicillin and cefaclor. *J Pediatr.* 1984;104:297–302

Syncope

John Willis, MD*

Objectives

After completing this article, readers should be able to:

1. Describe the steps involved in identifying the correct diagnosis of syncope.
2. Identify the only mandatory screening test in syncope.
3. Describe the ramifications of syncope with exercise.
4. Identify the most common diagnosis in syncope and why it is dangerous.
5. List the differential diagnosis and treatment of syncope.

Definition

Syncope is a transient loss of consciousness and muscle tone. Loss of cerebral oxygenation and perfusion is the usual mechanism. It often is benign but may cause injury (15% of cases). Syncope can be caused by serious cardiac disease, which should be suspected whenever syncope occurs with exercise.

Epidemiology

Up to 3% of emergency department visits by adults and 6% of hospital admissions are due to syncope. Among children, only 0.125% of emergency department visits are due to syncope. Nevertheless, 47% of college students report having fainted, and 15% of children suffer from syncope before the end of adolescence. The lay public realizes that healthy children who faint frequently are free of serious disease and may not require emergency medical attention. About 75% of children who faint have neurocardiac (vasovagal) syncope due to neurally mediated hypotension and bradycardia; most others have seizures, migraine, or cardiac disease.

Pathogenesis

The causes of syncope can be categorized as cardiac, noncardiac, and neurocardiac (Table).

CARDIAC SYNCOPE

Cardiac syncope is due to outflow obstruction (aortic stenosis, hypertrophic cardiomyopathy), myocardial dysfunction (cardiomyopathy, carditis, ischemia), or arrhythmias (ventricular tachycardia, long Q-T syndromes, Wolff-Parkinson-White syndrome). Cardiac disease is suggested when syncope accompanies exercise. Cardiac syncope is potentially fatal and always deserves careful evaluation and treatment.

NONCARDIAC SYNCOPE

This form of syncope includes many entities, some of which are distinguished easily by a careful history and are not true syncope. Seizures often manifest unusual eye or limb movements, may be prolonged, and—unlike syncope—usually are followed by postictal stupor. Seizures may result from cardiac or neurocardiac syncope if cerebral perfusion or oxygenation is sufficiently reduced, which is especially likely if the child is held upright during the syncopal episode. Epileptic seizures may cause cardiac disturbances, usually tachycardia. Many patients who have epilepsy have normal results on electroencephalography (EEG); diagnosis is made best by history.

Breathholding spells begin in infancy and resolve by school age. The history is stereotypical.

*Professor, Department of Psychiatry and Neurology; Clinical Professor of Pediatrics; Chief, Section of Child Neurology; Tulane University School of Medicine, New Orleans, LA.

The spells always begin with pain or anger, followed in order by a brief cry, holding of the breath (usually with the mouth open and a distressed expression), cyanosis or pallor (the latter if bradycardia occurs), possibly a loss of consciousness, and finally perhaps a brief tonic or clonic seizure. If the history is not perfectly typical, epilepsy or cardiac syncope should be suspected and these diagnoses pursued. If the history is typical, iron deficiency anemia, which is a possible cause, should be ruled out, and the parents should be reassured that breathholding is benign and will resolve. Antiepileptic medications should not be prescribed to breathholders unless the resulting seizure is lengthy. Seizures related to breathholding usually are brief and hypoxic and do not require treatment with antiepileptic medication. Breathholding is not a manipulative behavior. Its only sequel is a later propensity to neurocardiac syncope in 17% of patients. The best treatment is to keep the child horizontal and wait.

Migraine may cause syncope because of the pain or occasionally directly (brainstem migraine). The diagnosis can be made based on a history of associated severe headache with nausea, vomiting, photophobia, and relief by sleep. Family history is positive for migraine in 75% of cases.

Orthostatic hypotension is defined as a 20-mm Hg drop in systolic blood pressure upon assuming an upright posture. Patients should be monitored for at least 2 minutes upright with serial blood pressure measurements. Pregnancy should be considered as a cause in women of childbearing age. Dehydration, prolonged bedrest, drugs, and neuropathies may be predisposing factors.

Hyperventilation may produce sufficient cerebral vasoconstriction to cause syncope. An associated valsalva maneuver or chest compression can accentuate the cerebral hypoperfusion caused by hyperventilation.

Situational syncope can be caused by cough, micturition, defecation, neck stretching, hair grooming, venipuncture, or even swallowing in certain individuals. The diagnosis is based on the history.

Table 1. Etiologies of Syncope

Cardiac Syncope
- Outflow Obstruction
  - Valvular aortic stenosis
  - Pulmonary hypertension
  - Hypertrophic cardiomyopathy
  - Eisenmenger syndrome
- Myocardial Dysfunction
  - Dilated cardiomyopathy
  - Myocarditis
  - Neuromuscular disease (eg, Duchenne dystrophy)
  - Kawasaki disease
  - Anomalous coronary artery
- Arrhythmias
  - Long Q-T syndromes
  - Ventricular tachycardia
  - Arrhythmogenic right ventricular dysplasia
  - Supraventricular tachycardia (Wolff-Parkinson-White)
  - Sinus node dysfunction
  - Atrioventricular block

Appropriate Evaluations: Electrocardiography, cardiac echocardiography, chest radiography, creatine phosphokinase

Noncardiac Syncope
- Seizures
- Migraine
- Orthostatic hypotension
- Narcolepsy/cataplexy
- Familial dysautonomia
- Gastroesophageal reflux
- Spinal cord disease (autonomic instability)
- Metabolic disease (diabetes, hypoglycemia, endocrine)
- Situational (cough, micturition, neck stretching, hair grooming, venipuncture)
- Breathholding spells
- Toxins/drugs
- Hyperventilation
- Hysteria
- Fever (febrile delirium)
- Carotid sinus hypersensitivity

Appropriate Evaluations: Electroencephalography, blood glucose, toxic screen

Neurocardiac Syncope
Appropriate Evaluation: Electrocardiography

Narcolepsy may mimic syncope. Those who have narcolepsy go to sleep abruptly. Cataplexy (the abrupt intrusion of rapid eye movement sleep into waking) may be mistaken for syncope if a history of excessive daytime sleepiness is not sought. Cataplexy may produce loss of consciousness in response to emotional reactions such as laughter or anger. Narcolepsy is diagnosed by the sleep latency test. Narcolepsy is common in children, a fact that was not appreciated until recently.

Metabolic causes of syncope are rare, but hypoglycemia and electrolyte abnormalities should be considered because they could have serious consequences.

Hysterical syncope may be difficult to diagnose, but it should be suspected when the episode is prolonged, there is no change in vital signs or appearance, it does not raise concern in the patient, or the patient's recall or responsiveness during the event suggests that consciousness has been maintained.

NEUROCARDIAC SYNCOPE (VASOVAGAL)

This is the most common variety of syncope, and it can be diagnosed with a tilt table test, although this test is not perfectly sensitive or specific. Approximately 25% of cases are precipitated by acute illness and anemia or by such noxious stimuli as pain, fear, exhaustion, hunger, prolonged standing, or crowded/poorly ventilated rooms.

There usually are the following prodromal symptoms: nausea/vomiting, pallor, lightheadedness/vertigo, visual disturbances, sweating, and shortness of breath. After syncope, the patient may be fatigued, lightheaded, anxious, or nauseous or may complain of headache. The typical mental alertness following the episode is helpful in distinguishing syncope from seizures.

The pathophysiology of neurocardiac syncope is relatively well understood. Peripheral venous pooling leads to decreased ventricular filling and increased circulating catecholamines. The ventricle responds with vigorous contractions that stimulate mechanoreceptors (like hypertension) and produces a paradoxic withdrawal of sympathetic activity that causes hypotension, bradycardia, or both.

Clinical Aspects

The history is the key to diagnosis of syncope, and it must be obtained carefully both from the patient and from an eyewitness because the patient will be unreliable for observations during unconsciousness. Several points demand specific questioning:

● The *situation and antecedents* of the episode, which may identify precipitants (exercise suggests cardiac syncope)
● The *onset* of the episode, which may include epileptic activity that characterizes the event as a seizure (lateral eye movements, sensory hallucinations, focal or generalized motor activity)
● The *duration* of the episode (time expands with excitement, and comparison of the event with a common timed activity such as TV commercials will help to provide a clear picture of the duration)
● *Loss of consciousness,* which is presumed from unresponsiveness to the environment (voice, pain) and from amnesia, injury, or incontinence
● A *postictal state* of confusion, which suggests a seizure
● *Palpitations,* which suggest cardiac disease

The past history may reveal associated disease predisposing to syncope. Because many causes of syncope are familial, it is important to inquire carefully about a family history of syncope, sudden or early death, epilepsy and neurologic disease, heart disease, and deafness (Q-T syndromes may have familial deafness).

A general physical and neurologic examination must include measurement of vital signs and a cardiac evaluation. Approximately 90% of orthostatic hypotension occurs within 2 minutes of standing upright; such a finding provides an important clue to the diagnosis.

Electrocardiography is recommended for every case of unexplained syncope. Life-threatening cardiac disease is a first concern.

Other laboratory tests should be ordered according to findings from the history and physical examination. An EEG, video-EEG monitoring (if episodes are frequent), neuroimaging, or neurologic referral may help with suspected seizures. A multiple sleep latency test is used to diagnose narcolepsy. Determination of blood glucose or electrolyte concentrations or endocrinologic studies may be useful in selected cases. If cardiac disease is suspected, Holter or loop monitoring, chest radiography, echocardiography, exercise stress testing, or even invasive electrophysiologic testing may be pursued.

The tilt table test has made the diagnosis of neurocardiac syncope a positive one rather than simply one of exclusion. Protocols vary, but the patient is tilted upright for a time sufficient to reproduce symptoms and changes in cardiovascular function (hypotension or bradycardia). The tilt table test is not always specific or sensitive, and intravenous infusions of isoproterenol and other drugs may be confusing noxious stimuli. Nevertheless, this has become the gold standard for diagnosing neurocardiac syncope.

Management

Treatment of syncope is directed at the specific causative entity. Cardiac disease may require antiarrhythmics or surgery. Seizures may require anticonvulsants, with the choice depending on the exact type of seizure. Breathholding spells, which can be upsetting, necessitate reassurance of parents. A variety of acute and prophylactic medications are available for migraine. Hysteria in childhood merits psychiatric evaluation and the consideration of abuse. The sleepiness of narcolepsy is treated with stimulants (eg, methylphenidate hydrochloride 20 mg every morning) and brief naps; cataplexy is treated with tricyclic antidepressants (eg, imipramine 25 to 75 mg q hs). For situational syncope, the inciting stimulus should be avoided.

Neurocardiac syncope often can be managed with simple suggestions, such as lying down before losing consciousness, wearing elastic hose to prevent venous pooling in the legs, increasing salt and water intake, eating regularly, avoiding noxious stimuli that precipitate syncope, and intermittently contracting leg muscles when standing to increase venous return. Avoiding alcohol, beta-blockers, tricyclics, and isoproterenol may lessen the likelihood of neurocardiac syncope. Standard drug therapy includes mineralocorticoids (hydroflurocortisone 0.1 mg bid), atenolol (1 to 2 mg/kg per day), and pseudoephedrine (4 mg/kg per day qid). In truly refractory cases, cardiac pacing may be considered.

Prognosis

The outlook for syncope depends on the specific diagnosis. Neurocardiac syncope recurs in two thirds of cases, and syncope of other causes has a 90% or greater recurrence rate. Treatment often is effective once the condition is diagnosed. The outlook for many childhood epilepsies is benign. Migraine and narcolepsy usually are controlled by medication. Death can occur unexpectedly in cardiac syncope, and vigorous diagnostic evaluations are warranted whenever palpitations or exercise are associated with syncope.

Sugested Reading

Alehan DA, Celiker A, Ozme S. Head-up tilt test: a highly sensitive test for children with unexplained syncope. *Pediatr Cardiol*. 1996;17:86–90

Benditt DG, Ferguson DW, Grubb BP, et al. Tilt table test for assessing syncope. *J Am Coll Cardiol*. 1996;28:263–275

Driscoll DJ, Jacobsen SJ, Porter CJ, Wollan PC. Syncope in children and adolescents. *J Am Coll Cardiol*. 1997;29:1039–1045

Grubb BP, Kosinski D. Current trends in etiology, diagnosis, and management of neurocardiac syncope. *Curr Opin Cardiol*. 1996;11:32–41

McHarg ML, Shinnar S, Rascoff H, Walsh CA. Syncope in childhood. *Pediatr Cardiol*. 1997;18:367–371

Tanel RE, Walsh EP. Syncope in the pediatric patient. *Cardiol Clin*. 1997;15:277–293

Wolff GS. Unexplained syncope: clinical management. *PACE*. 1997;20:2043–2047

Treating Acne: A Practical Guide for Pediatricians

by Daniel P. Krowchuk, MD, FAAP

Acne vulgaris, more commonly termed acne, affects an estimated 17 million people in the United States, including 85% or more of adolescents and young adults. It is a chronic condition that may last for years and cause emotional distress and permanent scarring. Although there is no cure for acne, medications can control the disease and limit or prevent scar formation. Most adolescents with acne can be managed successfully by their pediatricians.

What Causes Acne?

Acne is a disorder of pilosebaceous follicles, comprised of a follicle or pore, sebaceous gland, and rudimentary or vellus hair. These specialized follicles are located on the face, chest, and back. Although the pathogenesis of acne has not been clearly defined, multiple factors contribute. Well-reasoned therapeutic choices require an understanding of these factors.

HORMONES

Androgens play an integral role in the causation of acne. At age 8 or 9 years, prior to the appearance of secondary sexual characteristics, the adrenal glands begin to produce increasing amounts of the androgen dehydroepiandrosterone sulfate (DHEAS) in a process called adrenarche. Rising levels of DHEAS cause sebaceous glands to enlarge and produce more sebum. In girls, DHEAS levels correlate with the presence of acne in pre-puberty and with the future severity of comedonal acne; analogous data do not exist for boys. In both females and males, the prevalence and severity of acne correlate with stage of sexual maturity.

Despite the importance of androgens in causing acne, most patients have normal hormone levels. In females, the picture is more complex; although hormone levels are usually normal, elevations of total and free testosterone, and DHEAS, and decreases in sex hormone-binding globulin (SHBG) may occur. One study of adolescent girls with severe disease (Lucky, Biro et al, 1997) demonstrated that only 29% had serum DHEAS concentrations above the 90th percentile.

SEBUM

Under the stimulation of adrenal and gonadal androgens, sebum secretion peaks during adolescence and begins to decline after age 20. In general, acne severity correlates with rates of sebum secretion. Sebum from patients with acne is deficient in linoleic acid, a factor that may increase desquamation of skin cells, contributing to obstruction within follicles.

Learning Objectives

After reading this article, pediatricians will be able to:
- discuss the causes of acne and how these relate to clinical findings and decisions regarding treatment;
- discuss currently available medications for the treatment of acne;
- design a treatment plan for adolescents with acne; and
- discuss criteria for referral to a dermatologist.

Daniel P. Krowchuk, MD, FAAP, is an associate professor in the Departments of Pediatrics and Dermatology and an associate in Sports Medicine at the Wake Forest University School of Medicine, Winston-Salem, North Carolina. Dr. Krowchuk is also an attending pediatrician at Brenner Children's Hospital of Wake Forest University Baptist Medical Center and associate director of the Pediatric Dermatology Clinic.

Adolescent Health Update, Vol 11, No. 1, October 1998

BACTERIA

Propionibacterium (P.) acnes is an anaerobic, gram-positive diptheroid that begins to colonize pilosebaceous follicles following increases in sebum production that accompany adrenarche. The organism appears to use sebum as a nutrient. Although *P. acnes* is a normal inhabitant of the skin, its levels are higher in patients with acne.

P. acnes appears to contribute to the causation of acne in two ways. First, it produces chemoattractant factors that cause polymorphonuclear neutrophils (PMNs) to enter pilosebaceous follicles. As PMNs ingest *P. acnes,* hydrolytic enzymes are released that may damage the follicular wall. Follicular contents can then enter the dermis, where they incite inflammatory reactions that are manifest as erythematous papules, pustules, or nodules. Second, within the follicle, *P. acnes* hydrolyzes triglycerides in sebum to free fatty acids (FFAs) which may contribute to the inflammatory process and increase follicular obstruction.

OBSTRUCTION WITHIN FOLLICLES

Pilosebaceous follicles are lined with squamous epithelium that is contiguous with the skin surface. In persons with acne, epithelial cells from the follicle lining are not shed properly and become more cohesive. The result is a collection of cells that cannot escape the follicle. This process, called comedogenesis, is essential for the development of acne. The trigger for comedogenesis has not been identified. One hypothesis suggests an abnormality in epidermal differentiation while another implicates the abnormal sebum composition discussed previously.

GENETICS

There appears to be a familial predisposition to severe acne. However, it is not possible to predict the severity of disease for an individual based on family history.

Clinical Manifestations

The pathologic processes described above have clinical correlates. Patients with acne may exhibit obstructive or inflammatory lesions, cysts, or scars.

OBSTRUCTIVE LESIONS

Initially, obstruction within the follicle is microscopic and cannot be perceived clinically; such lesions are termed microcomedones (singular microcomedo). As comedones enlarge, they become apparent as "blackheads" (open comedones) or "whiteheads" (closed comedones). Open comedones represent follicles with a widely dilated orifice. The black color characteristic of these lesions does not represent dirt; rather, it is hypothesized to be the result of oxidation of melanin, interference in transmission of light through compacted epithelial cells, or the presence of certain lipids in sebum. Closed comedones are small white papules without surrounding erythema. They represent follicles that have become dilated with cellular and lipid debris but possess only a microscopic opening to the skin surface.

INFLAMMATORY LESIONS

Patients with inflammatory forms of acne manifest erythematous papules, pustules, or nodules. Papules and pustules are small, measuring <5 mm in diameter, while nodules are larger.

SCARS AND CYSTS

Some patients with acne develop scars or cysts as inflammatory lesions resolve. In general, scarring is most likely in adolescents who develop large nodules. However, even small inflammatory lesions may produce scars. Most often, and particularly on the face, acne scars have the appearance of deep pits. On the trunk they usually look like small white spots. Rarely, patients develop hypertrophic or keloidal scars. Since scars may be irreversible, the pediatrician should be aggressive in the selection of therapeutic agents active against the inflammatory component of the disease. Less common residua of healing acne lesions are cysts and nodules that lack overlying inflammation.

Evaluation

The first step in the evaluation is to gather a history. Helpful questions and their rationale are presented in Table 1. At a minimum the examination should include the face, chest, and back. Examination of other systems will

Table 1. Key Elements of the History

Question

Which medications have been tried?

Is the patient using other products to treat acne?

Is there a history of other medical problems?

Is the patient receiving other medications?

Does the patient use cosmetics or hair greases?

Does the patient have recreational or occupational activities that may worsen acne?

For females:

Is the patient menstruating? Are there premenstrual flare-ups?

Is there a history of oligomenorrhea or hirsutism?

Is the patient sexually active?

Does she use hormonal contraception?

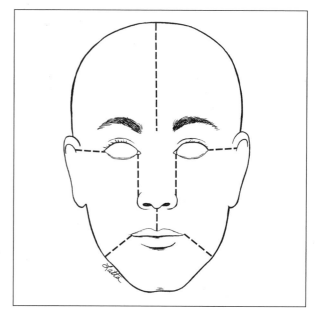

Figure 1. In each region, the physician records the number of open comedones (OC), closed comedones (CC), and inflammatory lesions (IL). (Diagram of face redrawn and reused with permission of Merck & Co., Inc.)

be dictated by the history. Routine measurement of serum androgens is not indicated. In females, hormone testing should be reserved for those with acne accompanied by other evidence of androgen excess (eg, irregular menses, hirsutism, or clitoromegaly).

To facilitate later comparison, an approximation of the number and types of lesions should be recorded for each geographic region. For the face, this may be accomplished using a diagram (see Figure 1). In each of the five areas in the diagram (excluding the nose), the clinician can estimate the number of inflammatory lesions, "blackheads," and "whiteheads." For the chest and back, one can also approximate the numbers and types of lesions present. Although this may seem tedious, it can be accomplished quickly and provides the clinician and patient with a valuable, objective assessment.

In addition to a "lesion count," it is helpful to make a global assessment of acne severity (eg, mild, moderate, or severe) that represents a synthesis of the number, size, and extent of lesions as well as the presence of scarring.

Treatment

Despite the potential negative impact of acne, some adolescents fail to voice concern about this problem during a clinical visit. Pediatricians should routinely ask patients if their acne is troublesome and if they desire treatment.

PATIENT EDUCATION

The clinician should briefly describe the causes of acne (see patient information sheet, page 288) and attempt to address and dispel commonly held myths.

● Acne is not caused by dirt and frequent washing will not improve the condition. In fact, frequent washing or the use of harsh soaps may irritate the skin and limit a patient's tolerance for topical medications. To control oily skin, patients may wash once or twice daily using a mild, nondrying soap.

● For most adolescents, diet plays no role in acne. Occasionally, a patient may observe an apparent relationship between a particular food and a flare-up. In such instances, common sense would limit the intake of this food.

Counsel the patient about those factors and behaviors that may worsen acne. The information contained in Table 1 may be of assistance in guiding this portion of the discussion.

- Picking at, wearing athletic gear over, or otherwise traumatizing acne lesions may increase inflammation, prolong resolution of lesions, and increase the likelihood of scar formation.
- Cosmetics and moisturizers, particularly those containing oils, may worsen acne. Advise the adolescent to take care to select cosmetics that are labeled oil-free, and noncomedogenic or nonacnegenic.
- A variant of cosmetic acne, known as pomade acne, may occur when greases used to style hair are inadvertently applied to the skin. Pomade acne is seen almost exclusively in African Americans and is characterized by the presence of comedones located on the forehead and temporal areas. To prevent such lesions, patients can be advised to keep hair care products away from their skin.
- Young women often experience premenstrual flare-ups that may be caused by androgenic effects of progesterone that is dominant during the second half of the menstrual cycle.
- Environmental factors may exacerbate acne among young people who come into contact with grease at work (eg, those employed in auto repair shops or fast-food restaurants). However, patients may be unwilling or unable to alter employment to accommodate concerns about acne.

Patients should be advised that acne treatment is a long-term process, taking 6 to 8 weeks before any therapeutic benefit is seen, and that when therapy is abandoned prematurely, the acne usually returns.

Medications

Medications to treat acne may be separated into topical and systemic preparations.

TOPICAL THERAPIES

Commonly employed topical preparations include benzoyl peroxide, antibiotics, retinoids, and salicylic acid. (See Table 2 for information on those most commonly used.)

Benzoyl peroxide: Benzoyl peroxide (BP) has antibacterial and anti-inflammatory effects. It may also decrease formation of free fatty acids, which would improve obstructive or comedonal disease. These two actions make it a useful first-line drug in the management of mild inflammatory or mixed (eg, inflammatory and comedonal) acne.

BP is available with or without a prescription in concentrations ranging from 2.5% to 10%. Over-the-counter products include creams, lotions, washes, or gels. Prescription forms generally employ a gel vehicle, a factor that enhances efficacy. A single daily application of a product containing a 5% concentration is adequate for most patients. Increasing the concentration of BP does not greatly enhance the therapeutic effect but does make skin irritation more likely.

BP is usually applied once daily, although twice-daily use may be beneficial for some patients. As with all topical medications, BP is applied as a thin coat to all acne-prone areas, not to individual lesions. When the entire face is to be treated, the patient may be instructed to dispense an amount the size of a pea onto a finger tip. To distribute the medication, the finger is touched to each side of the forehead, each cheek, and the chin. The medication is then spread to cover the entire face, avoiding the corners of the eyes, the alar folds, and the angles of the mouth. A BP wash that is applied during a bath or shower may be used to treat larger areas, such as the chest and back.

Adverse reactions resulting from the use of BP include stinging after application, and drying, redness, and peeling of the skin. These reactions often can be limited by selecting a water-based gel, or by reducing the concentration of BP. Contact dermatitis is an unusual complication characterized by erythema, small papules, and pruritus. To avoid this, patients using BP for the first time should apply a small amount of medication to the forearm. If there is no reaction after 48 to 72 hours, BP may be used on the face. Those who develop contact dermatitis should avoid BP and use an alternate product (eg, a topical antibiotic). Patients should be advised that BP may bleach clothing and bedding. It is safe for use during pregnancy.

Topical Antibiotics: Topical antibiotics kill *P. acnes*, reduce concentrations of mediators of

Table 2. Commonly Prescribed Topical Medications for the Treatment of Acne

Drug*	Formulation	Average Wholesale Price**	
Adapalene			
Differin	0.1% gel (15 gm, 45 gm)	15 gm	$23.63
	0.1% solution (30 ml)	30 ml	56.88
Antibiotics			
Clindamycin			
Cleocin T	1% gel (30 gm, 60 gm)	30 gm	23.58
	1% solution (30 ml, 60 ml)	30 ml	13.70
	1% pledgets (#60)	#60	32.24
	1% lotion (60 ml)	60 ml	32.79
Generic	1% solution (30 ml, 60 ml)	30 ml	10.97
Erythromycin			
Many products (generic)	2% gel (30 gm, 60 gm)	30 gm	19.11
	2% solution (60 ml)	60 ml	6.43
	2% swabs (#60)	#60	17.22
Erythromycin/benzoyl peroxide			
Benzamycin	3% erythromycin/5% benzoyl peroxide gel (23.3 gm, 46.6 gm)	23.3 gm	33.06
Azelaic acid			
Azelex	20% cream (30 gm)	30 gm	30.33
Benzoyl peroxide			
Many products (generic)	5% gel	45 gm	1.99
	2.5%–10% gel		
	5% liquid	4 oz	10.70
Tazarotene			
Tazorac	0.05% gel (30 gm, 100 gm)	30 gm	60.00
	0.1% gel (30 gm, 100 gm)	30 gm	63.75
Tretinoin			
Avita	0.025% cream (20 gm, 45 gm)	20 gm	27.12
Retin-A	cream: 0.025%, 0.05%, 0.1% (20 gm, 45 gm)	0.025%, 20 gm	29.34
	gel: 0.01%, 0.025% (15 gm, 45 gm)	0.01%, 15 gm	24.60
	micro: 0.1% (20 gm, 45 gm)	20 gm	31.08
	liquid: 0.05% (28 ml)	28 ml	45.54

* Use of trade names is for identification only and does not imply endorsement by the American Academy of Pediatrics.

**Medical Economics Inc. *1998 Drug Topics Red Book.* Montvale, NJ: Medical Economics, Inc.; 1998

inflammation, and may reduce FFA. As a result, these agents are most useful in the management of moderate inflammatory acne. However, the practical difficulties and cost associated with applying topical antibiotics to large areas limits their use to the treatment of facial acne. Products containing clindamycin or erythromycin are prescribed most often while tetracycline or meclocycline are used less frequently. All have comparable efficacy. Topical antibiotics are available in a variety of vehicles. As with other topical agents, lotions and creams are less drying than solutions or gels.

Products that combine agents enhance the therapeutic effect. For example, a formulation of BP 5% and erythromycin 3% (eg, Benzamycin) is more effective than either drug alone. Similarly, some formulations of erythromycin and zinc are more effective than erythromycin alone. The disadvantage of combination products is cost.

Topical retinoids: For adolescents with significant numbers of blackheads or whiteheads, topical retinoids are indicated. These drugs normalize the keratinization process within follicles, thereby reducing obstruction and the risk for follicular rupture. Retin-A (tretinoin) is the best known topical retinoid and is available in creams (0.025%, 0.05% and 0.1%), gels (0.01%, 0.025%), and a liquid (0.05%). The vehicle has an impact on efficacy; creams are less potent than gels which, in turn, are less potent than the liquid. A new formulation (Retin-A Micro 0.1%) is said to be as effective but less irritating than previous preparations. Tretinoin 0.25% cream is also marketed as Avita.

Many adolescents who use tretinoin experience irritation, redness or dryness. For African Americans, this inflammation may result in hypopigmentation that can last several months. To prevent or limit adverse effects, therapy is often begun with a 0.025% cream, the 0.1% micro preparation or adapalene (see below). Patients can be advised to use the medication every third night, progressing as tolerated over two to three weeks to a nightly application. Other adverse effects should be reviewed with the patient. About one-half of individuals experience an apparent, temporary, worsening of acne 2 to 3 weeks after starting tretinoin. Usually, this worsening results from increased photosensitivity caused by irritation. Because sensitivity to sunlight is increased, tretinoin should be applied at night and sunscreens used during the day. Applying too much tretinoin will worsen the irritant effect.

Because tretinoin is nearly identical in chemical structure to isotretinoin (eg, Accutane) some have raised concern about potential teratogenicity. There have been no reports of teratogenic effects in infants born to women who used tretinoin during pregnancy. Since *BP inactivates tretinoin,* the two drugs should not be applied simultaneously. Rather, BP may be applied in the morning and tretinoin at night.

Recently, two new topical retinoids have become available. Adapalene (eg, Differin) possesses retinoid-like activity and has been shown to be as effective as tretinoin but less irritating. It is available as a 0.1% alcohol-free gel or solution. The principles of use and potential adverse effects are the same as those of tretinoin. Tazarotene (eg, Tazorac) is formulated in 0.05% and 0.1% gels. Although proven effective in clinical studies, it is more expensive and may be more irritating than other retinoids and, therefore, is not widely prescribed for the treatment of acne.

Azelaic acid: Azelaic acid 20% (eg, Azelex) is both antibacterial and anticomedonal. It is applied twice daily and appears to be well tolerated, although some patients experience burning, irritation, erythema or dryness. No systemic toxicity has been reported. In one controlled trial, the drug was as effective as BP 5%, tretinoin 0.05%, or erythromycin 2%. Although clinical experience with azelaic acid is limited, it may be an alternative for patients with mild to moderate inflammatory and comedonal acne or for those with obstructive lesions who are unable to tolerate tretinoin.

Salicylic acid: Salicylic acid is available in prescription and nonprescription formulations. It reduces the formation of obstructive lesions but is less effective than tretinoin. Because it is less irritating, it may be useful for adolescents with obstructive acne who are unable to tolerate topical retinoids.

SYSTEMIC THERAPIES

Oral antibiotics: Oral antibiotics possess greater efficacy than topical preparations and, for this reason, are prescribed for patients with more severe or extensive inflammatory acne. Erythromycin and tetracycline are most often prescribed. Both drugs are effective and inexpensive. Depending on disease severity, both are initiated at a dose of 250 mg to 500 mg twice daily. The primary side effect of erythromycin is gastrointestinal upset that may be avoided by taking the medication with food. An additional concern is the possible development of erythromycin-resistant strains of *P. acnes.* Tetracycline is preferred by some clinicians. Although effective, it too has certain potential disadvantages. Tetracycline should not be taken with milk, it must be taken on an empty stomach, and, like erythromycin, it may cause gastrointestinal disturbances. Tetracycline should not be used during pregnancy or by patients under

9 years of age. Uncommon side effects include photosensitivity and esophageal ulceration. Finally, females taking tetracycline are more likely to develop vulvovaginal candidiasis.

For those who fail to respond to, or cannot tolerate, erythromycin or tetracycline, doxycycline is often effective. It is begun at a dose of 50 mg to 100 mg twice daily and can be taken with food. Unfortunately, doxycycline is even more likely than tetracycline to induce photosensitivity reactions. An alternative to doxycycline is minocycline, a drug favored by many dermatologists. Although effective, it is more expensive that other antibiotics and has uncommon but potentially permanent adverse effects, including pigmentation of skin, particularly in areas of scarring, and discoloration of teeth. Pigmentation is not necessarily irreversible; it may improve over time. Recent reports document minocycline-related hepatitis, arthritis, and a lupus erythematosus-like syndrome.

As with other acne therapies, 6 to 8 weeks are required before oral antibiotics produce a significant clinical effect. Once the appearance of new lesions has ceased or been satisfactorily reduced, the dose may be tapered gradually or eventually withdrawn. For example, if an adolescent's inflammatory acne has been controlled with erythromycin 250 mg twice daily, the dose may be decreased to 250 mg once daily. If control is sustained, the drug could be discontinued 1 to 2 months later in favor of topical therapy (eg, BP or a topical antibiotic). For some adolescents, however, attempts at tapering are unsuccessful and continued oral therapy may be required for months or years.

Concern often is raised that oral antibiotics may diminish oral contraceptive efficacy by decreasing enterohepatic recirculation of contraceptive steroids or by enhancing their hepatic degradation or renal excretion. Research fails to support this concern. However, packaging information provided with some oral contraceptives containing estrogen and progesterone states a "possible" reduction in efficacy during use of ampicillin or tetracyclines. Although "back-up" methods of birth control probably are not warranted, a final resolution of this issue is not likely to be forthcoming. Clinicians should advise

patients of this issue; based on this discussion, some patients may choose to employ a second form of contraception. For adolescents, however, the issue may be moot, since clinicians advise those using hormonal contraception to also employ a condom at all sexual encounters to protect against sexually transmitted infections.

13-cis-retinoic acid, isotretinoin (eg, Accutane) is an analogue of vitamin A that is highly effective for the treatment of severe or refractory inflammatory acne. Despite its efficacy, isotretinoin therapy may be associated with adverse effects, the most serious of which is teratogenicity. For this reason, the American Academy of Pediatrics Committee on Drugs has recommended that isotretinoin and other systemic retinoids should be prescribed "... only by those physicians with experience in the therapy ... of severe dermatological disorders." Thus, if a pediatrician believes that a patient is a candidate for isotretinoin, referral to a dermatologist is indicated. Some adolescents will take large doses of vitamin A to treat acne, believing it will be beneficial because of its relationship to isotretinoin. This practice should be discouraged, as it is ineffective and potentially harmful.

Hormonal therapy: Hormonal contraceptives may affect acne in several ways. Estrogen improves acne by increasing levels of SHBG, which decreases biologically active free testosterone and suppresses gonadotropin secretion, thereby reducing ovarian androgen production. The androgenic and antiestrogenic potential of the progestin component of an oral or other hormonal contraceptive also may influence acne severity. Thus, oral contraceptives containing progestins with low androgenic potential (eg, norethindrone or its acetate, ethynodiol diacetate, or a newer agent such as norgestimate) are considered to have the most favorable effects on acne. In contrast, the progestins in depot medroxyprogesterone acetate and long-acting progestin implants often worsen acne. Recent studies indicate that oral contraceptives containing newer progestins can improve inflammatory acne. These results notwithstanding, these agents are not generally viewed as a primary therapy for acne but as adjuncts. However, when selecting a hormonal contraceptive for an adolescent, particularly one who has acne, consideration should be given to its potential impact on the skin.

Adolescents with acne exacerbated by endocrine disorders may require treatment with other agents such as spironolactone (an androgen antagonist), low-dose glucocorticoids, or gonadotropin-releasing hormone agonists. Patients with these conditions are best managed in consultation with a specialist (eg, endocrinologist, gynecologist, or gynecologic endocrinologist).

Putting it Together

Deciding which medication(s) should be prescribed for an adolescent with acne is based on the types and numbers of lesions present, your impression of the severity of disease, the extent of acne, the patient's past experiences with medications, and personal preferences. Information contained in Table 3 is designed to assist you in developing rational treatment plans. Beyond this, however, there is an art to treating acne and two clinicians may differ in their approach to the same patient. Disturbingly, therapeutic choices may be governed by formulary restrictions. In some states, for example, prescription topical acne medications are not approved for Medicaid reimbursement.

Follow-up

A return visit is typically scheduled for 2 months following the initiation of therapy. However, adolescents should be encouraged to telephone sooner with questions or concerns regarding possible adverse effects. At the follow-up visit, one can determine the patient's impression of response to treatment, note the occurrence of adverse effects, and make an objective assessment of the effect of therapy. Based on the initial response, the pediatrician can determine and discuss the need to maintain or revise the therapeutic plan.

Table 3. Possible Management Options for Facial Acne

Acne Severity	Lesion Type	Initial Treatment	If No Response
Mild	Comedonal	Benzoyl peroxide gel 5% once daily	Substitute or combine with tretinoin cream 0.025%* once daily
	Inflammatory	Benzoyl peroxide gel 5% once daily	Increase benzoyl peroxide application to twice daily or substitute topical antibiotic twice daily
	Mixed	Benzoyl peroxide gel 5% once daily or azelaic acid twice daily	Add tretinoin cream 0.025%* once daily (for comedonal component), and/or substitute topical antibiotic twice daily (for inflammatory component)
Moderate	Comedonal	Tretinoin cream 0.025% once daily*	Increase strength of tretinoin to 0.05% cream
	Inflammatory	Topical antibiotic twice daily	Oral antibiotic (eg, erythromycin or tetracycline 250 mg) twice daily
	Mixed	Benzoyl peroxide gel 5% once daily and tretinoin cream 0.025%* once daily or azelaic acid, twice daily	Add oral antibiotic (eg, erythromycin or tetracycline, 250 mg twice daily) or substitute oral antibiotic for benzoyl peroxide. Continue tretinoin.
Severe	Comedonal	Tretinoin cream 0.025% once daily*	Increase strength of tretinoin to 0.05% cream
	Inflammatory	Oral antibiotic (eg, erythromycin or tetracycline) 250 mg–500 mg twice daily	Consider referral to dermatologist
	Mixed	Tretinoin cream 0.025%* once daily, and oral antibiotic (eg, erythromycin or tetracycline) 250 mg–500 mg twice daily	Consider referral to dermatologist

* Or another appropriate topical retinoid (eg, tretinoin gel 0.1% or adapalene)

When to Refer

Although most adolescents with acne have mild to moderate disease and can be managed effectively by their pediatrician, referral to a dermatologist occasionally is required. Common reasons for seeking consultation include refractory disease despite appropriate therapy, consideration for treatment with isotretinoin, the presence of cysts that may require intralesional injection of a corticosteroid, and management of acne scars.

Summary

Acne is the most common skin disorder that affects adolescents and one that pediatricians are frequently asked to treat. Although there is no cure for acne, the majority of patients will benefit from currently available medications, and most can be effectively managed by their pediatrician. By providing this care, pediatricians can reduce the emotional burden of acne and help prevent the permanent scarring so commonly seen in the past.

Acknowledgment

The editors would like to acknowledge technical review by Moise Levy, MD, FAAP, for the AAP Section on Dermatology.

Further Reading

Committee on Drugs, American Academy of Pediatrics. Retinoid therapy for severe dermatological disorders. *Pediatrics.* 1992;90:119–120

Helms SE, Brendle DL, Zajic J, Jarjoura D, Brodell RT, Krishnarao I. Oral contraceptive failure rates and oral antibiotics. *J Am Acad Dermatol.* 1997;36:705–710

Leyden JJ. Therapy for acne vulgaris. *N Eng J Med.* 1997;336: 1156–1162

Lucky AW, Biro FM, Simbarti LA, Morrison JA, Sorg NW. Predictors of severity of acne in young adolescent girls: Results of a five-year longitudinal study. *J Pediatr.* 1997;130:30–39

Lucky AW, Henderson TA, Olson WH, Robisch DM, Lebwohl M, Swinyer LJ. Effectiveness of norgestimate and ethinyl estradiol in treating moderate acne vulgaris. *J Am Acad Dermatol.* 1997;37:746–754

Miller DM, Helms SE, Brodell RT. A practical approach to antibiotic treatment in women taking oral contraceptives. *J Am Acad Dermatol.* 1994;30:1008–1011

Rothman KF, Lucky AW. Acne vulgaris. *Adv Dermatol.* 1993; 8:347–375

What You Should Know About Acne

Acne is a skin problem that begins about the time someone becomes a teenager and usually goes away as he or she gets older. Almost every teenager gets acne, but some people develop more pimples than others. During the time that a person has acne, it can be made better but it can't be cured. This means that medicines that can make acne better need to be used for a long time. This information sheet is meant to help you understand acne and how to make it better.

What causes acne?

Pimples begin in certain pores or openings in the skin. These pores have oil glands connected to them. At puberty, the time that you begin to grow into an adult, certain chemicals, called hormones, cause the oil glands to make more oil. You may have noticed that your skin became more oily before acne began. The oil and cells that line your pores stick together and cause a plug or block in the pore. The result is a blackhead or whitehead. The blackhead is not dirt and scrubbing or washing won't remove it. Whiteheads are the beginnings of larger pimples. The oil and other material in whiteheads may break through the pore wall and cause irritation under the skin—a pimple.

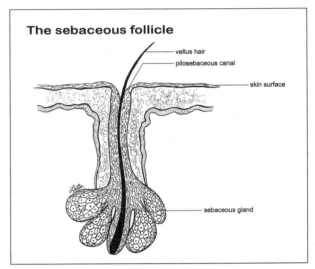

Original art adapted from Tunnessen, WW. "Help your acne patients help themselves," CONTEMPORARY PEDIATRICS, September 1984, Figure 1, page 12.

What makes acne worse?

- If you pinch, pop or pick at pimples you may cause them to become larger, take longer to disappear or scar.
- Washing too often or with harsh soaps may irritate the skin and make it hard to use the medicines that are prescribed by your doctor. To prevent this, wash only once or twice a day with a mild soap.
- Some makeups, cover-ups or hair greases may block pores and make your acne worse. If you use makeup or moisturizers, choose those that are oil-free and labeled as *non-acnegenic* or *noncomedogenic*. If you use a hair grease, try not to get it on the skin.
- Equipment (like helmets or chinstraps) or tight clothing that puts pressure on the skin may make acne worse in this area.
- Many young women notice a worsening of acne before a menstrual period. This is caused by changes in hormones.
- For some teenagers, stress may make acne worse.
- Foods like chocolate, other sweets or french fries almost never make acne worse.

How do we treat acne?

Acne does not go away overnight with treatment. *It takes time*—more time than you would like—to unblock the pores. In fact, it takes 6 to 8 weeks of using medicine before you see a change in your skin. Try to be patient. Don't give up too soon.

There are a number of medicines we may use. Some work better for some people than others. We need your help to tell us which ones work best for you. Sometimes we need to use more than one medicine.

Using topical medications (those placed on the skin):

Many of the medicines used to treat acne (like benzoyl peroxide, tretinoin and certain antibiotics) are placed on the skin. There are a few basic rules about using these medicines:

- Don't apply medication right after you wash your face. Waiting 20 to 30 minutes will help prevent drying and redness of your skin.
- Don't use too much medicine. A little bit is good, but a lot is NOT better. If too much medicine is used, your skin may become dry or red. To get the right amount, place a dab of medicine the size of a small pea on your finger. Dab the medicine on each side of your forehead, on each cheek, and on your chin. Then spread the medicine to make a thin coat over all areas where you get pimples. Some medicines are liquids that come with an applicator.
- Remember that the medicine should be placed over all problem areas and not just on pimples.

- If your skin becomes dry you may use an oil-free, nonacnegenic or noncomedogenic moisturizer. If it becomes too dry, red, or irritated, call your doctor.

How long must the medicines be used?

Even though acne usually goes away as one gets older, it can last for years. How long you will need to use medicines depends on your skin.

Your medicines:

The medicines that your doctor recommends that you use are written below along with directions on how to use them. We will want to see you in about two months to see how the medicines are working for you.

Name of Medicine   **How to Use the Medicine**

_____   _____

_____   _____

_____   _____

_____   _____

_____   _____

_____   _____

_____   _____

_____   _____

Content adapted from "Help your acne patients help themselves," by Walter W. Tunnessen, Jr., MD, CONTEMPORARY PEDIATRICS, September 1984, pages 17-18. Updated by the author and used with permission.

Pediatricians are welcome to photocopy this two-page patient education sheet for distribution to patients.

Important Information for Teens Who Get Headaches
Guidelines for Teens

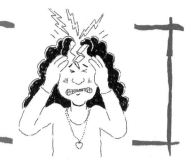

A headache is not a disease, but it may indicate that something is wrong. Headaches are common among teenagers and generally are not serious. In fact, 50% to 75% of all teens report having at least one headache per month. However, more frequent headaches can be upsetting and worrisome for you and your family. The most common headaches for teenagers are tension headaches and migraines. Sometimes these problems may be associated with health concerns that require a visit to your pediatrician.

What causes headaches?

Headaches are most commonly caused by:

Illness—Headaches often are a symptom of other illnesses. Viral infections, strep throat, allergies, sinus infections, and urinary tract infections can be accompanied by headaches. Fever may also be associated with headaches.

Skipping meals—Even if you're trying to lose weight, you still need to eat regularly. Fad diets can make you hungry and also can give you a headache. Not getting enough fluids—which leads to dehydration—also may cause a headache.

Drugs—Alcohol, cocaine, amphetamines, diet pills, and other drugs may give you a headache.

Often headaches are triggered by sleep problems, minor head injuries, or certain foods (dairy products, chocolate, food additives like nitrates, nitrites, and monosodium glutamate).

Sometimes, headaches can also be caused by prescribed medication, such as birth control pills, tetracycline for acne, and high doses of vitamin A.

Less commonly, headaches can be caused by a dental infection or abscess, and jaw alignment problems (TMJ syndrome). Although headaches are only rarely caused by eye problems, pain around the eyes—which can feel like a headache—can be caused by eye muscle imbalance or not wearing glasses that have been prescribed for you.

Only in **very** rare cases are headaches a symptom of a brain tumor, high blood pressure, or other serious problem.

Types of headaches

Tension headaches often feel like a tight band is around your head. The pain is dull and aching and usually will be felt on both sides of your head, but may be in front and back as well.

Pressure at school or at home, arguments with parents or friends, having too much to do, and feeling anxious or depressed can all cause a headache.

Migraines often are described as throbbing and usually are felt on only one side of your head, but may be felt on both. A migraine may make you feel light-headed or dizzy, and/or make your stomach upset. You may see spots or be sensitive to light, sounds, and smells. If you get migraines, chances are one of your parents or other family members also have had this problem.

A third, less common, type of headache is called a **psychogenic** headache. Psychogenic headaches are similar to tension headaches, but the cause is an emotional problem such as depression. Signs of depression include loss of energy, poor appetite or overeating, loss of interest in usual activities, change in sleeping patterns (trouble falling asleep, waking in the middle of the night or too early in the morning), and difficulty thinking or concentrating.

When should I see the pediatrician?

If you are worried about your headaches—or if this problem begins to disrupt your school, home, or social life—see your pediatrician. Other signs that may mean you should visit your pediatrician include:

Head injury—Headaches from a recent head injury should be checked right away—especially if you were knocked out by the injury.

Seizures/convulsions—Any headaches associated with seizures or fainting require immediate attention.

Frequency—You get more than one headache a week.

Degree of pain—Headache pain is severe and prevents you from doing activities you want to do.

Time of attack—Headaches that wake you from sleep or occur in early morning.

Visual difficulties—Headaches that cause blurred vision, eye spots, or other visual changes.

Other associated symptoms—If fever, vomiting, stiff neck, toothache, or jaw pain accompany your headache, you may require an examination—including laboratory or x-ray tests.

How are headaches treated?

Whichever type of headache you get, and whatever the cause, your pediatrician can explain why you get headaches and how they can be controlled. Be sure to ask any questions you may have.

If you get tension headaches or mild migraines, your pediatrician may suggest an aspirin or an aspirin substitute, such as acetaminophen or ibuprofen, and rest. If you get more severe headaches or classic migraines (when you have a visual disturbance called an "aura"), prescription medicine may be required. Your pediatrician may suggest that you keep a **headache diary** to help pinpoint information about what is causing the headaches. A headache diary helps you keep track of the following: when headaches occur, how long they last, what you were doing when the headaches start, what you had eaten, how much sleep you have had, and what seems to make the headaches better or worse.

If what you eat seems to trigger your headaches, your pediatrician will suggest that you eliminate certain foods from your diet. If stress is the culprit, your doctor can help you cope by suggesting special treatments such as relaxation exercises. Headaches that are caused by an emotional or psychological problem may require additional visits to your pediatrician or to other health care professionals to get to the cause of the problem. Sometimes entire families need counseling to eliminate the stress that is causing headaches.

It's important to know that, whatever the cause, headache pain is real. More importantly, with your pediatrician's help, you can identify the source of your headaches and get this problem under control.

The information contained in this publication should not be used as a substitute for the medical care and advice of your pediatrician. There may be variations in treatment that your pediatrician may recommend based on individual facts and circumstances.

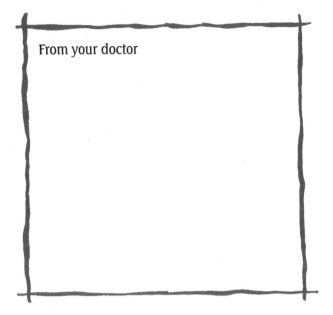

From your doctor

American Academy of Pediatrics

DEDICATED TO THE HEALTH OF ALL CHILDREN™

The American Academy of Pediatrics is an organization of 60,000 primary care pediatricians, pediatric medical subspecialists, and pediatric surgical specialists dedicated to the health, safety, and well-being of infants, children, adolescents, and young adults.

American Academy of Pediatrics
Web site — www.aap.org

Section II Further Reading

Feinberg AN, Lane-Davies A. Syncope in the adolescent. *Adolesc Med.* 2002;13:553–567

Hanna CE, LaFranchi SH. Adolescent thyroid disorders. *Adolesc Med.* 2002;13:13–35

Howenstine MS, Eigen H. Medical care of the adolescent with asthma. *Adolesc Med.* 2000;11:501–519

Kim HJ. Photoprotection in adolescents. *Adolesc Med.* 2001;12:181–193

Krowchuk DP, Lucky AW. Managing adolescent acne. *Adolesc Med.* 2001;12:355–374

Lewis DW. Migraine headaches in adolescents. *Adolesc Med.* 2002;13:413–432

Owens T. Chest pain in the adolescent. *Adolesc Med.* 2001;12:95–104

Pakalnis A. Nonmigraine headache in adolescents. *Adolesc Med.* 2002;13:433–442

Rowell HA, Evans BJ, Quarry-Horn JL, Kerrigan JR. Type 2 diabetes mellitus in adolescents. *Adolesc Med.* 2002;13:1–12

Schuen JN, Millard SL. Evaluation and treatment of sleep disorders in adolescents. *Adolesc Med.* 2000;11:605–616

Walsh CA. Syncope and sudden death in the adolescent. *Adolesc Med.* 2001;12:105–132

Ward MA. Lower respiratory tract infections in adolescents. *Adolesc Med.* 2000;11:251–262

White CB, Foshee WS. Upper respiratory tract infections in adolescents. *Adolesc Med.* 2000;11:225–249

Nutrition, Obesity, and Eating Disorders

Identifying and Treating Eating Disorders

Committee on Adolescence

ABSTRACT. Pediatricians are called on to become involved in the identification and management of eating disorders in several settings and at several critical points in the illness. In the primary care pediatrician's practice, early detection, initial evaluation, and ongoing management can play a significant role in preventing the illness from progressing to a more severe or chronic state. In the subspecialty setting, management of medical complications, provision of nutritional rehabilitation, and coordination with the psychosocial and psychiatric aspects of care are often handled by pediatricians, especially those who have experience or expertise in the care of adolescents with eating disorders. In hospital and day program settings, pediatricians are involved in program development, determining appropriate admission and discharge criteria, and provision and coordination of care. Lastly, primary care pediatricians need to be involved at local, state, and national levels in preventive efforts and in providing advocacy for patients and families. The roles of pediatricians in the management of eating disorders in the pediatric practice, subspecialty, hospital, day program, and community settings are reviewed in this statement.

ABBREVIATIONS. DSM-IV, *Diagnostic and Statistical Manual of Mental Disorders, Fourth Edition;* BMI, body mass index; *DSM-PC, Diagnostic and Statistic Manual for Primary Care.*

Introduction

Increases in the incidence and prevalence of anorexia and bulimia nervosa in children and adolescents have made it increasingly important that pediatricians be familiar with the early detection and appropriate management of eating disorders. Epidemiologic studies document that the numbers of children and adolescents with eating disorders increased steadily from the 1950s onward.[1-4] During the past decade, the prevalence of obesity in children and adolescents has increased significantly,[5,6] accompanied by an unhealthy emphasis on dieting and weight loss among children and adolescents, especially in suburban settings[7-10]; increasing concerns with weight-related issues in children at progressively younger ages[11,12]; growing awareness of the presence of eating disorders in males[13,14]; increases in the prevalence of eating disorders among minority populations in the United States[15-18]; and the identification of eating disorders in countries that had not previously been experiencing those problems.[3,4,19,20] It is estimated that 0.5% of adolescent females in the United States have anorexia nervosa, that 1% to 5% meet criteria for bulimia nervosa, and that up to 5% to 10% of all cases of eating disorders occur in males. There are also a large number of individuals with milder cases who do not meet all of the criteria in the *Diagnostic and Statistical Manual of Mental Disorders, Fourth Edition (DSM-IV)* for anorexia or bulimia nervosa but who nonetheless experience the physical and psychologic consequences of having an eating disorder.[21-25] Long-term follow-up for these patients can help reduce sequelae of the diseases; *Healthy People 2010* includes an objective (#18.5) seeking to reduce the relapse rates for persons with eating disorders including anorexia nervosa and bulimia nervosa.[26]

The Role of the Pediatrician in the Identification and Evaluation of Eating Disorders

Primary care pediatricians are in a unique position to detect the onset of eating disorders and stop their progression at the earliest stages of the illness. Primary and secondary prevention is accomplished by screening for eating disorders as part of routine annual health care, providing ongoing monitoring of weight and height, and paying careful attention to the signs and symptoms of an incipient eating disorder. Early detection and management of an eating disorder may prevent the physical and psychologic consequences of malnutrition that allow for progression to a later stage.[23,24]

Screening questions about eating patterns and satisfaction with body appearance should be asked of all preteens and adolescents as part of routine pediatric health care. Weight and height need to be determined regularly (preferably in a hospital gown, because objects may be hidden in clothing to falsely elevate weight). Ongoing measurements of weight and height should be plotted on pediatric growth charts to evaluate for decreases in both that can occur as a result of restricted nutritional intake.[27] Body mass index (BMI), which compares weight with height, can be a helpful measurement in tracking concerns; BMI is calculated as:

$$\text{weight in pounds} \infty 700/(\text{height in inches squared})$$

or

$$\text{weight in kilograms}/(\text{height in meters squared}).$$

Newly developed growth charts are available for plotting changes in weight, height, and BMI over time and for comparing individual measurements with age-appropriate population norms.[27] Any evidence of inappropriate dieting, excessive concern with weight, or a weight loss pattern requires further attention, as does a failure to achieve appropriate increases in weight or height in growing children. In each of these situations, careful assessment for the possibility of an eating disorder and close monitoring at intervals as frequent as every 1 to 2 weeks may be needed until the situation becomes clear.

A number of studies have shown that most adolescent females express concerns about being overweight, and many may diet inappropriately.[7-10] Most of these children and adolescents do not have an eating disorder. On the other hand, it is known that patients with eating disorders may try to hide their illness, and usually no specific signs or symptoms are detected, so a simple denial by the adolescent does not negate the possibility of an eating disorder. It is wise,

therefore, for the pediatrician to be cautious by following weight and nutrition patterns very closely or referring to a specialist experienced in the treatment of eating disorders when suspected. In addition, taking a history from a parent may help identify abnormal eating attitudes or behaviors, although parents may at times be in denial as well. Failure to detect an eating disorder at this early stage can result in an increase in severity of the illness, either further weight loss in cases of anorexia nervosa or increases in bingeing and purging behaviors in cases of bulimia nervosa, which can then make the eating disorder much more difficult to treat. In situations in which an adolescent is referred to the pediatrician because of concerns by parents, friends, or school personnel that he or she is displaying evidence of an eating disorder, it is most likely that the adolescent does have an eating disorder, either incipient or fully established. Pediatricians must, therefore, take these situations very seriously and not be lulled into a false sense of security if the adolescent denies all symptoms. Table 1 outlines questions useful in eliciting a history of eating disorders, and Table 2 delineates possible physical findings in children and adolescents with eating disorders.

Initial evaluation of the child or adolescent with a suspected eating disorder includes establishment of the diagnosis; determination of severity, including evaluation of medical and nutritional status; and performance of an initial psychosocial evaluation. Each of these initial steps can be performed in the pediatric primary care setting. The American Psychiatric Association has established *DSM-IV* criteria for the diagnosis of anorexia and bulimia nervosa (Table 3).[24] These criteria focus on the weight loss, attitudes and behaviors, and amenorrhea displayed by patients with eating disorders. Of note, studies have shown that more than half of all children and adolescents with eating disorders may not fully meet all *DSM-IV* criteria for anorexia or bulimia nervosa while still experiencing the same medical and psychologic consequences of these disorders[28]; these patients are included in another *DSM-IV* diagnosis, referred to as eating disorder-not otherwise specified.[24] The pediatrician needs

Table 1. Specific Screening Questions to Identify the Child, Adolescent, or Young Adult With an Eating Disorder

What is the most you ever weighed? How tall were you then? When was that?

What is the least you ever weighed in the past year? How tall were you then? When was that?

What do you think you ought to weigh?

Exercise: how much, how often, level of intensity? How stressed are you if you miss a workout?

Current dietary practices: ask for specifics—amounts, food groups, fluids, restrictions?
- 24-h diet history?
- Calorie counting, fat gram counting? Taboo foods (foods you avoid)?
- Any binge eating? Frequency, amount, triggers?
- Purging history?
- Use of diuretics, laxatives, diet pills, ipecac? Ask about elimination pattern, constipation, diarrhea.
- Any vomiting? Frequency, how long after meals?

Any previous therapy? What kind and how long? What was and was not helpful?

Family history: obesity, eating disorders, depression, other mental illness, substance abuse by parents or other family members?

Menstrual history: age at menarche? Regularity of cycles? Last menstrual period?

Use of cigarettes, drugs, alcohol? Sexual history? History of physical or sexual abuse?

Review of symptoms:
- Dizziness, syncope, weakness, fatigue?
- Pallor, easy bruising or bleeding?
- Cold intolerance?
- Hair loss, lanugo, dry skin?
- Vomiting, diarrhea, constipation?
- Fullness, bloating, abdominal pain, epigastric burning?
- Muscle cramps, joint paints, palpitations, chest pain?
- Menstrual irregularities?
- Symptoms of hyperthyroidism, diabetes, malignancy, infection, inflammatory bowel disease?

Table 2. Possible Findings on Physical Examination in Children and Adolescents With Eating Disorders

Anorexia Nervosa	Bulimia Nervosa
Bradycardia	Sinus bradycardia
Orthostatic by pulse or blood pressure	Orthostatic by pulse or blood pressure
Hypothermia	Hypothermia
Cardiac murmur (one third with mitral valve prolapse)	Cardiac murmur (mitral valve prolapse)
Dull, thinning scalp hair	Hair without shine
Sunken cheeks, sallow skin	Dry skin
Lanugo	Parotitis
Atrophic breasts (postpubertal)	Russell's sign (callous on knuckles from self-induced emesis)
Atrophic vaginitis (postpubertal)	Mouth sores
Pitting edema of extremities	Palatal scratches
Emaciated, may wear oversized clothes	Dental enamel erosions
Flat affect	May look entirely normal
Cold extremities, acrocyanosis	Other cardiac arrhythmias

Table 3. Diagnosis of Anorexia Nervosa, Bulimia Nervosa, and Eating Disorders Not Otherwise Specified, From *DSM-IV*[25]

Anorexia Nervosa

1. Intense fear of becoming fat or gaining weight, even though underweight.
2. Refusal to maintain body weight at or above a minimally normal weight for age and height (ie, weight loss leading to maintenance of body weight <85% of that expected, or failure to make expected weight gain during period of growth, leading to body weight <85% of that expected).
3. Disturbed body image, undue influence of shape or weight on self-evaluation, or denial of the seriousness of the current low body weight.
4. Amenorrhea or absence of at least 3 consecutive menstrual cycles (those with periods only inducible after estrogen therapy are considered amenorrheic).
   Types:
   Restricting—no regular bingeing or purging (self-induced vomiting or use of laxatives and diuretics).
   Binge eating/purging—regular bingeing and purging in a patient who also meets the above criteria for anorexia nervosa.

Bulimia Nervosa

1. Recurrent episodes of binge eating, characterized by:
   a. Eating a substantially larger amount of food in a discrete period of time (ie, in 2 h) than would be eaten by most people in similar circumstances during that same time period.
   b. A sense of lack of control over eating during the binge.
2. Recurrent inappropriate compensatory behavior to prevent weight gain; ie, self-induced vomiting, use of laxatives, diuretics, fasting, or hyperexercising.
3. Binges or inappropriate compensatory behaviors occuring, on average, at least twice weekly for at least 3 mo.
4. Self-evaluation unduly influenced by body shape or weight.
5. The disturbance does not occur exclusively during episodes of anorexia nervosa
   Types:
   Purging—regularly engages in self-induced vomiting or use of laxatives or diuretics.
   Nonpurging—uses other inappropriate compensatory behaviors; ie, fasting or hyperexercising, without regular use of vomiting or medications to purge.

Eating Disorder Not Otherwise Specified (those who do not meet criteria for anorexia nervosa or bulimia nervosa, per *DSM-IV*)

1. All criteria for anorexia nervosa, except has regular menses.
2. All criteria for anorexia nervosa, except weight still in normal range.
3. All criteria for bulimia nervosa, except binges <twice a wk or <3 times a mo.
4. A patient with normal body weight who regularly engages in inappropriate compensatory behavior after eating small amounts of food (ie, self-induced vomiting after eating 2 cookies).
5. A patient who repeatedly chews and spits out large amounts of food without swallowing.
6. Binge eating disorder: recurrent binges but does not engage in the inappropriate compensatory behaviors of bulimia nervosa.

---

to be aware that patients with eating disorders not otherwise specified require the same careful attention as those who meet criteria for anorexia or bulimia nervosa. A patient who has lost weight rapidly but who does not meet full criteria because weight is not yet 15% below that which is expected for height may be more physically and psychologically compromised than may a patient of lower weight. Also, in growing children, it is failure to make appropriate gains in weight and height, not necessarily weight loss per se, that indicates the severity of the malnutrition. It is also common for adolescents to have significant purging behaviors without episodes of binge eating; although these

patients do not meet the full *DSM-IV* criteria for bulimia nervosa, they may become severely medically compromised. These issues are addressed in the *Diagnostic and Statistical Manual for Primary Care (DSM-PC) Child and Adolescent Version*, which provides diagnostic codes and criteria for purging and bingeing, dieting, and body image problems that do not meet *DSM-IV* criteria.[29] In general, determination of total weight loss and weight status (calculated as percent below ideal body weight and/or as BMI), along with types and frequency of purging behaviors (including vomiting and use of laxatives, diuretics, ipecac, and over-the-counter or prescription diet pills as well as use of starvation and/or exercise) serve to establish an initial index of severity for the child or adolescent with an eating disorder.

The medical complications associated with eating disorders are listed in Table 4, and details of these complications have been described in several reviews.[23,24,30-34] It is uncommon for the pediatrician to encounter most of these complications in a patient with a newly diagnosed eating disorder. However, it is recommended that an initial laboratory assessment be performed and that this include complete blood cell count, electrolyte measurement, liver function tests, urinalysis, and a thyroid-stimulating hormone test. Additional tests (urine pregnancy, luteinizing and follicle-stimulating hormone, prolactin, and estradiol tests) may need to be performed in patients who are amenorrheic to rule out other causes for amenorrhea, including pregnancy, ovarian failure, or prolactinoma. Other tests, including an erythrocyte sedimentation rate and radiographic studies (such as computed tomography or magnetic resonance imaging of the brain or upper or lower gastrointestinal system studies), should be performed if there are uncertainties about the diagnosis. An electrocardiogram should be performed on any patient with bradycardia or electrolyte abnormalities. Bone densitometry should be considered in those amenorrheic for more than 6 to 12 months. It should be noted, however, that most test results will be normal in most patients with eating disorders, and normal laboratory test results do not exclude serious illness or medical instability in these patients.

The initial psychosocial assessment should include an evaluation of the patient's degree of obsession with food and weight, understanding of the diagnosis, and willingness to receive help; an assessment of the patient's functioning at home, in school, and with friends; and a determination of other psychiatric diagnoses (such as depression, anxiety, and obsessive-compulsive disorder), which may be comorbid with or may

Table 4. Medical Complications Resulting From Eating Disorders

Medical Complications Resulting From Purging

1. Fluid and electrolyte imbalance; hypokalemia; hyponatremia; hypochloremic alkalosis.
2. Use of ipecac: irreversible myocardial damage and a diffuse myositis.
3. Chronic vomiting: esophagitis; dental erosions; Mallory-Weiss tears; rare esophageal or gastric rupture; rare aspiration pneumonia.
4. Use of laxatives: depletion of potassium bicarbonate, causing metabolic acidosis; increased blood urea nitrogen concentration and predisposition to renal stones from dehydration; hyperuricemia; hypocalcemia; hypomagnesemia; chronic dehydration. With laxative withdrawal, may get fluid retention (may gain up to 10 lb in 24 h).
5. Amenorrhea (can be seen in normal or overweight individuals with bulimia nervosa), menstrual irregularities, osteopenia.

Medical Complications From Caloric Restriction

1. Cardiovascular

   Electrocardiographic abnormalities: low voltage; sinus bradycardia (from malnutrition); T wave inversions; ST segment depression (from electrolyte imbalances). Prolonged corrected QT interval is uncommon but may predispose patient to sudden death. Dysrhythmias include supraventricular beats and ventricular tachycardia, with or without exercise. Pericardial effusions can occur in those severely malnourished. All cardiac abnormalities except those secondary to emetine (ipecac) toxicity are completely reversible with weight gain.
2. Gastrointestinal system: delayed gastric emptying; slowed gastrointestinal motility; constipation; bloating; fullness; hypercholesterolemia (from abnormal lipoprotein metabolism); abnormal liver function test results (probably from fatty infiltration of the liver). All reversible with weight gain.
3. Renal: increased blood urea nitrogen concentration (from dehydration, decreased glomerular filtration rate) with increased risk of renal stones; polyuria (from abnormal vasopressin secretion, rare partial diabetes insipidus). Total body sodium and potassium depletion caused by starvation; with refeeding, 25% can get peripheral edema attributable to increased renal sensitivity to aldosterone and increased insulin secretion (affects renal tubules).
4. Hematologic: leukopenia; anemia; iron deficiency; thrombocytopenia.
5. Endocrine: euthyroid sick syndrome; amenorrhea; osteopenia.
6. Neurologic: cortical atrophy; seizures.

be a cause or consequence of the eating disorder. Suicidal ideation and history of physical or sexual abuse or violence should also be assessed. The parents' reaction to the illness should be assessed, because denial of the problem or parental differences in how to approach treatment and recovery may exacerbate the patient's illness. The pediatrician who feels competent and comfortable in performing the full initial evaluation is encouraged to do so. Others should refer to appropriate medical subspecialists and mental health personnel to ensure that a complete evaluation is performed. A differential diagnosis for the adolescent with symptoms of an eating disorder can be found in Table 5.

Several treatment decisions follow the initial evaluation, including the questions of where and by whom the patient will be treated. Patients who have minimal nutritional, medical, and psychosocial issues and show a quick reversal of their condition may be treated in the pediatrician's office, usually in conjunction with a registered dietitian and a mental health practitioner. Pediatricians who do not feel comfortable with issues of medical and psychosocial management can refer these patients at this early stage. Pediatricians can choose to stay involved even after referral to the team of specialists, as the family often appreciates the comfort of the relationship with their long-term care provider. Pediatricians comfortable with the ongoing care and secondary prevention of medical complications in patients with eating disorders may choose to continue care themselves. More severe cases require the involvement of a multidisciplinary specialty

Table 5. Differential Diagnosis of Eating Disorders

- Malignancy, central nervous system tumor
- Gastrointestinal system: inflammatory bowel disease, malabsorption, celiac disease
- Endocrine: diabetes mellitus, hyperthyroidism, hypopituitarism, Addison disease
- Depression, obsessive-compulsive disorder, psychiatric diagnosis
- Other chronic disease or chronic infections
- Superior mesenteric artery syndrome (can also be a consequence of an eating disorder)

team working in outpatient, inpatient, or day program settings.

The Pediatrician's Role in the Treatment of Eating Disorders in Outpatient Settings

Pediatricians have several important roles to play in the management of patients with diagnosed eating disorders. These aspects of care include medical and nutritional management and coordination with mental health personnel in provision of the psychosocial and psychiatric aspects of care. Most patients will have much of their ongoing treatment performed in outpatient settings. Although some pediatricians in primary care practice may perform these roles for some patients in outpatient settings on the basis of their levels of interest and expertise, many general pediatricians do not feel comfortable treating patients with eating disorders and prefer to refer patients with anorexia or bulimia nervosa for care by those with special expertise.[35] A number of pediatricians specializing in adolescent medicine have developed this skill set, with an increasing number involved in the management of eating disorders as part of multidisciplinary teams.[23,36] Other than the most severely affected patients, most children and adolescents with eating disorders will be managed in an outpatient setting by a multidisciplinary team coordinated by a pediatrician or subspecialist with appropriate expertise in the care of children and adolescents with eating disorders. Pediatricians generally work with nursing, nutrition, and mental health colleagues in the provision of medical, nutrition, and mental health care required by these patients.

As listed in Table 4, medical complications of eating disorders can occur in all organ systems. Pediatricians need to be aware of several complications that can occur in the outpatient setting. Although most patients do not have electrolyte abnormalities, the pediatrician must be alert to the possibility of development of hypokalemic, hypochloremic alkalosis resulting from purging behaviors (including vomiting and laxative or diuretic use) and hyponatremia or hypernatremia resulting from drinking too much or too little fluid as part of weight manipulation. Endocrine abnormalities, including hypothyroidism, hypercortisolism, and hypogonadotropic hypogonadism, are common, with amenorrhea leading to the potentially long-term complication of osteopenia and, ultimately, osteoporosis.[37-40] Gastrointestinal symptoms caused by abnormalities in intestinal motility resulting from malnutrition, laxative abuse, or refeeding are common but are rarely dangerous and may require symptomatic relief. Constipation during refeeding is common and should be treated with dietary manipulation and reassurance; the use of laxatives in this situation should be avoided.

The components of nutritional rehabilitation required in the outpatient management of patients with eating disorders are presented in several reviews.[23,24,41-44] These reviews highlight the dietary stabilization that is required as part of the management of bulimia nervosa and the weight gain regimens that are required as the hallmark of treatment of anorexia nervosa. The reintroduction or improvement of meals and snacks in those with anorexia nervosa is generally done in a stepwise manner, leading in most cases to an eventual intake of 2000 to 3000 kcal per day and a weight gain of 0.5 to 2 lb per week. Changes in meals are made to ensure ingestion of 2 to 3 servings of protein per day (with 1 serving equal to 3 oz of cheese, chicken, meat, or other protein sources). Daily fat intake should be slowly shifted toward a goal of 30 to 50 g per day. Treatment goal weights should be individualized and based on age, height, stage of puberty, premorbid weight, and previous growth charts. In postmenarchal girls, resumption of menses provides an objective measure of return to biological health, and weight at resumption of menses can be used to determine treatment goal weight. A weight approximately 90% of standard body weight is the average weight at which menses resume and can be used as an initial treatment goal weight, because 86% of patients who achieve this weight resume menses within 6 months.[45] For a growing child or adolescent, goal weight should be reevaluated at 3- to 6-month intervals on the basis of changing age and height.

Behavioral interventions are often required to encourage otherwise reluctant (and often resistant) patients to accomplish necessary caloric intake and weight gain goals. Although some pediatric specialists, pediatric nurses, or dietitians may be able to handle this aspect of care alone, a combined medical and nutritional team is usually required, especially for more difficult patients.[46]

Similarly, the pediatrician must work with mental health experts to provide the necessary psychologic, social, and psychiatric care.[47-49] The model used by many interdisciplinary teams, especially those based in settings experienced in the care of adolescents, is to establish a division of labor such that the medical and nutritional clinicians work on the issues described in the preceding paragraph and the mental health clinicians provide such modalities as individual, family, and group therapy. It is generally accepted that medical stabilization and nutritional rehabilitation are the most crucial determinants of short-term and intermediate-term outcome. Individual and family therapy, the latter being especially important in working with younger children and adolescents, are crucial determinants of the long-term prognosis.[50-53] It is also recognized that correction of malnutrition is required for the mental health aspects of care to be effective. Psychotropic medications have been shown to be helpful in the treatment of bulimia nervosa and prevention of relapse in anorexia nervosa in adults.[54-56] These medications are also used for many adolescent patients and may be prescribed by the pediatrician or the psychiatrist, depending on the delegation of roles within the team.

The Role of the Pediatrician in Hospital and Day Program Settings

Criteria for the hospitalization of children and adolescents with eating disorders have been established by the Society for Adolescent Medicine[23] (Table 6). These criteria, in keeping with those published by the American Psychiatric Association,[24] acknowledge that hospitalization may be required because of medical or psychiatric needs or because of failure of outpatient treatment to accomplish needed medical, nutritional,

Table 6. Criteria for Hospital Admission for Children, Adolescents, and Young Adults With Eating Disorders

Anorexia Nervosa

- <75% ideal body weight, or ongoing weight loss despite intensive management
- Refusal to eat
- Body fat <10%
- Heart rate <50 beats per minute daytime; <45 beats per min nighttime
- Systolic pressure <90
- Orthostatic changes in pulse (>20 beats per min) or blood pressure (>10 mm Hg)
- Temperature <96°F
- Arrhthymia

Bulimia Nervosa

- Syncope
- Serum potassium concentration <3.2 mmol/L
- Serum chloride concentration <88 mmol/L
- Esophageal tears
- Cardiac arrhythmias including prolonged QTc
- Hypothermia
- Suicide risk
- Intractable vomiting
- Hematemesis
- Failure to respond to outpatient treatment

or psychiatric progress. Unfortunately, many insurance companies do not use similar criteria, thus making it difficult for some children and adolescents with eating disorders to receive an appropriate level of care.[57-59] Children and adolescents have the best prognosis if their disease is treated rapidly and aggressively[36] (an approach that may not be as effective in adults with a more long-term, protracted course). Hospitalization, which allows for adequate weight gain in addition to medical stabilization and the establishment of safe and healthy eating habits, improves the prognosis in children and adolescents.[60]

The pediatrician involved in the treatment of hospitalized patients must be prepared to provide nutrition via a nasogastric tube or occasionally intravenously when necessary. Some programs use this approach frequently, and others apply it more sparingly. Also, because these patients are generally more malnourished than those treated as outpatients, more severe complications may

need to be treated. These include the possible metabolic, cardiac, and neurologic complications listed in Table 2. Of particular concern is the refeeding syndrome that can occur in severely malnourished patients who receive nutritional replenishment too rapidly.[61] The refeeding syndrome consists of cardiovascular, neurologic, and hematologic complications that occur because of shifts in phosphate from extracellular to intracellular spaces in individuals who have total body phosphorus depletion as a result of malnutrition. Recent studies have shown that this syndrome can result from use of oral, parenteral, or enteral nutrition.[62-64] Slow refeeding, with the possible addition of phosphorus supplementation, is required to prevent development of the refeeding syndrome in severely malnourished children and adolescents.

Day treatment (partial hospitalization) programs have been developed to provide an intermediate level of care for patients with eating disorders who require more than outpatient care but less than 24-hour hospitalization.[65-68] In some cases, these programs have been used in an attempt to prevent the need for hospitalization; more often, they are used as a transition from inpatient to outpatient care. Day treatment programs generally provide care (including meals, therapy, groups, and other activities) 4 to 5 days per week from 8 or 9 am until 5 or 6 pm. An additional level of care, referred to as an "intensive outpatient" program, has also been developed for these patients and generally provides care 2 to 4 afternoons or evenings per week. It is recommended that intensive outpatient and day programs that include children and adolescents should incorporate pediatric care into the management of the developmental and medical needs of their patients. Pediatricians can play an active role in the development of objective, evidence-based criteria for the transition from one level of care to the next. Additional research can also help clarify other questions, such as the use of enteral versus parenteral nutrition during refeeding, to serve as the foundation for evidence-based guidelines.

The Role of the Pediatrician in Prevention and Advocacy

Prevention of eating disorders can take place in the practice and community setting. Primary care pediatricians can help families and children learn to apply the principles of proper nutrition and physical activity and to avoid an unhealthy emphasis on weight and dieting. In addition, pediatricians can implement screening strategies (as described earlier) to detect the early onset of an eating disorder and be careful to avoid seemingly innocuous statements (such as "you're just a little above the average weight") that can sometimes serve as the precipitant for the onset of an eating disorder. At the community level, there is general agreement that changes in the cultural approaches to weight and dieting issues will be required to decrease the growing numbers of children and adolescents with eating disorders. School curricula have been developed to try to accomplish these goals. Initial evaluations of these curricula show some success in changing attitudes and behaviors, but questions about their effectiveness remain, and single-episode programs (eg, 1 visit to a classroom) are clearly not effective and may do more harm than good.[69–74] Additional curricula are being developed and additional evaluations are taking place in this field.[75] Some work has also been done with the media, in an attempt to change the ways in which weight and dieting issues are portrayed in magazines, television shows, and movies.[76] Pediatricians can work in their local communities, regionally, and nationally to support the efforts that are attempting to change the cultural norms being experienced by children and adolescents.

Pediatricians can also help support advocacy efforts that are attempting to ensure that children and adolescents with eating disorders are able to receive necessary care. Length of stay, adequacy of mental health services, and appropriate level of care have been a source of contention between those who treat eating disorders on a regular basis and the insurance industry.

Work is being done with insurance companies and on legislative and judicial levels to secure appropriate coverage for the treatment of mental health conditions, including eating disorders.[77,78] Parent groups, along with some in the mental health professions, have been leading this battle. Support by pediatrics in general, and pediatricians in particular, is required to help this effort.

Recommendations

1. Pediatricians need to be knowledgeable about the early signs and symptoms of disordered eating and other related behaviors.
2. Pediatricians should be aware of the careful balance that needs to be in place to decrease the growing prevalence of eating disorders in children and adolescents. When counseling children on risk of obesity and healthy eating, care needs to be taken not to foster over-aggressive dieting and to help children and adolescents build self-esteem while still addressing weight concerns.
3. Pediatricians should be familiar with the screening and counseling guidelines for disordered eating and other related behaviors.
4. Pediatricians should know when and how to monitor and/or refer patients with eating disorders to best address their medical and nutritional needs, serving as an integral part of the multidisciplinary team.
5. Pediatricians should be encouraged to calculate and plot weight, height, and BMI using age- and gender-appropriate graphs at routine annual pediatric visits.
6. Pediatricians can play a role in primary prevention through office visits and community- or school-based interventions with a focus on screening, education, and advocacy.
7. Pediatricians can work locally, nationally, and internationally to help change cultural norms conducive to eating disorders and proactively to change media messages.
8. Pediatricians need to be aware of the resources in their communities so they can coordinate care of various treating professionals, helping to create a seamless system between inpatient and outpatient management in their communities.
9. Pediatricians should help advocate for parity of mental health benefits to ensure continuity of care for the patients with eating disorders.

10. Pediatricians need to advocate for legislation and regulations that secure appropriate coverage for medical, nutritional, and mental health treatment in settings appropriate to the severity of the illness (inpatient, day hospital, intensive outpatient, and outpatient).

11. Pediatricians are encouraged to participate in the development of objective criteria for the optimal treatment of eating disorders, including the use of specific treatment modalities and the transition from one level of care to another.

COMMITTEE ON ADOLESCENCE, 2002–2003

David W. Kaplan, MD, MPH, Chairperson
Margaret Blythe, MD
Angela Diaz, MD
Ronald A. Feinstein, MD
*Martin M. Fisher, MD
Jonathan D. Klein, MD, MPH
W. Samuel Yancy, MD

CONSULTANT
*Ellen S. Rome, MD, MPH

LIAISONS
S. Paige Hertweck, MD
    American College of Obstetricians and
    Gynecologists
Miriam Kaufman, RN, MD
    Canadian Paediatric Society
Glen Pearson, MD
    American Academy of Child and Adolescent
    Psychiatry

STAFF
Tammy Piazza Hurley

*Lead authors

References

1. Whitaker AH. An epidemiological study of anorectic and bulimic symptoms in adolescent girls: implications for pediatricians. *Pediatr Ann.* 1992;21:752–759

2. Lucas AR, Beard CM, O'Fallon WM, Kurland LT. 50-year trends in the incidence of anorexia nervosa in Rochester, Minn.: a population-based study. *Am J Psychiatry.* 1991;148:917–922

3. Hsu LK. Epidemiology of the eating disorders. *Psychiatry Clin North Am.* 1996;19:681–700

4. Dorian BJ, Garfinkel PE. The contributions of epidemiologic studies to the etiology and treatment of the eating disorders. *Psychiatry Ann.* 1999;29:187–192

5. Troiano RP, Flegal KM, Kuczmarski RJ, Campbell SM, Johnson CL. Overweight prevalence and trends for children and adolescents: the National Health and Nutrition Examination Surveys, 1963 to 1991. *Arch Pediatr Adolesc Med.* 1995;149:1085–1091

6. Troiano RP, Flegal KM. Overweight children and adolescents: description, epidemiology, and demographics. *Pediatrics.* 1998;101(suppl):497–504

7. Strauss RS. Self-reported weight status and dieting in a cross-sectional sample of young adolescents: National Health and Nutrition Examination Survey III. *Arch Pediatr Adolesc Med.* 1999;153:741–747

8. Fisher M, Schneider M, Pegler C, Napolitano B. Eating attitudes, health risk behaviors, self-esteem, and anxiety among adolescent females in a suburban high school. *J Adolesc Health.* 1991;12:377–384

9. Stein D, Meged S, Bar-Hanin T, Blank S, Elizur A, Weizman A. Partial eating disorders in a community sample of female adolescents. *J Am Acad Child Adolesc Psychiatry.* 1997;36:1116–1123

10. Patton GC, Carlin JB, Shao Q, et al. Adolescent dieting: healthy weight control or borderline eating disorder? *J Child Psychol Psychiatry.* 1997;38:299–306

11. Krowchuk DP, Kreiter SR, Woods CR, Sinal SH, DuRant RH. Problem dieting behaviors among young adolescents. *Arch Pediatr Adolesc Med.* 1998;152:884–888

12. Field AE, Camargo CA Jr, Taylor CB, et al. Overweight, weight concerns, and bulimic behaviors among girls and boys. *J Am Acad Child Adolesc Psychiatry.* 1999;38:754–760

13. Andersen AE. Eating disorders in males. In: Brownell KD, Fairburn CG, eds. *Eating Disorders and Obesity: A Comprehensive Handbook.* New York, NY: Guilford Press; 1995:177–187

14. Carlat DJ, Camargo CA Jr, Herzog DB. Eating disorders in males: a report on 135 patients. *Am J Psychiatry.* 1997;154:1127–1132

15. Robinson TN, Killen JD, Litt IF, et al. Ethnicity and body dissatisfaction: are Hispanic and Asian girls at increased risk for eating disorders? *J Adolesc Health.* 1996;19:384–393

16. Crago M, Shisslak CM, Estes LS. Eating disturbances among American minority groups: a review. *Int J Eat Disord.* 1996;19:239–248

17. Gard MC, Freeman CP. The dismantling of a myth: a review of eating disorders and socioeconomic status. *Int J Eat Disord.* 1996;20:1–12

18. Pike KM, Walsh BT. Ethnicity and eating disorders: implications for incidence and treatment. *Psychopharmacol Bull.* 1996;32:265–274

19. Lai KY. Anorexia nervosa in Chinese adolescents—does culture make a difference? *J Adolesc.* 2000;23:561–568

20. le Grange D, Telch CF, Tibbs J. Eating attitudes and behaviors in 1435 South African Caucasian and non-Caucasian college students. *Am J Psychiatry.* 1998;155:250–254

21. Becker AE, Grinspoon SK, Klibanski A, Herzog DB. Eating disorders. *N Engl J Med.* 1999;340:1092–1098

22. Steiner H, Lock J. Anorexia nervosa and bulimia nervosa in children and adolescents: a review of the past 10 years. *J Am Acad Child Adolesc Psychiatry.* 1998;37:352–359

23. Fisher M, Golden NH, Katzman DK, et al. Eating disorders in adolescents: a background paper. *J Adolesc Health.* 1995;16:420–437

24. American Psychiatric Association, Work Group on Eating Disorders. Practice guideline for the treatment of patients with eating disorders (revision). *Am J Psychiatry.* 2000;157(1 suppl):1–39

25. American Psychiatric Association. *Diagnostic and Statistical Manual of Mental Disorders, 4th ed (DSM-IV).* Washington, DC: American Psychiatric Association; 1994

26. US Department of Health and Human Services. Mental health and mental disorders. In: *Healthy People 2010.* Vol II. Washington, DC: US Public Health Service, US Department of Health and Human Services; 2000. Available at: http://www.health.gov/healthypeople/document/html/volume2/18mental.htm. Accessed September 4, 2002

27. Kuczmarski RJ, Ogden CL, Grummer-Strawn LM, et al. *CDC Growth Charts: United States.* Hyattsville, MD: National Center for Health Statistics; 2000. Available at: http://www.cdc.gov/growthcharts/. Accessed February 26, 2002

28. Bunnell DW, Shenker IR, Nussbaum MP, et al. Subclinical versus formal eating disorders: differentiating psychological features. *Int J Eat Disord.* 1990;9:357–362

29. Wolraich ML, Felice ME, Drotar D, eds. *The Classification of Child and Adolescent Mental Diagnoses in Primary Care: Diagnostic and Statistical Manual for Primary Care (DSM-PC) Child and Adolescent Version.* Elk Grove Village, IL: American Academy of Pediatrics; 1996

30. Palla B, Litt IF. Medical complications of eating disorders in adolescents. *Pediatrics.* 1988;81:613–623

31. Fisher M. Medical complications of anorexia and bulimia nervosa. *Adolesc Med.* 1992;3:487–502

32. Rome ES. Eating disorders in adolescents and young adults: what's a primary care clinician to do? *Cleveland Clin J Med.* 1996;63:387–395

33. Mehler PS, Gray MC, Schulte M. Medical complications of anorexia nervosa. *J Womens Health.* 1997;6:533–541

34. Nicholls D, Stanhope R. Medical complications of anorexia nervosa in children and young adolescents. *Eur Eat Disord Rev.* 2000;8:170–180

35. Fisher M, Golden NH, Bergeson R, et al. Update on adolescent health care in pediatric practice. *J Adolesc Health.* 1996;19:394–400

36. Kreipe RE, Golden NH, Katzman DK, et al. Eating disorders in adolescents. A position paper of the Society for Adolescent Medicine. *J Adolesc Health.* 1995;16:476–479

37. Wong JCH, Lewindon P, Mortimer R, Shepherd R. Bone mineral density in adolescent females with recently diagnosed anorexia nervosa. *Int J Eat Disord.* 2001;29:11–16

38. Grinspoon S, Thomas E, Pitts S, et al. Prevalence and predictive factors for regional osteopenia in women with anorexia nervosa. *Ann Intern Med.* 2000;133:790–794

39. Castro J, Lazaro L, Pons F, Halperin I, Toro J. Predictors of bone mineral density reduction in adolescents with anorexia nervosa. *J Am Acad Child Adolesc Psychiatry.* 2000;39:1365–1370

40. Golden NH, Shenker IR. Amenorrhea in anorexia nervosa: etiology and implications. *Adolesc Med.* 1992;3:503–518

41. Schebendach J, Nussbaum MP. Nutrition management in adolescents with eating disorders. *Adolesc Med.* 1992;3:541–558

42. Rock CL, Curran-Celentano J. Nutritional disorder of anorexia nervosa: a review. *Int J Eat Disord.* 1994;15:187–203

43. Rock CL, Curran-Celentano J. Nutritional management of eating disorders. *Psychiatry Clin North Am.* 1996;19:701–713

44. Rome ES, Vazquez IM, Emans SJ. Nutritional problems in adolescence: anorexia nervosa/bulimia nervosa for young athletes. In: Walker WA, Watkins JB, eds. *Nutrition in Pediatrics: Basic Science and Clinical Applications.* 2nd ed. Hamilton, Ontario: BC Decker Inc; 1997:691–704

45. Golden NH, Jacobson MS, Schebendach J, Solanto MV, Hertz SM, Shenker IR. Resumption of menses in anorexia nervosa. *Arch Pediatr Adolesc Med.* 1997;151:16–21

46. Kreipe R, Uphoff M. Treatment and outcome of adolescents with anorexia nervosa. *Adolesc Med.* 1992;3:519–540

47. Yager J. Psychosocial treatments for eating disorders. *Psychiatry.* 1994;57:153–164

48. Powers PS. Initial assessment and early treatment options for anorexia nervosa and bulimia nervosa. *Psychiatry Clin North Am.* 1996;19:639–655

49. Robin AL, Gilroy M, Dennis AB. Treatment of eating disorders in children and adolescents. *Clin Psychol Rev.* 1998;18:421–446

50. Russell GF, Szmukler GI, Dare C, Eisler I. An evaluation of family therapy in anorexia nervosa and bulimia nervosa. *Arch Gen Psychiatry.* 1987;44:1047–1056

51. Eisler I, Dare C, Russell GF, Szmukler G, le Grange D, Dodge E. Family and individual therapy in anorexia nervosa: a 5-year follow-up. *Arch Gen Psychiatry.* 1997;54:1025–1030

52. North C, Gowers S, Byram V. Family functioning in adolescent anorexia nervosa. *Br J Psychiatry.* 1995;167:673–678

53. Geist R, Heinmaa M, Stephens D, Davis R, Katzman DK. Comparison of family therapy and family group psycho-education in adolescents with anorexia nervosa. *Can J Psychiatry.* 2000;45:173–178

54. Jimerson DC, Wolfe BE, Brotman AW, Metzger ED. Medications in the treatment of eating disorders. *Psychiatry Clin North Am.* 1996;19:739–754

55. Walsh BT, Wilson GT, Loeb KL, et al. Medication and psychotherapy in the treatment of bulimia nervosa. *Am J Psychiatry.* 1997;154:523–531

56. Strober M, Freeman R, De Antonio M, Lampert C, Diamond J. Does adjunctive fluoxetine influence the post-hospital course of restrictor-type anorexia nervosa? A 24-month prospective, longitudinal follow up and comparison with historical controls. *Psychopharmacol Bull.* 1997;33:425–431

57. Silber TJ, Delaney D, Samuels J. Anorexia nervosa. Hospitalization on adolescent medicine units and third-party payments. *J Adolesc Health.* 1989;10:122–125

58. Silber TJ. Eating disorders and health insurance. *Arch Pediatr Adolesc Med.* 1994;148:785–788

59. Sigman G. How has the care of eating disorder patients been altered and upset by payment and insurance issues? Let me count the ways [letter]. *J Adolesc Health.* 1996;19:317–318

60. Baran SA, Weltzin TE, Kaye WH. Low discharge weight and outcome in anorexia nervosa. *Am J Psychiatry.* 1995;152:1070–1072

61. Solomon SM, Kirby DF. The refeeding syndrome: a review. *JPEN J Parenter Enteral Nutr.* 1990;14:90–97

62. Birmingham CL, Alothman AF, Goldner EM. Anorexia nervosa: refeeding and hypophosphatemia. *Int J Eat Disord.* 1996;20:211–213

63. Kohn MR, Golden NH, Shenker IR. Cardiac arrest and delirium: presentations of the refeeding syndrome in severely malnourished adolescents with anorexia nervosa. *J Adolesc Health.* 1998;22:239–243

64. Fisher M, Simpser E, Schneider M. Hypophosphatemia secondary to oral refeeding in anorexia nervosa. *Int J Eat Disord.* 2000;28:181–187

65. Kaye WH, Kaplan AS, Zucker ML. Treating eating-disorder patients in a managed care environment. Contemporary American issues and Canadian response. *Psychiatry Clin North Am.* 1996;19:793–810

66. Kaplan AS, Olmstead MP. Partial hospitalization. In: Garner DM, Garfinkel PE, eds. *Handbook of Treatment for Eating Disorders.* 2nd ed. New York, NY: Guilford Press; 1997:354–360

67. Kaplan AS, Olmstead MP, Molleken L. Day treatment of eating disorders. In: Jimerson D, Kaye WH, eds. *Bailliere's Clinical Psychiatry, Eating Disorders.* Philadelphia, PA: Bailliere Tindall; 1997:275–289

68. Howard WT, Evans KK, Quintero-Howard CV, Bowers WA, Andersen AE. Predictors of success or failure of transition to day hospital treatment for inpatients with anorexia nervosa. *Am J Psychiatry.* 1999;156:1697–1702

69. Killen JD, Taylor CB, Hammer LD, et al. An attempt to modify unhealthful eating attitudes and weight regulation practices of young adolescent girls. *Int J Eat Disord.* 1993;13:369–384

70. Neumark-Sztainer D, Butler R, Palti H. Eating disturbances among adolescent girls: evaluation of a school-based primary prevention program. *J Nutr Educ.* 1995;27:24–31

71. Neumark-Sztainer D. School-based programs for preventing eating disturbances. *J Sch Health.* 1996;66:64–71

72. Carter JC, Stewart DA, Dunn VJ, Fairburn CG. Primary prevention of eating disorders: might it do more harm than good? *Int J Eat Disord.* 1997;22:167–172

73. Martz DM, Bazzini DG. Eating disorder prevention programs may be failing: evaluation of 2 one-shot programs. *J Coll Stud Dev.* 1999;40:32–42

74. Hartley P. Does health education promote eating disorders? *Eur Eat Disord Rev.* 1996;4:3–11

75. Story M, Neumark-Sztainer D. Promoting healthy eating and physical activity in adolescents. *Adolesc Med.* 1999;10:109–123

76. Becker AE, Hamburg P. Culture, the media, and eating disorders. *Harv Rev Psychiatry.* 1996;4:163–167

77. Andersen AE. Third-party payment for inpatient treatment of anorexia nervosa. *Eat Disord Rev.* 1997;7:1, 4–5

78. Stein MK. House bill aims to raise eating disorder awareness. *Eat Disord Rev.* 2000;11:1–2

All policy statements from the American Academy of Pediatrics automatically expire 5 years after publication unless reaffirmed, revised, or retired at or before that time.

'Just Dieting' or an Eating Disorder? A Practical Guide for the Clinician

by Janice K. Hillman, MD, FACP

More than 75% of adolescent girls report that they "want to lose weight." This striking statistic underscores the importance of maintaining a high index of suspicion for eating disorders when caring for adolescents.

Disordered eating is a progressive condition and proper patient management will take into account a spectrum of symptoms and signs. The American Psychiatric Association's *Diagnostic and Statistical Manual of Mental Disorders, Fourth Edition, Text Revision (DSM-IV-TR)* offers two diagnoses to describe disordered eating: *anorexia nervosa* and *bulimia nervosa*. A third category, *eating disorder not otherwise specified (EDNOS)*, accounts for eating disorders that do not meet criteria for a diagnosis of anorexia or bulimia. EDNOS includes the clinically important group of patients who have been labeled "pre-anorexia," "anorexia at-risk," or "subthreshold anorexia." For these patients, who suffer from physical and emotional stresses similar to those of patients with eating disorders, prompt intervention may halt progression.

Epidemiology of Eating Disorders

The prevalence of *anorexia nervosa*, estimated to be between 0.3% and 3% of adolescent and young adult females, has doubled in the last 20 years. While 90% of patients are white adolescent and young adult females, the incidence and recognition of eating disorders in teenage males, non-white populations, and lower socioeconomic groups appears to be increasing. It is more common among those who participate in sports and hobbies such as gymnastics, ice-skating, ballet, and modeling, where size and body shape are critical to success. Patients with anorexia nervosa are usually of normal weight at the outset; only 1/3 are overweight. Males represent between 5% and 15% of patients with eating disorders.

The typical age range at presentation is 10 to 25 years. There is a bimodal distribution for age of onset—14 years and 18 years—corresponding to the development of final secondary sexual characteristics and the start of college or work. There is often a pinpoint onset when seemingly benign comments by family, friends, or coaches trigger disordered eating. Events that signal a loss to the patient, such as parents' divorce or getting cut from a sports team, can also prompt anorexia nervosa.

Bulimia nervosa is more common than anorexia, with a prevalence of 0.5% to 5% of adolescent

Learning Objectives

After reading this article, pediatricians will understand their role in the recognition and management of patients who are diagnosed with anorexia nervosa, bulimia nervosa, or variants of these disorders. Pediatricians will be able to describe

- The epidemiology of eating disorders
- Criteria for diagnosis
- Typical clinical presentations
- Patient evaluation when an eating disorder is suspected
- Considerations for office-based management
- The role of the multidisciplinary treatment team
- Indications for referral and hospitalization
- Considerations for anticipatory guidance

Janice K. Hillman, MD, FACP, is a clinical assistant professor of pediatrics, University of Pennsylvania Health System, Philadelphia. Dr. Hillman is an attending physician for the University of Pennsylvania Clinical Care Associates, and maintains a private practice specializing in adolescent medicine and eating disorders.

and young adult females. It is more common in females and among whites. Patients with bulimia are generally older than those with anorexia nervosa, ranging in age from 12 years to middle-aged adults. Interestingly, one-third of patients with bulimia nervosa have a previous diagnosis of anorexia nervosa. A possible explanation for this association is a dysregulation of the hunger threshold. Patients resort to binge eating to satisfy their overwhelming hunger, and cannot depend upon the usual satiety cues to stop eating.

EDNOS is felt to be even more prevalent than anorexia nervosa and bulimia nervosa; it may be at least twice as common as anorexia nervosa. Since many of the associated behaviors (cutting out fat, exercising frequently) are considered healthy measures, it is difficult for the physician and family to decide what is "too much" or "not healthy."

Etiology

While the exact etiology of eating disorders is not known, five areas are being studied: genetic, neurochemical, psychodevelopmental, family dynamic-related, and sociocultural. There appears to be a genetic predisposition to the development of eating disorders; we see a four-fold increased risk when there is a first degree relative with an eating disorder. Mother-daughter and sister-sister dyads are being seen with more frequency in clinical practice.

Neurotransmitters such as serotonin, which play a role in the regulation of hunger and satiety, may be etiologically relevant; this is under study. Leptin, a hormone produced by fat cells that may play a role in satiety, is also the subject of ongoing research.

Psychological profiles often portray a young, perfectionist female who has low self-esteem and may have conflicts about her identity or sexuality. Patients often describe a feeling of loss of control, and say that making their own decisions about eating and elimination helps them to feel more in control. A history of abuse (sexual, physical, verbal, or emotional) is found in a significant proportion of patients. Families are sometimes described as overinvolved, enmeshed, and over-protective. Also relevant are sociocultural norms that favor extreme thinness and often show overt prejudice against obesity.

Although anorexia nervosa and bulimia nervosa appear to share a similar etiology, patients with bulimia do appear to have a greater incidence of borderline personality disorder and more problems with impulse control and high-risk behaviors.

Anorexia Nervosa

Table 1 presents criteria for a diagnosis of anorexia nervosa as described in the *DSM-IV-TR*. The typical clinical presentation is a teenage girl with profound weight loss, amenorrhea, and a

Table 1. Diagnostic Criteria for 307.1 Anorexia Nervosa

A. Refusal to maintain body weight at or above a minimally normal weight for age and height (eg, weight loss leading to maintenance of body weight less than 85% of that expected; or failure to make expected weight gain during period of growth, leading to body weight less than 85% of that expected).

B. Intense fear of gaining weight or becoming fat, even though underweight.

C. Disturbance in the way in which one's body weight or shape is experienced, undue influence of body weight or shape on self-evaluation, or denial of the seriousness of the current low body weight.

D. In postmenarcheal females, *amenorrhea,* ie, the absence of at least three consecutive menstrual cycles. (A woman is considered to have amenorrhea if her periods occur only following hormone, eg, estrogen, administration.)

Specify type:

Restricting Type: during the current episode of anorexia nervosa, the person has not regularly engaged in binge-eating or purging behavior (ie, self-induced vomiting or the misuse of laxatives, diuretics, or enemas)

Binge-Eating/Purging Type: during the current episode of anorexia nervosa, the person has regularly engaged in binge eating or purging behavior (ie, self-induced vomiting or the misuse of laxatives, diuretics, or enemas)

Reprinted with permission from the *Diagnostic and Statistical Manual of Mental Disorders, Fourth Edition, Text Revision.*
Copyright 2000 American Psychiatric Association.

distorted body image. Most adolescent girls are in the "restricting" subcategory, typified by the intake of limited calories and minimal fat (eg, rice cakes, water and diet soda). Some patients do engage in cycles of bingeing and purging in addition to frequent fasting.

EVALUATION

When an eating disorder is suspected, ask the patient to return for follow up within the next few weeks. (The urgency will be determined by your index of suspicion.) Several visits may be required to establish a diagnosis. Some patients will have lost more weight at the time of the next visit, which provides evidence that the problem is serious and treatment is needed.

The diagnosis of anorexia nervosa rests on clinical information and can be difficult to establish. Interview questions must be direct and focused on both the eating-disordered thinking and the eating-disordered behavior. Table 2 suggests a number of ways to approach this subject in the clinical interview. Screening tools are available (eg, the Eating Attitude Test) but they are not often used due to time constraints.

Physical examination

The physical examination is often normal unless there is significant weight loss. Height and weight should be measured to determine the patient's body mass index and ideal body weight. Vital signs may reveal orthostasis, bradycardia, or hypothermia. In severe cases, there may be hypotension. Dry skin, lanugo hair, or an orange cast to the skin (carotenemia) may be seen. Peripheral edema, acrocyanosis, or diminished capillary refill also occur. A distended bladder can be found in patients who "water load" to falsely elevate their weight. Finally, signs of purging (eg, eroded tooth enamel, scars on knuckles, or parotid enlargement), or self-injury (ie, cutting), are more common in patients with eating disorders.

Laboratory

Laboratory tests are not diagnostic; they are employed to assess medical complications. The laboratory workup should include a complete blood count, chemistry panel, serum magnesium, calcium, phosphate, urinalysis, and erythrocyte sedimentation rate (ESR). Hyponatremia may

---

Talking Points

When your patient "feels fat," explain that you can't "feel" fat. Ask her what she means or what she is feeling.

"I feel fat today," is often code for "I feel sad," "I feel angry," or "I feel worried." Reassure your patients that many teens and adults want to be thin. Don't dismiss a desire to lose weight as "silly." Your task as clinician is to teach body image awareness and the risks of eating disorders. Emphasize healthy behaviors. Encourage patients to have healthy eating habits, to exercise for fitness, to feel that their bodies are strong.

Table 2. A Guide to the Clinical Interview When an Eating Disorder is Suspected

If an eating disorder is suspected, ask the patient these questions:

- How has your eating behavior begun to interfere with your life?
- Do your thoughts about eating and/or your body interfere with your life?
- How do you feel about your size and shape? Are there certain parts of your body that you are unhappy about?
- Does your weight affect the way you feel about yourself?
- How many diets have you been on? Are there foods you won't eat anymore?
- How often do you weigh yourself?
- Do you feel guilty or anxious after eating a high-fat food?
- How much would you like to weigh?

If binge/purging behavior is suspected, ask the patient these questions as well:

- How often do you binge? How much do you eat? Where does the bingeing occur?
- What are the triggers to bingeing? Certain foods? Certain situations, such as being alone? Certain feelings?
- Have you ever used vomiting to counteract the binge? Diet pills? Laxatives? Water pills? Exercise?
- Do you still exercise despite illness, injury, or bad weather? How stressed are you if you can't exercise?
- How often does purging occur? Where does the purging occur? How do you purge?
- After the purge, how do you feel?
- Have you ever vomited blood?

reflect excess water intake or inappropriate regulation of antidiuretic hormone. Critical levels of hypoglycemia (eg, glucose levels of 30 to 40 mg/dl) are not uncommon. A low serum phosphate suggests severe malnutrition and requires periodic monitoring or replacement, as levels may drop further during refeeding and compromise cardiac function. Hematologic abnormalities may include leukopenia, thrombocytopenia, and anemia. A normal-to-low ESR is expected, and helps to rule out other causes, eg, inflammatory bowel disease. Workup of secondary amenorrhea may include pregnancy test, thyroid function test, prolactin, LH, and FSH. An estradiol level in the "postmenopausal" range can sometimes be used to show patients how hormonally depleted they have become. A euthyroid sick syndrome (normal thyroxine levels and a normal-to-low TSH) is sometimes seen. If there is significant bradycardia (eg, heart rate <50) an EKG should

be done to rule out potential cardiac conduction disturbances (eg, prolonged QTc interval, or dysrhythmia related to electrolyte disturbances).

Finally, if the clinical presentation does not arouse a high suspicion for an eating disorder, rule out other potential causes for weight loss, such as cancer, inflammatory bowel disease, tuberculosis, Addison's disease, and HIV infection.

If a patient has been amenorrheic for more than 6 months, a dual energy x-ray absorptiometry (DEXA) scan can be used to determine bone density. Given that adolescents have not usually achieved their adult bone density, the finding of "osteopenia" should be interpreted with caution; DEXA results should be compared with age-matched standards. DEXA scans are most helpful in two areas. First, they offer clear evidence to patients that their bones are osteopenic and vulnerable, reinforcing the need for nutritional balance. Second, if repeated annually, DEXA scans will reflect nutritional changes. An improvement in bone density affirms the patient's work to recover from the eating disorder, while worsening osteopenia can be used to mobilize the patient to action.

INDICATIONS FOR HOSPITALIZATION

It is essential to assess the patient's medical stability. Indications for hospitalization are presented in Table 3. Hospitalization at a center that specializes in eating disorders is preferable. Sometimes patients must first be stabilized on a medical unit, as when there is severe bradycardia or dysrhythmia, electrolyte imbalance, or diagnostic uncertainty.

OFFICE-BASED MANAGEMENT

If the patient is medically and psychiatrically stable, an outpatient team can be created, consisting of an individual therapist, a dietitian, and the primary care clinician. Family therapy may be provided by the team therapist or a separate family therapist. It is important to identify professionals who are skilled in treating eating disorders. The pediatrician's role on the team is to provide guidance, limit setting, medical safety, and coordination of care in collaboration with other members of the therapeutic team.

Table 3. Indications for Hospitalization in an Adolescent With an Eating Disorder

Any one or more of the following would justify hospitalization:

1. Severe malnutrition
   Weight <75% ideal body weight
2. Dehydration
3. Electrolyte disturbances
4. Cardiac dysrhythmia
5. Physiological instability
   Severe bradycardia
   Hypotension
   Hypothermia
   Orthostatic changes
6. Arrested growth and development
7. Failure of outpatient treatment
8. Acute food refusal
9. Uncontrollable bingeing and purging
10. Acute medical complications of malnutrition (eg, syncope, seizures, cardiac failure, pancreatitis, etc)
11. Acute psychiatric emergencies (eg, suicidal ideation, acute psychosis)
12. Comorbid diagnosis that interferes with the treatment of the eating disorder (eg, severe depression, obsessive compulsive disorder, severe family dysfunction)

Reprinted by permission of Elsevier Science from, "Eating Disorders in Adolescents: A Background Paper," by Fisher M, Golden NH, Katzman DK, Kreipe RE, Rees J, Schebendach J, et al. *Journal of Adolescent Health*, Vol 16, pp 420–437. Copyright 1995 by The Society for Adolescent Medicine.

Evaluation of concomitant psychiatric illness and assessment of suicide risk is essential. Accompanying anxiety, depression and obsessive-compulsive disorder are not uncommon. The use of psychotropic medications in the treatment of anorexia nervosa is generally not indicated unless there are comorbid psychiatric disorders, such as depression.

It is sometimes helpful to recommend that patients reduce extracurricular activities and eliminate team sports, gym, or other exercise. When physiologically appropriate, a possible return to sports participation can motivate patients to achieve their weight goals.

Support groups may be located through local eating disorders programs; American Anorexia/Bulimia Association (AABA) groups are often helpful.

Nutritional Counseling

Nutritional counseling usually starts with a dietary history. Questions typically seek to elicit a 24-hour dietary recall, descriptions of a typical "good day" or "bad day," the patient's perception of foods that are "safe" to eat versus foods that are not, and information on fluid intake. Remember that caloric needs for young teens (ages 11 to 14) are greater than those for older teens (15 to 18). Until the teen can be seen by the dietitian, the pediatrician might suggest that the patient add beverage calories. (Four cups of milk or juice can add about 500 calories in "safe" foods.)

Intervention

Clinicians are often confronted with treatment roadblocks. Sometimes the patient will not gain weight, or continually tries to deceive the family and treatment team. Suggested approaches include the following:

- Call a team meeting. This helps patients understand that they are part of a team and are expected to honor their commitment. The treatment plan is then presented as a group decision.
- Declare an impasse. Calling for crisis management helps to convince the patient and family that there is a problem and action is required.
- Write a contract with clear limits. For example, if the patient achieves her weight goal, she may return to sports participation. If her weight drops, she will be hospitalized.
- Consider referral to an eating disorder treatment center.

Monitoring and follow-up

Patients with anorexia nervosa need to be seen frequently, usually every 1 to 2 weeks. Close monitoring reinforces the message that there is a problem and supports the patient in the difficult process of gaining weight. Weights should be standardized as much possible. The patient should always be weighed in a gown, on the same scale, and after voiding. When weighing patients, be sensitive to the fact that they do not want to be weighed; avoid comments or judgments about weight gain or loss. Be aware that patients may try to falsely elevate weight or hide their cachexia by taping weights to their bodies, water-loading, or wearing bulky clothing. It is best to ask patients to avoid weighing themselves at home, at school, or at the gym. Blind weights (that is, turning the patient around during weighing) are helpful for patients, especially as they gain weight.

The weight gain should be slow, about 1 pound per week. Rarely, a too-rapid weight gain can precipitate a refeeding syndrome, characterized by a rapid drop in phosphate that can lead to seizures,

---

Talking Points

If you are worried about your patients, don't hesitate to say so.

Show evidence to support your concerns. If you suspect that a patient may have an eating disorder, ask him or her to return for follow up. Be prepared for a negative reaction, but be firm in your plan. Remember that the earlier the diagnosis, the better the prognosis. Prompt intervention can help to prevent a lifetime of chronic body dissatisfaction and dysfunctional eating. Teach your patients to be independent, intuitive eaters. Teach a simple three-step eating plan: 1) Eat only when hungry, not bored or depressed, 2) Make healthy food choices and portion sizes, and 3) Stop eating when full.

congestive heart failure, or death. Patients are afraid that they will get fat and a slow pace will help to reassure them. It is helpful to repeat, often, that they "will not get fat," and to remind patients that although they may not want to gain weight, they must do so in order to avoid medical complications.

Setting a Target Weight

Establishing an exact target weight can be very difficult, and should be done in consultation with the therapeutic team, especially the dietitian. It is less important to set a target weight than to ascertain a weight range in which the patient will be medically and emotionally safe.

The target weight range should clearly reflect the patient's premorbid body habitus; it is useful to know how much the patient weighed before she became amenorrheic. Standardized tables are helpful, but not sufficient. Determining the target weight range is probably best postponed until the patient has shown that she is willing to participate in her treatment plan.

Progressive weight goals are helpful in determining the weight at which hospital discharge can occur and the weight necessary for return to sports or school. They also reinforce the concept that just as the eating disorder developed progressively, treatment and recovery will be progressive. Ask your patients what weight they want to be. Their answers will help you assess their mindset, determine how realistic their thinking is, and set the stage for a discussion of attitudes about body weight.

Amenorrhea and Osteopenia

The resumption of menses is often used as a hallmark of "recovery," an assumption that adequate nutrition and weight gain have been achieved. It is also viewed as an emotional milestone. This is why the prevailing opinion discourages treatment of amenorrhea; it is thought best to allow menses to resume without hormonal therapy. Menses are sometimes delayed despite seemingly adequate weight gain. The delay may be due to inadequate body fat, excessive exercise, medications, or psychological factors. Just as menarche most likely will not occur until the patient has at least 22%

body fat, resumption of menses after prolonged amenorrhea probably requires adequate and similar body fat stores.

The most serious consequence of prolonged amenorrhea is bone loss. Bone loss is caused not only by estrogen deficiency, but also by nutritional deficiencies, hypercortisolism, and a direct inhibitory effect of undernutrition on bone formation and osteoblast function. Since the accrual of bone is at its peak during adolescence, eating disorders are associated not only with loss of existing bone, but also loss of this maximum bone deposition.

The decision to treat amenorrhea must be individualized; indications for hormonal treatment include refractory low weight, severe estrogen deficiency (signified by menopausal symptoms), and worsening osteopenia/osteoporosis. Oral contraceptive pills are used most commonly, although recent studies have suggested that the use of supplemental estrogen may not significantly improve bone density or prevent osteopenia. In addition, daily supplementation of elemental calcium (1200–1500 mg), and Vitamin D (400 IU), is necessary.

COMPLICATIONS AND PROGNOSIS

Multiple complications may occur in addition to amenorrhea and osteopenia. Cardiovascular complications range from dysrhythmias to cardiomyopathy and heart failure. Cerebral atrophy seen with significant weight loss may not be reversible. Fertility may be impaired unless the hormonal imbalance is corrected. Hematologic abnormalities include leukopenia, anemia, thrombocytopenia, and impaired cellular and humoral immunity. Renal failure, kidney stones, and electrolyte abnormalities have been reported. Finally, if the patient vomits, hematemesis, gastric dysmotility, reflux, and dental erosions may occur.

The prognosis for teens is generally good, and is felt to be better than the prognosis for adults. Using outcome measures of weight restoration, resumption of menses, and psychosocial functioning, about 50% of patients with anorexia nervosa achieve a full recovery, and 30% achieve a partial recovery. In 20% there is no substantial improvement. Reported mortality rates range from 0% to

22%, averaging about 5%. Causes of death include cardiac dysfunction and/or electrolyte imbalances.

Anorexia nervosa has significant psychosocial consequences, including negative impact on self image, relationships, school, and job performance. Good prognostic indicators include early age of onset, supportive family, and good initial "ego strength." Poor prognosis is linked to comorbidity with other psychiatric illnesses and a diagnosis of binge eating-purging subtype.

BULIMIA NERVOSA

Bulimia nervosa is an eating disorder character-ized by frequent binge eating and subsequent compensatory behavior to "get rid of the food or weight gain." While most patients believe that vomiting is the key feature of bulimia nervosa, the primary feature is binge eating.

The *DSM-IV-TR* recognizes two subtypes. (See Table 4) Purging type involves use of vomit-ing, laxatives, diuretics, diet pills, or enemas as counter-regulatory measures for the binge eating. Nonpurging type involves fasting or exercise as ways to lose or maintain weight. During a binge, the patient consumes a large amount of food quickly, impulsively, and usually alone. Patients describe a feeling of numbness, a loss of control. Binges can be triggered by certain foods, situa-tions, or feelings.

Talking Points

Teach your patients to avoid the bathroom scale.

For patients with eating disorders, the bath-room scale is highly provocative. In an instant, a number on the scale can diminish self-esteem, create self-doubt, and provoke inappropriate responses. Teach patients that they should be confident about their smart choices, their healthy eating, and healthy exercise. Patients who abandon the scale talk about how "liber-ated" they feel, how it is a relief to be free of the morning weigh-in. During a recent Eating Disorders Awareness week, students celebrated the affirmation "Don't weigh your self esteem...It's what's inside that counts."

EVALUATION

History-taking for patients with bulimia nervosa should incorporate the eating and body image questions discussed earlier, and also more directed questions about the binge eating-purging activity. It should also include an in-depth exploration of psychiatric symptoms, especially depression, par-ticipation in high-risk activities, impulsivity, and social functioning in areas of school, peers, and family. Examples of questions to frame the inter-view are presented in Table 2.

Table 4. Diagnostic Criteria for 307.51 Bulimia Nervosa

A. Recurrent episodes of binge eating. An episode of binge eating is characterized by both of the following:
>   (1) eating, in a discrete period of time (eg, within any 2-hour period), an amount of food that is definitely larger than most people would eat during a similar period of time and under similar circumstances
>   (2) a sense of lack of control over eating during the episode (eg, a feeling that one cannot stop eating or control what or how much one is eating)

B. Recurrent inappropriate compensatory behavior in order to prevent weight gain, such as self-induced vomiting; misuse of laxatives, diuretics, enemas, or other medications; fasting; or excessive exercise.

C. The binge eating and inappropriate compensatory behaviors both occur, on average, at least twice a week for 3 months.

D. Self-evaluation is unduly influenced by body shape and weight.

E. The disturbance does not occur exclusively during episodes of anorexia nervosa.

Specify type:

Purging Type: during the current episode of bulimia nervosa, the person has regularly engaged in self-induced vomiting or the misuse of laxatives, diuretics, or enemas.

Nonpurging Type: during the current episode of bulimia nervosa, the person has used other inappropriate compensatory behaviors, such as fasting or excessive exercise, but has not regularly engaged in self-induced vomiting or the misuse of laxatives, diuretics, or enemas.

Reprinted with permission from the *Diagnostic and Statistical Manual of Mental Disorders, Fourth Edition, Text Revision.* Copyright 2000 American Psychiatric Association.

Adolescents are being diagnosed more frequently as "exercise bulimics" or clinical variants of the female athlete triad (disordered eating, amenorrhea, osteopenia). These patients exercise compulsively despite bad weather, illness, or injury.

Physical Examination

On physical examination, patients are usually normal weight or overweight. Clinicians should be alert for signs of purging activity and self-injury. Bilateral parotid enlargement is common. Perimyolysis (loss of dentin) is best seen on the lingual and occlusal surfaces of the upper teeth (the edges of the teeth appear translucent). Calluses may be present on the backs of knuckles (Russell sign) when patients use their fingers to induce emesis. Finally, look for signs of self-mutilation (scars from cutting and cigarette burns) on arms, abdomen, legs, and buttocks.

Laboratory Evaluation

The laboratory evaluation is similar to that for patients with anorexia nervosa. Certain findings, such as electrolyte levels and electrocardiographic abnormalities, are useful to monitor the patient for complications.

MANAGEMENT

Create a multidisciplinary treatment team analogous to that employed in the management of anorexia nervosa. Treatment should focus on the binge eating behaviors and strategies to help patients recognize early symptoms of hunger, avoid potential triggers, make safe food choices, and practice relaxation techniques to reduce the anxiety associated with eating. If patients can accept a comfortable feeling of fullness, the risk of purging may lessen. Cognitive behavioral therapy is the approach of choice in the treatment of bulimia nervosa. It helps to identify the cognitive distortions (eg, "I am fat, therefore I am no good," "Either none of the cake or all of the cake") and to teach the behavioral skills (eg, relaxation breathing) to help avoid binge/purge activity.

Dental care is critical for patients with the purging subtype of bulimia. Patients should see their dentist at least every 4 to 6 months. Patients may be advised that after purging they should quickly rinse their mouth and avoid brushing their teeth for 30 minutes in order to avoid greater enamel erosion.

Psychotropic medications may be helpful in controlling the binge-eating behavior and the associated feelings of anxiety and depression. The best-studied of these agents is fluoxetine; doses of up to 60 mg/day may be required. Buproprion hydrochloride (Wellbutrin) is contraindicated for patients with anorexia nervosa and bulimia nervosa because of the risk of seizures.

COMPLICATIONS AND PROGNOSIS

The overall prognosis in bulimia nervosa is felt to be similar to that of anorexia nervosa. Associated morbidity is usually related to the purging activity. Chronic reflux esophagitis, esophageal dysmotility and esophageal tears may occur. The mortality in bulimia nervosa is low. Poor prognostic indicators are comorbidity with other psychiatric illnesses, especially borderline personality disorder.

Eating Disorder Not Otherwise Specified (EDNOS)

The typical presentation for the young female with anorexia nervosa is profound weight loss. Pediatricians more often see young women who do not quite meet the criteria for this diagnosis. Weight loss may be minimal, or there is no weight loss but only marginal weight gain or growth. Perhaps there have been only one or two missed periods, or menarche is delayed. Such patients are now classified in the DSM-IV-TR as having EDNOS.

EDNOS is a very important diagnostic category for several reasons. First, it represents a large group of patients who often go unrecognized because their symptoms and signs are less pronounced. Second, patients with EDNOS who begin treatment earlier may avoid morbidity or progression to anorexia nervosa. Finally, these patients may have a better outcome than patients with anorexia nervosa, especially if the condition is detected early.

The work-up and management of EDNOS is similar to that for anorexia nervosa and bulimia nervosa.

Conclusion

Eating disorders command our attention because they are prevalent and have serious physical and emotional consequences. Making a specific diagnosis is not as important as recognizing that the spectrum of signs and symptoms overlap significantly, and that early diagnosis and treatment will lead to a better prognosis.

Diagnosis is further complicated by the considerable "overlap" between many eating disordered behaviors and culturally acceptable practices (eg, going on a diet, eating low-fat foods, and routine exercising). It is critical that clinicians seek "teachable moments" to educate patients and families about eating disorders and their early warning signs. When an eating disorder is suspected, share concerns promptly with patient and family.

Bibliography

American Dietetic Association. Position Statement of the ADA: Nutrition intervention in the treatment of anorexia nervosa, bulimia nervosa, and binge eating. *J Am Diet Assoc.* 1994;8:902–907

American Psychiatric Association. *Diagnostic and Statistical Manual of Mental Disorders, Fourth Edition, Text Revision.* Washington, DC: American Psychiatric Association; 2000

Becker AE, Grinspoon SK, Klibanski A, Herzog DB. Eating disorders. *N Engl J Med.* 1999;340:1092–1098

Brownell KD, Fairburn CG, eds. *Eating Disorders and Obesity: A Comprehensive Handbook.* New York, New York: Guilford Press; 1995

Garner DM, Garfinkel PE. The Eating Attitudes Test: An index of the symptoms of anorexia nervosa. *Psychol Med.* 1979;9:273–279

Kreipe RE, Golden NH, Katzman DK, Fisher M, Rees J, Tonkin RS, et al. Eating Disorders in Adolescents. A position paper of the Society for Adolescent Medicine. *J Adolesc Health.* 1995;16:476–479

Skiba A, Loghmani E, Orr DP. Nutritional Screening and Guidance for Adolescents. *Adolescent Health Update.* 1997;9(2):1–8

Stashwick C. When you suspect an eating disorder. *Contemp Pediatr.* 1996;340:124–153

Acknowledgment

The editors would like to acknowledge technical review by Ellen S. Rome, MD, for the AAP Committee on Adolescence.

Resources for Patients and Families

Frequently Asked Questions About Eating Disorders

WHAT IS AN EATING DISORDER?

When a person has an eating disorder, his or her life seems to revolve around what they eat and how fat they believe they look. Some people with eating disorders eat almost nothing; others have "binge" episodes, when they eat a large amount of food in a short time (about 2 hours).They sometimes over-exercise, force themselves to vomit, or use laxatives, diet pills, water pills, or enemas to "get rid of " what they eat. We don't know why someone develops an eating disorder, but we do know that the causes are complicated and the medical consequences can be very serious. Eating disorders affect 5 million Americans each year, 90% of whom are teenaged and young adult females.

WHAT ARE THE WARNING SIGNS OF AN EATING DISORDER?

A person who has an eating disorder, or might be developing one, might:
- Diet all the time
- Think about food a lot
- Worry about body image (wear baggy clothes, avoid activities like swimming or gym class)
- Avoid eating in social situations
- Dislike being weighed (or weigh himself or herself all the time)
- Spend a lot of time in the bathroom, especially after eating
- Exercise a lot
- Withdraw from family and friends
- Seem to have mood swings

A person with an eating disorder might experience:
- Significant weight loss or gain
- Dizziness, fainting spells
- Menstrual periods that have not started, are unpredictable, or have stopped entirely

Resources*

Patients and parents interested in learning more about eating disorders might look to these resources.

Books

Hunger Pains by Mary Pipher, PhD. Random House, Inc., New York,New York. Rev ed. 1997

Surviving an Eating Disorder. Perspectives and Strategies for Family and Friends by Michelle Siegel PhD, Judith Brisman PhD, and Margot Weinshel PhD. HarperCollins Publishers, Toronto, Canada, Rev ed. 1997

Gürze 2001 Eating Disorders Resource Catalogue. Lists tapes, books, videos, associations, treatment facilities, and basic facts about eating disorders. Order from Gürze Books, Carlsbad California: 800-756-7533

Websites

Gürze Books, a resource for materials on eating disorders recovery, research, education, advocacy and prevention
www.bulimia.com

Eating Disorders Awareness & Prevention, Inc., a source of education and prevention materials for patients, families, and educators. EDAP organizes media campaigns and maintains a toll-free information and resource line (800-931-2237)
www.edap.org

The **American Anorexia/Bulimia Association,** a source on support groups, speakers, help lines, and school outreach projects
www.aabainc.org

The **Academy for Eating Disorders,** a resource for eating disorders treatment professionals
www.acadeatdis.org

* These resources are included as sources of general information only. Their content has not been reviewed or endorsed by the American Academy of Pediatrics.

Pediatricians are encouraged to photocopy this page for distribution to patients and parents.

- Constant fatigue
- Coldness all the time
- Hair loss

I think my child has an eating disorder. What do I do?

_Do:_

Do talk with your child

Do share your concerns

Do be firm

Do get help

Don't:

Don't threaten—(don't say "if you don't eat, you will go to the hospital")

Don't negotiate —(don't say, "if you eat, you can go to the party or the game")

Don't try to monitor—(don't weigh your child at home)

Don't be deceived by excuses

Nutrition in Adolescence

Giuseppina DiMeglio, MD, The University of Rochester Medical Center, Rochester, NY

Nutritional Requirements During Adolescence. Story M. In: McAnarney E, Kreipe REK, Orr DP, Comerci GD, eds. *Textbook of Adolescent Medicine.* Philadelphia, Penn: WB Saunders; 1992

http://www.nal.usda.gov/fnic/Dietary/drv.html

http://www.nal.usda.gov/fnic/Dietary/Chartls.gif

Food Intakes of United States Children and Adolescents Compared With Recommendations. Munoz KA, Krebs-Smith SM, Ballard-Barbash R, Cleveland LE. *Pediatrics.* 1997;100:323–329

Nutritional Supplements. Fact vs Fiction. Johnson WA, Landry GL. *State of the Art Reviews: Adolescent Medicine.* 1998;9:501–514

Adolescence is a time of remarkable growth. During this time, 20% of final adult height and 50% of adult weight are attained. Bone mass increases by 45%, and dramatic bone remodeling occurs. Soft tissues, organs, and even red blood cell mass increase in size. As a result, nutritional requirements peak in adolescence. Deficits in macronutrients or micronutrients can impair growth and delay sexual maturation. Requirements for the individual are impossible to estimate because of considerable variation in the rate and amount of growth. Population-based estimates include the reference daily intake (RDI), which estimates average requirements, and the recommended dietary allowance (RDA), which estimates the intake that meets the needs of most of the population. Eating a varied diet, with foods chosen from all the food groups in the proportion recommended on the United States Department of Agriculture's (USDA) Food Pyramid virtually insures meeting micronutrient requirements. Adolescents who meet these recommendations do not require nutritional supplements.

Adolescents often have chaotic eating patterns that do not conform to dietary recommendations. Fewer than 2% of adolescents consume adequate amounts of all the food groups, and almost 20% of females and 7% of males do not consume an adequate number of portions of any of the food groups. The vast majority of adolescents eat too much fat and saturated fat and too few vegetables and fruits. Fried potato is the number one vegetable they eat. The USDA recommends that no more than 30% of a person's calories come from fat and that cholesterol intake be limited to 300 mg/d.

Growth parameters provide a good estimate of the adequacy of energy intake. Caloric requirements vary highly from individual to individual, but in general, adolescent girls require 2,500 kcal and boys need 2,500 to 3,000 kcal. Adolescents who are obese are taking in more calories than they expend, and they may need assistance in substituting high-calorie foods with lower calorie alternatives. Teens should be encouraged to eat regular meals and snacks. Frequently they skip breakfast or lunch in an effort to lose weight, which impairs school performance in the early morning and contributes to chaotic and excessive eating later in the day. They should avoid very restrictive diets, especially during the growth spurt, because these may interfere with linear growth and sexual maturation. Although calorie restriction can affect short-term weight reduction, exercise is more likely to produce long-term gains.

Most teens, especially girls, experiment with diets, which are generally short-lived. Teens who have anorexia nervosa often will experience amenorrhea prior to becoming significantly underweight. Early identification and nutritional counseling are recommended because at the very low caloric intakes that these young women maintain, it is difficult to meet requirements for any of the vitamins, minerals, or even essential fatty acids. Bone mineral density often declines. Magnetic resonance imaging of the brains of young women who have anorexia also has shown decreases in white matter and gray matter volume during starvation. It is unclear whether these changes are completely reversible with improved nutrition. Zinc deficiency brought on by restrictive eating can contribute to the anorexia.

The teen who has bulimia nervosa "cycles" between bingeing and purging. Purging activities can include self-induced vomiting, laxative abuse, excessive exercise, or restriction of intake. Affected teens often are of normal weight, but the quality of their diets is poor; food consumed during binges tends to be high in fat and low in nutrients. Hypokalemia and alkalosis can occur due to vomiting.

As noted previously, considerable bone mass accretion occurs during adolescence. Although most of this occurs during the adolescent growth spurt, further bone mass is laid down throughout adolescence. The adolescent RDA for calcium (1,200 mg/d) exceeds that for every other stage of life except pregnancy, yet the average adolescent calcium intake is 800 mg/d, and adolescent girls tend to have a lower calcium intake than boys. Pregnant and lactating adolescents, whose requirement for calcium is higher (1,500 mg/d), are at even greater risk for calcium deficiency. It is unclear whether a calcium deficit in adolescence can be recouped in adulthood or whether such a deficit puts the individual at greater risk for osteoporosis in later life. Adolescents who are unable to meet their calcium requirements through their diet should take a calcium supplement.

Adolescents also are at risk for iron deficiency anemia. Iron is used to increase muscle mass and circulating red blood cell mass. Although both boys and girls have increased needs, adolescent girls also experience a monthly loss of total iron stores through the menses and are at greater risk for anemia. Adolescents living in poverty also are more likely to be anemic. Adolescents should be screened for iron deficiency anemia during health supervision visits every 2 years, and those found to be anemic should receive supplements.

Clinical vitamin deficiencies are rare in the United States. Munoz et al note that even adolescents who do not eat adequate amounts of any of the food groups are likely to have an adequate intake of most vitamins except B6, and adequate intake of any one of the food groups results in sufficient amounts of this vitamin. Other studies have identified subclinical deficiencies in folate, riboflavin, thiamine, and B6 stores, particularly among adolescents living in poverty. Folate deficiency is of particular concern because a substantial number of adolescents become pregnant each year, and subclinical folate deficiency has been correlated with a higher incidence of neural tube defects in the fetus. Teens often present for prenatal care late in the first trimester, when the sensitive period for neural tube fusion already has occurred, so some experts have advocated universal supplementation with folate. Certainly, teens who are trying to get pregnant and those who are identified as being pregnant in a setting that does not provide prenatal care should be started on folate.

Vegetarianism is gaining favor among adolescents and adults. Parents often are concerned that this type of diet is deficient in protein, vitamins, and minerals. However, even with a strict vegan diet, in which no animal-derived protein is consumed, including dairy, protein requirements are met easily with tofu, nuts, seeds, grains, and legumes. More importantly, riboflavin and B_{12} are harder to get on a strict vegan diet, and supplementation should be considered, especially in teens who describe a diet that has little variety. Vitamins free of animal products are available in health food stores.

Adolescent athletes have higher energy needs than their more sedentary peers. In general, 2 hours of active participation in athletics requires intake of an additional 800 to 1,700 kcal/d. Additional calories that are predominantly complex carbohydrates (60%), with 25% fats and 15% protein, meet the higher protein and micronutrient requirements. Nutritional supplements such as creatinine, carnitine, amino acids, and dehydroepiandrosterone sulfate have not been shown to enhance performance. All athletes should pay particular attention to hydration to maintain performance and avoid heat injury.

Female gymnasts and dancers often experience pressure to restrict calories severely to maintain a svelte physique. Such restriction can delay puberty and cause primary amenorrhea. Wrestlers have been known to purge to meet weight categories for a meet. This can hinder performance. Carbohydrate loading also has been used to improve performance in athletes. Although carbohydrate meals 3 to 6 hours before competition can improve performance by creating easily accessible glycogen stores, athletes should be cautioned against the severe calorie restriction that often precedes the loading phase, which can affect performance adversely.

It is important to involve parents in nutrition counseling for young teens because they often are still in control of the adolescent's diet. Teens can be provided with a copy of the Food Pyramid and encouraged to use it to guide their nutrition choices. Finally, it can be helpful to cultivate a relationship with a nutritionist who is comfortable with teens and to maintain a low threshold for referral for nutrition counseling. Good adolescent dietary habits can lead to a lifetime of good nutrition.

Overweight Adolescents: Clinical Challenges and Strategies

by Richard E. Kreipe, MD, FAAP

Clinical intervention for overweight adolescents can be one of the most complex challenges in pediatric practice. The adolescent who is overweight or at risk of becoming overweight because of rapid weight gain or genetic predisposition, should be able to rely upon the pediatrician for a treatment plan.

The term "obesity" refers to excess adiposity, while "overweight" refers to excess body weight for height, sex and age. Unfortunately, there are no universally accepted criteria to identify either obesity or overweight. Because most clinicians do not measure body fat, and because the term "obese" often has negative connotations for patients and their families, the term "overweight" can be used in discussing obesity.

This issue of *Adolescent Health Update* will address office-based management of adolescents who are overweight because their energy intake far exceeds energy output (ie, due to exogenous causes). Primary (ie, endogenous) causes of obesity, listed in Table 1, occur in <1% of obese patients. These should be detected with a comprehensive history and physical examination. The medical evaluation of the overweight adolescent, in almost all cases, consists of a history and physical examination. (Laboratory evaluation is discussed later.)

Concepts and Themes

The pediatrician's clinical approach should incorporate awareness of lifelong health risks associated with being overweight, family dynamics, and the adolescent's developmental status. Key concepts include the following:

- *Overweight is not a single entity*, but a final common pathway in which caloric intake exceeds expenditure.
- *Treatment should be flexible*, recognizing that no single approach is universally successful.
- *The energy imbalance which causes obesity may have biological, psychological, and social causes which are not readily modified.* Resultant weight gain has effects of its own, which may exacerbate the weight problem.
- *Overweight is best considered a chronic condition, not a curable disease.*
- *Comprehensive approaches are more likely to succeed than dieting alone.*
- *Overweight adolescents and their parents are subject to social disapproval*, and may blame others for their condition. This can intensify the normal adolescent/parent conflict.
- *Parental involvement is essential for successful treatment.*
- *If one or both parents are overweight, the family may be pessimistic* about the adolescent's ability to control weight. Data regarding limited

Learning Objectives

The goal of this article is to give the practicing pediatrician skills and information required for the diagnosis and management of overweight adolescents. After reading this paper, clinicians should be comfortable in discussing the causes of overweight, employing body mass index as an indicator of obesity, and implementing effective strategies to identify, assess, and manage their adolescent patients' weight control needs.

Richard E. Kreipe, MD, FAAP, is an associate professor of pediatrics and chief, Division of Adolescent Medicine, Department of Pediatrics, University of Rochester Medical Center, Rochester, New York. Dr. Kreipe is also director of the Adolescent Eating Disorders Program and the Maternal and Child Health Bureau Interdisciplinary Adolescent Health Training Program at the University of Rochester Medical Center.

long-term success of obesity treatment in adults may further discourage them. Yet it is clear that behavioral changes can ameliorate genetic influences.

- *Patients and parents may expect either a medical diagnosis ("I think it's her thyroid; she doesn't eat that much and I only have healthy foods in the house") or an easy solution ("I was reading about this pill...").*
- *Some health insurance policies will not pay for treatment.*
- *Peer support programs and comprehensive structured approaches have been helpful to many patients.*

Identifying Overweight Adolescents

Body weight for height at >120% of normal for gender and age (corresponding to approximately the 95th percentile on standard growth charts) has traditionally been used as the screening criterion for adolescent overweight and obesity. A more reliable measure is the body mass index (BMI). Although BMI does not assess body fat directly, it corresponds reasonably well to adiposity for adolescents. If weight is measured in pounds and height in inches, the formula is:

$$\frac{\textbf{weight in pounds x 700}}{\textbf{height in inches}^2}$$

The majority of patients with a BMI greater than 30 (the 95th percentile) will be overweight. Within that group, however, there may be individuals (eg, adolescent athletes) who are overweight but not obese.

An expert panel has recommended a two-level procedure (see Himes and Dietz) which employs body mass index to identify patients who are overweight (BMI>95th percentile or >30 kg/m^2) and those at risk of becoming overweight (BMI 85th to 95th percentile). In-depth medical assessment is recommended for overweight adolescents. Second-level screening is recommended for those at risk of becoming overweight (eg, family history, blood pressure and total cholesterol, as well as assessment of weight velocity or concerns about weight). Those patients with positive findings on the second-level screen are candidates for in-depth assessment and appropriate intervention.

Figure 1 presents a graph to chart BMI for males and females. This chart distinguishes between overweight and at-risk for overweight and shows how this value normally increases with age. Figure 2 presents a shorthand method to estimate BMI from patient height and weight.

For clinical purposes, adolescents over age 14 who are 20% above the ideal weight for height generally have a BMI of approximately 27 and are classified as overweight. Those who are 30% above ideal weight are classified as obese and have a BMI of approximately 30. Morbid obesity exists when body weight is 100% greater than ideal and translates into a BMI of at least 45. The February 1997 *Adolescent Health Update* (Vol 9:2) discusses body mass index in detail and provides a diagnostic algorithm to detect adolescents at nutritional risk.

If grids and charts are not available, the clinician can make a quick assessment by observing that the 95th percentile BMI in males is approximately the age in years + 14, while the 95th percentile BMI for females is approximately the age in years + 13. [For example, a 12-year-old boy with a BMI of >26 (ie, 12+14) is overweight and in need of further evaluation.]

Triceps skinfold thickness (TST) is a more direct measure of body fat, but requires the use of specialized equipment in the hands of an experienced examiner and is not practical for the typical overweight adolescent. Such an evaluation may be useful for patients who appear to be overweight, yet not overfat.

Other body fat measurement techniques (eg, bioelectric impedance analysis, dual energy x-ray absorptiometry, underwater weighing, etc) are impractical in daily practice. Even the BMI and TST are superfluous in most cases, where excess adiposity is readily identifiable on clinical examination.

Epidemiology

Obesity is second only to tobacco as a cause of adult morbidity and mortality in the United States. Although most medical complications of overweight will present in adulthood, some problems do become evident in adolescence, when habits contributing to obesity are frequently

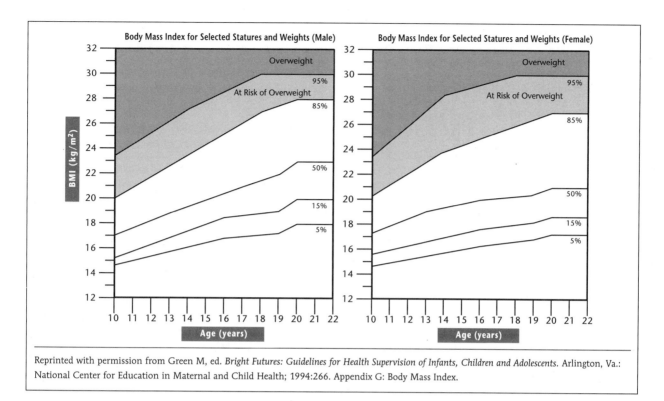

Reprinted with permission from Green M, ed. *Bright Futures: Guidelines for Health Supervision of Infants, Children and Adolescents.* Arlington, Va.: National Center for Education in Maternal and Child Health; 1994:266. Appendix G: Body Mass Index.

Figure 1. Graph to Chart Body Mass Index

Body mass index (BMI) is calculated either as [weight in pounds ∞ 700/(height in inches)^2] or [weight in kilograms/(height in meters)^2]. Once the BMI is calculated (or derived from the chart shown as Figure 2) it can be plotted on the gender-specific graph above and made a part of the patient record. The adolescent's percentile BMI can guide the pediatrician in determining what further evaluation or counseling may be indicated.

established. Forty percent of overweight children remain overweight as adults; about three in four overweight adolescents will find that the condition persists into adulthood.

Temporal trends in nutrient intake data for adolescents indicate that energy and fat intake among adolescents has been fairly constant over the past 20 to 30 years. However, physical activities have declined significantly throughout this period. Gortmaker and colleagues analyzed a large national data set of both normal-weight and overweight children and adults to track weight gain in a group of normal-weight 10-year-old children. Using a threshold of ≥85th percentile to define overweight, data revealed an 18% cumulative incidence of overweight by the time these normal-weight 10-year-old children were 14 years old. Sixty percent of those newly-overweight adolescents reported spending more than 2 hours per day watching television or playing video games.

Evaluation

Office evaluation of an overweight adolescent includes several components: a targeted clinical assessment to identify medical causes or complications, a family assessment to identify associated lifestyle factors, a full physical examination, and specific laboratory tests as indicated.

TARGETED CLINICAL HISTORY

The clinical history for adolescent obesity should identify conditions that suggest endogenous causes and complications that indicate a need for weight reduction. (See Tables 1 and 2)

The clinician should determine whether acute or potentially life-threatening complications of obesity exist, such as right heart failure associated with sleep apnea. The presence of such complications implies an urgent need for treatment. Questions that assess for evidence of sleep apnea (such as daytime somnolence), and congestive heart failure, should be included. An in-depth discussion

Stature m (in)

Weight kg (lb)	1.24 (49)	1.27 (50)	1.30 (51)	1.32 (52)	1.35 (53)	1.37 (54)	1.40 (55)	1.42 (56)	1.45 (57)	1.47 (58)	1.50 (59)	1.52 (60)	1.55 (61)	1.57 (62)	1.60 (63)	1.63 (64)	1.65 (65)	1.68 (66)	1.70 (67)	1.73 (68)	1.75 (69)	1.78 (70)	1.80 (71)	1.83 (72)	1.85 (73)	1.88 (74)	1.90 (75)	1.93 (76)
20 (45)	13	13	12	12	11	11	10	10	10	9	9	9	8															
23 (50)	15	14	13	13	12	12	12	11	11	10	10	10	9	9	9	9	8											
25 (55)	16	15	15	14	14	13	13	12	12	12	11	11	10	10	10	9	9	9										
27 (60)	18	17	16	16	15	15	14	13	13	13	12	12	11	11	11	10	10	10	9	9								
29 (65)	19	18	17	17	16	16	15	15	14	14	13	13	12	12	12	11	11	10	10	10	10							
32 (70)	21	20	19	18	17	17	16	16	15	15	14	14	13	13	12	12	12	11	11	11	10	10						
34 (75)	22	21	20	20	19	18	17	17	16	16	15	15	14	14	13	13	12	12	12	11	11	11	10					
36 (80)	24	22	21	21	20	19	19	18	17	17	16	16	15	15	14	14	13	13	13	12	12	11	11	11				
39 (85)	25	24	23	22	21	21	20	19	18	18	17	17	16	16	15	15	14	14	13	13	13	12	12	12	11			
41 (90)	27	25	24	23	22	22	21	20	19	19	18	18	17	17	16	15	15	14	14	14	13	13	13	12	12	12		
43 (95)	28	27	25	25	24	23	22	21	20	20	19	19	18	17	17	16	16	15	15	14	14	13	13	13	12	12		
45 (100)	29	28	27	26	25	24	23	22	22	21	20	20	19	18	18	17	17	16	16	15	15	14	14	14	13	13	13	12
48 (105)	31	30	28	27	26	25	24	24	23	22	21	21	20	19	19	18	17	17	16	16	16	15	15	14	14	13	13	13
50 (110)	32	31	30	29	27	27	25	25	24	23	22	22	21	20	19	19	18	18	17	17	16	16	15	15	15	14	14	13
52 (115)	34	32	31	30	29	28	27	26	25	24	23	23	22	21	20	20	19	18	18	17	17	16	16	16	15	15	14	14
54 (120)	35	34	32	31	30	29	28	27	26	25	24	24	23	22	21	21	20	20	19	19	18	17	17	17	16	16	15	15
57 (125)	37	35	34	33	31	30	29	28	27	26	25	25	24	23	22	22	21	21	20	20	19	19	18	17	17	17	16	15
59 (130)	38	37	35	34	32	31	30	29	28	27	26	26	25	24	23	22	22	21	20	20	19	19	18	18	17	17	16	16
61 (135)	40	38	36	35	34	33	31	30	29	28	27	27	25	25	24	23	22	22	21	20	20	19	19	18	18	17	17	16
64 (140)	41	39	38	36	35	34	32	31	30	29	28	27	26	26	25	24	23	22	22	21	21	20	20	19	19	18	18	17
66 (145)	43	41	39	38	36	35	34	33	31	30	29	28	27	27	26	25	24	23	23	22	21	21	20	20	19	19	18	18
68 (150)	44	42	40	39	37	36	35	34	32	31	30	29	28	28	27	26	25	24	24	23	22	21	21	20	20	19	19	18
70 (155)	46	44	42	40	39	37	36	35	33	33	31	30	29	29	27	26	26	25	24	23	23	22	22	21	21	20	19	19
73 (160)	47	45	43	42	40	39	37	36	35	34	32	31	30	29	28	27	26	25	24	24	23	22	22	21	21	20	20	19
77 (170)	50	48	46	44	42	41	39	38	37	36	34	33	32	31	30	29	28	27	27	26	25	24	24	23	23	22	21	21
79 (175)		49	47	46	44	42	40	39	38	37	35	34	33	32	31	30	29	28	27	27	26	25	24	24	23	22	22	21
82 (180)		51	48	47	45	44	42	40	39	38	36	35	34	33	32	31	30	29	28	27	27	26	25	24	24	23	23	22
84 (185)			50	48	46	45	43	42	40	39	37	36	35	34	33	32	31	30	29	28	27	26	26	25	25	24	23	23
86 (190)				49	47	46	44	43	41	40	39	37	36	35	34	32	32	31	30	29	28	27	27	26	25	24	24	23
88 (195)				51	49	47	45	44	42	41	39	38	37	36	35	33	32	31	31	30	29	28	27	26	26	25	25	24
91 (200)					50	48	46	45	43	42	40	39	38	37	35	34	33	32	31	30	30	29	28	27	27	26	25	24
93 (205)						50	47	46	44	43	41	40	39	38	36	35	34	33	32	31	30	29	29	28	27	26	26	25
95 (210)							49	47	45	44	42	41	40	39	37	36	35	34	33	32	31	30	29	28	28	27	26	26
98 (215)							50	48	46	45	43	42	41	40	38	37	36	35	34	33	32	31	30	29	28	28	27	26
100 (220)								49	47	46	44	43	42	40	39	38	37	35	35	33	33	31	31	30	29	28	28	27
102 (225)								51	49	47	45	44	42	41	40	38	37	36	35	34	33	32	31	30	30	29	28	27
104 (230)									50	48	46	45	43	42	41	39	38	37	36	35	34	33	32	31	30	30	29	28
107 (235)										49	47	46	44	43	42	40	39	38	37	36	34	34	33	32	31	30	30	29
109 (240)										50	48	47	45	44	43	41	40	39	38	36	36	34	34	33	32	31	30	29
111 (245)											49	48	46	45	43	42	41	39	38	37	36	35	34	33	32	31	31	30
113 (250)											50	49	47	46	44	43	42	40	39	38	37	36	35	34	33	32	31	30
116 (255)												50	48	47	45	44	42	41	40	39	38	37	36	35	34	33	32	31
118 (260)													49	48	46	44	43	42	41	39	39	37	36	35	34	33	33	32
120 (265)													50	49	47	45	44	43	42	40	39	38	37	36	35	34	33	32
122 (270)														50	48	46	45	43	42	41	40	39	38	37	36	35	34	33
125 (275)															49	47	46	44	43	42	41	39	38	37	36	35	35	33
127 (280)															50	48	47	45	44	42	41	40	39	38	37	36	35	34
129 (285)															50	49	47	46	45	43	42	41	40	39	38	37	36	35
132 (290)																50	48	47	46	44	43	42	41	39	38	37	36	35
134 (295)																50	49	47	46	45	44	42	41	40	39	38	37	36
136 (300)																	50	48	47	45	44	43	42	41	40	39	38	37

Figure 2. Guidelines for Adolescent Preventive Services Body Mass Index for Selected Weights and Statures

of the medical causes and complications of obesity is beyond the scope of this paper.

FAMILY ASSESSMENT

Since an adolescent's nutrition and activity behaviors are learned, parental involvement is essential to successful weight management. Information best elicited directly from the parents includes the following: What foods do they purchase for home? How are they prepared? Do they more often fry foods or bake them? Are the parents themselves overweight? Do they model healthy eating behaviors for their children? Do they skip meals? Do they eat to relieve stress? Are meals planned for nutritional balance? What kinds of snacks are in the home? Is regular exercise a part of family recreation? Are high-calorie snacks associated with routine activities whether or not anyone is hungry? What observations can they share about the adolescent's eating and exercise habits? Have they attempted to encourage any changes in those behaviors? With what results?

Some pediatricians may choose to present these items in a questionnaire distributed to parents at the time of the initial evaluation.

PHYSICAL EXAMINATION

Comprehensive physical assessment of the overweight adolescent includes measurement of height and weight, blood pressure, pulse, and respiratory rate. Weight velocity (the rate of weight gain over the previous 6 to 12 months) will help to identify those who are gaining weight rapidly and are at increased risk of becoming overweight. Height charts will often identify overweight adolescents who require evaluation for an underlying medical problem; these patients are generally short for their age (ie, below the fifth percentile for height), as opposed to those with exogenous obesity, who typically are normal height for their age. In addition, patients with obesity due to hyperadrenalism, hypothyroidism or other medical conditions usually have abnormal findings on history and physical examination and a decline in the rate of linear growth.

The physical examination should focus on the skin, cardiopulmonary, musculoskeletal, and neurological systems. Acanthosis nigricans may indicate insulin resistance. Overweight adolescents

Table 1. Medical Causes of Obesity

Genetic Syndromes
- Laurence-Moon-Biedl
- Prader-Willi

Hypothalamic
- trauma
- tumors
- inflammatory lesions
    - tuberculosis
    - sarcoidosis

Endocrine
- hypopituitarism
- hypothyroidism
- hypercortisolism
- hyperinsulinemia

Medications
- tricyclic antidepressants
- antipsychotics
- anticonvulsants
- corticosteroids

Table 2. Adverse Consequences of Adolescent Obesity

Medical Complications

Short-term
- sleep apnea with daytime somnolence
- slipped capital femoral epiphysis
- hypertension (also long-term)
- pseudotumor cerebri
- glucose intolerance
- hyperlipidemia (also long-term)

Long-term
- coronary artery disease
- cerebrovascular disease
- gallstones
- tibia vara
- osteoarthritis
- increased cancer risk in males (colon, rectum, prostate)
- diabetes mellitus

Psychosocial Complications
- depression
- low self-esteem
- work difficulties
- social difficulties

may experience intertrigo, redness, and erosions in skin folds that are the result of moisture and frictional forces. Striae are common in adolescents with obesity, and unless pigmented, rarely indicate hypercortisolism. Cardiopulmonary function should be assessed for evidence of hypertension, congestive heart failure, or cor pulmonale. Musculoskeletal examination should assess for joint disease due to degeneration of the medial tibial epiphysis, or slipped capital femoral epiphysis.

LABORATORY STUDIES

Laboratory studies are of limited value in the evaluation of overweight adolescents, except to identify those who might have glucose intolerance or hyperlipidemia. Adolescents whose BMI is ≥ the 85th percentile should be assessed for fasting glucose and lipid profile. Laboratory assessment for adrenal and thyroid function is rarely helpful in the absence of clinical indicators of disease. Laboratory studies to assess cardiopulmonary function (eg, electrocardiogram, echocardiogram), chest x-rays, and sleep studies should be considered for those with morbid obesity.

Management

Despite inherent challenges, there is cause for optimism about successful treatment of adolescent overweight. Many of these patients are motivated. Recent studies in adults show that a weight loss of as little as 10% translates into significantly decreased morbidity and increased sense of well-being. Pediatricians who care for such patients need to take a long-range view, akin to the treatment of hypertension or other chronic conditions. Case management for overweight adolescents is premised on lifestyle change: creating good habits and making sound choices about exercise and nutrition.

IMPEDIMENTS TO CHANGE

In obtaining a history, the pediatrician can identify impediments to change and lay the groundwork for management. Some adolescents and families may not view their weight as a problem, or recognize the medical consequences they are experiencing. Others may believe that they are incapable of changing unhealthy habits.

Tailor the interview to address apparent impediments. For example:

● When a mother talks about all the things that she has attempted to encourage change in the past, suggest: "You've certainly done a lot, yet we sometimes find it helps to change just one thing at a time and give it a chance to work. Then we can add something else. It can be confusing and hard to adjust to too many changes at once."

● When a father reports attempts to control what the adolescent eats, remind the parents that while *they* are in charge of what is offered at a meal or available in the house, *the adolescent* is in charge of what he or she consumes.

● When the adolescent says dejectedly, "I've tried everything and nothing works," your response might be, "I know it's hard, yet I've found that my patients may need several attempts before they finally find something that works. Don't give up on yourself, because I'm not going to."

One of the most difficult challenges is the family or cultural system that does not acknowledge being overweight as a health problem. These cases require more extensive psychosocial intervention. The Stages of Change Model developed by Prochaska and DiClemente, described in the two most recent issues of *Adolescent Health Update* (Vol. 9:3, 10:1) can be employed to guide the patient and family through the process of acknowledging a need to change behavior, deciding how that should be done, and taking responsibility for it.

A variety of successful, structured weight management programs are available. Both the patient and family should understand that success builds on experience. Previous unsuccessful attempts at weight loss do not portend failure; rather, they may help in the design of more appropriate approaches.

PREPARING FOR SUCCESSFUL INTERVENTION

Although overweight patients may desire weight loss, more pressing issues, such as family dysfunction, may need to be resolved first. If these or other significant underlying emotional factors need to be addressed, referral to a mental health professional with experience in adolescent and family therapy may be appropriate. When overweight adolescents face impediments to change, it is sometimes helpful to say that they are in "pretreatment," a time when they identify solutions to these barriers.

EFFECTIVE STRATEGIES

If a weight loss program is indicated, the history should include questions about previous attempts. Williams and colleagues have identified five key elements in pediatric office management of obesity:

- setting realistic weight goals (an initial goal of a 10% reduction of weight is suggested)
- teaching the adolescent to decrease intake by about 500 calories/day with a low-fat and high-fiber diet
- identifying realistic ways to increase activity or decrease sedentary time
- engaging parental involvement
- providing support to modify lifestyle behaviors related to eating and activity

All of these are important, and the more that can be incorporated into treatment, the better.

The life skills model to help adolescents change provides a strategy called guided decision-making, discussed in the February 1993 issue of *Adolescent Health Update* (Vol 4:2). The steps in the model include:

- Defining the problem
- Brainstorming possible solutions
- Evaluating pros and cons of each option
- Committing to a strategy
- Implementing the plan
- Evaluating the outcome of the plan

Ideally, the adolescent takes the initiative. A patient who does not acknowledge a weight problem is not likely to succeed in a weight management program. In guided decision-making, the adolescent determines the nature, cause, extent, and evolution of the excessive weight gain, then explores possible solutions with the pediatrician. (See Table 3.) Finally, the adolescent evaluates advantages, disadvantages, and likely effectiveness of the potential solutions.

For example, an adolescent male who thinks that increased activity alone will enable him to lose weight could be informed that exercise has

Table 3. Beliefs, Experiences, and Perceptions of Adolescent and Family

The targeted clinical history in adolescent overweight covers personal perceptions that will influence the success of treatment. The following areas might be addressed.

- How does overweight occur?
- Why is this now perceived to be a problem?
- Who is blamed for it?
- What solutions have been tried?
- When and why have those solutions worked?
- Do you believe that you can implement effective solutions?

been shown to be more useful for weight maintenance than weight loss, and that reduced calorie intake will be required as well. Similarly, an adolescent female who decides to eliminate breakfast to "save calories" can be advised that breakfast is the most important meal to include in a weight loss plan, and that any plan should include behaviors that can be continued into the maintenance phase.

The pediatrician also can help the patient set concrete and realistic goals. For example, we recently saw a 14-year-old female who weighed 330 pounds and had a goal weight of 125 pounds. We suggested that 299 pounds was a more realistic target; this represented a 10% reduction and was below 300 pounds. She appeared to be relieved to have a more attainable goal.

Specific Components of Management

Once the adolescent and family have made a commitment, a tailored weight loss program will be based on behavior modification, with emphasis on meal planning and exercise.

BEHAVIOR MODIFICATION

Behavior modification is a mainstay of effective weight loss and weight management. As in any comprehensive behavior modification, some recidivism is to be expected. Setbacks are common during weight loss efforts. The pediatrician can help parents and patients accept this occurrence as part of the process and help them to collaborate in building constructive coping skills. When setbacks occur, they should be regarded as temporary and cues to schedule a follow-up visit, perhaps to refine the treatment plan.

DIETARY HISTORY

Studies of overweight patients consistently show underreporting of energy intake and overreporting of physical activity. Many overweight patients will benefit from an increased awareness and a careful clinical evaluation of their actual energy balance.

Weekly food, beverage and activity journals can improve awareness of actual intake. Ask the patient to record the amount of time devoted to exercise and television or video games. Talk about how accurate perceptions about diet and exercise are based on carefully collected evidence, then explain that behavior cannot be changed until it is first understood. In a year's time, a 2% deviation in a 2500-calorie daily intake will result in a five pound weight change for an adolescent otherwise in balance. Talk about how a 2% decrease in intake can be achieved, by switching to skim milk, for example, or by eliminating one pat of butter each day. Such information may help patients see how minor increases in energy output (exercise) and decreases in energy intake can lead to weight reduction.

MEAL PLANNING

Meal planning for effective weight management involves both the adolescent and adults who have a role in the purchase, preparation and availability of foods and beverages in the home. Characterization of foods as "good" and "bad" should be avoided; instead, focus on balance and the larger picture of daily intake over the course of a week. For many patients, the word "diet" connotes restriction. "Healthy eating" is a better term.

Once the pediatrician, patient and family have discussed the approach, referral to a registered dietitian for meal planning is indicated.

EXERCISE

Exercise may be perceived as an enjoyable way to increase energy expenditure or an unpleasant burden. The latter is more likely if exercise has been associated with physical distress or social rejection. In either case, exercise alone rarely results in significant weight loss. Most successful weight loss programs achieve reduced intake and sedentary time through behavior modification. It is key that the adolescent choose an enjoyable activity. Those who passively agree to a prescribed exercise method are less likely to persist long-term. Approaches for patients who are averse to exercise regimens may more productively focus on reduction in sedentary time. Obese adolescents may have orthopedic problems that preclude some activities.

MEDICATIONS

Drugs have little role in routine management of adolescent overweight. The Food and Drug Administration has recently recalled appetite suppressants (eg, fenfluramine and dexfenfluramine) because of their association with primary pulmonary hypertension and cardiac valve abnormalities in adults. Phentermine is still available, but its use should be restricted to adolescents at least 16 years old with morbid obesity.

ADJUNCTIVE THERAPIES

In rare cases of morbid obesity (>200 percentile) with life-threatening medical complications such as congestive heart failure, initial rapid weight loss may be essential. In these cases, it may be appropriate to refer the patient to a facility that provides a medically-supervised protein sparing modified fasting program for initial, short-term management.

Some adolescents will benefit from age-appropriate (and, less often, adult oriented) community-based peer support, nutrition and exercise programs. Available proprietary programs for adolescents are based on changing behaviors related to daily energy balance and specifically address emotional factors. These programs focus primarily on attitudes, relationships and lifestyle changes that will facilitate changes in exercise and nutrition patterns, rather than on obesity itself. The pediatrician should be familiar with resources available in the community, know what is likely to appeal to adolescents, and be aware of programs that are medically safe and those that are not.

Maintenance

Patients should be monitored for adequate caloric and micronutrient intake. Follow-up every 2 to 4 weeks will offer opportunities to provide support, encouragement and continuing nutritional assessment. The pediatrician, in conjunction with the dietitian, can determine when new interventions are required, such as additional calcium or iron, and vitamins. The rate of weight loss should not exceed more than five pounds per month and frequently may be only a pound or two. The goals of treatment and the measure of success are not determined by the scales alone. If a patient is able to simultaneously stop weight gain and increase linear height, weight management has been achieved.

Prevention

Although weight problems are ideally identified and addressed in early childhood, effective prevention can take place in adolescence. The pediatrician is ideally suited to provide comprehensive assessment and effective management of adolescent obesity.

Pediatricians can help children to adopt life-long healthy eating and exercise habits by providing effective preventive services, such as those recommended in the American Academy of Pediatrics' *Guidelines for Health Supervision III.* School health and community-based wellness programs welcome the support of pediatricians, who can introduce and share resources.

Summary

This overview of adolescent obesity provides an approach to evaluation and treatment. Although the complex challenges presented in treatment of adolescent obesity may be daunting, the increasing prevalence and severity of overweight among adolescents requires a response from professionals who provide care for them.

Adolescent clinical preventive services guidelines recommend screening for obesity throughout childhood and adolescence so it can be identified and treated as early as possible. An initial screen using body mass index (BMI) differentiates those who are overweight (BMI>30 or at the 95th percentile for age and sex, whichever is smaller), and those at risk for overweight (BMI between the 85th and 95th percentile).

For overweight adolescents and those at risk of becoming overweight, comprehensive interventions address not only factors causing the energy imbalance resulting in weight gain, but also lifestyle and emotional factors that fuel those habits. The "success" of a weight management program should not be evaluated on the basis of weight loss alone. A multifaceted approach that accepts small improvements, especially if assimilated into daily patterns, can have a powerful influence on the health of adolescents.

Bibliography and Further Resources

American Academy of Pediatrics Committee on Nutrition. Kleinman, Ronald E, ed. *Pediatric Nutrition Handbook.* Elk Grove Village, IL: American Academy of Pediatrics; 1998. In press.

Anglin TM. Life Skills Training for Adolescent Health Promotion. *Adolescent Health Update.* 1993;5:2

Centers for Disease Control and Prevention, National Center for Chronic Disease Prevention and Health Promotion, Division of Nutrition and Physical Activity Web site: (http://www.cdc.gov/nccdphp/divinpa.htm)

Dietz WH, Robinson TN. Assessment and treatment of childhood obesity. *Pediatrics in Review.* 1993;14:337–344

Division of Health Statistics, National Center for Health Statistics, Division of Nutrition and Physical Activity, National Center for Chronic Disease Prevention and Health Promotion. Update: Prevalence of Overweight Among Children, Adolescents and Adults—United States, 1988–1994. *MMWR.* 1997;46:199–202

Forbes GB. Diet and exercise in obese subjects: Self-report versus controlled measurements. *Nutrition Reviews.* 1993; 51:296–300

Gortmaker SL, Must A, Sobol AM, Peterson K, Colditz GA, Dietz WH. Television viewing as a cause of increasing obesity among children in the United States, 1986–1990. *Arch Peds and Adolescent Med.* 1996;150:356–362

Helping Your Overweight Child. The Weight-Control Information Network. 1 Win Way, Bethesda, MD 20892-3665. 1-800/846-8098

Himes JH, Dietz WH. Guidelines for overweight in adolescent preventive services: Recommendations from an expert committee. *Am J Clin Nutr.* 1994;59:556–559

Kolata G. Obese children: A growing problem. *Science.* 1986;232:20–21

Mellin LM. *Shapedown.* San Anselmo, Cal: Balboa Publishing; 1991

Meredith CN, Fontera WR. Adolescent fitness. *Adolescent Medicine: State of the Art Reviews.* 1992;3:391–404

Rosenbaum M, Leibel RL, Hirsch J. Obesity. *NEJM.* 1997;337:396–407

Schlicker SA, Borra ST, Regan C. The weight and fitness status of United States children. *Nutrition Reviews.* 1994;52:11–17

Skiba A, Loghmani E, Orr DP. Nutritional Screening and Guidance for Adolescents. *Adolescent Health Update.* 1997;9:3

Teenage Health Teaching Modules: *Protecting Oneself and Others. Tobacco, Alcohol, and Other Drugs.* Newton, Mass: Educational Development Center, Inc; 1991

Troiano RP, Flegal KM, Kuczmarski RJ, Campbell SM, Johnson CL. Overweight prevalence and trends for children and adolescents: The National Health and Nutrition Examination Surveys, 1963 to 1991. *Arch Peds and Adolescent Med.* 1995; 149:1085–1091

Whitaker RC, Wright JA, Pepe MS, Seidel KD, Dietz WH. Predicting obesity in young adulthood from childhood and parental obesity. *NEJM.* 1997;337:869–873

Williams CL, Bollella M, Carter BJ. Treatment of childhood obesity in pediatric practice. *Ann NY Acad Sci.* 1993;669: 207–219

Prevention of Pediatric Overweight and Obesity

Committee on Nutrition

ABSTRACT. The dramatic increase in the prevalence of childhood overweight and its resultant comorbidities are associated with significant health and financial burdens, warranting strong and comprehensive prevention efforts. This statement proposes strategies for early identification of excessive weight gain by using body mass index, for dietary and physical activity interventions during health supervision encounters, and for advocacy and research.

ABBREVIATION. BMI, body mass index.

Introduction

Prevention is one of the hallmarks of pediatric practice and includes such diverse activities as newborn screenings, immunizations, and promotion of car safety seats and bicycle helmets. Documented trends in increasing prevalence of overweight and inactivity mean that pediatricians must focus preventive efforts on childhood obesity, with its associated comorbid conditions in childhood and likelihood of persistence into adulthood. These trends pose an unprecedented burden in terms of children's health as well as present and future health care costs. A number of statements have been published that address the scope of the problem and treatment strategies.[1-6]

The intent of this statement is to propose strategies to foster prevention and early identification of overweight and obesity in children. Evidence to support the recommendations for prevention is presented when available, but unfortunately, too few studies on prevention have been performed. The enormity of the epidemic, however, necessitates this call to action for pediatricians using the best information available.

Definitions and Description of the Problem

Body mass index (BMI) is the ratio of weight in kilograms to the square of height in meters. BMI is widely used to define overweight and obesity, because it correlates well with more accurate measures of body fatness and is derived from commonly available data—weight and height.[7] It has also been correlated with obesity-related comorbid conditions in adults and children. Clinical judgment must be used in applying these criteria to a patient, because obesity refers to excess adiposity rather than excess weight, and BMI is a surrogate for adiposity. The pediatric growth charts for the US population now include BMI for age and gender, are readily available online (http://www.cdc.gov/growthcharts), and allow longitudinal tracking of BMI.[8]

BMI between 85th and 95th percentile for age and sex is considered at risk of overweight, and BMI at or above the 95th percentile is considered overweight or obese.[9,10] The prevalence of childhood overweight and obesity is increasing at an alarming rate in the United States as well as in other developed and developing countries. Prevalence among children and adolescents has doubled in the past 2 decades in the United States. Currently, 15.3% of 6- to 11-year olds and 15.5% of 12- to 19-year-olds are at or above the 95th percentile for BMI on standard growth charts based on reference data from the 1970s, with even higher rates among subpopulations of minority and economically disadvantaged children.[10,11] Recent data from the Centers for Disease Control and Prevention also indicate that children younger than 5 years across all ethnic groups have had significant increases in the prevalence of overweight and obesity.[12,13] American children and adolescents today are less physically active as a group than were previous generations, and less active children are more likely to be overweight and to have higher blood pressure, insulin and cholesterol concentrations and more abnormal lipid profiles.[14,15]

Obesity is associated with significant health problems in the pediatric age group and is an important early risk factor for much of adult morbidity and mortality.[15,16] Medical problems are common in obese children and adolescents and can affect cardiovascular health (hypercholesterolemia and dyslipidemia, hypertension),[14,17-19] the endocrine system (hyperinsulinism, insulin resistance, impaired glucose tolerance, type 2 diabetes mellitus, menstrual irregularity),[20-22] and mental health (depression, low self-esteem).[23,24] Because of the increasing incidence of type 2 diabetes mellitus among obese adolescents and because diabetes-related morbidities may worsen if diagnosis is delayed, the clinician should be alert to the possibility of type 2 diabetes mellitus in all obese adolescents, especially those with a family history of early-onset (younger than 40 years) type 2 diabetes mellitus.[25] The psychologic stress of social stigmatization imposed on obese children may be just as damaging as the medical morbidities. The negative images of obesity are so strong that growth failure and pubertal delay have been reported in children practicing self-imposed caloric restriction because of fears of becoming obese.[26] Other important complications and associations include pulmonary (asthma, obstructive sleep apnea syndrome, pickwickian syndrome),[27-32] orthopedic (genu varum, slipped capital femoral epiphysis),[33,34] and gastrointestinal/hepatic (nonalcoholic steatohepatitis)[35] complications. All these disturbances are seen at an increased rate in obese individuals and have become more common in the pediatric population. The probability of childhood obesity persisting into adulthood is estimated to increase from approximately 20% at 4 years of age to approximately 80% by adolescence.[36] In addition, it is probable that comorbidities will persist into adulthood.[16,37] Thus, the potential future health care costs associated with pediatric obesity and its

comorbidities are staggering, prompting the surgeon general to predict that preventable morbidity and mortality associated with obesity may exceed those associated with cigarette smoking.[10,38]

Although treatment approaches for pediatric obesity may be effective in the short term,[39-44] long-term outcome data for successful treatment approaches are limited.[45,46] The intractable nature of adult obesity is well known. Therefore, it is incumbent on the pediatric community to take a leadership role in prevention and early recognition of pediatric obesity.

Risk Factors

Development of effective prevention strategies mandates that physicians recognize populations and individuals at risk. Interactions between genetic, biological, psychologic, sociocultural, and environmental factors clearly are evident in childhood obesity. Elucidation of hormonal and neurochemical mechanisms that promote the energy imbalance that generates obesity has come from molecular genetics and neurochemistry. Knowledge of the genetic basis of differences in the complex of hormones and neurotransmitters (including growth hormone, leptin, ghrelin, neuropeptide Y, melanocortin, and others) that are responsible for regulating satiety, hunger, lipogenesis, and lipolysis as well as growth and reproductive development will eventually refine our understanding of risk of childhood overweight and obesity and may lead to more effective therapies.[47,48]

Genetic conditions known to be associated with propensity for obesity include Prader-Willi syndrome, Bardet-Biedl syndrome, and Cohen syndrome. In these conditions, early diagnosis allows collaboration with subspecialists, such as geneticists, endocrinologists, behavioralists, and nutritionists, to optimize growth and development while promoting healthy eating and activity patterns from a young age. For example, data suggest that growth hormone may improve some of the signs of Prader-Willi syndrome.[49-51]

It has long been recognized that obesity "runs in families"—high birth weight, maternal diabetes, and obesity in family members all are factors—but there are likely to be multiple genes and a strong interaction between genetics and environment that influence the degree of adiposity.[47,48,52,53] For young children, if 1 parent is obese, the odds ratio is approximately 3 for obesity in adulthood, but if both parents are obese, the odds ratio increases to more than 10. Before 3 years of age, parental obesity is a stronger predictor of obesity in adulthood than the child's weight status.[54] Such observations have important implications for recognition of risk and routine anticipatory guidance that is directed toward healthy eating and activity patterns in families.

There are critical periods of development for excessive weight gain. Extent and duration of breastfeeding have been found to be inversely associated with risk of obesity in later childhood, possibly mediated by physiologic factors in human milk as well as by the feeding and parenting patterns associated with nursing.[55-58] Investigations of dietary factors in infancy, such as high protein intake or the timing of introduction of complementary foods, have not consistently revealed effects on childhood obesity. It has been known for decades that adolescence is another critical period for development of obesity.[59] The normal tendency during early puberty for insulin resistance may be a natural cofactor for excessive weight gain as well as various comorbidities of obesity.[60] Early menarche is clearly associated with degree of overweight, with a twofold increase in rate of early menarche associated with BMI greater than the 85th percentile.[61] The risk of obesity persisting into adulthood is higher among obese adolescents than among younger children.[54] The roles of leptin, adiponectin, ghrelin, fat mass, and puberty on development of adolescent obesity are being actively investigated. Data suggest that adolescents who engage in high-risk behaviors, such as smoking, ethanol use, and early sexual experimentation also may be at greater risk of poor dietary and exercise habits.[62]

Environmental risk factors for overweight and obesity, including family and parental dynamics, are numerous and complicated. Although clinical interventions cannot change these factors directly, they can influence patients' adaptations to them, and the physician can advocate for change at the community level. Food insecurity may contribute to the inverse relation of obesity prevalence with socioeconomic status, but the relationship is a complex one.[63] Other barriers low-income families may face are lack of safe places for physical activity and lack of consistent access to healthful food choices, particularly fruits and vegetables. Low cognitive stimulation in the home, low socioeconomic status, and maternal obesity all predict development of obesity.[64] In research settings, there is accumulating evidence for the detrimental effects of overcontrolling parental behavior on children's ability to self-regulate energy intake. For example, maternal-child feeding practices, maternal perception of daughter's risk of overweight,[65] maternal restraint, verbal prompting to eat at mealtime, attentiveness to noneating behavior, and close parental monitoring[66] all may promote undesired consequences for children's eating behaviors. Parental food choices influence child food preferences,[67] and degree of parental adiposity is a marker for children's fat preferences.[68] Children and adolescents of lower socioeconomic status have been reported to be less likely to eat fruits and vegetables and to have a higher intake of total and saturated fat.[69-71] Absence of family meals is associated with lower fruit and vegetable consumption as well as consumption of more fried food and carbonated beverages. Although our understanding of the development of eating behaviors is improving, there are not yet good trials to demonstrate effective translation of this knowledge base into clinical practices to prevent obesity. At a minimum, however, pediatricians need to proactively discuss and promote healthy eating behaviors for children at an early age and empower parents to promote children's ability to self-regulate energy intake while providing appropriate structure and boundaries around eating.

Widespread and profound societal changes during the last several decades have affected child rearing, which in turn has affected childhood patterns of physical activity as well as diet. National survey data indicate that children are currently less active than they have been in previous surveys. Leisure activity is increasingly sedentary, with wide availability of entertainment such as television, videos, and computer games. In addition, with increasing urbanization, there has been a decrease in frequency and duration of physical activities of daily living for children, such as walking to school and doing household chores. Changes in availability and requirements of school physical education programs have also generally decreased children's routine physical activity, with the possible exception of children specifically enrolled in athletic programs. All these factors play a potential part in the epidemic of overweight.[72]

National survey data indicate that 20% of US children 8 to 16 years of age reported 2 or fewer bouts of vigorous physical activity per week, and more than 25% watched at least 4 hours of television per day.[73] Children who watched 4 or more hours of television per day had significantly greater BMI, compared with those watching fewer than 2 hours per day.[73] Furthermore, having a television in the bedroom has been reported to be a strong predictor of being overweight, even in preschool-aged children.[74] Some cross-sectional data have found significant correlation between obesity prevalence and television viewing,[75-77] but others have not.[78,79] The results of a randomized trial to decrease television viewing for school-aged children has provided the strongest evidence to support the role of limiting television in prevention of obesity. In this study, decreasing "media use" without specifically promoting more active behaviors in the intervention group resulted in a significantly lower increase in BMI at the 1-year follow-up, compared with the control group.[80] Additional support for the importance of decreasing television viewing comes from controlled investigations that demonstrated that obese children who were reinforced for decreasing sedentary activity (and following an energy-restricted diet) had significantly greater weight loss than those who were reinforced for increasing physical activity.[42] These findings have important implications for anticipatory guidance and provide additional support for recommendations to limit television exposure for young children.[2]

Early Recognition

Routine assessments of eating and activity patterns in children and recognition of excessive weight gain relative to linear growth are essential throughout childhood. At any age, an excessive rate of weight gain relative to linear growth should be recognized, and underlying predisposing factors should be addressed with parents and other caregivers. The Centers for Disease Control and Prevention percentile grids for BMI are important tools for anticipatory guidance and discussion of longitudinal tracking of a child's BMI. Significant changes on growth patterns (eg, upward crossing of weight for age or BMI percentiles) can be recognized and addressed before children are severely overweight.[81] An increase in BMI percentiles should be discussed with parents, some of whom may be overly concerned and some of whom may not recognize or accept potential risk.[82]

Although data are extremely limited, it is likely that anticipatory guidance or treatment intervention before obesity has become severe will be more successful. Discussions to raise parental awareness should be conducted in a nonjudgmental, blame-free manner so that unintended negative impact on the child's self-concept is avoided.[24] Data from adult patient surveys indicate that those who were asked by their physician about diet were more likely to report positive changes.[83] Similarly, the efficacy of physicians discussing physical activity,[84] breastfeeding,[85] and smoking prevention[86] is well documented. Thus, pediatricians are strongly encouraged to incorporate assessment and anticipatory guidance about diet, weight, and physical activity into routine clinical practice, being careful to discuss habits rather than focusing on habitus to avoid stigmatizing the child, adolescent, or family.

Advocacy

Abundant opportunities exist for pediatricians to take a leadership role in this critical area of child health, including action in the following areas: opportunities for physical activity, the food supply, research, and third-party reimbursement.

Change is desperately needed in opportunities for physical activity in child care centers, schools, after-school programs, and other community settings. As leaders in their communities, pediatricians can be effective advocates for health- and fitness-promoting programs and policies. Foods that are nutrient rich and palatable yet low in excess energy from added sugars and fat need to be readily available to parents, school and child care food services, and others responsible for feeding children. Potential affordable sources include community gardens and farmers' market projects. Advertising and promotion of energy-dense, nutrient-poor food products to children may need to be regulated or curtailed. The increase in carbonated beverage intake has been linked to obesity[87]; therefore, the sale of such beverages should not be promoted at school. Pediatricians are encouraged to work with school administrators and others in the community on ways to decrease the availability of foods and beverages with little nutritional value and to decrease the dependence on vending machines, snack bars, and school stores for school revenue. Regarding physical activity, advocacy is sorely needed for physical education programs that emphasize and model learning of daily activities for personal fitness (as opposed to physical education limited to a few team sports).

New initiatives for pilot projects to test prevention strategies have been funded by the National Institutes of Health and other organizations, but a long-term commitment of substantial funds from many sources and to many disciplines will be needed to attack this serious, widespread, and potentially intractable problem. Support for development and testing of primary prevention strategies for the primary care setting will be critical. Likewise, investment of substantial resources will be required for development of effective treatment approaches for normalizing or improving body weight and fitness and for determining long-term effects of weight loss on comorbidities of childhood obesity. Collaboration and coalitions with nutrition, behavioral health, physical therapy, and exercise physiology professionals will be needed. Working with communities and schools to develop needed counseling services,

physical activity opportunities, and strategies to reinforce the gains made in clinical management is also important.

Pediatric referral centers will need to develop specialized programs for treatment of complex and difficult cases, and for research into etiology and new methods of prevention and treatment. Efforts are needed to ensure adequate health care coverage for preventive and treatment services. Even when serious comorbidities are documented, insurance reimbursement is limited.[88] Lack of reimbursement is a disincentive for physicians to develop prevention and treatment programs and presents a significant barrier to families seeking professional care.

Summary/Conclusions

1. Prevalence of overweight and its significant comorbidities in pediatric populations has rapidly increased and reached epidemic proportions.
2. Prevention of overweight is critical, because long-term outcome data for successful treatment approaches are limited.
3. Genetic, environmental, or combinations of risk factors predisposing children to obesity can and should be identified.
4. Early recognition of excessive weight gain relative to linear growth should become routine in pediatric ambulatory care settings. BMI (kg/m^2 [see http://www.cdc.gov/growthcharts]) should be calculated and plotted periodically.
5. Families should be educated and empowered through anticipatory guidance to recognize the impact they have on their children's development of lifelong habits of physical activity and nutritious eating.
6. Dietary practices should be fostered that encourage moderation rather than overconsumption, emphasizing healthful choices rather than restrictive eating patterns.
7. Regular physical activity should be consciously promoted, prioritized, and protected within families, schools, and communities.
8. Optimal approaches to prevention need to combine dietary and physical activity interventions.

9. Advocacy is needed in the areas of physical activity and food policy for children; research into pathophysiology, risk factors, and early recognition and management of overweight and obesity; and improved insurance coverage and third-party reimbursement for obesity care.

Recommendations

1. Health supervision
   a. Identify and track patients at risk by virtue of family history, birth weight, or socioeconomic, ethnic, cultural, or environmental factors.
   b. Calculate and plot BMI once a year in all children and adolescents.
   c. Use change in BMI to identify rate of excessive weight gain relative to linear growth.
   d. Encourage, support, and protect breast-feeding.
   e. Encourage parents and caregivers to promote healthy eating patterns by offering nutritious snacks, such as vegetables and fruits, low-fat dairy foods, and whole grains; encouraging children's autonomy in self-regulation of food intake and setting appropriate limits on choices; and modeling healthy food choices.
   f. Routinely promote physical activity, including unstructured play at home, in school, in child care settings, and throughout the community.
   g. Recommend limitation of television and video time to a maximum of 2 hours per day.
   h. Recognize and monitor changes in obesity-associated risk factors for adult chronic disease, such as hypertension, dyslipidemia, hyperinsulinemia, impaired glucose tolerance, and symptoms of obstructive sleep apnea syndrome.

2. Advocacy
   a. Help parents, teachers, coaches, and others who influence youth to discuss health habits, not body habitus, as part of their efforts to control overweight and obesity.
   b. Enlist policy makers from local, state, and national organizations and schools to support a healthful lifestyle for all children, including proper diet and adequate opportunity for regular physical activity.
   c. Encourage organizations that are responsible for health care and health care financing to provide coverage for effective obesity prevention and treatment strategies.
   d. Encourage public and private sources to direct funding toward research into effective strategies to prevent overweight and obesity and to maximize limited family and community resources to achieve healthful outcomes for youth.
   e. Support and advocate for social marketing intended to promote healthful food choices and increased physical activity.

Committee on Nutrition, 2002–2003
*Nancy F. Krebs, MD, Chairperson
Robert D. Baker, Jr, MD, PhD
Frank R. Greer, MD
Melvin B. Heyman, MD
Tom Jaksic, MD, PhD
Fima Lifshitz, MD

*Marc S. Jacobson, MD
  Past Committee Member

Liaisons
Donna Blum-Kemelor, MS, RD
  US Department of Agriculture
Margaret P. Boland, MD
  Canadian Paediatric Society
William Dietz, MD, PhD
  Centers for Disease Control and Prevention
Van S. Hubbard, MD, PhD
  National Institute of Diabetes and Digestive and Kidney Diseases
Elizabeth Yetley, PhD
  US Food and Drug Administration

Staff
Pamela Kanda, MPH

*Lead authors

References

1. American Academy of Pediatrics, Committee on Sports Medicine and Fitness. Promotion of healthy weight-control practices in young athletes. *Pediatrics.* 1996;97:752–753

2. American Academy of Pediatrics, Committee on Public Education. Children, adolescents, and television. *Pediatrics.* 2001;107:423–426

3. American Dietetic Association. Position of the American Dietetic Association. Dietary guidance for healthy children aged 2 to 11 years. *J Am Diet Assoc.* 1999;99:93–101

4. Gidding SS, Leibel RL, Daniels S, Rosenbaum M, Van Horn L, Marx GR. Understanding obesity in youth. A statement for healthcare professionals from the Committee on Atherosclerosis and Hypertension in the Young of the Committee on Cardiovascular Disease in the Young and Nutrition Committee, American Heart Association. *Circulation.* 1996;94:3383–3387

5. American Medical Association, Council on Scientific Affairs. *Obesity as a Major Public Health Problem.* Chicago, IL: American Medical Association; 1999. Available at: http://www.ama-assn.org/meetings/public/annual99/reports/csa/rtf/csa6.rtf. Accessed September 4, 2002

6. Barlow SE, Dietz WH. Obesity evaluation and treatment: expert committee recommendations. The Maternal and Child Health Bureau, Health Resources and Services Administration and the Department of Health and Human Services. *Pediatrics.* 1998;102(3). Available at: http://www.pediatrics.org/cgi/content/full/102/3/e29

7. Pietrobelli A, Faith MS, Allison DB, Gallagher D, Chiumello G, Heymsfield SB. Body mass index as a measure of adiposity among children and adolescents: a validation study. *J Pediatr.* 1998;132:204–210

8. Kuczmarski RJ, Ogden CL, Grummer-Strawn LM, et al. CDC growth charts: United States. *Adv Data.* 2000 Jun 8;(314):1–27

9. Himes JH, Dietz WH. Guidelines for overweight in adolescent preventive services: recommendations from an expert committee. *Am J Clin Nutr.* 1994;59:307–316

10. US Dept Health and Human Services. *The Surgeon General's Call to Action to Prevent and Decrease Overweight and Obesity.* Rockville, MD: US Department of Health and Human Services, Public Health Service, Office of the Surgeon General; 2001

11. Ogden CL, Flegal KM, Carroll MD, Johnson CL. Prevalence and trends in overweight among US children and adolescents, 1999–2000. *JAMA.* 2002;288:1728–1732

12. Mei Z, Scanlon KS, Grummer-Strawn LM, Freedman DS, Yip R, Trowbridge FL. Increasing prevalence of overweight among US low-income preschool children: The Centers for Disease Control and Prevention Pediatric Nutrition Surveillance, 1983 to 1995. *Pediatrics.* 1998;101(1). Available at: http://www.pediatrics.org/cgi/content/full/101/1/e12

13. Ogden CL, Troiano RP, Breifel RR, Kuczmarski RJ, Flegal KM, Johnson CL. Prevalence of overweight among preschool children in the United States, 1971 through 1994. *Pediatrics.* 1997;99(4). Available at: http://www.pediatrics.org/cgi/content/full/99/4/e1

14. Gidding SS, Bao W, Srinivasan SR, Berenson GW. Effects of secular trends in obesity on coronary risk factors in children: the Bogalusa Heart Study. *J Pediatr.* 1995;127:868–874

15. Freedman DS, Dietz WH, Srinivasan SR, Berenson GS. The relation of overweight to cardiovascular risk factors among children and adolescents: the Bogalusa heart study. *Pediatrics.* 1999;103:1175–1182

16. Must A, Jacques PF, Dallal GE, Bajema CJ, Dietz WH. Long-term morbidity and mortality of overweight adolescents. A follow-up of the Harvard Growth Study of 1922 to 1935. *N Engl J Med.* 1992;327:1350–1355

17. Clarke WR, Woolson RF, Lauer RM. Changes in ponderosity and blood pressure in childhood: the Muscatine Study. *Am J Epidemiol.* 1986;124:195–206

18. Johnson AL, Cornoni JC, Cassel JC, Tyroler HA, Heyden S, Hames CG. Influence of race, sex and weight on blood pressure behavior in young adults. *Am J Cardiol.* 1975;35:523–530

19. Morrison JA, Laskerzewski PM, Rauh JL, et al. Lipids, lipoproteins, and sexual maturation during adolescence: the Princeton Maturation Study. *Metabolism.* 1979;28:641–649

20. Shinha R, Fisch G, Teague B, et al. Prevalence of impaired glucose tolerance among children and adolescents with marked obesity. *N Engl J Med.* 2002;346:802–810

21. Pinhas-Hamiel O, Dolan LM, Daniels SR, Standiford D, Khoury PR, Zeitler P. Increased incidence of non-insulin-dependent diabetes mellitus among adolescents. *J Pediatr.* 1996;128:608–615

22. Richards GE, Cavallo A, Meyer WJ III, et al. Obesity, acanthosis nigricans, insulin resistance, and hyper-androgenemia: pediatric perspective and natural history. *J Pediatr.* 1985;107:893–897

23. Strauss RS. Childhood obesity and self-esteem. *Pediatrics.* 2000;105(1). Available at: http://www.pediatrics.org/cgi/content/full/105/1/e15

24. Davison KK, Birch LL. Weight status, parent reaction, and self-concept in five-year-old girls. *Pediatrics.* 2001;107:46–53

25. Mitchell BD, Kammerer CM, Reinhart LJ, Stern MP. NIDDM in Mexican-American families. Heterogeneity by age of onset. *Diabetes Care.* 1994;17:567–573

26. Pugliese MT, Lifshitz F, Grad G, Fort P, Marks-Katz M. Fear of obesity. A cause of short stature and delayed puberty. *N Engl J Med.* 1983;309:513–518

27. American Academy of Pediatrics, Section on Pediatric Pulmonology, Subcommittee on Obstructive Sleep Apnea Syndrome. Clinical practice guideline: diagnosis and management of childhood obstructive sleep apnea syndrome. *Pediatrics.* 2002;109:704–712

28. Rodriguez MA, Winkleby MA, Ahn D, Sundquist J, Kraemer HC. Identification of population subgroups of children and adolescents with high asthma prevalence: findings from the Third National Health and Nutrition Examination Survey. *Arch Pediatr Adolesc Med.* 2002; 156:269–275

29. Riley DJ, Santiago TV, Edelman NH. Complications of obesity-hypoventilation syndrome in childhood. *Am J Dis Child.* 1976;130:671–674

30. Boxer GH, Bauer AM, Miller BD. Obesity-hypoventilation in childhood. *J Am Acad Child Adolesc Psychiatry.* 1988; 27:552–558

31. Mallory GB Jr, Fiser DH, Jackson R. Sleep-associated breathing disorders in obese children and adolescents. *J Pediatr.* 1989;115:892–897

32. Silvestri JM, Weese-Mayer DE, Bass MT, Kenny AS, Hauptman SA, Pearsall SM. Polysomnography in obese children with a history of sleep-associated breathing disorders. *Pediatr Pulmonol.* 1993;16:124–129

33. Dietz WH, Gross WL, Kirkpatrick JA Jr. Blount disease (tibia vara): another skeletal disorder associated with childhood obesity. *J Pediatr.* 1982;101:735–737

34. Loder RT, Aronson DD, Greenfield ML. The epidemiology of bilateral slipped capital femoral epiphysis. A study of children in Michigan. *J Bone Joint Surg.* 1993;75: 1141–1147

35. Rashid M, Roberts EA. Nonalcoholic steatohepatitis in children. *J Pediatr Gastroenterol Nutr.* 2000;30:48–53

36. Guo SS, Chumlea WC. Tracking of body mass index in children in relation to overweight in adulthood. *Am J Clin Nutr.* 1999;70(suppl):145S–148S

37. Wisemandle W, Maynard LM, Guo SS, Siervogel RM. Childhood weight, stature, and body mass index among never overweight, early-onset overweight and late-onset overweight groups. *Pediatrics.* 2000;106(1). Available at: http://www.pediatrics.org/cgi/content/full/106/1/e14

38. Wolf AM, Colditz GA. Current estimates of the economic cost of obesity in the United States. *Obes Res.* 1998;6: 97–106

39. Becque MD, Katch VL, Rocchini AP, Marks CR, Moorehead C. Coronary risk incidence of obese adolescents: reduction by exercise plus diet intervention. *Pediatrics.* 1988;81:605–612

40. Sothern MS, von Almen TK, Schumacher H, et al. An effective multidisciplinary approach to weight reduction in youth. *Ann N Y Acad Sci.* 1993;699:292–294

41. Jacobson MS, Copperman N, Haas T, Shenker IR. Adolescent obesity and cardiovascular risk: a rational approach to management. *Ann N Y Acad Sci.* 1993; 699:220–229

42. Epstein LH, Myers MD, Raynor HA, Saelens BE. Treatment of pediatric obesity. *Pediatrics.* 1998;101(suppl): 554–570

43. Harrell JS, Gansky SA, McMurray RG, Bangdiwala SI, Frauman AC, Bradley CB. School-based interventions improve heart health in children with multiple cardiovascular disease risk factors. *Pediatrics.* 1998;102:371–380

44. Willi SM, Oexamnn MJ, Wright NM, Collup NA, Key LL Jr. The effects of a high protein, low-fat, ketogenic diet on adolescents with morbid obesity: body composition, blood chemistries, and sleep abnormalities. *Pediatrics.* 1998;101:61–67

45. Epstein LH, Valoski A, Wing RR, McCurley J. Ten-year follow-up of behavioral family-based treatment for obese children. *JAMA.* 1990;264:2519–2523

46. Wadden TA, Foster GD, Letizia KA. One-year behavioral treatment of obesity: comparison of moderate and severe caloric restriction and the effects of weight maintenance therapy. *J Consult Clin Psychol.* 1994;62:165–171

47. Rosenbaum M, Leibel RL, Hirsch J. Obesity. *N Engl J Med.* 1997;337:396–407

48. Rosenbaum M, Leibel RL. The physiology of body weight regulation: relevance to the etiology of obesity in children. *Pediatrics.* 1998;101(suppl):525–539

49. Ritzen EM, Lindgren AC, Hagenas L, Marcus C, Muller J, Blichfeldt S. Growth hormone treatment of patients with Prader-Willi syndrome. Swedish Growth Hormone Advisory Group. *J Pediatr Endocrinol Metab.* 1999 Apr; 12(suppl 1):345–349

50. Whitman BY, Myers S, Carrel A, Allen D. The behavioral impact of growth hormone treatment for children and adolescents with Prader-Willi syndrome: a 2-year, controlled study. *Pediatrics.* 2002;109(2). Available at: http://www.pediatrics.org/cgi/content/full/109/2/e35

51. Carrel AL, Myers SE, Whitman BY, Allen DB. Sustained benefits of growth hormone on body composition, fat utilization, physical strength and agility, and growth in Prader-Willi syndrome are dose-dependent. *J Pediatr Endocrinol Metab.* 2001;14:1097–1105

52. Stunkard AJ, Harris JR, Pedersen NL, McClearn GE. The body mass index of twins who have been reared apart. *N Engl J Med.* 1990;322:1483–1487

53. Bouchard C, Tremblay A, Despres JP, et al. The response to long-term overfeeding in identical twins. *N Engl J Med.* 1990;322:1477–1482

54. Whitaker RC, Wright JA, Pepe MS, Seidel KD, Dietz WH. Predicting obesity in young adulthood from childhood and parental obesity. *N Engl J Med.* 1997;337:869–873

55. Agras SW, Kraemer HC, Berkowitz RI, Hammer LD. Influence of early feeding style on adiposity at 6 years of age. *J Pediatr.* 1990;116:805–809

56. von Kries R, Koletzko B, Sauerwald T, et al. Breast feeding and obesity: cross sectional study. *BMJ.* 1999;319:147–150

57. Gilman MW, Rifas-Shiman SL, Camargo CA Jr, et al. Risk of overweight among adolescents who were breastfed as infants. *JAMA.* 2001;285:2461–2467

58. Hediger ML, Overpeck MD, Kuczmarski RJ, Ruan WJ. Association between infant breastfeeding and overweight in young children. *JAMA.* 2001;285:2453–2460

59. Heald FP. Natural history and physiological basis of adolescent obesity. *Fed Proc.* 1966;25:1–3

60. Travers SH, Jeffers BW, Bloch CA, Hill JO, Eckel RH. Gender and Tanner stage differences in body composition and insulin sensitivity in early pubertal children. *J Clin Endocrinol Metab.* 1995;80:172–178

61. Adair LS, Gordon-Larsen P. Maturational timing and overweight prevalence in US adolescent girls. *Am J Public Health.* 2001;91:642–644

62. Irwin CE Jr, Igra V, Eyre S, Millstein S. Risk-taking behavior in adolescents: the paradigm. *Ann N Y Acad Sci.* 1997;817:1–35

63. Alaimo K, Olson CM, Frongillo EA Jr. Low family income and food insufficiency in relation to overweight in US children: is there a paradox? *Arch Pediatr Adolesc Med.* 2001;155:1161–1167

64. Strauss RS, Knight J. Influence of the home environment on the development of obesity in children. *Pediatrics.* 1999;103(6). Available at: http://www.pediatrics.org/cgi/content/full/103/6/e85

65. Birch LL, Fisher JO. Mothers' child-feeding practices influence daughters' eating and weight. *Am J Clin Nutr.* 2000;71:1054–1061

66. Klesges RC, Stein RJ, Eck LH, Isbell TR, Klesges LM. Parental influence on food selection in young children and its relationships to childhood obesity. *Am J Clin Nutr.* 1991;53:859–864

67. Ray JW, Klesges RC. Influences on the eating behavior of children. *Ann N Y Acad Sci.* 1993;699:57–69

68. Fisher JO, Birch LL. Fat preferences and fat consumption of 3- to 5-year-old children are related to parental adiposity. *J Am Diet Assoc.* 1995;95:759–764

69. Neumark-Sztainer D, Story M, Resnick MD, Blum RW. Correlates of inadequate fruit and vegetable consumption among adolescents. *Prev Med.* 1996;25:497–505

70. Krebs-Smith SM, Cook A, Subar AF, Cleveland L, Friday J, Kahle LL. Fruit and vegetable intakes of children and adolescents in the United States. *Arch Pediatr Adolesc Med.* 1996;150:81–86

71. Kennedy E, Powell R. Changing eating patterns of American children: a view from 1996. *J Am Coll Nutr.* 1997;16:524–529

72. Berkey CS, Rockett HR, Field AE, et al. Activity dietary intake, and weight changes in a longitudinal study of preadolescent and adolescent boys and girls. *Pediatrics.* 2000;105(4). Available at: http://www.pediatrics.org/cgi/content/full/105/4/e56

73. Anderson RE, Crespo CJ, Bartlett SJ, Cheskin LJ, Pratt M. Relationship of physical activity and television watching with body weight and level of fatness among children: results from the Third National Health and Nutrition Examination Survey. *JAMA.* 1998;279:938–942

74. Dennison BA, Erb TA, Jenkins PL. Television viewing and television in bedroom associated with overweight risk among low-income preschool children. *Pediatrics.* 2002;109:1028–1035

75. Pate RR, Ross JG. The National Children and Youth Fitness Study II: factors associated with health-related fitness. *J Physical Educ Recreation Dance.* 1987;58:93–96

76. Dietz WH Jr, Gortmaker SL. Do we fatten our children at the TV set? Obesity and television viewing in children and adolescents. *Pediatrics.* 1985;75:807–812

77. Gortmaker SL, Must A, Sobol AM, Peterson K, Colditz GA, Dietz WH. Television viewing as a cause of increasing obesity among children in the United States, 1986–1990. *Arch Pediatr Adolesc Med.* 1996;150:356–362

78. Tucker LA. The relationship of television viewing to physical fitness and obesity. *Adolescence.* 1986;21:797–806

79. Robinson TN, Hammer LD, Killen JD, et al. Does television viewing increase obesity and reduce physical activity? Cross-sectional and longitudinal analyses among adolescent girls. *Pediatrics.* 1993;91:273–280

80. Robinson T. Reducing children's television viewing to prevent obesity: a randomized controlled trial. *JAMA.* 1999;282:1561–1567

81. Miller LA, Grunwald G, Johnson SL, Krebs NF. Disease severity at time of referral for pediatric failure to thrive and obesity: time for a paradigm shift? *J Pediatr.* 2002;141:121–124

82. Jain A, Sherman SN, Chamberlin DL, Carter Y, Powers SW, Whitaker RC. Why don't low-income mothers worry about their preschoolers being overweight? *Pediatrics.* 2001;107:1138–1146

83. Nawaz H, Adams ML, Katz DL. Physician-patient interactions regarding diet, exercise, and smoking. *Prev Med.* 2000;31:652–657

84. Calfas KJ, Long BJ, Sallis JF, Wooten WJ, Pratt M, Patrick K. A controlled trial of physician counseling to promote the adoption of physical activity. *Prev Med.* 1996;25:225–233

85. Lu MC, Lange L, Slusser W, Hamilton J, Halfon N. Provider encouragement of breast-feeding: evidence from a national survey. *Obstet Gynecol.* 2001;97:290–295

86. Epps RP, Manley MW. The clinician's role in preventing smoking initiation. *Med Clin North Am.* 1992;76:439–449

87. Ludwig DS, Peterson KE, Gortmaker SL. Relation between consumption of sugar-sweetened drinks and childhood obesity: a prospective, observational analysis. *Lancet.* 2001;357:505–508

88. Tershakovec AM, Watson MH, Wenner WJ Jr, Marx AL. Insurance reimbursement for the treatment of obesity in children. *J Pediatr.* 1999;134:573–578

Additional Resources

American Academy of Pediatrics, Committee on Nutrition. Cholesterol in childhood. *Pediatrics*. 1998;101:141–147

American Academy of Pediatrics, Committee on Sports Medicine and Fitness and Committee on School Health. Physical fitness and activity in schools. *Pediatrics*. 2000;105:1156–1157

Centers for Disease Control and Prevention. 2000 CDC Growth Charts: United States. Atlanta, GA: Centers for Disease Control and Prevention; 2000. Available at: http://www.cdc.gov/growthcharts

Jacobson MS, Rees J, Golden NH, Irwin C. Adolescent nutritional disorders. *Ann N Y Acad Sci*. 1997;817

National Association for Sports and Physical Activity Web site. Available at: http://www.aahperd.org

National Institutes of Health, National Heart, Lung, and Blood Institute. *The Practical Guide: Identification, Evaluation, and Treatment of Overweight and Obesity in Adults*. Rockville, MD: National Heart, Lung, and Blood Institute; 2000. NIH Publ. No. 00-4084

Story M, Holt K, Sofka D, eds. *Bright Futures in Practice: Nutrition*. Arlington, VA: National Center for Education in Maternal and Child Health; 2000

US Department of Health and Human Services, Office of Public Health and Science, Office of Disease Prevention and Health Promotion, Public Health Foundation. *Healthy People 2010 Toolkit: A Field Guide to Health Planning*. Washington, DC: Public Health Foundation; 2002. Available at: http://www.health.gov/healthypeople/state/toolkit or by calling toll-free 877/252–1200 (Item RM-005)

Weight-control Information Network Web site. Available at: http://www.niddk.nih.gov/health/nutrit/win.htm

All policy statements from the American Academy of Pediatrics automatically expire 5 years after publication unless reaffirmed, revised, or retired at or before that time.

Vegetarianism

by Lori Clayton Pereyra, MFCS, RD, CDN, and Marcie Schneider, MD

Adolescents may cite a variety of motivations to practice vegetarianism. The most frequent reason given by teens is a desire to lose (or not gain) weight. Compassion for animals is another common incentive, particularly for vegans. And many teens choose a vegetarian diet because they believe it to be healthier.

The term "vegetarian" encompasses many different eating practices and philosophies (Table 1). At one end of the spectrum are semivegetarians, whose diet includes poultry and/or fish but not red meat. Lacto-ovo vegetarians consume eggs and dairy but no other animal products. Vegans avoid all foods containing any animal products. A macrobiotic diet is plant-based with occasional white fish and seafood; requirements are consistent with a new-age commitment to respect for the land and local agriculture. The most restrictive variations, raw foodist and fruitarian diets, are not recommended for adolescents.

Epidemiology

Data on adolescent vegetarianism are not readily available, in part because there are so many forms of vegetarian practice. However, studies indicate that up to 6% of American adolescents are self-described vegetarians. The majority of vegetarian adolescents follow a lacto-ovo vegetarian diet. Although only about 0.5% of adolescents follow a vegan diet, this alternative is becoming more popular. Between 50% and 80% of vegetarian teens are females and relatively few are members of minority groups. Vegetarianism is common among Buddhists, Hindus, and Seventh Day Adventists.

Health Effects

Health benefits from vegetarian diets include lower body mass index (BMI), lower serum cholesterol, less oxidation of low-density lipoprotein (LDL), lower blood pressure, and lower mortality rates. The mortality rate from ischemic heart disease among vegetarians is 24% lower than that seen in omnivores.

NUTRITIONAL BENEFITS

Vegetarians' diets include more whole grains, nuts and seeds, meat analogs, legumes, dark green and yellow vegetables, citrus, and dried fruit than

(continued on page 348)

Goals and Objectives

Goal: Pediatricians who have read this issue will be better prepared to counsel adolescents and their families about vegetarianism and to conduct an appropriate nutritional assessment for vegetarian patients.

Objectives: Reading this article will prepare pediatricians to:
- Recognize and discuss the range of vegetarian practices
- List the nutrients most likely to be deficient in vegetarian patients
- Develop a comprehensive assessment and management plan that will address any medical complications of vegetarianism
- Provide nutritional guidance to help teens achieve optimal nutrition as vegetarians
- Develop strategies to help vegetarian adolescents and their families negotiate compromises around eating choices

---

Lori Clayton Pereyra, MFCS, RD, CDN is a registered dietitian and certified nutritionist in private practice in Ridgefield and Norwalk, Connecticut. Ms Pereyra specializes in adolescent nutrition and eating disorders.

Marcie Schneider, MD, FAAP, FSAM, an adolescent medicine specialist, is the director of Greenwich Adolescent Medicine Services at Greenwich Hospital. Dr Schneider is on faculty at the Yale University School of Medicine.

Table 1. Types of Vegetarianism

Type of Vegetarianism	Description	Common Foods Eaten	Foods Avoided	Potential Nutritional Concerns
Lacto-Ovo Vegetarian	Plant-based diet that includes dairy and eggs but no other animal products.	Milk, yogurt, cheese, eggs, grains, legumes, fruits, vegetables, nuts, and seeds.	Animal flesh (eg, beef, lamb, veal, poultry, fish, seafood).	Little concern with varied diet. Saturated fat intake could be high if diet relies too heavily on high-fat dairy foods.
Lacto-Vegetarian	Plant-based diet that includes dairy foods but no other animal products.	Milk, yogurt, cheese, grains, legumes, fruits, vegetables, nuts, and seeds.	Eggs and foods made with eggs (eg, muffins, some veggie burgers), all animal flesh (eg, beef, veal, poultry, lamb, fish).	Little concern with varied diet. Saturated fat intake could be high if diet relies too heavily on high-fat dairy foods.
Ovo-Vegetarian	Plant-based diet that includes eggs but no dairy or animal products.	Eggs, grains, legumes, fruits, vegetables, nuts, and seeds.	Dairy foods, including milk, yogurt, cheese and foods made with these products, all animal flesh.	Calcium, vitamin D
Semivegetarian	Plant-based diets that include some animal flesh that may be consumed on a regular basis.	May or may not eat dairy or eggs, chicken and/or fish/seafood. Grains, legumes, fruits, vegetables, nuts, and seeds.	Beef, veal, lamb, and animal flesh with the exception of chicken and or fish/seafood.	Little concern with varied diet.
Pollo Vegetarian	Pollo—will eat chicken, but no other animal flesh, may or may not eat eggs or dairy.			
Pesca Vegetarian	Pesca—will eat fish and/or seafood, but no other animal flesh, may or may not eat eggs or dairy.			
Vegan	A diet that includes only plants and avoids all animal products, including foods that involve animals in the processing.	Grains, legumes, fruit, vegetables, nuts, seeds, soy analogs, nutritional yeast, blackstrap molasses.	All animal flesh, honey, white sugar, vinegar, beer, foods produced with whey and casein.	Calcium, iron, zinc, vitamins D, B-12, omega-3 fatty acids. Potential for high fiber intake.
Macrobiotic (formerly called "Zen Macrobiotic")	Plant-based diet incorporating lifestyle principles and practices. May include fish on an occasional basis and provides specific guidelines for food selection, preparation, and practices. Emphasizes locally grown foods and foods free from chemical additives.	Grains, legumes, nuts, seeds, unrefined sesame and corn oil, sea vegetables, locally grown vegetables, occasional use of locally grown fruits in season, occasional use in moderation of tofu and tempeh.	All animal flesh except some white fish and seafood (allowed for occasional use), dairy, eggs, unrefined and processed foods, sugars, tropical and subtropical fruits and vegetables, nightshade family vegetables (eggplant, asparagus, sweet potatoes, yams, bell peppers, avocado).	Calcium, vitamin D, B-12, zinc, iron, omega-3 fatty acids.
Fruitarian (not recommended for adolescents)	Plant-based diet allowing fruits, nuts and seeds.	Fruits, nuts, and seeds.	All animal products, grains, legumes, most vegetables.	Calcium, vitamin D, B-12, zinc, iron, protein, omega-3 fatty acids.
Raw Foodist (not recommended for adolescents)	Plant-based diet allowing only uncooked plant foods.	Uncooked fruits, vegetables, grains, legumes, nuts, and seeds.	All animal products, cooked plant foods.	Calcium, vitamin D, B-12, zinc, iron, protein, omega-3 fatty acids.

Table 2. Key Nutrients of Concern in Vegetarian Diets

Nutrient	Physiological Role	Adolescent RDA/AI (Recommended Dietary Allowance/Adequate Intakes)	Acceptable Vegetarian Food Sources
Calcium	Bone formation and bone health, blood clotting, muscle contraction and relaxation, nerve impulse transmission, absorption of vitamin B-12	1200–1300 mg (upper limit of safety–2500 mg) Many experts recommend a slightly higher calcium intake range (1200–1500 mg) during the teen years, due to its importance in bone formation.	For those who consume them, dairy products (milk, yogurt, cheese). For vegans, soy foods fortified with calcium such as fortified soy milk and soy yogurt, tofu set with calcium, tempeh, sesame tahini, calcium-fortified cereals, calcium-fortified juices, dried figs, bok choy (Chinese cabbage), dark leafy greens, such as collard or turnip greens and broccoli, blackstrap molasses, beans/legumes, figs, sea vegetables, almonds.
Iron	Component of hemoglobin needed for oxygen transport; key role in cell metabolism and immune system maintenance	Children ages 9-13: 8 mg (*16 mg for vegetarians, not to exceed 40 mg) Boys 14-18: 11 mg (*22 mg for vegetarians, not to exceed 45 mg) Girls 14-18: 15 mg (*30 mg for vegetarians, not to exceed 45 mg) *Increased amount reflects Institute of Medicine (IOM) recommendation that vegetarians' requirement be doubled to account for bioavailability of non-heme iron	Soybeans, tofu, tempeh, Adzuki beans, chick peas, lentils, pumpkin seeds, cashews, sesame tahini, fortified cereals, dried apricots, baked potato, mushrooms, quinoa, wheat germ, wax beans, potato, prunes/dried plums, blackstrap molasses, sea vegetables (kelp, nori, dulse)
Zinc	Involved in multiple enzyme reactions for growth, development, sexual maturation, wound healing, immune system, taste acuity, appetite maintenance	Children ages 9-13: 8 mg (*16 mg for vegetarians, not to exceed 23 mg) Boys 14-18: 11mg (*22 mg for vegetarians, not to exceed 34 mg) Girls 14-18: 9 mg (*18 mg for vegetarians, not to exceed 34 mg) *Increased amount reflects IOM recommendation that vegetarians' requirement be doubled to account for poor bioavailability of plant zinc	Adzuki beans, chick peas, lentils, tofu, tempeh, miso, tahini, cashews, almond, flax seeds, pumpkin seeds, wheat germ, quinoa, fortified cereals, corn, peas, beans/legumes, peanuts, dairy products
Vitamin B12	Coenzyme in nucleic acid metabolism, brain and spinal cord function, red blood cell maturation, amino acid metabolism, fatty acid metabolism, maintain myelin sheath, cellular division	Children ages 9-13: 1.8 μg Boys ages 14-18: 2.4 μg Girls ages 14-18: 2.4 μg	Fortified soy milk and soy yogurt, fortified cereals, Red Star brand nutritional yeast
Vitamin D	Bone mineralization, blood calcium and phosphorus level maintenance, calcium absorption	5 μg (200 IU), not to exceed 50 μg	Daily sunlight (10–15 minutes on face and arms without SPF protection; darker skin requires longer exposure of 30 minutes to up to 3 hours); fortified cereals, fortified soy and rice milk
Riboflavin (B2)	Energy metabolism, tissue maintenance, coenzyme in many cellular processes	Children ages 9-13: 0.9 mg Boys ages 14-18: 1.3 mg Girls ages 14-18: 1.0 mg	Red Star nutritional yeast, almonds, tahini, wheat germ, fortified cereals, broccoli, mushrooms, avocado, raspberries, beet greens, spinach, strawberries, beans, tofu, whole grains
Alpha Linolenic Acid (ALA)	A precursor to eicosapentaenoic acid (EPA) and docosahexaenoic acid (DHA), 2 important omega-3 fatty acids. Also affects growth and neurological development of infants, reduces inflammation response, and increases total omega-3 fatty acid content of cellular membranes to enhance cellular flexibility	Boys ages 9-13–1.1 mg ages 14-18–1.6 mg Girls ages 9-13–1.0 mg ages 14-18–1.1 mg	Ground flaxseeds, flax oil, canola oil, soybeans, walnuts. Fatty fish such as salmon and swordfish are sources of EPA and DHA, although swordfish should be avoided by pregnant and lactating women due to concerns about mercury content.
Protein	Supplies amino acids which are needed to synthesize the body's enzymes, hormones, cellular structure	Children 9-13: 34 gm (0.9 gm/kg body weight) Boys 14-18: 52 gm (0.85 gm/kg body weight) Girls 14-18: 46 gm (0.85 gm/kg body weight)	For those who consume them, dairy and egg products. For vegans, soy products such as tofu, tempeh, texturized soy protein, soy flour, soybeans, and soy milk products, meat analogs such as veggie deli slices (made from soy), soy burgers, beans/legumes, lentils, nuts, seeds, grains, seitan, aramath, barley, quinoa, millet, rice, oats, corn, nuts, seeds, vegetables.

those of nonvegetarians. They eat less white and fried potatoes, less saturated fat, and consume less fast food, sweet and salty snacks, and sugary drinks.

Data show that the caloric intake of adolescent vegetarians is significantly lower than that of nonvegetarians, with a higher percentage of calories from carbohydrates (60%). Vegetarians' fat intake approximates 25% of total calories, versus 33% for nonvegetarians. Vegetarians also tend to consume more calcium, phosphorus, iron, magnesium, copper, vitamins A, E, C, and folate than nonvegetarians, and twice as much fiber.

NUTRITIONAL RISKS

Nutrients of concern for vegetarians are the same as those for nonvegetarians: adequate calories, protein, fat, carbohydrates, fiber, calcium, iron, zinc, vitamin D, vitamin B-12, and omega-3 fatty acids. Research has shown that vegetarians consume diets higher in many of these nutrients than nonvegetarians, and clinical nutritional deficiencies are not common.

There is little concern about nutritional deficiencies with a lacto-ovo vegetarian diet when a variety of foods are consumed, although there can be an excess intake of saturated fats if the diet relies heavily on high-fat dairy products. Good planning can enable adolescents on vegan and macrobiotic diets to avoid potential nutritional deficiencies. Many cereals and soy products are fortified with calcium, vitamin D, and vitamin B-12. The risk for deficiency increases when entire categories of foods are omitted without increasing consumption of foods to replace the missing nutrients. Table 2 describes key nutrients that may be of concern in any teen following a vegetarian diet.

EFFECTS ON GROWTH AND PUBERTY

Vegetarian teens grow and develop well as long as their nutritional intake is adequate. There has been discussion in the literature of increased menstrual irregularity in vegetarians; however, the studies that are available are conflicting. There are also no definitive data on the question of decreased bone density among vegetarian teens.

Levels of Specific Nutrients

CALCIUM

While calcium is present in a variety of foods, dairy products account for 75% of calcium intake in the western world. Lacto-ovo vegetarians who consume adequate levels of dairy foods should get enough calcium, but this important nutrient is an issue for vegans and vegetarians who do not consume dairy products. (See *Targeted Counseling: Calcium*, left.)

The bioavailability of plant calcium is affected by several factors. Absorption is inhibited by oxalates (found in spinach, beet greens, Swiss chard, and chocolate), and phytates (found in whole grains, legumes and nuts and seeds). Sodium intake is thought to be the biggest factor in urinary excretion of calcium. There is some evidence that vegetarians, who have lower total protein intakes with fewer sulfur-containing amino acids, may have a lower calcium requirement. (Plant proteins, which are not high in sulfur-containing amino acids, create less calcium loss.) However data are lacking in this

---

Targeted Counseling: Calcium

Concrete examples will help vegetarian teens assure that they consume the 1200–1500 mg of calcium needed in their daily diet. Assess the calcium intake of vegetarian patients and talk about securing adequate intake through calcium-rich foods and beverages, calcium-fortified foods, and supplements if needed. Assure that the teen understands the role of supplements and the importance of avoiding excess intake. The vegetarian food guide pyramid can help guide the teen to make appropriate food choices.

Care should also be taken to assure that the teen gets enough calcium for bone growth but does not consume excessive amounts of calcium through overuse of fortified foods and supplements. The upper limit of safety for calcium has been set at 2,500 mg/day. Excessive intake can result in hypercalcemia, hypercalciuria, soft tissue calcification, renal failure, osteochondrosis, and even death.

area so it is important that vegetarian teens meet the RDA for calcium.

IRON

Iron is an important nutrient, particularly during adolescence. There are 2 types of iron present in food, heme iron and nonheme iron. Heme iron is found in red meat, chicken, fish, and eggs. Vegetarians consume nonheme (plant-based) iron, which is not as readily absorbed by the body. Nonheme iron absorption rates are affected by several dietary factors. (See *Targeted Counseling: Maximizing Iron and Zinc Absorption*, right.)

Vegetarian diets should be carefully planned to avoid iron deficiency. Vegetarians have been found to have lower heme stores with lower ferritin levels but no increase in iron deficiency anemia. This could be due to their higher intake of foods high in total iron and vitamin C, which compensates for the reduced bioavailability of nonheme iron.

ZINC

Zinc deficiency can be an issue for vegetarians. Lacto-ovo vegetarians can meet their zinc requirement with dairy products. Legumes, whole grains, nuts and seeds are rich in zinc, but they are also rich in phytates, which decreases zinc absorption. Calcium supplements and foods fortified with high levels of calcium can interact with phytates to bind zinc and prevent its absorption. Acidic foods enhance zinc absorption.

VITAMIN B-12

B-12 is available only in animal products. Lacto-ovo vegetarians can obtain adequate amounts of B-12 by eating dairy products and eggs. Vegans can avoid vitamin B-12 deficiency by consuming cereals, soymilk, and rice milk that are B-12 fortified, or by taking a supplement. Some foods, such as spirulina and sea vegetables, are advertised to contain B-12, but they do not contain an active form, and therefore cannot be reliable sources of the vitamin.

Targeted Counseling: Maximizing Iron and Zinc Absorption

Ascorbic acid, alcohol, and retinol enhance iron absorption while phytates, polyphenols, oxylates, soy protein, egg, antacids, and calcium and phosphate salts inhibit absorption. Instruct vegetarians to avoid drinking tea (black and green) and coffee with or directly after a meal. These beverages are high in polyphenols; tea has been shown to reduce nonheme iron absorption by 75%–83% and coffee to reduce nonheme iron absorption by 60%.

Advise vegetarians to take calcium supplements or highly fortified calcium foods between meals. High calcium foods consumed in the same meal as nonheme iron foods and zinc foods reduce both iron and zinc absorption.

Educate vegetarians on foods high in vitamin C and encourage intake with meals in order to enhance absorption of iron and zinc. Good sources of vitamin C include citrus fruits and juices, tomatoes, strawberries, kiwi, cantaloupe, bell peppers, broccoli and cauliflower.

Soaking legumes in water, roasting nuts, sprouting seeds, consuming yeast-leavened bread and fermenting soybeans are all ways to inactivate the phytates in these foods, which in turn, enhance zinc and iron absorption as well. Iron absorption can be enhanced through cooking with cast iron cookware, especially in the presence of acidic foods.

VITAMIN D

The primary dietary source of vitamin D is fortified milk. Lacto-ovo vegetarians who consume dairy products regularly will be able to meet their requirement for vitamin D. Vegans and vegetarians who do not consume adequate amounts of dairy foods are at risk for deficiency. Many soy and rice milks are fortified with vitamin D. When taken in conjunction with fortified foods, vitamin D supplements may provide too much vitamin D.

The body manufactures vitamin D when the skin is exposed to sunlight; 10 to 30 minutes' exposure daily on the face and arms is adequate for vitamin D biosynthesis. Persons with darker skin require longer sun exposure in order for

Guide to Clinical Interview

How to ensure teen consumes adequate nutrients

The clinical interview provides excellent opportunities to learn what your vegetarian patients are eating, why they have chosen a vegetarian diet, and whether their intake is nutritionally adequate. Some questions to ask include:

- Why did you become a vegetarian?
- How long have you been vegetarian?
- Are there foods that you will or won't eat? (Be aware that adolescent vegetarians may have eating-disordered behaviors and the vegetarianism may be a way to disguise them. Consistent avoidance of high-calorie foods and liquids may signal a need to probe further.)

   Ask the teen for a complete 24-hour diet recall, and discuss his or her choices. For example:

- What did you have for breakfast?
- (If cereal and milk) What type of cereal and milk? Was there any other drink with the meal? Any fruit?
- What snacks have you had since this time yesterday?
- How many snacks?

   Phrase questions thoughtfully. For example, instead of asking about a snack before practice, you might say, "What snack and drink did you have before your basketball practice to ensure you were well hydrated and had enough energy to participate?"

   Once you have determined the type of vegetarianism the teen is practicing, you might ask:

- What foods are you eating to give you protein, calcium, fat?
- What concerns do you have about being a vegetarian?
- Do you think you are getting all the nutrients you need?
- Where did you learn about being a vegetarian?
- Would you like resources for more information on following a vegetarian diet?
- Are you receiving support at home/from your friends about your choice to be a vegetarian?
- Do you take dietary supplements, herbs, herbal teas, homeopathic products? Which ones?

this to take place; the same is true during the winter months for those living at northern latitudes. Sunscreen with SPF above 8 will prevent biosynthesis.

OMEGA FATTY ACIDS

Two fatty acids are essential for humans: alpha-linolenic acid (an omega-3 fatty acid) and linoleic acid (an omega-6 fatty acid). These fatty acids are derived only from food as the body is not able to synthesize them. Omega-6 fatty acids are readily available in grains, legumes, nuts, and seeds; thus, a deficiency is not a concern for vegetarians. Omega-3 fatty acids are a concern for vegetarians in general and particularly vegans, as the most common dietary source for these fatty acids are fatty fish. Alpha-linolenic acid, found in ground flaxseeds, flax oil, canola oil, soybeans and walnuts, is the precursor for the other omega-3 fatty acids. Sufficient fat consumption may be an issue

for some vegans and for lacto-ovo vegetarians who consume only nonfat dairy foods.

PROTEIN

Proteins obtained from plant products are incomplete; they do not provide all of the essential amino acids required for all biological functions. At one time, experts believed that vegetarians needed special combinations of plant foods or "complementary proteins," at each meal in order to be sure that they were getting all the essential amino acids. The current understanding is that a vegetarian consuming a variety of foods over the course of a day can maintain an adequate level of essential amino acids. Protein in cereals and legumes is not digested as well as animal protein, so vegan protein requirements may need to be increased 15% to 20% to compensate. Lacto-ovo vegetarians can easily meet their protein needs with the inclusion of dairy and eggs.

Clinical Assessment

Aspects of nutritional assessment are addressed through the history, physical examination, and laboratory testing.

HISTORY

A thorough nutritional history and 24-hour dietary recall should be a part of each check-up. (See *Guide to Clinical Interview,* left.) A good dietary history informs and reassures the pediatrician, teen, and parents, and may reveal possible deficiencies. The history should also explore motivations for pursuing a vegetarian lifestyle. A comprehensive nutritional history should include questions about the use of vitamins or supplements as well as frequency of dieting behaviors. Ask teens if they or anyone in their household are on a diet: this can shed light on potential nutritional risks. If a patient reports avoiding certain foods without acceptable replacements, nutritional counseling should include appropriate replacement foods. Referral to a registered dietitian may be warranted. (See *Guidelines for Referral,* below.)

In the review of systems, ask about fatigue, neurological symptoms, menstrual irregularity, and other signs of general malnutrition including cold hands and feet, alopecia, muscle wasting, constipation, dry skin, and decreased concentration.

PHYSICAL EXAMINATION AND LABORATORY ASSESSMENT

A complete physical examination should be done at the initial assessment, to include height and weight plotted on growth charts and assessment for proper pubertal progression. Appropriate growth and development indicate that energy intake and nutritional quality are acceptable. Height or weight below expected levels may signify a nutritional concern that needs to be addressed. Pallor may indicate an iron deficiency; smooth tongue may suggest a B-12 deficiency. Any wounds should be examined for adequate healing, as slow healing may signal a zinc deficiency.

In terms of laboratory assessment, some clinicians might find it helpful to obtain blood work once a year including a complete blood count, ferritin and iron levels, B-12, and folate.

Management and Anticipatory Guidance

Patients who have adopted a vegetarian diet should be asked about motivation. If the motivation is weight loss, remind the teen that life-long healthy eating habits, and not quick fixes, are the key to optimal weight over time. Explain how fad diets can lead to deficiencies in macro- and micronutrients.

It is important to advise teens to make sure all food groups are represented in their diet, and that they are getting 12 to 15 servings of calcium-rich foods daily. The vegetarian food guide pyramid is a useful tool to illustrate healthful types of foods and serving amounts. Several versions of this pyramid are available; the one for North American vegetarians developed by Messina, Melina, and Mangels is particularly helpful, as it identifies recommended servings and lists high-calcium plant foods in each food group. The pyramid is an adaptation of this vegetarian food guide pyramid; recommended servings in each category are modified to reflect nutritional needs of adolescents. The pyramid shows liquids (eg, ½ cup milk, calcium-fortified soy milk, or

---

Guidelines for Referral

When to refer to a nutritionist

- When more guidance is needed to correct nutritional deficiencies.
- When help is needed for meal planning.
- When an eating disorder is suspected.

Referring to a qualified nutritionist will allow the physician to spend more time on medical issues. Choose a nutritionist who is a registered dietitian (RD). These professionals are required to complete a degree from an accredited university and an internship, pass a certifying examination, and maintain continuing education. More information is available from the American Dietetic Association at www.eatright.org.

calcium-fortified fruit juice), and foods (eg, ¾ oz cheese, 1 oz calcium-fortified breakfast cereal, or ½ cup tempeh) that provide a single serving of calcium. Plant sources of calcium are prominent in this pyramid, but clinicians should remember that most vegetarian teens are not vegans and will get their calcium from dairy and calcium-fortified foods.

Physicians can compare the teen's diet recall with the number of recommended servings of each food group on the pyramid to identify potential deficiencies and provide guidance for improving intake. Recommending a basic multi-vitamin with minerals (and iron for females) is not inappropriate, although not essential if nutrition is adequate. If further education is required, consider referring the teen and family to a registered dietitian.

VEGETARIANISM AND EATING DISORDERS

Studies have demonstrated that between 2.5% and 54% of patients with eating disorders are vegetarian. Although this is a wide range, it shows that some studies find a high incidence.

Vegetarian diets have more fiber, less fat, and fewer calories than omnivore diets. Teens, however, may cut out red meat because they hope to decrease their fat intake and lose weight, rather than because they have chosen to adopt a true vegetarian lifestyle. Eliminating red meat, then discontinuing other foods, may represent the onset of disordered eating. It may also be a "socially acceptable" way for a teen who has an eating disorder to mask the problem.

Teens with eating disorders may also cut out most fat and eat differently than most other teenage vegetarians. Ask vegetarians who are underweight or losing weight whether or not they eat nuts, seeds, eggs with the yolks, or cheese, and in what quantity. If the teen refuses to consume these foods, yet wants to follow a vegetarian diet, their reasons should be carefully examined.

Researchers have attempted to examine any associations between disordered eating and vegetarianism. In one study, when vegetarian teens with an eating disorder were asked about the timing of the former with respect to the latter,

only a small percentage of vegetarian patients with eating disorders became vegetarian first. More restrictive vegetarians who have avoided meat for a longer time have been found to be less involved with unhealthy weight behaviors than less restrictive vegetarians. Adolescent males who are vegetarian seem to be at high risk for unhealthy weight behaviors. Please see the *Checklist for the Clinical Encounter* (below) for more on exploring concerns about eating disorders through the history and dietary recall. In-depth information on eating disorders is available in the February 2001 edition of *Adolescent Health Update* (AHU 13:2), and the *Consultant's Corner* in this issue of *AAP News*.

HELPING FAMILIES ADAPT

Parents of vegetarians are often concerned that their teenager is not getting adequate nutrition. If the diet recall seems appropriate, there are no symptoms or physical complaints, growth and development are as expected, and laboratory tests are normal, the family and teen can be reassured that the teen is healthy.

Whether vegetarianism is a move for autonomy, a rebellion, a sign of disordered eating, a fad, or a healthy lifestyle choice will become clear over time. Whatever the reason, fitting it into the rest

---

Checklist for the Clinical Encounter

Clues to an eating disorder

- ❑ Eating habits used as an excuse to isolate from family and friends
- ❑ Minimal fat in the diet
- ❑ Proteins eaten are low in fat or nonfat
- ❑ History of menstrual irregularity or loss of periods
- ❑ Distortion of body image
- ❑ Excessive exercise with goal of weight loss
- ❑ Weight is lower than expected on the growth curve
- ❑ Patient doesn't see low weight as a problem
- ❑ Physical examination with signs of malnutrition, tooth erosion
- ❑ Use of stimulant laxatives, diet pills, diuretics, ipecac

of the family life is important. Making it a parent-teen battleground will not be helpful. If the vegetarianism is an act of rebellion or a fad, fighting will only prolong the behavior. If the vegetarianism is a healthful choice and everyone assumes a cooperative attitude, it should not be a source of discord. With proper planning, parents can support their adolescent's choice in a way that does not prompt stress or conflict.

Conclusion

Vegetarian diets that include a variety of nutrient-dense foods in adequate servings can enable adolescents to meet their requirements for day-to-day nutrition as well as long-term growth and development. By supporting a teen's decision for vegetarianism and providing guidance on appropriate food choices, with referrals to a registered dietitian when necessary, the physician can assure that the teen consumes a diet that meets the dietary guidelines for optimal health and longevity.

Acknowledgment

The editors would like to acknowledge technical review by Jatinder Bhatia, MD, for the AAP Committee on Nutrition.

Selective Bibliography

Herbold NH, Frates SE. Update of nutrition guidelines for the teen: trends and concerns. *Curr Opin Pediatr.* 2000;12:303–309

Messina V, Melina V, Mangels RA. A new food guide for North American vegetarians. *J Am Diet Assoc.* 2003;103:771–775

Neumark-Sztainer D, Story M, Resnick MD, Blum RW. Adolescent Vegetarians. A behavioral profile of a school-based population in Minnesota. *Arch Pediatr Adolesc Med.* 1997;151: 833–838.

Position of the American Dietetic Association and Dieticians of Canada. Vegetarian diets. *J Am Diet Assoc.* 2003;103: 748–765.

References and Resources

BOOKS

Messina V, Mangels R, Messina M. *A Dietitian's Guide to Vegetarian Diets: Issues and Applications.* 2nd ed. Sudbury, MA: Jones & Bartlett Publishers, Inc; 2004

Stepaniak J, Melina V. *Raising Vegetarian Children.* New York, NY: McGraw-Hill; 2002

Melina V, Davis B. *Becoming Vegan.* Summertown, TN: Book Publishing Company; 2000

INFORMATION ON THE WEB

http://www.vrg.org
Vegetarian Resources Group
A not-for-profit educational group that works to educate the public on vegetarianism and related issues.

http://www.nal.usda.gov/fnic/etext/000058.html
U.S.D.A. Food and Nutrition Information Center
Mostly consumer-oriented site with lots of good information and great links.

http://www.llu.edu/llu/vegetarian/
Loma Linda University Nutrition and Health Letter
Consumer information provided by the school of public health at Loma Linda University.

MAGAZINES

Vegetarian Times
Veggie Life
Eating Well

Nutrition Notes

Planning to reduce your meat consumption? Here's what you need to know

by Lori Clayton Pereyra, MFCS, RD, CDN

Moving toward a more plant-based diet is not difficult! The key is to remember that animal products are an entire food group, and when an entire food group is eliminated, you need to find other foods to replace the missing nutrients. Animal products are good sources of many necessary nutrients such as protein, fat, iron, zinc, calcium, and vitamins D and B-12. So when you eat less meat you need to eat more whole grains, beans, nuts, and soy foods like tofu or tempeh.

The entire family can benefit from eating less meat, especially when the meat is replaced with whole grains, legumes, vegetables, and fruits. Eating more plant foods can help prevent heart disease, high blood pressure, diabetes, obesity, and possibly some cancers. Teens can help the family eat less meat by finding meatless recipes and helping cook the meals.

WHAT SHOULD I EAT?

Beans! Try kidney beans, black beans, pinto beans and chick peas. Beans are great sources of protein, iron, zinc, plus lots of healthy fiber. Try them in soups, casseroles, salads, and pasta dishes.

Soy foods! Soy beans can be prepared in lots of different ways—tofu, tempeh, soy "hot dogs," soy "burgers," and soy "lunch meat." Soy can be baked, grilled, or stir-fried. It soaks up the flavors of the foods it is cooked with.

Low-fat dairy foods! Milk, yogurt and cheese are great sources of calcium and other nutrients growing teens need for bone development and health. Try low-fat milk in cereal, low-fat yogurt in smoothies, and cheese in veggie pizza, veggie lasagna, and cheese quesadillas.

HOW CAN I BE SURE I'M STILL GETTING ALL THE NUTRITION MY BODY NEEDS?

If you eat a variety of foods in healthy quantities and you still eat eggs and dairy foods such as milk, yogurt and cheese, you can be sure you are getting all the nutrients you need. If your diet does not include eggs and dairy, good planning can assure that you get all of nutrients your body needs from plant foods. Eat a variety of foods daily from each food group. The vegetarian food guide pyramid shows how much of each food

---

Where can I get more information?

Magazines
Vegetarian Times
Eating Well

Books
The Moosewood Restaurant cookbooks (various titles and authors)
The Whole Soy Cookbook (Patricia Greenburg, Helen Newton Hartung)
The Vegetarian Way (Mark Messina, Virginia Messina)
The Complete Idiot's Guide to Being Vegetarian (Suzanne Havala)
Becoming Vegetarian: The Complete Guide to Adopting a Healthy Vegetarian Diet (Vesanto Melina, Brenda Davis, Victoria Harrison)

Web sites
Vegetarian Resource Group: www.vrg.org
American Dietetic Association: www.eatright.org
International Vegetarian Union: www.ivu.org

LORI CLAYTON PEREYRA, MFCS, RD, CDN is a registered dietitian and certified nutritionist in private practice in Ridgefield and Norwalk, Connecticut who specializes in adolescent nutrition and eating disorders.

This patient education sheet is distributed in conjunction with the October 2004 issue of Adolescent Health Update, *published by the American Academy of Pediatrics.*

The information in this publication should not be used as a substitute for the medical care and advice of your pediatrician. Comments and suggestions on Nutrition Notes should be forwarded to Marc Jacobson, MD, FAAP (jacobson@lij.edu).

Pediatricians are encouraged to photocopy this page for distribution to patients and parents.

group you need. If you think your diet is lacking in some nutrients, talk to your doctor to see if you need to take a vitamin or mineral supplement.

DID YOU KNOW?

- Vegetarians easily get enough protein in their diet by eating beans, nuts, soy, whole grains, and vegetables.
- Most vegetarians follow a lacto-ovo vegetarian diet (they consume eggs and milk, but no meat).
- Vitamin B-12 is an important nutrient found only in animal products. Vegans, who consume no meat or dairy products, need to supplement their diet with vitamin B-12 or eat foods fortified with vitamin B-12.
- Consuming foods high in vitamin C with a meal will increase the body's absorption of the iron in the meal.
- The rates of anemia (low blood iron) are no higher among vegetarians than among nonvegetarians.

Better Health and Fitness Through Physical Activity
Guidelines for Teens

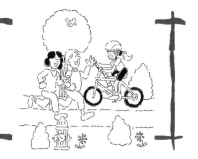

What exactly is physical fitness? Being fit means you have more energy to do daily tasks, can be more active, and do not tire as easily during the day. Being fit also helps you build a positive self-image and feel better about yourself.

You do not have to spend hours in a gym to be physically active. Every time you throw a softball, swim a lap, or climb up a flight of stairs, you are improving your health and fitness level.

The American Academy of Pediatrics has developed this brochure to help you understand what physical fitness is and to give you ideas on how you can become more physically active.

Benefits of physical activity

Physical activity has many proven benefits. When you are physically fit, you feel and look better, and you stay healthier. Physical activity can help you to:

- Prevent high blood pressure
- Strengthen your bones
- Ward off heart disease and other medical problems
- Relieve stress
- Stay active as an adult
- Maintain or achieve an appropriate weight for your height and body build

A major benefit of physical activity is that it helps reduce stress. Learning to cope with stress is an important part of healthy living. Family problems, conflicts with friends, and school pressures can cause stress. Major changes in your life, such as moving to a new home or breaking up with someone, are also sources of stress. Exercise helps you relax by causing physical changes inside your body that help it react to and handle stress.

Physical activity also has many other health benefits, such as helping to ward off heart disease. Coronary heart disease is the leading cause of death in the United States. Research has shown that your risk factors as an adult for developing heart disease start during your childhood. A lack of physical activity is one of the major risk factors influencing heart disease, such as high blood pressure, and other medical illnesses.

Physical fitness is a balance of many areas

To be physically fit, you must work on all aspects of fitness, including the following:

Cardiorespiratory endurance (aerobic fitness)—This is the ability of the heart, lungs, and circulatory system to deliver oxygen and nutrients to all areas of your body. When you are active, you breathe harder and your heart beats faster so that your body is able to get the oxygen it needs. If you are not fit, your heart and lungs have to work extra hard during physical activity.

Body composition (body fat)—This is the percentage of body weight that is fat. Overweight people have more body fat in relation to the amount of bone and muscle in their bodies than do people who are physically fit. Overeating, not exercising enough, or both often lead to more body fat. Being overweight increases your risk of diabetes, high blood pressure, and heart attacks.

Muscle strength and endurance—This is the amount of work and the amount of time that your muscles are able to do a certain activity before they get tired, such as lifting heavy objects or in-line skating.

Flexibility—Flexibility is the ability to move joints and stretch muscles through a full range of motion. For example, people who are very flexible can bend over and touch the floor easily. A person with poor flexibility is more likely to get hurt during physical activity.

What can I do to become more fit?

First, you have to make the commitment to become more physically active. Try to do some physical activity every day, whether it is through physical education classes in school or an activity on your own. Exercise should be a routine part of your day, just like brushing your teeth, eating, and sleeping. It may help to plan a physical activity with a friend or family member. Most people find that it is more fun to exercise with someone else. More importantly, though, is that you like the exercise or activity. You are more apt to stay in the habit of doing whatever activity you choose if it is one that you enjoy.

Now is a good time to pick a "life sport" that you enjoy. Unlike a competitive team sport like football or baseball, a life sport is any kind of physical exercise or activity that you can do throughout your life. Examples of life sports are:

- Swimming
- Golf
- Bicycling
- Jogging
- Tennis
- Walking
- Skating

Regular exercise should include aerobic activity. Aerobic activity is continuous. It makes you breathe harder and increases your heart rate. This type of exercise increases your fitness level and makes your heart and lungs work more efficiently. It also helps you maintain a normal weight by burning off excess fat. Examples of aerobic activities are brisk walking, basketball, bicycling, swimming, in-line or ice skating, soccer, jogging, and taking an aerobics or step class. Baseball and football do not involve as much continuous exercise because you are not active the whole time.

In general, the more aerobic an activity, the more calories—and eventually fat—you will burn. The chart at the end of this brochure gives you an estimate of the aerobic level of many different activities. You will notice that all physical activities burn more calories than sitting does.

Choose any activity you enjoy. If you like the exercise, you will want to keep doing it. Anything that involves movement qualifies as exercise. You do not have to be on a sports team, have expensive athletic clothes or shoes, or be good at sports to become more fit. Any type of regular, physical activity is good for your body. Household chores, such as mowing the lawn, vacuuming, or scrubbing, involve exercise and may have fitness benefits, depending on how vigorously you do the chores. The most important thing is that you keep moving.

Be sure to include stretching exercises in your daily routine. Before you do any physical activity, you should stretch out your muscles. This warms them up and helps protect against injury. Stretching makes your muscles and joints more flexible, too. It is also important to stretch out after you exercise to cool down your muscles. Exercise videotapes, programs on television, and magazines can show you examples of how to stretch out different muscle groups, as well as different exercises you can do.

Just about any physical activity will improve fitness. For example, walking is better than riding in a car, and using the stairs is better than taking an elevator. Making small changes like these in your everyday life can make you more physically fit.

Is it safe to train with weights?

You may want to include strength training as part of your regimen of physical activity, along with some form of aerobic exercise. Strength training, also called "weight training" or "resistance training," is where you use free weights and/or weight machines to increase muscle strength and muscle endurance.

When you strength train, it is more important to focus on proper technique and number of repetitions than on the amount of weight you are lifting If you decide to strength train or weight train, make sure you use the proper safety measures. You should always have a trained adult supervise you.

You should avoid weight lifting, power lifting, and body building until your body has reached full adult development (usually between the ages of 15 and 18) because these sports can result in serious injury. Your pediatrician can help determine your stage of development.

How Often Should I Exercise?

Make exercise a part of your lifestyle. Your goal should be to do some type of exercise every day, or at the very least, three to four times a week. Try to do some kind of aerobic activity that requires continuous physical activity without stopping for at least 20 to 30 minutes each time. Do the activity as often as possible, but do not exercise to the point of pain because this can lead to injury.

Like all things, exercise can be overdone. You may be exercising too much if:

- Your weight falls below what is normal for your age, height, and build
- It starts to interfere with your normal school and other activities
- Your muscles become so sore that you risk injuring yourself

If you notice any of these signs, talk with your parents or pediatrician before health problems occur.

Exercise is only one part of living healthy

Besides the physical and mental health benefits, regular physical activity can also help you become more self-confident, organize your time better, learn new skills, and meet people with similar interests. To make more time for exercise, limit the amount of time you watch television or play computer or video games.

Whenever possible, eat three healthy meals a day, including at least two to four servings of fruit and three to five servings of vegetables each day. Limit your intake of fat, cholesterol, salt, and sugar. Also, get enough sleep and take time to do things you enjoy. For even better health, don't smoke, drink alcohol, or do other drugs.

Physical activity is just one important part of preventive health care, which should be a part of your daily lifestyle. The activities you decide to do should be enjoyable, use a variety of muscle groups, and include some weight-bearing exercises. If you are not exercising much now, increase your level of activity gradually and have fun! Exercise for a better today and a healthier tomorrow!

Fitness Activity Chart

Activity	Calories Burned During 10 Minutes of Continuous Activity	
	77-lb Person (35 kg)	**132-lb Person (60 kg)**
Basketball (game)	60	102
Cross Country Skiing	23	72
Bicycling (9.3mph or 15 km/h)	36	60
Judo	69	118
Running (5 mph or 8 km/h)	60	90
Sitting (complete rest)	9	12
Soccer (game)	63	108
Swimming (30 m/min or 33 yd)		
Breaststroke	34	58
Freestyle	43	74
Tennis	39	66
Volleyball (game)	35	60
Walking (2.5 mph or 4 km/h)	23	34
3.7 mph or 6km/h	30	43

kg = kilogram; mph = miles per hour

km = kilometer; m = meter

Modified from Bar-Or O. Pediatric Sports Medicine for the Practitioner. New York, NY: Springer-Verlag; 1983: 349-350.

Ferguson JM. Habits, Not Diets. Palo Alto, CA: Bull Publishing Co; 1988.

The information contained in this publication should not be used as a substitute for the medical care and advice of your pediatrician. There may be variations in treatment that your pediatrician may recommend based on individual facts and circumstances.

American Academy of Pediatrics
DEDICATED TO THE HEALTH OF ALL CHILDREN™

The American Academy of Pediatrics is an organization of 60,000 primary care pediatricians, pediatric medical subspecialists, and pediatric surgical specialists dedicated to the health, safety, and well-being of infants, children, adolescents, and young adults.

American Academy of Pediatrics
Web site — www.aap.org

Copyright © 1996
American Academy of Pediatrics

Calcium and You
Facts for Teens

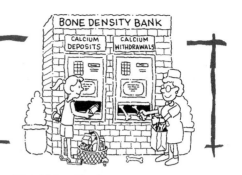

As you grow, you need calcium to build a healthy body. It keeps you strong so you can do well at things like sports, dancing, and school activities.

Getting plenty of calcium while you are young also makes you strong and keeps you looking good for your entire lifetime.

In fact, your body's need for calcium is very high between the ages of 9 and 18 years. However, most young people in the United States do not get enough calcium in their diets.

What is calcium?

Calcium is a mineral that many parts of your body require. Its main job is **to build strong bones and teeth.** About 99% of your body's calcium is in your bones and teeth. A very small amount of calcium is in body fluids such as blood. But this small amount performs vital functions, including the following:

- Keeping a strong heart beat
- Controlling blood pressure
- Making muscles move
- Helping blood clot
- Sending nerve messages

If you make the right choices, the food you eat will provide the calcium you need. If you do not get enough calcium, your body will take calcium from your bones to support other vital functions, weakening the bones.

Why do my bones need calcium?

Bones provide the basic support structure (skeleton) for your body and protect vital organs such as your heart and lungs.

Although bones may appear lifeless, they are alive and growing. Existing bone constantly is being renewed through a process called remodeling. Your body needs a good supply of calcium to fuel this process.

The "bone bank"

Bones serve as a "bank" for calcium. When you are young, your body can deposit calcium in your "bone bank" by increasing your **bone density.** Density means how closely packed together the materials in your bones are. Dense bones are strong bones.

As you get older, you lose the ability to bank calcium. By the time you reach about 30 years of age, your bones reach their **peak bone density.** That means your bones are as dense (or packed with calcium) as they will get — for life.

After that time, **you can no longer deposit extra calcium in your bone bank.** Instead your body withdraws calcium from your bone bank.

Why should I bank calcium?

Having a good supply of calcium stored in your bones means that there will be plenty for growing, rebuilding bones, and performing the many body functions that require it. You are much less likely to break bones that are packed with calcium.

In addition, you are saving calcium that you will need to withdraw from the bone bank when you are older. People who do not store enough calcium when they are young are at high risk for getting diseases such as osteoporosis later in life.

Osteoporosis is a disease of older people that can make bones so fragile that they can break from the stress of merely bending over. It can result in a hunched-over appearance. People with osteoporosis may not realize they have the disease until 1 or more bones fracture. By this time, it is usually too late to undo the bone damage.

Is calcium all I need for strong bones?

Calcium does not work alone. After you eat or drink foods that contain calcium, your body must absorb the calcium through your intestines. You need a small amount of **vitamin D** for this to happen. Rickets, a disease that softens bones, can develop if your body does not absorb enough calcium.

Sources of vitamin D include the following:

- Sunlight. (Your body makes vitamin D when your skin is exposed to sunlight.)
- Milk fortified with vitamin D.

In addition, some juices or other products may be fortified with vitamin D. Check nutrition labels to learn which foods are fortified with vitamin D.

Exercise is important as well. Studies show that regular, weight-bearing exercise helps you build strong bones. Combined with a balanced diet, exercise does the following:

- Helps your body make hormones that protect bones
- Generates electrical activity that promotes bone growth and repair
- Boosts the flow of blood and nutrients to your bones

How much calcium do I need?

The amount of calcium that your body needs varies according to age. The greatest need is during late childhood and the teenage years.

The American Academy of Pediatrics recommends the following daily intake of calcium:

TABLE 1. Daily calcium needs

Age	Calcium need (mg per day)	Servings of milk to meet need
4–8 years	800	3 servings
9–18 years	1,300	4 servings
19–50 years	1,000	3–4 servings

How can I get calcium?

The best way to get the calcium that you need is by **eating and drinking foods that naturally contain calcium.** Many foods contain calcium.

Milk and other dairy products are good sources of calcium. They naturally offer the most calcium per serving. For example, 1 cup of milk has about the same amount of calcium as 4 cups of broccoli.

Most teenagers can get the calcium they need with 4 daily servings of dairy products, plus some green vegetables. Keep the following tips in mind:

- Low-fat and nonfat dairy products are super sources of calcium.
- Chocolate (or any flavor) milk has as much calcium as plain milk.
- Dark green, leafy vegetables such as kale and turnip greens are low in calories and are high in calcium.
- Tofu, broccoli, chickpeas, lentils, canned sardines, salmon, and other fish with bones also are good sources of calcium.
- Calcium-fortified foods such as juices and cereals can help boost the calcium in your diet. However, remember to limit the amount of juice that you drink each day to 8 to 12 ounces (1½ cups).

The tables at the end of this brochure show the amount of calcium in a variety of foods.

Calcium supplements

Certain medical conditions, diets, or lifestyle choices can make it hard for you to get enough calcium by eating the right foods. In some cases, your pediatrician may recommend a calcium supplement, such as a daily dose of a calcium-containing antacid tablet or liquid.

Lactose intolerance

A few young people have lactose intolerance, which means they have trouble digesting lactose (the sugar in milk). Milk with reduced lactose is available to help these teens. Nondairy foods that are rich in calcium, as well as calcium-fortified foods, also can be good choices for people who have lactose intolerance. In some cases, your pediatrician may recommend a calcium supplement.

However, most of the people who have lactose intolerance have only partial lactose intolerance. They can digest dairy products in small amounts with a meal. Aged cheeses and yogurts in which the lactose is broken down can provide good sources of calcium for them. Lactase preparations that make the lactose easier to digest also are available.

Can I get too much calcium?

It is unlikely that you would get too much calcium through your diet. However, it is important to watch how much calcium you get if you take supplements and eat many calcium-fortified foods.

Calcium boosters

On the go

- Order milk or milk shakes instead of soda at restaurants or school cafeterias.
- Choose foods with cheese, such as pizza, tacos, cheeseburgers, or grilled cheese sandwiches.
- Top salads, chips, or soups with cheese.
- Select yogurt or ice cream.

At home

- Choose easy, calcium-rich snacks such as cheese sticks, chocolate milk, yogurt, and pudding.
- Create special drinks with milk. Add flavorings. Make shakes.
- Use low-fat yogurt — on its own or with fresh fruit — as a topping for pancakes or waffles, and in shakes, salad dressings, dips, and sauces.
- Add milk to soups and hot cereals.
- Eat calcium-rich vegetables with cheese or yogurt-based dips.
- Sprinkle cheese on pastas, chili, and popcorn.
- Top sandwiches with a slice of cheese.
- Rely on favorites such as macaroni and cheese, pizza, and tacos.

Calcium blockers

The amount of calcium that your body gets can be thrown out of balance by the following:

- **Drinking a lot of soda (pop or soft drinks)** — Studies show that this may make you more prone to bone fractures. That may be because of the high phosphorus content of sodas. (Phosphorus may make it difficult for your body to absorb calcium, even if you eat or drink enough.) It also may be because sodas are taking the place of calcium-rich drinks and foods in many teenagers' diets.
- **Fad diets** — Some diets do not provide enough calories or offer a variety of foods. This may keep your body from getting enough calcium as well as many other nutrients it needs.
- **Vegetarian diets** — Teens who choose vegetarian diets that exclude dairy products must be very careful to include enough calcium.
- **Excess alcohol** — This can reduce the absorption of calcium in your intestines. It also can damage your liver, decreasing your body's ability to use vitamin D.
- **Diseases of the pancreas, small intestine, or liver** — Diabetes is an example.
- **Certain medications** — Medications such as steroids, anticonvulsants, and antacids that contain aluminum can interfere with calcium absorption.
- **Excess protein, salt, or phosphorus in your diet** — These may block calcium absorption.

- Experiment with calcium-rich foods that may be new to you and your family. Try sardines, tofu, slivered almonds, and salmon with bones.
- Try calcium-fortified juice and calcium-fortified waffles or cereal for breakfast.

Making low-fat calcium choices

Watching how much fat you eat and drink is also important. While you need to include some fat in your diet, no more than 30% of your daily calorie intake should come from fat.

However, you can easily increase the calcium and lower the fat in your diet at the same time.

There are many good sources of calcium that are either low in fat or have no fat at all. The following are examples:

- Nonfat dairy products such as milk, yogurt, and cheese
- Low fat dairy products such as milk, yogurt, and cheese

How to read food labels

Nutrition labels can help you choose foods that are high in calcium. These labels are on food packages.

The labels list the amount of calcium in a serving as **"% Daily Value,"** not as **milligrams (mg).**

100% of the Daily Value = 1,000 mg of calcium per day

The Daily Value is an amount that applies mainly to adults. Remember, if you are between the ages of 9 and 18 years, you need 1,300 mg of calcium per day.

To find out how many milligrams (mg) of calcium are in a serving, place a "0" at the end of the number listed for the Daily Value. For example, a serving of calcium-fortified orange juice might list the amount of calcium as 30% of the Daily Value.

30% Daily Value = 300 mg calcium

In general, a food that lists a Daily Value of 20% or more for calcium is high in calcium. Any food that contains less than 5% of the Daily Value is low in calcium.

- Calcium-rich vegetables
- Calcium-fortified foods such as orange juice

Removing fat from a food does not take away calcium.

Making trade-offs in your food choices is another option to keep in mind. For example, if you go for a thick, chocolate milk shake, skip the fatty French fries.

Counting calcium

If you are between the ages of 9 years and 18 years, you need about **1,300 mg of calcium each day.** Keep track of what you eat for a few days to see if you are getting enough calcium.

If a medical condition or restricted diet may be keeping you from getting the calcium you need, talk to your pediatrician.

The following tables show the amount of calcium in a variety of foods from several food groups. Calcium amounts may vary. Check nutrition labels on products for exact amounts.

Milk Group	Calcium (mg)
* Milk, regular or low fat, 1 cup	300
Chocolate milk, 1 cup	300
Yogurt, 1 cup	300–415
American cheese, 2 oz	348
Cheddar cheese, 1½ oz	300
Cottage cheese, ½ cup	77
Mozzarella cheese, 1½ oz	275
Parmesan cheese, ¼ cup	338
Ricotta cheese, part skim, ½ cup	337
Swiss cheese, 1½ oz	408
Milk shake, 10 fl oz	319–344
Ice cream, ½ cup	88
Ice cream, soft-serve, ½ cup	113
Frozen yogurt, ½ cup	103
Pudding, instant, ½ cup	151
Soy milk, calcium-fortified, 1 cup	300
Rice milk, calcium-fortified, 1 cup	300

Prepared Foods	Calcium (mg) (Verify on label.)
Bean burrito	57
Cheese enchilada	324
Cheeseburger	182
Lasagna with meat, 2½" by 2½"	460
Macaroni & cheese, ½ cup	180
Pizza, cheese, 1 slice	220
Taco, 1 small	221

*Low-fat milk has as much or more calcium than whole milk.

Protein Group	Calcium (mg)
Almonds, chopped, 1 oz	66
White beans, ½ cup	113
Salmon, canned with bones, 2 oz	110
Sardines, 2 oz	248
Tofu, calcium-fortified, 1 cup	260

Fruits	Calcium (mg)
Orange juice, calcium-fortified	300
Orange, 1 medium	50
Prunes, dried, ¼ cup	22
Raisins, ¼ cup	22

Vegetables	Calcium (mg)
Bok choy (Chinese cabbage) ½ cup	79
Broccoli, cooked, ½ cup	35
Broccoli, raw, 1 cup	35
Carrots, raw, 1 medium	27
Kale, cooked, ½ cup	45
Mustard greens, cooked, ½ cup	64
Sweet potatoes, mashed, ½ cup	44
Turnip greens, cooked, ½ cup	98

Grains	Calcium (mg) (Verify on label.)
Bread, whole wheat, 1 slice	25
Cereal, ready-to-eat, 1 oz	48
Farina, enriched, ½ cup	95
Tortilla, corn, 1 medium	60
Waffle, enriched, 4-inch	77

The information contained in this publication should not be used as a substitute for the medical care and advice of your pediatrician. There may be variations in treatment that your pediatrician may recommend based on individual facts and circumstances.

From your doctor

American Academy of Pediatrics

DEDICATED TO THE HEALTH OF ALL CHILDREN™

The American Academy of Pediatrics is an organization of 60,000 primary care pediatricians, pediatric medical subspecialists, and pediatric surgical specialists dedicated to the health, safety, and well-being of infants, children, adolescents, and young adults.

American Academy of Pediatrics
Web site — www.aap.org

eating disorders: anorexia and bulimia

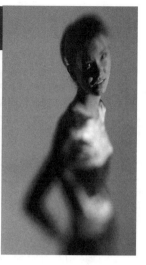

Most people enjoy eating.

But for people with an eating disorder, it brings about very different feelings. They become **obsessed** with thoughts of eating and have an intense fear of gaining weight. These thoughts disrupt their daily activities.

The 2 most well-known eating disorders are *anorexia nervosa* and *bulimia nervosa*. **Anorexia** is self-starvation. **Bulimia** is a disorder in which a person eats large amounts of food *(binges)* and then tries to undo the effects of the binge in some way, usually by ridding the body of the food that was eaten. Some people have symptoms of both anorexia and bulimia. (A quick note about people with **binge-eating disorder:** they eat large amounts of food in a short time and feel intense guilt afterward, but unlike people with bulimia, they don't purge themselves.)

What **causes** eating disorders?

There is **no single cause** of eating disorders. But many factors can lead to an eating disorder. Genetics are now felt to play an important role. Although each person's situation is different, people with eating disorders may **share many of the same traits,** such as

- Feeling insecure
- An **excessive desire** to be in **control**
- A **distorted** body image (feeling fat even when they're not)
- A family **history of depression** or an eating disorder
- Severe **family problems**
- A history of **sexual or physical abuse**
- **Pressure** from activities that place a high value on body size such as running, gymnastics, wrestling, or ballet

What is anorexia?

People with anorexia have a distorted image of their bodies and such an intense fear of becoming fat that they hardly eat and become **dangerously thin.** Many people with anorexia also vomit and overexercise, and they may abuse diet pills to keep from gaining weight. If the condition gets worse, they can die from suicide, heart problems, or starving to death.

People with anorexia focus all of their energy on staying thin. Much of their time is spent thinking about food. For example, people with anorexia may

- **Eat only a small number of "safe" foods,** usually those low in calories and fat.
- Cut up food into tiny pieces.
- Spend more time *playing with food* than eating it.
- Cook food for others but not eat it.

- Exercise compulsively.
- Wear baggy clothes to **hide their bodies,** or complain that normal clothes are too tight.
- Spend more time **alone** and **isolated** from friends and family.
- Become more withdrawn and *secretive.*
- Seem depressed or anxious.
- Have a decrease in activities, motivation, or energy level.
- Do things to keep their minds off their hunger, such as chewing food 30 times before swallowing.

What does anorexia do to the body?

Over time, anorexia can lead to kidney and liver damage, bone damage, and heart problems. When the **body is starved of food,** many physical changes occur like

- The constant feeling of being **cold** because the body has lost the fat and muscle it needs to keep warm. (People with anorexia may **exercise** even more to try to get warm).
- Dizziness, **fainting,** or near-fainting.
- **Bones sticking out** and skin shrinking around the bones. The stomach may look like it's sticking out (often causing anorexics to think they're still fat).
- Hair loss.
- *Brittle hair* and *fingernails.*
- Dry and rough skin.
- **Menstrual periods stopping** (or not starting at all if a girl developed anorexia before her first period). This condition is called **amenorrhea.**
- Stomach **pain,** constipation, and bloating.
- Stunted growth that could be permanent.
- **Anemia** (low red blood cells) causing tiredness, weakness, and dizziness.
- **Loss of sexual function** in *boys.*

Who is at risk of developing anorexia?

Most people with anorexia are **girls** in their teens or even younger. But **boys** can be anorexic, too. Teens who develop anorexia usually are good students, even overachievers. They get along well with others, tend to be **perfectionists,** and don't like to admit they need help with anything. They may appear to be in **control.** However, they actually are insecure, self-critical, and have **low self-esteem.** They are very concerned about being liked and focused on pleasing others.

Most people who develop anorexia start by dieting. Dieting becomes more severe and strict over time. They may think that losing weight will make them feel better about themselves. Dieting also might be a response to a major life change like puberty or going away to college. Because people with anorexia have low self-esteem, they have a hard time coping with these changes and feel like they're **losing control.** Over time, dieting is no longer about losing weight, but a way to feel in control.

When should a person get help?

It's important to know the **early signs of anorexia** before it's too late. The earlier an eating disorder is recognized, the better chance there is of recovery. If someone is having physical symptoms caused by weight loss or answers "yes" to any of the following, that person should get help right away.

- "I can't stop dieting, even though I've been told that I've lost too much weight."
- "Even though I've lost a lot of weight, when I look in the mirror, I still think I'm fat."
- "**I can't stop** exercising."

What is bulimia?

Bulimia is another eating disorder that is harmful to a person's physical and mental health. Bulimia and anorexia share some of the same symptoms.

- As with anorexia, food and staying thin become an obsession, but instead of avoiding food, people with bulimia eat large amounts of food in a short time (binge).
- Guilt and fear then cause them to **get rid of the food** (purge) by vomiting or other means such as overexercising.

People with bulimia have a difficult time controlling their eating behavior. They may be afraid to eat in public or with other people because they are afraid they won't be able to control their urges to **binge and purge.** Their fear may cause them to avoid being around people. They also may

- Become very **secretive** about eating food.
- Spend a lot of time thinking about and planning the next binge, set aside certain times to binge and purge, or avoid social activities to binge and purge.
- **Steal food or hide it** in strange places, like under the bed or in closets.
- Binge on **foods with distinct colors** to know when the food is later thrown up.
- Exercise to "purge" their bodies of food consumed.

People with bulimia often suffer from other problems as well, such as

- Depression and thoughts of suicide
- Substance abuse

What are bingeing and purging?

Bingeing

- During a binge, people with bulimia eat large amounts of food, often in less than a few hours.
- **Eating during a binge is almost mindless.** They eat without paying attention to what the food tastes like or if they are hungry or full.
- Binges usually end when there is no more food to eat, their stomachs hurt from eating, or something such as a phone call breaks their concentration on bingeing.

Purging

- After bingeing, people with bulimia **feel guilty** and are **afraid of gaining weight.** To ease their guilt and fear, they purge the food from their bodies by vomiting or other means.
- They also may turn to extreme exercise or strict dieting.
- This period of "control" lasts until the next binge, and then **the cycle starts again.** Bulimia becomes an attempt to control 2 very strong impulses—the desire to eat and the desire to be thin.

What does bulimia do to the body?

Like anorexia, bulimia damages the body. For example,

- Teeth start to **decay** from contact with stomach acids during vomiting.
- Weight goes up and down.
- Menstrual periods become irregular or stop.
- The face and throat look puffy and swollen.
- Periods of **dizziness** and blackouts occur.
- **Dehydration** caused by loss of body fluids occurs (treatment in a hospital may be needed).
- Constant upset stomach, constipation, and sore throat may be present.
- **Damage** to vital organs such as the liver and kidneys, heart problems, and death can occur.

Who gets bulimia?

Most people with bulimia are girls in their **teens** and **young adult women.** But **boys** can be bulimic, too. People with bulimia often have a hard time controlling impulses, stress, and anxieties. As with anorexia, people with bulimia aren't happy with their bodies and **think they are fat.** This leads to dieting. Then in response to anxiety and other emotions or hunger, they give in to their **impulses and cravings** for food by bingeing. People with bulimia may be underweight, overweight, or of average weight.

How are eating disorders **treated?**

The **earlier** an eating disorder is recognized, the higher the chances are of treatment working. Treatment depends on many things, including the person's willingness to make changes, **family support**, and the stage of the eating disorder.

Successful treatment of eating disorders involves a team approach. The team includes many health care professionals working together, each treating a certain aspect of the disorder. Treatment should begin with a visit to a pediatrician to see how the eating disorder has affected the body. If the effects are severe, the person may need medical treatment or even need to be hospitalized.

In treating anorexia, increasing the person's weight is crucial. If this person refuses to eat, hospitalization may be needed so that adequate nutrition can be ensured. People with bulimia also may need to be hospitalized to treat medical complications, replace needed nutrients in the body, or **stop the cycle** of bingeing and purging.

Counseling is an important part of treatment. Counseling helps people with eating disorders understand how they use food as a way to deal with problems and feelings. It helps them improve their self-images and develop the **confidence** to take control of their lives. Family therapy usually is needed to help **family** members understand the problem, how to be encouraging and supportive, and how to help manage the symptoms. Nutrition counseling with a registered dietitian also is recommended to assist patients and families in returning to healthy eating habits.

Living with an eating disorder is very hard on teens and their families! The wear and tear on the body is tremendous. Without help, a person with an eating disorder can have serious health problems, become very sick, and even die. However, with treatment, **a person can get well and go on to lead a healthy life.**

Where can I find more information?

National Eating Disorders Association
www.nationaleatingdisorders.org
800/931-2237

National Association of Anorexia Nervosa and Associated Disorders
www.anad.org
847/831-3438

American Anorexia/Bulimia Association
www.uvm.edu/~jlbrink/index.html
212/575-6200

From your doctor

Please note: Listing of resources does not imply an endorsement by the American Academy of Pediatrics (AAP). The AAP is not responsible for the content of the resources mentioned in this brochure. Phone numbers and Web site addresses are as current as possible, but may change at any time.

The information contained in this publication should not be used as a substitute for the medical care and advice of your pediatrician. There may be variations in treatment that your pediatrician may recommend based on individual facts and circumstances.

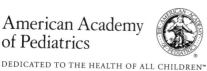

American Academy of Pediatrics

DEDICATED TO THE HEALTH OF ALL CHILDREN™

The American Academy of Pediatrics is an organization of 60,000 primary care pediatricians, pediatric medical subspecialists, and pediatric surgical specialists dedicated to the health, safety, and well-being of infants, children, adolescents, and young adults.

American Academy of Pediatrics
PO Box 747
Elk Grove Village, IL 60009-0747
Web site — http://www.aap.org

Section III Further Reading

Copperman N, Jacobson MS. Medical nutrition therapy of overweight adolescents. *Adolesc Med.* 2003;14:11–21

Kiess W, Boettner A. Obesity in the adolescent. *Adolesc Med.* 2002;13:181–190

Levine RL. Endocrine aspects of eating disorders in adolescents. *Adolesc Med.* 2002;13:129–143

Schneider M. Bulimia nervosa and binge-eating disorder in adolescents. *Adolesc Med.* 2003;14:119–131

Story M, Neumark-Sztainer D. Promoting healthy eating and physical activity in adolescents. *Adolesc Med.* 1999;10:109–123

Emotional, Behavioral, and Mental Health Concerns

Adolescent School Failure: Failure to Thrive in Adolescence

Michael I. Reiff, MD*

Important Points

1. School failure in adolescence is a strong predictor of other high-risk behaviors, including delinquency, substance abuse, and adolescent pregnancy.
2. Effective programs for prevention of school failure and dropout focus on the antecedents of school failure rather than on failure itself, include individualized attention to learners, and incorporate community support in meaningful ways.
3. The differential diagnosis of school failure in adolescence includes medical/neurologic, biobehavioral, and behavioral/emotional disorders. A systematic review of this differential diagnosis often can lead to the development of a successful intervention plan for adolescents failing in school.
4. A number of clinically useful "normed" and validated rating scales and questionnaires are available to pediatricians. With some experience, they can be scored easily and used to help gather information quickly and cost-effectively.
5. The pediatrician's role in prevention and treatment of adolescents at risk for school failure and dropout encompasses the pediatric/adolescent life span. It includes components of social and public health advocacy, preventive medicine, evaluation, treatment, and referral.

Introduction

Success in school is an excellent marker for general adolescent well-being; school failure in adolescence is a powerful indicator of other high-risk behaviors, such as delinquency, substance abuse, and pregnancy. It is estimated that about 17% of White non-Hispanic children in the United States are at high or very high risk for these behaviors compared with 51% of African-American children and 45% of Hispanic children.

It is difficult to consider any one of these high-risk behaviors in isolation because all can be antecedents to or consequences of any of the others. Lower grades, for example, are associated with substance abuse and early childbearing, and truancy and disruptive behavior at school are related to substance abuse and delinquency. Although there are many complex mitigating factors and pressures, most adolescents initially try hard drugs, commit a first delinquent act, or engage in unprotected intercourse as a personal decision at a given time and place.

In contrast, school failure is more insidious, resulting from an array of forces, many of which are outside the control of the adolescent. It occurs at the end of a long process rather than at its initiation. Because school progress frequently is measured through grades and group achievement testing, there are many opportunities for preventive interventions. The ultimate marker of school failure is dropping out. In a sense, school failure and dropout can be viewed as failure to thrive of adolescence. Many of the etiologies for adolescent school failure can be viewed in both public health and medical model frameworks.

---

*Director, Learning & Behavior Problems Clinic, Children's Hospital; Assistant Professor of Pediatrics, University of Minnesota, Minneapolis, MN.

A Public Health/ Epidemiologic Perspective

ANTECEDENTS OF SCHOOL FAILURE AND DROPOUT

Successful programs and interventions for adolescent high-risk behaviors largely address the antecedents to these behaviors rather than the behaviors themselves. The antecedents of school failure and subsequent dropping out, which are virtually the same, have been described by Dryfoos (see Suggested Reading) and are summarized in Table 1.

Demographics

Children who are 1 year older than classmates (behind 1 modal grade) have a 20% to 30% greater chance of dropping out of school, even when achievement, social status, and gender are controlled for. This should make clinicians skeptical of endorsing any recommendation for retention. Race and ethnicity cease to become factors in school dropout when social status is controlled for.

Personal

In addition to the factors listed in Table 1, low self-concept and an external locus of control (believing that the "winds of fate" control one's destiny rather than the individual being able to bring about change) are significant predictors of school failure. Children and adolescents who have low self-esteem about their academic ability should be provided with individualized successful academic experiences. Youths who have an external locus of control can be provided with mentored learning experiences that demonstrate the relationship between their positive behaviors (such as sticking to a structured study schedule) and academic outcomes (including getting more work turned in and better test scores).

Conduct, General Behavior, and Psychological Factors

The epidemiologic research (Table 1) cites conduct problems and "behavior"—referred to in the biobehavioral literature as externalizing behavior problems—as major predictors of school failure. At the same time, "psychological factors," including stress and depression, are characterized as predictors that only are "cited in selected sources" in the literature. This may be explained by reporting bias. Externalizing behavior problems (oppositional and defiant behavior and conduct problems) are easily recognizable in the classroom and affect the ability of teachers to teach and learners to learn as well as the "social ecology" of the entire classroom. Internalizing behaviors (anxiety and depression), on the other hand, are not easily identified by teachers and peers and do not often interfere with general classroom functioning. It is strongly incumbent on clinicians to ask about and identify any internalizing behavior problems in adolescents who are performing poorly in school because the health-care system may be the only professional interface outside of school used by adolescents and their families that is prepared to diagnose and treat these symptoms.

Family

The relationship between household composition and school failure is inconsistent. For example, it is unclear whether single-parent households are correlated with higher rates of school failure or dropping out.

School Quality

Children from disadvantaged homes have been found to succeed in excellent schools. On the other hand, some schools are so inadequate that success is the exception. In one recent survey, almost 70% of adolescents who had dropped out of school stated that they might have stayed if "teachers paid more attention to students" and if "we were not treated like inmates."

PREVENTING SCHOOL FAILURE

What Works?

Effective programs that prevent school failure and dropout share three major attributes:
- A focus on the antecedents of school failure rather than on failure itself
- Individualized attention to the learners

Table 1. Antecedents of School Dropout

Antecedent	Association with Dropping Out
Demographic	
Age	**Old for grade
Gender	*Males
Race and ethnicity	**Native American, Hispanic, black
Personal	
Expectations for education	**Low expectations, no plans for college
School grades	**Low grades
Basic skills	**Low test scores
School promotion	**Left back in early grades
Attitude toward school	**Strong dislike, bored
Conduct, general behavior	**Truancy, "acting out," suspension, expulsion
Peer influence	*Friends have low expectations for school
	**Friends drop out
School involvement	**Low interest, low participation
Involvement in other high-risk behaviors	*Early delinquency, substance use, early sexual intercourse
Social life	*Frequent dating, riding around
Conformity–rebelliousness	*Nonconformity, alienation
Psychological factors	*Stress, depression
Pregnancy	**High rates
Family	
Household composition	*Inconsistent data
Income, poverty status	**Family in poverty
Parental education	**Low levels of education
Welfare	*Family on welfare
Mobility	*Family moves frequently
Parental role, bonding, guidance	**Lack of parental support, authoritarian, permissive
Culture in home	*Lack of resources in home
Primary language	*Other than English
Community	
Neighborhood quality	*Urban, high-density area, poverty area, also rural
School quality	**Alternative or vocational school
	**Segregated school
	*Large schools, large classes
	*Tracking, emphasis on testing
	*Public (vs parochial)
Employment	*Higher rates of employment

* = Cited in selected sources.

** = Major predictor.

Adapted from Table 6.7, "Antecedents of School Dropout," from *Adolescents at Risk: Prevalence and Prevention* by Joy G. Dryfoos, copyright © 1991 by Joy G. Dryfoos. Used by permission of Oxford University Press, Inc.

● Incorporation of community support in meaningful ways

Early intervention programs such as Head Start and Early Childhood Special Education have focused successfully on the prevention of learning and developmental problems and educating parents in child development. Successful school-age programs have maintained a focus on basic academic skills and recognized the primary importance of a healthy school climate.

Several years ago Dr Michael Rutter studied students making the transition from primary schools to middle schools in London. He found that the best students often did poorly when moved into the worst schools, while the poorer students often did well when placed in the best schools. The "best" schools could be characterized as emphasizing academics; allowing teachers autonomy to meet the educational needs of individual students; and having programmatic flexibility, systems of incentives and rewards for students, and systems that allow students to take responsibility for their own behaviors. In the United States, Dr James Comer has established a model school-based management approach in inner-city New Haven, Connecticut, and other cities. These schools have advisory councils consisting of the principal, teachers, teacher aides, and parent groups. They also have school-based mental health teams, paid parent participation programs, and a flexible academic program.

Programs such as these provide for individualized attention and instruction for students and attract committed teachers who have high expectations. Links between learning and working (such as working in a nursing home and keeping a daily journal of this experience) have been found to be extremely effective in many programs. Some high-risk students require intensive, sustained counseling before they can take full advantage of these programs.

Adolescents who are successful despite extremely high-risk profiles have been found to have specific interests and been supported in pursuing them; often have had some mentoring relationship that has encouraged them to believe in themselves; and have been described as self-aware, self-directed, and committed to interpersonal relationships.

What Doesn't Work?

State-mandated promotion policies that rely solely on testing results are ineffective. Raising school standards without raising the quality of the schools simply encourages failure and dropout. Grouping classes by "ability" has uncertain benefits for the lowest achieving students at a potentially enormous psychological cost. Being labeled as "below average" can have a tremendously negative effect on students' self-concepts. Teachers often have low expectations of these students, and this can become self-fulfilling. Early intervention or basic skills programs without

follow-up are often unsuccessful. Programs in which adolescents are "scared straight" or "moralized to" almost always fail. The question should be: "How do schools fail adolescents?" rather than "How do adolescents fail school?"

A Bio-Psycho-Social Model: A Differential Diagnostic Approach

Factors contributing to school failure are among the most frequent problems presenting to primary care clinicians who see school-age children and adolescents. The public health model reviewed previously provides an important overview that is particularly helpful when formulating public policy. Although this model also can suggest some important areas to be pursued, it lacks the analysis of pathogenesis that is most helpful to clinicians in making a diagnosis and planning effective intervention for individual adolescents and their families. A differential diagnostic model for school failure in adolescents is presented in Table 2.

MEDICAL/NEUROLOGIC

Infants exposed to prenatal drugs and alcohol have an increased potential for school failure, particularly secondary to attentional disorders and lowered cognitive abilities. The same holds true for significant exposure to toxins such as lead. Serious hearing or vision impairment, particularly when unrecognized, can result in poor achievement and subsequent behavior problems. Chronic illness can result in significant school absence, as can "functional disorders" such as chronic recurrent abdominal pain or headaches. Neurologic

---

Table 2. Factors Contributing to Adolescent School Failure: Medical Model Differential Diagnosis

Medical/Neurologic	Biobehavioral Disorders	Behavioral/Emotional Disorders
Prenatal drug and alcohol exposure	Attention disorders (attention deficit hyperactivity disorder)	Externalizing behavior disorders
Exposure to toxins (including lead)	Learning challenges/disabilities	● Oppositional defiant disorder
Sensory impairment (hearing/vision)	Mental retardation	● Conduct disorder
Chronic illness	Pervasive developmental disorders	Internalizing behavior disorder
"Functional" disorders		● Depressive disorders
Seizure disorders		● Anxiety disorders
Neurodegenerative diseases		
Static and toxic encephalopathies		
Posttraumatic disorders		
Medication-induced cognitive changes		
Substance use and abuse		
Teenage pregnancy		

disorders such as seizure disorders, neurodegenerative diseases, static and toxic encephalopathies, and posttraumatic disorders may be accompanied by cognitive and attentional limitations.

In addition, certain medications, including some anticonvulsants and asthma medications, can lead to cognitive slowing and attentional problems in school. Adolescent substance use and abuse certainly can lead to school failure and truancy. Teenage pregnancy is another marker for all of the high-risk behaviors of adolescence. All of these conditions are likely to come to the attention of clinicians who care for adolescents, and a careful school history should be an integral part of these medical/neurologic evaluations.

BIOBEHAVIORAL DISORDERS

Biobehavioral disorders are associated with impaired production in school work, mild-to-severe learning problems, socialization and communication difficulties, and disruptive behavior in the classroom.

Attention Deficit Hyperactivity Disorder (ADHD)

ADHD is the most prevalent biobehavioral disorder of childhood and adolescence. The current *DSM-IV* formulation for ADHD is two-dimensional and has three subtypes: predominantly inattentive, predominantly hyperactive-impulsive, and combined. The latter two types are often brought to the attention of parents by teachers and subsequently to the attention of clinicians. The predominantly inattentive type often remains undetected. It manifests primarily through difficulties with school achievement and a slow work production speed and often occurs concomitantly with symptoms of anxiety or depression.

The number of children and adolescents diagnosed with ADHD is largely a function of the diagnostic criteria used. In a clinical sample, 15% more children and adolescents meet *DSM-IV* criteria for ADHD than met the former *DSM-III-R* criteria. In an epidemiologic sample (Wolraich), a comparison of teacher ratings of the same students on *DSM-III-R* and *DSM-IV* scales resulted in a 57% increase in diagnoses of ADHD, primarily due to identification of children who met the criteria for inattentive and hyperactive-impulsive types of ADHD.

ADHD presents differently in adolescence than it does in early and middle childhood. Hyperactivity often is diminished, and the condition is characterized more by continued impulsivity, poorer school performance, and school failure in adolescence. Previous social skills deficits are magnified as poor peer relationships become more obvious and prominent at a developmental stage where peer group acceptance increases in significance. Because of continuing impulsivity, the high-risk behaviors of childhood become the extraordinarily high-risk behaviors of adolescence. The challenges to minor rules or parental limit setting of early and middle childhood now become substance abuse, delinquency, early and unprotected sexual activity, and repeated antisocial behavior.

Diagnosing and treating attention disorders in adolescents is associated with several complicating factors. Because of the process of separation and adolescent individuation, parents may no longer be good sources of information about their adolescents. Feedback from and communication with teachers often is complicated by a student having multiple teachers, none of whom may know the student in the detail required to formulate specific learning needs. Finally, the signs and symptoms of attentional disorders usually are not evident during routine office visits.

Medication management of attentional disorders also may be more complicated and problematic with adolescents. Dosing is more variable among patients. Stimulant medications take on "street value." Afternoon and early evening doses of stimulant medications increase in importance as demands for producing school work increase. Adolescents who attributed little value to taking medications in early and middle childhood now may refuse to take them, which can lead to increased parent-adolescent conflict as well as escalating school failure.

Factors that support a favorable outcome for adolescents who have ADHD include: early evaluation and intervention; self-understanding and acceptance of problems and issues; a supportive family; an understanding and developmentally attuned school system; appropriate individual educational plans (IEPs) if indicated; and a willingness to engage in appropriate counseling, mentoring relationships, and "coaching" surrounding production and completion of work. High-risk factors for negative outcomes include: delayed diagnosis; an ongoing cycle of failure; serious behavior problems in school (oppositional, defiant, and conduct problems); significant substance abuse; medication refusal; and damaged self-esteem resulting from the adolescent's problems being viewed as "characterologic disorders" rather than as biobehavioral issues that are amenable to systematic interventions.

Learning Challenges and "Disabilities"

Learning disabilities generally are defined on a discrepancy model: significant discrepancies between cognitive skills (intelligence quotient [IQ]) and achievement, between achievement in different areas (eg, mathematics and reading), or between an individual's achievement and that of grade-mates. The *DSM-IV* recognizes learning disabilities in reading, mathematics, and written expression as well as communication disorders involving expressive language and mixed receptive and expressive language. Criteria for special educational services based on these disabilities vary from state to state.

Learning challenges and demands change significantly during adolescence. Demands on attention in adolescence require more consistent and sustained mental energy, more efficient processing of information, and a significantly increased ability to produce school work. Adolescents need more techniques for remembering, recalling, and summarizing new information, such as mnemonic devices and visual associations. New visual/spatial challenges include increased demands for nonverbal reasoning, visualizing strategies, and familiarity with interpretation and production of graphic representations of information.

At this developmental stage, it is assumed that sequential skills include the abilities to stage work appropriately, preview what is required to do the work, make realistic schedules for accomplishing long-term assignments, and organize

school work in the context of a busy life with increased social demands and outside activities. Language demands require a greater emphasis on abstract language, learning of a second language, more complex verbal reasoning, and a considerably increased demand for fluency in written language. Neuromotor skills call on abilities for speed-writing, note-taking, and keyboarding. If writing is not automatic or too slow, work production may be impaired severely. Increased cognitive demands include abilities in advanced problem-solving skills and a greater ability to handle abstract concepts.

Mental Retardation and Pervasive Developmental Disorders (PDD)

The majority of students who are mentally retarded (IQ <69 with commensurably delayed adaptive functioning) or have autism and more severe autistic-like disorders (PDD) should have been evaluated, diagnosed, and placed in special school programming well before adolescence. Adaptive programs that optimize life and vocational skills and minimize physical, emotional, and sexual exploitation should be well under way for these individuals by the time they reach mid-adolescence.

However, adolescents who have borderline intellectual functioning (IQ of 70 to 85) may not have been detected or may have been labeled as "slow learners." They may not qualify for special help in the school system because their academic achievement is not significantly discrepant from their cognitive abilities (IQ). These adolescents are particularly vulnerable to school failure when success demands a greatly increased ability to organize, plan, complete, and turn in work and depends on accessing and using many higher level cognitive skills.

Milder forms of PDD, including "high-functioning autism," Asperger syndrome, and nonspecific forms of PDD, also may not have been detected previously. Adolescents who have these disorders are at risk for increasing emotional trauma and rejection as their social awkwardness among peers becomes more evident and relationships take on increased significance.

BEHAVIORAL AND EMOTIONAL DISORDERS

Externalizing (Disruptive) Behavior Disorders: Oppositional Defiant Disorder (ODD) and Conduct Disorder (CD)

The disruptive behavior disorders are defined in the *DSM-IV* as ADHD, ODD, and CD. ODD is characterized by losing one's temper; arguing with adults; defying adult requests and rules; blaming others for one's own mistakes; using obscenity; and being touchy or easily annoyed, angry, resentful, spiteful, and vindictive. During adolescence these attributes may lead to increased conflict at school and at home as developmental individuation becomes prominent. With parents less able to exert control over behavior and issues such as homework production, school failure becomes more likely.

CD is characterized by stealing, running away from home, setting fires, lying, breaking into homes or cars, and physical and sexual aggression. Although patterns of CD may be well established before adolescence, during the adolescent years the behaviors are likely to be more serious and have more serious consequences. The prognosis for ADHD in adolescents is much poorer when CD is also present. Further, CD can be exacerbated by impulsivity, especially when it occurs concomitantly with ADHD. These adolescents may be easily influenced to become involved in delinquent acts when they succumb to peer pressure. CD may be helped by the same measures used to treat ADHD: stimulant medication, behavioral techniques, and cognitive-behavioral training.

Conduct-disordered behavior that is premeditated is much more difficult to treat, carries a much worse prognosis, and may be seen in adulthood as an antisocial personality disorder. Adolescents who exhibit conduct-disordered behavior are at significant risk for major depressive disorder, and this always should be ruled out or treated as indicated.

Internalizing Behavioral Disorders: Depressive and Anxiety Disorders

The disruptive behavior disorders are usually obvious at home and interfere significantly with classroom functioning. For these reasons, they often are brought to the attention of clinicians by parents and teachers. In contrast, the internalizing behavior disorders, depression and anxiety, often are unrecognized by parents and teachers and may present as nonspecific school failure and/or social isolation. The primary care clinician may be in a unique position as the only professional outside of the school system to interact with adolescents and their families about school-related issues. Symptoms and signs may not be apparent during an office visit, and adolescents may be reluctant to discuss these issues spontaneously. Depression and anxiety should be considered routinely whenever the issues of suboptimal school performance or school failure arise.

Evaluation and Treatment Planning

The clinician can link the public health and medical models for adolescent school failure. A format for planning an evaluation for school problems, failure, and dropout is presented in Table 3. It is important to recognize that the biobehavioral and behavioral/emotional diagnoses cannot withstand the rigors of the more "medical model" diagnostic approach. For example, ADHD and depressive disorders can be quite difficult to distinguish from each other by using any clinical data other than the diagnostic criteria. In addition, multiple diagnoses are more often the rule than the exception. For this reason, it may be more fruitful to generate a problem checklist based on functional limitations than to use a more formal diagnostic approach. This allows the generation of evidence-based treatment interventions for problems where an adolescent's behavior is *significantly* interfering with optimal functioning.

Evaluation of school-related problems can present a challenge. The gathering of information can be time-consuming, and insurance coverage for these labor-intensive and often lengthy

Table 3. Primary Care Evaluation Format

Dimension	Confirmatory Measures*	Treatment Implications*
Inattention Impulsivity Hyperactivity	History/Interview Behavior rating scales Continuous Performance Task (CPT)† Neurodevelopmental findings	Medication management Patient and parent education/mentoring Cognitive-behavioral strategies
Disruptive behavior	History/Interview Behavior rating scales	Parent training (behavior modification) School behavioral programs Medication management
Underachievement Learning disabilities	Cognitive testing (IQ) Achievement testing	Individual Education Plan (IEP) Learning style interventions
Mental retardation	Cognitive testing (IQ) Adaptive behavior measure	IEP Parent education and resources Medical evaluation and follow-up plan
Pervasive Developmental Disorders (PDD)	History/Interview Behavior rating scales Observation	IEP Parent education and resources Medical follow-up planning
Depressive symptoms Anxious symptoms	History/Interview Rating scales	Psychotherapy referral Medication management
Problematic family functioning	History/Interview Rating scales	Family therapy referral
Problematic social functioning Difficulty with self-modulation	History/Interview Rating scales	Cognitive behavioral therapy
Substance use or abuse	History/Interview Drug screen (after informed consent)	Treatment program referral
Suboptimal school quality	History/Interview	Counseling about locating more appropriate school setting

*Assessment and interventions should be individualized. Not all items are indicated for all individuals.

†Routine use remains controversial.

evaluations generally is suboptimal. Although it can be argued that early and comprehensive evaluation and treatment should be extremely cost-effective, this remains an unexamined and highly neglected area of clinical research.

Most of the target behaviors related to the etiology of school failure are not evident in the office and may require multiple measures, information from multiple observers, and at times, a multidisciplinary approach. Many rating scales that have been devised to help gather information efficiently also have been normed for reliability and validity (Table 4). Most scales cannot be used to make diagnoses, but they can be extremely helpful in gathering structured information from various sources in a manner that allows for quantitative comparison of adolescents with their peers. Recent reviews by Aylward and Kutcher of these and other rating scales can be found in the Suggested Reading.

Primary care clinicians should develop or use previously developed structured histories that can be filled out by parents and teachers before an initial evaluation visit and reviewed by the clinician prior to the visit. By using rating scales and prereviewed structured histories, a primary care evaluation visit that includes observations and interviews with parents and adolescents usually can be conducted in less than 1 hour of direct clinical time. The use of rating scales and structured histories allows the clinician to focus on the most important questions for a particular adolescent during the evaluation visit. Parent-adolescent dynamics and conflicts and affective

Table 4. Diagnostic Scales and Screening Tools

Screening Tool	Description	Where Available
Rating Scales for Externalizing Behaviors (ADHD, oppositional-defiant, conduct disorder)		
Conners Parent and Teacher Rating Scales	Several sets of widely used parent and teacher rating scales that are nondiagnostic	Multi-Health Systems, Inc. 908 Niagara Falls Blvd N. Tonawanda, NY 14120
ADHD Rating Scale IV	Normed and validated rating scale for ADHD based on DSM diagnostic criteria	George DuPaul, PhD Iacocca Hall, Room A-219 111 Research Drive Bethlehem, PA 18015
ACTeRS	Teacher rating scales measuring attention, hyperactivity, social skills, and oppositionality	Meritech, Inc. 111 N. Market St Champaign, IL 61820
ADDES	Parent and teacher rating scales standardized on a broad normative sample	Hawthorne Educational Services PO Box 7570 Columbia, MO 62505
Rating Scales for Internalizing Behaviors (depression, anxiety)		
Children's Depression Inventory (CDI)	A self-endorsed 27-item scale composed of statements regarding affective, cognitive, behavioral, and somatic symptoms of depression	Multi-Health Systems, Inc. 908 Niagara Falls Blvd N. Tonawanda, NY 14120
Revised Children's Manifest Anxiety Scale (RCMAS)	A self-endorsed 37-item scale yielding a total anxiety score and subscales for physiologic worry, over-sensitivity, social concerns, and concentration	Western Psychological Services 12031 Wilshire Boulevard Los Angeles, CA 90025
General Multidimensional Behavior Rating Scales		
Behavior Assessment Scales for Children (BASC)	A multimethod system that includes a self-report scale, a teacher rating scale, parent rating scales, a structured developmental history, and classroom observation forms	American Guidance Service Circle Pines, MN 55014-1796
Child Behavior Checklist (CBCL)	Parent and teacher scales measuring social competence and internalizing and externalizing behaviors	Thomas M. Achenbach, PhD Department of Psychiatry University of Vermont Burlington, VT 05401
Children's Global Assessment Scale (CGAS)	A clinician rating system for overall child functioning: Ten categories from superior functioning to needing constant supervision	*Archives of General Psychiatry* Vol 44 September, 1987
School Functioning		
Academic Performance Rating Scale	A 19-item teacher rating scale for academic productivity and accuracy, learning ability, impulse control, academic performance, and social withdrawal	George DuPaul, PhD Iacocca Hall, Room A-219 111 Research Drive Bethlehem, PA 18015
Family Functioning		
The Family Adaptability and Cohesion Scales (FACES) II	A 30-question self-endorsed questionnaire measuring family cohesion, adaptability, and communication	D. Olsen, PhD Family Social Science University of Minnesota St Paul, MN 55108
The Family Assessment Measure (FAM)	A series of 50 statements about family functioning rated by children and parents from strongly agree to strongly disagree	Multi-Health Systems, Inc. 908 Niagara Falls Blvd N. Tonawanda, NY 14120
The Parent-Adolescent Communication	A 20-item scale from strongly agree to strongly disagree in which an adolescent endorses items for each parent	D. Olsen, PhD Family Social Science University of Minnesota St Paul, MN 55108
Continuous Performance Tests		
Conners Continuous Performance Test (CCPT)	A 15-minute computerized test of attention and associated variables	Multi-Health Systems, Inc. 908 Niagara Falls Blvd N. Tonawanda, NY 14120
Gordon Diagnostic System	A self-contained computerized unit measuring the ability to inhibit responding, vigilance, and distractibility	GSI Publications PO Box 746 DeWitt, NY 13214
Structured Neurodevelopmental Examinations		
PEER, PEEX 2, PEERAMID 2 (Levine)	A series of structured neurodevelopmental examinations for ages 4 to 6, 6 to 9, 9 to 15. Training available.	Educators Publishing Service 75 Moulton St Cambridge, MA 02138

responses of the adolescent to family issues and other specific questions can be observed only during an effective interview.

In the clinical setting, private discussions should be initiated with preadolescents. A primary goal is to foster self-esteem and to promote self-efficacy and ownership of both strengths and vulnerabilities through education and support. Adolescents generally should be seen alone and identified as the "patient" where developmentally appropriate. They should participate in making decisions and take increasing responsibility for all interventions. However, clear communication with parents or guardians is also essential.

Problems with attention, impulsivity, and hyperactivity (the ADHD "triad") can be confirmed with a careful history, interview, and use of normed and validated rating scales. Physical and routine neurologic examinations usually are not helpful unless otherwise indicated. Neurodevelopmental findings can support the diagnosis of attentional disorders (particularly difficulties with short-term and active working memory and sequential organization) and suggest the presence of coexisting developmental and learning style problems, such as motor and language delays or processing difficulties. Examining general learning style issues, rather than problems related only to inattention and impulsivity, is critical.

The neurodevelopmental examination of an adolescent typically includes an examination of fine motor, gross motor, and graphomotor skills; language; visual-perceptual-motor functioning; temporal-sequential organization abilities; cognitive speed; and short-term memory skills. The role of computerized tests of attention (continuous performance tasks) in the evaluation and management of attentional disorders remains controversial. These tests never should be used alone for diagnosis, although they can be helpful in distinguishing the group of adolescents at highest risk for attentional disorders. Typical false-negative rates range from 15% to 35%, and false-positive rates are about 2%.

Interventions for the ADHD triad of symptoms include education about and demystification of the symptoms, medication management with stimulants or other agents such as certain antidepressants or alpha-2-adrenergics as indicated, and interventions related to specific learning style issues.

Disruptive behavior disorders also can be evaluated with a careful history and interview as well as normed and validated rating scales. Interventions include behavioral parent training for parents and the introduction or enhancement of behavioral management programs at school.

Underachievement can be evaluated by cognitive (IQ) and achievement testing performed by the school or a community child psychologist. An optimal assessment includes an analysis of where in the process of reading, writing, or mathematics the learning breaks down. Adolescents in whom there are significant findings are entitled to and should request a formal Individual Education Plan (IEP) through the school system.

The internalizing behaviors of depression and anxiety can be screened for by history, interview, and normed and validated rating scales. Screening tools include multidimensional rating scales such as the Child Behavior Checklist (Achenbach) and the Behavioral Assessment Scales for Children (BASC) as well as the more specific (but not truly categorical) scales of the Child Depression Inventory (CDI) and the Revised Children's Manifest Anxiety Scale (RCMAS). Referrals then can be made as indicated by results of screening. Adolescents at risk should be referred for appropriate evaluation. Interventions include medication management and psychotherapy.

Family functioning always should be assessed as part of the evaluation for school failure. Again, evaluation consists of a careful history and interview and may be enhanced using normed and validated scales for family stress and perceptions concerning family functioning. The primary intervention for significantly impaired family functioning is family therapy. Some families often cannot take advantage of the more behaviorally oriented parent training until they engage in family therapy.

Adolescent social functioning and the ability to self-modulate behavior adequately can be evaluated through history, interview, and rating scales. Effective interventions center on cognitive-behavioral (self-talk) techniques.

However substance abuse is addressed, a drug screen is strongly recommended. This can be performed ethically only with the adolescent's consent.

Assessing the match between the adolescent and the school and/or teachers is difficult for most primary care clinicians providing care to a geographically diverse population of adolescents. However, if a decline in school performance has been precipitous or it cannot be accounted for by the rest of the evaluation, a school/teacher and adolescent mismatch may be significant.

Because school-related problems are multidimensional, it is very helpful to primary care clinicians to develop a community referral network or become part of a community-based assessment team that might include a clinical psychologist (for evaluation of adolescents at risk for depression, anxiety, and other emotional concerns as well as provision of family and individual psychotherapy), an educational or school psychologist (for psychoeducational assessment), and school professionals, with additional consultants as indicated. Within this context, primary care clinicians should be able to diagnose attentional disorders and medically related problems and be able to screen for other problems and disorders.

Summary

The role of the primary clinician in dealing with school failure can be critical by linking the epidemiological with the clinical and encompassing the pediatric/adolescent life span. It includes components of social and public health advocacy, preventive medicine, evaluation, education, treatment, and referral. The most effective interventions are early and multifaceted. The primary care role includes: community advocacy; counseling about prenatal drug and alcohol abuse; early detection and treatment for attentional disorders, underachievement, and learning disabilities; interviews addressing multiple risk factors, grades, school attitudes, behavior, and friends; anticipatory guidance; education about individual learning style and good "learning hygiene"; early referral and intervention for preadolescent conduct problems and parent-child conflict; early referrals for family distress; and prevention of substance abuse and adolescent pregnancy.

Suggested Reading

Alyward GP. *Practitioner's Guide to Developmental and Psychological Testing.* New York, NY: Plenum Medical Book Company; 1994

Barkley RA, Fischer M, Edelbrock CS, Smallish L. The adolescent outcome of hyperactive children diagnosed by research criteria. An 8-year prospective study. *J Am Acad Child Adolesc Psychiatry.* 1990;29:546–557

Barkley RA, Anastopoulos AD, Guevrement DC, Fletcher KE. Adolescents with attention deficit hyperactivity disorder: mother-adolescent interactions, family beliefs and conflicts, and maternal psychopathology. *J Abnorm Child Psychol.* 1992;20:263–288

Bernstein GA, Borchardt CM, Perwien AR. Anxiety disorders in children and adolescents: a review of the past 10 years. *J Am Acad Child Adolesc Psychiatry.* 1996;35:1110–1119

Birmaher B, Ryan ND, Williamson DE. Childhood and adolescent depression: a review of the last 10 years. Part I. *J Am Acad Child Adolesc Psychiatry.* 1996;35:1427–1439

Birmaher B, Ryan ND, Williamson DE, Brent DA, Kaufman J. Childhood and adolescent depression: a review of the past 10 years. Part II. *J Am Acad Child Adolesc Psychiatry.* 1996; 35:1575–1583

Cantwell D. Attention deficit disorder: a review of the past 10 years. *J Am Acad Child Adolesc Psychiatry.* 1996;35:978–987

Culbert T, Banez GA, Reiff MI. Children who have attentional disorders: intervention. *Pediatrics in Review.* 1994;15:5–14

Diagnostic and Statistical Manual of Mental Disorders. 4th ed. Washington, DC: American Psychiatric Association; 1994

Dryfoos J. *Adolescents at Risk.* New York, NY: Oxford University Press; 1990

Dryfoos J. Adolescents at risk: a summation of work in the field—programs and policies. *J Adolesc Health.* 1991;12: 630–637

Faigel HC, Doak E, Howard SD, Sigel ML. Emotional disorders in learning disabled adolescents. *Child Psychiatry Hum Dev.* 1992;23:31–40

Fischer M, Barkley RA, Edelbrock CS, Smallish L. The adolescent outcome of hyperactive children diagnosed by research criteria: II. Academic, attentional, and neuropsychological status. *J Consult Clin Psychol.* 1990;58:580–588

Fox LC, Forbing SE. Overlapping symptoms of substance abuse and learning handicaps: implications for educators. *J Learn Dis.* 1991;24:24–31

Kutcher SP. *Child and Adolescent Psychopharmacology.* Philadelphia, Penn: WB Saunders Company; 1997

Levine M. *Developmental Demands Over Time: Some Evolving and Cumulative School-related Expectations.* Cambridge, Mass: Educators Publishing Service; 1994

Levine M. *Educational Care.* Cambridge, Mass: Educators Publishing Service, Inc; 1994

Mannuzza S, Klein RG, Bonagura N, Mallow P, Giampino TL, Addalli KA. Hyperactive boys almost grown up. V. Replication of psychiatric status. *Arch Gen Psychiatry.* 1991;48:77–83

Nunn GD, Parish TS. The psychosocial characteristics of at-risk high school students. *Adolescence.* 1992;27:435–440

Reiff M, Banez GA, Culbert TP. Children who have attentional disorders: diagnosis and evaluation. *Pediatrics in Review.* 1993; 14:455–465

Weiss G, Hechtman LT. *Hyperactive Children Grown Up.* New York, NY: Guilford Press; 1986

Weiss G, Hechtman L, Perlman T, Hopkins J, Wener A. Hyperactives as young adults: a controlled prospective ten-year follow-up of 75 children. *Arch Gen Psychiatry.* 1979;36: 675–681

Wolraich ML, Hannah JN, Pinnock TY, Baumgaertel A, Brown J. Comparison of diagnostic criteria for attention-deficit hyperactivity disorder in a county-wide sample. *J Am Acad Child Adolesc Psychiatry.* 1996;35:319–324

Attention-Deficit/Hyperactivity Disorder Among Adolescents: A Review of the Diagnosis, Treatment, and Clinical Implications

Mark L. Wolraich, MD*; Charles J. Wibbelsman, MD‡; Thomas E. Brown, PhD§; Steven W. Evans, PhD‖; Edward M. Gotlieb, MD¶; John R. Knight, MD#; E. Clarke Ross, DPA**; Howard H. Shubiner, MD‡‡; Esther H. Wender, MD§§; and Timothy Wilens, MD#

ABSTRACT. Attention-deficit/hyperactivity disorder (ADHD) is the most common mental disorder in childhood, and primary care clinicians provide a major component of the care for children with ADHD. However, because of limited available evidence, the American Academy of Pediatrics guidelines did not include adolescents and young adults. Contrary to previous beliefs, it has become clear that, in most cases, ADHD does not resolve once children enter puberty. This article reviews the current evidence about the diagnosis and treatment of adolescents and young adults with ADHD and describes how the information informs practice. It describes some of the unique characteristics observed among adolescents, as well as how the core symptoms change with maturity. The diagnostic process is discussed, as well as approaches to the care of adolescents to improve adherences. Both psychosocial and pharmacologic interventions are reviewed, and there is a discussion of these patients' transition into young adulthood. The article also indicates that research is needed to identify the unique adolescent characteristics of ADHD and effective psychosocial and pharmacologic treatments. *Pediatrics* 2005;115:1734–1746; *attention-deficit/hyperactivity disorder, ADHD, adolescents, diagnosis, treatment.*

ABBREVIATIONS. ADHD, attention-deficit/hyperactivity disorder; ADD, attention-deficit disorder.

Attention-deficit/hyperactivity disorder (ADHD) is the most common mental disorder in childhood,[1] and primary care clinicians provide a major component of the care for children with ADHD.[2] To improve the care of those children, the American Academy of Pediatrics developed practice guidelines for the diagnosis and treatment of ADHD among children 6 to 12 years of age who are evaluated by primary care clinicians.[2,3] However, because of limited available evidence, the guidelines did not include adolescents and young adults.

Contrary to early views of the disorder that indicated that it might represent a maturational lag and suggested that children would grow out of it,[4] it has become clear that, in most cases, ADHD does not resolve once children enter puberty. For the majority of children diagnosed with ADHD, as many as 65%,[5,6] the diagnosis persists into adolescence. When the diagnosis of ADHD is made during childhood, the task for clinicians is to continue treatment as long as needed. However, some adolescents present without having been diagnosed, and the symptoms of the disorder may be subtler during the teenage

From *University of Oklahoma Health Sciences Center, Oklahoma City, Oklahoma; ‡Kaiser Permenente San Francisco, San Francisco, California; §Yale University School of Medicine, New Haven, Connecticut; ‖James Madison University, Harrisonburg, Virginia; ¶Emory University Schools of Medicine and Nursing, Atlanta, Georgia; #Harvard Medical School, Cambridge, Massachusetts; **Children and Adults With Attention Deficit/Hyperactivity Disorder, Landover, Maryland; ‡‡Providence Hospital, Mobile, Alabama; and §§University of Washington, Seattle, Washington.

Accepted for publication Jan 24, 2005.

doi:10.1542/peds.2004-1959

Conflicts of interest: Dr Wolraich is a consultant for Lilly, Shire, and McNeil and receives research support from Shire and Lilly; Dr Brown receives research support from Lilly, GlaxoSmithKline, and McNeil, is a consultant for McNeil, Lilly, Novartis, and Shire, and is a speaker for Lilly, Janssen Cilag, McNeil, Novartis, Shire, and Wyeth; Dr Gotlieb receives research support from Shire and Novartis and is a speaker for Novartis and Lilly; Dr Schubiner is a consultant and speaker for McNeil, Lilly, and Shire; and Dr Wilens receives research support and is a speaker and consultant for Abbott, Alza/McNeil, Celltech, GlaxoSmithKline, Janssen, Lilly, Neurosearch, Novartis, Pfizer, Shire, National Institute on Drug Abuse, National Institute of Mental Health, and National Institute of Child Health and Human Development.

Address correspondence to Mark L. Wolraich, MD, Oklahoma University Child Study Center, 1100 NE 13th St, Oklahoma City, OK 73117. E-mail: mark-wolraich@ouhsc.edu

years. Therefore, it is important for clinicians who care for adolescents and young adults to be knowledgeable about diagnosing and treating ADHD. It is the intent of this article to review the current evidence about the diagnosis and treatment of adolescents and young adults with ADHD and to indicate how the information informs practice.

Clinical Picture

CLINICAL MANIFESTATIONS IN ADOLESCENCE

The most obvious adolescents to identify as needing treatment are those who were diagnosed with ADHD in childhood. Studies have shown repeatedly that the majority of those diagnosed with ADHD while in elementary school continue to have significant manifestations of ADHD throughout adolescence and continue to need treatment.[5,6] Many studies have also shown that the most salient manifestations of ADHD change during adolescence. Hyperactivity, although still present, becomes much less visible during this age period.[7] Academic problems that might have been less noticeable or were treated effectively during elementary school may become much more of a problem. In middle school and high school, cognitive demands increase significantly, and the adolescent is expected to become more independent of adult supervision.[8] Students are exposed to multiple teachers and classes, and the amount of assigned homework increases. Finally, problems with peer relationships become more obvious as the social environment changes with adolescence and peer interactions assume a new importance.

These changes in context, expectations, and maturation result in very different case presentations than among school-aged children. In fact, the diagnosis of ADHD may be missed if an adolescent has the predominantly inattentive subtype.[9] Although studies addressing differences between the subtypes with an adolescent population do not exist, it is our clinical impression that many of the differences reported for children persist in adolescence. For example, children with the inattentive subtype have been described by teachers as exhibiting less disruptive behavior but

higher degrees of social impairment, unhappiness, and anxiety or depression, compared with children with the combined type.[10] These problems may produce greater impairment in adolescence than in childhood because the demands for independence and the complexity of social functioning increase. Similarly, Milich et al[11] summarized data indicating that the age of referral and recognition of the problem is older for children with the inattentive type, compared with the combined type. These children are more likely to be female than are children with the combined type, although male students still outnumber female subjects.[11] The absence of disruptive behavior problems in this group disguises its identity, but these adolescents suffer significantly from problems such as disorganization, inability to follow through on academic tasks, and difficulty sustaining attention for extended academic projects.

OTHER CHARACTERISTICS OF ADOLESCENTS WITH ADHD

Adolescents with ADHD often seem emotionally immature, compared with their same-age peers.[12] They often do best when interacting with younger children or in the environment of adults who tolerate their immature behaviors. Adolescents and children with ADHD often display affect, both negative and positive, that is excessive for the situation.[13] The symptoms include becoming frustrated easily and having a "short fuse," with sudden outbursts of anger. In the extreme, the symptoms reflect co-occurring oppositional defiant disorder, as described below. Cognitive impairments become increasingly problematic during adolescence. These impairments may have widespread effects that often seem like behavioral problems and are not recognized as part of the ADHD. The adolescents procrastinate and, after having started, are distracted easily or have difficulty tracking and completing their projects, especially when the task requires a good deal of time and effort.[14]

Children with ADHD have been reported to have significant sleep disturbances, unrelated to medication status, that are characterized by dyssomnias, parasomnias, and sleep-related involuntary movements.[15] Sleep disturbances among adolescents with ADHD have not been studied as thoroughly as has been the case with children and are complicated by the fact that adolescence is a developmental period that often includes sleep disturbances.[16] Although stimulant medication does disrupt the sleep of adolescents with ADHD frequently,[16] it is important for prescribing physicians to establish a baseline of sleep behavior before initiating stimulant treatment, to provide a valid comparison for the determination of medication-induced sleep disturbances.

CO-OCCURRING DISORDERS

Between 25% and 75% of adolescents with ADHD also meet diagnostic criteria for oppositional defiant disorder or conduct disorder,[17] which results in significant additional impairment that increases the difficulty of treating these adolescents. Others reported similar increased risk for conduct disorder and increased risk for adolescents with ADHD to meet diagnostic criteria for a substance use disorder or mood disorder.[18] Long-term follow-up studies of children diagnosed with ADHD found that, in late adolescence and early adulthood, there is increased risk for antisocial personality disorder,[19-22] substance use disorders, and depression.[19] In a sample of 9- to 16-year-old subjects who met criteria for attention-deficit disorder (ADD) with or without hyperactivity,[23] 48% had comorbid depression/dysthymic disorder, 36% had comorbid oppositional defiant disorder/conduct disorder, and 36% had comorbid anxiety disorder. These incidence rates are comparable to the Multimodal Treatment Study of ADHD data for younger children regarding the comorbidity of anxiety and oppositional defiant disorder with ADHD but reflect a 12-fold increase in the reported incidence of depressive/dysthymic symptoms, with an incidence that is much closer to that found for depressive comorbidity in samples of adults with ADHD.[24] The high rate of comorbidity makes working with these comorbid disorders an inevitable part of treating adolescents with ADHD, leading to a need for assessment and treatment that target a range of impairments.

COGNITIVE DEFICITS

In addition, children and adolescents with mild to moderate degrees of mental retardation, for example, may have behavioral symptoms consistent with a diagnosis of ADHD and may also respond to medication and other ADHD treatments.[25] Although the *Diagnostic and Statistical Manual of Mental Disorders, Fourth Edition,*[9] excludes individuals with pervasive developmental disorders from having a co-occurring diagnosis of ADHD, children and adolescents with these disorders may also have symptoms of ADHD and may benefit from treatment for this condition as well as treatment for their pervasive developmental disorders.

OPPOSITIONAL DEFIANT DISORDER

The most noticeable psychiatric disorder that often occurs with ADHD in adolescence is oppositional defiant disorder. Adolescents with oppositional defiant disorder are chronically much more argumentative, negativistic, and defiant than most other adolescents, even most others with ADHD.[26] Although most adolescents with ADHD and oppositional defiant disorder do not manifest the more severe behavioral problems of conduct disorder, a serious pattern of delinquent behavior, those with oppositional defiant disorder often suffer significant problems in school, family, and social relationships. A central factor underlying this disorder is impairment in the adolescent's ability to modulate and to cope with the routine frustrations of daily life.

ANXIETY DISORDERS

Children with anxiety disorders may be tense and chronically anxious, quick to panic and often asking for reassurance, or they may tend to be socially phobic, extremely shy, and avoidant of unstructured interactions with any unfamiliar persons.[9] Others with ADHD may have obsessive-compulsive disorder, characterized by persistent obsessional fears that remain unspoken or tightly constrained by compulsive behaviors of checking, repeating, counting, cleaning, arranging, or hoarding that may be carried on only in private.[9] Adolescents with comorbid ADHD and anxiety may present a complicated clinical picture, because these disorders are characterized by thinking too little (ADHD) and thinking too much (anxiety). Careful assessment is important when attempting to diagnose these comorbid conditions.

MOOD DISORDERS

ADHD is also associated with an elevated risk of dysthymia, sometimes in combination with anxiety disorders or oppositional defiant disorder.[27] These disorders may be manifested by persistent profound unhappiness, with weeks and months of being unable to find any real pleasure, even in activities that once were enjoyable. The unhappiness may manifest as a persistently irritable mood. Dysthymic symptoms often are alleviated among adolescents who receive effective treatment for their ADHD but, in cases in which such symptoms persist despite effective ADHD interventions, specific counseling and medication treatment for depressive symptoms may be indicated.[28] Symptoms such as hypersomnia or hyposomnia, extremes of excessive or insufficient appetite, marked loss of energy, intense feelings of worthlessness, and persistent feelings of "not caring any more" may indicate the presence of comorbid major depressive disorder.[9] This is a potentially life-threatening comorbid condition, because the combination of depression and a disruptive behavior disorder has been identified as a particularly high-risk condition for a suicide attempt.[29] As a result, screening for depression among patients diagnosed as having ADHD is highly recommended. When signs of this morbid syndrome appear, careful assessment of depressive severity and the risk of self-injurious or life-threatening behaviors is needed, and conventional ADHD treatments alone are not likely to be sufficient.

There is a great deal of debate about the overlap of bipolar disorder and ADHD[30] and, until an accepted definition and diagnostic criteria appropriate for children and adolescents are developed, this debate will probably continue. Generally, bipolar disorder can be distinguished from severe ADHD by the presence of elated mood, grandiosity, flight of ideas or racing thoughts, and a decreased need for sleep.[31] Whenever possible, adolescents with complicated psychiatric presentations related to both ADHD and bipolar disorder should be referred to specialists in the area.

SUBSTANCE USE AND ABUSE

Children with ADHD are at increased risk for developing substance abuse as they grow older. Studies of adults with substance use disorders[9] show an overrepresentation of those with ADHD, with several reports indicating that between 15% and 25% of adults with substance use disorders have ADHD.[32,33] The presence of ADHD is also associated with greater severity of substance use disorders, including higher rates of substance-related motor vehicle accidents and treatment episodes.[33-35] One study found that the risk of developing substance use disorders over the lifespan for individuals with ADHD was twice that of individuals without ADHD.[36]

Prospective studies of children with ADHD found increased drinking and risk of substance use disorders during adolescence, which might be compounded by co-occurring conduct disorder or bipolar disorder.[34,37-39] In addition, individuals with ADHD start smoking at a younger age[40] and have higher rates of smoking than do individuals without ADHD.[41] Although adolescents with ADHD are at greater risk of substance use, the evidence suggests that appropriate treatment of ADHD, including the use of psychostimulant medication, does not increase that risk. A recent meta-analysis by Wilens,[42] which identified a total of 7 studies on this topic, found that stimulant pharmacotherapy was protective with respect to substance use disorders later in life (odds ratio: 1.9) and the effect was stronger among adolescents, compared with adults.

When the question of ADHD first arises during the adolescent years among individuals without previous diagnoses, the presence of substance use confounds the diagnostic process. Recurrent use of alcohol or drugs, including cannabis, may cause inattentiveness and other cognitive impairments.[43-46] Clinicians should therefore be cautious in making an ADHD diagnosis during adolescence when substance use is present and childhood symptoms are absent. It may be best to reassess an adolescent suspected of having ADHD after at least a 1-month period of abstinence from all psychoactive drugs.

Assessment and Diagnosis

Assessment of ADHD among adolescents is often more challenging than assessment among younger children. Students in preschool and early elementary grades are usually supervised closely by parents and, for most of the school day, by 1 teacher, who is able to observe much of the child's academic performance and social interaction. Observations by parents and the primary classroom teacher are usually a rich source of information to guide assessment for possible ADHD among younger children.

In contrast, adolescents usually have 5 to 7 different teachers, each of whom are responsible for 100 to 150 students and see each student for just a small portion of each school day. Outside school, adolescents are often involved in many activities where parents have very little direct contact to observe details of their strengths and problems. Parents can usually provide helpful information about homework patterns, school grades, and daily routines of their adolescent son or daughter but little direct information on school function, social interactions, and peer relationships.

A study by Mitsis et al[47] reported that parent-teacher agreement regarding the diagnosis of ADHD was only moderate (74%). Teachers tended to report a greater number of school symptoms than did parents, and parent reports of school behaviors were found to be influenced by their observations of behaviors in the home. The authors concluded that parent reports of ADHD behaviors in school settings are not an adequate substitute for direct teacher input. The subjects in that study were in elementary school, and parents frequently profess to know more about their child's behavior at the elementary school level than at the middle or high school level, which suggests that parent reports of school behaviors may be more inadequate in secondary schools than they were found to be in elementary school. Adolescents' needs for independence and privacy make it even more difficult for parents to obtain information about how their son or daugh-

ter is really doing in school, extracurricular activities, and social relationships.

Although obtaining assessment information from secondary school teachers may be important, there are many obstacles. First, teacher ratings do not provide information on symptoms and functioning manifested in less-structured settings such as the cafeteria, hallway, and bus. Second, inter-rater reliability is poor with secondary school teachers.[48] Agreement is best for questions pertaining to hyperactivity and academic progress and improves over the academic year from fall to spring semesters.[49] Given these problems, clinicians are encouraged to collect information from multiple teachers and from other sources such as counselors. If the adolescent has an individual education plan or 504 plan,[50] then it may be possible to receive help from the school in organizing the assessment effort.

Given the limitations of teacher and parent reports, it would be ideal if adolescents could provide reliable self-reports about symptoms and impairment; however, this does not seem to be the case. Consistent with studies reporting information for younger children, adolescents with ADHD tend to under-report dramatically their level of impairment and symptoms.[51-53] Interviewing adolescents and using self-report scales such as the Brown ADD Scales for Adolescents[54] or the Conners-Wells Adolescent Self-Report Scale[55] remain important components of the clinical evaluation. However, the information should be interpreted with the understanding that frequently it is an under-representation of impairment.

The presenting problems of adolescents continue to include many of the same behaviors as exhibited by children with ADHD. Their context, complexity, and potential for serious harm, however, change considerably. As a result, assessment and treatment must address not only the core symptoms of the disorder but also associated sequelae, including academic problems, impaired peer relationships, delinquent behavior, dangerous driving, substance use, impulsive sexual activity, and defiance.[8,56]

ADHD evaluation of an adolescent should include a review of recent report cards and school progress reports, especially noting patterns in teacher comments, and a review of psychoeducational testing results, if testing has already been completed. Reviewing previous school reports may be helpful in documenting problems before the age of 7 years. Psychoeducational testing cannot establish an ADHD diagnosis, but it may offer useful information. Results can indicate the range of an adolescent's cognitive abilities and can identify specific areas of strengths and weaknesses. Extensive batteries of neuropsychologic tests are usually not indicated for assessment of ADHD, unless there are questions about other neurologic impairments.

Adolescents with ADHD may be eligible for special education services under the category of "Other Health Impaired."[50] They are also at elevated risk for specific learning disorders involving reading, math, and/or written expression.[57] It can be helpful for clinicians to encourage parents to request, in writing, that the school complete a multidisciplinary evaluation if there are problems with their child at school. The process can be aided by a report from the clinician documenting the diagnosis of ADHD. If school personnel initiate the evaluation process, then they are likely to include an individually administered achievement test such as the Wechsler Individual Achievement Test-Second Edition or Woodcock-Johnson Achievement Tests-Third Edition, to be compared with the student's grades and ability, as measured with an individually administered IQ test, to determine the presence or absence of impairment. Definitions of impairment vary according to the state and school district, but some comparison of these scores is used frequently to determine impairment.

Adequate assessment for ADHD among adolescents requires screening for other psychiatric disorders. As noted above, individuals with ADHD have two- to fivefold greater risk of developing ≥1 additional psychiatric disorder at some point in their lives, and many have multiple disorders, with onsets at various points in the life cycle. Broad-based rating scales such as the Child Behavior Check List[58] or the Behavior Assessment System for Children[59] are standardized scales to screen for possible co-occurring disorders. The Brown ADD Diagnostic Form for Adolescents-Revised[54] and an interview outline in a book by Robin[60] provide probe questions that can be used to inquire about indicators of possible co-occurring disorders.

Evaluating clinicians should also ask the parents and, privately, the adolescent about risk-taking behaviors. These behaviors include the use of tobacco, marijuana, alcohol, and other drugs and association with others who tend to engage in illegal or dangerous behaviors. For those old enough to drive a motor vehicle, clinicians should inquire about attitudes and behaviors when driving (eg, speeding). Adolescents with ADHD are at increased risk of having car accidents associated with injuries.[61] To obtain adequate information about driving habits, pediatricians usually need to reassure adolescents that confidential disclosures will not be passed back to the parents.

Treatment

TREATMENT MODEL

The National Initiative for Children's Healthcare Quality, adapting a "chronic care model"[62,63] from the work of others, proposed that children with ADHD, including teens and adolescents, and their families require ≥6 supports in addition to an individualized and appropriate clinically based program.[62,63] These supports are (1) community resources and policies (such as schools), (2) health care systems and organizations (such as health insurance), (3) clinical information systems (such as public health community-based monitoring), (4) decision support, ie, application of evidence-based guidelines such as the American Academy of Pediatrics ADHD assessment and treatment guidelines, (5) delivery system design, ie, planned interventions by a coordinated, multidisciplinary, professional team, and (6) family and self-management support; families and individuals are those who must implement treatment interventions, and such individuals must be educated adequately about these treatments. The following review refers to these supports and is consistent with treatment characterized as a chronic care model.

EDUCATION AND ADHERENCE

All individuals with ADHD need a basic understanding of the disorder, including the fact that this is a neurobiological disorder. It may be helpful to "destigmatize" ADHD by comparing it with a less-stigmatizing condition such as poor eyesight or asthma. With these conditions, individuals are not deemed to be at fault for having the disorder, because they were born with it. However, individuals can be limited in life by the disorder unless it is treated. People who have these disorders need to be reminded frequently that they are not "bad," "damaged," "stupid," or "mentally deranged," just people who need help in certain areas. Having ADHD is no different. It is also critical to inform adolescents that having ADHD is not a reflection of their intelligence.

Adolescents with ADHD may have negative attitudes toward medication use and may be nonadherent with pharmacotherapies. In their longitudinal follow-up study of 358 clinic-referred children with ADHD, Pelham, Molina, and co-workers[64] reported that psychoactive medication usage decreased precipitously throughout adolescence, which indicates that stimulants or other psychoactive medications become an increasingly unpopular method of treatment as children mature beyond the elementary school period. In their sample, among the 87% of children who were medicated at some time in their lives, 27.9% had stopped taking medication by the age of 11 years and 67.9% had stopped by the age of 15 years. Starting medication in this age range was uncommon. Only 0.7% to 4.7% of the sample began taking medication between the ages of 11 and 15 years. Most individuals (86.5%) had started taking medication by the age of 10 years. Finally, one half of the participants in that study were in the adolescent age range at the time of their interviews (1998–2000), which suggests that recently improved, long-acting, stimulant preparations were available and might not ameliorate adolescent discontent with medication treatment for ADHD. In a separate, 3-year, longitudinal study,[65] it was reported that 48% of the children between the ages of 9 and 15 years had discontinued medication. Age was a significant moderator of adherence, such that older children were less likely to be continuing with their medication.

The lack of treatment adherence is not always obvious to prescribing physicians, because it may be manifested by the absence of visits. Unless the physician is monitoring the patient in such a way as to note omissions and to follow up actively when they occur, the discontinuation of therapies may go unnoticed. When children reach adolescence, they are better able to defy parent requests; this is accompanied frequently by a belief that they do not have a problem and therefore do not need treatment.

Physicians and parents can often be frustrated by a lack of adherence to prescribed regimens when they have a strong belief in the value of behavioral and medical interventions for ADHD but have little control over whether the adolescent will actually take the medications or follow behavioral contracts.[66] Important factors promoting adherence include self-concept,[67,68] family stability,[69-72] internal locus of control,[68,70,73] increased motivation,[74,75] simplified medication regimens,[76] lack of adverse effects,[70,77-79] and characteristics of the doctor-patient relationship, such as the physician's verbal and nonverbal communication skills and satisfaction of both the patient and the physician.[80] The use of motivational interviewing techniques by physicians can help adolescents feel in control and make their own decisions about the use of medications and behavioral interventions[81-85] (although the techniques have not been evaluated among adolescents with ADHD). This use can help diminish resistance and activate the motivation of the adolescents, 2 critical factors in successful treatment.[86] If an adolescent prefers to forego medication at a given time, it may be helpful to concur and then to develop a plan with the adolescent that helps him or her achieve goals through the use of tutors, behavioral interventions, organizational help, or whatever he or she thinks will help. A reevaluation of this plan in 2 to 4 weeks can identify whether it is working and what needs to be changed. If the adolescent chooses to start medication at a later time, it is at his or her request and the physician may then be seen as an ally, rather than as an enforcer and an authority figure.

MEDICATION

The pharmacologic management of ADHD relies on agents that affect dopaminergic and noradrenergic neurotransmission, namely, the stimulants, antidepressants, and antihypertensives.[87-88] A new agent, a noradrenergic reuptake inhibitor, has also become available.

The most commonly used stimulants are methylphenidate (Ritalin, Ritalin LA, Ritalin SR, Concerta, Focalin, Methylin, Methylin ER, Metadate ER, and Metadate CD) and amphetamine compounds (Adderall, Adderall XR, Dexedrine, Dexedrine Spansule, and DextroStat). Stimulants have been shown to be effective for ~70% of adolescents and seem to operate in a dose-dependent manner in improving cognition and behavior.[89,90] The beneficial effects of stimulants are of similar quality and magnitude for adolescents of both genders and for younger and older children.[91] Immediate-release preparations of methylphenidate and amphetamine are available in generic form. The extended-release formulations provide longer durations of action, resulting in the need for fewer daily administrations, elimination of school administrations, and thus fewer adherence issues and less potential for diversion and abuse. The extended-release preparations of the stimulants have durations of action that start ~30 minutes after dosing and last 8 hours (Ritalin LA and Metadate CD) to 12 hours (Concerta and Adderall XR). Dosing starts at the lowest dose available. Doses exceeding those approved by the Food and Drug Administration have been used clinically. A recent multisite study of OROS methylphenidate with adolescents demonstrated that one third of the participants experienced the best efficacy with 72 mg daily, with good tolerability.[92]

There seems to be a dose-response relationship for both behavioral and cognitive effects of the stimulants among youths with ADHD,[89,93] as well as for the most commonly reported short-term adverse effects, such as appetite suppression, sleep disturbances, and abdominal pain.[89,94,95]

Long-term adverse effects remain controversial, with mixed literature findings indicating only a weak association with motor tic development and variable results regarding height/weight decrement among prepubertal youths with ADHD.[88,94,96]

Survey studies suggest that diversion of stimulants, especially immediate-release preparations, continues to be noteworthy.[97-99] Medications may be abused orally or by grinding them into powder and then administering them through nasal insufflation. Psychostimulant medications may also be diverted to peers, either as a "favor" to friends or for financial profit. For example, in a survey of junior and senior high students who were prescribed stimulants,[100] 7% had sold (diverted) their medications. Similarly, diversion of stimulants to young adults presumably without ADHD seems problematic.[101] Survey studies with college students indicated that ~11% of students without ADHD reported using methylphenidate or amphetamine recreationally (including intranasally).[102] Recently Wilens[97] presented data indicating that 11% of older adolescents and collegeaged students were diverting their stimulants. Interestingly, diversion was exclusively with immediate-release but not extended-release stimulants and was confined largely to those with concurrent substance abuse or conduct disorder. More disturbingly, Low and Gendaszek[98] reported that, in a survey study of 150 undergraduate students (ADHD status not assessed) at Bates College, 4% had misused amphetamine compounds, 7% methylphenidate, and 24% both (total of 36%). As a comparison with another abused substance, one third of subjects in that sample also admitted using cocaine. However, as noted above, recently published evidence indicates that pharmacotherapy of ADHD does not increase the risk for substance abuse among individuals with ADHD but seems to reduce the risk for substance abuse by one half.[99]

Atomoxetine (Strattera) is a recently approved, nonstimulant agent that has been approved for adolescents with ADHD. Atomoxetine is a highly specific, noradrenergic reuptake inhibitor with efficacy for ADHD.[100,101] Moreover, atomoxetine seems to have efficacy for ADHD plus co-occurring disorders such as anxiety, tics, and depression. Atomoxetine has been shown to have similar efficacy and tolerability (side-effect profile) among adolescents, relative to more prototypic school-aged children with ADHD. In addition, long-term data indicate continued effectiveness with normal growth in height and weight and no unexpected adverse events occurring over 2 years.[101]

Atomoxetine demonstrates no abuse liability and is unscheduled by the Drug Enforcement Administration. Atomoxetine can be dosed once or twice daily; it should be initiated at a dose no higher than 0.5 mg/kg per day and increased to 1.2 mg/kg per day in 2 weeks. The peak efficacy of the medication seems to develop over 2 to 6 weeks. If adolescents continue to manifest symptoms, then the dose of atomoxetine can be increased to 1.4 mg/kg per day (100 mg per day) (Food and Drug Administration-approved dosing) to 1.8 mg/kg per day (maximal dose evaluated in clinical studies).[100,101] The effects of atomoxetine are more gradual than those experienced primarily with stimulant medications.

Adverse effects of atomoxetine among adolescents (as among younger children) include sedation (usually noted during initial titration), appetite suppression, nausea, vomiting, and headaches. Most short-term adverse effects can be managed by changing the time of administration of the medication. Most recently, rare occurrences of hepatotoxicity that resolves when the medication is stopped have been reported (Lilly, personal communication). Data on the long-term adverse effects of atomoxetine are limited. There do not seem to be drug interactions with the stimulants, a combination that might be very helpful in refractory cases of ADHD. Case reports of this combination have been published,[102] but there have been no formal studies of the effects of combined therapy. Atomoxetine doses should be reduced if the drug is administered with agents that inhibit the cytochrome P450 microsomal enzyme system, such as paroxetine (Paxil). Until additional evidence defines its safety and efficacy, the drug should be considered for adolescents with conditions unresponsive to stimulants, those with a preference for a nonstimulant, and those

for whom there is concern about abuse by the patient or family members.

The antidepressants are off-label and are considered second-line medications for ADHD. The tricyclic antidepressants, eg, imipramine (Tofranil), desipramine (Norpramine), and nortriptyline (Pamelor), block the reuptake of neurotransmitters including norepinephrine. Tricyclic antidepressants are effective in controlling behavioral problems and improving cognitive impairments associated with ADHD but are less effective than the majority of stimulants, particularly for cognitive impairments.[88] Desipramine and nortriptyline were shown in published reports to have both short-term and long-term effects among adolescents.[103,104] The tricyclic antidepressants should be considered only when adequate trials with both stimulant medications (amphetamine compounds and methylphenidate) have failed, atomoxetine is ineffective, and behavioral interventions have been tried. Dosing of the tricyclic antidepressants starts with 25 mg daily and is titrated upward slowly to a maximum of 5 mg/kg per day (2 mg/kg per day for nortriptyline).[104] Common adverse effects among adolescents include sedation, weight gain, dry mouth, constipation, and headache. Four deaths among children with ADHD (including 1 adolescent) who were treated with desipramine were reported.[105] However, independent evaluation of those cases failed to support a causal link.[106] Because minor increases in heart rate and the electrocardiographic intervals are predictable with tricyclic antidepressants, electrocardiographic monitoring at baseline and at the therapeutic dose is suggested (although not mandatory).[107]

The novel dopaminergic antidepressant bupropion (Welbutrin) has been reported to be effective and well tolerated in the treatment of ADHD,[108] although it remains untested among adolescents with ADHD under controlled conditions and therefore is a second-line treatment. One open-label study among depressed adolescents showed improvement in both ADHD and depression.[109] Bupropion should be started at 100 mg and slowly titrated upward, with beneficial effects for ADHD being noted generally at 300 to 400 mg daily.

The antihypertensive agent clonidine (Catapres) has been used increasingly as a second-line medication for the treatment of ADHD, particularly among adolescents with hyperactivity and aggressiveness.[110] Although the effect of clonidine on ADHD is not as robust as that of stimulants, a meta-analysis suggested a moderate effect size (0.58) for this agent on symptoms of ADHD co-occurring with tics, aggression, or conduct disorder.[110] Clonidine is a short-acting agent, with daily doses ranging from 0.05 mg to 0.6 mg, given in divided doses up to 4 times daily. Clonidine is commonly used clinically in addition to stimulants and antidepressants. Short-term adverse effects include sedation (which tends to subside with continued treatment), dry mouth, depression, confusion, electrocardiographic changes, and hypertension with abrupt withdrawal. A recent multisite study demonstrated the usefulness of clonidine alone and in combination for the treatment of ADHD among children with tics.[111] Abrupt withdrawal of clonidine has been associated with rebound; therefore, slow tapering is advised. Guanfacine (Tenex) has also been used to treat ADHD, alone or in combination with tic disorders, among preadolescent children.[112] Dosing of guanfacine generally starts at 0.5 mg per day and is increased as necessary to a maximum of 4 mg per day, in 2 or 3 divided doses.

Although the serotonin reuptake inhibitors (for example, Prozac) are not useful for treatment of ADHD, venlafaxine (Effexor), because of its noradrenergic reuptake inhibition, may have mild efficacy for ADHD.[113] Monoamine oxidase inhibitors (Nardil and Parnate) have been shown to be effective among adolescents with ADHD.[114] However, the potential for hypertensive crises associated with tyramine-containing foods (such as most cheeses) and interactions with prescribed, illicit, and over-the-counter drugs (pressor amines, most cold medicines, and amphetamines) limit its usefulness. Provigil and cholinergic agents remain untested among adolescents.

PSYCHOSOCIAL INTERVENTIONS

Types of Treatments

Psychosocial treatments encompass a broad set of interventions, including behavior therapy, academic interventions, family therapy, and care coordination. Relatively little research has been conducted on psychosocial treatments for adolescents with ADHD,[53] compared with the vast amount of treatment outcome research completed for children with the disorder.[115] Nevertheless, there are important practice implications for adolescents that can be surmised from this work.

School Problems

Problems at school tend to be the most common complaints of parents of adolescents with ADHD.[116] These usually include poor performance on tests and quizzes, missing assignments, careless work, and poor writing. Psychosocial interventions targeting these areas include behavioral techniques addressing organization and academic interventions, including training in note-taking and study skills, that focus on underachievement.[60,117,118] These interventions tend to be labor intensive and are provided frequently by teachers and other school personnel. School districts' willingness to provide these interventions to adolescents varies. Some schools prioritize these services and provide them when the problems are recognized. Receiving these services in other districts can be enhanced by having a child identified as eligible to receive services under Section 504 of the Rehabilitation Act or in the "Other Health Impaired" category of the Individuals with Disabilities Education Act.[50] Although a diagnosis of ADHD does not by itself qualify a student for these services, an adolescent with ADHD is likely to be found eligible if the ADHD is accompanied by significant academic impairment. Physicians may facilitate this process by educating parents about these services (www.ideapractices.org/index) and providing documentation of the diagnosis and impairment.

Substance Use

Because substance abuse becomes a prominent issue among adolescents, educating parents and patients about the risks and informing them about appropriate local prevention and intervention resources may be very helpful. The data suggest that this should be performed at a relatively young age (<11 years), because youths with ADHD begin their experimentation earlier than do children without the disorder.[35,119] Some parents may request that their physician conduct random drug screens. Although parents may want to know the truth about their child's experimentation and use of illegal drugs, conducting these screens against the wishes of the adolescent can affect family relationships seriously. For example, parents who request a drug screen communicate to their child that they no longer trust him or her. Although this may be obviously true in some families, in others this message may disrupt family functioning seriously. Furthermore, it can lead to power struggles and defiance by adolescents who refuse to comply with these screens. Adolescents also may find ways to defeat the validity of the screens, by drinking excessive amounts of water or using products that are readily available via the Internet. Depending on the age of the adolescent and the consent laws in the state, the child's consent may be needed to conduct the screens, and the American Academy of Pediatrics recommends that drug screening not be performed without a child's knowledge and consent except in cases of medical necessity.[120] In addition, parents need to know what to do if the test results are positive. Parents wonder frequently how to respond to this news, and counterproductive responses are not uncommon. Pediatricians conducting drug screens should consult with a toxicologist or addiction professional at the time the test is ordered, to avoid false-positive and false-negative tests.

Family Stress

In addition to concerns about substance use, the cumulative effect of the chronic stress of raising a child with moderate to severe ADHD can take a serious toll on parents.[121] Parents respond to this stress in many different ways, and some of these reactions may affect the adolescent, the parents, and the siblings negatively. Simple recognition and assessment of parents' stress and coping can be a useful psychosocial intervention for many parents. Parents may need supportive services, and physician encouragement and appropriate referrals can facilitate this need being met. Although early reports indicate that parent training and family therapy are not as effective for adolescents with ADHD and their families as they have been for children with ADHD,[122] these interventions can be helpful for some parents and should be considered for families exhibiting significant distress. Furthermore, some forms of family therapy that have not been assessed directly with families of adolescents with ADHD have been found to be effective with families of adolescents with problems such as substance abuse and should be evaluated with this population.[123]

Social Impairment

The social impairment reported frequently to accompany ADHD among children continues into adolescence.[124] The consequences of these problems may be even greater for adolescents than for children, because the cruelty of peer rejection and bullying can be greatest in the young adolescent years. In addition, social impairment with ADHD increases the risk for substance use and other problems.[125] Effective psychosocial treatments for adolescents with social impairment have not been reported, although modest results were observed in initial studies of comprehensive and intensive psychosocial treatment programs.[117] These interventions incorporated novel techniques, including videotape reviews of naturally occurring social behavior, and emphasized strategies to facilitate generalization. Many traditional social skills interventions fail to generalize to natural settings and have minimal impact on social functioning[126,127] or have not been evaluated with adolescents.[128]

Driving

The data describing automobile accidents and traffic violations involving adolescents with ADHD are likely to lead many parents of these young drivers to ask their physicians for guidance.[61] Unfortunately, there are no reports of effective psychosocial interventions for this problem and only preliminary information on the potential benefits of medication.[129] Parent management strategies related to the use of an automobile have implications for this difficult area. Parents may restrict the peers who can ride with their adolescent driver, limit the time of day the car can be used, and provide close monitoring. The risks associated with driving problems are increased significantly if the adolescent is experimenting with drugs or alcohol.[129] Parents should be encouraged to discuss this topic regularly with their teenager and to follow up aggressively on any suspicions. In some situations, maintaining driving privileges may be contingent on demonstrating responsible behavior in other settings, such as home and school, and possibly participating in laboratory testing for drugs. For some adolescents with ADHD, it may be important to plan medication dosing so that the adolescents have coverage during periods in which they are likely to be driving.

Primary care physicians are being incorporated increasingly into important roles in the delivery of universal and selective psychosocial mental health services.[130,131] Implementing these basic psychosocial interventions in a busy pediatric practice is likely to be a challenge. Because of the wide range of impairment among adolescents with ADHD, care is often provided by a variety of professionals. As other providers become involved, the coordination of care becomes a central issue and can be facilitated by the sharing of information about the services and measures of progress. This system is part of the medical home concept.[132] Collaborating with a qualified psychologist or mental health counselor with expertise working with adolescents and behavioral techniques can be a practical solution; however, there are many communities without providers with expertise in these areas. Counselors and teachers at secondary schools may provide many of these services and may be very interested in collaborating with a physician practice.

Transition to Adulthood

INSURANCE COVERAGE

The peer-reviewed medical literature about the transition from secondary education for young people with ADHD is sparse. It is clear, however, that the move to increasing independence and postsecondary training is fraught with difficulties for all adolescents with chronic medical conditions.[133] Before they can begin to consider training and other issues, they would benefit from finding ways to continue medical care and maintain at least the semblance of a medical home.

Even in childhood, health insurance for individuals with ADHD is limited. A survey of Children and Adults with Attention-Deficit/Hyperactivity Disorder members[134] found that 82% of health insurance policies held by a sample of members contained assessment of ADHD limitations and 24% of health policies did not cover the treatment of ADHD; of the 76% of policies that covered the treatment of ADHD, 83% contained treatment limits. In addition, the out-of-pocket obligations were higher than for other health conditions and were similar to those for other psychiatric conditions.

The insurance coverage issues are magnified when a child becomes an adult. At a time when many of the family structures that have supported them through their school careers begin to change and become more tenuous, adolescents' ability to obtain and fund medical care decreases precipitously. Young adults, 18 to 24 years of age, are more likely than any other age group to be uninsured.[135] Of Americans between the ages of 18 and 24 years, 31.6% are without medical insurance, compared with 12.0% for those ≤18 years of age.[136] Many commercial policies no longer cover young people under their parents' policies, particularly if the young people are not enrolled full-time in college or other advanced training.[136] Because the median costs of health care for individuals with ADHD are twice those for individuals without ADHD,[137] obtaining private health insurance on their own before they are employed full-time is likely to be difficult for individuals with

ADHD. Government health care programs also cease after age 18 for unmarried people without children.[138] The ability to pay for continuing medical care and medication therefore becomes a critical issue for young adults with ADHD, which is complicated by preexisting-condition exclusions present in many policies.

ACCESS TO CARE

After reaching the age of majority, fewer young people are cared for by pediatricians, and family and adult physicians may be less comfortable dealing with young people with ADHD. Although some patients continue care for ADHD through the services of the psychiatric community, the inability of these physicians to provide comprehensive medical services would preclude their replacing a medical home model for their patients,[139,140] which would be provided ideally by the patient's pediatrician. College health services may provide support for individuals who are enrolled in college, but such services cannot be expected to offer comprehensive care when the student is home or outside the school calendar. Whenever possible, it is important to have a plan on how to transition these individuals into the adult health care system.

ANTICIPATORY GUIDANCE

The need for pediatricians and other health professionals to provide anticipatory guidance to their graduating patients with ADHD is important. Adolescents with ADHD who are leaving home for what may be the first time are particularly vulnerable to the consequences of sudden diminution of parental supervision. In preparing students with ADHD for being away at school, physicians need to caution them about the increased risk of their becoming smokers[141] and their increased risk of driving-related morbidities.[56] In addition to a general warning to college-bound students to avoid binge drinking, students with ADHD need to know that they have an increased long-term risk of alcohol and illicit drug use if they are not receiving appropriate treatment.[142] Individuals preparing for college need to become aware of how to navigate the complexities of dealing with college scheduling and course planning, acquiring study skills, and learning to access any special services for students with ADHD that their college may offer. They also need to deal with the more basic problems of following a schedule on their own and taking their medication reliably. There are several educational materials that may be useful for them to read.[143-145] They should be reminded of the potential for theft in keeping a controlled substance in their dormitory rooms and the hazards of sharing or selling controlled substances to their peers.[146]

TESTING ACCOMMODATIONS

Both the SAT[147] and ACT[148] have processes in place to allow students with ADHD to apply for special accommodations, including extended testing time. However, there are strict requirements for the type and timing of documentation required. Details are available at the Educational Testing Service Web site (www.ets.org/disability/adhdplcy.html). Both testing services have subscribed to the basic tenets established by the Consortium on ADHD Documentation[149] and have ceased flagging tests taken with special accommodations.[150] For consideration for military service, each enlistee must take and pass the Armed Services Vocational Aptitude Battery, a timed test for which no accommodations are permitted.[143]

MILITARY ENLISTMENT

Enlistment in the military is uncertain for those with ADHD. The reasons for rejection for appointment, enlistment, or induction include a history of immaturity and impulsiveness, a chronic history of academic skill deficits that interfere with work or school after age 12, and the current use of medication to improve or to maintain academic skills. Under certain circumstances, individual military services may grant waivers to individuals who do not meet the basic eligibility criteria. Demonstrating success in either school or work for a certain period of time without the use of medication is basic in whether a waiver will be granted.[143]

Planning for the Future

Planning for the future is complicated for all graduating high school students but offers special challenges for those with ADHD. Educational attainment is less for patients with ADHD, and their future occupational outcomes are of lower ranking than those of their cohorts.[151] Young people who have ADHD, predominantly inattentive type, or ADHD, combined type, have fewer years of school and are less likely to graduate from college, compared with young people without ADHD. Furthermore, youths with the combined type of ADHD have higher rates of oppositional defiant disorder, suicide attempts, and arrests than do those with the inattentive type.[152]

High school, college, and other counselors have made themselves available to help such students, and vocational tests are available to help assess likely job satisfaction, but the usefulness of such assistance for this population is not well documented in the medical literature. Anecdotally, special services programs provided by colleges seem to fulfill real needs for students with ADHD, including providing late course-dropping dates, special registration assistance, adaptive equipment such as computers, and note-takers for qualifying students.[153] Some communities offer support for students with ADHD through state vocational rehabilitation services or through ADHD coaching services.[154] Although there is little research in this area, there are a number of organizations, publications, and websites offering information, encouragement, and support to adolescents making the transition from secondary school to work or postsecondary education.[155-162]

Future Research

Although much progress has been made in our understanding of the diagnosis and treatment of ADHD, much has yet to be researched, particularly for adolescents. It is clear that the current diagnostic criteria, although valid for children, may need to be modified for adolescents and adults, to reflect the developmental changes that take place as children approach adulthood. How the subtypes change in the transition from childhood to adolescence and how the patterns of comorbidities change need to be identified more clearly. The recent pressure and incentives that the government has placed on the pharmaceutical industry have increased the number of pharmaceutical company-sponsored studies among adolescents. However, additional studies are required to clarify how medication needs, types, dosages, and frequencies of administration differ among adolescents and adults, compared with children. Given the developmental significance of social functioning, additional studies of the development and evaluations of psychosocial interventions targeting these behaviors are greatly needed. The unique aspects of obtaining adolescents' adherence to treatment are important factors requiring clarification. Lastly, longitudinal studies examining the outcomes for adolescents and adults are required to identify more clearly the course of the disorder and the impact of treatment.

Acknowledgments

This study was supported in part by the National Resource Center on AD/HD, a program of Children and Adults with Attention-Deficit/Hyperactivity Disorder. The National Resource Center is funded by the Centers for Disease Control and Prevention under cooperative agreement R04-CCR321831.

We thank Edward Zimmerman, Karen Wanatowicz, and Regina Martinez for help with preparation of the manuscript.

References

1. Olfson M. Diagnosing mental disorders in office-based pediatric practice. *J Dev Behav Pediatr.* 1992;13:363–365
2. Rappley MD, Gardiner JC, Jetton JR, Houang RT. The use of methylphenidate in Michigan. *Arch Pediatr Adolesc Med.* 1995;149:675–679
3. Ruel JM, Hickey P. Are too many children being treated with methylphenidate? *Can J Psychiatry.* 1992;37:570–572
4. Bakwin H, Bakwin R. *Clinical Management of Behavior Disorders in Children.* Philadelphia, PA: WB Saunders; 1966
5. Biederman J, Farone S, Milberger S, et al. A prospective 4-year follow-up study of attention-deficit hyperactivity and related disorders. *Arch Gen Psychiatry.* 1996;53:437–446
6. Ingram S, Hechtman L, Morgenstern G. Outcome issues in ADHD: adolescent and adult long-term outcome. *Ment Retard Dev Disabil Res Rev.* 1999;5:243–250

7. Milich R, Loney J. The role of hyperactivity and aggressive symptomatology in predicting adolescent outcome among hyperactive children. *J Pediatr Psychol.* 1979;4: 93–112

8. Barkley R, Anastopoulos A, Buevremont DC, et al. Adolescents with ADHD: patterns of behavioral adjustment, academic functioning, and treatment utilization. *J Am Acad Child Adolesc Psychiatry.* 1991;30:752–761

9. American Psychiatric Association. *Diagnostic and Statistical Manual of Mental Disorders.* 4th ed, text rev. Washington, DC: American Psychiatric Association; 2000

10. Carlson C, Mann M. Sluggish cognitive tempo predicts a different pattern of impairment in the attention deficit hyperactivity disorder, predominantly inattentive type. *J Clin Child Adolesc Psychol.* 2002;31:123–129

11. Milich R, Balentine AC, Lynam DR. ADHD combined type and ADHD predominantly inattentive type are distinct and unrelated disorders. *Clin Psychol Sci Pract.* 2001;8:463–488

12. Hoy E, Weiss G, Minde K, Cohen N. The hyperactive child at adolescence: emotional, social, and cognitive functioning. *J Abnorm Child Psychol.* 1978;6:311–324

13. Barkley R, Anastopoulos AD, Guevremont DC, Fletcher KE. Adolescents with attention deficit hyperactivity disorder: mother-adolescent interactions, family beliefs and conflicts, and maternal psychopathology. *J Abnorm Child Psychol.* 1992;20:263–288

14. Stewart M, Mendelson W, Johnson NE. Hyperactive children as adolescents: how they describe themselves. *Child Psychiatry Hum Dev.* 1973;4:3–11

15. Corkum P, Moldofsky H, Hogg-Johnson S, et al. Sleep problems in children with attention-deficit/hyperactivity disorder: impact of subtype, comorbidity, and stimulant medication. *J Am Acad Child Adolesc Psychiatry.* 1999;38: 1285–1293

16. Stein D, Pat-Horenczyk R, Blank S, et al. Sleep disturbances in adolescents with symptoms of attention-deficit/hyperactivity disorder. *J Learn Disabil.* 2002;35: 268–275

17. Barkley R. *Attention Deficit Hyperactivity Disorder: A Handbook for Diagnosis and Treatment.* New York, NY: Guilford Press; 1998

18. Fergusson D, Horwood LJ, Lynskey MT. Prevalence and comorbidity of DSM-III-R diagnoses in a birth cohort of 15 year olds. *J Am Acad Child Adolesc Psychiatry.* 1993; 32:1127–1134

19. Fischer M, Barkley RA, Smallish L, Fletcher K. Young adult follow-up of hyperactive children: self-reported psychiatric disorders, comorbidity, and the role of childhood conduct problems and teen CD. *J Abnorm Child Psychol.* 2002;30:463–475

20. Manuzza S, Klein RG, Bessler A, et al. Adult outcomes of hyperactive boys. *Arch Gen Psychiatry.* 1993;50:565–576

21. Rasmussen P, Gillberg C. Natural outcome of ADHD with developmental coordination disorder at age 22 years: a controlled, longitudinal, community-based study. *J Am Acad Child Adolesc Psychiatry.* 2000;39:1424–1431

22. Weiss G, Hechtman LT. *Hyperactive Children Grown Up.* New York, NY: Guilford Press; 1986

23. Bird H, Gould MS, Staghezza BM. Patterns of diagnostic comorbidity in a community sample of children aged 9 through 16 years. *J Am Acad Child Adolesc Psychiatry.* 1993;32:361–368

24. Kessler R. Prevalence of adult ADHD in the United States: results from the National Comorbidity Study Replication (NCS-R). Presented at the 157th annual meeting of the American Psychiatric Association; May 1–6, 2004; New York, NY

25. Pearson D, Santos CW, Casat CD, et al. Treatment effects of methylphenidate on cognitive functioning in children with mental retardation and ADHD. *J Am Acad Child Adolesc Psychiatry.* 2004;43:677–685

26. American Psychiatric Association. *Diagnostic and Statistical Manual of Mental Disorders.* 4th ed. Washington, DC: American Psychiatric Association; 1994

27. Connor D, Edwards G, Fletcher KE, et al. Correlates of comorbid psychopathology in children with ADHD. *J Am Acad Child Adolesc Psychiatry.* 2003;42:193–200

28. Gammon G, Brown T. Fluoxetine and methylphenidate in combination for treatment of attention deficit disorder and comorbid depressive disorder. *J Child Adolesc Psychopharmacol.* 1993;3:1–10

29. Lewinsohn P, Rohde P, Seeley JR. Adolescent psychopathology, III: the clinical consequences of comorbidity. *J Am Acad Child Adolesc Psychiatry.* 1995;34:510–519

30. Faraone S, Biederman J, Wozniak J, et al. Is comorbidity with ADHD a marker for juvenile-onset mania? *J Am Acad Child Adolesc Psychiatry.* 1997;36:1046–1055

31. Geller B, Zimmerman B, Williams M, et al. DSM-IV mania symptoms in a prepubertal and early adolescent bipolar disorder phenotype compared to attention-deficit hyperactive and normal controls. *J Child Adolesc Psychopharmacol.* 2002;12:11–25

32. Wilens T. Alcohol and other drug use and attention deficit hyperactivity disorder. *Alcohol Health Res World.* 1998;22:127–130

33. Schubiner H, Tzelepis A, Milberger S. Prevalence of attention deficit hyperactivity disorder and conduct disorder among substance abusers. *J Clin Psychiatry.* 2000;61: 244–251

34. Biederman J, Wilens T, Mick E, et al. Is ADHD a risk factor for psychoactive substance use disorders? Findings from a four-year prospective follow-up study. *J Am Acad Child Adolesc Psychiatry.* 1997;36:21–29

35. Carroll K, Rounsaville BJ. History and significance of childhood attention deficit disorder in treatment-seeking cocaine abusers. *Compr Psychiatry.* 1993;34:75–82

36. Biederman J, Wilens T, Mick E, et al. Psychoactive substance use in adults with attention deficit hyperactivity disorder (ADHD): effects of ADHD and psychiatric comorbidity. *Am J Psychiatry.* 1995;52:1652-1658

37. Molina B, Pelham W. Childhood predictors of adolescent substance use in a longitudinal study of children with ADHD. *J Abnorm Psychol.* 2003;112:497-507

38. Satterfield J, Hoppe C, Schell A. A prospective study of delinquency in 110 adolescent boys with attention deficit hyperactivity disorder and 88 normal adolescent boys. *Am J Psychiatry.* 1982;139:795-798

39. Katusic S, Barbaresi W, Colligan R. Substance abuse among ADHD cases: a population-based birth cohort study. Presented at the annual meeting of the Pediatric Academic Societies; May 3-6, 2003; Seattle, WA

40. Hartsough C, Lambert NM. Pattern and progression of drug use among hyperactives and controls: a prospective short-term longitudinal study. *J Child Psychol Psychiatry.* 1987;28:543-553

41. Lambert N, Hartsough C. Prospective study of tobacco smoking and substance dependence among samples of ADHD and non-ADHD subjects. *J Learn Disabil.* 1998; 31:533-544

42. Faraone SV, Wilens T. Does stimulant treatment lead to substance use disorders? *J Clin Psychiatry.* 2003; 11(suppl 64):9-13

43. Kempel P, Lampe K, Parnefjord R, et al. Auditory-evoked potentials and selective attention: different ways of information processing in cannabis users and controls. *Neuropsychobiology.* 2003;48:95-101

44. Parrot A. Cognitive deficits and cognitive normality in recreational cannabis and ecstasy/MDMA users. *Hum Psychopharmacol.* 2003;18:89-90

45. Fried P, Watkinson B, James D, Gray R. Current and former marijuana use: preliminary findings of a longitudinal study of effects on IQ in young adults. *CMAJ.* 2002;166:887-891

46. Ehrenreich H, Rinn T, Kunert H. Specific attentional dysfunction in adults following early start of cannabis use. *Psychopharmacology.* 1999;142:295-301

47. Mitsis EM, McKay KE, Schulz KP, et al. Parent-teacher concordance for DSM-IV attention-deficit/hperactivity disorder in a clinic-referred sample. *Child Adolesc Psychiatry.* 2000;39:308-313

48. Molina B, Pelham WE, Blumenthal J, Galiszewski EG. Agreement among teachers' behavior ratings of adolescents with a childhood history of attention deficit hyperactivity disorder. *J Clin Child Psychol.* 1998;27:330-339

49. Evans SW, Allen J, Moore S, Strauss V. Measuring symptoms and functioning of youth with ADHD in middle schools. *J Abnorm Child Psychol.* In press

50. Davila RR, Williams ML, MacDonald JT. Memorandum on clarification of policy to address the needs of children with attention deficit disorders within general and/or special education. In: Parker HC, ed. *The ADD Hyperactivity Handbook for Schools.* Plantation, FL: Impact Publications; 1991:261-268

51. Kramer TL, Phillips SD, Hargis MB, et al. Disagreement between parent and adolescent reports of functional impairment. *J Child Psychol Psychiatry.* 2004;45:248-259

52. Romano E, Tremblay RE, Vitaro F, et al. Prevalence of psychiatric diagnoses and the role of perceived impairment: findings from an adolescent community sample. *J Child Psychol Psychiatry.* 2001;42:451-462

53. Smith B, Pelham WE Jr, Gnagy E, et al. The reliability, validity, and unique contributions of self-report by adolescents receiving treatment for attention-deficit/hyperactivity disorder. *J Consult Clin Psychol.* 2000; 68:489-499

54. Brown TE. *Brown ADD Scales for Children and Adolescents.* San Antonio, TX: Psychological Corp; 2001

55. Conners C, Wells K. *Conners-Wells Adolescent Self-Report Scale.* North Tonowanda, NY: Multi-Health Systems; 1997

56. Barkley R, Murphy K, Kwasnik D. Motor vehicle driving competencies and risks in teens and young adults with attention deficit hyperactivity disorder. *Pediatrics.* 1996; 98:1089-1095

57. Tannock R, Brown T. Attention deficit disorders with learning disorders in children and adolescents. In: Brown T, ed. *Attention Deficit Disorders and Comorbidities in Children, Adolescents and Adults.* Washington, DC: American Psychiatric Press; 2000

58. Achenbach T, Edelbrock L. *Manual for the Child Behavior Checklist 4-18 and 1991 Profile.* Burlington, VT: University of Vermont; 1991

59. Reynolds C, Kamphouse R. *BASC: Behavior Assessment System for Children Manual.* Circle Pines, MN: American Guidance Service; 1992

60. Robin A. *ADHD in Adolescents: Diagnosis and Treatment.* New York, NY: Guilford; 1998

61. Barkley R. Driving impairments in teens and adults with attention-deficit/hyperactivity disorder. *Psychiatr Clin North Am.* 2004;27:233-260

62. Bodenheimer T, Wagner EH, Grumbach K. Improving primary care for patients with chronic illness. *JAMA.* 2002;288:1775-1779

63. Bodenheimer T, Wagner EH, Grumbach K. Improving primary care for patients with chronic illness: the chronic care model, part 2. *JAMA.* 2002;288:1909-1914

64. Charach A, Ickowicz A, Schachar R. Stimulant treatment over five years: adherence, effectiveness, and adverse effects. *J Am Acad Child Adolesc Psychiatry.* 2004;43:559-567

65. Thiruchelvam D, Charach A, Schachar RJ. Moderators and mediators of long-term adherence to stimulant treatment in children with ADHD. *J Am Acad Child Adolesc Psychiatry.* 2001;40:922-928

66. Anderson R, Funnell M. Compliance and adherence are dysfunctional concepts in diabetes care. *Diabetes Educ.* 2000;26:597–604

67. Lindeman M, Behm K. Cognitive strategies and self-esteem as predictors of bracewear noncompliance in patients with idiopathic scoliosis and kyphosis. *J Pediatr Orthopediatr.* 1999;19:493–499

68. Litt I, Cuskey W, Rosenberg A. Role of self-esteem and autonomy in determining medication compliance among adolescents with juvenile rheumatoid arthritis. *Pediatrics.* 1982;69:15–17

69. Thompson S, Auslander W, White N. Influence of family structure on health among youths with diabetes. *Health Social Work.* 2001;26:7–14

70. Emans S, Grace E, Wood E. Adolescents' compliance with the use of oral contraceptives. *JAMA.* 1987;257:3377–3381

71. Martinez J, Bell D, Camacho R. Adherence to antiviral drug regimens in HIV infected adolescent patients engaged in care in a comprehensive adolescent and young adult clinic. *J Natl Med Assoc.* 2000;92:55–61

72. Korsch B, Fine R, Negrete V. Noncompliance in children with renal transplants. *Pediatrics.* 1978;61:872–876

73. Tebbi C. Treatment compliance in childhood adolescence. *Cancer.* 1993;71:3441–3449

74. Creer T, Burns K. Self-management training for children with chronic bronchial asthma. *Psychother Psychosom.* 1979;32:270–278

75. Friedman I, Litt I. Promoting adolescents' compliance with therapeutic regimens. *Pediatr Clin North Am.* 1986;33:955–973

76. Cramer J, Mattson R, Prevey M. How often is medication taken as prescribed: a novel assessment technique. *JAMA.* 1989;261:3273–3277

77. Cromer B, Steinberg K, Gardner L. Psychosocial determinants of compliance in adolescents with iron deficiency. *Am J Disord Child.* 1989;143:55–58

78. Lloyd A, Horan W, Borgaro W. Predictors of medication compliance after hospital discharge in adolescent psychiatric patients. *J Child Adolesc Psychopharmacol.* 1998;8:133–141

79. Slack M, Brooks A. Medication management issues for adolescents with asthma. *Am J Health Syst Pharm.* 1995;52:1417–1421

80. Fotheringham M, Sawyer M. Adherence to recommended medical regimens in childhood and adolescence. *J Pediatr Health.* 1995;31:72–78

81. Barnett N, Monti P, Wood M. Motivational interviewing for alcohol-involved adolescents in the emergency room. In: Wagner E, Waldron H, eds. *Innovations in Adolescent Substance Abuse Interventions.* Philadelphia, PA: Elsevier; 2001:143–168

82. Colby S, Monti P, Barnett N. Brief motivational interviewing in a hospital setting for adolescent smoking: a preliminary study. *J Consult Clin Psychol.* 1998;66:574–578

83. Dunn C, Deroo L, Rivara F. The use of brief interventions adapted from motivational interviewing across behavioral domains: a systematic review. *Addiction.* 2001;96:1725–1742

84. Lawendowski L. A motivational intervention for adolescent smokers. *Prev Med.* 1998;27:39–46

85. Miller W, Rollnick S. *Motivational Interviewing: Preparing People for Change.* New York, NY: Guilford Press; 2002

86. Brown R, Border K, Cingerman S. Adherence to methylphenidate therapy in a pediatric population: a preliminary investigation. *Psychopharmacol Bull.* 1998;21:192–211

87. Garland E. Pharmacotherapy of adolescents with attention deficit disorder: challenges, choices and caveats. *J Psychopharmacol.* 1998;12:385–395

88. Spencer T, Biederman J, Wilens T. Pharmacotherapy of attention deficit/hyperactivity disorder: a life span perspective. 1998

89. Evans S, Pelham WE, Smith BH, et al. Dose-response effects of methylphenidate on ecologically-valid measures of academic performance and classroom behavior in adolescents with ADHD. *Exp Clin Psychopharmacol.* 2001;9:163–175

90. Biederman J, Spencer T, Wilens T. Evidence-based pharmacotherapy for ADHD. *Int J Neuropsychopharmacol.* 2004;7:77–91

91. Smith B, Pelham WE, Gnagy E, Yudell RS. Equivalent effects of stimulant treatment for attention-deficit hyperactivity disorder during childhood and adolescence. *J Am Acad Child Adolesc Psychiatry.* 1998;37:314–321

92. Wilens T. Safety and efficiency of OROS methylphenidate in adolescents with ADHD. Presented at the annual meeting of the American Psychiatric Association; 2004

93. Rapport M, Jones J, DuPaul G, et al. Attention deficit disorder and methylphenidate: group and single-subject analysis of dose effects on attention in clinic and classroom settings. *J Clin Psychol.* 1987;16:329–338

94. Greenhill L, Pliszka S, Dulcan M, et al. Practice parameter for the use of stimulant medications in the treatment of children, adolescents, and adults. *J Am Acad Child Adolesc Psychiatry.* 2002;41:26–49

95. Swanson J, Greenhill L, Pelham W, et al. Initiating Concerta (OROS methylphenidate HCl) qd in children with attention-deficit hyperactivity disorder. *J Clin Res.* 2000;3:59–76

96. MTA Cooperative Group. National Institute of Mental Health Multimodal Treatment Study of ADHD follow-up: changes in effectiveness and growth after the end of treatment. *Pediatrics.* 2004;113:762–769

97. Wilens T. Subtypes of ADHD at risk for substance abuse. Presented at the 157th annual meeting of the American Psychiatric Association; May 1–6, 2004; New York, NY

98. Low K, Gendaszek AE. Illicit use of psychostimulants among college students: a preliminary study. *Psychol Health Med.* 2002;7:283–287

99. Wilens T, Faraone S, Biederman J, Gunawardene S. Does stimulant therapy of ADHD beget later substance abuse: a metanalytic review of the literature. *Pediatrics.* 2003;111:179–185

100. Michelson D, Faries D, Wernicke J, et al. Atomoxetine in the treatment of children and adolescents with attention deficit hyperactivity disorder: a randomized, placebo-controlled, dose-response study. *Pediatrics.* 2001;108(5). Available at: www.pediatrics.org/cgi/content/full/108/5/e83

101. Michelson D, Allen AJ, Busner J, et al. Once-daily atomoxetine treatment for children and adolescents with attention deficit hyperactivity disorder: a randomized, placebo-controlled study. *J Psychiatry.* 2002; 159:1896–1901

102. Brown T. Atomoxetine and stimulants in combination for treatment of attention deficit hyperactivity disorder: four case reports. *J Child Adolesc Psychophamacol.* 2004; 1:129–136

103. Daly J, Wilens T. The use of tricyclic antidepressants in children and adolescents. *Pediatr Clin North Am.* 1998;45:1123–1135

104. Prince J, Wilens T, Biederman J, et al. A controlled study of nortriptyline in children and adolescents with attention deficit hyperactivity disorder. *J Child Adolesc Psychopharmacol.* 2000;10:193–204

105. Riddle M, Geller B, Ryan N. Another sudden death in a child treated with desipramine. *J Am Acad Child Adolesc Psychiatry.* 1993;32:792–797

106. Varley C. Sudden death related to selected tricyclic antidepressants in children: epidemiology, mechanisms and clinical implications. *Paediatr Drugs.* 2001;3:613–627

107. Perrin JM, Stein MT, Amler RW, et al. Clinical practice guideline: treatment of the school-aged child with attention-deficit/hyperactivity disorder. *Pediatrics.* 2001;108:1033–1044

108. Conners CK, Casat CD, Gualtieri TC, et al. Buprorion hydrochloride in attention deficit disorder with hyperactivity. *J Am Acad Child Adolesc Psychiatry.* 1996;35: 1314–1321

109. Davis W, Bentivoglio P, Racusin R, et al. Bupropion SR in adolescents with combined attention deficit hyperactivity disorder and depression. *J Am Acad Child Adolesc Psychiatry.* 2001;40:307–314

110. Conner D, Fletcher K, Swanson J. A meta-analysis of clonidine for symptoms of attention deficit hyperactivity disorder. *J Am Acad Child Adolesc Psychiatry.* 1999;58:1551–1559

111. Kurlan R. Treatment of ADHD in children with tics: a randomized controlled trial. *Neurology.* 2002;58:527–536

112. Scahill L, Chappell P, Kim Y, et al. A placebo-controlled study of guanfacine in the treatment of children with tic disorders and attention deficit hyperactivity disorder. *Am J Psychiatry.* 2001;158:1067–1074

113. Reimherr F, Hedges D, Strong R, Wender P. An open trial of venlafaxine in adult patients with attention deficit hyperactivity disorder. Presented at the annual meeting of the New Clinical Drug Evaluation Unit Program; 1995

114. Zametkin A, Rapaport J, Murphy D, et al. Treatment of hyperactive children with monoamine oxidase inhibitors, I: clinical efficacy. *Arch Gen Psychiatry.* 1985;42:962–966

115. Pelham WEJ, Wheeler T, Chronis A. Empirically supported psychosocial treatments for attention deficit hyperactivity disorder. *J Clin Child Psychol.* 1998;27: 190–205

116. Robin A. Training families with ADHD adolescents. In: Barkley R, ed. *Attention Deficit Hyperactivity Disorder: A Handbook for Diagnosis and Treatment.* New York, NY: Guilford Press; 1990:462–467

117. Evans S, Axelrod JL, Langberg JM. Efficacy of a school-based treatment program for middle school youth with ADHD: pilot data. *Behav Modif.* 2004;28:528–547

118. Evans S, Pelham W, Grudberg M. The efficacy of notetaking to improve behavior and comprehension of adolescents with attention deficit hyperactivity disorder. *Exceptionality.* 1995;5:1–17

119. Wilens T, Biederman J, Mick E, et al. Attention deficit hyperactivity disorder (ADHD) is associated with early onset substance use disorders. *J Nerv Ment Dis.* 1997;185:475–482

120. American Academy of Pediatrics, Committee on Substance Abuse. Testing for drugs of abuse in children and adolescents. *Pediatrics.* 1996;98:305–307

121. Johnston C, Mash E. Families of children with attention deficit hyperactivity disorder: review and recommendations for future research. *Clin Child Family Psychol.* 2001;4:183–207

122. Barkley R, Edwards G, Laneri M, et al. The efficacy of problem solving communication training alone, behavior management training alone, and their combination for parent adolescent conflict in teenagers with ADHD and ODD. *J Consult Clin Psychol.* 2001;69:926–941

123. Waldron H, Slesnick N, Brody JL, et al. Treatment outcomes for adolescent substance abuse at 4- and 7-month assessments. *J Consult Clin Psychol.* 2001;69:802–813

124. Bagwell C, Molina B, Pelham W, Hoza B. Attention deficit hyperactivity disorder and problems in peer relations: predictions from childhood to adolescence. *J Am Acad Child Adolesc Psychiatry.* 2001;40:1285–1292

125. Greene R, Biederman J, Faraone S, et al. Further validation of social impairment as a predictor of substance use disorders: findings from a sample of siblings of boys with and without ADHD. *J Clin Child Psychol.* 1999; 28:349–354

126. Evans S, Langberg J, Williams J. Treatment generalization in school based mental health. In: Weist M, Evans S, Lever N, eds. *Handbook of School Mental Health: Advancing Practice and Research.* New York, NY: Kluwer/Plenum; 2003

127. Gresham F. Social skills training: should we raise, remodel, or rebuild? *Behav Disord.* 1998;24:19–25

128. Pfiffner LJ, McBurnett K. Social skills training with parent generalization: treatment effects for children with attention deficit disorder. *J Couns Clin Psychol.* 1997;65:749–757

129. Cox D, Merkel R, Penberthy J, et al. Impact of methylphenidate delivery profiles on driving performance of adolescents with attention deficit/hyperactivity disorder: a pilot study. *J Am Acad Child Adolesc Psychiatry.* 2004; 43:269–275

130. Alfano C, Zbikowski S, Robinson L, et al. Adolescent reports of physician counseling for smoking. *Pediatrics.* 2002;109:1–6

131. Sanders M, Markie-Dadds C, Turner K. Theoretical, scientific and clinical foundations of the Triple P-Positive Parenting Program: a population approach to the promotion of parenting competence. *Parenting Res Pract Monogr.* 2003;1:1–24

132. American Academy of Pediatrics, Medical Home Initiatives for Children With Special Needs Project Advisory Committee. Policy statement: organizational principles to guide and define the child health care system and/or improve the health of all children. *Pediatrics.* 2004;113(suppl):1545–1547

133. Blum R. Improving transitions for adolescents with special health care needs from pediatric to adult centered health care. *Pediatrics.* 2002;110:1301–1335

134. Ross E. CHADD members document health insurance problems. *Attention.* 2002;9:8–9

135. Newachek P. Trends in private and public health insurance for adolescents. *JAMA.* 2004;2001:60–66

136. White P. Access to health care: health insurance consideration for young adults with special health care needs/disabilities. *Pediatrics.* 2002;110:1328–1333

137. Leibson C, Katusic S, Barbaresi W. Use and costs of medical care for children and adolescents with and without attention deficit hyperactivity disorder. *JAMA.* 2001;285:60–66

138. Social Security Administration, Office of Disability. Understanding SSI Disability for Children. Baltimore, MD: Social Security Administration; 2002

139. American Academy of Pediatrics, Medical Home Initiatives for Children With Special Needs Project Advisory Committee. The medical home. *Pediatrics.* 2002;110:184–186

140. Kelly A. Implementing transitions for youth with complex chronic conditions using the medical home model. *Pediatrics.* 2002;110:1322–1327

141. Milberger S, Biederman J, Faraone SV, et al. ADHD is associated with early initiation of cigarette smoking in children and adolescents. *J Am Acad Child Adolesc Psychiatry.* 1997;36:37–44

142. Applegate B, Lahey BB, Hart E, et al. Validity of the age-of-onset criterion for ADHD: a report from the DSM-IV field trials. *J Am Acad Child Adolesc Psychiatry.* 1997;36:1211–1221

143. National Resource Center on AD/HD. ADHD and the military. Available at: www.ets.org/disability/adhdplcy. html. Accessed April 14, 2005

144. Bramer J. *Succeeding in College with Attention Deficit Disorders.* Plantation, FL: Specialty Press; 1996

145. Dendy C. *After High School: What's Next? Teenagers with ADD: A Parents' Guide.* Bethesda, MD: Woodbine House; 1995:287–313

146. Teter C, McCabe SE, Boyd CJ, Guthrie SK. Illicit methylphenidate use in an undergraduate student sample: prevalence and risk factors. *Pharmacother Ther.* 2003;23:609–617

147. Educational Testing Service, Office of Disabilities and Testing. *Policy Statement for Documentation of Attention Deficit Hyperactivity Disorder in Adolescents and Adults.* Princeton, NJ: Educational Testing Service; 1999

148. ACT. *ACT Policy for Documentation to Support Requests for Testing Accommodations on the ACT Assessment.* Iowa City, IA: ACT; 2004. Available at: www.act.org/aap/disab/ policy.html. Accessed April 14, 2005

149. Consortium on ADHD Documentation. *Guidelines for Documentation of Attention Deficity Hyperactivity Disorder in Adolescents and Adults.* Consortium on ADHD Documentation; 2004. Available at: www.act.org/ aap/disa/appx.html. Accessed April 14, 2005

150. College Board Services for Students with Disabilities. *Nonstandard Designation Removal.* New York, NY: The College Board; 2004. Available at: http://apcentral. collegeboard.com/article/0,3045,149-0-0-21272,00.html. Accessed April 14, 2005

151. Mannuzza S, Klein RG, Bessler A, et al. Educational and occupational outcome of hyperactive boys grown up. *J Am Acad Child Adolesc Psychiatry.* 1997;36:1222–1227

152. Murphy K, Barkley RA, Bush T. Young adults with attention deficit hyperactivity disorder: subtype differences in comorbidity, educational and clinical history. *J Nerv Ment Dis.* 2002;190:147–157

153. National Resource Center on ADHD. *College Issues for Students with ADHD.* Landover, MD: National Resource Center on ADHD; 2004

154. Attention Deficit Disorder Association, Subcommittee on ADD Coaching. *The ADDA Guiding Principles for Coaching Individuals with Attention Deficit Disorder.* Pottstown, PA: Attention Deficit Disorder Association; 2002

155. CHADD: Children and Adults with Attention-Deficit/ Hyperactivity Disorder. Home page. Available at: www.chadd.org

156. National Resource Center on ADHD. Educational issues. Available at: www.help4adhd.org/en/education/college

157. Attention Deficit Disorders Association. Home page. Available at: www.add.org

158. Dendy CAZ. *Teenagers with ADD: A Parents' Guide.* Bethesda, MD: Woodbine House; 1995

159. Bramer JS. *Succeeding in College with Attention Deficit Disorders.* Plantation, FL: Specialty Press; 1996

160. Nadeau KG, Littman EB, Quinn PO. *Understanding Girls with AD/HD.* Silver Spring, MD: Advantage Books; 1999

161. Taymans JM, West LL. *Selecting a College for Students with Learning Disabilities or Attention Deficit Hyperactivity Disorder (ADHD): ERIC Digest.* Arlington, VA: ERIC Clearinghouse on Disabilities and Gifted Education; 2001

162. Dendy CAZ, Zeigler A. *A Bird's-Eye View of Life with ADD and ADHD: Advice from Young Survivors.* Cedar Bluff, AL: Cherish the Children; 2003

The Central Serotonin Syndrome: Paradigm for Psychotherapeutic Misadventure

Donald H. Arnold, MD, FAAP*

Case Presentation 1

Sharon is a 16-year-old adolescent well known to you since you became her pediatrician in early childhood. Sunday morning at 3 AM you receive an urgent call from the emergency department at your community hospital where she presented after collapsing while dancing at a local "rave" party. You are informed that she is agitated, confused, and disoriented; has a high fever; and is having seizures. The emergency department physician has administered intravenous lorazepam and rectal acetaminophen and requests your presence immediately.

You arrive at the emergency department as quickly as possible. The physician who called you notes that the seizure activity diminished after two doses of lorazepam, but he is preparing to administer fosphenytoin because she continues to jerk her arms and legs. You obtain a brief history from her parents, who arrived several minutes before you.

The parents remind you that Sharon has been treated with sertraline 150 mg/d for generalized anxiety disorder. They state that she has been otherwise happy, healthy, and on no other medications. She recently obtained her driving permit and was allowed to go out with several friends earlier in the evening.

Sharon's vital signs are: temperature, 106.7°F (41.5°C); heart rate, 145 beats/min; respiratory rate, 20 breaths/min; blood pressure, 162/96 mm Hg; and SaO$_2$, 99%. She is agitated and diaphoretic. There are coarse, nonpurposeful jerking motions and hypertonia of the extremities. The pupils are equal and reactive, and there are no asymmetric or localizing neurologic abnormalities.

At this moment, determining a unifying process that would explain the abrupt onset of altered mental status, the extreme hyperthermia and other vital sign abnormalities, and the myoclonic seizurelike activity and hypertonia is a tremendous challenge. Your differential diagnosis includes toxic ingestion, infectious encephalitis, and closed-head trauma.

Sharon's boyfriend has been waiting in the triage area, and you speak with him. He states that at the "rave," Sharon collapsed while dancing and began shaking. After you emphasize the critical importance of knowing any recreational drugs used, he informs you that she tried her first dose of ecstasy (MDMA) about 2 hours before her collapse.

You immediately consult the toxicologist at the regional poison control center and learn that the toxic syndrome associated with ecstasy is believed possibly to represent "serotonin syndrome." She assists in planning diagnostic tests and treatment. Because the hyperthermia has not and is not expected to respond to antipyretics, nondepolarizing neuromuscular paralysis and endotracheal intubation are undertaken, and external cooling with cooling blankets is initiated.

While preparations are being made for transfer to the pediatric intensive care unit at a nearby children's hospital, diagnostic studies are obtained. Results include normal head computed tomography, sinus tachycardia and mildly peaked T waves on electrocardiography, negative urine human chorionic gonadotropin, and negative urine drug screen. The salicylate level is less than 5 mg/dL (0.36 mmol/L), creatine kinase (CK) is 1,550 U/L, serum sodium is 135 mEq/L (135 mmol/L), potassium is 5.4 mEq/L (5.4 mmol/L), chloride is 112 mEq/L (112 mmol/L), bicarbonate is 16 mEq/L (16 mmol/L), glucose is 110 mg/dL (6.1 mmol/), and alanine aminotransferase is

*Assistant Professor, Departments of Emergency Medicine and Pediatrics, Vanderbilt University School of Medicine, Nashville, TN
Pediatrics in Review, *Vol 23, No. 12, December 2002*

110 U/L. Results of a complete blood count and screening studies for disseminated intravascular coagulation are normal.

Paralysis and assisted ventilation are continued as well as intravenous fluids and diuresis for presumed rhabdomyolysis. The following evening, approximately 18 hours after her initial presentation, a normal body temperature is maintained without external cooling measures, serum potassium is 3.6 mEq/L (3.6 mmol/L), and CK is 940 U/L. She is weaned from paralysis, sedation, and assisted ventilation the following morning, at which time muscle tone and mental status are normal. CK continues to decrease over the ensuing 48 hours, and renal function is normal.

Case Presentation 2

Will, a 9-year-old boy seen by one of your associates in conjunction with a child psychiatrist, has been maintained on fluvoxamine 100 mg/d for obsessive-compulsive disorder (OCD) with good result. On a Saturday afternoon in November, you receive a frantic call from his father, who explains that Will has not been able to walk since mid-morning. They did not want to bother you initially because he has had the flu, and they thought he was having muscle cramps. When his fever began to exceed 105°F (40.5°C) and he appeared agitated, they realized the seriousness of the situation.

Because you do not know the patient well, you question the parent in detail and are told that, except for the boy's history of OCD, he has been well. He has not received aspirin and, except for two doses of dextromethorphan syrup for cough at 3 AM and 9 AM, has not received other medications. You ask them to meet you at the emergency department immediately and request that they bring all of Will's medications.

As you discuss this case with the emergency department physician, you see Will being assisted to a bed by the triage nurse and his parents. He ambulates with difficulty, appearing to shiver and to be stiff. As the nurse obtains vital signs, you review the history with Will and his parents. The boy is anxious and mildly agitated, but he can tell you that he has not ingested any other medicines except his daily medication and the cough

medicine. You inspect the latter, noting that it contains dextromethorphan and guaifenesin but no sympathomimetic or antihistamine. His parents insist that he was behaving normally the prior evening and that there has been no head trauma.

Will's vital signs are: temperature, 105.8°F (41°C); heart rate, 160 beats/min; respiratory rate, 26 breaths/min; blood pressure, 142/96 mm Hg; and SaO_2, 100%. He appears anxious and somewhat agitated and has coarse shivering of the extremities and bright red facial flushing. His pupils are dilated to 6 mm but briskly and equally reactive. Although there are no localizing neurologic findings, you do note hyperactive tendon reflexes and bilateral ankle clonus. Results of the remainder of the examination are normal. You wonder if the fever, tachycardia, tachypnea, hypertension, muscle stiffness, and facial rash are from influenza or due to Reye syndrome.

You order rectal acetaminophen, intravenous access, and screening laboratory tests, including complete blood count, blood cultures, and an ammonia level, results of which subsequently are reported as normal. A rapid nasal influenza test is positive for influenza A. While awaiting these results and with Will's medications in hand, you speak with the on-call pharmacist. After reviewing a drug interaction database, he reports that serotonin syndrome has been reported after dextromethorphan administration to patients who are receiving selective serotonin reuptake inhibitors (SSRIs). You consult the regional poison control center for further assistance in diagnosis and management.

You obtain additional recommended laboratory studies, which all have normal results, including an initial CK measurement. External cooling measures, including mist, fans, and cooling blankets, are instituted, and intravenous fluids are administered at 1.5 times maintenance with good urine output. Because Will can swallow oral medications safely, you administer doses of clonazepam and cyproheptadine. Over the next 8 hours, the shivering and stiffness appear to diminish, and his temperature is maintained at approximately 104°F (40°C). The following morning, Will is afebrile and appears to have returned to his normal baseline. A CK level that afternoon of 960 U/L decreases to normal levels over the subsequent 36 hours, and serum blood urea nitrogen and creatinine concentrations and urinalysis results remain normal. Outpatient management includes follow-up with his psychiatrist with the goal of adequately managing Will's OCD while avoiding future medication complications.

Background

Central serotonin syndrome (CSS) is an iatrogenic complication resulting from the use of drugs and dietary supplements that have central nervous system (CNS) serotonin (5-HT) activity. CSS is a constellation of signs and symptoms that may be confused with other disorders, including those for which the medications are being used. It is believed to result from excess stimulation of 5-HT_{1A} and possibly 5-HT_{2A} receptors in the CNS. It is distinctly different from carcinoid syndrome and other disorders resulting from the peripheral actions of 5-HT and most frequently results when two or more drugs that have serotonergic activity are combined. It occurs infrequently after single drug use.

Serotonin is one of the most widely distributed substances in the animal and plant kingdoms both as a biologically active amine and as a venom. Initially isolated from 30 kg of octopus salivary glands, 5-HT was isolated in humans by Rapport in 1948 and identified as a vasoconstrictor released by platelets and involved in blood clotting. The concurrent development of antituberculosis drugs with monoamine oxidase inhibitor (MAOI) activity (iproniazid) and their use with serotonergic drugs (meperidine) occasionally resulted in drug reactions now recognized as the CSS, some of which were fatal.

An epidemic of eosinophiliamyalgia syndrome in 1989 appeared to result from a contaminant in imported L-tryptophan sold as a dietary supplement. Although temporarily removed from the market, this serotonergic agent is being sold again. Additionally, the continued use of tricyclic antidepressants, the increasing use of other serotonergic agents (SSRIs, SRIs), and the improved recognition of CSS have resulted in an acceleration of reported cases. It is important for clinicians to be familiar with and to recognize CSS because the condition is potentially fatal, altered 5-HT function underlies many medical and psychiatric conditions, many medications interact with 5-HT receptors or with other serotonergic medications, and recognition and management of CSS depend on an awareness of central 5-HT function.

Neuropharmacology of 5-HT

Only 2% of total body 5-HT is located in the CNS; approximately 90% and 8% are in the enterochromaffin cells of the gastrointestinal tract and in platelets, respectively. 5-HT does not cross the blood-brain barrier, and it is synthesized within the CNS serotonergic neurons from the essential amino acid tryptophan. The latter crosses the blood-brain barrier, enters the neuron, and is hydroxylated to 5-HT. 5-HT is stored in vesicles and, on neuronal stimulation, is released into the synapse whereupon it binds to pre- and postsynaptic receptors. Synaptic 5-HT is pumped back into the neuron where it is recycled into vesicles or metabolized by MAO enzyme residing on mitochondrial membranes. Stimulation of presynaptic 5-HT_{1A} and 5-HT_{1D} receptors limit further 5-HT release.

Serotonergic CNS neuronal cell bodies are located in nuclei in the midline brainstem, with axonal projections superior to the thalamus and cortex and inferior to the medulla and spinal cord. Unlike the other CNS monoamine neurotransmitter systems (norepinephrine, dopamine), 5-HT generally functions as a slow modulator and inhibitor of CNS function, influencing affect, personality, sleep, appetite, sexual function, aggression, pain perception, learning, and probably other as yet unrecognized functions. Seven classes and fifteen subclasses of 5-HT receptors have been identified, accounting in part for the protean effects of this neurotransmitter system.

Theory of CSS Causation

With the development and clinical introduction of tricyclic antidepressants, MAOI agents, and more recently SSRI/SRIs, clinicians noted a delay in their antidepressant effects, generally of several weeks' duration. This phenomenon was not consistent with their immediate biochemical action of increasing synaptic 5-HT. Researchers hypothesized that changes in pre- and postsynaptic receptor density and sensitivity accounted for these delayed effects. As applied to 5-HT, the "serotonin receptor neurotransmitter hypothesis" at least partially accounts for CSS and its development most frequently after the addition of a second serotonergic agent. This theory holds that:

1. In the depressed patient, there is a relative state of 5-HT deficiency, resulting in upregulation of 5-HT_{1A} presynaptic autoreceptors and postsynaptic receptors.

2. Introduction of an SSRI or other reuptake blocker initially predominantly affects the presynaptic inhibitory autoreceptor, causing downregulation of these inhibitory autoreceptors over days to weeks.

3. This downregulation results in increased neuronal impulse flow and increased synaptic 5-HT release.

4. Increased synaptic 5-HT causes postsynaptic 5-HT receptor downregulation and elevated mood.

5. In this milieu of altered receptor physiology, the addition of a second serotonergic medication may increase synaptic 5-HT and postsynaptic 5-HT_{1A} stimulation rapidly, resulting in manifestations of CSS.

The multiple steps in 5-HT synthesis, distribution, and metabolism are reflected in the numbers of serotonergic medications, any of which has the potential to precipitate CSS (Table 1).

As of 1995, the most frequent combinations of agents leading to CSS involved an MAOI plus an SSRI, tricyclic antidepressant, meperidine, dextromethorphan, or L-tryptophan. However, with the increasing use of newer SSRIs, a trend toward cases involving these agents has been noted.

Although several hundred cases have been reported, the incidence of CSS is not well defined, in part due to lack of recognition of mild cases (*formes frustes*), misdiagnosis, and confusion with other similar disorders. More than 20 deaths and a mortality rate of 11% to 15% due to CSS have been reported. Of particular concern are cases of CSS and deaths resulting from the use of ecstasy (MDMA).

Table 1. Serotonergic Medications

Increase 5-HT Synthesis
- L-tryptophan

Increase Synaptic Release
- Amphetamine
- Cocaine
- Ecstasy (MDMA)
- Fenfluramine
- Mescaline
- Psilocin
- L-dopa/carbidopa

Serotonin Agonists
- Lithium
- LSD

Inhibit Reuptake
- Selective serotonin reuptake inhibitors
- Serotonin reuptake inhibitors
- Tricyclic antidepressants
- Meperidine
- Dextromethorphan (DM)
- MDMA

Inhibit Breakdown
- Monoamine oxidase inhibitors
- MDMA

Clinical Manifestations

The triad of cognitive/behavioral, autonomic, and neuromuscular abnormalities characterizes CSS. Both the pathogenesis and clinical presentation are distinct from those of SSRI or tricyclic antidepressant overdose and from the peripheral manifestations of serotonin excess (carcinoid syndrome). The diagnosis is based on the exclusion of other processes (in particular, neuroleptic malignant syndrome and other toxic and metabolic encephalopathies), on a compatible drug history, and on fulfillment of criteria. A review of 127 patients reported in the literature provides insight to potential presentations (Table 2).

Although criteria suggested by Sternbach are useful (Table 3), it must be recognized that many cases of CSS are incomplete or mild and do not fully satisfy these criteria. Recognition of these *formes frustes* allows appropriate patient treatment.

Table 2. Clinical Manifestations of Central Serotonin Syndrome

Cognitive/Behavioral	
Confusion/disorientation	54%
Agitation/irritability	35%
Coma	28%
Anxiety	16%
Hypomania/seizures/hallucinations	15%
Autonomic	
Hyperthermia	46%
Diaphoresis	46%
Sinus tachycardia	41%
Hypertension	33%
Tachypnea/mydriasis	27%
Neuromuscular	
Myoclonus	57%
Hyperreflexia	50%
Muscle rigidity/tremor	49%
Hyperactivity/restlessness	42%
Ataxia	38%

Adapted from Mills, 1997.

Differential Diagnosis

Because the CSS consists of a syndromic cluster of signs and symptoms, difficulty in diagnosis may result from failure to consider CSS or from confusion with other diagnostic entities (Table 4). A comprehensive medication history is vital.

Neuroleptic malignant syndrome (NMS) is perhaps the most frequently confused entity, at least in part because certain features and even aspects of the neurotransmitter causes of NMS and CSS overlap. Blockade of dopamine (D_2) receptors in the basal ganglia is believed to precipitate NMS, and 5-HT decreases dopamine secretion. Conversely, dopamine enhances 5-HT release. However, the two syndromes generally can be distinguished according to presenting features (Table 5).

Ecstasy (MDMA): A Special Note

Particular reference should be made of ecstasy (MDMA), a recreational "club drug" popularized for its purported beneficial effects, including "entactogenesis" (all is right and good with the world) and "empathogenesis" (emotional closeness to others and to oneself). MDMA generally is regarded as safe by the lay public and is a frequent part of "raves." Users dance for prolonged periods in a warm environment and consume amino acid drinks to enhance the experience. Unfortunately, the heat and the tryptophan in these drinks, combined with MDMA, enhance the likelihood of CSS. Multiple cases in the medical literature report morbidity and mortality from MDMA and encompass extreme hyperthermia, muscle rigidity leading to rhabdomyolysis and myoglobinuric renal failure, coagulopathy, autonomic instability, and status epilepticus. That MDMA is both a potent stimulus for 5-HT release and an inhibitor of reuptake may account for the recognition that many of these cases represent MDMA-induced

Table 3. The Sternbach Criteria

Criteria A, B, and C required for diagnosis.

A. Coincident with the addition of or increase in a known serotonergic agent to an established medication regimen, at least three of the following clinical features are present:
1. Mental status changes (confusion, hypomania)
2. Agitation
3. Myoclonus
4. Muscle rigidity (usually lower extremities predominating)
5. Hyperreflexia
6. Diaphoresis
7. Shivering
8. Tremor
9. Diarrhea
10. Incoordination
11. Fever

B. Other causes (eg, infectious, metabolic, substance abuse or withdrawal) have been ruled out.

C. A neuroleptic agent had not been started or increased in dosage prior to the onset of the signs and symptoms listed previously.

Table 4. Partial List of Conditions for the Differential Diagnosis of CSS

Toxic syndromes
- Ingestions
  - Anticholinergics
  - Sympathomimetics
  - Salicylates
- Withdrawal states
  - Barbiturates
  - Ethanol
  - Sedative-hypnotics

Infections
- Central nervous system
- Sepsis-systemic inflammatory response syndrome

Neuroleptic malignant syndrome (NMS)

Table 5. Comparison of Central Serotonin Syndrome (CSS) and Neuroleptic Malignant Syndrome (NMS)

	CSS	NMS
Cause	5-HT$_{1A/2A}$ agonists	D$_2$ antagonists
Symptom onset after drug change	Minutes to hours	Days to weeks
Symptom resolution	<24 h	7 to 10 d
Hyperthermia	46%	>90%
Altered mental status	54%	>90%
Autonomic changes	50% to 90%	>90%
Muscle rigidity	49% (legs > arms)	>90% (lead pipe)
Myoclonus/hyperreflexia	57%	Rare

Adapted from Brent, 2001.

CSS. The significance of this association must be recognized because cases of MDMA toxicity may respond to measures used in the management of CSS.

Management

Perhaps the most important consideration in evaluation and management is to be aware of the possibility of CSS in any patient who is taking or has access to serotonergic medications. The contributions of laboratory evaluation are limited. Drug levels usually are within therapeutic ranges, rarely are available on a timely basis, and almost never assist in management. Other laboratory tests (eg, electrocardiography, aspirin and other toxin screens, and measurement of electrolytes) primarily are used to exclude other diagnoses. If muscles are rigid, serum CK levels should be monitored; urine globin screens are inadequate for this purpose.

Treatment begins with discontinuation of serotonergic agents and provision of supportive care and monitoring that includes airway, breathing, and circulation (ABCs); intravenous fluids; and hemodynamic monitoring. It is important to anticipate and treat complications. Hyperthermia is due to muscle rigidity and may indicate a poor prognosis. It must be treated aggressively with external cooling measures (antipyretics are not effective), benzodiazepines (particularly clonazepam) and, if necessary, nondepolarizing paralysis and endotracheal intubation/ventilation.

Myoclonus may respond to clonazepam. Seizures should be treated with benzodiazepines and phenobarbital. Patients should be monitored for rhabdomyolysis/myoglobinuria, disseminated intravascular coagulation, and metabolic acidosis and treated accordingly. It may be appropriate to consider administration of antiserotonergic medications. Propranolol offers specific 5-HT$_{1A}$ postsynaptic receptor blockade, although results of propranolol treatment are not conclusive. Some authors recommend intravenous propranolol followed by oral cyproheptadine when tolerated. Cyproheptadine offers nonspecific postsynaptic 5-HT$_{1A}$ and 5-HT$_2$ blockade. Multiple case reports support its potential benefit.

To prevent future recurrence of CSS, it is important to assess the need for future serotonergic drug treatment. Many of these medications have long half-lives and require a washout period before introducing other serotonergic medications (MAOIs require 4 weeks of washout). Clinicians always should obtain a careful, comprehensive drug history and avoid using multiple drugs that have serotonergic activity or interactions (eg, MAOIs, tricyclic antidepressants, SSRIs, meperidine, dextromethorphan).

Outcome

CSS is associated with a mortality rate of 11% to 15%. Morbidity can be reduced substantially with aggressive diagnostic and management measures. Most cases of CSS resolve within 24 hours of drug discontinuation. However, most cases also can be prevented if practitioners keep in mind the possibility of CSS resulting from serotonergic medications, particularly when more than one such agent is used.

Suggested Reading

Ames D, Wirshing WC. Ecstasy, the serotonin syndrome, and neuroleptic malignant syndrome—a possible link? *JAMA.* 1993; 269:869–870

Barbey JT, Roose SP. SSRI safety in overdose. *J Clin Psychiatry.* 1998;59(suppl):42–48

Brent J. Serotonin reuptake inhibitors, newer antidepressants, and the serotonin syndrome. In: Ford MD, ed. *Clinical Toxicology.* 1st ed. Philadelphia, Pa: WB Saunders; 2001:522–531

Cargone JR. The neuroleptic malignant and serotonin syndromes. *Emerg Med Clin North Am.* 2000;18:317–325

Coyle JT. Drug treatment of anxiety disorders in children. *N Engl J Med.* 2001;34:1326–1327

Lappin RI, Auchincloss EL. Treatment of the serotonin syndrome with cyproheptadine. *N Engl J Med.* 1994;331: 1021–1022

LoCurto MJ. The serotonin syndrome. *Emerg Med Clin North Am.* 1997;15:665–675

Mills KC. Serotonin syndrome. *Crit Care Clin.* 1997;13: 763–783

Mills KC. Serotonin toxicity: a comprehensive review for emergency medicine. *Top Emerg Med.* 1993;15:54–73

Mullins ME, Horowitz BZ. Serotonin syndrome after a single dose of fluvoxamine. *Ann Emerg Med.* 1999;34:806–807

Nierenberg DW, Semprebon M. The central nervous system serotonin syndrome. *Clin Pharmacol Ther.* 1993;53:84–88

Rushon JL, Whitmire JT. Pediatric stimulant and selective serotonin reuptake inhibitor prescription trends 1992 to 1998. *Arch Pediatr Adolesc Med.* 2001;155:560–565

Sanders-Bush E, Mayer SE. 5-Hydroxytryptamine (serotonin) receptor agonists and antagonists. In: Hardman J, Limbird L, ed. *Goodman and Gilman's The Pharmacological Basis of Therapeutics.* 9th ed. New York, NY: McGraw Hill; 1996: 249–263

Sporer KA. The serotonin syndrome. Implicated drugs, pathophysiology and management. *Drug Safety.* 1995;13:94–104

Stahl SM. *Essential Psychopharmacology. Neuroscientific Basis and Practical Applications.* Cambridge, United Kingdom: Cambridge University Press; 1996

Sternbach H. The serotonin syndrome. *Am J Psychiatry.* 1991;148:705–713

Wolraich ML. Increased psychotropic medication use. Are we improving mental health care by drugging our kids? *Arch Pediatr Adolesc Med.* 2001;155:545

Zito JM, Safer DJ, dosReis S, Gardner JF, Boles M, Lynch F. Trends in the prescribing of psychotropic medications to preschoolers. *JAMA.* 2000;283:1025–1030

Children and Adolescents Who Have Schizophrenia

Adriana E. Groisman, MD, and Martha L. Seminatore, MD

Practice Parameter for the Assessment and Treatment of Children and Adolescents with Schizophrenia. McClellan J, Werry J, and the Work Group on Quality Issues of the AACAP. *J Am Acad Child Adolesc Psychiatry.* 2001;40(suppl):4S–23S

Symptom Factors in Early-Onset Psychotic Disorders. McClellan J, McCurry C, Speltz ML, Jones K. *J Am Acad Child Adolesc Psychiatry.* 2002;41:791–798

Substance Abuse and Emergency Psychiatry. Zealberg JJ, Brady KT. *Psychiatr Clin North Am.* 1999;22:808–817

Diagnostic and Statistical Manual of Mental Disorders. 4th ed (*DSM-IV*). Washington, DC: American Psychiatric Association; 1994:273–315

Schizophrenia is a chronic disorder associated with deficits in cognition, affect, and social functioning. The onset of illness can occur rarely as early as 5 years of age, but after the age of 13 years, the incidence increases steadily.

Early-onset (before age 18 y) and very early-onset (before age 13 y) schizophrenia are diagnosed by using the same criteria as in adults, and these forms appear to be continuous with the adult form of the disorder. Youths who have schizophrenia are predominantly males, have high rates of premorbid abnormalities and higher ratings on negative and positive symptoms, and often exhibit poor outcome.

Schizophrenia is a phasic disorder, with individual variability. The phases are:

Prodrome Phase: Period of deteriorating function that includes social isolation, idiosyncratic or bizarre preoccupations, unusual behaviors, academic problems, and deteriorating self-care skills.

Acute Phase: Period dominated by positive psychotic symptoms (hallucinations, delusions, formal thought disorder, bizarre psychotic behavior) and functional deterioration.

Recovery Phase: At this point, active psychosis begins to remit, but some psychotic symptoms are present, and there may be confusion, disorganization, or dysphoria.

Residual Phase: In this phase, positive psychotic symptoms are minimal, but negative symptoms are still present (social withdrawal, apathy, amotivation, flat affect).

Chronic Impairment Phase: In some patients, symptoms persist and do not respond to treatment.

According to the *DSM-IV* diagnostic criteria, at least two of the following symptoms should be present for a significant period of time during a 1-month period:

- Delusions
- Hallucinations
- Disorganized speech
- Grossly disorganized or catatonic behavior
- Negative symptoms such as flat affect and paucity of thought or speech

Only one symptom is needed if the delusions are bizarre, hallucinations include a voice providing running commentary on the person's behavior or thinking, or two or more voices are conversing with each other.

Another criterion is the deterioration of social, occupational, and self-care functioning below the level achieved before onset. For children and adolescents, this includes the failure to achieve age-appropriate levels of interpersonal, academic, or occupational development. The disturbances also must be present for at least 6 months.

Conditions in the differential diagnosis must be excluded, such as mood disorders (especially bipolar disorder), pervasive developmental disorders, nonpsychotic emotional and behavioral disturbances (including posttraumatic stress

Jacobi Medical Center, Albert Einstein College of Medicine, Bronx, NY
Pediatrics in Review, *Vol 24, No. 10, October 2003*

disorder), and organic conditions. The list of potential organic causes is vast and encompasses: seizure disorders, central nervous system lesions (eg, brain tumors, head trauma), neurodegenerative disorders (eg, Huntington chorea, lipid storage disorders), metabolic disorders (eg, endocrinopathies, Wilson disease), developmental disorders (eg, velocardiofacial syndrome), toxic encephalopathies (eg, abuse of substances such as amphetamines, cocaine, hallucinogens, phencyclidine, alcohol, marijuana, and solvents; medications such as stimulants, corticosteroids, or anticholinergic agents; and other toxins such as heavy metals), and infectious diseases (eg, encephalitis, meningitis, or human immunodeficiency virus-related syndromes).

Intoxication or withdrawal from drugs or alcohol can mimic nearly every psychiatric disorder, including mania, schizophrenia, or other psychotic disorders. Physiologic manifestations and urine drug screening are critical in diagnosing a substance-induced psychosis, but substance use disorders also are common among patients who have schizophrenia. As many as 50% of affected patients have a history of alcohol or illicit drug dependency. For this reason, urine drug screening is critical to evaluate the cause of psychotic exacerbation. If psychotic symptoms persist for more than 1 week after drug detoxification, a primary psychotic disorder is more likely.

Laboratory and neuroimaging procedures are not helpful in diagnosing schizophrenia, but they are used to rule out other neurologic or medical problems. They should be justified on the basis of the clinical presentation and findings in either the history or the physical examination.

Once the diagnosis is established, it needs to be reassessed longitudinally because misdiagnosis at the time of onset is common. Most children who have hallucinations do not have schizophrenia.

The treatment of schizophrenia in children and adolescents combines psychopharmacologic agents and psychosocial interventions. Therapies vary, depending on the individual patient characteristics and the stage of the disorder. Both factors are specific for the symptomatology (positive and negative) of the disorder and general in relation to the psychological, social, educational, and cultural needs of the child and the family.

Comment: Schizophrenia rarely occurs before age 13 years, but the onset increases steadily during adolescence, peaking between ages 15 and 30 years. It is believed to be a neurodevelopmental disorder; there is no evidence of causation from psychological or social factors. Adult schizophrenia is associated with perinatal complications, abnormal brain structure and size, minor physical anomalies, and disruption of fetal neural development (especially in the second trimester of gestation). Early developmental delays, including cognitive, language, and communication delays, and neurobiological abnormalities (deficits in smooth pursuit eye movements, autonomic responsivity, and neuroimaging findings) may be early manifestations of the disorder. Approximately 10% to 20% of children who have schizophrenia have intelligence quotients in the borderline to mentally retarded range. Outcome is predicted best by premorbid and cognitive functioning, negative symptoms, and behavioral problems. The risk of self-inflicted and unintentional injury related to psychotic thinking is high and is associated with high rates of mortality.

Psychopharmacology includes traditional neuroleptics that block dopamine receptors and atypical antipsychotics that have a variety of effects, such as antagonism of serotonergic receptors. Psychoeducational therapy for patients and families include education about the illness and social skills training for the patient. Unfortunately, studies on the effectiveness of these interventions in children are limited.

The Practice Parameter for the Assessment and Treatment of Children and Adolescents with Schizophrenia of the American Academy of Child and Adolescent Psychiatry referenced previously is important reading for care of these patients.

Tina L. Cheng, MD, MPH
Associate Editor, In Brief

Delinquent Behavior

J. David Hawkins, PhD, * *Brian H. Smith, MSW,* * *Richard F. Catalano, PhD* *

Objectives

After completing this article, readers should be able to:

1. Describe the general pattern of delinquency prevalence in the child and adolescent populations. ·
2. Explain the significance and characteristics of chronic offending delinquents.
3. Describe the co-occurrence of other problem behaviors with delinquency.
4. Identify common risk and protective factors predictive of delinquency.
5. Identify examples of effective and ineffective interventions.

Introduction

Juvenile delinquency, a major public concern in the United States, refers to illegal acts committed by youth younger than age 18 years. A subset of chronic juvenile offenders is responsible for a majority of juvenile crime. These juveniles are products of interactions between individual and environmental factors, and their lives often are characterized by the presence of other problems, including drug use, mental health problems, and school failure. This article is a guide to assessing the potential significance of involvement in delinquent behavior. It also summarizes current knowledge about the developmental epidemiology of delinquency, the antecedent risk and protective factors predictive of delinquency, and effective approaches to prevention and treatment that can be used in pediatric practice.

Epidemiology

Two sources of data on juvenile delinquency are available: official reports of arrests and referrals to juvenile court and self-reports of behavior. Most juveniles report committing at least one delinquent act, and many are involved in some type of delinquent behavior each year. This appears to be relatively constant over time and across geographic areas. Even though a majority of youths self-report involvement in chargeable offenses, only about one third of all adolescents are arrested. Arrest data are limited to offenders who are apprehended by the police. In a multiethnic sample drawn from high-crime neighborhoods in Seattle, 33.8% of youths were referred to juvenile court for at least one delinquent offense compared with 86.3% of youths who self-reported involvement in delinquent acts. Research has shown that police policies and behavior are important determinants of who is arrested and may mask the underlying delinquent behavior. Self-report measures provide an important epidemiologic alternative to arrest measures. Although both urban and rural youth report nearly equal levels of involvement in delinquent behaviors, urban juveniles are significantly more likely to be arrested. Similarly, studies comparing arrest records with self-report data have shown that African-American juveniles involved in delinquency are substantially more likely to be arrested than European-American juveniles. These data caution against relying only on a juvenile's arrest history when assessing involvement in delinquent behavior.

Social Development Research Group, School of Social Work, University of Washington, Seattle, WA.

Drs. Hawkins and Catalano are consultants to the Channing Bete Company, distributor of the Preparing for the Drug-Free Years, the Preparing for School Success curricula, and SOAR training materials. These programs were tested in the intervention described in this article.

Generally low levels of delinquent behavior are observed among children prior to age 10 years, but this is followed by increasing prevalence from age 10 to 16 years and a subsequent declining prevalence to age 21 years. The pattern for serious violent behavior appears to be a similar inverted U-shaped curve, with prevalence peaking slightly later (age 17), then rapidly falling to prevalence levels of 12- to 13-year-olds by age 21 to 24 years and decreasing further in the late twenties. Thus, for most forms of delinquent behavior, there is a clear pattern of growth during early adolescence followed by a predictable decline in the late teens and into the twenties.

Only a small proportion of offenders commits the majority of juvenile offenses. Both self-report studies and studies of arrest records have found that 6% to 8% of youths involved in delinquent behavior are responsible for 50% to 70% of the crimes committed by young people and 60% to 85% of the serious and violent crimes. The lives of chronic juvenile offenders tend to be marked by problems in multiple domains, and these individuals are disproportionately victims of violence themselves. About 50% of chronic offenders begin their delinquency before age 12 years, and most have begun committing serious offenses by age 14 years. Youths involved in serious delinquency at early ages show a high rate of continued serious offending, but others who were involved only in minor delinquency before age 13 years also commit serious offenses in late adolescence. This latter group constitutes the majority of serious delinquent offenders, indicating that early initiation of serious offending is not a prerequisite for later serious delinquency.

Males account for more than two thirds of juvenile arrests overall, but arrests of female juveniles have increased relative to males in recent years. Juvenile females comprised 22% of the arrests for aggravated assault in 1999; they accounted for more than 50% of the juvenile arrests for running away from home. Males, once arrested, are more than twice as likely as females to be arrested again while still younger than age 18 years and almost four times as likely to accumulate four or more juvenile arrests. Male delinquents also are approximately three times as likely as females to be arrested for a serious offense.

Gang membership is an important factor in delinquency. Although associating with other delinquents is one of the strongest predictors of delinquent behavior, gang members commit a disproportionate number of both nonviolent and violent offenses, even when compared with other youths who have delinquent friends. In 1996, the National Youth Gang Survey estimated that gangs were active in more than 4,700 United States cities. Gangs have moved beyond their urban origins and are becoming more common in rural areas, suburbs, and small towns. Although females sometimes are involved, youth gangs are 90% male.

Delinquent behavior overlaps with other forms of health-compromising behaviors. A large proportion of those engaged in delinquent behavior also has problems with school, substance use, risky sexual behavior, and mental health. Rates of alcohol use and illicit drug use are higher for youths who report general delinquent involvement, and among delinquents, they are higher for those who commit more serious offenses compared with those who commit minor offenses. Youth who evidence school problems, drug and alcohol use, risky sexual behavior, delinquency, or mental health concerns should be assessed for other co-occurring problems. The nature of the relationships among co-occurring problems is the subject of continuing research. For example, depression has been found to be highly correlated with delinquency, and some research suggests that early conduct problems often precede and even may contribute to depression in adolescents and young adults. Importantly, many of these co-occurring adolescent health, mental health, and behavior problems are predicted by common factors that can be observed earlier in development and addressed as they are recognized to prevent the emergence of these problems. These predictors are described in the next section.

Causes

Multiple predictors of delinquency have been identified in longitudinal studies. These factors either increase the likelihood of future delinquency (risk factors) or decrease the likelihood of future delinquency by either moderating or mediating risk exposure (protective factors). The risk factors that have been found to predict problem behaviors are detailed in the Table.

A number of factors commonly believed to predict juvenile crime have not been substantiated by research. Although often considered to be a cause of delinquency, impulsivity and inattention are weakly predictive of delinquent behavior by themselves and only become strong risk factors when combined with early physical aggression. Similarly, studies have shown that learning disabilities alone do not lead to increased offending. Although low self-esteem commonly has been thought to underlie a host of adolescent problems, the research on this topic indicates otherwise. Longitudinal studies clearly show that low self-esteem is not a risk factor for crime, delinquency, violence, or drug use, although it is a risk factor for suicide attempts, depression, and eating disorders.

Given the proportion of crimes committed by chronic and serious offenders, it is important to consider the specific risk factors that characterize this group. From ages 6 to 11 years, youths who become chronic offenders are more likely to exhibit persistent behavior problems, aggression, and substance use and to come from families of low socioeconomic status that include antisocial parents. From ages 10 to 12 years, later chronic offending is predicted by aggressive behavior, having antisocial peers, having low commitment and attachment to school, and living in a

Table. Adolescent Problem Behaviors

Risk Factors	Substance Abuse	Teen Delinquency	School Pregnancy	Drop-Out	Violence
Family					
Family history of the problem behavior	✓	✓	✓	✓	✓
Family management problems	✓	✓	✓	✓	✓
Family conflict	✓	✓	✓	✓	✓
Favorable parental attitudes and involvement in the problem behavior	✓	✓			✓
School					
Early and persistent antisocial behavior	✓	✓	✓	✓	✓
Academic failure beginning in late elementary school	✓	✓	✓	✓	✓
Lack of commitment to school	✓	✓	✓	✓	✓
Individual/Peer					
Alienation and rebelliousness	✓	✓		✓	
Friends who engage in the problem behavior	✓	✓	✓	✓	✓
Favorable attitudes toward the problem behavior	✓	✓	✓	✓	
Early initiation of the problem behavior	✓	✓	✓	✓	✓
Constitutional factors	✓	✓			✓
Community					
Availability of drugs	✓				✓
Availability of firearms		✓			✓
Community laws and norms favorable toward drug use, firearms, and crime	✓	✓			✓
Media portrayals of violence					✓
Transitions and mobility	✓	✓		✓	
Low neighborhood attachment and community disorganization	✓	✓			✓
Extreme economic deprivation	✓	✓	✓	✓	✓

neighborhood where drugs are available. The strongest predictors that distinguish chronic offenders by ages 12 to 14 years are involvement with antisocial peers; lack of social ties; nonserious delinquent acts; and low school commitment, attachment, and achievement.

Research on populations exposed to multiple risk factors has identified subgroups of individuals who negotiate risk exposure successfully without serious involvement in delinquency or violence. This research has led to studies of the factors that protect against risk exposure. Protective factors predict successful outcomes even in the face of risk. Three types of protective factors and three protective processes have been identified. Protective factors include individual factors (eg, high intelligence, a positive social orientation, and a resilient temperament), social bonding (eg, warm, supportive, affective relationships in families or with other positive adults and school commitment or investment in the future), and healthy beliefs and clear standards for behavior (eg, valuing educational success and healthy development and holding norms or standards opposed to crime and violence). Protective processes include opportunities for active involvement in socializing institutions of family, school, and community; the development of competencies or skills (cognitive, social, emotional, and behavioral); and reinforcement for positive behavior and moderate, consistent punishment for negative behavior.

Several generalizations are evident from longitudinal research on risk and protective factors for juvenile delinquency and violence. First, no single risk or protective factor accounts for the majority of juvenile delinquency and violence; rather, exposure to increasing numbers of risk factors contributes to an increasing likelihood of delinquency and violence. Second, risk and protective factors are found in multiple socialization domains, including community, family, school, and peer group, as well as within the individual. Third, risk and protection exposure is developmental. Different risk and protective factors become important predictors at different points developmentally from before conception through adolescence. Fourth, common risk and

protective factors appear to predict diverse problems. In addition to predicting delinquency and violence, these same risk and protective factors have been found to predict other adolescent problems, including substance use, school drop-out, and teen pregnancy. Fifth, risk and protective factors appear to operate similarly in different cultural and ethnic groups, despite varying levels of exposure to risk. Finally, protective factors appear to mediate or moderate the effects of risk exposure.

Prevention and Treatment

Effective prevention efforts focus on reducing risk and enhancing protective factors. To be most effective, risk and protective factors should be prioritized for preventive interventions based on a diagnosis or assessment of the individual's or community's profile of risk and protection. In recent years, a range of prevention interventions targeting risk and protective factors throughout development have been developed and proven effective.

The American Medical Association (AMA) *Guidelines for Adolescent Preventive Services* (GAPS) explicitly recommend that physicians increase their emphasis on preventive services, targeting social morbidities as well as biomedical problems. The guidelines suggest that parents be provided information during their children's adolescence regarding parenting and how to help adolescents avoid potentially harmful behaviors. Risk and protective factor research highlights the importance of parents providing clear standards for behavior and consistent consequences as well as monitoring the activities and whereabouts of their children. Parenting programs that provide parents with information about developmental changes and appropriate skills to protect their children from risk and to enhance protection, such as Preparing for the Drug Free Years, have been shown to promote developmentally appropriate parenting skills among parents of elementary through high school-age children and to reduce adolescent alcohol use and delinquent behaviors.

The AMA guidelines suggest that practitioners assess their patients' use of alcohol and other substances as well as any learning or school problems and recommend further assessment of the psychosocial functioning for any patients experiencing these problems. The high level of co-occurrence of problem behaviors discussed earlier further emphasizes the importance of a broad assessment for youths who report difficulties in any of the areas discussed previously.

When a child or youth is identified as involved in problem behavior, the pediatrician can use a risk and protection-focused approach to move toward intervention. The AMA guidelines direct the practitioner to follow up on assessment by determining the patient's readiness to change, helping him or her weigh the pros and cons of different solutions, and identifying both opportunities and barriers to successful intervention. A technique developed and proven successful in the substance abuse field, Motivational Interviewing, provides a set of tools for this process. Motivational Interviewing is a brief technique designed to avoid raising defenses through confrontation. Instead, it seeks to understand and weigh patients' concerns about their behavior and increase their intrinsic motivation to change. The practitioner works to highlight the discrepancy between patients' behaviors and their goals while supporting their sense of self-efficacy to move in a new direction.

Once the problem is identified, risks and protective factors assessed, and motivation enhanced, the practitioner can move the patient toward an appropriate evidence-based intervention. The GAPS encourage practitioners to enhance their patients' behavioral health through participating in the coordination of guidance and support provided by families, schools, and the community. Significant progress has been made even within the past 10 years in developing and testing effective delinquency interventions. There is good evidence of both interventions that work and are cost-effective and approaches that are not effective. For children whose risk profiles indicate the presence of early conduct problems, The Incredible Years offers a videotape and training-based series of interventions appropriate at preschool and early elementary school ages that work effectively with parents, teachers, and children. Two family-oriented interventions for adolescent

delinquents have been found to be effective: Multisystemic Family Therapy and Functional Family Therapy. Information on these programs is available through Blueprints for Violence Prevention (http://www.colorado.edu/cspv/blueprints/model). Other effective delinquency interventions are Aggression Replacement Training, the Adolescent Diversion Project, and Multidimensional Treatment Foster Care. For serious offenders, successful intervention requires a multimodal approach that addresses problems in several areas, including substance use and abuse, school, and family problems as well as delinquent behavior. In addition to having been proven efficacious, all these programs have been shown to be cost-effective, with measurable benefits that strongly outweigh the costs of the program. In communities or settings where tested effective interventions are not in place, the physician's role may include advocating for the development of appropriate services.

Research also has shown that some commonly used approaches do not work to prevent or reduce delinquency. These include juvenile boot camps, wilderness or challenge programs, deterrence-oriented programs, and generally, individual therapy, although there is limited evidence that individual therapy may be effective with some more serious offenders. The heightened developmental salience of peer influence in adolescence has led many to treat youths who have problems in group-based interventions. Recent research argues against this practice. Several studies have found undesired effects for peer-group treatment programs, with long-term negative behavior outcomes increased for program participants compared with control youths.

Conclusion

The pediatrician can play an important role in both prevention and early intervention to reduce the delinquency of patients. For many families, the pediatrician is the single most credible source of information on children's health. Knowledge of those factors that place young people at risk and of those that can protect against delinquency is the foundation for assessment, diagnosis, prevention, and early intervention. A healthy, open relationship with children and families and an understanding of normal development allow the physician to assess existing and emerging risks for delinquency.

Pediatricians also can provide knowledge and access to effective prevention programs for parents. Increasingly, effective approaches for reducing specific risks and enhancing protection have been identified and tested. These programs are available in many forms and have been used effectively with parents in health maintenance organizations. The potential to intervene before problems arise is an opportunity to promote the health of children.

Suggested Reading

Hawkins JD. Risk and protective factors and their implications for preventive interventions for the health care professional. In: Schydlower M, ed. *Substance Abuse: A Guide for Health Professionals.* 2nd ed. Elk Grove Village, Ill: American Academy of Pediatrics; 2002:1–19

Hawkins JD, Herrenkohl T, Farrington DP, Brewer D, Catalano RF, Harachi TW. A review of predictors of youth violence. In: Loeber R, Farrington DP, eds. *Serious and Violent Juvenile Offenders: Risk Factors and Successful Interventions.* Thousand Oaks, Calif: Sage; 1998:106–146

Herrenkohl TI, Maguin E, Hill KG, Hawkins JD, Abbott RD, Catalano RF. Developmental risk factors for youth violence. *J Adolesc Health.* 2000;26:176–186

Howell JC, Hawkins JD. Prevention of youth violence. In: Tonry M, Moore MH, eds. *Crime and Justice: A Review of Research: Vol. 24. Youth Violence.* Chicago, Ill: University of Chicago Press; 1998:263–315

Diagnosis and Treatment of Depression in Adolescence

by Jennifer Hagman, MD

In September 2000, US Surgeon General David Satcher, MD, PhD, called a national conference to focus on children's mental health. The main findings of his report, released in January 2001, emphasize that the efficacy of mental health treatment is well documented and that a range of treatments exist for most mental disorders. The report issues a call to action, and underscores the urgent need for providers to be able to identify and initiate treatment or referral for depression and other mental illnesses in children and adolescents.

In May 2001, Dr Satcher announced a national campaign to prevent suicide and urged that suicide risk screening become part of every primary health care practice. The surgeon general's data demonstrate that the incidence of suicide attempts peaks during midadolescent years. He also observes that suicide is the third leading cause of death in adolescents, following closely behind accidents and homicide. It is estimated that one in ten teens contemplate suicide, and nearly a half-million teens in the United States make a suicide attempt each year.

Mood disorders significantly increase the risk of suicide. The hormonal changes of puberty are widely believed to be associated with parallel changes in brain neurochemistry. Increased prevalence rates for mood disorders and other mental illnesses after puberty are thought to be related to these changes. The onset of puberty leads to increasing rates of depression; the prevalence of depression in adolescence is around 8%. The rate of depression in females begins to approach adult levels by age 15. The lifetime risk of depression ranges from 10% to 25% for women, and 5% to 12% for men.

Role of the Pediatrician

Individuals with depression almost always present initially to their primary care physician. Thus, it is important that pediatricians are able to identify patients with depression and initiate evaluation and treatment. It is not uncommon for the pediatrician to be the first person who has the opportunity to diagnose depression, and it is increasingly common for primary care physicians to be responsible for the medication management of depressive disorders. Many patients will go undiagnosed and untreated if their clinicians are not prepared to consider the diagnosis of mental illness.

Learning Objectives

After reading this article, pediatricians will understand their role in the diagnosis and management of depression. They will be able to:
- Describe the epidemiology and natural history of depression in adolescence
- Discuss approaches to screening for depression
- Recognize common clinical presentations, differential diagnosis, and comorbidities of adolescent depressive disorders
- List *DSM-IV-TR* criteria for diagnosis of major depressive disorders
- Discuss criteria for referral and/or hospitalization of the depressed adolescent
- Describe the pediatrician's role in management of depression, including use of medications

---

Jennifer Hagman, MD, is an associate professor of psychiatry at the University of Colorado Health Sciences Center. She is the medical director of clinical services and codirector of the eating disorders treatment program at The Children's Hospital in Denver, Colorado. Dr. Hagman is board certified in general psychiatry as well as child and adolescent psychiatry.

The diagnosis and treatment of depression during adolescence can be challenging. A depressive episode in adolescence can significantly impair social, emotional, and academic potential at a critical point in development. Children and adolescents are more likely to present with somatic symptoms and school avoidance due to stomachaches, headaches, fatigue, and other generalized physical complaints, than to present with awareness of a clinical depression.

Some families may be reluctant to seek help from a therapist or psychiatrist, or to accept the need for a referral, due to perceptions that mental illness carries a stigma, or that a record of treatment for mental illness could have an adverse effect on future opportunities in education or employment. The pediatrician can be helpful in providing information to decrease anxiety about the diagnosis and potential interventions.

Assessment and Screening

Adolescents struggle to define themselves within their peer groups, families, and communities as they adjust to the changes of puberty and the social interactions that come with the teen years. Sorting through changes in mood, attitude, and behavior that characterize adolescence to determine the nature of a suspected mental health problem can be a challenge for parents and clinicians. Adolescents usually tell their friends more than they tell their parents, and are often reluctant to talk with adults about their inner thoughts.

All of these factors, combined with hormonal changes, place the adolescent at increased risk for depression. Persistent change in mood lasting more than 2 weeks should alert the family and physician to screen for the presence of a depressive episode.

Because the pediatric office visit is often short, the method used to screen must be brief yet effective. Questionnaires support the screening process, but they should not take the place of direct assessment. If the pediatrician identifies symptoms that may indicate a depressive disorder during the course of a routine pediatric visit (Table 1), further assessment is required. If this cannot be accomplished during the scheduled

Table 1. Screening Questions

- Have you lost interest in things you used to enjoy?
- Have you had any change in your sleep patterns?
- Have you had any thoughts about hurting yourself?
- Have you been feeling sad, down, or depressed much of the time?

visit, a longer office visit should be arranged within 7 days.

Screening must include assessment for current suicidal ideation, and intent of self-harm if suicidal thoughts are present. A more thorough assessment by a mental health professional is immediately warranted for adolescents who report current thoughts about killing themselves (suicidal ideation), or someone else (homicidal ideation). A history of suicide attempts, aggressive behavior, or substance abuse increases the risk that a patient will act upon these thoughts.

Talking Points

How to ask about suicidal ideation
In the context of assessing for depression, it is important to ask, "Have you had any thoughts about not wanting to be alive?" If there is an affirmative response, continue with, "Have you had any thoughts about suicide, or about hurting yourself?" Also explore how they would hurt themselves, or, if they have contemplated suicide, what ways they have thought about attempting it.

Patients who have thought *specifically* about how to hurt or kill themselves present a psychiatric emergency. Teens who are actively suicidal should be evaluated the same day at the nearest emergency room. If the teen is in therapy, the parent and physician should contact the therapist to make them aware of the situation. Whether or not the crisis is immediate, it is important to let the teen know that you are concerned and that you want to help. The guardian should be made aware of the teen's suicidal thinking and further assessment should be urgently arranged. Confidentiality must be breached in this circumstance.

Emergency assessment of suicidal or homicidal ideation can be accomplished by referral to the closest emergency room. Pediatricians should be aware of the services available for psychiatric crisis assessment in the community. Awareness of the mental health provisions of patients' insurance coverage will facilitate referrals for further evaluation and treatment and can be helpful in preparing the family for the crisis assessment process.

DIFFERENTIAL DIAGNOSIS

Underlying physical disease or illness that can produce depressive symptoms should be ruled out. The clinical assessment may include laboratory studies for hypo- or hyperthyroidism, anemia, and mononucleosis, in addition to any other conditions suggested by physical symptoms. Substance abuse, specifically marijuana and opiate abuse, can also lead to symptoms of depression. Stimulants, cocaine, and certain "club drugs," such as Ecstasy (MDMA), can cause a depressive syndrome following episodes of use. Teens may also try to "self-medicate" depressive symptoms with alcohol or drugs.

SYMPTOMS OF DEPRESSION

If screening raises suspicion about the possibility of depression and the physician's examination has ruled out other causes, further assessment of symptoms and contributing factors is required. A significant decline in quality of academic work and grades often indicates a mental health problem. Environmental stressors, such as family problems, moves, troubled peer relationships, traumatic experiences, and abuse may also cause problems at school.

Changes in sleep, appetite, social interactions, concentration, self-esteem, and mood are core symptoms of depressive disorders. Decreased sleep is associated with lying awake in bed for more than 1 hour, often preoccupied and worried, frequent awakenings through the night, and early morning awakening. Increased sleep may be described by teens as a feeling that they could sleep all day.

Depressed adolescents often withdraw from family and friends and spend increasing amounts of time alone. They become less interested in activities they used to enjoy and may seem apathetic. Lowered self-esteem is reflected in negative comments about themselves, decreased attention to hygiene, and a pessimistic view of the future. Suicidal ideation (eg, "it would be easier to be dead") often evolves in the context of a depressive episode.

DIAGNOSIS OF DEPRESSION AND OTHER MOOD DISORDERS

The *Diagnostic and Statistical Manual of Mental Disorders, Fourth Edition, Text Revision (DSM-IV-TR)*, published by the American Psychiatric Association, provides the diagnostic criteria for mood disorders and other mental illnesses. The American Academy of Pediatrics' guide, *Diagnostic and Statistical Manual for Primary Care: Child and Adolescent Version (DSM-PC: Child and Adolescent Version)* is also an excellent diagnostic reference.

Major depressive disorder, dysthymic disorder, adjustment disorder with depressed mood, and depression not otherwise specified (NOS) are the four most common mood disorder diagnoses found in the adolescent age group, followed by bipolar disorder and mood disorder NOS.

A *DSM-IV-TR* diagnosis of major depression requires that five of nine symptoms be present most of the day every day for 2 weeks (Table 2). Dysthymic disorder is a depressive condition of lesser intensity, present for at least 1 year in children and adolescents (2 years in adults). Adjustment disorders develop in response to a specific stressor and do not last longer than 6 months. Diagnoses of depression NOS and mood disorder NOS can be used when there is clearly a mood disorder present, but the *DSM-IV-TR* criteria are not fully met or do not cluster in the required patterns. The criteria for bipolar mood disorder requires the occurrence of a manic episode. Individuals with bipolar mood disorder often have had one or more major depressive episodes prior to the onset of manic symptoms.

It is always important to screen for bipolar affective disorder in an adolescent whom you believe may be depressed. Up to 30% of those diagnosed with child-onset and adolescent-onset depression (also known as early-onset depression) may develop the spectrum of symptoms diagnosed

Table 2. Criteria for Major Depressive Episode

A. Five (or more) of the following symptoms have been present during the same 2-week period and represent a change from previous functioning; at least one of the symptoms is either (1) depressed mood or (2) loss of interest or pleasure.
 Note: Do not include symptoms that are clearly due to a general medical condition, or mood-incongruent delusions or hallucinations.

 (1) depressed mood most of the day, nearly every day, as indicated by either subjective report (eg, feels sad or empty) or observation made by others (eg, appears tearful). **Note:** In children and adolescents, can be irritable mood.

 (2) markedly diminished interest or pleasure in all, or almost all, activities most of the day, nearly every day (as indicated by either subjective account or observation made by others)

 (3) significant weight loss when not dieting or weight gain (eg, a change of more than 5% of body weight in a month), or decrease or increase in appetite nearly every day. **Note:** In children, consider failure to make expected weight gains

 (4) insomnia or hypersomnia nearly every day

 (5) psychomotor agitation or retardation nearly every day (observable by others, not merely subjective feelings of restlessness or being slowed down)

 (6) fatigue or loss of energy nearly every day

 (7) feelings of worthlessness or excessive or inappropriate guilt (which may be delusional) nearly every day (not merely self-reproach or guilt about being sick)

 (8) diminished ability to think or concentrate, or indecisiveness, nearly every day (either by subjective account or as observed by others)

 (9) recurrent thoughts of death (not just fear of dying), recurrent suicidal ideation without a specific plan, or a suicide attempt or a specific plan for committing suicide

B. The symptoms do not meet criteria for a mixed episode.

C. The symptoms cause clinically significant distress or impairment in social, occupational, or other important areas of functioning.

D. The symptoms are not due to the direct physiological effects of a substance (eg, a drug of abuse, a medication) or a general medical condition (eg, hypothyroidism).

E. The symptoms are not better accounted for by bereavement, ie, after the loss of a loved one, the symptoms persist for longer than 2 months or are characterized by marked functional impairment, morbid preoccupation with worthlessness, suicidal ideation, psychotic symptoms, or psychomotor retardation.

Reprinted with permission from the *Diagnostic and Statistical Manual of Mental Disorders, Fourth Edition, Text Revision.*
Copyright 2000 American Psychiatric Association.

as bipolar affective disorder (Strober et al, 1993). A mixed manic phase of bipolar disorder in childhood or adolescence is likely to present with irritability, hyperactivity, decreased sleep and grandiose thinking or psychotic symptoms. The possibility of bipolar disorder is increased for the child or adolescent who presents with depression, a family history of bipolar affective disorder, a personal history of attention deficit/hyperactivity disorder (ADHD), and the presence of psychotic symptoms. These cases warrant referral to a child psychiatrist for further assessment and diagnostic clarification.

Some individuals with unsuspected bipolar affective disorder may experience agitation, decreased sleep, and even manic episodes when treated with an antidepressant. If the pediatrician suspects that the episode is related to undiagnosed bipolar disorder, the antidepressant should be stopped and treatment with a mood stabilizer (such as lithium, valproate or carbamazepine) may be indicated. This usually warrants a consultation with a child psychiatrist.

OTHER MENTAL HEALTH DIAGNOSES ASSOCIATED WITH DEPRESSION

Comprehensive assessment should include consideration of comorbid conditions in addition to the primary diagnosis of depression. Another mental illness may be present in up to 40% of adolescents diagnosed with a depressive disorder. Potential mental health comorbidities include anxiety disorders, substance use disorders, disruptive behavior disorders, eating disorders, and ADHD. Another 30% of adolescents with depression may later develop bipolar disorder.

Management

Interventions for the treatment of depression in adolescence include psychotherapy, medication, and careful attention to school, home, peer, and work-related stressors. Interventions should be designed to address the depressive diagnosis, severity of episode, and the specific needs of the child and family.

If a diagnosis of depression is suspected or supported, the pediatrician must decide whether the patient requires referral to a mental health specialist. This decision depends on the pediatrician's comfort level with diagnosing and treating depression. Optimal treatment for the adolescent with a diagnosis of depression is counseling combined with assessment for possible treatment with medication (Table 3). Not all adolescents will require medication. Ideally, the pediatrician will have access to child psychiatrists with whom he or she can confer regarding referrals and medication management. The assessment of severity of depression and response to therapy should be ongoing through the course of treatment. In some cases, antidepressants are started when mood symptoms have not significantly improved with psychotherapy.

If psychotic symptoms are present (auditory or visual hallucinations and/or paranoia), referral to a psychiatrist is strongly recommended. Psychotic symptoms can be associated with substance use, depression, schizophrenia, bipolar disorder, and post-traumatic stress disorder. Thorough assessment to clarify the differential diagnosis is essential to initiate appropriate interventions when psychotic symptoms are present. Common reasons for referral are presented in Table 4.

Consideration of a higher level of care is necessary when symptoms include suicidal ideation or the adolescent is unable to function as a result of the depressive episode. Options include inpatient hospitalization and day treatment.

INDIVIDUAL AND FAMILY PSYCHOTHERAPY

A referral for psychotherapy should be made for all adolescents who are diagnosed with depression. Once a referral is made, it is imperative that the managing physician communicate regularly with the therapist.

Psychiatrists, psychologists, social workers, licensed professional counselors, and clinical nurse specialists may provide individual, family, or group therapy. It is important, whenever possible, to be familiar with the training of each provider, and to be knowledgeable about their experience relevant to the treatment of children and adolescents.

The chance that a family will follow through with the referral for therapy is greatly increased if the pediatrician makes referrals to therapists that he or she knows, or can review the managed care provider list and make recommendations.

Individual therapy can help the teen develop increased understanding of his or her skills to cope with the depressive episode and related life stressors or circumstances. *Family therapy* facilitates improved communication patterns within the family structure. If dynamics between the parents are contributing to the teen's symptoms and impeding recovery, *marital counseling* may be recommended, or individual therapy for one or both parents. *Group therapy,* sometimes available at school, can be a helpful component of care for depressed adolescents, who may see themselves as alone and their problems as unique, with no one else who can understand. *School counselors* can provide support in the school environment and assist with assessment of academic functioning and school-based peer relationships during the depressive episode and recovery process.

Education is often necessary to help families understand the depression diagnosis so they can help in the recovery process. A discussion about what the depression diagnosis means, combined

Table 3. Interventions for the Treatment of Depression

Adjustment Disorder	refer for psychotherapy	medications usually not needed
Mild Depression	refer for psychotherapy	medications may not be needed
Moderate Depression	refer for psychotherapy	consider antidepressant medication
Severe Depression	refer for psychotherapy	strongly encourage antidepressant medication

Table 4. When to Consider Consultation With a Psychiatrist?

Diagnosis is not clear
Pediatrician feels further assessment is needed
Pediatrician believes medications may be needed, but will not be prescribing
Pediatrician has started medications and needs further psychopharmacologic consultation
Individual, family, and/or group psychotherapy is needed
Psychotic symptoms (hallucinations, paranoia) are present
Bipolar affective disorder is suspected.

Immediate referral for crisis assessment is needed:
Current suicidal thoughts are present
Current homicidal intent is present

---

with handouts on the diagnosis and references for additional information, is helpful to parents, siblings, and to the teenager (See resource page for families).

RATING SCALES

Rating scales, such as the Beck Depression Inventory®-II (BDI®-II) and the Reynolds Adolescent Depression Scale (RADS), provide an objective assessment of depressive symptoms. Scales are useful tools to monitor symptom severity and improvement over the course of treatment. Scales are also helpful to patients who can use them to follow how their symptoms have changed over time.

MEDICATION

The natural course of an untreated depressive episode can range from 9 months to 2 years. The effective use of antidepressant medications can lead to remission of symptoms within 1 month or less. In general, antidepressants are recommended for all moderate to severe cases of major depression, and should be considered for diagnoses of dysthymic disorder. Medication is generally not required for the treatment of adjustment disorder. Treatment of mood disorder NOS and depression NOS require further assessment, initiation of psychotherapy, and monitoring of symptoms over time to determine if an antidepressant or mood stabilizer is needed.

Studies examining the use of tricyclic antidepressants (TCAs) for the treatment of depression in children and adolescents have not demonstrated efficacy compared to placebo. The TCAs are also cardiotoxic, and thus quite dangerous in overdose situations, and they require medical monitoring of EKG, blood pressure, pulse, and blood levels. The continued development of the noradrenergic system during the adolescent years is thought to be the reason for the lack of efficacy of these medications in children and adolescents. The serotonergic system is thought to be relatively stable throughout development, thus leading to what appear to be more positive results in psychopharmacologic studies of selective serotonin reuptake inhibitors (SSRIs) in this age group. (Findling et al, 1998; Friedman et al, 1998).

Due to greater comparative efficacy and safety, the SSRIs have replaced tricyclic antidepressants as the primary agents prescribed for the treatment of major depression in adolescents. Agents that target primarily serotonergic and noradrenergic systems (eg, buproprion, mirtazapine, nefazodone and venlafaxine) are generally second-line choices. Although no antidepressants are approved by the Food and Drug Administration for treatment of major depressive disorders in children or adolescents, studies supporting the use, safety, and efficacy of SSRIs in adolescence have been published.

SSRIs are generally well tolerated, treatment is relatively easy to start, and therapy is not complex to monitor. The most common side effects include nausea, diarrhea, headache, insomnia, psychomotor activation, and decreased libido. Taking the medication in the morning with breakfast can minimize these side effects. No blood levels are required and there are no cardiac, renal, hepatic, or hematologic indices to follow. The SSRIs are not lethal in overdose and there have been no reported deaths due to SSRIs alone. SSRIs are relatively potent inhibitors of the cytochrome P450 isoenzymes in the liver, which metabolize many medications. If an SSRI is given in combination with a medication that is metabolized by the P450 system, metabolism of the other medication will be decreased (Table 5)

Table 5. Examples of Medications Metabolized by Cytochrome P450-2D6

Beta Blockers
Antiarrhythmics
Codeine
Amphetamines
Methylphenidate
Desipramine
Nortriptyline
Venlafaxine

leading to higher blood levels of the other medication. This is a consideration in the case of the patient who is on more than one medication. The order of potency of P450 2D6 binding is: paroxetine>fluoxetine>sertraline>fluvoxamine>citalopram.

The SSRIs are usually started at half the recommended adult dose and titrated upward in 1 week intervals as necessary for optimal therapeutic response. Table 6 offers guidelines and maximum doses of each medication. The average effective dose for each medication varies with the individual. Once at the target dose, improvement in symptoms should be expected within 2 to 4 weeks. If there is not significant improvement in depressive symptoms at 4 weeks, the dose should be increased, a different medication considered, or referral made to a specialist for further assessment. It is important to educate the adolescent and family about the delayed onset of symptom improvement and the need to continue the antidepressant for 6 to 9 months.

Selecting and managing medications

Choice of medication is based upon symptom profile, history of positive or negative response to other psychopharmacologic agents, family history, and reliability of the person taking the medication and those monitoring it.

The SSRIs, although largely comparable, have slightly different side effect profiles, and patients may tolerate one better than another. None of the SSRIs or alternative antidepressants are addictive. Sedation may occur in up to 10% of patients treated with an SSRI. Paroxetine may be more sedating, and thus better tolerated when taken at bedtime. Fluoxetine has the longest half-life.

Table 6. Medications Used to Treat Depression in Adolescents

The SSRIs are usually given once a day in the morning with breakfast. One in ten individuals may experience sedation and prefer to take the medication at bedtime. The alternative antidepressants and fluvoxamine are usually given in BID dosing. Buproprion and venlafaxine are now available in a sustained/extended release form.

Generic	Trade name	Adolescent Starting dose	Target dose (Average effective dose)	Maximum dose
SSRIs				
Citalopram	Celexa	20 mg QAM	20 mg QAM	40 mg QAM
Fluoxetine*	Prozac	10 mg QAM	20 mg QAM	60 mg QAM
Fluvoxamine*	Luvox	50 mg QHS	100-150 mg QD	100 mg BID
Paroxetine*	Paxil	10 mg QAM	20 mg QAM	60 mg QAM
Sertraline*	Zoloft	25 mg QAM	50 mg QAM	150 mg QAM
Alternative Antidepressants				
Buproprion*	Wellbutrin	75 mg QAM	150 mg BID	200 mg BID
Buproprion SR	Wellbutrin SR	100 mg QAM	100 mg BID	150 mg BID
Mirtazapine	Remeron	7.5 mg QHS	15 mg QHS	30 mg QHS
Nefazodone	Serzone	50 mg QHS	100 mg BID	300 mg BID
Venlafaxine	Effexor	37.5 mg QAM	75 mg BID	150 mg BID
Venlafaxine XR	Effexor XR	37.5 mg QAM	150 mg QD	225 mg QD

*Published studies support the use of these medications in adolescents, although no antidepressants have FDA approval for treatment of major depression in this age group.

Alternative antidepressants are generally recommended after two SSRIs have been tried and remission of symptoms has not been achieved (Hughes et al, 1999). Comorbid diagnoses may also influence the selection of antidepressant. Fluvoxamine has FDA approval for the treatment of adult and pediatric obsessive-compulsive disorder. Sertraline has FDA approval for treatment of adult depression, post-traumatic stress disorder and panic disorder, and pediatric and adult obsessive-compulsive disorder. Fluoxetine has FDA approval for the treatment of adults for bulimia nervosa and premenstrual dysphoric disorder, in addition to depression. Paroxetine has FDA approval for treatment of depression and panic disorder in adults. Buproprion has FDA approval for the treatment of depression and smoking cessation in adults. Buproprion should not be prescribed for individuals with eating disorders due to increased risk of seizure in these individuals.

When possible, it is optimal to let the adolescent participate in the decision about which medication to take. If insurance or formulary issues are not a concern and an SSRI is the medication category of choice, the pediatrician can present several choices. A teen who knows that his or her parent or a friend has been treated for depression with a particular medication may select or decline a medication on that basis alone.

Antidepressants should be continued for at least 6 to 9 months after a therapeutic response occurs. Patients should be specifically told not to unilaterally discontinue their medication once they are feeling better. On the other hand, some people are reluctant to stop taking an antidepressant when it appears to be an appropriate time to do so. It is best to discuss a plan for stopping medications. It is wise to discontinue medications during a time of minimal psychosocial stress, such as during a school vacation. This makes it easier to assess sustained improvement or relapse, and reduces the potential impact of a recurrence of depressive symptoms. Sertraline and paroxetine have relatively short half-lives and should be tapered by reducing the dose by one-half every 5 to 10 days, based on the patient's tolerance.

Some patients report dizziness and flu-like symptoms when stopping an SSRI abruptly.

When medication is decreased or stopped, it is critical to educate the teen and family on how to monitor for return of depressive symptoms. Early intervention can prevent the descent into an incapacitating major depressive episode. Over 50% of individuals with childhood or adolescent onset depression will experience another depressive episode later in life.

Informed consent

Informed consent is complicated in child and adolescent psychopharmacology due to the lack of safety and efficacy data for many medications. Information to be shared regarding side effects and efficacy is often based on the available data from studies primarily on adults, or on studies of the medication used for other diagnoses in pediatric age groups. The clinician's experience with the medication can also be shared when discussing efficacy and side effects.

Informed consent involves explaining and discussing possible common side effects and any possible side effects that should be closely monitored. This should be documented in the patient record. The expected benefit of the medication and time frame in which benefit should be expected should also be discussed. How long the medication should be taken, and the basis for an eventual decision to discontinue it, should be reviewed as well. It is especially important to discuss the course of a depressive episode, in order to give the patient and family a basis for realistic expectations for recovery. Those who understand the expected course will be more motivated to comply with the medication regimen to prevent relapse. Dulcan's (1999) book, which features medication information handouts for psychotropic medications prescribed for children and adolescents, is a useful resource in counseling adolescents and families.

State laws vary regarding the age for providing informed consent. Regardless of state law, both the adolescent and the guardian should understand the risks and benefits of the proposed medication, agree to the treatment regimen, and provide informed consent.

Managed Care Issues

Almost all managed care plans have "carved out" mental health benefits. This means that mental health and medical benefits are managed differently. Often a different managed care organization manages the mental health benefit. Because of variations in reimbursement based on geography, practice structure, capitation, etc, primary care physicians providing mental health services should consult local experts and investigate strategies for obtaining reimbursement for services they provide. Many states have established "parity" for some mental disorders. Parity mandates that the same benefits are available for the treatment of mental illness as for physical illness. In many states, major depression and bipolar disorder, which are both established as biologically based illnesses, are included under parity.

Summary

Thousands of children and adolescents suffer with undiagnosed and untreated depression each year. Suicide is directly linked to depression and is a preventable cause of death in adolescence. It is essential that pediatricians be able to identify depression and suicidal ideation and organize appropriate treatment. More pediatricians are becoming comfortable initiating psychopharmacologic interventions with an antidepressant while making a referral for further assessment and therapy. It is important that the pediatrician know when to make a referral and how to continue the psychopharmacologic intervention if started by a consulting psychiatrist.

Acknowledgements:

The author would like to thank David Kaplan, MD, Harriet Stern, MD, and Deborah Mulkey, PNP, for their editorial assistance in preparing this article.

The editors would like to acknowledge technical review by W. Sam Yancy, MD, for the Committee on Adolescence.

Recommended Reading

American Academy of Pediatrics. *Surviving: Coping with Adolescent Depression and Suicide. Guidelines for Parents.* (Brochures available from the Academy in packets of 100. 1-888-227-1770)

American Psychiatric Association. *Diagnostic and Statistical Manual of Mental Disorders, Fourth Edition, Text Revision.* Washington, DC: American Psychiatric Assn; 2000

Beck AT, Steer RA, Brown GK. *Beck Depression Inventory®-II.* San Antonio, TX: The Psychological Corporation. (1-800-872-1726 or www.psychcorp.com)

Dulcan MK, Benton T, eds. *Helping Parents, Youth, and Teachers Understand Medications for Behavioral and Emotional Problems: A Resource Book of Medication Information Handouts.* (Includes CD-ROM) Washington, DC: American Psychiatric Press, Inc; 1999

Findling RL, Blumer JL, guest eds. Child and Adolescent Psychopharmacology. *Pediatr Clin North Am.* 1998;45 (theme issue):1021–1278

Friedman SB, DeMaso DR, guest eds. Adolescent Psychiatric and Behavioral Disorders. *Adolescent Medicine: State of the Art Reviews.* 1998;9(theme issue):197–414

Hughes CW, Emslie GJ, Crismon ML, et al. The Texas Children's Medication Algorithm Project: Report of the Texas Consensus Conference Panel on Medication Treatment of Childhood Major Depressive Disorder. *J Am Acad Child Adolesc Psychiatry.* 1999;38:1442–1454

Insurance coverage of mental health and substance abuse services for children and adolescents: A consensus statement. *Pediatrics.* 2000;106:860–862

Practice parameters for the assessment and treatment of children and adolescents with depressive disorders. *J Am Acad Child Adolesc Psychiatry.* 1998;37(10 suppl):63S–83S

Report of the Surgeon General's Conference on Chidren's Mental Health: A National Action Agenda. Rockville, MD: US Dept. of Health and Human Services; 2001.

Reynolds WM. Reynolds Adolescent Depression Scale (RADS). Lutz, Florida: PAR-Psychological Assessment Resources, Inc. (1-800-331-8378 or www.parinc.com)

Strober M, Lampert C, Schmidt S, Morrell W. The course of major depressive disorder in adolescents: I. Recovery and risk of manic switching in a follow-up of psychotic and nonpsychotic subtypes. *J Am Acad Child Adolesc Psychiatry.* 1993;32:34–42

Walkup JT, Labellarte MJ, Riddle MA, et al. Fluvoxamine for the treatment of anxiety disorders in children and adolescents. *N Engl J Med.* 2001:1279–1285

CHILD AND ADOLESCENT PSYCHOPHARMA-COLOGY TEXTBOOKS AND NEWSLETTERS

Green WH. *Child and Adolescent Psychopharmacology.* 3rd ed. Baltimore, MD: Lippincott, Williams and Wilkins; 2001

Leonard HL, ed. *The Brown University Child and Adolescent Psychopharmacology Update.* (monthly newsletter) Providence, RI: Manisses Communications Group, Inc; (800-333-7771).

Rosenberg DR, Holttum J, Gershon S. *Textbook of Pharmacotherapy for Child and Adolescent Psychiatric Disorders.* Philadelphia, PA: Brunner/Mazel Publishers; 1994

Rosenberg DR, et al. *Pocket Guide for the Textbook of Child and Adolescent Psychiatric Disorders.* Washington DC: Taylor & Francis; 1998

Information and Resources for Families

What are the symptoms of depression in adolescence?

- Frequent sadness, tearfulness, crying
- Decreased interest in activities or inability to enjoy previously favorite activities
- Persistent boredom
- Low energy
- Social isolation, poor communication
- Low self esteem, hopelessness, and guilt
- Extreme sensitivity to rejection or failure
- Increased irritability, anger, or hostility

- Difficulty with relationships
- Frequent complaints of physical illnesses such as headaches and stomachaches
- Frequent absences from school or poor performance in school
- Poor concentration
- A major change in eating and/or sleeping patterns
- Talk of (or attempts to) run away from home
- Thoughts or expressions of suicide or self-destructive behavior.

What should I do if I think my child is depressed?

- Ask your child if he or she has been feeling sad or depressed.
- Tell them if you have noticed a change in mood or behavior
- Be supportive and nonjudgmental
- Schedule an appointment with your pediatrician
- Tell the physician you think your child might be depressed
- Learn more about depression

Sources of Further Information*

WEB SITES:

American Academy of Child and Adolescent Psychiatry
www.aacap.org
General information for parents and families on developmental, behavioral, emotional and mental disorders affecting children and adolescents. See especially the "Facts for Families" page, which offers brief and concise information sheets on a wide spectrum of illnesses and concerns. Also available in Spanish.

American Psychiatric Association
www.psych.org
Site is primarily for mental health professionals, but offers some general information and links on mental health and public policy

American Psychological Association
www.helping.apa.org
General information for patients and families on mental health, when and how to seek help

National Alliance for the Mentally Ill
www.nami.org
Good information for families of the mentally ill on support, education, advocacy, and research

National Institute of Mental Health
www.nimh.nih.gov
General information in mental health, including current research

National Mental Health Association
www.nmha.org
General information on mental health for patients and families

Report of the Surgeon General's Conference on Children's Mental Health
www.surgeongeneral.gov/cmh/childreport.htm
A summary of findings and call to action resulting from a September 2000, national conference convened by the US Surgeon General

BOOKS:

Pruitt D, ed. *Your Adolescent. Emotional, Behavioral and Cognitive Development from Early Adolescence Through the Teen Years.* American Academy of Child and Adolescent Psychiatry. New York, NY: Harpercollins; 2000

Wilens, TE. *Straight Talk About Psychiatric Medications for Kids.* New York, NY: Guilford Publications; 1998

*These resources are included as sources of general information only. Their content has not been reviewed or endorsed by the American Academy of Pediatrics.

Pediatricians are encouraged to photocopy this page for distribution to patients and parents.

Issues of Adolescent Psychological Development in the 21st Century

Margaret E. Gutgesell, MD, PhD, * *Nancy Payne, MD†*

Objectives

After completing this article, readers should be able to:

1. Describe outside influences on adolescent psychological development.
2. Explain why cognitive development advances during adolescence should be assessed before initiating counseling.
3. Describe the relationship between risk-taking behaviors of adolescents and cognitive maturity.
4. Explain how visible and nonvisible health conditions affect the adolescent's view of self.
5. Discuss how physicians can help improve compliance in an adolescent.

Introduction

Dealing with adolescents always has been a challenge for both parents and clinicians. In today's society, adolescence is a prolonged developmental stage that lasts approximately 10 years, nominally described as between the ages of 11 and 22 years. An adolescent progresses through stages of biologic development as well as changes in psychological and social functioning. It is in this period that a person becomes both physically and psychologically mature and capable of independent living. Although some recent data show that 75% of adolescents and their families have a transitional experience that is trouble-free, many have described this period as one of "storm and stress." Physicians caring for adolescents need to know how the influences of family and the adolescent peer group affect teenagers as they progress through the early (11 to 14 y), middle (15 to 17 y), and late (18 to 21 y) stages of development. Although the outcome might be the same (eg, a healthy and independent adult), individual variation in the progression through these stages can be substantial; adolescence is a highly variable and somewhat asynchronous process. Progression through the various stages does not follow the same timelines for each adolescent. Finally, physicians need to know how to address the major issues of sexuality, risk-taking, and other health-related concerns of adolescents. This article will help the pediatrician manage these issues of adolescence, especially in the setting of the United States. However, many of these issues also pertain to adolescents in other countries.

The Family and the Adolescent Peer Group

Children, including teenagers, learn what they live. The physician who cares for adolescents must recognize the importance of understanding family dynamics and the potential impact of such dynamics on symptoms of an individual adolescent. This issue is particularly important when the physician is assessing an adolescent's psychological status. Is this a traditional family with the father as the breadwinner and the mother "at home," are both parents employed outside of the home, or is it a single-parent home? And if the latter, what is the role of the other parent? Does the teenager's health problems mimic those of the parents? School truancy may be modeled from a parent's work habits (eg, the alcoholic who has frequent Monday absences). The obese teenager generally has obese parents who have little time or interest in providing home-cooked meals and exercise activities.

*Associate Professor of Pediatrics and Psychiatric Medicine.

†Assistant Professor of Pediatrics, University of Virginia Health System, Charlottesville, VA.

Understanding the socioeconomic status and the culture of each family also may help the pediatrician understand the adolescent's developmental process. This is reflected in the type of leisure activities, including dating, that the adolescent may pursue. Upper-class youth may have more travel experience and cultural activities as well as community activities; middle-class adolescents frequently participate in activities such as sports and youth-groups; lower-class youth may not have any structured activities. Certain cultures have less apparent parent-youth conflict throughout this developmental phase. In addition, cultures that are less technology-oriented may have less conflict.

Increasing numbers of youth are computer-literate. Although most use such technology for information and social reasons (e-mail), many are involved with the "dark side" of the Internet, which may lead to asocial or pathologic behavior. Many adolescents are unsupervised in their computer and Internet use, with parents being totally unfamiliar with this world. Parents can place the family computer in a central gathering place to monitor Internet use and engage blocking devices to limit access.

The process of pubertal maturation requires role readjustments among and between family members, often resulting in increased stress and conflict. Parents may not feel as important in their child's life as they once were because the adolescent no longer sees them as all-powerful. In the first part of adolescent development, teens may seek out other adult authority figures. Most adolescents feel that their parents love them but do not necessarily understand them.

Parents need to realize that some actions of their teenage children may be hard to control and that adolescents have certain legal rights. These rights vary among states, and physicians should know the laws of the state in which they practice. In most states, a minor can be treated for sexually transmitted diseases, pregnancy, family planning, and outpatient substance abuse or mental illness without parental permission. It can be frustrating for a parent to bring a teenager to a clinician, demanding that the child be screened for drug use, only to be told that the child has the right to refuse such drug testing. Similarly, the adolescent who has a sexually transmitted disease has the right to privacy. Although the presence of an adolescent can be inherently stressful for a family, there often are other sources of family stress. It is essential that the physician identify changes and stresses for each family. Parental marital problems or frequent absence of one parent, employment or financial insecurity, substance use, mental illness, or incarceration of a family member can have serious consequences on the adolescent's mental health and coping skills.

The physician needs to identify sources of stress within families and the predominant methods of coping with such stress. Does the family set aside at least one evening or a similar time each week to review such issues or conflict management? Is the family involved in a religious or community organization that offers support in stressful situations? Do the parents seek out school guidance counselors when school personnel suggest that the adolescent is having difficulty coping at school?

In addition to the family, peers are important influences for the adolescent. The young adolescent begins separation from family members in an attempt to demonstrate independent thought. Initially, this separation is manifested by an interest in finding peers of the same gender who have similar dress, grooming, and behavioral standards. Early teens strive to find acceptance within such peer groups, thus forming new "family" units. These friendships entail responsibilities unlike those of earlier years. The teen is finding self-expression and forming moral thought while struggling with an emerging image of self in society.

Amid these years of turmoil in body changes, adolescents look to their peers for acceptance, importance, and unity. Peers, not parents, generally first grant autonomy to the adolescent. Jobs, dating, and parenting tasks require interaction on equal grounds. Most adult emotional experiences begin in relationships with peers. Within the context of building peer relations, adolescents learn loyalty, empathy, criticism, and rejection.

Family conflict often ensues with the development of peer friendships. Dress choice, for example, may appear to make rebellious statements toward parents, but actually may be an attempt to show free choice or find acceptance within a group. In building peer relationships, most teens do not intentionally strive to isolate parents. Nonetheless, parents should expect heightened demands for privacy and decreased time spent in family activities from their adolescent children.

Peers have a powerful daily influence on the adolescent's healthy and unhealthy behaviors. Alcohol, cigarette, and illicit drug use frequently are encountered initially among peers. Both peer selection and peer influence contribute to adolescent behaviors. For example, cigarette use may be encouraged by covert peer pressure or an adolescent's wish to project a seemingly sophisticated image. Peer influence extends past substance use to other unhealthy behaviors of risk-taking, such as carrying a weapon to school or unsafe use of motor or recreational vehicles. Peers also can promote early sexual behaviors or encourage negative school attitudes. Peers who disregard the value of education may promote school truancy or failure. Decreased parental involvement, poor communication with parents, and poor parental discipline contribute to the degree of influence that peers have on a young adolescent. Pediatricians should advise parents of their important role in minimizing negative peer influence and encourage the parents and family to foster a positive self-image in an adolescent through praise and acceptance. Praise should be directed not only at the teenager, but also at others in his or her life, such as peers and teachers. Adolescents need to hear parents speak positively about other people in general; intolerance frequently is learned at home.

Finally, parental acceptance of an adolescent's separation from the family often enables the adolescent to return psychologically to the family. Parents need to learn how to increase the teenager's independence gradually from the shelter of home in a manner that is not too restrictive. As the adolescent and the family learn that the teen can handle dating, driving, or outside employment responsibly, the adolescent also will learn how to interact with the family as an adult. Many adolescents appreciate their parents more after separation has occurred.

Stages of Adolescent Development

EARLY ADOLESCENCE

The period from 11 to 14 years of age is characterized by marked physical changes that make adolescents extremely vulnerable to perceptions of how they appear to others. In addition, behavioral changes are common with the onset of early adolescence and include fatigue, increased sleeping, irritability, secretiveness, and easy embarrassment. Fatigue and increased sleeping may be related to the physical changes of a growth spurt. The parent needs to recognize the increased sleep demands, encourage regular bedtimes, and minimize distractions in the bedroom (televisions, computer games, and telephones). The marked physical changes, which include growth of body hair and genital development, sometimes can be a source of embarrassment (eg, the inconsistent voice changes of a teenage male or an outbreak of acne before a major social event). Each adolescent responds differently to bodily changes and consequential psychological effects, but family and peer relationships can help guide this development.

Cognitive skills in adolescents also show broad change, as described by Jean Piaget. With concrete thinking, an early adolescent understands issues as absolute truths such as right and wrong. Concrete thinkers may understand simple cause and effect and relate this to themselves egocentrically. This rigid framework gives way to abstract reasoning and the understanding of complex interrelationships that Piaget described as formal operative thought. Although the onset of formal operative thought may come in early adolescence, refinement of these cognitive skills occurs throughout adolescence. As an outcome of this developmental process, the late adolescent applies hypothetical and deductive reasoning skills for consideration of multiple viewpoints, critical decision-making, and contemplation of long-term consequences. Because of the early adolescent's restricted ability for complex abstract thought, physicians must recognize the limited ability of a young teenager to consider long-range health risks (eg, cholesterol in diet, sedentary lifestyle). Similarly, sexual behavior can be affected by stages of cognitive development, with risk-taking by the early adolescent (eg, no condom use) and the development of more mature, intimate relationships in late adolescence. Paramount to this theory is that cognitive age does not equal chronologic age. Children, therefore, must be assessed through open conversation during the health supervision visit for the physician to match anticipatory guidance with cognitive thought.

Experience and environment can influence cognitive development. Although parents and schools take responsibility for shaping the mental growth of a teen, the variety of sources from which teens learn proactively are no less important. Television and the Internet are technological sources from which adolescents learn about society. Volunteer groups, sports teams, recreational activities, and religious groups are social avenues in which teens gain knowledge of self and society. As the adolescent participates in these groups, he or she may develop "crushes" on adult authority figures, which are not uncommon in early and mid-adolescent social development.

Summer reading or trips to museums can improve a child's vocabulary, thinking, and reasoning skills. Community sports teams and mentoring programs can teach cooperation, loyalty, and respect (moral thinking). In contrast, adolescents who join a street gang can learn distortions of these skills with detrimental effects. Negative influences also are promoted heavily by media and advertising campaigns.

Sexuality and violent behavior frequently are glamorized, misrepresenting consequences for risk-taking behaviors and promoting false themes regarding punishment. Media and advertising portrayals can lead to poor body image and acceptance of poor school performance. Physicians should be acquainted with policy statements and recommendations from the American Academy of Pediatrics about the media's influence on children.

MIDDLE ADOLESCENCE

The physiologic changes that characterize early adolescence generally are completed by 15 to 17 years (middle adolescence) for girls, whereas boys still are maturing during this phase. However, most adolescents are secure in their sexual identities. They are better able to understand relationships as well as expectations and their roles in society. As mentioned previously, participation in a variety of extracurricular activities helps them achieve this understanding. High school academic performance may be stressful. Physicians need to help teenagers learn to deal with such stress.

LATE ADOLESCENCE

Although late adolescence is characterized by formal operative thinking (abstract thought), it is important to realize that a person in this stage is not always consistent in his or her thought process. The goal of independence dominates thinking; vocational, educational, and personal issues are major decisions. Health care practitioners need to instruct parents to encourage their adolescents in independent decision-making (Table 1).

Table 1. Anticipatory Guidance for Parents of Adolescents

Early Adolescent	Middle Adolescent	Late Adolescent
Spend time with adolescent	Same as early adolescent plus...	Same as early and middle adolescent plus...
Praise positive behavior	Discuss dangers of drinking and driving	Encourage adolescent in independent decision-making
Respect adolescent's need for privacy	Insist on seat belts	Encourage designated drivers (or calling for a ride) if drinking
Establish limits and consequences for breaking them	Discuss sexuality and disease prevention	
Discuss sexuality		
Model good behavior, including health promotion		

Data from Green M, Palfrey JS—Bright Futures.

Risk-taking, Sexuality, and Other Health-related Concerns of Adolescents

Only through open-ended questioning can the physician gain insight into the teenager's understanding of health, disease, and risk-taking. However, before the patient encounter, physicians should review routinely their working knowledge of the risk-taking behaviors of adolescents and the consequences of these behaviors. The following statistics elaborate on some of the core issues that currently face adolescents.

Motor vehicle accidents remain the leading cause of serious injury and death among adolescents between 16 and 20 years of age, especially males. For every adolescent killed in a motor vehicle crash, about 100 nonfatal injuries occur, with crashes representing a leading cause of disability related to head and spinal cord injuries in this age group. A 16-year-old driver is 20 times more likely to have a crash as is the general population of drivers. Risk-taking behavior and lack of driving experience account for this increased risk of crashing. Risk-taking behavior includes nighttime driving, use of alcohol and other drugs such as marijuana, and low rate of seat belt usage. The physician must recognize the limited ability of an early adolescent to link cause and effect in regard to health behavior (eg, smoking, overeating, use of alcohol or drugs, reckless driving). In addition, the inability to think in the abstract influences the early adolescent's concept of immortality ("It won't happen to me") as a factor in risk-taking behavior (eg, use of alcohol or drugs, reckless driving, nonuse of a seat belt). Risk-taking and testing of limits are part of achieving independence and self-identity for the adolescent, but the physician can suggest safe ways of achieving such goals. Homicide and suicide are the other major causes of death in 15- to 19-year-old youth. Physician inquiries of both parents and teens regarding gun ownership and access are mandatory.

Risk-taking behavior in adolescents includes sexual behavior. Nearly two thirds of high school seniors have had sexual intercourse, one half are currently sexually active, and one fifth of adolescents have had four or more partners. Factors associated with early initiation of sexual intercourse include early puberty, sexual abuse, and poverty. Factors associated with later initiation of sexual activity include parental consistency and firmness in discipline and high academic achievement. Of those adolescents who are sexually active, 25% become infected with a sexually transmitted disease each year. Female adolescents in the United States have one of the world's highest teenage pregnancy rates. The younger the age of an adolescent girl's first intercourse, the more likely that she has had involuntary or forced sex. Allowing access to condoms in school-based clinics does not affect rates of sexual activity but does increase the use of condoms with intercourse. Physicians caring for adolescents need to be familiar with current contraceptive practices and treatment of sexually transmitted diseases.

During the adolescent years, many youths engage in sexual experimentation, which may include homosexual behavior. Transient homosexual experimentation is not uncommon in early and mid-adolescent social development; such behavior does not predict future sexual orientation. Not all adolescents who are emotionally attracted to a member of the same gender engage in any sexual activity. Adolescents struggling with issues of sexual preference should be reassured that they gradually will form their own identities. This is extremely important because approximately 30% of gay youths have attempted suicide at least once.

In the same manner that struggles with sexual identity may produce a negative self-concept, health issues that affect the outward appearance of an adolescent may interfere with achieving a positive self-image. Early adolescents place confidence in their external features, so any physical feature that is viewed as suboptimal will affect the teen's view of self substantially. Acne or orthodontics, for example, can contribute to a poor self-image. The potential psychological complications of having a large facial birthmark, an arm contracted by hemiparesis, or the disfiguring scar of a burn will be even more severe. Similarly, nonvisible health conditions may have associated emotional problems. Because of therapies, restrictions, or other ways of obviously not fitting a norm, children who have diabetes, epilepsy, a learning disability, or other chronic illness may encounter isolation and have a poor self-image.

In addition to self-image, the goal of achieving independence also may suffer. Illnesses such as juvenile rheumatoid arthritis, diabetes, and asthma require medications and routine physician visits. In a stage of life where gaining independence shapes a person's definition of self, it is difficult to accept emotional and physical constraints of an illness, such as reduced physical endurance, pain, dependence on medical specialists, physical assistance, and treatments. The disease itself or the treatment may be the aggravating factor. If the disease interferes with growth and physical maturation, added "disfigurement" could occur. Because physical attractiveness is increasingly important, variations from society's standards are considered unacceptable. Temporary social withdrawal may result from illness and treatment that interferes with engaging fully in peer activity. Isolation from peers and teasing that occurs from differences can engender poor socialization. Depression, aggression, or antisocial behaviors are some of the potential consequences. It is important for the clinician to understand the relationship between chronic illness and psychopathology in adolescence.

Due to the fight for independence and social acceptance, an adolescent may show poor compliance with health regimens. Features of an illness that worsen compliance include lack of symptoms and lack of perceived seriousness of the illness. For example, the silent disease of hypertension occurs in some adolescents and without treatment may lead to serious complications. The same sense of invulnerability that leads to risk-taking behaviors in adolescents can prompt disregard of treatments.

Physicians should recognize that rejection of authority and risk-taking tendencies of adolescents also may include rejection of previously accepted medical advice and treatment. The child who has asthma and once was interested in maintaining health for adult approval may stop using preventive medicines and begin cigarette smoking as an early adolescent. Parents and physicians should not attempt to regain authority over the child's behavior. Instead, guidance based on the teen's cognitive level should be offered.

Additionally, adverse effects of the treatment, multiple doses of a medication, or multiple treatment requirements may be perceived as restrictive. The later cognitive development in adolescence will allow the teen to understand how limited and shortsighted this thought is. However, not every person matures to such higher cognitive function; for those who do not, the consequences of noncompliance already may be manifest.

Physicians' efforts to promote quality health care should include careful interviewing of the adolescent to assess cognitive skills and developmental maturity with respect to illness. Advice or an explanation by a physician will be more effective if it is adapted to the developmental phase of the adolescent receiving it (Table 2). Consider the athlete who has concerns that his or her illness may affect social function or limit performance. Matching the teen's cognitive level and addressing these concerns will be more effective than simply

Table 2. Anticipatory Guidance for Adolescents

Early Adolescent	Middle Adolescent	Late Adolescent
Sleep 8 hours every night	Same as early adolescent plus...	Same as early and middle adolescent plus...
Engage in 30 minutes of moderately strenuous activity at least 3 d/wk	Seek help if you feel angry	Take on new challenges to increase your self-confidence
Learn about yourself	Accept who you are	Continue to develop your sense of identity
Develop skills in conflict resolution	Learn how to deal with stress	Ride with a designated driver (or call for a ride) if drinking
Learn ways to resist sexual pressures	Set reasonable but challenging goals	
Do not drink alcohol or smoke cigarettes	Understand that sexual feelings are normal but that having sex is a major decision	
Wear a seat belt in cars	Drive responsibly	

Data from Green M, Palfrey JS—Bright Futures.

explaining the symptoms and long-term consequences of a disease. On the other hand, an adolescent who does not understand how symptoms are a part of a disease requires instruction before healthy behavioral changes can be made.

Behavioral techniques that may enhance patient compliance should be sought. For example, sustained-release methylphenidate preparations allow home dosing of medication, facilitating privacy and minimizing the labeling of a child as hyperactive or inattentive. Medical calendars, dosing in synchrony with a patient's regular activity, and allowing medical appointments or routine hospitalizations that do not interfere with the adolescent's school and extracurricular activities can facilitate improved compliance. Taking daily medication at the same time as brushing one's teeth helps to establish compliance. Use of intramuscular depot medroxyprogesterone may be useful in teens unable to take daily medication consistently. Developmentally appropriate parental involvement, taking into account the adolescent's capacity for self-care and emerging need for autonomy, may improve compliance.

Physicians also must understand that chronic disease necessitates an element of increased social maturation to achieve best compliance. The already difficult task of finding acceptance is worsened, for example, in the case of the child who has asthma when faced with competing demands of experimentation to gain peer acceptance and avoidance of smoking behaviors for best health. Encouraging the patient's strengths and promoting self-reliance and early independence of care within the adolescent's abilities should be part of routine counseling. Physicians also need to help older adolescents, especially those who have chronic illness, identify clinicians who can provide medical care and advice at college or in the community.

In addition, the focus of intervention must shift from the isolated patient to the social setting in which the patient lives to provide the best care for adolescents. Families can help by showing support, assisting with needs, and developing problem-focused decision-making and coping skills. Parents need to model good health and lifestyle behaviors for the adolescent to learn such. Through the use of peer educators, other adolescents can be instructed in disease education and take active roles in support and interest in the patient's health. Physicians should remember their responsibilities in providing the adolescent, family members, and the community with information that will promote well-being for the adolescent during these difficult transition years.

Suggested Reading

AAP Committee on Adolescence. Condom use by adolescents. *Pediatrics.* 2001;107:1463–1469

AAP Committee on Adolescence. Contraception and adolescents. *Pediatrics.* 1999;104:1161–1166

AAP Committee on Adolescence. Homosexuality and adolescence. *Pediatrics.* 1993;92:631–634

AAP Committee on Communications. Children, adolescents, and advertising. *Pediatrics.* 1995;95:295–297

AAP Committee on Injury and Poison Prevention and Committee on Adolescence. The teenage driver. *Pediatrics.* 1996;98:987–990

AAP Committee on Public Education. Children, adolescents, and television. *Pediatrics.* 2001;107:423–426

AAP Committee on Public Education. Sexuality, contraception, and the media. *Pediatrics.* 2001;107:191–194

Fisher L, Weihs K. Can addressing family relationships improve outcomes in chronic disease? Report of the National Working Group on Family-Based Interventions in Chronic Disease. *J Fam Pract.* 2000;49:561–566

Green M, Palfrey JS, eds. *2000: Bright Futures: Guidelines for Health Supervision of Infants, Children, and Adolescents.* 2nd ed. Arlington, Va: National Center for Education in Maternal and Child Health; 2000

Henricson C, Roker D. Support for the parents of adolescents: a review. *J Adolesc.* 2000;23:763–783

Hoyert DL, Freedman MA, Strobino DM, Guyer B. Annual summary of vital statistics: 2000. *Pediatrics.* 2001;108:1241–1255

Kyngas HA, Kroll T, Duffy ME. Compliance in adolescents with chronic diseases: a review. *J Adolesc Health.* 2000;26:379–388

Sexual Orientation and Adolescents

Barbara L. Frankowski, MD, MPH; and the Committee on Adolescence

ABSTRACT. The American Academy of Pediatrics issued its first statement on homosexuality and adolescents in 1983, with a revision in 1993. This report reflects the growing understanding of youth of differing sexual orientations. Young people are recognizing their sexual orientation earlier than in the past, making this a topic of importance to pediatricians. Pediatricians should be aware that some youths in their care may have concerns about their sexual orientation or that of siblings, friends, parents, relatives, or others. Health care professionals should provide factual, current, nonjudgmental information in a confidential manner. All youths, including those who know or wonder whether they are not heterosexual, may seek information from physicians about sexual orientation, sexually transmitted diseases, substance abuse, or various psychosocial difficulties. The pediatrician should be attentive to various potential psychosocial difficulties, offer counseling or refer for counseling when necessary and ensure that every sexually active youth receives a thorough medical history, physical examination, immunizations, appropriate laboratory tests, and counseling about sexually transmitted diseases (including human immunodeficiency virus infection) and appropriate treatment if necessary.

Not all pediatricians may feel able to provide the type of care described in this report. Any pediatrician who is unable to care for and counsel nonheterosexual youth should refer these patients to an appropriate colleague. *Pediatrics* 2004;113:1827–1832; *sexual orientation, adolescents, homosexuality, gay, lesbian, bisexual.*

ABBREVIATIONS. STD, sexually transmitted disease; HIV, human immunodeficiency virus; AAP, American Academy of Pediatrics; AIDS, acquired immunodeficiency syndrome.

Introduction

Pediatricians are being asked with increasing frequency to address questions about sexual behavior and sexual orientation. It is important that pediatricians be able to discuss the range of sexual orientation with all adolescents and be competent in dealing with the needs of patients who are gay, lesbian, bisexual, or transgendered or who may not identify themselves as such but who are experiencing confusion with regard to their sexual orientation. Young people whose sexual orientation is not heterosexual can have risks to their physical, emotional, and social health, primarily because of societal stigma, which can result in isolation.[1,2] Because self-awareness of sexual orientation commonly occurs during adolescence, the pediatrician should be available to youth who are struggling with sexual orientation issues and support a healthy passage through the special challenges of the adolescent years. Pediatricians may be called on to help parents, siblings, and extended families of nonheterosexual youth. Also, nonheterosexual youth and adults are part of peer groups with whom all pediatric patients and their parents spend time in the neighborhood, at school, or at work. Thus, pediatricians may be called on to help promote better understanding of issues involving nonheterosexual youth.

Gay, lesbian, and bisexual people in the United States have unique health risks. The US Department of Health and Human Services has identified 29 *Healthy People 2010* objectives in which disparities exist between homosexual or bisexual persons and heterosexual persons. These focus areas include access to care, educational and community-based programs, family planning, immunization and infectious disease, sexually transmitted diseases (STDs) including human immunodeficiency virus (HIV) infection, injury and violence prevention, mental health and mental disorders, substance abuse, and tobacco use.[3]

PEDIATRICS (ISSN 0031 4005). Copyright © 2004 by the American Academy of Pediatrics.

Definitions

Sexual orientation[4,5] refers to an individual's pattern of physical and emotional arousal toward other persons. Heterosexual individuals are attracted to persons of the opposite sex, homosexual individuals are attracted to persons of the same sex, and bisexual individuals are attracted to persons of both sexes. Homosexual males are often referred to as "gay"; homosexual females are often referred to as "lesbian." In contrast, gender identity is the knowledge of oneself as being male or female, and gender role is the outward expression of maleness or femaleness. Gender identity and gender role usually conform to anatomic sex in both heterosexual and homosexual individuals. Exceptions to this are transgendered individuals and transvestites. Transgendered individuals feel themselves to be of a gender different from their biological sex; their gender identity does not match their anatomic or chromosomal sex. Transvestites are individuals who dress in the clothing of the opposite gender and derive pleasure from such actions; their gender role does not match societal norms. Transgendered individuals and transvestites can be heterosexual, homosexual, or bisexual.

Sexual orientation is not synonymous with sexual activity or sexual behavior (the way one chooses to express one's sexual feelings). Certain sexual behaviors can put individuals of any sexual orientation at risk of pregnancy (penile-vaginal sexual intercourse) and/or certain diseases (penile-vaginal, oral, and anal sexual intercourse). Especially during adolescence, individuals may participate in a variety of sexual behaviors. Many homosexual adults report having relationships and sexual activity with persons of the opposite sex as adolescents,[6,7] and many adults who identify themselves as heterosexual report sexual activity with persons of the same sex during adolescence.[8-10] Also, many youth label themselves as gay, lesbian, or bisexual years after labeling their attractions as such.[11] In addition, adolescents may also self-identify as nonheterosexual without ever being sexually active. Pediatricians need to understand that they should inquire about sexual attraction or orientation even when youth do not report being gay or lesbian.

Etiology and Prevalence

Homosexuality has existed in most societies for as long as recorded descriptions of sexual beliefs and practices have been available.[4] Societal attitudes toward homosexuality have had a decisive effect on the extent to which individuals have hidden or made known their sexual orientation.

Human sexual orientation most likely exists as a continuum from solely heterosexual to solely homosexual. In 1973, the American Psychiatric Association reclassified homosexuality as a sexual orientation or expression and not a mental disorder.[12] The mechanisms for the development of a particular sexual orientation remain unclear, but the current literature and most scholars in the field state that one's sexual orientation is not a choice; that is, individuals do not choose to be homosexual or heterosexual.[8,11]

A variety of theories about the influences on sexual orientation have been proposed.[5] Sexual orientation probably is not determined by any one factor but by a combination of genetic, hormonal, and environmental influences.[2] In recent decades, biologically based theories have been favored by experts. The high concordance of homosexuality among monozygotic twins and the clustering of homosexuality in family pedigrees support biological models. There is some evidence that prenatal androgen exposure influences development of sexual orientation, but postnatal sex steroid concentrations do not vary with sexual orientation. The reported association in males between homosexual orientation and loci on the X chromosome remains to be replicated. Some research has shown neuroanatomic differences between homosexual and heterosexual persons in sexually dimorphic regions of the brain.[5] Although there continues to be controversy and uncertainty as to the genesis of the variety of human sexual orientations, there is no scientific evidence that abnormal parenting, sexual abuse, or other adverse life events influence sexual orientation.[4,5] Current knowledge suggests that sexual orientation is usually established during early childhood.[1,2,4,5]

The estimated proportion of Americans who are homosexual is imprecise at best, because surveys are hampered by the stigmatization and the climate of fear that still surround homosexuality.

Past studies asked more often about sexual behavior and not sexual orientation. Kinsey et al,[9,13] from their studies in the 1930s and 1940s, reported that 37% of adult men and 13% of adult women had at least 1 sexual experience resulting in orgasm with a person of the same sex and that 4% of adult men and 2% of adult women are exclusively homosexual in their behavior and fantasies. A more recent review of various US studies estimated that 2% of men are exclusively homosexual and 3% are bisexual.[14] Other current studies conclude that somewhere between 3% and 10% of the adult population is gay or lesbian, and perhaps a larger percentage is bisexual.[4,5] Sorenson[15] surveyed a group of 16- to 19-year-olds and reported that 6% of females and 17% of males had at least 1 sexual experience with a person of the same sex. Remafedi et al,[10] in a large, population-based study of junior and senior high school students performed in the late 1980s that measured sexual fantasy, emotional attraction, and sexual behavior, found that more than 25% of 12-year-old students felt uncertain about their sexual orientation. This uncertainty decreased with the passage of time and increasing sexual experience to only 5% of 18-year-old students. Only 1.1% of students reported themselves as predominantly homosexual or bisexual. However, 4.5% reported primary sexual attractions to persons of the same sex, which better reflects actual sexual orientation. The Garofalo et al study,[16] based on the 1995 Massachusetts Youth Risk Behavior Survey, found that 2.5% of youth self-identified as gay, lesbian, or bisexual.

These data illustrate the complexity of labeling sexual orientation in adolescents. Health care professionals should be aware that a large number of adolescents have questions about their sexual feelings; some are attracted to and may have sexual relations with people of the same sex, and a small number may know themselves to be gay or lesbian.

Special Needs of Nonheterosexual and Questioning Youth

The overall goal in caring for youth who are or think they might be gay, lesbian, or bisexual is the same as for all youth: to promote normal adolescent development, social and emotional well-being, and physical health. If their environment is critical of their emerging sexual orientation, these adolescents may experience profound isolation and fear of discovery, which interferes with achieving developmental tasks of adolescence related to self-esteem, identity, and intimacy.[17,18] Nonheterosexual youth often are subjected to harassment and violence; 45% of gay men and 20% of lesbians surveyed were victims of verbal and physical assaults in secondary school specifically because of their sexual orientation.[1,19]

Nonheterosexual youth are at higher risk of dropping out of school, being kicked out of their homes, and turning to life on the streets for survival. Some of these youth engage in substance use, and they are more likely than heterosexual peers to start using tobacco, alcohol, and illegal drugs at an earlier age.[20] Nonheterosexual youth are more likely to have had sexual intercourse, to have had more partners, and to have experienced sexual intercourse against their will,[20] putting them at increased risk of STDs including HIV infection. In a recent study of HIV seroprevalence, 7% of 3492 15- to 22-year-old males who have sex with males living in 7 US cities were HIV-seropositive. Among adolescent males who have sex with males, HIV seroprevalence rates in descending order were highest among black adolescents, then "mixed race or other" adolescents, and then Hispanic adolescents and were lowest among Asian and white adolescents.[21] Women having sex with women have the lowest risk of any STD, but lesbian adolescents remain at significant risk because they are likely to have had sexual intercourse with males. Youth in high school who identify themselves as gay, lesbian, or bisexual; engage in sexual activity with persons of the same sex; or report same-sex romantic attractions or relationships are more likely to attempt suicide, be victimized, and abuse substances.[20,22] Although only representing a portion of youth who someday will self-identify as gay, lesbian, or bisexual, school-based studies have found that these adolescents, compared with heterosexual peers, are 2 to 7 times more likely to attempt suicide,[16,19,23,24] are 2 to 4 times more likely to be threatened with a weapon at school,[16,23] and are more likely to engage in frequent and heavy use of alcohol, marijuana, and cocaine. It is important to note that these psychosocial problems and suicide attempts in non-heterosexual youth are neither universal nor attributable to homosexuality per se, but they are significantly associated with stigmatization of gender nonconformity, stress, violence, lack of support, dropping out of school, family problems, acquaintances' suicide attempts, homelessness, and substance abuse.[2,25] In addition to suicidality, young gay and bisexual men might also suffer body image dissatisfaction and disordered eating behaviors for some of the same reasons.[26]

Nonheterosexual youth are represented within all populations of adolescents, all social classes, and all racial and ethnic groups. Ethnic minority youth who are nonheterosexual are required to manage more than one stigmatized identity, which increases their level of vulnerability and stress.[27] They retain their minority status when they seek help in the predominately white gay and lesbian support communities. In addition, sexual minority youth are represented among handicapped adolescents, homeless adolescents, and incarcerated youth.[1]

Most nonheterosexual youths are "invisible" and will pass through pediatricians' offices without raising the issue of sexual orientation on their own. Therefore, health care professionals should raise issues of sexual orientation and sexual behavior with all adolescent patients or refer them to a colleague who can. Such discussions normalize the notion that there is a range of sexual orientation. The portrayal of openly gay or lesbian characters in media is starting to change how adolescents view these differences. Even adolescents who are quite sure of their own heterosexuality are likely to have friends, relatives, teachers, etc whom they know or suspect to be gay or lesbian or who are struggling with questions about their sexual orientation. Rather than asking patients whether they have a "boyfriend" or "girlfriend," pediatricians could ask, "Have you ever had a romantic relationship with a boy or a girl?" or "When you think of people to whom you are sexually attracted, are they men, women, both, neither, or are you not sure yet?" By doing so, pediatricians open the door to additional communication and start to break down stereotypes and stigmatization. It implies that any of the options is possible and that an adolescent may not be sure of his or her sexual orientation. If these issues are addressed, specifically targeted medical screening, medical treatment, and anticipatory guidance can be provided to adolescents who need it. Pediatricians can have an important positive effect on young people and their families by addressing sexual orientation and sexual behavior on several levels: office and hospital policies, clinical care, and community advocacy.[2]

Office Practice: Ensure a Safe and Supportive Environment

A pediatric encounter may give adolescents a rare opportunity to discuss their concerns about their sexual orientation and/or activities. Adolescents' level of comfort in the pediatric office sets the tone for their other health care interactions. The way sexuality and other important personal issues are discussed also sets an example for all adolescents and their parents. In the office, pediatricians are encouraged to[28]:

1. Assure the patient that his or her confidentiality is protected.[29]
2. Implement policies against insensitive or inappropriate jokes and remarks by office staff.
3. Be sure that information forms use gender-neutral, nonjudgmental language.
4. Consider displaying posters, brochures, and information on bulletin boards that demonstrate support of issues important to nonheterosexual youth and their families (eg, the American Academy of Pediatrics [AAP] brochure "Gay, Lesbian, and Bisexual Teens: Facts for Teens and their Parents").
5. Provide information about support groups and other resources to nonheterosexual youth and their friends and families if requested.

Comprehensive Health Care for All Adolescents

Pediatricians are not responsible for labeling or even identifying nonheterosexual youth. Instead, the pediatrician should create a clinical environment in which clear messages are given that sensitive personal issues including sexual orientation can be discussed whenever the adolescent feels ready to do so. A major obstacle to effective medical care is adolescents' misunderstanding of their right to confidential care.[30] The pediatrician should be ready to raise and discuss issues of sexual orientation with all adolescents, particularly those in distress or engaged in high-risk behaviors. The pediatrician should be able to explore the adolescent's understanding and concerns about sexual orientation, dispel any misconceptions, provide appropriate medical care and anticipatory guidance, and connect the adolescent to appropriate supportive community resources. Pediatricians are encouraged to[29,31]:

1. Be aware of the special issues surrounding the development of sexual orientation.[29]
2. Assure the patient that his or her confidentiality is protected.[29]
3. Discuss emerging sexuality with all adolescents.[32]
   - Be knowledgeable that many heterosexual youth also may have sexual experiences with people of their own sex. Labeling as homosexual an adolescent who has had sexual experiences with persons of the same sex or is questioning his or her sexual orientation could be premature, inappropriate, and counterproductive.
   - Use gender-neutral language in discussing sexuality; use the word "partner" rather than "boyfriend" or "girlfriend," and talk about "protection" rather than just "birth control."
   - Give evidence of support and acceptance to adolescents questioning their sexual orientation.
   - Provide information and resources regarding gay, lesbian, and bisexual issues to all interested adolescents.
   - Ask all adolescents about risky behaviors, depression, and suicidal thoughts.
   - Encourage abstinence, discourage multiple partners, and provide "safer sex" guidelines to all adolescents.[33] Discuss the risks associated with anal intercourse for those who choose to engage in this behavior, and teach them ways to decrease risk.
   - Counsel all adolescents about the link between substance use (alcohol, marijuana, and other drugs) and unsafe sexual intercourse.
   - Ask all adolescents about personal experience with violence including sexual or intimate-partner violence.

   Provide additional screening and education as indicated for each adolescent's sexual activity:
   - STD testing from appropriate sites[34]
   - HIV testing with appropriate support and counseling[35]
   - Pregnancy testing and counseling[36,37]
   - Papanicolaou testing
   - Hepatitis B and, when appropriate, hepatitis A immunization
4. Ensure that colleagues to whom adolescents are referred or with whom you consult are respectful of the range of adolescents' sexual orientation.

Special Considerations for Non-Heterosexual Youth

For adolescents who self-identify as gay, lesbian, or bisexual, pediatricians should be particularly aware of several points:

1. Be prepared to refer adolescents' care if you have personal barriers to providing such care. Many individuals have strong negative attitudes about homosexuality or may simply feel uncomfortable with the subject. Even discomfort expressed through body language can send a very damaging message to nonheterosexual youth. It is an ethical and professional obligation to make an appropriate referral in these situations for the good of the child or adolescent.

2. Assure the patient that his or her confidentiality is protected.[29] Discuss with adolescents and, if appropriate, their parents whether they wish to have their sexual orientation recorded in office and hospital charts. Many nonheterosexual adults prefer to have this information recorded so that health care professionals will not assume heterosexuality.

3. Help the adolescent think through his or her feelings carefully; strong same-sex feelings and even sexual experiences can occur at this age and do not define sexual orientation.

4. Carefully identify all risky behaviors (sexual behaviors; use of tobacco, alcohol, and drugs; etc) and offer advice and treatment if indicated.

5. Ask about mental health concerns and evaluate or refer patients with identified problems.

6. Offer support and advice to adolescents faced with or anticipating conflicts with families and/or friends.

7. Encourage transition to adult health care when age-appropriate.

Pediatricians should be aware that the revelation of an adolescent's homosexuality (also called disclosure or "coming out") has the potential for intense family discord.[1,2,28] In many families, it precipitates physical and/or emotional abuse or even expulsion. The pediatrician can advise the adolescent to use certain language that may be helpful at the time of disclosure, such as "I am the same person, you just know one more thing about me now." However, there is no one disclosure technique that will preclude negative reactions. Parents, siblings, and other family members may require professional help to deal with their confusion, anger, guilt, and feelings of loss, and professionals who work with adolescents may be required to intervene on the adolescent's behalf. If the pediatrician has a relationship with the parents from ongoing primary care, he or she can be an important initial source of support and information. However, adolescents should be counseled to think carefully about the consequences of disclosure and to take their time in sharing information that could have many repercussions.[1]

With regard to parents of nonheterosexual adolescents, pediatricians are encouraged to:

1. Advise adolescents about whether, when, and how to disclose their nonheterosexuality to their parents. If unsure, assist the adolescent in finding a knowledgeable professional who can help.

2. Be knowledgeable about the process of disclosure.

3. Be supportive of parents of adolescents who have disclosed that they are not heterosexual. Most states have chapters of Parents and Friends of Lesbians and Gays (PFLAG) to which interested families may be referred.

4. Remind parents and adolescents that gay and lesbian individuals can be successful parents themselves.[38–41]

5. Be prepared to refer parents if you do not feel personally comfortable accepting this responsibility.

Community Advocacy

Despite AAP statements issued in 1983[42] and 1993[43] urging excellent clinical care for nonheterosexual adolescents, these patients still experience many risks to their physical and mental health and safety that occur outside the scope of usual office practice. Some pediatricians may wish to take a broader role in their communities to help decrease these risks. Pediatricians could model and provide opportunities for increasing awareness and knowledge of homosexuality and bisexuality among school staff, mental health professionals, and other community leaders. They can make themselves available as resources for community HIV and acquired immunodeficiency syndrome (AIDS) education and prevention activities. It is critical that schools find a way to create safe and supportive environments for students who are or wonder about being nonheterosexual or who have a parent or other family member who is nonheterosexual. Support from respected pediatricians can facilitate these efforts greatly. Pediatricians who choose to be active on these issues may wish to[2,28]:

1. Help raise awareness among school and community leaders of issues relevant to nonheterosexual youth.

2. Help with the discussion of when and how factual materials about sexual orientation should be included in school curricula and in school and community libraries.

3. Support the development and maintenance of school- and community-based support groups for nonheterosexual students and their friends and parents.

4. Support HIV and AIDS prevention and education efforts.

5. Develop and/or request continuing education opportunities for health care professionals related to issues of sexual orientation, nonheterosexual youth, and their families.

Summary of Physician Guidelines

The AAP reaffirms the physician's responsibility to provide comprehensive health care and guidance in a safe and supportive environment for all adolescents, including nonheterosexual adolescents and young people struggling with issues of sexual orientation. Some pediatricians might choose to assume the additional role of advocating for nonheterosexual youth and their families in their communities. The deadly consequences of HIV and AIDS, the damaging effects of violence and ostracism, and the increased prevalence of adolescent suicidal behavior underscore the critical need to address and seek to prevent the major physical and mental health problems that confront nonheterosexual youths in their transition to a healthy adulthood.

COMMITTEE ON ADOLESCENCE, 2002–2003
David W. Kaplan, MD, MPH, Chairperson
Angela Diaz, MD
Ronald A. Feinstein, MD
Martin M. Fisher, MD
Jonathan D. Klein, MD, MPH
W. Samuel Yancy, MD

PAST COMMITTEE MEMBERS
Luis F. Olmedo, MD
Ellen S. Rome, MD, MPH

LIAISONS
S. Paige Hertweck, MD
American College of Obstetricians and Gynecologists
Glen Pearson, MD
American Academy of Child and Adolescent Psychiatry
Miriam E. Kaufman, MD
Canadian Paediatric Society
Barbara L. Frankowski, MD, MPH
Past Liaison to Section on School Health
Diane G. Sacks, MD
Past Liaison From Canadian Paediatric Society

CONSULTANT
Ellen C. Perrin, MD

STAFF
Karen S. Smith

References

1. Ryan C, Futterman D. *Lesbian and Gay Youth: Care and Counseling.* New York, NY: Columbia University Press; 1998

2. Perrin EC. *Sexual Orientation in Child and Adolescent Health Care.* New York, NY: Kluwer Academic/Plenum Publishers; 2002

3. Sell RL, Becker JB. Sexual orientation data collection and progress toward Healthy People 2010. *Am J Public Health.* 2001;91:876–882

4. Friedman RC, Downey JI. Homosexuality. *N Engl J Med.* 1994;331:923–930

5. Stronski Huwiler SM, Remafedi G. Adolescent homosexuality. *Adv Pediatr.* 1998;45:107–144

6. Bell AP, Weinberg MS. *Homosexualities: A Study of Diversity Among Men and Women.* New York, NY: Simon and Shuster; 1978

7. Jay K, Young A. *The Gay Report: Lesbians and Gay Men Speak Out About Their Sexual Experiences and Lifestyles.* New York, NY: Summitt Books; 1979

8. Rowlett JD, Patel D, Greydanus DE. Homosexuality. In: Greydanus DE, Wolraich ML, eds. *Behavioral Pediatrics.* New York, NY: Springer-Verlag; 1992:37–54

9. Kinsey AC, Pomeroy WB, Martin CE. *Sexual Behavior in the Human Male.* Philadelphia, PA: WB Saunders Co; 1948

10. Remafedi G, Resnick M, Blum R, Harris L. Demography of sexual orientation in adolescents. *Pediatrics.* 1992;89:714–721

11. Savin-Williams RC. Theoretical perspectives accounting for adolescent homosexuality. *J Adolesc Health Care.* 1988;9:95–104

12. American Psychiatric Association. *Diagnostic and Statistical Manual of Mental Disorders.* 3rd ed. Revised. Washington, DC: American Psychiatric Association; 1987

13. Kinsey AC, Pomeroy WB, Martin CE. *Sexual Behavior in the Human Female.* Philadelphia, PA: WB Saunders Co; 1953

14. Seidman SN, Reider RO. A review of sexual behavior in the United States. *Am J Psychiatry.* 1994;151:330–341

15. Sorenson RC. *Adolescent Sexuality in Contemporary America.* New York, NY: World Publishing; 1973

16. Garofalo R, Wolf RC, Wissow LS, Woods ER, Goodman E. Sexual orientation and risk of suicide attempts among a representative sample of youth. *Arch Pediatr Adolesc Med.* 1999;153:487–493

17. Kreiss JL, Patterson DL. Psychosocial issues in primary care of lesbian, gay, bisexual, and transgender youth. *J Pediatr Health Care.* 1997;11:266–274

18. Remafedi G. Adolescent homosexuality: psychosocial and medical implications. *Pediatrics.* 1987;79:331–337

19. Russell ST, Franz BT, Driscoll AK. Same-sex romantic attraction and experiences of violence in adolescence. *Am J Public Health.* 2001;91:903–906

20. Garofalo R, Wolf RC, Kessel S, Palfrey SJ, DuRant RH. The association between health risk behaviors and sexual orientation among a school-based sample of adolescents. *Pediatrics.* 1998;101:895–902

21. Valleroy LA, MacKellar DA, Karon JM, et al. HIV prevalence and associated risks in young men who have sex with men. *JAMA.* 2000;284:198–204

22. Remafedi G, Farrow JA, Deisher RW. Risk factors for attempted suicide in gay and bisexual youth. *Pediatrics.* 1991;87:869–875

23. Faulkner AH, Cranston K. Correlates of same-sex sexual behavior in a random sample of Massachusetts high school students. *Am J Public Health.* 1998;88:262–266

24. Remafedi G, French S, Story M, Resnick MD, Blum R. The relationship between suicide risk and sexual orientation: results of a population-based study. *Am J Public Health.* 1998;88:57–60

25. Remafedi G. Sexual orientation and youth suicide. *JAMA.* 1999;282:1291–1292

26. French SA, Story M, Remafedi G, Resnick MD, Blum RW. Sexual orientation and prevalence of body dissatisfaction and eating disordered behaviors: a population-based study of adolescents. *Int J Eat Disord.* 1996;19:119–126

27. Savin-Williams RC, Cohen KM. *The Lives of Lesbians, Gays, and Bisexuals: Children to Adults.* Fort Worth, TX: Harcourt Brace College Publishing; 1996

28. Perrin EC. Pediatricians and gay and lesbian youth. *Pediatr Rev.* 1996;17:311–318

29. American Academy of Pediatrics. Confidentiality in adolescent health care. *AAP News.* April 1989:9. Reaffirmed January 1993

30. Allen LB, Glicken AD, Beach RK, Naylor KE. Adolescent health care experience of gay, lesbian, and bisexual young adults. *J Adolesc Health.* 1998;23:212–220

31. Ryan C, Futterman D. Caring for gay and lesbian teens. *Contemp Pediatr.* 1998;15:107–130

32. American Academy of Pediatrics, Committee on Psychosocial Aspects of Child and Family Health and Committee on Adolescence. Sexuality education for children and adolescents. *Pediatrics.* 2001;108:498–502

33. American Academy of Pediatrics, Committee on Adolescence. Condom use by adolescents. *Pediatrics.* 2001;107:1463–1469

34. American Academy of Pediatrics, Committee on Adolescence. Sexually transmitted diseases. *Pediatrics.* 1994;94:568–572

35. American Academy of Pediatrics, Committee on Pediatric AIDS and Committee on Adolescence. Adolescents and human immunodeficiency virus infection: the role of the pediatrician in prevention and intervention. *Pediatrics.* 2001;107:188–190

36. American Academy of Pediatrics, Committee on Adolescence. Counseling the adolescent about pregnancy options. *Pediatrics.* 1998;101:938–940

37. American Academy of Pediatrics, Committee on Adolescence. Adolescent pregnancy—current trends and issues: 1998. *Pediatrics.* 1999;103:516–520

38. Gold MA, Perrin EC, Futterman D, Friedman SB. Children of gay or lesbian parents. *Pediatr Rev.* 1994;15:354–358

39. Perrin EC. Children whose parents are lesbian or gay. *Contemp Pediatr.* 1998;15:113–130

40. American Academy of Pediatrics, Committee on Psychosocial Aspects of Child and Family Health. Coparent or second-parent adoption by same-sex parents. *Pediatrics.* 2002;109:339–340

41. Benkov L. *Reinventing the Family: The Emerging Story of Lesbian and Gay Parents.* New York, NY: Crown Publishers; 1994

42. American Academy of Pediatrics, Committee on Adolescence. Homosexuality and adolescence. *Pediatrics.* 1983;72:249–250

43. American Academy of Pediatrics, Committee on Adolescence. Homosexuality and adolescence. *Pediatrics.* 1993;92:631–634

All clinical reports from the American Academy of Pediatrics automatically expire 5 years after publication unless reaffirmed, revised, or retired at or before that time.

Somatization Disorders in Children and Adolescents

Tomas Jose Silber, MD, * Maryland Pao, MD†*

Objectives

After completing this article, readers should be able to:

1. Describe the various manifestations of somatization disorders in children and adolescents.
2. Delineate the association of psychosomatic disorders with stress, parental anxiety, or pressure for a child to perform.
3. Distinguish between primary and secondary gain.
4. Explain why school attendance should be assessed with every recurrent complaint.
5. Explain why pediatricians should establish a partnership with patients and their parents when addressing their symptoms.
6. Develop a cost-effective investigation of suspected somatoform disorders and an approach to insurance companies regarding reimbursement of services.

Introduction

The diagnosis and treatment of children and adolescents who have somatization disorders constitute a challenge for pediatricians: On one hand, they raise the specter of "missing something"; on the other, any "false step" in explaining the condition risks alienating both the patient and the family. Many clinicians rise to the challenge, but many more are baffled by the onslaught of symptoms, become annoyed by the time consumed in caring for patients who are "not really sick," or feel frustrated by the never-ending recurrent complaints.

To make matters worse, these disorders have been scantly researched; neither meta-analysis nor evidence-based medicine has contributed significantly to the field. Paradoxically, although somatoform disorders in children have been defined as psychiatric disorders, psychiatrists seldom see these patients except for the most extreme, unusual, and bizarre cases. Most children and adolescents who have functional symptoms are seen by primary care physicians. This review, therefore, focuses on understanding and assessing somatization as well as developing strategies for the day-to-day management of these conditions.

Definition and Classification

Somatization has been defined as the occurrence of one or more physical complaints for which appropriate medical evaluation reveals no explanatory physical pathology or pathophysiologic mechanism. Somatization also can coincide with a physical illness. Somatization is deemed to exist in conjunction with a physical illness whenever the physical complaints resulting in impairment are grossly in excess of what would be expected from the known illness or findings. Thus, the central feature of somatoform disorders is that they present with symptoms suggestive of an underlying medical condition, yet such a condition either is not found or does not fully account for the level of functional impairment.

The diagnostic criteria for somatoform disorders originally were established for adults and are applied to children because no child-specific alternative system has been developed. This is

Professor, Department of Pediatrics, The George Washington University School of Medicine and Health Sciences; Director, Adolescent Medicine Fellowship Program, Children's National Medical Center, Washington, DC.

†*Office of the Clinical Director, National Institute of Mental Health, National Institutes of Health; Clinical Assistant Professor of Psychiatry, The George Washington University School of Medicine and Health Sciences, Washington, DC.*

unfortunate because the current classification lacks a pediatric research base. Nevertheless, some progress has been made with a recent classification of child and adolescent mental diagnosis in primary care, which takes into account developmentally appropriate considerations. This review focuses on somatic complaint variation, somatic complaint problem, undifferentiated somatoform disorder, pain disorder, and conversion disorders (Table 1). Factitious disorder (300.16), which sometimes is included in the classification, does not fit very well because the signs and symptoms presented to the physician have been staged deliberately, rather than experienced, by the patient.

Epidemiology

Somatoform disorders seem to follow a developmental sequence. Children appear to experience affective distress in the form of somatic sensations. Initially, these are monosymptomatic, with recurrent abdominal pain and headaches predominating in early childhood. Limb pain, neurologic symptoms, insomnia, and fatigue tend to emerge with increasing age. The prevalence of somatic symptoms is high in the pediatric population: Recurrent abdominal pain accounts for 5% of pediatric office visits, and headaches have been reported to affect 20% to 55% of all children. During adolescence, 10% of teenagers report frequent headaches, chest pain, nausea, and fatigue. A general teenage population survey (ages 12 to 16 y) found that distressing somatic symptoms were present in 11% of girls and 4% of boys. This gender disparity seems to persist into adulthood. There is a higher rate of somatization among lower socioeconomic groups.

Pathogenesis: Genetic and Family Factors

Information on the genetics of somatoform disorders is limited. However, recent genetic studies have shown that somatoform disorders are concordant in twins. They also cluster in families in which there is attention deficit disorder and alcoholism above what would be expected by chance.

Table 1. Current Classification of Somatization Disorders in Children and Adolescents

- Somatic complaint variation (v 65.49)
- Somatic complaint problem (v 40.3)
- Somatization disorder (300.82)
- Somatoform disorder (undifferentiated) (300.82)
- Somatoform disorder, not otherwise specified (300.82)
- Pain disorder (307.8)
- Conversion disorders (300.6)

From Wolraich ML, Felice ME, Drotar D. The classification of child and adolescent mental diagnosis in primary care. In: *Diagnostic and Statistical Manual for Primary Care (DSM-PC) Child and Adolescent Versions.* Elk Grove Village, Ill: American Academy of Pediatrics; 1996

More commonly, clinicians consider somatization to be a learned behavior. It probably begins with the experience that children's somatic complaints are more acceptable in many households than is the expression of strong feelings. When children cannot get attention for emotional distress, they may gain attention for the physical symptoms that often accompany the disturbed emotional state. This reinforcing "psychosomatic pathway" can manifest through a spectrum of somatization disorders, ranging from the mild "somatic complaint variation" (transient complaints that do not interfere with normal functioning) to the severe "somatoform disorder" (associated with significant social and academic problems).

The importance of psychosocial factors in the family of origin is highlighted by the finding that if a family member had a chronic physical illness, there were more somatic symptoms among the children. Even more striking is the finding that somatizing children often live with family members who complain of similar physical symptoms. Theoretic contributions stemming from systemic family therapy also indicate the importance of the family. The symptoms are proposed to be displayed by the child as a way of protecting distressed parents who, when galvanized into caring for their suffering child, are distracted from their own personal concerns. Stress has been implicated as a triggering factor that often is bound to parental anxiety. The most common form of stress consists of pressure on the child to perform. Finally, adolescents who have histories of physical or sexual abuse often present with somatic complaints, develop a somatization disorder, and score higher on measures of somatizations than do controls.

Clinical Aspects

Children and adolescents readily report pain and somatic complaints in their sick visits. These complaints often result from a disease such as tonsillitis, gastroenteritis, or urinary tract infection. However, they can voice similar complaints in the absence of physical disease, and these reports must be approached as possible somatization. The diagnosis of a somatization disorder involves a continuum that ranges from everyday aches and pains to disabling "functional symptoms." Symptoms are spontaneous and not feigned (which distinguishes them from malingering and factitious disorder) and are not better explained by another mental illness (such as depression or anxiety disorder).

SOMATIC COMPLAINT VARIATION

This variation involves discomfort and complaints that do not interfere with everyday functioning. It is a universal experience. In infancy, the complaints probably manifest as transient gastrointestinal distress. In childhood, classic recurrent abdominal pain, headaches, and "growing pains" make their appearance. Adolescents may experience menstrual discomfort and other transient aches and pains, but these characteristically do not impair their ability to function. Females report more somatic complaints after puberty.

SOMATIC COMPLAINT PROBLEM

This consists of one or more physical complaints that do cause sufficient distress and impairment (physical, social, or school) to be considered a problem. In infancy, this would occur when gastrointestinal symptoms seriously interfere with feeding and sleep. In childhood, it entails avoiding or refusing to undertake expected activities (eg, increased school absences). As adolescence approaches, in addition to the somatic complaints, more emotional distress, social withdrawal, and academic difficulties begin to appear. More severe complaints may result in refusal to attend school, aggressive behavior, and recurrent pain syndromes.

UNDIFFERENTIATED SOMATOFORM DISORDER

This condition emerges during adolescence, causing significant impairment. Multiple severe symptoms of at least 6 months' duration are required to make the diagnosis. They include, but are not limited to, pain syndromes, gastrointestinal or urogenital complaints, fatigue, loss of appetite, and pseudoneurologic symptoms. To qualify for this diagnosis, the symptoms should not be explained better by another mental disorder, such as a mood or anxiety disorder, and should not be feigned or intentionally produced. A more severe form, the classic somatization disorder, usually is an adult condition.

SOMATOFORM DISORDER, NOT OTHERWISE SPECIFIED

This classification encompasses adolescents who have somatoform symptoms that do not meet the criteria for any specific somatoform disorder, such as pseudocyesis, in which the false belief of being pregnant often is accompanied by endocrine changes. Another common example is unexplained physical complaints (eg, fatigue, weakness) of fewer than 6 months' duration.

PAIN DISORDER

There are three types of pain disorder: pain associated with psychological factors, pain associated with both a psychological and general medical condition, and pain associated with a general medical condition. The onset of pain may be related to psychological stressors or avoidance of something threatening. Pain disorders frequently begin as a mild pain syndrome. Pain can worsen due to the inadvertent secondary gain achieved by avoiding stress or academic pressures. These symptoms may be associated with frequent visits to the pediatrician and parental pressure for unnecessary testing and interventions.

CONVERSION DISORDERS

In conversion disorders, one or more symptoms or deficits affects a sensory or voluntary motor function (eg, blindness, paresis), suggesting a medical or neurologic condition, yet the findings are not consistent with any known neuroanatomic/pathophysiologic explanation. The symptoms tend to have a "symbolic meaning," dealing with an unsolved and unconscious conflict (often relating to themes of aggression or sexuality). The symptoms appear to be an attempt to resolve the conflict (primary gain), although they often result in increased attention for the patient (secondary gain). This form of somatization disorder frequently, but not always, is accompanied by "la belle indifference," an attitude of disinterest by the patient despite the serious symptoms experienced. Although the symptoms are usually self-limited, resolving within 3 months, they may be associated with chronic sequelae, such as contractures. There is frequently a model for the symptoms, with the patient sometimes serving as his or her own model, as is the case with pseudoseizures in patients who have epilepsy. However, over time, up to one third of patients in whom conversion disorder is diagnosed develop a neurologic disorder.

The fourth edition of the *Diagnostic and Statistical Manual of Mental Disorders (DSM-IV)* from the American Psychiatric Association includes additional disorders in the list of somatization disorders: hypochondriasis (preoccupation with the idea of having a serious disease) and body dysmorphic disorder (overpreoccupation with an imagined or exaggerated defect in physical appearance). They are uncommon and seen primarily during adolescence and young adulthood.

It is beyond the scope of this review to address specifically the large variety of common symptoms that may have a psychogenic origin or component, such as constipation and encopresis, enuresis, vomiting, headaches, syncope, and fainting. All have been reviewed in detail in *Pediatrics in Review* (see Suggested Reading).

Psychiatric Disorders and Somatic Complaints

Psychiatric disorders such as depression and anxiety disorder often present initially with physical complaints such as poor concentration; fatigue; weight loss; and an increase in headaches, stomachaches, and chest pains. They must be considered as primary or possibly comorbid conditions in the evaluation of somatoform disorders. This is important to look for because epidemiologic studies show that 14% to 20% of American children have one or more moderate-to-severe psychiatric disorders, with the overall prevalence rising.

Evaluation

Establishing the diagnosis of a somatoform illness evolves over time along three simultaneous tracks: 1) Ruling out an organic disease as the cause of the symptoms, 2) Identifying psychosocial dysfunction, and 3) Containing and alleviating stressors. A concomitant biopsychosocial assessment by itself is therapeutic and often is followed by improvement and sometimes even resolution of symptoms. It also is important to highlight that the differential diagnosis is not based solely on a process of exclusion, but incorporates instead a set of positive findings (Table 2).

It can be unclear whether a particular complaint eventually will be functional or reflect an underlying disease. Therefore, it is important to consider explicitly psychosomatic etiology in the initial patient evaluation. This will make any future "disclosure" easier.

Findings that are highly suggestive of a somatization disorder include a history of multiple somatic complaints, multiple physician visits and specialty consultations, a family member who has chronic and recurrent symptoms, and dysfunction in the primary areas of life (family, peers, and school). Additional inquiry should

Table 2. Differential Diagnosis in Pediatric Somatization

- Unrecognized physical disease
- Unrecognized psychiatric disorder (eg, depression, anxiety)
- Factitious disorder/by proxy
- Psychological factors affecting medical condition

include: Does the parent have any concern about the child's behavior or emotional well-being? Is there a family history of psychiatric disorder or "bad nerves"? A detailed school history that reviews each year and the numbers of days missed is essential.

In the process of evaluating somatic complaints, the clinician should avoid the temptation to perform unnecessary, repetitive, or extensive testing in an attempt to demonstrate to the family that the presenting complaint is of psychosomatic origin.

A cost-effective method of determining the extent of laboratory and radiographic evaluation is to base it on the presence of "red flags"; that is, the detection of complaints and findings that suggest an organic pathology, such as syncope on exercise, asymmetric location of pain, anemia, or weight loss. When the history and physical examination findings are suggestive of somatization, a basic laboratory screening consisting of a complete blood count, an erythrocyte sedimentation rate or assessment of C-reactive protein, a urine dipstick evaluation, and sometimes a blood chemistry and occult blood stool test is sufficient. More extensive assessments are reserved for the "red flags."

Eventually, the clinician needs to "bite the bullet," so it is important to present initially to the family a differential diagnosis that includes the possibility that the symptoms may be related to stress, temperamental sensitivity, anxiety, or whatever term may be tolerated by the family to accept a behavioral intervention or even a request for psychological assessment. The best method of persuasion is to precede any disclosure with a clear demonstration that one has taken the complaint very seriously. This is best accomplished with a careful history and a detailed physical examination of much longer duration than the patient has been used to. The aim is to convey a sense of specialness to the child and family, which may serve as a buffer to the narcissistic injury stemming from having to recognize that "something is wrong" in the child's life. Finally, it is necessary to reassess the course of illness and remain alert to the presence of the most common psychiatric disorders, which frequently

present initially to the pediatrician. Therefore, pediatricians treating children who have recurrent somatic complaints need to become familiar with screening for anxiety disorder, depression, attentiondeficit/hyperactivity disorder, substance use disorder, and conduct disorder.

Management/Disclosure

Correct identification of somatization disorders may not be sufficient to provide help to patients and families, who often are reluctant to accept the explanation. Therefore, successful communication about the condition and the needed treatment is a crucial but sometimes elusive goal (Table 3). In preparation for disclosure of concerns about a possible somatization disorder, it is very important to ask the child and family about their fear or "fantasy of disease." This may elicit surprising answers, such as fear that the child may have cancer or heart disease. Conversely, the reply may convey an already harbored suspicion or understanding of the problem, such as "It may be stress or nerves." In any case, patients will be willing to listen to the pediatrician only if he or she first listens to them. A clear, supportive, matter-of-fact explanation also should assure families that the pediatrician will be available to help with the onslaught of feelings that many families experience at the time of diagnosis.

It is important for pediatricians to recognize their own response to the family resistance and

Table 3. Principles of Treatment of Pediatric Somatization

- Form an alliance with the patient and family
- Be direct; avoid deception in explanations and treatments
- Offer reassurance when appropriate
- Use cognitive and behavioral interventions
- Use a rehabilitative approach
- Use positive and negative reinforcement
- Teach self-monitoring techniques (eg, hypnosis, relaxation, biofeedback)
- Consider family and group therapies
- Improve communications between clinicians and school
- Consolidate care when possible
- Aggressively treat comorbid psychiatric conditions
- Consider psychopharmacologic interventions
- Monitor outcome

Adapted from Campo and Fritz, 2001.

reluctance to lay aside the "search for disease" and not inadvertently transmit their own frustration about the difficult and time-consuming task they are facing.

A primary reason that patients are angry and reject the diagnosis of somatization disorder is that they feel disrespected and not believed: "You think it is all in my head, but I know I hurt and that there is something wrong." In part, this relates to the unfortunate term "psychosomatic," which conveys the mistaken notion of a body-mind duality, and for some still has the connotation of craziness ("psycho"). Therefore, it is important to explain that a "functional versus organic" paradigm is old-fashioned and does not reflect current thinking, which suggests a more complex interplay of multiple factors underlying the patient's symptoms.

Essentially, the pediatrician must convey understanding that the patient's pain is real. That is, the doctor has learned that pain is due to a neural nociceptive component and an affective component, both processed by the central nervous system and influenced by personal experience, genetics, and the environment.

To help patients and parents become more open to the concept of somatization, they can be reminded of how themes in language acknowledge the connection between emotions and bodily processes. For example, we talk about having a "gut reaction," having "butterflies in my stomach," feeling "all choked up," and that something "makes me vomit." In addition, we also note that embarrassment can manifest as blushing, fear as cold sweat, and anger as stiffening muscles and clenching teeth, thus facilitating explanations such as "blushing of the gut" and "spastic colon." Another strategy is to help them view somatization as a sensitivity, a phenomenon of "amplification" of otherwise normal body sensations.

Treatment

At the center of any successful program is the untiring effort to motivate patients and parents toward a partnership in dealing with the symptoms and complaints. It could be argued that the risk of antagonizing patients with a diagnosis of somatization and the subsequent running away

and "doctor shopping" calls for simply helping patients by medicating them with analgesics, tranquilizers, anxiolytics, and other agents from the pharmacopeia, including placebos. Although this may be tempting and certainly is easier, such an approach should be avoided when possible because it may reinforce the search for the "magic pill" and a never-ending pursuit of a technological solution. At a deeper level, the reason for informing patients and families of the nature of the disorder involves the principle of respect for persons; it is an ethical duty, with few exceptions, to share with patients our understanding of their situation. The primary exception to this rule, which allows for justified paternalism and "face-saving" suggestive therapies, is patients who have conversion disorders and cannot make use of the information. This may be due to the nature of the disorder, which often does not allow them to realize that they are experiencing stress or that their response to the stressor is dysfunctional.

The diagnosis of somatization never should lead a patient or parent to the perception that this diagnosis will be raised as a barrier to preempt future complaints. Instead, it should become clear that the diagnosis is made in the spirit of offering an interpretation that may call for newer and more effective treatments such as stress management and individual or family counseling. Somatoform disorders do respond to treatment and rehabilitation. Cognitive and behavioral interventions; use of positive and negative reinforcements; and self-monitoring techniques such as hypnosis, relaxation, and biofeedback have been proven successful. Family counseling and good communication between the clinician and the school often can "turn things around."

An important consideration when treating patients who have somatization disorders is that although the presence of a concomitant psychiatric disease is much lower in children than in the adult population, children can be afflicted by comorbidities such as mood disorders, anxiety disorders, and substance abuse, which should be sought to assure successful treatment. Patients who have a comorbid condition do not respond to treatment unless the psychiatric condition is addressed. Conversely, a patient not responding to intensive treatment should be evaluated for the possibility of comorbidity.

Judicious use of psychopharmacologic treatment in somatoform disorders may be appropriate when comorbid depression or anxiety is suspected or the severity of symptoms has led to significant and prolonged impairment (>3 mo). If the pediatrician can convince the patient and family to seek additional treatments such as therapy and evaluation for the use of medication, it is important that the consulting psychiatrist be asked to provide feedback directly to the pediatrician. Families often otherwise report that the psychiatrist said there was "nothing wrong, it was all medical." The consultant should be expected to tell the referring pediatrician what services will be provided and what the pediatrician is expected to monitor. For pediatricians who are sophisticated in the use of psychotropic medications, a psychiatric referral might not be necessary.

Often families worry that the diagnosis of somatization will be followed by abandonment by the physician. This concern can be dispelled by arranging frequent follow-up visits, which have the potential to "preempt" the frequent emergence of new symptoms, prevent emergency department visits, and ease the overall management of symptoms. It is helpful to emphasize that all forthcoming symptoms will be examined with the attention they deserve because somatizing under stress is very common and does not "provide immunity" against appendicitis, lupus, diabetes, and other conditions. Most families, even when disagreeing with their physicians, can accept (albeit grudgingly) treatment recommendations if they are assured of an attentive, open-minded, and regularly scheduled follow-up.

Administrative Issues

The structure of medical services conspires against optimal care for patients afflicted by somatization disorders, in part because procedural interventions historically have been valued above spending time with patients and in part because many organizations "carve out" these types of disorders for treatment through the mental health coverage. Frequently, such "carve outs" mean that patients have to pay their pediatrician out of pocket or from their mental health benefits. At other times, services simply go unpaid.

Depending on contractual arrangements, pediatricians currently have three less-than-satisfying options: 1) accept the rate of reimbursement for their services and bill the rest to the family, 2) refer the family to a consultant and coordinate care, or 3) negotiate directly with the payer about the case (armed with the *DSM-IV*).

Prognosis

With appropriate intervention, the prognosis for most somatization disorders in children and adolescents is very good. However, many untreated children risk continuous somatization as adults. On occasion, somatization is the proverbial "tip of the iceberg" that calls attention to a psychiatric disorder that requires mental health consultation and treatment. The most severe form, the undifferentiated somatoform disorder, probably is related closely to personality disorders, is of long duration, and has a persistent course, continuing into adulthood.

From a professional development perspective, advocacy work must continue to emphasize that changes in medical economics and the recognition of the financial impact of somatization on utilization call for increased funding for research and training in this area.

Suggested Reading

Ali-Hanna A, Lake AM. Constipation and encopresis in childhood. *Pediatr Rev*. 1998;18:24

Alfven G. The covariation of common psychosomatic symptoms among children from socio-economically differing residential areas. An epidemiological study. *Acta Paediatr*. 1993;82:484–487

American Psychiatric Association. *Diagnostic and Statistical Manual of Mental Disorders*. 4th ed. Washington, DC: American Psychiatric Press; 1994

American Psychiatric Association. *Diagnostic and Statistical Manual of Mental Disorders Primary Care Version*. 4th ed. Washington, DC: American Psychiatric Press; 1996

Arnhold RD, Callos ER. Composition of a suburban pediatric office practice: an analysis of patient visits during one year. *Clin Pediatr*. 1966;5:722–727

Atlas JA, Wolfson MA, Lipschitz DS. Dissociation and somatization in adolescent inpatients with and without history of abuse. *Psychol Rep.* 1995;76:1101–1102

Barsy AJ, Goodson JD, Lane RS, Cleary PD. The amplification of somatic symptoms. *Psychosom Med.* 1988;50:510–519

Bass C, Murphy M. Somatoform and personality disorders: syndromal co-morbidity and overlapping developmental pathways. *J Psychosom Research.* 1995;39:403–427

Bernal P, Estroff DB, Aboudarham JF, Murphy M, Keller A, Jellinek MS. Psychosocial morbidity: the economic burden in a pediatric health maintenance organization sample. *Arch Pediatr Adolesc Med.* 2000;154:261–266

Berntsson LT, Kohler L. Long-term illness and psychosomatic complaints in children aged 2–17 years in the five Nordic countries. Comparison between 1984 and 1996. *Eur J Public Health.* 2001;11:35–42

Berntsson LT, Gustafsson JE. Determinants of psychosomatic complaints in Swedish schoolchildren aged seven to twelve years. *Scand J Public Health.* 2000;28:283–293

Borres MP, Tanaka H, Thulesius O. Psychosomatic and psychosocial symptoms are associated with low blood pressure in Swedish schoolchildren. *Psychother Psychosom.* 1998;67:88–93

Brown RT. Adolescents with psychosomatic problems. *Compr Ther.* 1996;22:810–816

Campo JV, Fritz G. A management model for somatization. *Psychosomatics.* 2001;42:467–476

Cohen P, Pine DS, Must A, Kasen S, Brook J. Prospective associations between somatic illness and mental illness from childhood to adulthood. *Am J Epidemiol.* 1998;147:232–239

Dutta S, Mehta M, Verma IC. Recurrent abdominal pain in Indian children and its relation with school and family environment. *Indian Pediatr.* 1999;36:917–920

Dvonch VM, Bunch WH, Siegler AH. Conversion reactions in pediatric athletes. *J Pediatr Orthop.* 1991;11:770–772

Forsyth R, Farrell K. Headache in childhood. *Pediatr Rev.* 1999;20:39–45

Friedrich WN, Schafer LC. Somatic symptoms in sexually abused children. *J Pediatr Psychol.* 1995;20:661–670

Fritz GK, Fritsch S, Hagino O. Somatoform disorders in children and adolescents: a review of the past 10 years. *J Am Acad Child Adolesc Psychiatry.* 1997;36:1329–1337

Garralda ME. Psychosomatic illness in children. *Practitioner.* 1992;236:621–622

Gooch JL, Wolcott R, Speed J. Behavioral management of conversion disorder in children. *Arch Phys Med Rehabil.* 1997;78:264–268

Greene JW, Walker LS. Psychosomatic problems and stress in adolescence. *Pediatr Clin North Am.* 1997;44:1557–1572

Haugland S, Wold B, Stevenson J, Aaroe LE, Woynarowska B. Subjective health complaints in adolescence. A cross-national comparison of prevalence and dimensionality. *Eur J Public Health.* 2001;11:4–10

Hodgman CH. Conversion and somatization in pediatrics. *Pediatr Rev.* 1995;16:29–34

Hyams JS, Hyman PE. Recurrent abdominal pain and the biopsychosocial model of medical practice. *J Pediatr.* 1998;133:473–478

Kinzl JF, Traveger C, Biebl W. Family background and sexual abuse associated with somatization. *Psychother Psychosom.* 1995;64:82–87

Murray KF, Christie DL. Vomiting. *Pediatr Rev.* 1998;19:237

Narchi H. The child who passes out. *Pediatr Rev.* 2000;21:384

Offord DR, Boyle MH, Szatmari P, et al. Ontario Child Health Study. II: six month prevalence of disorder and rates of service utilization. *Arch Gen Psychiatr.* 1987;44:832–836

Olness K. Hypnosis and biofeedback with children and adolescents; clinical, research, and educational aspects. Introduction. *J Dev Behav Pediatr.* 1996;17:299

Orr D. Adolescence, stress, and psychosomatization. *J Adol Health Care.* 1986;7:97S–108S

Reese A, Strasburger VC. Is it "real" or is it "psychosomatic?" Basic principles of psychosomatic medicine in children and adolescents. In: Greydanus DE, Wolraich ML, eds. *Behavioral Pediatrics.* New York, NY: Springer Verlag; 1992

Rickert VI, Jay MS. Psychosomatic disorders: the approach. *Pediatr Rev.* 1994;15:448–454

Schmitt BD. Nocturnal enuresis. *Pediatr Rev.* 1997;18:183

Selbst SM, Ruddy RM, Clark BJ, et al. Pediatric chest pain: a prospective study. *Pediatrics.* 1988;82:319–323

Sherry DD, McGuire T, Mellins E, Salmonson K, Wallace CA, Nepom B. Psychosomatic musculoskeletal pain in childhood: clinical and psychological analyses of 100 children. *Pediatrics.* 1991;88:1093–1099

Starfield B, Gross E, Wood M, et al. Psychosocial and psychosomatic diagnoses in primary care of children. *Pediatrics.* 1980;66:159–167

Steinhauer PD. Resistances to the biopsychosocial approach: individual, familial and systemic. *Behavior Pediatr.* 1990;11:330–332

Sugarman LI. Hypnosis: teaching children self-regulation. *Pediatr Rev.* 1996;17:5–11

Tanaka H, Tamai H, Terashima S, Takenaka Y, Tanaka T. Psychosocial factors affecting psychosomatic symptoms in Japanese schoolchildren. *Pediatr Int.* 2000;42:354–358

Torgersen S. Genetics of somatoform disorders. *Arch Gen Psychiatry.* 1986;43:502–505

Walker LS, Greene JW. Children with recurrent abdominal pain and their parents: more somatic complaints, anxiety, and depression than other patient families? *J Pediatr Psychol.* 1989;14:231–243

Wender PH, Klein DF. *Mind, Mood and Medicine.* New York, NY: Meridian; 1981

Weyrer S, Castell R, Biener A, et al. Prevalence and treatment of psychiatric disorders in 3- to 14-year-old children: results of representative field study in the small town rural region of Traunstein, Upper Bavaria. *Acta Psychiatr Scand.* 1988;77: 290–296

Willis J. Syncope. *Pediatr Rev.* 2000;21:201

Wolraich ML, Felice MD, Drotar D. *The Classification of Child and Adolescent Mental Diagnoses in Primary Care.* In: *Diagnostic and Statistical Manual for Primary Care (DSM-PC) Child and Adolescent Version.* Elk Grove Village, Ill: American Academy of Pediatrics; 1996

Zuckerman B, Stevenson J, Bailey V. Stomach and headaches in a community sample of preschool children. *Pediatrics.* 1987; 79:677–682

Appendix: Sections of the Relevant Criteria of the *Diagnostic and Statistical Manual of Mental Disorders (DSM-IV)*

The purpose of this appendix is to provide details on the diagnostic categories for the *DSM-IV* disorders pertinent to children. The disorders are listed in alphabetical order.

DIAGNOSTIC CRITERIA FOR CONVERSION DISORDER 300.11

A. One or more symptoms or deficits affecting voluntary motor or sensory function that suggest a neurologic or other general medical condition.

B. Psychological factors are judged to be associated with the symptom or deficit because the initiation or exacerbation of the symptom or deficit is preceded by conflicts or other stressors.

C. The symptom or deficit is not intentionally produced or feigned (as in factitious disorder or malingering).

D. The symptom or deficit cannot, after appropriate investigation, be fully explained by a general medical condition, or by the direct effects of a substance, or as a culturally sanctioned behavior or experience.

E. The symptom or deficit causes clinically significant distress or impairment in social, occupational, or other important areas of functioning or warrants medical evaluation.

F. The symptom or deficit is not limited to pain or sexual dysfunction, does not occur exclusively during the course of somatization disorder, and is not better accounted for by another mental disorder.

> *Specify* type of symptom or deficit:
> With Motor Symptom or Deficit
> With Sensory Symptom or Deficit
> With Seizures or Convulsions
> With Mixed Presentation

DIAGNOSTIC CRITERIA FOR PAIN DISORDER 307.80

A. Pain in one or more anatomical sites is the predominant focus of the clinical presentation and is of sufficient severity to warrant clinical attention.

B. The pain causes clinically significant distress or impairment in social, occupational, or other important areas of functioning.

C. Psychological factors are judged to have an important role in the onset, severity, exacerbation, or maintenance of the pain.

D. The symptom or deficit is not intentionally produced or feigned (as factitious disorder or malingering).

E. The pain is not better accounted for by a mood, anxiety, or psychotic disorder, and does not meet criteria for dyspareunia.

> Specify if:
> Acute: duration of less than 6 months
> Chronic: duration of 6 months or longer

307.89 PAIN DISORDER ASSOCIATED WITH BOTH PSYCHOLOGICAL FACTORS AND A GENERAL MEDICAL CONDITION

Both psychological factors and a general medical condition are judged to have important roles in the onset, severity, exacerbation, or maintenance of the pain. The associated general medical condition or anatomical site of the pain is coded.

> Specify if:
> Acute: duration of less than 6 months
> Chronic: duration of 6 months or longer
> Note: The following is not considered to be a mental disorder and is included here to facilitate differential diagnosis.

PAIN DISORDER ASSOCIATED WITH A GENERAL MEDICAL CONDITION

A general medical condition has a major role in the onset, severity, exacerbation, or maintenance of the pain. (If psychological factors are present, they are not judged to have a major role in the onset, severity, exacerbation, or maintenance of the pain.) The diagnostic code for the pain is selected based on the associated general medical condition if one has been established or on the anatomical location of the pain if the underlying general medical condition is not yet clearly established—for example, low back **(724.2)**, sciatic **(724.3)**, pelvic **(625.9)**, headache **(784.0)**, facial **(784.0)**, chest **(786.50)**, joint **(719.4)**, bone **(733.90)**, abdominal **(789.0)**, breast **(611.71)**, renal **(788.0)**, eye **(379.91)**, throat **(784.1)**, tooth **(525.9)**, and urinary **(788.0)**.

DIAGNOSTIC CRITERIA FOR SOMATIZATION DISORDER 300.82

A. A history of many physical complaints beginning before age 30 years that occur over a period of several years and result in treatment being sought or significant impairment in social, occupational, or other important areas of functioning.

B. Each of the following criteria must have been met, with individual symptoms occurring at any time during the course of the disturbance:
(1) *Four pain symptoms:* a history of pain related to at least four different sites or functions (eg, head, abdomen, back, joints, extremities, chest, rectum, during menstruation, during sexual intercourse, or during urination)
(2) *Two gastrointestinal symptoms:* a history of at least two gastrointestinal symptoms other than pain (eg, nausea, bloating, vomiting other than during pregnancy, diarrhea, or intolerance of several different foods)
(3) *One sexual symptom:* a history of at least one sexual or reproductive symptom other than pain (eg, sexual indifference, erectile or ejaculatory dysfunction, irregular menses, excessive menstrual bleeding, vomiting throughout pregnancy)

(4) *One pseudoneurological symptoms:* a history of at least one symptom or deficit suggesting a neurologic condition not limited to pain (conversion symptoms such as impaired coordination or balance, paralysis or localized weakness, difficulty swallowing or lump in throat, aphonia, urinary retention, hallucinations, loss of touch or pain sensation, double vision, blindness, deafness, seizures; dissociative symptoms such as amnesia; or loss of consciousness other than fainting)

C. Either (1) or (2):
(1) After appropriate investigation, each of the symptoms in criterion B cannot be fully explained by a known general medical condition or the direct effects of a substance (eg, a drug of abuse, a medication).
(2) When there is a related general medical condition, the physical complaints or resulting social or occupational impairment are in excess of what would be expected from the history, physical examination, or laboratory findings.

D. The symptoms are not intentionally produced or feigned (as in factitious disorder or malingering).

DIAGNOSTIC CRITERIA FOR SOMATOFORM DISORDER, NOT OTHERWISE SPECIFIED 300.82

This category includes disorders with somatoform symptoms that do not meet the criteria for any specific somatoform disorder. Examples include:

(1) Pseudocyesis: a false belief of being pregnant that is associated with objective signs of pregnancy, which may include abdominal enlargement (although the umbilicus does not become everted), reduced menstrual flow, amenorrhea, subjective sensation of fetal movement, nausea, breast engorgement and secretions, and labor pains at the expected date of delivery. Endocrine changes may be present, but the syndrome cannot be explained by a general medical condition that causes endocrine changes (eg, a hormone-secreting tumor).

(2) A disorder involving nonpsychotic hypochondriacal symptoms of less than 6 months' duration.

(3) A disorder involving unexplained physical complaints (eg, fatigue or body weakness) of less than 6 months' duration that are not due to another mental disorder.

DIAGNOSTIC CRITERIA FOR UNDIFFERENTIATED SOMATOFORM DISORDER 300.82

A. One or more physical complaints (eg, fatigue, loss of appetite, gastrointestinal or urinary complaints)

B. Either (1) or (2):

(1) After appropriate investigation, the symptoms cannot be fully explained by a known general medical condition or the direct effects of a substance (eg, a drug of abuse, a medication).

(2) When there is a related general medical condition, the physical complaints or resulting social or occupational impairment is in excess of what would be expected from the history, physical examination, or laboratory findings.

C. The symptoms cause clinically significant distress or impairment in social, occupational, or other important areas of functioning.

D. The duration of the disturbance is at least 6 months.

E. The disturbance is not better accounted for by another mental disorder (eg, another somatoform disorder, sexual dysfunction, mood disorder, anxiety disorder, sleep disorder, or psychotic disorder).

F. The symptom is not intentionally produced or feigned (as in factitious disorder or malingering).

Suicide and Suicide Attempts in Adolescents

Committee on Adolescence

ABSTRACT. Suicide is the third leading cause of death for adolescents 15 to 19 years old.[1] Pediatricians can help prevent adolescent suicide by knowing the symptoms of depression and other presuicidal behavior. This statement updates the previous statement[2] by the American Academy of Pediatrics and assists the pediatrician in the identification and management of the adolescent at risk for suicide. The extent to which pediatricians provide appropriate care for suicidal adolescents depends on their knowledge, skill, comfort with the topic, and ready access to appropriate community resources. All teenagers with suicidal symptoms should know that their pleas for assistance are heard and that pediatricians are willing to serve as advocates to help resolve the crisis.

The number of adolescent deaths from suicide in the United States has increased dramatically during the past few decades. In 1997, there were 4186 suicides among people 15 to 24 years old, 1802 suicides among those 15 to 19 years old, and 2384 among those 20 to 24 years old.[1] In 1997, 13% of all deaths in the 15- through 24-year-old age group were attributable to suicide.[1] The true number of deaths from suicide actually may be higher, because some of these deaths are recorded as "accidental."[3]

From 1950 to 1990, the suicide rate for adolescents in the 15- to 19-year-old group increased by 300%.[4] Adolescent males 15 to 19 years old had a rate 6 times greater than the rate for females.[1] The ratio of attempted suicides to completed suicides among adolescents is estimated to be 50:1 to 100:1, and the incidence of unsuccessful suicide attempts is higher among females than among males.[5] Suicide affects young people from all races and socioeconomic groups, although some groups seem to have higher rates than others. Native American males have the highest suicide rate, African American women the lowest.

A statewide survey of students in grades 7 through 12 found that 28.1% of bisexual and homosexual males and 20.5% of bisexual and homosexual females had reported attempting suicide.[6] The National Youth Risk Behavior Survey of students in grades 9 through 12 indicated that nearly one fourth (24.1%) of students had seriously considered attempting suicide during the 12 months preceding the survey, 17.7% had made a specific plan, and 8.7% had made an attempt.[7]

Firearms, used in >67% of suicides, are the leading cause of death for males and females who commit suicide.[8] More than 90% of suicide attempts involving a firearm are fatal because there is little chance for rescue. Firearms in the home, regardless of whether they are kept unloaded or stored locked up, are associated with a higher risk for adolescent suicide.[9,10] Parents must be warned about the lethality of firearms in the home and be advised strongly to remove them from the premises.[11] Ingestion of pills is the most common method among adolescents who attempt suicide.

Youth, who seem to be at much greater risk from media exposure than adults, may imitate suicidal behavior seen on television.[12] Media coverage of a teenage suicide may lead to cluster suicides, additional deaths from suicides in youths within a 1- to 2-week period afterward.[12-14]

Adolescents at Increased Risk

Although no specific tests are capable of identifying suicidal persons, specific risk factors exist. Adolescents at higher risk commonly have a history of depression, a previous suicide attempt, a family history of psychiatric disorders (especially

PEDIATRICS (ISSN 0031 4005).

depression and suicidal behavior), family disruption, and certain chronic or debilitating physical disorders or psychiatric illness.[15] Alcohol use and alcoholism indicate high risk for suicide.[16] Alcohol use has been associated with 50% of suicides.[17] Living out of the home (in a correctional facility or group home) and a history of physical or sexual abuse are additional factors more commonly found in adolescents who exhibit suicidal behavior.[18] Psychosocial problems and stresses, such as conflicts with parents, breakup of a relationship, school difficulties or failure, legal difficulties, social isolation, and physical ailments (including hypochondriacal preoccupation), commonly are reported or observed in young people who attempt suicide. These precipitating factors often are cited by youths as reasons for attempting suicide. Gay and bisexual adolescents have been reported to exhibit high rates of depression and have been reported to have rates of suicidal ideation and attempts 3 times higher than other adolescents. Studies of twins show that monozygotic twins show significantly higher concordance for suicide than dizygotic twins.[16] Long-term high levels of community violence may contribute to emotional and conduct problems and add to the risk of suicide for exposed youth.[19] Adolescent and parent questionnaires that cover those risk factors listed above, may be useful in the office setting to assist in obtaining a complete history.[20]

Approaching the Adolescent

All adolescents with symptoms of depression should be asked about suicidal ideation, and an estimation of the degree of suicidal intent should be made. No data indicate that inquiry about suicide precipitates the behavior. In fact, adolescents often are relieved that someone has heard their cry for help. For most adolescents, this cry for help represents an attempt to resolve a difficult conflict, escape an intolerable living situation, make someone understand their desperate feelings, or make someone feel sorry or guilty. Suicidal thoughts or comments should never be dismissed as unimportant. Adolescents must be told by pediatricians that their plea for assistance has been heard and that they will be helped.

Serious depression in adolescents may manifest in several ways. For some adolescents, symptoms may be similar to those in adults, with signs, such as depressed mood almost every day, crying spells or inability to cry, discouragement, irritability, a sense of emptiness and meaninglessness, negative expectations of self and the environment, low self-esteem, isolation, a feeling of helplessness, markedly diminished interest or pleasure in most activities, significant weight loss or weight gain, insomnia or hypersomnia, fatigue or loss of energy, feelings of worthlessness, and diminished ability to think or concentrate.[21] However, it is more common for an adolescent with serious depression to exhibit psychosomatic symptoms or behavioral problems. Such a teenager may seek care for recurrent or persistent complaints, such as abdominal pain, chest pain, headache, lethargy, weight loss, dizziness and syncope, or other nonspecific symptoms.[22] Behavioral problems that may be manifestations of masked depression include truancy, deterioration in academic performance, running away from home, defiance of authorities, self-destructive behavior, vandalism, alcohol and other drug abuse, sexual acting out, and delinquency.[23] Episodic despondency leading to self-destructive acts can occur in any adolescent, including high achievers. These adolescents may believe that they have failed or disappointed their parents and family and perceive suicide as their only option. Other adolescents may believe that suicide is a better option than life as they experience it.

One approach to initiate an inquiry into suicidal thoughts or concerns is to ask a general question, such as "Have you ever felt so unhappy or depressed that you thought about killing yourself or wished you were dead?" If the response is positive, the pediatrician should inquire about thoughts of death, thoughts of suicide, suicide plans (eg, method, time, and place), securing the available means (eg, guns and ropes), previous attempts (and whether the attempts were discovered), and the response of the family. These basic questions can help pediatricians construct an assessment of suicidal risk. In addition, they should assess individual coping resources, accessible support systems, and attitudes of the adolescent and family toward intervention and follow-up.[24]

Although confidentiality is important in adolescent health care, for adolescents at risk to themselves or others, confidentiality must be breached. Pediatricians need to inform the appropriate persons when they believe an adolescent is at risk of suicide. In all cases, determination of the sequence of events that preceded the threat, identification of current problems and conflicts, and assessment of the degree of suicidal intent must be completed.

Management of the Suicidal Adolescent

Adolescents with a well-thought-out plan that includes method, place, time, and clear intent are at high risk. The degree of intent can be inferred from the actual and perceived lethality of the intended means. Use of firearms, for example, has a high degree of lethality and poor chance of rescue. An adolescent who takes pills in the presence of others, however, has a good chance of rescue (Table 1).[25] Even adolescents who initially may seem at low risk, joke about suicide, or seek treatment for repeated somatic complaints may be asking for help the only way they can. Their concerns should be assessed thoroughly and follow-up arranged for additional evaluation and treatment. For adolescents who seem to be at moderate or high risk for suicide or have attempted suicide, a mental health professional should be consulted immediately during the office visit. Options for immediate evaluation include hospitalization, transfer to an emergency department, or an appointment the same day with a mental health professional.

The safest course of action is hospitalization, placing the adolescent in a safe and protected environment. An inpatient stay will allow time for a complete medical and psychiatric or psychologic evaluation and initiation of therapy in a controlled setting. The choice of hospital unit depends on available facilities in the area, health

Table 1. Examples of Adolescents at Low, Moderate, and High Risk for Suicide

Low risk

Took 5 ibuprofen tablets after argument with girlfriend

Impulsive; told mother 15 minutes after taking pills

No serious problems at home or school

Occasionally feels "down" but has no history of depression or serious emotional problems

Has a number of good friends

Wants help resolving problems and is no longer considering suicide after interview

Moderate risk

Suicidal ideation precipitated by recurrent fighting with parents and failing grades in school

Wants to "get back" at parents

Cut both wrists while at home alone; called friend 30 minutes later

Parents separated, changed school this semester, history of attention-deficit hyperactivity disorder

Symptoms of depression for the last 2 months, difficulty controlling temper

Binge drinking on the weekends

Answers all the questions during the interview, agrees to see a therapist if parents get counseling, will contact the interviewer if suicidal thoughts return

High risk

Thrown out of house by parents for smoking marijuana at school, girlfriend broke up with him last night, best friend killed in auto crash last month

Wants to be dead; sees no purpose in living

Took father's gun; is going to shoot himself where "no one can find me"

Gets drunk every weekend and uses marijuana daily

Hates parents and school; has run away from home twice and has not gone to school for 6 weeks

Hospitalized in the past because he "lost it"

Does not want to answer many of the questions during the interview and hates "shrinks" and mental health insurance, and managed care policies. Adolescent medicine units must be staffed to manage the medical and psychiatric needs of suicidal adolescents.[26] Proper medical intervention and treatment are essential for stabilization and management of patients' conditions. After the adolescent's condition has been stabilized medically, a comprehensive emotional and psychosocial assessment must be initiated before discharge. Inquiry should be made into the events that preceded the attempt, the adolescent's current problems, and the presence of current or previous psychiatric illness and self-destructive behavior. In addition to an in-depth psychological evaluation of the adolescent, family members should be interviewed to obtain additional information to help explain the adolescent's suicidal thoughts or attempt. This information includes detailed questions about the adolescent's medical, emotional, social, and family history with special attention to signs and symptoms of depression, stress, and substance abuse. With parental permission and adolescent assent, teachers and family friends also may provide useful information if confidentiality is not breached.

Intervention should be tailored to the adolescent's needs. Adolescents with a responsive intact family, good peer relations and social support, hope for the future, and a desire to resolve conflicts may require only brief crisis-oriented intervention.[27] In contrast, adolescents who have made previous attempts, exhibit a high degree of intent to commit suicide, show evidence of serious depression or other psychiatric illness, are abusing alcohol and other drugs, and have families who are unwilling to commit to counseling are at high risk and may require psychiatric hospitalization.

All adolescents who attempt suicide need a comprehensive outpatient treatment plan before discharge. Specific plans are needed because compliance with outpatient therapy often is poor. Most adolescents examined in emergency rooms and referred to outpatient facilities fail to keep their appointments. This is especially true when the appointment is made with someone other than the family pediatrician or the person who performed the initial assessment.[28] Continuity of care is, therefore, of paramount importance.

Pediatricians can enhance continuity and compliance by maintaining contact with suicidal adolescents even after referrals are made. All firearms should be removed from the home because adolescents may still find access to locked guns stored in the home.

Adolescents judged not to be at high risk for suicide should be followed up closely, referred for mental health evaluation in a timely manner, or both.

Recommendations

1. Pediatricians need to know the risk factors (eg, signs and symptoms of depression) associated with adolescent suicide and serve as a resource for parents, teachers, school personnel, clergy, and community groups that work with youth about the issue of adolescent suicide.

2. Pediatricians should ask questions about depression, suicidal thoughts, and other risk factors associated with suicide in routine history-taking throughout adolescence.

3. During routine evaluations, pediatricians need to ask whether firearms are kept in the home and discuss with parents the risks of firearms as specifically related to adolescent suicide. Specifically for adolescents at risk of suicide, parents should be advised to remove guns and ammunition from the house.

4. Pediatricians should recognize the medical and psychiatric needs of the suicidal adolescent and work closely with families and health care professionals involved in the management and follow-up of youth who are at risk or have attempted suicide.

5. Pediatricians should become familiar with community, state, and national resources that are concerned with youth suicide, including mental health agencies, family and children's services, crisis hotlines, and crisis intervention centers. Working relationships should be developed with colleagues in child and adolescent psychiatry, clinical psychology, and other mental health professions to manage the care of adolescents at risk for suicide optimally. Because mental and physical health services are often provided through different systems

of care, extra effort is necessary to assure good communication, continuity, and follow-up.

6. Pediatricians should advocate for benefit packages in health insurance plans to assure that adolescents have access to preventive and therapeutic mental health services that adequately cover the treatment of clinically significant mental health disorders.

COMMITTEE ON ADOLESCENCE, 1999–2000
David W. Kaplan, MD, MPH, Chairperson
Ronald A. Feinstein, MD
Martin M. Fisher, MD
Jonathan D. Klein, MD, MPH
Luis F. Olmedo, MD
Ellen S. Rome, MD, MPH
W. Samuel Yancy, MD

LIAISON REPRESENTATIVES
Paula J. Adams Hillard, MD
    American College of Obstetricians
    and Gynecologists
Diane Sacks, MD
    Canadian Paediatric Society
Glen Pearson, MD
    American Academy of Child and
    Adolescent Psychiatry

SECTION LIAISON
Barbara L. Frankowski, MD, MPH
    Section on School Health

References

1. Centers for Disease Control and Prevention/National Center for Health Statistics. *Death Rates From 72 Selected Causes by 5-Year Age Groups, Race, and Sex: United States, 1979-1997.* Atlanta, GA: Centers for Disease Control and Prevention/National Center for Health Statistics; 1999. Table 291A

2. American Academy of Pediatrics, Committee on Adolescence. Suicide and suicide attempts in adolescents and young adults. *Pediatrics.* 1988;81:322–324

3. Committee on Adolescence, Group for the Advancement of Psychiatry. *Adolescent Suicide.* Washington, DC: American Psychiatric Press; 1996

4. Centers for Disease Control and Prevention. Programs for prevention of suicide among adolescents youth adults. *Morb Mortal Wkly Rep CDC Surveill Summ.* 1994;43:1–7. No RR-6

5. Husain SA. Current perspective on the role of psychological factors in adolescent suicide. *Psychiatr Ann.* 1990; 20:122–127

6. Remafedi G, French S, Story M, Resnick MD, Blum R. The relationship between suicide risk and sexual orientation: results of a population-based study. *Am J Public Health.* 1998;88:57–60

7. Centers for Disease Control and Prevention. Youth risk behavior surveillance: United States, 1995. *Morb Mortal Wkly Rep CDC Surveill Summ.* 1996;45(SS-4):1–84

8. Kachur SP, Potter LB, James SP, Powell KE. *Suicide in the United States: 1980-1992: Violence Surveillance.* Atlanta, GA: National Center for Injury Prevention and Control; 1995:12. Summary Series 1

9. Brent DA, Perper JA, Allman CJ, et al The presence and accessibility of firearms in the home of adolescent suicides: a case-control study. *JAMA.* 1991;266:2989–2995

10. American Academy of Pediatrics, Committee on Injury and Poison Prevention. Firearm injuries affecting the pediatric population. *Pediatrics.* 1992;89:788–790

11. American Academy of Pediatrics, Committee on Adolescence. Firearms and adolescents. *Pediatrics.* 1992;89:784–787

12. Bollen KA, Phillips DP. Imitative suicides: a national study of the effects of television news stories. *Am Sociol Rev.* 1982;47:802–809

13. Gould MS, Wallenstein S, Kleinman M. Time-space clustering of teenage suicides. *Am J Epidemiol.* 1990; 131:71–78

14. Phillips DP, Carstenson LL. Clustering of teenage suicides after television news stories about suicide. *N Engl J Med.* 1986;315:685–689

15. Bennett DS. Depression among children with chronic medical problems: a meta-analysis. *J Pediatr Psychol.* 1994;19:149–169

16. Roy A, Segal NL, Centerwall BS, Robinette CD. Suicide in twins. *Arch Gen Psychiatry.* 1991;48:29–32

17. Frances RJ, Franklin J, Flavin DK. Suicide and alcoholism. *Am J Drug Alcohol Abuse.* 1987;13:327-341

18. Hodgman CH, McAnarney ER. Adolescent depression and suicide: rising problems. *Hosp Pract (Off Ed).* 1992; 27:73–76,81,84–85

19. Cooley-Quille MR, Turner SM, Beidel DC. Emotional impact of children's exposure to community violence: a preliminary study. *J Am Acad Child Adolesc Psychiatry.* 1995;34:1362–1368

20. Remafedi G, Farrow JA, Deisher RX. Risk factors for attempted suicide in gay and bisexual youth. *Pediatrics.* 1991;87:869–875

21. American Psychiatric Association. *Diagnostic and Statistical Manual of Mental Disorders.* 4th ed. Washington, DC: American Psychiatric Association; 1994

22. Wolraich ML, Felice ME, Drotar D, eds. *The Classification of Child and Adolescent Mental Diagnoses in Primary Care: Diagnostic and Statistical Manual for Primary Care (DSM-PC) Child and Adolescent Version.* Elk Grove Village, IL: American Academy of Pediatrics; 1996

23. McIntire MS, Angle CR, Wikoff RL, Schlicht ML. Recurrent adolescent suicidal behavior. *Pediatrics.* 1977;60:605–608

24. Gispert M, Wheeler K, Marsh L, Davis MS. Suicidal adolescents: factors in evaluation. *Adolescence.* 1985; 20:753–762

25. Jellinek MS, Snyder JB. Depression and suicide in children and adolescents. *Pediatr Rev.* 1998;19:255–264

26. Marks A. Management of the suicidal adolescent on a nonpsychiatric adolescent unit. *J Pediatr.* 1979;95: 305–308

27. Hodgman CH, Roberts FN. Adolescent suicide and the pediatrician. *J Pediatr.* 1982;101:118–123

28. Hawton K. *Suicide and Attempted Suicide Among Children and Adolescents.* Beverly Hills, CA: Sage Publications; 1986

Gay, Lesbian, and Bisexual Teens:
Facts for Teens and Their Parents

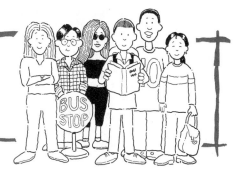

The teenage years are filled with new experiences, changes, and a growing sense of who you are. But for teenagers who feel "different" from their peers, these years can be confusing, frustrating, and even scary.

It is important for everyone to understand more about the diversity in people's sexual orientation. If you are a teenager, this brochure provides information to help as you discover more about yourself, your friends, and your place in the world. There also is information that may help your parents understand you better.

"Am I gay?"

Many gay and lesbian adults remember their late childhood or early teenage years as the time when they first began to wonder about their sexual orientation. Unfortunately, because we live in a society that is not always accepting of gay, lesbian, and bisexual people, dealing with the possibility that they may be gay can be a very difficult thing for teens.

How do you know if you are gay? Many young people go through an anxious stage during which they wonder, "Am I gay?" It is normal to feel this way as your sexual identity is taking shape. Maybe you feel attracted to someone of the same gender or you have had some same-sex activity. This is normal and does not necessarily mean that you are gay, lesbian, or bisexual.

Sexual *behavior* is not always the same as sexual *orientation*. Many people have had same-sex experiences but do not consider themselves gay, lesbian, or bisexual. Others call themselves gay without having had any sexual experience.

Sexual orientation develops as you grow and experience new things. It may take time to figure it all out. Do not worry if you are not sure. If over time you find you feel romantic attraction to members of the same sex, and these feelings continue to grow stronger as you get older, you probably are gay or bisexual. It is not a bad thing, it is just who you are.

Definitions

Gay (or *homosexual*): People who have sexual and/or romantic feelings for people of the same gender. Men are attracted to men and women are attracted to women.

Lesbian: Gay woman.

Straight (or *heterosexual*): People who have sexual and/or romantic feelings for people of the opposite gender. Men are attracted to women and women are attracted to men.

Bisexual (or *bi*): People who have sexual and/or romantic feelings for both men and women.

Sexual orientation: How an individual is physically and emotionally attracted to other males and females.

You are not alone

Some estimates say that about 10% of the population is gay. You cannot tell by looking at people whether they are gay. Gay people are all shapes, sizes, and ages. They have many types of racial and ethnic backgrounds.

Pay no attention to stereotypes. Just because a boy has some feminine qualities or a girl acts somewhat masculine does not mean that he or she is gay. Most gay males and females look and act just like their straight peers.

"Am I normal?"

First, homosexuality is not a mental disorder. The American Psychiatric Association confirmed this in 1974. The American Psychological Association and the American Academy of Pediatrics agree that homosexuality is not an illness or disorder, but a form of sexual expression.

No one knows what causes a person to be gay, bisexual, or straight. There probably are a number of factors. Some may be biological. Others may be psychological. The reasons can vary from one person to another. The fact is, you do not choose to be gay, bisexual, or straight.

Talking about it

Most people find that it is hard to start talking about their sexual feelings and attractions, but in the long run it feels better if you do not keep these important feelings a secret. You do not have to *know* that you are lesbian, gay, or bisexual before you talk to people about your feelings. Remember that the process of sharing what you are feeling is different for every person. Start with people you trust the most. This may include the following:

- Close friends
- Gay, lesbian, or bisexual friends
- Parents
- Close family members
- Your pediatrician
- A teacher, school counselor, coach, or other adult mentor
- A minister, priest, rabbi, or spiritual advisor
- A local gay, lesbian, and bisexual support group

The important thing is to find someone you trust with whom you can talk about your thoughts and worries.

Coming out

Because of the negative feelings some people have about homosexuality, "coming out of the closet," or revealing your sexual orientation, can be difficult. Some people wrestle with revealing their identity for years before finally deciding to do so. Others keep their sexual orientation a secret for their entire lives.

Talk to other gay friends about their "coming out" experiences. This may help you know what to expect. Gay youth organizations also can be a great source of support. See the end of this brochure for a list of such groups.

If you do know that you are gay, lesbian, or bisexual, do not feel pressured to "come out" before you are ready. On the other hand, keeping your identity a secret can be a burden. It is up to you to decide the best time to share your sexual orientation with your family and friends.

Telling your family and friends that you are gay probably will not be easy. Your family may respond well. But most parents picture a traditional future for their child. News that their child is gay may require them to rethink a whole new future.

Choose a good time and place to tell your family. If this information comes out during a family conflict or crisis, it may be even harder for your parents to accept it.

Be prepared for a variety of reactions including shock, denial, anger, guilt, sadness, and even rejection. Remember, you have had time to accept your identity. Give your family and friends time, too. Keep in mind that you can help them by being open, honest, and patient.

Often family and friends will be relieved that you have helped them to understand you better. Whether right away, or after some time, they may be happy to help you sort out your sexual orientation and how it affects your life.

Health concerns for gay and lesbian youth

Gay, lesbian, and bisexual teens are not the only ones who need to be concerned about their health. All teens need to be aware of what can happen if they are sexually active, use drugs, or engage in other risky behaviors.

Sexual activity: You do not have to have sex to be aware of your sexual identity. Most teenagers, whether they are gay, lesbian, bisexual, or straight, are not sexually active. In fact, not having sex is the *only* way to protect yourself completely against sexually transmitted diseases (STDs). But if you choose to have sex, make sure you know the risks and how to protect yourself.

- Gay and bisexual males must be particularly careful and always use latex condoms. Using condoms is the only way to protect against human immunodeficiency virus (HIV)/acquired immune deficiency syndrome (AIDS) and many other diseases that are spread during anal, vaginal, or oral intercourse. Condoms also help to prevent pregnancy during vaginal intercourse.
- Lesbians and bisexual females also must *always* use protection such as latex dental dams and condoms to avoid sexually transmitted diseases and unplanned pregnancies.
- Avoid risky sexual practices like using alcohol and drugs before or during sex, having unknown sexual partners, or having sex in unfamiliar or public places.
- Regular health examinations are crucial. Ask your pediatrician if you have questions or concerns about STDs or other health issues.
- Make sure all of your immunizations are up-to-date. Check that you have had three doses of the hepatitis B vaccine. Hepatitis B is a virus that can make you very sick. It can be spread through contact with infected blood or other body fluids. This can happen during sexual intercourse or when drug users share needles.

Substance use: Being a gay or lesbian teen in our society can be very difficult. Avoid using drugs or alcohol to relieve depression, anxiety, and low self-esteem. Doing so can lead to addiction.

In many communities, bars are popular places for gay and lesbian people to socialize. This increases the pressure to drink and use other drugs. Drug and alcohol use can lead to unsafe sex. Adopt a drug-free lifestyle and look for other ways to socialize and meet new people.

Mental health: Isolation, peer rejection, ridicule, harassment, depression, and thoughts of suicide — any teen may feel these things at some time. However, gay and lesbian youth are more than twice as likely to attempt suicide than straight teenagers. About 30% of those who try to kill themselves actually die.

A message to parents: when your teenager is gay, lesbian, or bisexual

Each year some parents learn that their son or daughter is gay, lesbian, or bisexual. This news is sometimes difficult. Most parents dream that their child's future will include a traditional marriage and grandchildren. Keep in mind that your son or daughter still can find lifelong companionship and become a parent.

Parents also often have to deal with their own guilt. They may ask themselves questions like, "Did I do anything to cause this?" "Should we have done something differently when he was a child?" "Is it my fault?" Questions like these are common, but do not help.

Rejecting your child also is not a good response. When gay, lesbian, and bisexual teens make their sexual orientation known, some families reject them. Perhaps that is how you think you would react. But that is the wrong response. It may be very difficult for your teenager to come to terms with her or his sexuality. Your child may find it devastating if you reject her or him at the same time. Your child needs you very much!

So take a deep breath and think. Take a little time to come to grips with your child's sexual orientation. You may need to readjust your dreams for your child's future. You may have to deal with your own negative stereotypes of gay, lesbian, and bisexual people. But you must not reject your teenager for his or her sexual orientation. He or she is still your child and needs your love and support.

Many parents find that it helps to talk to other parents whose children are lesbian, gay, or bisexual. Check the end of this brochure for information about support groups for parents.

Your teenager did not choose to be gay, lesbian, or bisexual. Accept her or him and be there to help with any problems that arise. Your pediatrician may be able to help you with this new challenge or suggest a referral for counseling.

Gay and lesbian youth who fear rejection or discovery may not know whom to turn to for support. Try your pediatrician, parents, a trusted teacher, or a counselor. Members of the gay, lesbian, and bisexual community, or gay and lesbian youth groups, also can be helpful. They can be a real source of support and a place to find healthy role models.

Counseling may be helpful for you if you feel confused about your sexual identity. Avoid any treatments that claim to be able to change a person's sexual orientation, or treatment ideas that see homosexuality as a sickness.

Discrimination and violence: Gay and lesbian youth are at high risk for becoming victims of violence. Studies have found that 30% to 70% of gay youth have experienced verbal or physical assaults in school. They also may be called names, harassed by others, or rejected by friends and family.

There are things you can do to avoid becoming a victim of violence, especially at school.

- Talk to a trusted school counselor, administrator, or teacher about any harassment or violence you have experienced at school. You have the right to attend a safe school that is free from discrimination, harassment, violence, and abuse.
- Get involved in gay/straight alliances at your school (or help form one). These groups can help promote better understanding between gay, lesbian, and bisexual youth, and other students and teachers.
- Join a gay youth support group in your community.
- Encourage your parents to join a support group for parents and family members of gay and lesbian teenagers.

Resources

Hetrick-Martin Institute for the Protection of Gay and Lesbian Youth
2 Astor Pl
New York, NY 10003
212/674-2400
www.hmi.org

Lambda Youth OUTreach
www.lambda.org

National Gay and Lesbian Task Force
1700 Kalorama Rd NW
Washington, DC 20009-2624
202/332-6483
www.ngltf.org

National Youth Advocacy Coalition
1638 R St NW
Suite 300
Washington, DC 20009
202/319-7596
Fax: 202/319-7365
www.nyacyouth.org

OutProud, the National Coalition for Gay, Lesbian, Bisexual and
    Transgender Youth
369 Third St
Suite B-362
San Rafael, CA 94901-3581
www.outproud.org

Parents, Families and Friends of Lesbiansand Gays (PFLAG)
1726 M St NW
Suite 400
Washington, DC 20036
202/467-8180
www.pflag.org

Youth Guardian Services, Inc
8665 Sudley Rd
#304
Manassas, VA 20110-4588
877/270-5152
www.youth-guard.org

Youth Resource
A Project of Advocates for Youth
1025 Vermont Ave NW
Suite 200
Washington, DC 20005
202/347–5700
www.youthresource.com

The information contained in this publication should not be used as a substitute for the medical care and advice of your pediatrician. There may be variations in treatment that your pediatrician may recommend based on individual facts and circumstances.

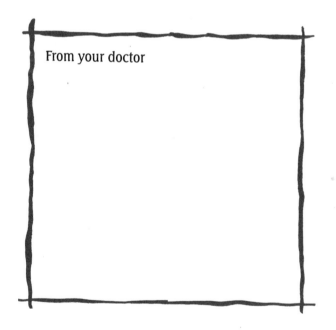

From your doctor

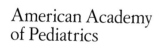

American Academy
of Pediatrics

DEDICATED TO THE HEALTH OF ALL CHILDREN™

The American Academy of Pediatrics is an organization of 60,000 primary care pediatricians, pediatric medical subspecialists, and pediatric surgical specialists dedicated to the health, safety, and well-being of infants, children, adolescents, and young adults.
American Academy of Pediatrics
Web site — www.aap.org

Learning Disabilities and Young Adults

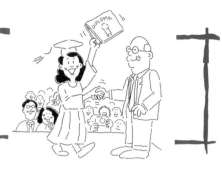

Experts estimate that as many as 12 percent of all school-aged youths in elementary, junior high and high school have some type of learning problem. These students may have emotional problems, poor hearing or vision problems; they also could be developmentally delayed. Other young people who do not face these obvious stumbling blocks still fail to do well in school or at work. These teens and young adults may have an unrecognized learning disability.

This brochure explains some of the different types of learning disabilities and how to help your learning-disabled teen or young adult cope with these problems. It also explains the training and education options that are available so your son or daughter can learn valuable job skills and work around a disability.

What is a learning disability?

Experts say that learning disabilities are due to problems with the way the brain handles information. Having a disability means that learning is difficult despite a person's best attempts. The good news is that many of these problems can be overcome by using different skills. Many learning-disabled people have made their mark in science, the arts and other fields. Albert Einstein is a good example. He learned new skills to solve problems.

Many learning-disabled youths may have normal or above-average intelligence. However, these teens may have a hard time working with written figures, spoken ideas, or certain letters and words. A student may have a hard time knowing how letters make up words, how words combine to create sentences and how sentences express thoughts. This can lead to problems with reading, spelling, writing and math.

What causes a learning disability?

A number of different factors may lead to a learning disability, such as inherited (genetic) health problems, low birth weight in ill babies or harmful environmental conditions. However, the causes are often unknown. Despite these problems, children with a disability can lead a normal life.

Experts look for early signals of a disability, including:

- failing to follow directions and appearing to "forget" what a parent or teacher says
- constant daydreaming or taking an unusually long time to finish a task
- problems organizing work at home and school

Some learning-disabled people may have several disabilities that combine to worsen the problem. For example, these students may:

- fail to learn facts and information
- handle assignments poorly
- have problems relating with peers
- not understand jokes, subtle responses or facial expressions
- have trouble paying attention or may be overactive
- feel bad about themselves

As a result, they could become unsure or uneasy in school. On the job, these workers may:

- fail to finish projects that require reading or math skills
- seem to "forget" what people say
- not understand a request
- clash with other workers

If your teen or young adult has problems like these, you should contact teachers, your pediatrician or other professionals who can help. Experts can identify the problem and find ways to help.

Building on strengths

Your teen has special talents as well as weaknesses. He may be good at math, music or sports, or he could be skilled at art or working with tools. Finding special strengths, and learning to use them, is hard work. It may be difficult for him to accept and work around a weak point. Encourage your son to use his strengths to explore and meet new challenges. This can help him develop new skills.

Developing social skills

The teen years are an awkward time of change. A learning disability can make growing up even harder, because being like other youths is important for your teen. Disabilities combined with the pain of growing up can make your teen sad, angry or withdrawn. Talking about the problem may be difficult.

In groups, a learning-disabled worker or student may be shy. Many learning-disabled youths have above average intelligence and special skills that others may not have. Your family can help by pointing out that a learning disability is not tied to how smart she is. Family members also can help by finding clubs and teams that stress friendship and fun, instead of just winning.

Your teen's pediatrician can help with tests that identify a disability. The doctor also may refer your teen to other medical specialists. Depending on what your teen's needs are, she may be referred to a pediatric neurologist, a behavioral pediatrician, a psychiatrist, a psychologist or an educator. Look for local groups in your state for support and information on learning disabilities.

Look for opportunities

Start planning for adulthood. Your child must make career and education choices during the school years. Most schools have special classes to teach your learning-disabled youth the right skills for the work force and/or higher education.

Find a specialist who can help. Teachers, employers, and college and job counselors can encourage your son or daughter to tap into special skills and cope with weak points.

Look for career search programs. These programs teach the skills that are necessary for teens to succeed in the workplace. Many career search programs include aptitude tests to help youths find the right talents and choose a career. A good program teaches useful job skills and also shows the value of self-esteem and decision-making skills.

Vocational programs. These programs teach young people how to apply for a job, accept directions, and get along with family, friends and coworkers.

Some high schools and colleges have programs to help learning-disabled students learn new skills. Counselors can direct students to tutors, study groups or graduate assistants who are willing to help.

Types of learning disabilities

Dyslexia is a term that describes serious problems with reading. With this problem, your child may not understand letters, groups of letters, sentences or paragraphs.

At the beginning of first grade, children may occasionally reverse and rotate the letters they read and write. This may be normal when first learning to read. By the middle of first grade (and with maturity) these problems disappear.

However, a young student with dyslexia (reading disabilities) may not overcome these problems. The difficulty can continue as the student gets older.

- To her, a "b" may look like a "d."
- She may write "on," when she really means "no."
- Your daughter may reverse a "6" to make "9."

This is not a vision problem. The problem involves how the brain interprets the information it "sees."

Dysgraphia is a term for problems with writing. With this problem, your teen may not form letters correctly, and there is difficulty writing within a certain space. Writing neatly takes time and effort. But despite the extra effort, handwriting still may be hard to read.

A teacher may say that a learning-disabled student can't finish written tests and assignments on time. Supervisors may find that written tasks are always late or incomplete.

Dyscalculia is a term for problems doing math. With this problem, your teen may not grasp math concepts. He may do well in history and language, but he may fail tests involving fractions and percentages. Math is difficult for many students. But with dyscalculia, a young person may have a much more difficult time doing math than others his age. Dyscalculia may prevent your teen from solving basic math problems that others his age complete with no difficulty.

Auditory memory and processing disabilities is a term for problems understanding and remembering words or sounds. Your daughter may hear normally, but she may not remember key facts because her memory does not store and interpret facts correctly. This is not caused by a hearing problem. It happens when the brain fails to understand words or sounds the right way.

Parents, teachers and pediatricians usually detect learning disabilities during the school years, but a problem may not surface until the teen years. It's important to remember that it's never too late to get help.

Communication is the key that opens the door to the working world. You can help your young adult land that first job by helping him practice for interviews, choose the right clothes to wear and maintain a positive point of view. With a little coaching, he can build self-esteem and become a successful worker.

Coping on the job

Choose the right career. Your young adult can find and hold a good job. Landing the right job increases her chance of success—especially if the work is rewarding. Handling on-the-job tasks will help her deal with problem situations and build self-esteem.

Ask for help. Hiding a disability can make a situation worse. It pays to ask questions. When your teen asks at work—and a supervisor is willing to help—a job can open new doors of opportunity.

It's the law. Federal law forbids discrimination against disabled persons in the workplace. Some employers know that it's good business to provide the help that learning-disabled people need. During an interview, an employer may ask to see written proof of a disability from a pediatrician or some other professional.

Continuing education

Learning disabilities are not tied to intelligence, which is why some learning-disabled students can perform well in high school and college. If your teen has not completed high school, he should try to obtain the Graduate Equivalency Diploma (GED). Ask a counselor for help. A counselor may be able to recommend a tutor who works with the learning disabled. Passing the GED test will make a learning-disabled youth confident during job interviews and help him land a good job. Some young adults choose to attend a trade school or junior college after high school. Other students may complete a two-year community college program and then move on to a four-year school. Many learning-disabled students can meet the entrance requirements for a four-year college. These schools usually expect all young adults to meet the same standards. This includes high school grade point averages and ACT and/or SAT scores.

Some colleges have special testing and admissions policies for the learning disabled, such as SAT or ACT tests that are not timed. To apply to special college programs, students usually need written proof of a disability and recommendations from teachers and counselors.

College is hard work. Your young adult can meet this challenge by carefully arranging schedules and asking others for help. Tutors usually are available for specific classes, and more and more colleges have writing clinics to help students develop communications skills.

It's also very important to notify the admissions counselor if your son or daughter has a disability. Ask about special classes for the learning disabled. Many community colleges have programs aimed at skills, such as aviation technology, auto mechanics, computer technology, electronics and cosmetology. In these programs, students learn valuable skills that help them find a job. With all the facts, a student can decide if the college has the right programs and services for him or her.

Support from friends and family is vital

Whether at work or school, it's important to praise your son or daughter for doing a good job. But if he or she fails, coaching and support from family and friends is very important.

Coping with a learning disability is a lifelong job. It's a full-time job for your teen's friends and family members, too. With the right support from friends and family, your teen can build a positive self-esteem despite the occasional setbacks. Without support, a learning disability is much harder to cope with.

Friends and family can help by working on new solutions, providing new challenges, offering praise when it is due and encouraging learning disabled teens.

Written reminders, quiet study areas and scheduled study times are great ways to learn the right skills for the workplace.

Hard work leads to success

People from all walks of life have overcome disabilities to become very successful. Some of the success stories include singer/actress Cher; actors Harry Anderson and Tom Cruise; inventor Thomas Edison; former Vice President Nelson Rockefeller; baseball pitcher Nolan Ryan; Olympic diver Greg Louganis; and former British Prime Minister Winston Churchill.

Your pediatrician, together with educators and other professionals, can help with early detection of a learning disability. Contact a pediatrician if you have other questions, and remember the following tips:

- Promote a positive self-image.
- Emphasize your teen's best assets.
- Work with your child to help him/her develop compensation skills.
- Be patient, and never demand that your teen complete a task that is too difficult for him/her.
- Work with useful aids such as calculators, word processors, tape recorders and typewriters.
- Know what kind of help is available through schools and employers.
- Practice skills at home.
- Find a tutor or a training program
- Seek a quiet, distraction-free place to study.
- Talk to counselors and set reasonable goals.
- Learn what rights a disabled person has under the law.
- Don't be afraid to ask questions or find help; it's never too late.

For more information on learning disabilities, refer to the following resources:

- Learning Disabilities Association of America
  4156 Library Rd
  Pittsburgh, PA 15234
  412/341-1515
- HEATH Resource Center
  (The National Clearinghouse on
  Postsecondary Education for Individuals With Disabilities)
  One Dupont Circle
  Suite 800
  Washington, DC 20036
  800/544-3284
- National Information Center for Children and Youths With Disabilities (NICHCY)
  PO Box 1492
  Washington, DC 20013
  800/999-5599
- Mangrum CT, Strichart SS, Peterson's Guide to Colleges With Programs for Learning-Disabled Students, Peterson's Guide, Inc., Princeton, NJ: 1988.

The information contained in this publication should not be used as a substitute for the medical care and advice of your pediatrician. There may be variations in treatment that your pediatrician may recommend based on individual facts and circumstances.

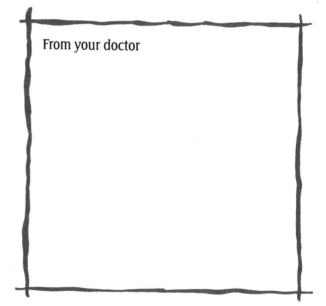

From your doctor

American Academy of Pediatrics

DEDICATED TO THE HEALTH OF ALL CHILDREN™

The American Academy of Pediatrics is an organization of 60,000 primary care pediatricians, pediatric medical subspecialists, and pediatric surgical specialists dedicated to the health, safety, and well-being of infants, children, adolescents, and young adults.

American Academy of Pediatrics
Web site — www.aap.org

Surviving: Coping With Adolescent Depression and Suicide
Guidelines for Parents

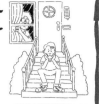

A 19-year-old college sophomore finished his term paper, asked his roommate to hand it in, and then drove himself to a park and rigged his car's exhaust pipe with a hose to the inside of his car. He died of carbon monoxide poisoning, leaving a note that asked his family for forgiveness because he "could not go on."

Like many other teens he seemed happy, well-adjusted, and high achieving. But inside him was an unhappiness and depression so great that the only solution he could see was suicide.

This is not an isolated incident. Children, teenagers, and young adults are killing themselves at rising rates. Suicide is the third leading cause of death among young people 15 to 24 years old, and it appears to be on the rise. According to a 1991 Centers for Disease Control and Prevention study, 27% of high school students thought about suicide, 16% had a plan, and 8% made an attempt. The Alcohol, Drug Abuse and Mental Health Administration has declared adolescent suicide as a national mental health problem.

Why do teens kill themselves? Experts cite divorce, family violence, the breakdown of the family unit, stress to perform and achieve, and even the threat of AIDS as factors that contribute to the higher suicide rate. More than 50% of teens who commit suicide also have a history of alcohol and drug use. Stressful life events, such as the loss of a significant person or school failure, often trigger suicides among teens.

Depression plays a role

To better understand the cause of adolescent suicide, one must look past the surface to figure out what is going on inside the suicidal teen's head. Many teens who are considering suicide suffer from depression. People who work with depressed teens see a common theme of unhappiness, as well as feelings of inner turmoil, chaos, and low self-worth. Also hopelessness and anger often contribute to adolescent suicide.

One study found that 90% of suicidal adolescents believed that their families did not understand them. These teens felt alone and anonymous. They also believed that their parents either denied or ignored their attempts to communicate feelings of unhappiness, frustration, or failure. Some parents view depression and complaining as weaknesses, so they encourage their children to be strong and not to show their emotions. Suicidal teens often feel that their emotions are played down, not taken seriously, or met with hostility by the people around them.

One pediatrician who counsels suicidal adolescents said they often talk about how hopeless everything seems. They often feel that they are not in control, as an example, not in control over the direction of their lives.

Depressed teens may be drawn to others who feel as they do forming a bond of hopelessness and despair. Some popular music reflects these feelings of alienation, self-destructive rage, and thoughts about suicide.

Adolescents need to learn that with treatment, depression ends. However, a teen who is experiencing deep depression for the first time may not be able to focus on that. Something that may seem trivial to a parent or teacher may crush an adolescent who is already in a fragile emotional state—so much so that he or she is unable to think clearly and see a way out of the problem. The teen may then see suicide as the only choice.

Adolescent suicide is treatable and preventable

People who are depressed and thinking about suicide often show changes in their behavior. These changes in behavior are usually an outgrowth of depression and are warning signs. If your teen shows these warning signs, please talk to her about her concerns and have her get help if the warning signs continue.

- Noticeable changes in eating or sleeping habits
- Unexplained, or unusually severe, violent or rebellious behavior
- Withdrawal from family or friends
- Running away
- Persistent boredom and/or difficulty concentrating
- Drug and/or alcohol abuse
- Unexplained drop in the quality of schoolwork
- Unusual neglect of appearance
- Drastic personality change
- Complaints of physical problems that are not real
- A focus on themes of death
- Giving away prized possessions
- Talking about suicide or making plans, even jokingly
- Threatening or attempting to kill oneself

Before committing suicide, people often threaten to kill themselves. These threats should always be taken seriously, as should previous suicide attempts. Most people who commit suicide have made at least one previous attempt.

Asking your teen whether he is depressed or is thinking about suicide lets him know that someone cares. You're not putting thoughts of suicide into his head. Instead you're giving your teen the chance to talk about his problems.

Remember that depression and suicidal feelings are treatable mental disorders. The first step is to listen to your adolescent. A professional must then diagnose your teen's illness and determine a proper treatment plan. Your teen needs to share her feelings, and many suicidal teens are pleading for help in their own way. Your teen needs to feel that there is hope-that people will listen, that things will get better, and that she can overcome her problems.

Parents and friends can help a depressed teen through the following strategies:

1. Talk, ask questions, and be willing to really listen. Don't dismiss your teen's problems as unimportant. Parents and other influential adults should never make fun of or ignore an adolescent's concerns, especially if they matter a great deal to her and are making her unhappy.
2. Be honest. It you're worried about your teen, say so. You will not spark thoughts of suicide just by asking about it.

3. Share your feelings. Let your teen know he's not alone. Everyone feels sad or depressed at times.

4. Get help for your teen and yourself. Talk to your pediatrician, teacher, counselor, clergy, or other trained professional. Don't wait for the problem to "go away." Although feelings of sadness and depression can disappear as quickly as they came, they can also build to the point that an adolescent thinks of suicide as the only way out. Be careful not to assume that your teen's problems have been so easily solved.

A teen attempting suicide should immediately be taken to a hospital emergency room for a psychiatric evaluation. If a depressed adolescent is assessed to be safe to go home, it's a good idea to remove from your home any lethal, accessible means to commit suicide, such as medications, firearms, razors, knives, etc.

Sources of help

There are many sources of information to help troubled teens and their families. Often a pediatrician, who has charted the adolescent's physical and emotional progress since infancy, is in the best position to detect and help treat adolescent depression. Your teen may, however, need additional counseling.

Check the *Yellow Pages* in your city for the phone numbers of local suicide hot lines, crisis centers, and mental health centers.

The following organizations can also supply information on suicide prevention:

American Academy of Child and Adolescent Psychiatry
3615 Wisconsin Ave, NW,
Washington, DC 20016
202/966-7300

American Association of Suicidology
4201 Connecticut Ave, NW, Suite 310,
Washington, DC 20008
202/237-2280

American Psychiatric Association
1400 K St, NW, Suite 501,
Washington, DC 20005
202/682-6000

American Psychological Association
750 1st St, NE,
Washington, DC 20002
202/336-5700

National Mental Health Association
1021 Prince St,
Alexandria, VA 22314-2971
800/969-6642

With professional treatment and support from family and friends, teens who are suicidal can become healthy again.

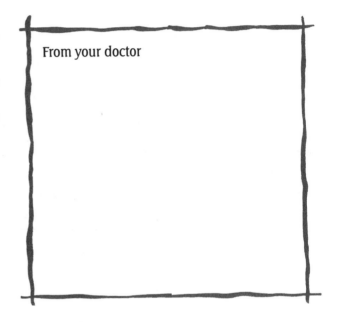

From your doctor

**American Academy
of Pediatrics**

DEDICATED TO THE HEALTH OF ALL CHILDREN™

The American Academy of Pediatrics is an organization of 60,000 primary care pediatricians, pediatric medical subspecialists, and pediatric surgical specialists dedicated to the health, safety, and well-being of infants, children, adolescents, and young adults.

American Academy of Pediatrics
Web site—www.aap.org

Copyright ©1990, Rev 2/95
American Academy of Pediatrics

what about medicines for ADHD?
questions from teens who have ADHD

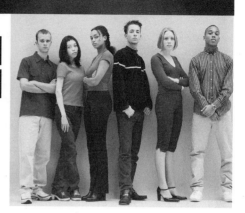

Q: What can I do besides taking medicines?

A: Medicines and **behavior therapies** are the only treatments that have been shown by scientific studies to work consistently for ADHD. Medicines are prescribed by a doctor, while behavior therapies usually are done with a counselor. These 2 treatments are probably best used together, but you might be able to do well with one or the other. You **can't rely on other treatments** such as biofeedback, allergy treatments, special diets, vision training, or chiropractic because there isn't enough evidence that shows they work.

Counseling may help you learn how to cope with some issues you may face. And there are things **YOU** can do to help yourself. For example, **things that may help you stay focused** include using a daily planner for schoolwork and other activities, making to-do lists, and even getting enough sleep.

Q: How can medicines help me?

A: There are several different ADHD medicines. They work by causing the brain to have more *neurotransmitters* in the right places. Neurotransmitters are chemicals in the brain that help us focus our attention, control our impulses, organize and plan, and stick to routines. Medicines for ADHD **can help you focus your thoughts and ignore distractions** so that you can reach your full potential. They also can help you control your emotions and behavior. Check with your pediatrician.

Q: Are medicines safe?

A: For most teens with ADHD, stimulant medicines are safe and effective if taken as recommended. However, like most medicines, there **could be side effects.** Luckily, the side effects tend to happen early on, are usually mild, and don't last too long. If you have any side effects, tell your pediatrician. Changes may need to be made in your medicines or their dosages.

- **Most common side effects** include decreased appetite or weight loss, problems falling asleep, headaches, jitteriness, and stomachaches.

- **Less common side effects** include a bad mood as medicines wear off (called the rebound effect) and facial twitches or tics.

Q: Will medicines change my personality?

A: Medicines won't change who you are and should not change your personality. If you notice changes in your mood or personality, **tell your pediatrician.** Occasionally when medicines wear off, some teens become more irritable for a short time. An adjustment of the medicines by your pediatrician may be helpful.

Q: Will medicines affect my growth?

A: Medicines will **not** keep you from growing. Significant growth delay is a very rare side effect of some medicines prescribed for ADHD. Most scientific studies show that taking these medicines has little to no long-term effect on growth in most cases.

Q: Do I need to take medicines at school?

A: There are 3 types of medicines used for teens with ADHD: **short acting** (immediate release), **intermediate acting,** and **long acting.** You can avoid taking medicines at school if you take the intermediate- or long-acting kind. Long-acting medicines usually are taken once in the morning or evening. Short-acting medicines usually are taken every 4 hours.

Q: Does taking medicines make me a drug user?

A: No! Although you may need medicines to help you stay in control of your behavior, medicines used to treat **ADHD do not lead to drug abuse. In fact, taking medicines as prescribed by your pediatrician and doing better in school may help you avoid drug use and abuse.** (But **never** give or share your medicines with anyone else.)

Q: Will I have to take medicines **forever**?

A: In most cases, ADHD continues later in life. Whether you need to keep taking medicines as an adult **depends on your own needs. The need for medicines may change over time.** Many adults with ADHD have learned how to **succeed in life** without medicines by using behavior therapies.

The information contained in this publication should not be used as a substitute for the medical care and advice of your pediatrician. There may be variations in treatment that your pediatrician may recommend based on individual facts and circumstances.

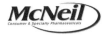

Supported by a grant from McNeil Consumer & Specialty Pharmaceuticals and partially funded by the CHADD National Resource Center on AD/HD.

From your doctor

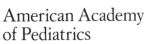

American Academy of Pediatrics

DEDICATED TO THE HEALTH OF ALL CHILDREN™

The American Academy of Pediatrics is an organization of 60,000 primary care pediatricians, pediatric medical subspecialists, and pediatric surgical specialists dedicated to the health, safety, and well-being of infants, children, adolescents, and young adults.

American Academy of Pediatrics
PO Box 747
Elk Grove Village, IL 60009-0747
Web site — http://www.aap.org

Copyright © 2005   American Academy of Pediatrics

what is ADHD anyway?
questions from teens

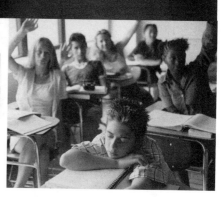

Attention-deficit/hyperactivity disorder

(ADHD) is a condition of the brain that **makes it difficult for people to concentrate.** The following are quick answers to some common questions:

Q: What causes ADHD?

A: There isn't just one cause. Research shows that

- **ADHD is a medical condition** caused by small changes in how the brain works. It seems to be related to 2 chemicals in your brain called *dopamine* and *norepinephrine*. These chemicals help send messages between nerve cells in the brain—especially those areas of the brain that control attention and activity level.
- **ADHD most often runs in families.**
- In a few people with ADHD, being *born prematurely* or being *exposed to alcohol during the pregnancy* can contribute to ADHD.
- Immunizations and eating too much sugar **do NOT cause** ADHD. And there **isn't enough evidence that shows** allergies and food additives cause ADHD.

Q: How can you tell if someone has ADHD?

A: You can't tell if someone has ADHD just by looks. People with ADHD don't look any different, but *how they act may make them stand out* from the crowd. Some people with ADHD are very hyperactive (they move around a lot and are not able to sit still) and have behavior problems that are obvious to everyone. Other people with ADHD are quiet and more laid back on the outside, but on the inside struggle with schoolwork and other tasks. They are distracted by people and things around them when they try to study; they may have trouble organizing schoolwork or forget to turn in assignments.

Q: Can ADHD cause someone to act up or get in trouble?

A: Having ADHD can cause you to struggle in school or have problems controlling your behavior. Some people may say or think that your struggles and problems are because you are bad, lazy, or not smart. **But they're wrong.** It's important that you get help so your impulses don't get you into serious trouble.

Q: Don't little kids who have ADHD outgrow it by the time they are teens?

A: Often kids with the hyperactive kind of ADHD get less hyperactive as they get into their teens, but usually they still have **a lot of difficulty paying attention,** remembering what they have read, and getting their work done. They may or may not have other behavior problems. Some kids with ADHD have never been hyperactive at all, but usually their attention problems also continue into their teens.

Q: If I have trouble with homework or tests, do I have ADHD?

A: There could be many reasons why a student struggles with schoolwork and tests. **ADHD could be one reason.** It may or may not be, but your pediatrician is the best person to say for sure. Kids with ADHD often say it's hard to concentrate, focus on a task (for example, schoolwork, chores, or a job), manage their time, and finish tasks. This could explain why they may have trouble with schoolwork and tests. Whatever the problem, **there are many people willing to help you.** You need to find the approach that works best for you.

Q: Does having ADHD mean a person is not very smart?

A: Absolutely not! People who have trouble paying attention may have problems in school, but that doesn't mean they're not smart. In fact, some people with ADHD are very smart, *but may not be able to reach their potential in school until they get treatment.*

ADHD is a common problem. Teens with ADHD have the potential to do well in school and live a normal life with the right treatment.

Q: Is it just a guy thing?

A: ADHD is **more common in guys than girls.** About 3 times more guys than girls are diagnosed with ADHD. But **more girls are being identified with ADHD.**

Q: What do I do if I think I have ADHD?

A: Don't be afraid to talk with your parents or other adults that you trust. Together you can meet with your pediatrician and find out if you really have ADHD. If you do, **your pediatrician will help you** learn how to live with ADHD and find ways to deal with your condition.

The information contained in this publication should not be used as a substitute for the medical care and advice of your pediatrician. There may be variations in treatment that your pediatrician may recommend based on individual facts and circumstances.

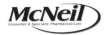

Supported by a grant from McNeil Consumer & Specialty Pharmaceuticals and partially funded by the CHADD National Resource Center on AD/HD.

From your doctor

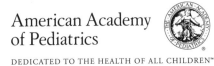

American Academy
of Pediatrics

DEDICATED TO THE HEALTH OF ALL CHILDREN™

The American Academy of Pediatrics is an organization of 60,000 primary care pediatricians, pediatric medical subspecialists, and pediatric surgical specialists dedicated to the health, safety, and well-being of infants, children, adolescents, and young adults.

American Academy of Pediatrics
PO Box 747
Elk Grove Village, IL 60009-0747
Web site — http://www.aap.org

Section IV Further Reading

Albrecht MA, Naugle AE. Psychological assessment and treatment of somatization: adolescents with medically unexplained neurologic symptoms. *Adolesc Med.* 2002;13:625–641

Beasley PJ, Beardslee WR. Depression in the adolescent patient. *Adolesc Med.* 1998;9:351–362

Hack S, Jellinek MS. Early identification of emotional and behavioral problems in a primary care setting. *Adolesc Med.* 1998;9:335–350

McGregor RS. Chronic complaints in adolescence: chest pain, chronic fatigue, headaches, abdominal pain. *Adolesc Med.* 1997;8:15–31

Pratt HD. Neurodevelopmental issues in the assessment and treatment of deficits in attention, cognition, and learning during adolescence. *Adolesc Med.* 2002;13:579–598

Robin AL. Attention deficit hyperactivity disorder. *Adolesc Med.* 1998;9:373–383

Steinman S, Petersen V. The impact of parental divorce for adolescents: a consideration of intervention beyond the crisis. *Adolesc Med.* 2001;12:493–507

Health Risk Behaviors/Adolescents at Risk

Adolescent Violence

by Robert D. Sege, MD, PhD, FAAP

Violence is a leading cause of injury, death, and mental health problems in adolescents. The violence affecting adolescents takes many forms, including peer and dating violence. This issue of *Adolescent Health Update* will describe roles for pediatricians and other clinicians caring for adolescents who are involved in, or affected by, violence.

Most opportunities for clinical intervention occur either during the course of routine health care or at the time of treatment for a violence-related injury. The most effective approaches require knowledge of risk factors and protective factors, an understanding of factors that affect behavioral change, and knowledge of community-based resources. Anticipatory guidance about violence prevention should not wait until adolescence. This aspect of preventive care begins in childhood, and is well within the pediatrician's sphere.

A policy statement from the AAP Task Force on Violence, published in the January 1999 issue of *Pediatrics*, discusses ways to approach violence issues that affect pediatric patients. The policy statement can be accessed via the AAP Web site (www.aap.org).

Epidemiology of Youth Violence

The United States has the highest homicide rate of any developed country, exceeding the next-highest country by a factor of four. Within the United States, adolescents and young adults are at the highest risk of death due to homicide. Black youth are at a ten-fold higher risk of homicide than are white youth. Poverty and low socioeconomic status are associated with high rates of violent death; thus, poor white youth are also at increased risk.

While homicide rates rose dramatically between 1985 and 1995, the late 1990s have seen a national decline in the rates of youth homicide. Overall, while violence-related injuries have continued to increase, motor vehicle crashes — the other leading cause of death and injury for adolescents — have also shown a decline. Centers for Disease Control and Prevention authorities estimate that, within the next few years, firearm-related injury will surpass motor vehicle crashes as the leading cause of death for young Americans.

Learning Goal and Objectives

Goal. Pediatricians will understand how violence affects adolescents and their families.

Objectives. After reading this article, pediatricians will be able to:

● Discuss epidemiology and risk factors for involvement in peer violence

● Obtain a violence-related history during a primary care and acute care/injury office visit, including risk and resiliency factors

● Identify patients and families at risk as victims or perpetrators of violence and provide office-based practical primary prevention and intervention for adolescents and parents

● Counsel and refer patients when peer violence or dating violence is identified

● Utilize community resources which provide services for patients and families at risk of violence

● Advocate for community programs and legislative proposals to protect youth who are, or are at risk of becoming, victims or perpetrators of violence

---

Robert D. Sege, MD, PhD, is director of the Pediatric and Adolescent Health Research Center at the Floating Hospital for Children in Boston, Massachusetts, and assistant professor of pediatrics, Tufts University School of Medicine.

The number of victims of violence increases dramatically when psychological sequelae are considered. Children and young adults who witness violence, or who are themselves victims of violence, are at increased risk for depression, poor school performance, and post-traumatic stress disorder (PTSD). While national data are not available, smaller studies bear this out. Nearly one third of inner city children attending a summer day camp near Washington DC had PTSD, as did nearly 25% of Detroit-area HMO members in their early 20s. Community surveys of youth in some of America's poorest cities show a high prevalence of PTSD, often associated with violence.

Risk Factors

Young people learn about violence through experience, both personal and vicarious. Certain events or conditions in preadolescence are associated with the subsequent use of violence. Three childhood and adolescent risk factors have been most clearly validated:

1. *Exposure to violence in the home.* Violent homes—those with domestic violence or child abuse—appear to promote violent behavior among adolescents even if the family violence occurred years earlier. When encountering young people with a history of fights, assaults, or dating violence, the possibility of current or previous domestic violence should be explored.
2. *Parental reliance on corporal punishment.* Numerous studies have demonstrated an association between parental reliance on corporal punishment and subsequent violence as adults. In recognition of this substantial association, the American Academy of Pediatrics released a statement encouraging pediatricians to counsel parents about alternatives to corporal punishment.
3. *Exposure to violence through television.* Television is perhaps the best-studied environmental risk factor for violence, and has been the subject of several AAP policy statements. While the best available data appear to suggest that young children are particularly vulnerable, violent mainstream media productions have demonstrated measurable short-term effects on adolescents. The effects of today's extremely popular and violent video and computer games have not been well studied.

Individual risk factors are further discussed at right ("Adolescent Violence: Myth Versus Reality").

Medical Roles

Potential interventions occur in at least three contexts: (1) primary prevention for youth and their families; (2) identification and assessment of youth at risk; and (3) intervention for injured adolescents and their parents. In general, extensive psychosocial intervention for children and youth at high risk falls outside of the expertise of most pediatricians. Pediatricians should be familiar with resources in their communities for consultation or referral.

PRIMARY PREVENTION

Parents should be advised to limit their adolescents to no more than 2 hours per day of total screen time: videos, TV, and video games. In addition, young adolescents should be restricted from viewing particularly violent movies. When their teenager watches graphic media violence, or sees news reports that are especially disturbing, parents can either turn the television off or help them put the violence into context by talking with them. Parents who disapprove of the violence on television can express their objection, or ask their teen: "Why do you think there is so much violence on TV? What would happen if people in the real world behaved like that?"

Although many parents purchase handguns believing that this will increase the safety of their families, available evidence indicates that having a handgun in the home increases the risk that a family member will be involved in a homicide or suicide. Pediatricians can disseminate this information to parents. Teens appear to be at particular risk of suicide when there is a gun in the home.

See Table 1 and page 486 for advice about counseling parents on warning signs that their teen may be at risk for involvement in violence, and tips for parents trying to talk to their adolescents about it.

Adolescent Violence: Myth Versus Reality

Popular media portray most adolescent victims of violence as gang members, drug dealers, or victims of predatory criminals, which encourages a tendency to describe violence-involved youth as either victims or perpetrators. However, review of medical records and other evidence suggests that the difference between victim and perpetrator is less clear. Respective roles may be more closely related to the exact circumstances of a particular event than to any factor of personality or behavior. After an injury, the criminal justice system identifies victims and perpetrators.

The majority of violent injuries involving adolescents grow out of fights or disagreements among friends, acquaintances, or other young adults who know each other. Use of weapons escalates with age. Those who carry weapons or who report being threatened with a weapon are at increased risk of more serious injury, either because they are members of a social group that condones weapon-carrying or because they are unable to avoid dangerous situations. Three salient observations about adolescent injuries place the issues of risk and resilience in context.

- In studies of young adolescent violent offenders conducted in the late 1980's, Slaby and Guerra demonstrated that these youngsters have habits of thought that promote violent interactions. In assessing situations of potential conflict, violent youngsters are more likely to feel threatened than their less violent peers. Also, they have more difficulty in arriving at nonviolent solutions to conflicts. Other reports have confirmed that the most violent adolescents conceptualize two possible solutions: fight or be a "sucker." Their less violent peers more often use strategies that involve information gathering, humor, or understanding to de-escalate tense situations.

- As the title of Geoffrey Canada's book, *Fist, Stick, Knife, Gun,* suggests, there is a progression toward increasing use of weapons among adolescents involved in violence. Adolescents who arm themselves in order to feel safer may then allow themselves to venture into more dangerous circumstances that are more likely to lead to violent confrontations.

- Recent surveillance reports suggest that the gender gap in fighting-related injury is shrinking. Emergency department and primary care visits for female adolescents injured in fights with other young women appear to account for about one in three violence-related injuries.

IDENTIFICATION

Some teens are able to avoid violent situations more easily than others. Those who lack the skills to de-escalate a situation are more likely to get hurt. Evidence suggests that adolescents at greatest risk for violence and violence-related injury are those who have engaged in other health risk behaviors and also report a history of fighting. Analyses by DuRant of National Youth Risk Behavior Survey data demonstrated an association between drug use, number of sexual partners, and recent fights. Other studies have suggested that failing in school or not being in school at age 16 should be added to these clustered factors or risk behaviors. A specific violence-related history may be obtained by following the FISTS mnemonic (Table 2).

RISK ASSESSMENT

Once a violence history has been obtained, determine whether the adolescent is at low, moderate or high risk for violence.

Validate the behavior of low-risk teens, defined as those who have not been in a fight in the past year, are passing their courses in school, and do not report any drug use. (*EG, That's terrific; you've really learned to handle yourself. Sometimes I see other teens who live in the same neighborhood as you do, but find themselves getting into a lot of fights. I worry about them. What would you tell them if you were me?*)

Adolescents at moderate risk, defined as those who report recent fights, are failing in school, or have other associated risk factors, should receive developmentally appropriate counseling. One useful avenue is to ask about the most recent fight,

Table 1. Teen Violence: Facts for Parents

FACT: *Most kids who are hurt in a fight have been fighting with a friend or someone they know.*

TIP: Teach your teen how to walk away from a fight. If you are unsure how to do this, ask for help from people who work with kids.

TIP: Get to know your teen's friends. Tell your adolescent why you want to know them.

FACT: *Adolescents tend to get into trouble after school and before supper. This is when fights start, drugs are used, and pregnancies begin.*

TIP: Know where your adolescent is after school.

TIP: Help your adolescent to get involved with an organized sport or other adult-supervised activity. Ask your friends, neighbors, teachers, and school counselors to recommend good local programs.

FACT: *Adolescents with other problems such as truancy, drug use, or behavioral and emotional problems often also get hurt in fights.*

TIP: If you have noticed any of these problems in your adolescent, ask to speak with the nurse, social worker, or your adolescent's pediatrician. They can refer you to someone in your community who can help.

FACT: *Guns do not make you (or your adolescent) safer.*

TIP: If you have teenagers at home, make sure there are no guns at home. If this is impossible, keep your guns locked, unloaded, and separate from the ammunition—which should also be kept in a locked place. **Guns can turn adolescent troubles into tragedy!**

TIP: Talk to your adolescent about the truth of carrying a gun. When carrying a gun, people feel bold, resulting in foolish behaviors. If another person sees the gun, that person may shoot first. Carrying a gun gives a false sense of protection and may actually make a young person less safe!

Adapted with permission from Sege RD. Your Child Has Been Injured in a Fight: What Parents Need to Know. In: Sege RD, ed. *Violence Prevention for Children and Youth: Parent Education Cards.* 2nd ed. Waltham, MA: Massachusetts Medical Society. In press.

and help the patient find moments when it could have been de-escalated. They should leave with some ability to defuse tense situations.

For those in early and middle adolescence, concrete skill-building is important. It may help to give teenagers specific words that they can use to de-escalate tense situations. (*I've talked with lots of young people who live around here. I've learned a few things about how to avoid fights. Sometimes, you just need to look the other person in the eye and say, "This isn't worth fighting about." Do you think this would work for you? What could you say if someone tried to pick a fight with you?*)

Teens at high risk, those who report more than four physical fights in the past year, who have dropped out of school or are in danger of failing at school, and those who carry a weapon, (even for "self-defense") require further intervention. These interventions may not be in the province of the primary care provider.

Potential resources to consider include school counselors, counselors associated with an after-school or Boys and Girls Club program, community outreach programs, church ministers, or the social work department within the health care setting. For younger adolescents, it is often appropriate

to include the parent(s) in the discussion, and enlist their support in engaging the patient in further interventions. For older adolescents, particularly those out of school, the primary contact will be the adolescent. Experience suggests that having an initial contact within the context of an office visit enhances patient follow-through.

INTERVENTION FOLLOWING AN INJURY

Once an adolescent has been injured in a fight, the risk of re-injury increases. This increase is due to at least two different mechanisms. First, the conflict that led to the injury may not be resolved, and the youth may become re-involved, seeking revenge for the index injury. Second, the youth may be involved in a peer group that condones or values violence, may be involved in illegal drug use, or may not have learned the skills to extricate himself or herself from situations of potential conflict. Prevention focuses on reducing both of these types of risks.

When providing medical care for an adolescent who has been injured in a fight, the pediatrician has an important opportunity for intervention. Prior to sending a young person home, ask him or her:

Table 2. The FISTS Mnemonic

The device shown below may be employed to screen for health risk behaviors that suggest increased risk for violence-related injury.

Fighting: *How many fights have you been in during the past year? When was your last fight?* Those adolescents who report that they have been in more than two physical fights in the past year are at substantially increased risk for future violence-related injury. For those adolescents who disclose a recent fight, it is important to get a more detailed account of the incident itself. Pay careful attention to how it started, what motivated your patient to fight, who else was there, and whether a weapon was involved. Explore whether there could have been a resolution, other than fighting, and assess their ability to resolve conflict peacefully.

Injuries: *Have you ever been injured in a fight? Have you ever injured someone else in a fight?* These two questions help the clinician elicit an estimate of the severity of previous fights. Patients who have been injured may be more likely to carry a weapon in the future.

Sex: *Has your partner ever hit you? Have you hit (hurt) your partner? Have you ever been forced to have sex against your will? Do you think that couples can stay in love when one partner makes the other one afraid?*

Threats: *Has someone carrying a weapon ever threatened you? What happened? Has anything changed since then to make you feel safer?*

Self-defense: *What do you do if someone tries to pick a fight with you? Have you ever carried a weapon in self-defense?* Asking about weapons in the context of self-defense facilitates a more candid response. In all cases carrying a firearm indicates high risk. Knife-carrying is not as clear. Adolescents who carry a small pocket knife, for example, may or may not be at increased risk.

Adapted with permission from the Association of American Medical Colleges, "Interpersonal violence and the education of physicians," Alpert E, Sege R, Bradshaw Y; *Academic Medicine.* 1997:72(suppl):S41–S50.

- Is the conflict settled?
- Do you feel safe leaving the clinical setting?
- Is there a safe place to go while things cool off?
- What plans do you have involving the other individual(s) involved in the violent incident? Are you thinking about further violence involving the other person? Carrying or using a weapon?
- Is there an adult who can help mediate the dispute, or is there a peer mediation program in the school or community?

When available, a social worker or other mental health professional can assist in crisis intervention, identification of co-occurring risk factors, (for example, family violence, drug use, or school failure) and facilitation of patient access to community agencies for mental health support.

Advocacy

Successful violence intervention requires a coordinated response from all sectors of society, particularly those institutions that interact directly with youth: health care personnel, media, schools, law enforcement, religious, and community organizations. Cities that have successfully mobilized these institutions have experienced a decline in the rates of youth violence in the 1990s. Several aspects are worthy of advocacy at the individual and professional level.

Improved adolescent access to mental health services is critical.

GUNS

Pediatricians need to continue to advocate for strict enforcement of laws, and educate parents about the importance of locking up guns in the home. The availability of guns in the home is a risk factor for homicide and suicide, and adolescents are vulnerable. Academy policy statements ("Firearms and Adolescents" and "Firearm Injuries Affecting the Pediatric Population") are relevant in this regard.

There are a number of programs which claim success in reducing the willingness or ability of adolescents to obtain weapons. Speakers' kits for violence prevention talks and other materials for media initiatives are available through the Academy. Television and cable stations can join with local health care organizations to promote antiviolence messages. While community-wide gun buybacks remove only a small proportion of weapons from circulation, the campaign itself offers visibility for the issue and provides a positive role for youth in reducing this danger.

Early efforts to reduce gun violence focused on regulations designed to make it more difficult or expensive to obtain weapons and ammunition. This led to successful campaigns for background

Dating Violence

Surveys of teenagers demonstrate that one in ten is involved in dating violence, which may be verbal, physical, or psychological. It is important to avoid gender stereotypes in caring for adolescents who have been victimized. Be alert to abuse of young men by their female partners.

The pediatrician's essential message must be simple and emphatic: **No behavior on the part of the victim justifies the use of physical force.** Romantic relationships should never be dangerous.

Pregnant adolescents are at high risk of violence. Personal safety should be addressed in all encounters with these young women.

Intervention, which is indicated when a patient has been involved in a violent relationship, begins with an assessment of severity. For example:

- Mild abuse: The partner has persuaded your patient to drop out of ordinary activities and has begun to select his or her clothes and friends.
- Moderate abuse: The partner exhibits jealousy and rage, screaming, swearing or belittling your patient, who fears physical violence. The patient should be referred for counseling.
- Severe abuse: The partner has used physical force, forced sex, and the threat of force to control your patient, who wants to end the relationship but is afraid to do so. This case should be discussed with parents and, if possible, a social worker. School intervention, police involvement, or a restraining order may be needed.

Follow-up is essential for all patients involved in dating violence to re-assess the initial problem and to determine whether outside referral appointments have been made or kept.

TEEN DATING VIOLENCE: TIPS FOR PARENTS

Dating violence can happen in families of all cultures, income levels, and educational backgrounds. More than one in ten adolescents experience physical violence in a dating relationship. Here are tips to help you know if your adolescent is the victim of dating violence, and some advice for you to share with your teen.

Warning signs

Some of the following are just part of being a teenager. But when these changes happen suddenly, or without explanation, there may be cause for concern:

- Sudden changes in clothing or makeup
- Bruises, scratches or other injuries
- Failing grades or dropping out of school activities
- Avoiding friends
- Sudden changes in mood or personality, "crying jags" or "getting hysterical"
- Constantly thinking about dating partner
- Pregnancy (some teenagers believe that having a baby will help make things better; some young women are forced to have sex).

What you can say to your teen

"I care about what happens to you. I love you and I want to help."

"If you feel afraid, it may be abuse. Pay attention to your gut feelings"

"The abuse is not your fault. You are not to blame, no matter how guilty the person doing this to you makes you feel. Your partner should not be doing this to you."

"It is the abuser who has the problem, not you. It is not your responsibility to help this person change."

Remember to focus on your adolescent, not on the partner.

Point out how unhappy your adolescent seems to be. Love should not be like that!

WARNING SIGNS OF A POTENTIALLY VIOLENT PARTNER

- Wants to get serious quickly, and will not take "NO" for an answer;
- Often loses his or her temper
- Is possessive or jealous: wants to choose the partner's friends and activities, to know where the partner is at all times
- Blames the victim: "You make me get so mad"
- Apologizes for outbursts, promising never to do it again
- May drink, use drugs, or get involved in violence outside the relationship as well

"Teen Dating Violence: Tips for Parents," and "Warning Signs of a Potentially Violent Partner," are adapted with permission from Sousa CA. Teen Dating Violence: What Parents Need to Know. In: Sege RD, ed. Violence Prevention for Children and Youth: Parent Education Cards. *Waltham, MA: Massachetts Medical Society, 1997. Copies of the card are available from the Massachusetts Medical Society (1-800/322-2303) for distribution to parents.*

checks on purchasers, cooling-off waiting periods before a gun could be brought home, regulations requiring the use of trigger locks and safe storage, and restrictions on sales of military assault weapons. Strict enforcement of regulations prohibiting the sale of handguns to minors will prevent the legal purchase of weapons. However, many weapons continue to be acquired illegally, or through so-called "straw man" purchases, which occur when an adult legally purchases a handgun for sale to a minor.

Current efforts are designed to further restrict the illegal gun trade. Regulations limiting purchasers to one gun per month are an attempt to prevent the purchase of weapons in some states for import into states or localities with stricter regulations. Some local governments have attempted to make gun manufacturers and distributors liable for gun deaths under some circumstances. These lawsuits are modeled after the successful anti-tobacco litigation.

Table 3 lists sources of information and referral that may be useful to pediatricians who are interested in antiviolence advocacy.

SCHOOL PROGRAMS FOR VIOLENCE PREVENTION AND PEER MEDIATION

Antiviolence curricula developed for school systems teach anger management, conflict resolution, and dating violence prevention in the context of school health classes. Most such programs employ active learning and role-playing exercises. Studies have demonstrated the effectiveness of these programs. Peer mediation programs offer young people nonviolent yet socially acceptable methods for resolving conflicts in the school setting.

Pediatricians can be effective advocates for the incorporation of these methods in local curricula. At the same time, they can advise against programs developed by advocacy groups that familiarize students with firearms and their use. These programs have never been proven effective in reducing accidental injuries, or useful in teaching young people that firearm ownership and use is a major health hazard for adolescents.

Conclusion

Violence prevention is an essential element of pediatric care. In early childhood, the pediatrician offers anticipatory guidance for parents about firearms in the home and corporal punishment. In adolescence, primary prevention and intervention for adolescents affected by violence may be required. In the event that office-based preventive education and intervention is not sufficient, the pediatrician should be prepared to refer patients for mental health and other support services. Advocacy for access to needed mental health services, as well as legislative and regulatory measures to counter violence, are important roles for pediatricians.

Table 3. Sources of Information and Referral

The American Academy of Pediatrics Web site (www.aap.org) is an excellent resource for pediatricians who are interested in learning more about how violence affects their patients and what they can do about it. Options on the site are listed below.
- Academy policy statements
- Links to professional groups active in violence prevention
- Brochures for patient and parent anticipatory guidance

To access the Web site, go to www.aap.org, click on "Advocacy" and then "Violence Prevention Resources."

The Children's Safety Network (http://www.edc.org/HHD/csn/) is a clearinghouse funded by the federal Maternal and Child Health Bureau. This site contains up-to-date references on violence prevention programs, including school curricula and publications for use in education programs.

The Massachusetts Medical Society, in cooperation with the Massachusetts chapter of the AAP, has published parent education cards for use in physician offices. *Violence Prevention for Children and Youth: Parent Education Cards* are available from the Massachusetts Medical Society, 1-800-322-2303, ext. 1015.

Further Reading

American Academy of Pediatrics, Committee on Psychosocial Aspects of Child and Family Health. Guidance for effective discipline. *Pediatrics.* 1998;101:723–728

American Academy of Pediatrics Task Force on Violence. The role of the pediatrician in youth violence prevention in clinical practice and at the community level. *Pediatrics.* 1999;103:173–181

Annest J, Mercy J, Gibson D, Ryan G. National estimates of nonfatal firearm-related injuries: Beyond the tip of the iceberg. *JAMA.* 1995;273:1749–1754

Apfel RJ, Simon B. *Minefields in Their Hearts.* New Haven, CT: Yale University Press; 1996:244

Canada G. *Fist, Stick, Knife, Gun: A Personal History of Violence in America.* Boston, MA: Beacon Press; 1995

Centers for Disease Control and Prevention. Deaths Resulting from Firearm and Motor Vehicle-Related Injuries—United States, 1968-1991. *MMWR.* 1991;43:37–42

Centers for Disease Control and Prevention. *Mortality Trends, Causes of Death, and Related Risk Behaviors Among US Adolescents.* Atlanta, GA: 1995

Dietz WH, Strasburger VC. Children, adolescents and television. *Current Problems in Pediatrics.* 1991;21:8–31

DuRant RH, Kahn J, Beckford PH, Woods ER. The association of weapon carrying and fighting on school property and other health risk and problem behaviors among high school students. *Arch Pediatr Adolesc Med.* 1997;151:360–366

DuRant RH, Cadenhead C, Pendergrast RA, Slavens G, Linder CW. Factors associated with the use of violence among urban black adolescents. *Am J Public Health.* 1994;84:612–616

Fingerhut LA, Kleinman JC. International and interstate comparisons of homicide among young males. *JAMA.* 1990; 263:3292–3294

Foshee VA, Bauman KE, Arriaga XB, Helms RW, Koch GG, Linder GF. An evaluation of Safe Dates, an adolescent dating violence prevention program. *Am J Public Health.* 1998;88: 45–50

Osofsky JD. *Children in a Violent Society.* New York, NY: Guilford Press; 1997:338

Sege RD. Peer violence. In: Dershewitz R, ed. *Ambulatory Pediatric Care.* 3rd ed. New York, NY: Lippincott-Raven; 1998:155–160

Sege R, Stigol LC, Perry C, Goldstein R, Spivak H. Intentional injury surveillance in a primary care pediatric setting. *Arch Pediatr Adolesc Med.* 1996;150:277–283

Sege R, Stringham P, Short S, Griffith J. Ten years after: Examination of adolescent screening questions that predict future violence-related injury. *J Adolesc Health.* 1999;24: 395–402

Slaby RG, Guerra NG. Cognitive mediators of aggression in adolescent offenders. 1. Assessment. *Dev Psychol.* 1988;24: 580–588

Spivak H, Harvey B, eds. The role of the pediatrician in violence prevention: A call to action. *Pediatrics.* 1994;94:577–651

Stone DA, Kharasch SJ, Perron C, Wilson K, Jacklin B, Sege RD. Comparing pediatric intentional injury surveillance data with data from publicly available sources: Consequences for a public health response to violence. *Injury Control.* 1999;5: 136–141

Straus MA, Sugarman DB, Giles-Sims J. Spanking by parents and subsequent antisocial behavior of children. *Arch Pediatr Adolesc Med.* 1997;151:761–767

Acknowledgment

The editors would like to acknowledge technical review by Howard Spivak, MD, FAAP, who served as chair of the now-retired AAP Task Force on Violence.

Clinical Evaluation of Substance Abuse

Paritosh Kaul, MD, * *Susan M. Coupey, MD†*

Objectives

After completing this article, readers should be able to:

1. Identify the percentage of United States high school seniors who have used an illicit drug and name the most common drug used.
2. Discuss coexisting mental health disorders and other findings that are prevalent among adolescents who have substance use disorders.
3. Describe the steps in diagnosing substance use disorder or dependence.
4. Characterize the effects of frequent prolonged use of most illicit drugs.
5. Describe the usefulness of laboratory testing for drugs of abuse.

Case Report

An 18-year-old man was admitted to the adolescent inpatient unit with a history of 2 days of abdominal pain, vomiting, and diarrhea. He was dehydrated and was treated with intravenous fluids. Over the following 2 days, the diarrhea and vomiting resolved, but the abdominal pain persisted. Approximately 48 hours after admission, the patient became irritable, complained of palpitations, and expressed a strong desire to leave the hospital. On the third day, his irritability increased, he developed chills but no fever, and he complained of aching all over his body.

A detailed psychosocial history revealed that both of the young man's parents were dead, and he felt responsible for his two younger brothers. He admitted to smoking between 5 and 10 "blunts" (large marijuana cigars) a day for "at least" the past year. He admitted that he sold drugs to finance his habit and help support his brothers, although he had never been arrested.

His treating physicians agreed that the admitting diagnosis was gastroenteritis with dehydration, but a secondary diagnosis of cannabis dependence with acute withdrawal syndrome was made on the third hospital day, based on the psychosocial history and the timing of the "flu-like" symptoms.

Introduction

Substance use and abuse continue to threaten the health and well-being of adolescents and young adults. Whether sporadic intoxication leads to unintentional trauma or frequent substance use impairs health, development, and learning, the morbidity is considerable. In addition, substance use contributes to many deaths from injuries, homicide, and suicide, the three leading causes of mortality in this age group. Pediatricians caring for adolescents must identify substance users, assess the effect that substance use has on the patient's overall health and development, plan appropriate interventions with patients and parents, and monitor the effectiveness of the interventions.

In this article, we review the epidemiology of illicit drug use and discuss identification of the at-risk adolescent. In addition, we address the process of screening for and diagnosing substance use disorders in the adolescent. Finally, we provide an overview of the major classes of illicit drugs and the use of laboratory screening tests. We do not discuss tobacco or alcohol because they will be covered in other

*Postdoctoral Fellow in Adolescent Medicine.

†Professor of Pediatrics, Associate Director, Adolescent Medicine, Children's Hospital at Montefiore Medical Center, Albert Einstein College of Medicine, Bronx, NY.

articles this year. Similarly, the management of substance abuse in adolescents is the subject of a future article.

Epidemiology

Patterns of illicit drug use are in a state of continuous evolution and change in response to fluctuating drug popularity and perceptions of harm. In the 1990s, for example, there was a decline in the use of cocaine, in part due to widespread publicity about the drug's harmful effects, but a simultaneous increase in use of amphetamines, thus exchanging one dangerous stimulant drug for another. Use of marijuana by high school students increased throughout most of the 1990s, and nasal inhalation of heroin began to become more popular in the latter part of the decade. Data collected in 2000 show a sharp increase in use of "ecstasy," 3, 4-methylenedioxymethamphetamine (MDMA), among young people in the United States.

For the past 25 years, the University of Michigan's Institute for Social Research has been documenting youth drug use patterns in its *Monitoring the Future* study, which surveys nationally representative samples of high school students in 8th, 10th, and 12th grades. In the 2000 survey, 54% of 12th-grade students reported ever using an illicit drug. However, only 29% had ever used an illicit drug other than marijuana. This underscores that marijuana is the most commonly used illicit drug, with 40% of 10th-grade and 49% of 12th-grade students reporting having tried it (Table 1). Ecstasy now is used by more American adolescents than cocaine. Approximately 1 in 10 12th-grade students have used this drug.

Data from the *Monitoring the Future* survey are confirmed by another nationally representative series of surveys of high school students conducted by the Centers for Disease Control and Prevention entitled the Youth Risk Behavior Surveillance (YRBS). In the most recent 1999 survey, 47% of high school seniors reported using marijuana at least once in their lifetime, and 27% had used this drug in the 30 days prior to the survey. Initiation of marijuana use before age 13 years was reported by 11% of students. In

Table 1. Prevalence of Use of Selected Illicit Drugs Among United States High School Seniors—2000*

Drug	Lifetime Use (%)	Past Year (%)	Past 30 Days (%)
Marijuana	48.8	36.5	21.6
Amphetamines	15.6	10.5	5.0
MDMA (Ecstasy)	11.0	8.2	3.6
Barbiturates	9.2	6.2	3.0
Hallucinogens	13.0	8.1	2.6
Tranquilizers	8.9	5.7	2.6
Inhalants	14.2	5.9	2.2
Cocaine	8.6	5.0	2.1
Heroin	2.4	1.5	0.7

*See Johnson, Suggested Reading

the 1999 YRBS, boys were more likely than girls to report lifetime and current marijuana use; current cocaine use; and lifetime heroin, anabolic steroid, and injection drug use. This survey also asked students if they had been sold, offered, or given an illegal drug on school property during the past year; 30% responded positively, indicating that the illicit drug trade has become commonplace on many high school campuses.

Identification of At-risk Adolescents

The quest for autonomy and independence is a major psychosocial task of adolescent development. A normal and necessary aspect of this stage of development is experimentation with new and different experiences. The initiation of illicit drug use often starts as a form of experimentation for recreational purposes, as a social lubricant, for thrill-seeking, or as a way to bond with peers. Experimentation may be followed by more frequent drug use, and a small number of young people may progress to more serious abuse or addiction. The etiology of substance abuse is multifactorial and best conceptualized in a biopsychosocial framework. Many risk factors have been found to be important for the onset and persistence of illicit drug use among young people.

Early behavior problems are risk factors for some teenagers who abuse drugs. A follow-up study of young adult males (mean age, 18 y) who had been diagnosed as having attention deficit hyperactivity disorder (ADHD) in childhood found that the 31% of boys whose ADHD persisted in adolescence and who also had a conduct disorder were at very high risk for a substance use disorder. Other studies have shown that depression, conduct disorders, and antisocial personality disorders are prevalent among adolescents who abuse drugs. Thus, the likelihood of coexisting mental health disorders, often called "comorbidity" in the psychiatric literature, should be kept in mind when diagnosing substance abuse. Kandel and colleagues, in the Methods for the Epidemiology of Child and Adolescent Mental Disorders (MECA) study of a probability sample of 401 adolescents in the community, found that adolescents who had current substance use disorder had much higher rates of comorbid mood and disruptive behavior disorders than adolescents who did not. Youth who have psychiatric disorders may use illicit drugs to "self-medicate." The initial effect may be to improve symptoms of the disorder, which perpetuates the substance use, but as substance abuse persists, the adolescent's symptoms almost always worsen. Timely diagnosis and treatment of psychiatric disorders in adolescents may help to decrease rates of substance abuse.

A study of the relationship among substance use patterns and physical and sexual abuse was conducted in Minnesota in 1995. More than 100,000 public school students in the 6th, 9th, and 12th grades were surveyed. Study findings showed that a history of either physical or sexual abuse was significantly associated with substance use. This was true for both boys and girls in all three grades that were surveyed. Adolescents who had been abused were more likely to use multiple substances and initiate substance use at a younger age compared with their nonabused peers. For those 6th grade students who reported both physical and sexual abuse, the risk of multiple substance abuse was elevated by a factor of more than 50. Routine screening for abuse experiences should be part of every comprehensive adolescent medical visit.

Multifactorial genetic risk factors for substance abuse vary from inherited personality factors (eg, poor impulse control, risk-seeking) to variability in drug metabolism. Apart from genetic factors, family attitudes and behavior

play an important role in adolescent drug use. Many studies have shown that adolescents from families in which there is poor supervision, a chaotic environment, or parental drug use are at risk for drug abuse. One key influential variable is the degree to which parents monitor the adolescent's activities and whereabouts. Steinberg and colleagues surveyed more than 6,000 primarily middle and professional class high school students in California and Wisconsin by asking five questions about parental monitoring: "How much do your parents REALLY know about. . . . . . Who your friends are? Where you go at night? How you spend your money? What you do with your free time? Where you are most afternoons after school?". Students responded on a three-point scale: don't know, know a little, know a lot. Both boys and girls who reported less parental monitoring were significantly more likely to be involved in substance abuse than their peers. In a survey of the same students 1 year later, boys who initially reported heavy substance use but relatively high parental monitoring were significantly more likely to have decreased their substance use than their less monitored peers. These findings strongly support parent education aimed at improving monitoring skills. Indeed, the office of National Drug Control Policy through its Partnership for a Drug Free America sponsors public service advertisements addressing this point.

One of the strongest predictors of substance use is association with peers who use substances. The study of high school students cited previously, like others, found that the more involved an adolescent was in substance use, the more likely that his or her peers also were involved. In addition, not surprisingly, adolescents are more likely to use drugs if they live in communities where drugs are easily available. Thus, interventions that aim to reduce drug availability in a school or community are likely to reduce adolescent substance use. Lack of after-school supervision and poverty are additional factors that increase the risk of adolescent drug use.

Data about media influences on substance use have focused on alcohol and tobacco and indicate that the media play a powerful role in shaping adolescent behaviors related to these two substances. Influence of the media on illicit drug use has not been studied extensively. However, because rap artists and rock musicians serve as role models for adolescents, the many references to illicit drug use by such performers undoubtedly glamorize the lifestyle and encourage emulation by adolescent fans.

Although there is no single "resilient factor" that protects young people from substance abuse problems, those who grow up in supportive family environments that include positive role models and in communities that have good schools appear to be better equipped to avoid becoming involved with illicit drugs. A cross-sectional analysis of data from the National Longitudinal Study of Adolescent Health, in which more than 12,000 students in the 7th to 12th grades in schools across the United States were interviewed, found that 25% had smoked marijuana and about 6% of both boys and girls were heavy users. Family context variables explained 6% to 9% of the variability in marijuana use, with high levels of parent-family connectedness and a greater frequency of parental presence in the home associated with less frequent use. School variables explained 5% to 6% of the variability in marijuana use, with high levels of school connectedness associated with less frequent use.

Making the Diagnosis

Most often, the teenager does not present to the clinician exhibiting physical signs or medical complications of substance abuse. Regular screening by history during routine health care visits is the best method of identifying and diagnosing substance use disorders. Given the preceding discussion of risk and protective factors, it is clear that this historical screening must include not only detailed questions about substance use, but also questions about affect and mood, family and school functioning, and experiences of abuse. It is essential to provide a safe, nonthreatening environment for the adolescent to discuss these sensitive issues, and confidentiality always should be stressed. However, when a problem is identified, it may be necessary to obtain information from parents, school authorities, and sometimes law enforcement officers to help with diagnosis and treatment.

The Substance Use History

THE ADOLESCENT

The doctor-patient relationship is tested to its limits when dealing with substance abuse. Clinicians must be aware of their own biases and beliefs and strive to be patient-centered, nonthreatening, and nonjudgmental. Reading about interviewing techniques, discussing the issues with colleagues, and attending continuing medical education courses all can help in achieving success in this area. Questions related to illicit drug use should be asked in private without parents present. Every state authorizes minors to consent for care related to substance abuse, including diagnosis, testing, and at least short-term intervention. Professional ethics and state and federal laws protect the privacy of doctor-adolescent communication and medical records related to substance abuse.

When introducing the topic of substance use in the medical interview with adolescents, it can be less threatening to use a tangential approach. Instead of asking, "Do you smoke marijuana?", the clinician can say, "I know that marijuana is used by lots of kids. How about your friends and people you know, do any of them smoke marijuana?" This type of questioning elicits information on the adolescent's environment and peer group and provides an easy segue into the young person's personal views and experiences with marijuana. If the patient acknowledges trying marijuana, follow-up questions about the frequency of use, the setting in which use occurs, and any social and educational disruption that the drug use may have caused are mandatory to assess the degree of risk to the patient's health. Marijuana has been shown to be a "gateway" drug and is virtually always the initial illicit drug a teen will use. Accordingly, it should be specifically asked about first. If the response to marijuana use is positive, use of other illicit drugs should be specifically and individually surveyed, including hallucinogens and club drugs (with ecstasy specifically mentioned by name), cocaine and amphetamines, sedatives and tranquilizers (downers), inhalants, and opiates. For every positive response, frequency of use, route of administration (pills, smoking, nasal inhalation [snorting], intravenous injection), and negative health and social consequences should be explored.

The American Psychiatric Association *Diagnostic and Statistical Manual of Mental Disorders (DSM-IV)* criteria for substance use disorders are shown in Table 2 and suggest the type of questioning required to establish whether any social consequences of drug use have occurred. For example, school attendance and any suspensions or expulsions should be asked about specifically. In addition, the adolescent should be asked whether he or she ever has been stopped by the police or arrested. Asking about parents' and friends' responses to the adolescent's drug use can help establish if the use is exacerbating interpersonal problems.

THE PARENTS

Whenever possible, it is beneficial to involve parents in the medical care of their adolescents. However, the clinician should discuss with the young person in advance exactly what information regarding his or her substance use will and will not be shared with the parents. As a routine part of health supervision, parents should be encouraged to talk about drug use with their children. Also, as mentioned previously, the clinician should encourage parents to monitor their adolescents and know where and with whom they are spending time.

When a substance use disorder is diagnosed, parents usually need to be informed so that appropriate treatment can be initiated. In addition, it often is essential to interview the parents without the adolescent present to hear their observations about their child's problem. One of the most delicate negotiating tasks a clinician must face is gaining the trust of all involved so that these objectives are accomplished without alienating either the adolescent or the parents. Taking the time to try to persuade the adolescent to tell the parents him- or herself is the best solution. The clinician can offer to help by convening a meeting with all parties and can role play with

Table 2. *DSM-IV* Diagnostic Criteria for Substance Use Disorders*

Criteria for Substance Abuse

1. A maladaptive pattern of substance use leading to clinically significant impairment or distress, as manifested by one or more of the following occurring within a 12-month period:
   1. Recurrent substance use resulting in failure to fulfill major role obligations at work, school, or home (eg, absences, suspensions, or expulsions from school)
   2. Recurrent substance use in situations in which it is physically hazardous (eg, driving when impaired)
   3. Recurrent substance-related legal problems
   4. Continued substance use despite having persistent or recurrent social or interpersonal problems caused or exacerbated by the effects of substance use
2. The symptoms have never met the criteria for Substance Dependence for this class of substance.

Substance Dependence

Similar criteria to those for Substance Abuse, but include evidence for development of tolerance and withdrawal symptoms. In addition, important activities are given up and a great deal of time is spent in activities necessary to obtain the substance, use it, and recover from its effects.

Dependence is often accompanied by a persistent desire to cut down or control substance use.

*Adapted from American Psychiatric Association *Diagnostic and Statistical Manual of Mental Disorders*. 4th ed. Washington, DC: American Psychiatric Association; 2000.

the adolescent about how to approach the task. It is not necessary to disclose all the specific details of the adolescent's drug use to the parents, and it is important to allow the teenager to retain some control and privacy by letting him or her specify some aspects of the behavior that will not be revealed to parents if he or she chooses. However, the clinician should not lie either to the parents or the adolescent; this is the surest way to undermine the therapeutic relationship and lose the trust of all concerned. Several visits may be required to complete the negotiations before referral and treatment can be initiated.

THE SCHOOL AND LAW ENFORCEMENT

Often information from school personnel, probation officers, or others outside the family is helpful in providing optimal care to the substance-abusing adolescent. However, all such information should be gathered only after enlisting the consent of the teenager and informing the parents. Teachers or guidance counselors frequently have a different perspective on the adolescent's behavior than the parents and, of course, can educate the clinician about the general culture of the school and the extent of drug problems in the student body.

Physical Examination

As mentioned previously, in a primary care setting, the history and not the physical examination will be the most important part of the medical visit when diagnosing substance abuse. However, certain physical findings might be present either with intoxication or chronic substance use. Evaluation of the teenager who presents with signs of intoxication or altered mental status is beyond the scope of this article. Physical signs that have been associated with chronic illicit drug use are described in Table 3. Adolescents who have sexually transmitted infections, including human immunodeficiency virus, should be questioned about substance abuse because these infections are more prevalent among substance-abusing adolescents.

Major Classes of Illicit Drugs

Knowing some specifics about the commonly abused drugs allows the clinician to discuss their effects knowledgeably with the drug-using adolescent and his or her parents. The neurochemistry of addiction is becoming better understood, and there have been important new research findings in the past decade. In addition, knowing how different illicit drugs are metabolized is essential for accurate interpretation of toxicologic screening.

MARIJUANA

The effects of marijuana are related to the content of delta-9-tetrahydrocannabinol (THC) and other cannabinoids in the leaves and buds of the hemp plant. Present-day marijuana is much more potent than that available 2 decades ago. Due to selective plant breeding, concentrations of THC have been increased between 5 and 15 times. Marijuana is a euphoriant that is used to produce feelings of relaxation and well-being. Effects begin within seconds after inhalation of the smoke or

Table 3. Selected Physical Signs of Illicit Drug Use

Physical Sign	Drug of Abuse
Increased heart rate	Amphetamine, cocaine, marijuana
Increased blood pressure	Amphetamine, cocaine, phencyclidine
Pinpoint pupils	Heroin, morphine, other opiates
Sluggish pupillary response	Barbiturates
Irritation/ulceration of nasal mucosa	Intranasal cocaine, heroin, glue sniffing
Cutaneous scars ("tracks")	Intravenous use
Subcutaneous fat necrosis	Intravenous and intradermal use
Tattoos in antecubital fossa	Intravenous use
Skin abscesses and cellulitis	Intravenous and intradermal use
Icterus	Intravenous use

within 30 to 60 minutes following oral ingestion. Initially, blood levels of THC are high, but they fall rapidly over the first 30 minutes after inhalation. However, the drug and its metabolites are lipid-soluble and are stored in fatty tissue and released slowly. Elimination of THC and metabolites occurs primarily in feces but also in urine and may take up to 1 month to be complete. Thus, urine tests can remain positive for a substantial time, especially among chronic smokers.

Marijuana behaves in the brain like other addictive drugs of abuse. There is a specific receptor for cannabinoids, and in 1990, the gene for the receptor was cloned. The past 10 years have witnessed an explosion of research into the neurochemistry of THC. It is becoming increasingly clear that when high doses are smoked frequently, physiologic addiction with a withdrawal syndrome similar to the opiate withdrawal syndrome occurs. Adolescents who are daily marijuana smokers report a clinical withdrawal syndrome beginning within 24 to 48 hours of discontinuation of the drug, characterized by a flu-like illness and drug craving. The cannabis withdrawal syndrome has been well described, with symptoms peaking in intensity by the fourth or fifth day and gradually resolving in approximately 2 weeks. One article suggests trazodone as an effective treatment for the insomnia that can be disabling (see Duffy in the Suggested Reading).

STIMULANTS

Amphetamines and cocaine are the prototypical stimulant drugs of abuse. Other stimulants, the amphetamine "look alikes," such as phenyl-propanolamine, ephedrine, pseudoephedrine, Ma Huang (an ephedrine-like herbal drug), and caffeine, are sold over-the-counter or by mail order and are widely available. When taken in sufficiently large quantities, they are capable of producing both the "high" and the adverse effects associated with the amphetamines. In addition, methylphenedate is sold on the illegal market and can be abused by adolescents. Many stimulants are taken orally as pills, but cocaine and methamphetamine may be inhaled nasally and taken intravenously. Smokable forms of cocaine ("crack") and methamphetamine ("ice") generate an instantaneous and extremely intense but relatively short-lived euphoria or "rush." Stimulants can be detected in blood and urine, but because they are rapidly metabolized, the outside time limit for detection is about 48 hours after the last dose.

When used intermittently, cocaine stimulates the release and inhibits the reuptake of dopamine and norepinephrine in selected areas of the brain and has a peripheral sympathomimetic effect. Chronic use leads to depletion of dopamine and other neurotransmitters. Amphetamines also have peripheral sympathomimetic effects and affect the norepinephrine- and dopamine-mediated systems of the brain. Mild toxic effects of stimulants include irritability, insomnia, tremor, hyperreflexia, diaphoresis, dilated pupils, and flushing. Severe toxicity can result in hypertensive crises, dysrhythmias, seizures, coma, cardiovascular collapse, and death. Tolerance and physical dependence occur with regular use of stimulants, and an abstinence syndrome occurs on cessation of use. Depression and severe drug cravings that peak 2 to 3 days after the last dose are the most prominent manifestations of stimulant drug withdrawal.

HALLUCINOGENS

Hallucinogens include such naturally occurring compounds as mescaline (found in peyote cactus) and psilocybin (found in "magic mushrooms") as well as synthetic compounds such as lysergic acid diethylamide (LSD), phencyclidine (PCP), and the club drug ecstasy, a derivative of amphetamine. All of the hallucinogens are ingested orally, and most take 30 to 60 minutes for the effects to be noticed. They generally cause visual hallucinations and distortions of sense of time. PCP causes a feeling of disinhibition and euphoria and, in large doses, can produce psychosis that is difficult to differentiate from schizophrenia. LSD is the most potent hallucinogen; it is effective orally in doses of 20 to 50 mcg and has a wide therapeutic index. Some of the hallucinogens are detectable in urine. The enzyme-multiple immunoassay technique (EMIT) test for PCP is widely available. Routine urine toxicology screens will fail to detect ecstasy unless very large quantities were ingested, in which case the test will be positive for amphetamines.

LSD and psilocybin increase serotonin (5-hydroxytryptamine [5-HT]) levels in the brain by binding with specific 5-HT$_2$ receptors. Mescaline and ecstasy are catechol-type hallucinogens that interact with catecholamine-type neurotransmitters such as norepinephrine. Other hallucinogens act on the neurotransmitter acetylcholine.

OPIATES

Opiates are naturally occurring or synthetic sedative analgesic drugs whose effects are similar to opium. This class of drugs includes morphine, heroin, codeine, methadone, fentanyl, meperidine, and hydromorphone. Most adolescents use heroin by nasal inhalation (snorting, sniffing) rather than by injection. The heroin available now is of much higher purity than in the past, which allows those who inhale it to achieve the desired "rush" formerly achieved only by intravenous injection. Opiates can be used orally, intranasally, subcutaneously, intramuscularly, and intravenously. In addition, opium and heroin freebase can be smoked. Opiates are metabolized in the liver and excreted in the urine. Although 90% of heroin is cleared from the body within

24 hours after administration, methadone, a long-acting opiate, has a plasma half-life of approximately 22 hours. In addition to a direct analgesic effect, the opiates produce an altered psychological response to pain, suppression of anxiety, and sedation, all of which contribute to their abuse. Consequences of chronic opiate abuse are related not only to the pharmacologic action of the drug but also (and even more frequently) to the method of drug administration and the lifestyle of the abuser. Intravenous use is associated with the most serious complications. Urine testing for the presence of opiates is widely available in most medical centers. Both thin-layer chromatography and radioimmunoassay techniques detect opiate metabolites for several days after the last use.

The range and intensity of the pharmacologic effects of each different opiate drug depend on its relative binding affinity to the four major central nervous system opioid receptors. Receptors in the nucleus accumbens activate the brain's "reward" pathways, thus fostering dependence and addiction. Dependence develops within approximately 3 to 4 weeks of regular use of heroin or morphine, but it can develop very rapidly with short-acting opiates such as fentanyl.

SEDATIVES

The most common sedative drugs subject to abuse are the barbiturates. Barbiturates are classified as long-acting (eg, phenobarbital), short-acting (eg, secobarbital, pentobarbital), and, ultra short-acting (eg, thiopental). Long-acting barbiturates have a low potential for abuse because although rapidly absorbed after oral ingestion, it takes some time for them to affect the brain. Short-acting barbiturates are more lipid-soluble and cross the blood-brain barrier relatively quickly. They produce a feeling of sedation and anxiety reduction within 15 to 30 minutes of ingestion and have a high potential for abuse. The barbiturates are either detoxified in the liver or excreted unchanged in the urine. Sedatives produce effects that may be mistaken for alcohol inebriation, such as slurred speech, an unsteady gait, impaired judgment, and poor impulse control. Mild toxicity is manifested by nystagmus, ataxia, emotional lability, and mental confusion. Large overdoses result in coma,

which may be followed by respiratory and cardiovascular collapse and death.

Barbiturates exert their action on the central nervous system by enhancing the action of gamma-aminobutyric acid (GABA), the primary inhibitory neurotransmitter. They are highly addictive; on average, addiction develops within 1 to 2 months of regular daily use. The abstinence syndrome is similar to delirium tremens (the alcohol withdrawal syndrome) and can be life-threatening. Plasma and urine testing are widely available for the detection of barbiturates.

TRANQUILIZERS

Although diazepam is one of the most widely abused tranquilizers, flunitrazepam, a drug that is not licensed for sale in the United States but is sold legally in many other countries, is the benzodiazepine currently favored for abuse by adolescents. Flunitrazepam is 10 times more potent than diazepam and is used to heighten the effect of alcohol and other drugs. The small white pills dissolve easily in liquid and are odorless, colorless, and tasteless; thus, it is easy to see why this tranquilizer is also known as the "date rape drug."

Benzodiazepines exert their pharmacologic effects by activating GABA (A) receptors in the brain. This class of drugs possesses all of the characteristics of addictive substances, including development of a serious withdrawal syndrome after regular use. The abstinence syndrome may begin as long as 5 to 8 days after the last dose of the longer half-life forms and continue for several weeks.

INHALANTS

Inhalant abuse is popular among young adolescents, particularly among aboriginal children living in isolated areas. Substances such as airplane glue, gasoline, spray paints, aerosols, and cleaning fluids are inexpensive and readily available. The substance can be inhaled by pouring or spraying the volatile substance into a plastic bag and inhaling from the bag. Soaked rags placed over the mouth and nose can be used to inhale the vapors of liquid hydrocarbons such as solvents or cleaning fluids. Inhalants are rapidly absorbed in the lungs and produce an altered mental state within seconds, but the effects last for only about 5 to 15 minutes. Specific testing for most inhalants is difficult because of their rapid elimination and volatility. These substances frequently cause hepatic, renal, and hematologic damage; gasoline sniffers can develop lead toxicity.

Laboratory Testing

A parent may ask the clinician to test the adolescent's urine for drugs without his or her consent. This request needs to be handled sensitively yet firmly. The parent should be made aware that neither is it ethical for the clinician to test the adolescent covertly nor will it foster a positive relationship between the adolescent and the clinician. At the same time, the clinician should attempt to discover why the parent is worried about the adolescent and offer to assess the teenager. Framing the clinician's role as a partnership with the parents in assuring the adolescent's well-being is helpful. The American Academy of Pediatrics in 1996 stated, "Involuntary testing is not appropriate in adolescents with decisional capacity even with parental consent and should be performed only if there are strong medical or legal reasons to do so." Drug tests may be very helpful as an adjunct to treatment and relapse prevention of adolescents who are known drug abusers. In addition, they aid in the diagnosis of youth whose mental status is altered. Nonmedical uses of drug screening tests help to deter illicit drug use in sports and in the workplace.

There are two different types of laboratory drug testing: screening and confirmatory. The former has a high sensitivity and is relatively inexpensive; the latter has a high specificity but is expensive and not available in all laboratories (Table 4). Most tests are performed on urine, but blood tests are available for some drugs. Screening tests include thin-layer chromatography, which detects micrograms of drug metabolites, and immunoassay tests, which detect nanograms of drug metabolites. Both methods may be influenced by adulterants, making confirmatory tests necessary. Highly sophisticated and accurate confirmatory tests are performed by gas chromatography or mass spectrometry; they are

Table 4. Comparison of Screening and Confirmatory Drug Tests

Screening Tests	Confirmatory Tests
High sensitivity	High specificity
Thin-layer chromatography/ Immunoassay	Gas chromatography/ Mass spectrometry
Inexpensive but influenced by adulterants	Expensive but accurate
Used in emergency and substance abuse treatment	Used for forensic analysis and government-mandated workplace testing

used for forensic analysis and for United States government-mandated workplace drug testing.

URINE COLLECTION TECHNIQUE

A screening drug test should be performed on a teenager with his or her knowledge and consent. A same-gender monitor should be available to observe the act of micturition and ensure that the sample is not adulterated. If possible, the urine sample should be collected on a Sunday or Monday morning because weekend drug use is more likely. An early morning sample will have the highest concentration of drug.

Common methods of adulteration are use of liquids with the color of urine, such as tea, Mountain Dew, or apple juice. Patients also may add other substances, such as toilet water, soap, salt, acids, and alkali to interfere with the accuracy of the test. The specimen should have the appearance of a freshly voided sample. Once the sample is collected, it should be carefully sealed, accurately labeled, and correctly stored prior to transportation to the laboratory. The approximate duration of detection of selected drugs is given in Table 5.

Conclusion

Pediatricians and other clinicians caring for adolescents have a responsibility to provide anticipatory guidance to teens and their parents regarding the direct and indirect effects of substance use. Screening of all adolescent patients for evidence of psychiatric disorders, physical or sexual abuse, and substance use disorder is imperative because

Table 5. Approximate Duration of Detection of Selected Illicit Drugs in Urine

Drug	Approximate Duration of Detection* (Days)
Amphetamines	2
Barbiturates (short-acting)	1
Cannabinoids—single use	3
Cannabinoids—moderate use (3∞/wk)	5
Cannabinoids—heavy use (6∞/wk)	10
Cannabinoids—chronic heavy use	21 to 27
Cocaine metabolites	2 to 3
Methamphetamine	2
Morphine	3
Phencyclidine	3 to 8

*These are general guidelines only. Interpretation of the duration of detection must take into account many variables, such as drug metabolism and half-life, the subject's physical condition, fluid balance and state of hydration, and route and frequency of drug administration. Adapted from Schonberg SK, ed. *Substance Abuse: A Guide for Health Professionals.* Elk Grove Village, Ill: American Academy of Pediatrics; 1988.

of the high prevalence and high comorbidity of these conditions. Creating an atmosphere of privacy and trust during the medical interview with the adolescent is essential for accurate diagnosis. When a substance use disorder is suspected, several visits with the patient and parents may be required to complete the evaluation and negotiate treatment.

Suggested Reading

Alcohol, Drug Abuse, and Mental Health Administration. Cannabinoid receptor gene cloned. *JAMA.* 1990;264:1389

American Academy of Pediatrics Committee on Substance Abuse. Testing for drugs of abuse in children and adolescents. *Pediatrics.* 1998;98:305–307

Centers for Disease Control and Prevention. Youth risk behavior surveillance—United States, 1999. *Morbid Mortal Wkly Rep MMWR.* 2000;49(SS 05):1–96

Coupey SM. Barbiturates. *Pediatr Rev.* 1997;18:260–265

Coupey SM. Interviewing adolescents. *Pediatr Clin North Am.* 1997;44:1349–1364

Crowley TJ, MacDonald MJ, Whitmore EA, Mikulich SK. Cannabis dependence, withdrawal, and reinforcing effects among adolescents with conduct symptoms and substance use disorders. *Drug Alcohol Depend.* 1998;50:27–37

Duffy A, Milin R. Case study: withdrawal syndrome in adolescent chronic cannabis users. *J Am Acad Child Adolesc Psychiat.* 1996;35:1618–1621

Farrar HC, Kearns GL. Cocaine: clinical pharmacology and toxicology. *J Pediatr.* 1989;115:665–675

Gittelman R, Mannuzza S, Shenker R, Bonagura N. Hyperactive boys almost grown up. *Arch Gen Psychiatry.* 1985;42:937–947

Harrison PA, Fulkerson JA, Beebe TJ. Multiple substance use among adolescent physical and sexual abuse victims. *Child Abuse Neglect.* 1997;21:529–539

Johnson LD, O'Malley PM, Bachman JG. *Monitoring the Future Study.* Washington, DC: United States Department of Health and Human Services; 2000. Available at www.monitoringthefuture. org

Kandel DB, Johnson JG, Bird HR, et al. Psychiatric comorbidity among adolescents with substance use disorders: findings from the MECA study. *J Am Acad Child Adolesc Psychiatry.* 1999;38:693–696

Neumark YD, Delva J, Anthony JC. The epidemiology of adolescent inhalant involvement. *Arch Pediatr Adolesc Med.* 1998;152:781–786

Pentel P. Toxicity of over-the-counter stimulants. *JAMA.* 1984;252:1898–1903

Resnick MD, Bearman PS, Blum RW, et al. Protecting adolescents from harm: findings from the national longitudinal study on adolescent health. *JAMA.* 1997;278:823–832

Rickert VI, Wiemann CM, Berenson AB. Prevalence, patterns, and correlates of voluntary flunitrazepam use. *Pediatrics.* 1999;103:e6–e9. Available at http://www.pediatrics.org/cgi/content/full/103/1/e6

Schwartz R. Testing for drugs of abuse: controversies and techniques. *Adolesc Med.* 1993;4:353–370

Schwartz RH. LSD: its rise, fall, and renewed popularity among high school students. *Pediatr Clin North Am.* 1995;42:403–413

Steinberg L, Fletcher A, Darling N. Parental monitoring and peer influence on adolescent substance use. *Pediatrics.* 1994;93:1060–1064

Strasburger VC, Donnerstein E. Children, adolescents, and the media in the 21st century. *Adolesc Med.* 2000;11:51–68

Tanda G, Pontieri FE, Di Chiara G. Cannabinoid and heroin activation of mesolimbic dopamine transmission by a common mu1 opioid receptor mechanism. *Science.* 1997;276:2048–2050

Weisbeck GA, Schuckit MA, Kalmijn JA, et al. An evaluation of the history of a marijuana withdrawal syndrome in a large population. *Addiction.* 1996;91:1469–1478

Counsel Kids on Permanence of Tattoos, Body Piercings

Jessica Little, Correspondent

As tattoos and body piercings become more mainstream in popular youth culture, pediatricians should counsel patients about the potential health problems they present, say AAP pediatricians.

Although the Academy has yet to take an official stance on tattoos and piercings, Tom Saari, M.D., FAAP, AAP Committee on Infectious Diseases member, discourages his patients from getting tattoos and piercings because of the health risks involved.

Infections

"The more worrisome risks are HIV infection and hepatitis B," Dr. Saari says.

Even though these risks are relatively small, they are reason enough to not get tattooed or pierced, Dr. Saari says. And if Dr. Saari needs more reasons to encourage patients to avoid the needle, he looks to the recent controversy centered on the hepatitis C virus (HCV).

HCV can be transmitted through contact with contaminated needles, contaminated dyes, the operator's hands or cloths the operator uses.

A controversial study printed March 2001 found that having a tattoo increases one's risk for HCV (Haley RW, Fischer PR. *Medicine.* 2001;80:134–151[Medline]). The authors found that commercially acquired tattoos accounted for 41% of HCV infections in their study.

Further, the study found that about 22% of people with tattoos were seropositive for HCV. About 32% of people who got their tattoos at a commercial parlor were seropositive.

Researchers got their information from interviews with 626 consecutive patients undergoing medical evaluation for spinal problems. The patients then were screened for HCV, and 43 were seropositive.

But this study hasn't convinced the U.S. Centers for Disease Control and Prevention (CDC) of the connection between tattooing and HCV. In its "Position on Tattooing and HCV Infection," the CDC says that it is not sure whether this study can be generalized to the whole population (http://www.cdc.gov/ncidod/diseases/hepatitis/c/tattoo.htm).

According to the CDC statement, "During the past 20 years, less than 1% of persons with newly acquired hepatitis C reported to the CDC's sentinel surveillance system gave a history of being tattooed."

The CDC is conducting its own study to determine whether tattooing is a risk for HCV.

Robert Haley, M.D., author of the *Medicine* study and chief of epidemiology at the University of Texas Southwestern Medical Center, says the CDC surveillance system only notes acute hepatitis cases, but HCV is mostly asymptomatic.

"A very small percentage of people who are HCV positive remember a jaundice episode," Dr. Haley says. "Most people believe the acute cases aren't really relevant. That doesn't seem to be a good decision to say that tattooing does not transmit hepatitis."

"I don't think there's any question that tattooing has been associated with the transmission of hepatitis B and C," Dr. Saari says. "The debate has to do with how often it actually occurs."

Transmission doesn't occur as frequently at reputable, professional tattoo shops, says Dennis Dwyer, executive director of the Alliance of Professional Tattooists, a national tattoo organization founded to address the health and safety issues facing the tattoo industry.

"There are risks involved in passing hepatitis C through tattooing, but most of the tattoo shops are really adhering to the standard of universal precautions," Dwyer says. "These people don't want to lose their jobs or hurt people."

This controversy concerns David Kaplan, M.D., FAAP, chair of the AAP Committee on Adolescence.

"I am really worried about whether or not the prevalence is high enough that we need to do something about it immediately," Dr. Kaplan says. "We need much more data."

Dr. Haley recommends that pediatricians encourage their tattooed patients to get a hepatitis C test. If patients already have the virus, pediatricians should counsel them to protect their livers by avoiding alcohol.

"We know that alcohol greatly speeds up the occurrence of liver disease," Dr. Haley says. "Abstinence can greatly put off the occurrence and maybe eliminate the risk. I guarantee when teens get to be 50, they don't want to have cirrhosis or liver cancer."

Other Potential Problems

While hepatitis C may be a concern for adolescents who have tattoos, body piercings don't seem to carry as great a risk.

Dr. Kaplan considers getting body piercings an almost normative adolescent behavior.

"Honestly, I don't see many complications," Dr. Kaplan says. "Even kids with their tongue pierced, I rarely see kids with an infection or any kind of seriously concerning complications."

From an infection standpoint, Dr. Kaplan is concerned, however, about adolescents who share needles to pierce or tattoo themselves and their friends. Those who self-pierce or self-tattoo do not always sterilize their oftentimes makeshift equipment. If people share their needles, they open themselves up to a host of infections.

Even as body piercings have become more commonplace and tattoo artists continue to make efforts to sterilize their practices, some people still experience complications.

One of the most common complications is an infection at the site of the piercing or tattoo. The ear is still the most common site for a piercing (Marcoux D. *Dermatol Clin.* 2000;18:667–672 [Medline]). Infections are more common when the upper ear, or the cartilaginous helix, is pierced, according to the report. Bacterial infections can destroy cartilage, causing permanent deformities, Dr. Saari says. Piercings at these sites also take longer to heal. The navel, however, takes the longest to completely heal after a piercing, sometimes requiring nine months. *Staphylococcus aureus* is the most common infection-causing organism, according to the report. Adolescents should keep pierced and tattooed areas clean until they have completely healed.

Keloids, or excess scar tissue, also can be a problem for adolescents who scar easily, according to a U.S. Food and Drug Administration (FDA) fact sheet (http://vm.cfsan.fda.gov). Keloids can erupt around the site of the piercing or underneath a new tattoo. More commonly, keloids can form after a tattoo removal has been attempted.

Allergic reactions also are common side-effects to piercings and tattoos, experts say. Nickel in body rings can cause allergies, and different types of tattoo dyes can cause reactions.

The immune system responds to nickel like it does to poison ivy, says Laurie Smith, M.D., FAAP, chair of the AAP Section on Allergy and Immunology. Nickel can cause allergic contact dermatitis.

"They estimate that 90% of people are allergic to poison ivy," Dr. Smith says. "With nickel, it's up there in the top three or four contact synthesizers."

Oftentimes, according to the *Dermatologic Clinics* study, people who react to nickel also will react to nickel-free jewelry. One alternative is to use titanium studs as opposed to other metals that may contain nickel.

Tattoos come with their own allergic reactions. Many people are hypersensitive to the red tattoo pigment, called cinnabar, and photosensitivity reactions to cadmium, sometimes used in yellow pigment (Montgomery DF, Parks D. *J Pediatr Health Care.* 2001;15:14–19[Medline]).

Parents and patients should be informed that the FDA does not regulate tattoo inks. Local laws may or may not regulate tattoo inks, and according to the FDA, many of the pigments in tattoo inks should not even come in contact with the skin.

According to Dwyer and the Alliance of Professional Tattooists, the inks are safe. Dwyer says cadmium hasn't been used in inks for years. The reputable tattoo artists use pigments from one of only a few manufacturers.

"There really [are] not any data or indication that the pigments are a risk or have been a risk," Dwyer says.

Regulations and health codes for tattoo and piercing shops vary from state to state, Dwyer says. Most of them do not regulate the types of pigments used. In Arizona, for example, the only law for tattoo shops is that minors cannot be tattooed without parental consent. Most of the states have age restrictions and require a business license, says Dwyer.

The Alliance of Professional Tattooists does not recommend tattooing for anyone under the age of 18. "I don't think anyone under the age of 18 is mature enough to make a decision that would last a lifetime," Dwyer says.

Many adolescents have turned to temporary tattoos as a means to express themselves without breaking state regulations. But pediatricians should advise adolescents to be careful of the types of temporary tattoos they use.

While henna, a plant paste that temporarily stains the skin, is generally safe, black and blue henna has caused severe skin reactions. Black and blue henna may contain phenylenediamine, which has been associated with severe contact dermatitis, according to the *Dermatologic Clinics* study.

Pediatric Office Procedures

In response to the complications associated with ear piercing, a few doctors have begun piercing patients' ears in their offices. Dr. Saari and Dr. Kaplan do not pierce in their offices.

Parents commonly request to have a medical professional pierce their children's ears, Dr. Saari says. He discourages parents from having their young child's ears pierced.

"Infants' ears are small, and they will grow substantially," Dr. Saari says. "To be able to place an earring expecting it to be in the same position 12 years from now is a risk and a gamble."

If he knows parents will have their children's ears pierced regardless of his advice, Dr. Saari encourages parents to wait until their child has received vaccines for tetanus and hepatitis B. However, the risk of tetanus and hepatitis is quite small, Dr. Saari says.

Because there are so many risks involved with tattooing and piercing, Dr. Saari says it's important to communicate these potential risks to young patients.

"As an adult, you can digest all this information and not do it [get pierced or tattooed] as a peer activity," he says. "The pediatrician must put this into perspective."

Delinquent Youth in Corrections: Medicaid and Reentry Into the Community

ABBREVIATION. SCHIP, State Children's Health Insurance Program.

In general, states and public agencies acting as custodians for youth in the corrections branch of the juvenile justice system are responsible for ensuring that such youth receive access to timely and appropriate physical and mental health care. However, to date, health care for youth in the juvenile justice system has generally been considered inadequate. Note that in this article "health care" refers to the treatment of both physical and mental health problems. The American Academy of Pediatrics and others have issued policy statements in the past 2 decades that stress the need for better health care for juvenile offenders in correctional facilities.[1-4] In response, correctional facilities have put in place enhanced acute care services for children and adolescents in juvenile justice.

Although such services are almost certainly needed, these efforts are likely to be deficient on at least 2 counts. First, many of these youth suffer not only from acute medical and psychiatric problems but also chronic ones including substance abuse and other psychiatric disorders. Second, with an estimated 88 000 youth being released from juvenile commitment facilities each year,[5] the need for ongoing medical treatment after parole and reentry into the community is high. However, care often stops when the juveniles leave the system, with little or no reintroduction to community services.[6] Pediatricians and other primary care clinicians have a central role to play in establishing a medical home for these youth and expediting access to critical medical and behavioral services.

This review will provide an overview of the juvenile justice system, present the extant literature on the chronic health problems found in incarcerated youth, and discuss how the absence of care after release from the juvenile justice system impacts public health and society. We argue that Medicaid financing could be used as an immediate measure to ameliorate part of this problem and outline recommendations for future interventions.

Juvenile Justice System

It is estimated that 2.4 million juveniles were arrested in 2000, accounting for 17% of all arrests in the United States.[7] Approximately 2 million cases are handled by US juvenile courts each year. In 1999, there were 80 400 committed youth in juvenile facilities, of which 88% were male. Because no current data exist, it is estimated that 88 000 youth are released from juvenile facilities each year.[5] Among these, the number afflicted with chronic illnesses is small but represents an important subgroup, because they are a high-risk, high-cost group, prone to recidivate. Although the rate of juvenile crime steadily fell between 1994 and 2001, arrests of juvenile females, although only comprising 28% of all juvenile arrests in 2001, are increasing more than those of males in most offense categories including aggravated assault, drug-abuse violations, and simple assault.[7] Minorities and youth of low socioeconomic status are also overrepresented in the juvenile justice population.[5,8]

Accepted for publication Aug 23, 2004. doi:10.1542/peds.2004-0776

No conflict of interest declared.

Reprint requests to (K.K.) Office of Clinical Sciences, Columbus Children's Research Institute, 700 Children's Dr, Suite J1401, Columbus, OH 43205. E-mail: kellehek@pediatrics.ohio-state.edu

An arrested youth may be brought home without charges or detained in a detention facility. Postadjudication, the youth may be sentenced to a correctional facility, assigned to a community program, or admitted to a mental health treatment facility or program. The focus of this article is youth in correctional facilities. Specifically, we are interested in the outcomes of youth with chronic health problems postrelease.[9,10] Youth are released from correctional facilities by either being placed on parole or completing their sentence. Parole is the supervised released of a prisoner from imprisonment with certain conditions. A violation of parole, such as not maintaining regular contact with parole or probation officers, truancy, substance use, or failure to attend treatment, can result in reimprisonment.[9]

Health Status

Research to date has focused on the health of youth in detention facilities. Few studies have investigated these issues in incarcerated youth. In addition, we are not aware of any studies that have addressed the health of youth postrelease.

Detained youth present with higher rates of substance abuse, acute illnesses, sexually transmitted diseases, unplanned pregnancies, and psychiatric disorders. In 1 study, 46% of detained youth had medical problems including drug use, chronic liver infections, and gonorrhea.[11] Another study of adolescents being admitted to a detention center reported that 16.5% had a history of hospitalization for a medical or surgical reason; the same percentage received previous treatment for mental illness by a psychiatrist or therapist, and 11% were found to have a condition that needed close medical supervision after release.[12] These conditions can be attributed to their high-risk behaviors, challenging social environments, and lack of previous health care.[4] Although many detained youth have chronic physical health problems, there is also a high prevalence of psychiatric disorders among this population. Teplin et al[13] report that even after excluding conduct disorder, almost three fifths of male juvenile detainees and more than two thirds of females met the criteria for ≥1 psychiatric disorders. It is reported that as many as 60% of youth in detention meet the criteria for conduct disorder, 20% for a major depressive disorder, and 18% for attention-deficit/hyperactivity disorder.[14] This compares with 37% of youth in the community reported to have at least 1 psychiatric disorder.[15,16] One specific category of mental disorders that affects this population are trauma disorders. These youth are not only perpetrators but victims of trauma. As Cauffman[17] reports, 43% of females and 40% of males present with traumatic experiences.

A large proportion of youth already incarcerated are afflicted with chronic illnesses that require ongoing medical attention. A survey of Washington State correctional facilities found that youth in long-term correctional facilities tend to have more chronic medical conditions than youth in short-term facilities. Dental problems were reported in 65.9% of youth, 44.1% had dermatological problems, 35.6% had respiratory problems, and 33.7% had substance-use problems.[18] According to the 2001 National Household Survey on Drug Abuse, 10.8% of youth 12 to 17 years old were current illegal-drug users.[19] In long-term facilities, 68% of males have a mental health disorder. Anywhere from 21% to 45% have a disruptive-disorder diagnosis, 20% to 50% have a substance-abuse diagnosis, and 7% to 36% have an anxiety diagnosis.[20-25] Although specific information on the physical health status of female offenders could not be found, the rate of mental health disorders is higher for females in the juvenile justice system than for males.[5,26]

Although physical and mental health problems are common both before and during incarceration, no studies have examined aftercare services or medical/behavioral services provided after reentry into the community for these extremely high-risk youth. There is reason to be concerned. First, any abrupt discontinuity in the care received while incarcerated puts the youth at significant risk for relapse.[27] Second, many questions remain about challenges to enrollment, eligibility for benefits, and identification of treatment facilities for youth released from juvenile justice facilities. Third, not only should the percentage of youth in the juvenile justice system with chronic illnesses be alarming, but the lack of services being received by this population should be of concern.

The Costs of Inaction

In addition to the ethical argument that all children with chronic illness are deserving of care, any delay in receiving treatment after release may not only lead to increased morbidity and mortality but also may contribute to public health and legal problems such as increased spread of infection, continuation of antisocial behavior, higher health care use, and commitment of repeat offenses (criminal recidivism). Moreover, ignoring this problem may have dire consequences for the next generation of children.

Youth involved in the juvenile justice system are more likely to engage in high-risk behaviors such as substance abuse and sexual activities. Detained juveniles report high rates of behaviors that could be detrimental to their health. Ninety-three percent of these youth claim to have had sexual intercourse, and the prevalence of sexually transmitted diseases was nearly double that of a comparison group of high-school youth.[28] Nearly all youth have engaged in alcohol drinking by age 15, and 40% have used marijuana >40 times.[28] After release, it is likely that these youth continue to engage in high-risk behaviors, thereby communicating diseases through many avenues including sexual contact and drug use. In this instance, this "revolving-door" effect of spreading disease both inside the prison and inside the community after release can occur.[29]

Although research has been performed on recidivism and its prediction, not much has been conducted on recidivism among persons who have received psychiatric services in jail[30] or in children and adolescents. Although untreated physical illnesses are not likely to contribute to the rate of recidivism, in the absence of adequate treatment, mental illnesses (attention-deficit/hyperactivity disorder, conduct disorder) have been shown to be predictors of recidivism.[31,32] Thus, it is likely that by maintaining a continuum of high levels of care for youth leaving a correctional facility, a drop in the rate of recidivism may be achieved.

In a study of incarcerated female juvenile offenders, 47% had used mental health services in the past, and 63% were repeat offenders.[26] The Bureau of Justice Statistics states that 80% of youth under the age of 18 years that were released

in 1994 were rearrested.[33] As Draine et al[30] conclude, those who do not get appropriate, effective treatment after release are more likely to return to jail. From this we can determine that mental illness plays a role in the higher arrest (and rearrest) rates of those with mental illnesses,[34] showing that mental health care must be provided to this population. In addition, Hammett et al[6] present the idea that many individuals deliberately return to incarceration because they receive better care in correctional facilities than after release. No studies, however, could be found on the effect of postrelease mental health services on recidivism rates.

Lack of follow-up care also places an inordinately high burden on the health care system. Because of a lack of insurance and access to health care, juveniles are forced to use emergency departments as their usual source of care. Wilson and Klein[35] report that 1.5 million adolescents in the United States reported using the emergency department as their usual source of health care. This places an enormous burden on the health system, because emergency departments are required to treat patients without the ability to pay. This cost, however, is absorbed by the system and is translated to higher costs of medical care for everyone, including those using Medicaid. Although the emergency department may be an immediate solution to an immediate problem, it does not provide adolescents with preventive screening or counseling, nor does it provide routine check-ups. Therefore, the emergency department is not considered an appropriate source of primary care.[35] Although no research could be found in this area, it is hypothesized that youth involved in the juvenile justice system use the emergency department as a primary source of care at a higher percentage than youth not involved with the juvenile justice system. This usage of emergency departments as primary care facilities is preventable by providing access to proper care.

The financial costs of crimes committed by a typical juvenile delinquent is estimated to be $80 000 to $335 000 between the ages of 14 and 17 years alone. An adult career criminal can add an extra $1.4 million. It can be estimated that by preventing a high-risk youth from embarking on a criminal life path, a savings of $1.7 to $2.3 million can be generated.[36] Costs to the victim, including direct financial losses and pain and suffering, compose a majority of these costs. For crimes committed by juveniles, the annual victim costs (based on 1–4 crimes per year) is estimated to be $15 000 to $62 000.[36] Many of these youth might be prevented from traveling such a path if provided proper health care, especially mental health treatment. There are studies that show that mental health treatment reduces crime[37–42]; therefore, based on existing research we can infer that mental health treatment also reduces associated costs.

As previously stated, there are many youth released from the juvenile justice population that do not have health insurance but are Medicaid eligible. It is estimated that it costs Medicaid approximately $1600 per year, on average, to provide health services to each Medicaid-eligible child.[43] Comparing this figure to the financial costs of crimes committed by a juvenile, the potential for savings seems great.

Policy Issues and Barriers to Care

However clear it is that health and mental health care should be provided to youth released from correctional facilities (and detention centers) with chronic health problems, numerous hurdles to adequate aftercare services remain, including complex societal issues such as generally inadequate support for mental health services, stigma, and discrimination. However, specific financing issues seem particularly relevant and remediable. Although Medicaid is the most likely source of insurance for health coverage after release, enrollment in Medicaid is often terminated after the youth is placed in a detention center, prison, or jail. Thus, youth leaving correctional facilities on parole are often uninsured and not eligible for immediate benefits. One of the main barriers to receiving medical care is not having medical insurance, because the uninsured are more likely to not have a usual source of care than insured individuals.[44] As Aday and Andersen[44] show, the percentage of individuals with Medicaid coverage who had seen a physician in the last year was very close to the number who had some form of

private insurance. Kasper et al[45] also report on the outcomes of individuals who gained insurance coverage after not having any initially. Their research shows that those who gained insurance coverage had an increase in access to medical care "across all indicators of access." Over the course of the study, the percentage of subjects who reported having no usual source of care dropped from 33% to 20% after gaining insurance.

In addition to funding, other barriers are related to enrollment difficulties, such as the lengthy eligibility-determination process. In the following section, various financing issues and barriers are discussed and solutions are presented.

FUNDING

There are 2 major sources of funding available to delinquent youth: private and public funds. Private insurance plans generally pay for most medical expenses but frequently have upper limits on the amount of money that they will pay for most services. Although an individual may have medical insurance, many times the copayments or deductibles for visits or medications can prove to be prohibitive. Parents and their youth then must either pay for the remaining expenses out-of-pocket or attempt to obtain help through the public sector.[46] However, as a result of their socioeconomic status, most youth released from correctional facilities do not have private health insurance and cannot afford to pay for the repeated physician visits required by chronic illnesses such as mental disorders. Even when their parents have adequate private insurance, their juvenile justice record and activities may have severed ties with their family, making them functionally uninsured. This leads them to seek public assistance to pay for medical care.

Public funds are primarily available in the form of Medicaid and the State Children's Health Insurance Program (SCHIP). In 2002, Medicaid became the largest health insurance program in the United States, with expenditures totaling $259 billion.[47] In federal fiscal year 2000, this federal-state program covered 44 million Americans, 24 million of which were children.[43] To receive Medicaid benefits, a youth must apply and be found to be eligible for benefits, that is, she or he must meet certain requirements set by the state using federal guidelines. Once eligibility is determined, benefits cannot be paid until a youth has been enrolled successfully.

Although no studies could be found that report the insurance status or Medicaid eligibility of youth released from correctional facilities, it is suspected that a large portion of this population may be eligible for Medicaid or SCHIP programs. Many of these youth may have participated previously in these programs but may no longer be enrolled, because most states terminate program benefits for the youth after incarceration.

Although we cannot be sure why states are choosing this course of action, anecdotal reports provide several possible reasons. First, many states may not be aware of other options available to them such as the suspension, rather than termination, of benefits. In addition, stiff penalties are given to states that bill Medicaid inappropriately. To avoid any possibility of billing Medicaid for an incarcerated youth, states may find it easier to terminate the youth's benefits. If a state is found to have billed Medicaid for an incarcerated youth, a possible fraud investigation may ensue, which again can be avoided by terminating enrollment. As a result, many states may find it is easier to terminate rather than suspend a youth's Medicaid benefits after incarceration.

States justify this termination of benefits by citing CFR §416.211,[48] which states that Medicaid benefits cannot be paid for any month throughout which an individual is a resident of a public institution. In addition, §1905(a)(A) of the Social Security Act[49] also excludes federal financial participation for medical care to inmates of a federal institution. Applied equally to juveniles and adults, these laws exclude federal financial participation in "care or services for any individual who is an inmate of a public institution" unless the inmate is in a medical institution. Although federal law does not require termination of eligibility,[50] most states automatically terminate participation because of this misunderstanding of current policies.[27]

In a letter to all state Medicaid directors, the Centers for Medicare and Medicaid Services encouraged all states to "'suspend' and not 'terminate' Medicaid benefits while a person is in a public institution."[51] The letter goes on to clarify that the eligibility of an individual for Medicaid is not affected by their status as a resident of a public institution. In addition, states are urged to place an eligible inmate in a "suspended status" so that the individual may begin receiving Medicaid benefits immediately after release.[51] However, many youth that are eligible for Medicaid benefits after release are no longer enrolled and thus cannot receive any benefits. Although it is not a complete solution, Medicaid could be used to pay for health benefits for a large portion of these youth after release.

Although there is no clear-cut solution for solving the funding issue, Congress did provide 1 option when it passed the Balanced Budget Act of 1997. Presumptive eligibility allows states to give health care providers and community-based organizations the authority to "presumptively" enroll children in Medicaid or SCHIP programs who seem eligible based on age and family income.[52] This enrollment greatly decreases the waiting time of getting health insurance and allows youth to receive needed care immediately rather than waiting for eligibility to be completely determined. To keep coverage, however, families must be found eligible for Medicaid or SCHIP through the regular eligibility-determination process by the end of the month after the initial application.[53]

Although presumptive eligibility would immediately make health insurance (and subsequently health care) available to many more youth, as of August 2002 only 10 states had adopted presumptive eligibility in Medicaid and 5 had adopted presumptive eligibility as part of the SCHIP program. A contributing factor to why many states may not have adopted presumptive eligibility is the additional costs (administrative and programmatic) associated with covering and enrolling more people into state-funded health insurance programs. One major concern is that the state may end up paying health care costs for individuals who are found later to be ineligible for health coverage.[53]

Medicaid provides retroactive payments to individuals who received services before enrollment and pays providers for services rendered only if the individual is determined to have been eligible during that time.[53] The problem with this, especially when dealing with the juvenile population, is that many youth and families of youth cannot afford to take the risk of being found ineligible, causing them to be responsible for payments to service providers. With the inability to pay medical expenses, care is not sought by youth. Therefore, it is necessary to provide coverage during the period in which eligibility is being determined. Presumptive eligibility allows a child to receive services while guaranteeing that the provider will be paid for those services, even if he or she is found to be ineligible for Medicaid or SCHIP. The law also allows the state to designate any entity to determine presumptive eligibility,[53] which means that the ability to determine eligibility can be given to state juvenile correctional facilities, and delinquent youth can be deemed eligible on the day of their release.

Another option to providing Medicaid coverage immediately after release is that states can suspend a youth's enrollment after incarceration. To suspend Medicaid coverage would result in the youth remaining eligible for Medicaid after discharge, but no benefits would be paid during incarceration.[54] Although many states may not have a system in place for suspending eligibility,[50] the development of such a system would certainly be beneficial in the long run. Aside from providing immediate funding for health care, benefits include no waiting time for the resumption of coverage and the elimination of a potentially lengthy reenrollment process.

ENROLLMENT

According to a policy report from the Urban Institute,[55] knowledge gaps such as not being aware of public-assistance programs is a primary barrier to enrolling 32% of all low-income uninsured children. The authors also state administrative hassles as a primary barrier to enrolling another 10% of all low-income uninsured children. It can be assumed that these numbers apply equally, if not to a greater extent, to youth released from the juvenile justice system, because low socioeconomic status is a risk factor for involvement in the juvenile justice system.[8]

Once an application has been submitted successfully, it is not unusual for there to be a processing time of ≥60 days before a youth becomes eligible for benefits.[56] This delay of access to community treatment services can potentially undo any stabilization the individual gained while incarcerated.[27] The gap between submission of the application and access to benefits can result in a large gap of time, during which the youth has no available medical care. Many states do not allow the application process to begin until after release.[6]

States could reduce the time required to enroll delinquent youth in Medicaid in 3 ways: improving enrollment efficiency, providing release planning, and allowing the application to start before a youth is released. Enrollment efficiency can be attained in several ways. For example, enrollment times can be reduced by eliminating the face-to-face interview, permitting mail-in applications, and allowing the self-verification of income.[55] Federal law (42 CFR 435.916) also allows states to use simplified procedures to determine a youth's eligibility after release from correctional facilities.[57]

Release planning is becoming more important in helping to make the transition between jail and the community easier. Services provided through a release-planning program should include plans for social services (housing, food, vocational rehabilitation) as well as mental and physical health services.[58] Wolff et al[59] report that 71% of New Jersey jails believe release planning is "very" or "extremely" important, yet almost all the jails reported providing "no real release planning." Providing contact to postrelease medical services and insurance coverage, especially mental health services, is important in maintaining continuity of care while youth make the difficult transition. Because many inmates are unaware of their Medicaid eligibility and lack knowledge about the application process, they are delayed further in receiving program enrollment. Release planning can provide invaluable assistance in ensuring the timely restoration of medical insurance benefits by educating youth about Medicaid and assisting inmates in completing applications and getting their paperwork in order.

In addition to simplifying the application process and providing release planning, states can enroll delinquent youth in Medicaid more rapidly by allowing the application process to begin while the youth is still committed. Generally, the determination process begins after a youth is released.[50] If states would allow the processing of applications to start before release, for example, after parole has been approved or 2 months before the release date, youth could be approved for and enrolled in Medicaid on the day they are released.

Combining simplified enrollment procedures, release planning, and an earlier application process can greatly reduce the amount of time and hassle it takes to enroll a youth in Medicaid, which would lead to a higher percentage of youth on parole having health insurance that, one would hope, would lead to better treatment of their chronic illnesses.

Recommendations

Improving the aftercare for youth released from corrections with chronic physical and mental illnesses is a daunting task because of financial and nonfinancial barriers that exist. However, clinicians, researchers, and lawmakers can reduce these barriers to care. Here we outline some possible improvements in the current system.

Clinicians should:

1. Have a higher index of suspicion of psychiatric disorders during evaluation of these youth. Because of the prevalence of chronic illnesses in this population, clinicians must be more vigilant in identifying these conditions during evaluations regardless of whether the youth are seen in emergency departments, primary care clinics, or urgent care settings.

2. Assess barriers to community reentry and health services. When receiving medical care, it is not enough for these youth to be provided a referral or prescribed medication without first ensuring that they have the resources available to receive the recommended care. If the resources are not available, appointments with community health organizations should be made or assistance provided to help the youth apply for Medicaid or other forms of health insurance.

3. Act as a "medical home" for managing and coordinating all of a youth's care and preventative services for all medical needs.

4. Use their powerful community voice to act as advocates to encourage change, increase access to services, and decrease stigmas.

Researchers should:

1. Describe the aftercare or medical/behavioral services received by youth on reentry into the community after release from long-term correctional facilities. The focus of this work should be on those youth with chronic (physical and mental) health problems, because these youth have the greatest need for health care.

2. Investigate the factors associated with recidivism and desistance and apply those data to the creation of new transition programs for aftercare services.

3. Determine the usual source of care (if any) for uninsured youth.

4. Collect data on how many youth are eligible for public insurance (Medicaid, SCHIP, Social Security Insurance) after release from correctional facilities and identify the barriers they face to obtaining coverage.

5. Investigate the relationship between mental health treatment and a decrease in crime and associated costs.

Policy makers should:

1. Adopt presumptive eligibility as an immediate solution to providing health benefits to eligible youth released from corrections until a permanent solution can be developed.

2. Develop a structured, streamlined system by which youth can apply for public insurance while they are still incarcerated so that they can have insurance benefits immediately available to them after release from correctional facilities.

3. Reduce the time taken to determine eligibility and enroll youth into public insurance programs by eliminating the face-to-face interview, permitting mail-in applications, and allowing the self-verification of income.

4. Implement a system to suspend Medicaid benefits as an alternative to terminating them after a youth's incarceration.

5. Collect data on the insurance status or Medicaid eligibility of youth released from correctional facilities.

6. Provide better release planning to youth in correctional facilities, which is important in helping to make the transition between jail and the community easier. These services should include social services, as well as mental and physical health services.

RAVINDRA A. GUPTA, BS
Office of Clinical Sciences
Columbus Children's Research Institute
Columbus, OH 43205

KELLY J. KELLEHER, MD, MPH

KATHLEEN PAJER, MD, MPH

JACK STEVENS, PhD
Department of Pediatrics
Ohio State University and Columbus Children's
Research Institute
Columbus, OH 43205

ALISON CUELLAR, PhD
Department of Health Policy and Management
Columbia University
New York, NY 10032

Acknowledgments

Support for this article was provided by the John D. and Catherine T. MacArthur Foundation and the Children's Research Institute of Columbus Children's Hospital.

We thank Janet Chiancone of the Office of Juvenile Justice and Delinquency Prevention and Lisa Blackwell of Columbus Children's Hospital for their research efforts.

References

1. American Academy of Pediatrics, Committee on Adolescence. Health care for children and adolescents in the juvenile correctional care system. *Pediatrics.* 2001;107:799–803

2. National Association of State Mental Health Program Directors. *Position Statement on Mental Health Services in a Juvenile Justice Population.* Alexandria, VA: National Association of State Mental Health Program Directors; 2001

3. Joseph-DiCaprio J, Farrow J, Feinstein RA, et al. Health care for incarcerated youth: position paper of the Society for Adolescent Medicine. *J Adolesc Health.* 2001;27(1): 73–75

4. American Medical Association, Council on Scientific Affairs. Health status of detained and incarcerated youths. *JAMA.* 1990;263:987–991

5. Snyder HN. An empirical portrait of the youth reentry population. *Youth Violence Juv Justice.* 2004;2:39–55

6. Hammett TM, Roberts C, Kennedy S. Health-related issues in prisoner reentry. *Crime Delinq.* 2001;47:390–409

7. Snyder HN. *Juvenile Arrests 2001.* Washington, DC: Office of Juvenile Justice and Delinquency Prevention; 2003

8. Messner SF, Raffalovich LE, McMillan R. Economic deprivation and changes in homicide arrest rates for white and black youths, 1967–1988: a national time-series analysis. *Criminology.* 2001;39:591–613

9. Hill G, Hill K. Real life dictionary of the law. Available at: http://dictionary.law.com/default2.asp?selected=1451&bold=||||. Accessed April 6, 2004

10. Office of Juvenile Justice and Delinquency Prevention. Census of juveniles in residential placement. Available at: http://ojjdp.ncjrs.org/ojstatbb/cjrp/. Accessed April 6, 2004

11. Hein K, Cohen MI, Litt IF, et al. Juvenile detention: another boundary issue for physicians. *Pediatrics.* 1980;66:239–245

12. Feinstein RA, Lampkin A, Lorish CD, Klerman LV, Maisiak R, Oh MK. Medical status of adolescents at time of admission to a juvenile detention center. *J Adolesc Health.* 1998;22:190–196

13. Teplin LA, Abram KM, McClelland GM, Dulcan MK, Mericle AA. Psychiatric disorders in youth in juvenile detention. *Arch Gen Psychiatry.* 2002;59:1133–1143

14. Pliszka SR, Sherman JO, Barrow MV, Irick S. Affective disorder in juvenile offenders: a preliminary study. *Am J Psychiatry.* 2000;157:130–132

15. Costello EJ, Mustillo S, Erkanli A, Keeler G, Angold A. Prevalence and development of psychiatric disorders in childhood and adolescence. *Arch Gen Psychiatry.* 2003; 60:837–844

16. Goodman SH, Hoven CW, Narrow WE, et al. Measurement of risk for mental disorders and competence in a psychiatric epidemiologic community survey: the National Institute of Mental Health Methods for the Epidemiology of Child and Adolescent Mental Disorders (MECA) Study. *Soc Psychiatry Psychiatr Epidemiol.* 1998;33:162–173

17. Cauffman E. A statewide screening of mental health symptoms among juvenile offenders in detention. *J Am Acad Child Adolesc Psychiatry.* 2004;43:430–439

18. Anderson B, Farrow JA. Incarcerated adolescents in Washington State. *J Adolesc Health.* 1998;22:363–367

19. Department of Health and Human Services. *Results from the 2001 National Household Survey on Drug Abuse: Vol I. Summary of Findings.* Rockville, MD: Department of Health and Human Services; 2002

20. Atkins D, Pumariega A, Rogers K. Mental health and incarcerated youth. I: prevalence and nature of psychopathology. *J Child Fam Stud.* 1999;8:193–204

21. Duclos CW, Beals J, Novins DK, Martin C, Jewett CS, Manson SM. Prevalence of common psychiatric disorders among American Indian adolescent detainees. *J Am Acad Child Adolesc Psychiatry.* 1998;37:866–873

22. Garland AF, Hough RL, McCabe KM, Yeh M, Wood PA, Aarons GA. Prevalence of psychiatric disorders in youths across five sectors of care. *J Am Acad Child Adolesc Psychiatry.* 2001;40:409–418

23. Randall J, Henggeler SW, Pickrel SG, Brondino MJ. Psychiatric comorbidity and the 16-month trajectory of substance-abusing and substance-dependent juvenile offenders. *J Am Acad Child Adolesc Psychiatry.* 1999; 38:1118–1124

24. Teplin LA, Abram KM, McClelland GM. Comorbidity among detained females: implications for policy in the juvenile justice and mental health systems. Presented at: American Society of Criminology Conference; November 6–10, 2001; Atlanta, GA

25. Wasserman GA, McReynolds LS, Lucas CP, Fisher P, Santos L. The voice DISC-IV with incarcerated male youths: prevalence of disorder. *J Am Acad Child Adolesc Psychiatry.* 2002;41:314–321

26. Kataoka SH, Zima BT, Dupre DA, Moreno KA, Yang X, McCracken JT. Mental health problems and service use among female juvenile offenders: their relationship to criminal history. *J Am Acad Child Adolesc Psychiatry.* 2001;40:549–555

27. SAMHSA Jail Diversion Knowledge Development and Application Initiative. *Maintaining Medicaid Benefits for Jail Detainees with Co-Occurring Mental Health and Substance Abuse Disorders.* Delmar, NY: National Gains Center for People With Co-Occurring Disorders in the Justice System; 1999

28. Morris RE, Harrison EA, Knox GW, Tromanhauser E, Marquis DK, Watts LL. Health risk behavioral survey from 39 juvenile correctional facilities in the United States. *J Adolesc Health.* 1995;17:334–344

29. Adams DL, Leath BA. Correctional health care: implications for public health policy. *J Natl Med Assoc.* 2002;94:294–298

30. Draine J, Solomon P, Meyerson A. Predictors of reincarceration among patients who received psychiatric services in jail. *Hosp Community Psychiatry.* 1994;45:163–167

31. Cottle CC, Lee RJ, Heilbrun K. The prediction of criminal recidivism in juveniles: a meta-analysis. *Crim Justice Behav.* 2001;28:367–394

32. Vermeiren R. Psychopathology and delinquency in adolescents: a descriptive and developmental perspective. *Clin Psychol Rev.* 2003;23:277–318

33. Langan PA, Levin DJ. *Recidivism of Prisoners Released in 1994, Bureau of Justice Statistics Special Report.* Washington, DC: Bureau of Justice Statistics; 2002

34. Schellenberg EG, Wasylenki D, Webster CD. A review of arrests among psychiatric patients. *Int J Law Psychiatry.* 1992;15:251–264

35. Wilson KM, Klein JD. Adolescents who use the emergency department as their usual source of care. *Arch Pediatr Adolesc Med.* 2000;154:361–365

36. Cohen MA. The monetary value of saving a high-risk youth. *J Quant Criminol.* 1998;14:5–33

37. Chamberlain P, Reid JB. Comparison of two community alternatives to incarceration for chronic juvenile offenders. *J Consult Clin Psychol.* 1998;66:624–633

38. Cuellar AE, Markowitz S, Libby AM. Mental health and substance abuse treatment and juvenile crime. *J Ment Health Policy Econ.* 2004;7:59–68

39. Foster EM, Qaseem A, Connor T. Can better mental health services reduce the risk of juvenile justice system involvement? *Am J Public Health.* 2004;94:859–865

40. Henggeler SW, Clingempeel WG, Brondino MJ, Pickrel SG. Four-year follow-up of multisystemic therapy with substance-abusing and substance-dependent juvenile offenders. *J Am Acad Child Adolesc Psychiatry.* 2002;41: 868–874

41. Henggeler SW, Cunningham PB, Pickrel SG, Schoenwald SK, Brondino MJ. Multisystemic therapy: an effective violence prevention approach for serious juvenile offenders. *J Adolesc.* 1996;19:47–61

42. Klein NC, Alexander JF, Parsons BV. Impact of family systems intervention on recidivism and sibling delinquency: a model of primary prevention and program evaluation. *J Consult Clin Psychol.* 1977;45:469–474

43. American Academy of Pediatrics, National Association of Children's Hospitals and Related Institutions. United States Medicaid facts. Available at: www.aap.org/advocacy/washing/elections/mfs_us.pdf. Accessed March 25, 2003

44. Aday LA, Andersen R. Insurance coverage and access: implications for health policy. *Health Serv Res.* 1978; 13:369–377

45. Kasper JD, Giovannini TA, Hoffman C. Gaining and losing health insurance: strengthening the evidence for effects on access to care and health outcomes. *Med Care Res Rev.* 2000;57:298–318

46. US Department of Health and Human Services. *Mental Health: A Report of the Surgeon General—Executive Summary.* Rockville, MD: US Department of Health and Human Services, Substance Abuse and Mental Health Services Administration, Center for Mental Health Services, National Institutes of Health, National Institute of Mental Health; 1999

47. Iglehart JK. The dilemma of Medicaid. *N Engl J Med.* 2003;348:2140–2148

48. Medicare program: changes to the inpatient hospital prospective payment system and fiscal year 1991 rates. 55 *Fed Regist* 35990 (1990). Codified at CFR §416.211

49. Social Security Act, §1905(a)(A), 42 USC §1396d

50. Lipton L. Medicaid eligibility termination plagues former inmates. *Psychiatr News.* 2001;26:8

51. Stanton G, Centers for Medicare and Medicaid Services. Ending chronic homelessness. Letter to all state Medicaid directors. May 25, 2004

52. Ross DC. Presumptive eligibility for children: a promising new strategy for enrolling uninsured children in Medicaid. Available at: www.cbpp.org/presum.htm. Accessed April 6, 2004

53. Klein R. Presumptive eligibility. *Future Child.* 2003;13: 230–237

54. Judge David L. Bazelon Center for Mental Health Law. Building bridges: an act to reduce recidivism by improving access to benefits for individuals with psychiatric disabilities upon release from incarceration. Available at: www.bazelon.org/issues/criminalization/publications/buildingbridges. Accessed January 28, 2005

55. Kenney GM, Haley JM. Why aren't more uninsured children enrolled in Medicaid or SCHIP? 2001. No. B-35 in a series. Available at: www.urban.org/url.cfm?ID=310217. Accessed January 28, 2005

56. Lipton L. Gap in Medicaid benefits curtails access, treatment. *Psychiatr News.* 2000. Available at: www.psych.org/pnews/00-03-03/medicaid.html

57. Kelly S, Division of Medicaid and State Operations, Department of Health and Human Services. Letter responding to inquiries regarding Medicaid eligibility for detainees and inmates in the New York City jail system. September 14, 2000

58. Committee on Persons With Mental Illness Behind Bars and the Committee on Continuity of Care and Discharge Planning of the American Association of Community Psychiatrists. Position statement on postrelease planning. 2001. Available at: www.wpic.pitt.edu/aacp/finds/postrelease.html. Accessed January 28, 2005

59. Wolff N, Plemmons D, Veysey B, Brandli A. Release planning for inmates with mental illness compared with those who have other chronic illnesses. *Psychiatr Serv.* 2002;53:1469–1471

Increasing the Screening and Counseling of Adolescents for Risky Health Behaviors: A Primary Care Intervention

Elizabeth M. Ozer, PhD*; Sally H. Adams, PhD*; Julie L. Lustig, PhD*; Scott Gee, MD‡;
Andrea K. Garber, PhD, RD*; Linda Rieder Gardner, MPH*; Michael Rehbein, MD‡;
Louise Addison, MD‡; and Charles E. Irwin, Jr, MD*

ABSTRACT. *Objective.* To determine whether a systems intervention for primary care providers resulted in increased preventive screening and counseling of adolescent patients, compared with the usual standard of care.

Methods. The intervention was conducted in 2 outpatient pediatric clinics; 2 other pediatric clinics in the same health maintenance organization served as comparison sites. The intervention was implemented in 2 phases: first, pediatric primary care providers attended a training workshop (*N* = 37) to increase screening and counseling of adolescents in the areas of tobacco, alcohol, drugs, sexual behavior, and safety (seatbelt and helmet use). Second, screening and charting tools were integrated into the intervention clinics. Providers in the comparison sites (*N* = 39) continued to provide the usual standard of care to their adolescent patients. Adolescent reports were used to assess changes in provider behavior. After a well visit, 13- to 17-year olds (*N* = 2628) completed surveys reporting on whether their provider screened and counseled them for risky behavior.

Results. Screening and counseling rates increased significantly in each of the 6 areas in the intervention sites, compared with rates of delivery using the usual standard of care. Across the 6 areas combined, the average screening rate increased from 58% to 83%; counseling rates increased from 52% to 78%. There were no significant increases in the comparison sites during the same period. The training component seems to account for most of this increase, with the tools sustaining the effects of the training.

Conclusions. The study offers strong support for an intervention to increase clinicians' delivery of preventive services to a wide age range of adolescent patients. *Pediatrics* 2005;115:960–968; *primary care, adolescents, risk behavior, preventive services, quality improvement, managed care.*

ABBREVIATIONS. GAPS, Guidelines for Preventive Services; HMO, health maintenance organization; AROV, Adolescent Report of the Visit; ANCOVA, analysis of covariance.

The majority of adolescent morbidity and mortality is preventable and associated with behaviors such as substance use and abuse, unsafe sexual practices, and risky vehicle use.[1] Accidents and unintentional injuries account for the greatest number of adolescent deaths and often involve use of alcohol.[2-4] Sexually transmitted diseases are the most common infectious diseases among adolescents; among older adolescents, pregnancy and childbirth are the leading causes of hospitalization.[5]

Current trends in adolescent morbidity and mortality have turned greater attention to the preventive role of the health care system. The majority of adolescents visit a health care provider once a year,[6] providing an ideal opportunity to integrate prevention into clinical encounters. To facilitate screening and counseling for risky health behaviors, guidelines specifically targeting the delivery of adolescent clinical preventive services have been developed.[7-13] However, despite the existence of guidelines, rates of screening and counseling consistently are lower than recommended.[12,14,15] Although primary care providers often screen adolescents for some

---

From the *Division of Adolescent Medicine, Department of Pediatrics, and Research and Policy Center for Childhood and Adolescence, University of California, San Francisco, California; and ‡Department of Pediatrics, Kaiser Permanente of Northern California, California.
Accepted for publication Jul 28, 2004.
doi:10.1542/peds.2004-0520
This work was presented in part at the annual research meeting of Academy Health; June 29, 2003; Nashville, TN.
No conflict of interest declared.
Reprint requests to (E.O.) Division of Adolescent Medicine, Department of Pediatrics, Box 0503, LH 245, University of California, San Francisco, CA 94143. E-mail: eozer@itsa.ucsf.edu

risky behavior,[15,16] there is inconsistency in screening across various risk areas.[15]

Barriers to guideline implementation include physician knowledge, physician attitudes, and external factors.[17,18] Physician factors, such as knowledge and attitudes, may be linked to training. For example, almost half (45%) of primary care clinicians who see adolescent patients cited insufficient training as the most significant barrier to the delivery of health care to adolescents,[19] yet even with adequate knowledge and attitudes, external barriers, such as a lack of tools or reminder systems, can affect a provider's ability to follow recommendations. Recent reviews cite the lack of appropriate screening tools as a major barrier to the delivery of preventive services.[18] When tools do exist, they often are too lengthy to be feasible for use in the context of a primary care visit, or, if shorter, they tend to focus on only a single risk behavior.[20] Thus, both clinician and external/system barriers need to be overcome to implement guidelines effectively.

The manner in which guidelines are incorporated into a system also influences the delivery of services. Effective components include educational outreach, feedback and reminders, interactive educational/clinical workshops, involving local opinion leaders, and reaching local consensus.[21] In addition, combining 2 or more modalities (eg, combination of training, feedback, and resources at the systems level such as tools) leads to greater success in improving professional practice.[22-25]

Evidence of the feasibility of systemwide implementation of adolescent preventive guidelines is limited, and experimental research evaluating the process of implementation is scarce. In 1 study of the implementation of Guidelines for Preventive Services (GAPS) in community health centers, Klein et al[26] found that when health center staff were trained to implement GAPS and were provided patient questionnaires, resource materials, and clinician manuals, adolescents received more screening and counseling. However, even after implementation of GAPS, screening rates across the various areas ranged from a low of 21% to a high of 48%. In the only study to implement and evaluate the delivery of adolescent preventive

services in managed care, we found that the provision of provider training, customized screening and charting tools, and preventive services support staff (health educator) resulted in very high rates of screening and counseling of adolescents by primary care providers.[27] Although provider training resulted in significant increases in screening and counseling rates,[28] it was the subsequent addition of screening and charting forms, as well as the resources of a health educator, that resulted in markedly higher rates of preventive services delivery.[27]

This research indicates that interventions that provide the major components of (1) training and (2) screening and charting tools may be particularly effective in increasing delivery of services to adolescents. However, a limitation of our previous research[27] is that it is not possible to separate the effects of tools from the effect of adding a health educator to help facilitate the process because both components were implemented at the same time. It therefore is not clear how great an increase in provider delivery of services can be expected by introducing training and tools into the health care system. Furthermore, no study of the implementation of adolescent preventive services has included comparison sites in the design. This is an essential next step in determining the most effective way to provide adolescent preventive services. The primary objective of this study was to determine the percentage increase in provider delivery of adolescent preventive services that will result from a systems intervention involving provider training and the utilization of screening and charting tools.

We used the Precede/Proceed Model as a framework to assist in the development of this training and tools systems intervention.[29,30] The model posits that predisposing factors, enabling factors, and reinforcing factors influence clinician behavior in preventive care. Predisposing factors relate to the necessary attitudes and motivation to perform a behavior; enabling factors include the competence, skills, and resources necessary to perform the behavior; and reinforcing factors are those that support or reward the behavior.[29,31]

Training clinicians in the delivery of preventive services addresses predisposing variables such as knowledge, attitudes, and self-efficacy to deliver preventive services; enabling factors such as skill in communicating with adolescents; and reinforcing factors such as feedback and support from colleagues. Implementing screening and charting tools should also address predisposing, enabling, and reinforcing factors that impede or enhance delivery of preventive services. For example, tools address predisposing factors such as providers' competence to screen and counsel by facilitating their ability to deliver services efficiently. Tools also enable providers to screen and counsel adolescents by providing prompts, cues, and charting forms. The need to document screening and counseling provides a form of accountability and monitoring that serves as a reinforcing factor.

The goal of this intervention was to increase clinicians' screening and brief counseling of adolescents in the targeted health risk areas of tobacco, alcohol and drug use, sexual behavior, seatbelt use, and helmet use. Our primary hypothesis was:

1. A systems-level intervention, consisting of training and tools to facilitate the delivery of adolescent clinical preventive services, will result in significantly higher rates of provider delivery of services in 6 targeted risk areas, compared with rates of delivery using the usual standard of care.

A secondary set of hypotheses to test the additive effects of the 2 components of the system level intervention were:

2a. Training alone (component 1 of systems-level intervention) will result in significantly higher rates of provider delivery of services in 6 targeted risk areas, compared with rates of delivery using the usual standard of care.

2b. The provision of tools (component 2 of systems-level intervention) will result in significantly higher rates of provider delivery of services in 6 targeted risk areas, compared both with the results of training alone and with rates of delivery using the usual standard of care.

Methods

DESIGN

The study was conducted in 4 outpatient pediatric clinics within a large health maintenance organization (HMO) throughout Northern California; 2 clinics served as intervention sites, and 2 served as comparison sites. The clinic-wide systems intervention focused on increasing the delivery of preventive services during routine well visits. In the intervention sites, 2 components were implemented in 2 separate phases: the first phase consisted of training for primary care providers in the delivery of preventive services; and the second phase consisted of the integration of screening and charting forms into the clinics. The comparison sites continued to deliver the usual standard of care. There were 3 separate assessment time periods in the clinics: (1) a pretraining baseline period (T0), (2) a posttraining period (T1), and (3) a posttools full implementation period (T2). Data were collected at both the intervention and the comparison sites throughout the 3 periods.

Providers' screening and counseling behaviors during adolescent well visits, as reported by adolescents who attended the visits, served as the basis for the evaluation of the intervention. These independent adolescent reports of provider behavior were obtained immediately after well visits in both the intervention and the comparison clinics during the 3 assessment periods. The health behaviors targeted in the intervention included tobacco use, alcohol use, drug use, sexual behavior, and safety (seatbelt and helmet use). All procedures were approved by the internal review boards at the University of California, San Francisco, and at the participating HMO.

CLINICIAN PARTICIPANTS

Clinics were selected on the basis of their provision of care to large numbers of adolescents and their agreement to participate in a study of clinical preventive services to adolescents. Our selection of sites into intervention versus comparison group was based on factors such as size and location of clinic, balancing ethnicity of the adolescents, and previous use of adolescent screening tools. Providers were eligible to participate in the study when they saw adolescents for well visits in the clinic, and all eligible providers agreed to participate in the study.

The original provider sample consisted of 86 participants, 42 from the 2 intervention clinics and 44 from the 2 comparison clinics. Ten providers (5 from the intervention and 5 from the comparison clinics) were excluded from the present analyses because we lacked sufficient evaluation data (at least 2 adolescent well visits per phase). Thus, the present sample consisted of 37 providers in the intervention group and 39 in the comparison group, for a total of 76 providers. Providers in the intervention group were similar to those in the comparison group in terms of gender, age, and proportion of nurse practitioners to physicians. In the provider intervention sample, 62.2% were female, the mean age was 41.2, and 4 were nurse practitioners. In the comparison sample, 64.1% were female, the mean age was 44.1, and 4 were nurse practitioners. The majority of providers were either white or Asian. There were significantly more black providers in the intervention group than in the comparison group. There were no other significant differences in provider characteristics between the intervention and comparison groups (Table 1).

Table 1. Provider Demographics

Demographic Variables	Intervention (n = 37)	Comparison (n = 39)
Age, y (SD)	41.4 (8.67)	44.1 (9.06)
Gender, % female	62	64
Ethnicity, %		
White	41.2	54.5
Black*	11.8	0
Hispanic	2.9	12.1
Asian-Pacific Islander	41.2	30.3
Other	2.9	3
% MD vs nurse practitioner	89	89
Years since graduation (SD)	14 (9.3)	15 (9.2)

*Note: Percentage of black providers in intervention group is significantly greater than in comparison group ($F = 4.2$, $P < .05$).

PREVENTIVE SERVICES INTERVENTION

The preventive services intervention was composed of clinician trainings in adolescent preventive services and the later implementation of screening and charting forms customized for this study (see below for description). The intervention focused on the targeted risk areas of tobacco, alcohol, drugs, sexual behavior, and safety (helmet and seatbelt use). All clinicians participated in the training, and the tools were implemented on a clinic-wide basis. Thus, we expected that all adolescents who were 13 to 17 years of age and attended well visits would receive screening and counseling in the targeted risk areas. Adolescents met with their primary care provider for a well visit that lasted 20 to 30 minutes. The amount of time allocated for a well visit was consistent with the usual standard of care in the health care system.

At each intervention clinic, either the chief or assistant chief of pediatrics served as a physician "champion" who promoted the study and served as the primary contact with the study investigators. Clinicians and administrative staff also participated in committees that collaborated on the methods of data collection and the plans for implementation of the clinical tools into the clinics.

Component 1: Training

The training workshops for providers focused on increasing clinicians' knowledge, attitudes, self-efficacy, and skills to conduct preventive services and were based on social cognitive theory.[32,33] This training model had been developed and evaluated previously and had been shown to be effective.[28] Minor modifications were implemented to address specific needs in the intervention clinics. The provider training was conducted by an expert panel of adolescent medicine specialists from the University of California, San Francisco, and the participating HMO, with consultation from our clinician committees in the intervention clinics. In addition, we used actors from an educational theater program within the HMO to portray adolescent patients in the demonstration and interactive practice role plays.

The 8-hour workshop focused on adolescent health, confidentiality, screening, and conducting a brief office-based intervention that included anticipatory guidance/brief counseling for the 6 risk behaviors. As suggested by the review of effective interventions for health professionals,[24] the workshops contained 4 components: (1) didactic presentations, (2) discussion, (3) demonstration role plays, and (4) interactive role plays. The didactic component included

presentations of the following: adolescent health and risk behavior statistics, adolescent development, the role of primary care providers in health and risk prevention, interviewing adolescents, confidentiality, screening and brief counseling, and prioritizing in clinical visits. The second component included discussion and question-and-answer sessions based on the presentations. The third component included demonstration role plays conducted by the expert panel with the theater actors playing adolescents; and in the fourth component, providers had the opportunity to practice screening and counseling, using the theater actors. All nonprovider staff attended a 1-hour lunchtime training that focused on general topics of adolescent development and adolescent priorities in the health care setting.

Component 2: Adolescent Health Screening Questionnaire and Charting Forms Implementation

Before this study, the Regional Health Education Department of the HMO had developed 2 forms for use in adolescent well visits: (1) an adolescent health screening questionnaire and (2) a provider charting form. On the basis of our earlier work,[27] we modified these region forms for use in this study. These modifications, intended to facilitate the delivery of preventive services in the targeted risk areas, were made in collaboration with Regional Health Education, with feedback from the clinicians at the intervention sites.

Before this study, only 1 of the study intervention sites was using the region's screening form. Furthermore, the site was not using the screening form consistently with all teenagers before well visits. The process of implementing tools was enhanced in several ways at the intervention clinics. First, we collaborated with clinicians and staff in both intervention sites to develop a system for distributing the modified adolescent screening questionnaires. Second, we assisted administrators and clinicians in establishing a process for providing an area for adolescents to complete the form confidentially and for retrieving them when completed. Third, we conducted 1-hour lunch meetings with clinicians and staff to introduce the forms and explain the implementation procedures.

Adolescent Screening Questionnaire

The region's original adolescent health screening form included questions about risk engagement in a broad variety of areas. We modified the form to include the following: (1) addition of follow-up questions in the target areas of sexual behavior, tobacco use, and alcohol and drug use; (2) addition of a screening question regarding helmet use; and (3) addition of prompts and cues in the target areas reminding providers to screen and to deliver brief counseling messages. Providers were cued to give adolescents positive reinforcement if they reported that they were engaging in healthy behavior. Examples of healthy behavior include not using tobacco or always using a bicycle helmet when riding. Providers were cued to express concern to adolescents if they reported engaging in risky behavior, such as using tobacco or alcohol.

Provider Charting Form

Both intervention clinics were already using the charting form previously developed by the HMO region, and modifications made for the study to the region's charting form were minor. They included placing an asterisk next to the behavior areas that were targeted in the intervention. The asterisks referred to a boxed area at the bottom of the page, reminding clinicians to screen and counsel in those areas.

EVALUATION OF THE PREVENTIVE SERVICES INTERVENTION

Adolescent Reporters

Adolescents completed the Adolescent Report of the Visit (AROV), an independent survey of provider behavior, immediately after well visits (see below). The survey was distributed by trained research or clinic staff, who approached adolescents as they left examination rooms and asked them to complete the assessment. To have a representative array of adolescents per provider, we obtained reports from as many adolescents as possible across all providers. We focused on collecting data from a wide age range of adolescent patients (13–17 years of age) and from both male and female patients. (In cases in which we did not achieve broad representation for a provider, it tended to be female providers who saw very few adolescent male patients, or vice versa.) Data collection took place in 3 of the clinics on a daily basis and in the fourth clinic 2 to 3 days per week. This was necessary because of staffing limitations and physical location of the clinic. Parent consent and adolescent assent were not required because adolescents completed the AROV anonymously. On the basis of clinic schedules of completed visits in the intervention sites, we estimate that 75% of the adolescents who were asked to complete questionnaires agreed to do so. The adolescents were similar in age and gender in the intervention and comparison samples. See Table 2 for detailed description of the adolescent-reporter demographic characteristics.

Adolescents completed the AROV during each of the 3 evaluation periods in both the intervention and comparison clinics. Each of the periods lasted ~4 months: pretraining (T0) data collection included 226 intervention and 246 comparison adolescents; posttraining (T1) data collection began immediately after the training and included 551 intervention adolescents and 260 comparison adolescents. The T2 data collection began immediately after the implementation of tools into the clinics and included 940 intervention and 405 comparison adolescents. (The adolescent sample from the comparison sites was smaller than the sample from the intervention sites for 2 reasons: (1) In the intervention sites, the reception and medical assistant staff were involved with implementing the intervention. They were interested in the research and made an effort to help our research staff track prospective adolescent reporters as they left exam rooms. The adolescents then were approached and asked to complete the AROV. (2) In 1 of the comparison sites, our research assistant was not present on a full-time basis, thus limiting data collection opportunities. We adjust for these differences in sample size as needed in the analyses.)

Table 2. Adolescent Reporter Demographics

Demographic Variables	Intervention (n = 1717)	Comparison (n = 911)
Age, y (SD)	14.8 (1.31)	14.8 (1.34)
Gender, % female	53	59
Ethnicity, %		
White	38.3	28.4
Black	17.3	22.1
Hispanic	22.4	27.0
Asian-Pacific Islander	13.0	14.7
Native American/ Alaskan Native	5.0	3.9
Other	4.0	4.0

There were larger numbers of adolescents during T2 implementation because of the seasonal increase in well visits during the summer months. (We examined correlations among the numbers of adolescents seen per provider at each phase and found that providers who saw a higher number of patients at T0 tended to see a higher number during T1 and T2 implementation. Thus, the potential bias as a result of uneven numbers of adolescents seen across phases in terms of provider characteristics was minimized.) Across all phases, the full intervention sample size was 1717; the full comparison sample size was 911, for a total of 2628 adolescents reporting on their providers' behaviors.

Assessment of Clinician Practices

The AROV is a 45-item patient-report measure that includes questions about whether clinicians screen and offer brief counseling messages for each of the 6 target risk areas. Adolescent-based assessments of provider behavior yield an appraisal of clinician practices that is free of the confounding influences of provider self-report and social desirability biases and have been shown to be a valid indicator of delivery of services.[26] The AROV has been used previously and possesses adequate construct validity.[27,28] An example of a screening question is, "Did your doctor ask if you smoke or chew tobacco?" Items that assessed counseling differed, by skip patterns, depending on whether an adolescent was engaging in a particular risk behavior and whether she or he had informed the clinician about engagement in the risk behavior. An example of a counseling question for adolescents who were not engaging is, "Did your doctor encourage you to remain a nonsmoker or nontobacco user?" An example of a counseling question for adolescents who were engaging in a risky behavior is, "Did your doctor express concern that you use tobacco?" Similar screening and counseling questions were asked for each of the 6 risk areas. The response categories were dichotomous: yes or no. On average, adolescents completed the measure in 3 to 5 minutes.

Each adolescent questionnaire identified the provider who conducted the visit. A provider's score for each screening and counseling area was obtained by taking the average of the individual items for that area, summed across all of the adolescent questionnaires available for that provider. The resulting score for each item (eg, screening for tobacco use) represented the percentage of the time a provider performed screening or counseling in that area. For example, if a provider saw 4 adolescents during the T0 period in the study and 2 of them reported that they were asked whether they used tobacco and 2 reported that they were not asked, then that provider's score for screening in tobacco use for T0 would be 0.50. Thus, each provider had a mean score representing his or her screening rate across adolescent reports for each behavior area and each time period.

ANALYSIS PLAN

The primary focus of the evaluation was to assess providers' rates of screening and counseling in the intervention group, in relation to providers' rates of screening and counseling in the comparison group. The 6 targeted areas of screening and counseling were tobacco, alcohol, drugs, sexual behavior, and seatbelt and helmet use. The unit of analysis was the provider. Rates of screening and counseling for each provider were obtained on the basis of reports from their adolescent patients. Each behavioral risk area was evaluated individually for screening and counseling rates (eg, screening for tobacco use, counseling for tobacco use).

First, we present descriptive statistics for the adolescent reports that comprise the provider screening and counseling means. Second, we present rates of clinic-wide tools implementation. Third, we present provider screening and counseling means for each of the 3 phases separately for the intervention and comparison groups. Fourth, we present analysis of covariance (ANCOVA) to compare screening and counseling rates between the intervention and comparison groups.

Results

DESCRIPTIVE STATISTICS: NUMBER OF ADOLESCENT REPORTERS SEEN FOR WELL VISITS

The mean number of adolescent reporters per provider during T0 was 6.6 (SD: 3.8) for the intervention group and 6.6 (SD: 4.2) for the comparison group. During T1, the mean number of adolescent reporters per provider was 14.9 (SD: 6.0) for the intervention group and 6.7 (SD: 3.9) for the comparison group. During T2, the mean number of adolescents seen per provider was 25.4 (SD: 10.6) for the intervention and 10.4 (SD: 5.6) for the comparison groups. The number of adolescents was uneven across the time periods and between the intervention and comparison groups. To evaluate potential bias, we examined correlations between number of adolescent reporters per provider during each period and screening and counseling rates. This allowed us to determine whether providers who conducted a greater number of well visits tended to screen or counsel at higher or lower rates during those visits. In >80% of the screening and counseling behaviors, the number of adolescent reporters was not significantly correlated with screening or counseling rates. In the cases in which the number of adolescent reporters was significantly correlated with screening or counseling rates, the number of adolescent reporters per provider was included as a covariate in the ANCOVA for that behavior. (The number of adolescent reporters per provider was positively correlated with counseling for drug use at T2 and with helmet screening and counseling at both T1 and T2.)

ASSESSMENT OF TOOLS IMPLEMENTATION

During T2, we monitored the integration of the study screening form into the intervention clinics through questions on the AROV. Ninety-seven percent of the adolescents reported that they received the Health Screening Questionnaire, 80% reported that they had time to complete the

questionnaire, and 89% reported that they were able to fill it out privately.

DESCRIPTIVE STATISTICS: PROVIDER SCREENING AND COUNSELING RATES IN THE INTERVENTION GROUP

Table 3 presents the screening and counseling rates for the intervention group at each of the 3 phases: T0, T1, and T2. Analyses of change in the rates are presented in the ANCOVA sections that follow the descriptive statistics. At T0 in the intervention group, providers' average screening rates ranged from 42% for helmet use to 71% for tobacco use (Table 3). During this phase, the screening rates for seatbelt and helmet use were considerably lower than screening rates for substance use or sexual behavior. At T1, screening rates ranged from 70% for helmet use to 85% for tobacco use. At T2, screening rates tended to remain stable from posttraining rates.

Counseling rates across the 3 phases in the intervention group followed a similar pattern. At T0, average counseling rates ranged from 39% for helmet counseling to 65% for tobacco counseling. At T1, counseling rates ranged from 71% for helmet use to 83% for tobacco use. At T2, the pattern of the counseling rates remained relatively stable from posttraining rates.

DESCRIPTIVE STATISTICS: PROVIDER SCREENING AND COUNSELING RATES IN THE COMPARISON GROUP

In the comparison group, providers delivered the usual standard of care during each of the 3 phases. T0 screening rates in the comparison sites ranged from 30% for helmet use to 65% for tobacco use (Table 3). Screening rates in the comparison group tended to remain stable at T1 and T2, with the lowest rate of screening in the area of helmet use and the highest rate in the area of tobacco use. Counseling rates followed a similar pattern to those for screening during each phase.

ANCOVA TO TEST HYPOTHESES

We conducted ANCOVA to test the differences in screening and counseling rates between the intervention and comparison groups. We tested a separate model for each screening and for each

Table 3. Descriptive Statistics and ANCOVA Results: Intervention and Comparison Provider Screening and Counseling Rates During Each Phase

Variable	Intervention Means (SD) (n = 37)			Comparison Means (SD) (n = 39)			ANCOVA: Full Intervention (T0–T2)	ANCOVA: Training Phase Only (T0–T1)
	T0	T1	T2	T0	T1	T2	F	F
Screening								
Tobacco	0.71 (0.24)	0.85 (0.16)	0.85 (0.16)	0.65 (0.30)	0.69 (0.27)	0.60 (0.27)	28.34*	8.54†
Alcohol	0.67 (0.22)	0.82 (0.17)	0.83 (0.19)	0.60 (0.34)	0.64 (0.30)	0.60 (0.26)	17.81*	8.26†
Drugs	0.65 (0.24)	0.84 (0.16)	0.84 (0.17)	0.61 (0.34)	0.66 (0.30)	0.62 (0.29)	17.11*	16.60*
Sexual behavior	0.57 (0.27)	0.81 (0.16)	0.81 (0.18)	0.54 (0.34)	0.57 (0.34)	0.52 (0.28)	36.23*	12.24*
Seatbelt	0.43 (0.26)	0.82 (0.20)	0.82 (0.21)	0.51 (0.31)	0.53 (0.36)	0.47 (0.30)	49.36*	22.86*
Helmet	0.42 (0.30)	0.70 (0.23)	0.81 (0.22)	0.30 (0.29)	0.28 (0.25)	0.30 (0.29)	52.21*	25.56*
Total Screening	0.58 (0.20)	0.81 (0.16)	0.83 (0.17)	0.53 (0.27)	0.56 (0.24)	0.52 (0.23)		
Counseling								
Tobacco	0.65 (0.26)	0.83 (0.16)	0.88 (0.16)	0.56 (0.32)	0.67 (0.26)	0.67 (0.20)	23.08*	7.01†
Alcohol	0.59 (0.29)	0.77 (0.17)	0.81 (0.18)	0.46 (0.32)	0.54 (0.32)	0.55 (0.23)	25.37*	10.76†
Drugs	0.62 (0.28)	0.81 (0.16)	0.85 (0.17)	0.49 (0.29)	0.58 (0.33)	0.54 (0.28)	25.36*	9.93†
Sexual behavior	0.52 (0.28)	0.76 (0.20)	0.78 (0.18)	0.48 (0.33)	0.54 (0.34)	0.50 (0.25)	27.77*	9.89†
Seatbelt	0.44 (0.24)	0.79 (0.23)	0.81 (0.20)	0.46 (0.31)	0.52 (0.34)	0.46 (0.29)	48.48*	18.30*
Helmet	0.39 (0.28)	0.71 (0.24)	0.80 (0.21)	0.35 (0.32)	0.28 (0.24)	0.33 (0.30)	58.68*	31.62*
Total Counseling	0.54 (0.22)	0.78 (0.17)	0.82 (0.17)	0.46 (0.25)	0.52 (0.23)	0.51 (0.19)		

* $P < .001$

† $P < .01$.

counseling behavior (eg, screening for tobacco; counseling for tobacco). We took into account several sources of potential bias in each analysis. To control for differences in baseline levels of screening and counseling, we entered the baseline level of screening and counseling as a covariate in each model. To control for the potential influence of unequal numbers of adolescent reporters per provider, we entered the number of adolescent reporters into the model when it was significantly correlated with the level of screening or counseling in a specific time period. To control for individual provider and adolescent characteristics, we included as covariates the age, gender, and ethnicity of provider or adolescent when they were correlated with screening or counseling levels.

We also examined the possibility that provider screening and counseling rates within an individual site could account for effects (eg, that one intervention site might be intrinsically different from the other intervention site). Controlling for the baseline values, we conducted post hoc analyses using Tukey b to test for the influence of site on the screening and counseling outcomes. We used this method, rather than hierarchical linear modeling, to examine the effects of clinic site, as the present study included only 2 sites in the intervention group and 2 sites in the comparison group. Therefore, multilevel analyses were not feasible.

Hypothesis 1: ANCOVA Results Testing the Full Intervention of Training and Tools: Intervention Versus Comparison Groups

Our primary hypothesis was that, after implementation of the full intervention, consisting of both provider training and tools, provider screening and counseling rates would be significantly higher in our intervention group than in our comparison group. We conducted ANCOVA to test the differences in screening and counseling rates between the intervention and comparison groups.

Screening

ANCOVA results indicated that screening rates after the implementation of the full intervention (training plus tools) were significantly higher for each of the 6 target areas in the intervention group than in the comparison group, controlling for baseline levels of screening and other covariates. Fs ranged from 17.11 for drug screening to 52.21 for helmet screening (all $P < .000$; Table 3). The effect sizes (η^2) ranged from 0.19 for drug screening to 0.43 for helmet screening, all considered large effects.

Counseling

ANCOVA results indicated that counseling rates after the implementation of the full intervention (training plus tools) were significantly higher for each of the 6 target areas, compared with the comparison group, controlling for baseline counseling levels and other covariates. Fs ranged from 23.08 (df 1,75) for tobacco counseling to 58.68 (df 1,75) for helmet counseling (all $P < .001$; Table 3). The effect sizes (η^2) were large, ranging from 0.24 for tobacco counseling to 0.46 for helmet counseling.

Hypothesis 2a: ANCOVA Results Testing the Effect of Training Alone: Intervention Versus Comparison Groups

We hypothesized that training alone (component 1 of systems-level intervention) would result in significantly higher rates of provider delivery of services in 6 targeted risk areas, compared with rates of delivery using the usual standard of care.

Screening

ANCOVA results indicated that rates of screening during T1 were significantly higher in the intervention group than in the comparison group in each of the 6 areas after taking into account baseline and other covariates. Fs ranged from 8.26, (df 1,75; $P < .01$) for alcohol screening to 25.56 (df 1,75; $P < .001$) for helmet screening (Table 3). The η^2 ranged from 0.11 (medium effect size) for alcohol screening to 0.27 (large effect size) for helmet screening.

Counseling

ANCOVA results indicated that counseling rates were significantly higher in each of the 6 target areas in the intervention group compared with the comparison group after the training. This was after controlling for baseline counseling level and other covariates. Fs ranged from 7.01, (df 1,74; $P < .01$) for tobacco counseling to

31.62 (df 1,75; $P < .001$) for helmet counseling (Table 3). The η^2 ranged from 0.09 (medium effect size) for tobacco counseling to 0.31 (large effect size) for helmet counseling.

Hypothesis 2b: ANCOVA Results Testing the Effect of the Addition of Tools: Intervention Versus Comparison Groups

We hypothesized that the addition of the tools component of the intervention would result in additional increases in screening and counseling rates in the intervention group, in relation to the comparison group. We conducted repeated measures ANCOVA to test the effect of adding the tools component in the intervention group. To determine whether screening and counseling rates increased significantly in the intervention group after the addition of the tools component, we examined the interaction between group (intervention vs comparison) and the repeated measure (the screening rates at the T1 and T2). There were no significant interactions in the ANCOVAs, indicating that screening and counseling rates did not increase significantly from T1 to T2 in the intervention group, in relation to the comparison group.

SUMMARY OF ANCOVA RESULTS

The results of the ANCOVAs demonstrated that (1) screening and counseling rates were significantly higher in the intervention group than in the comparison group after the full implementation of the intervention (T2); (2) screening and counseling rates were significantly higher in the intervention group than in the comparison group after the training component alone (T1); and (3) screening and counseling rates did not increase significantly in the intervention group, in relation to the comparison group, after the addition of the tools component. Our analyses of effect of site indicated that provider screening and counseling rates within the 2 intervention sites and within the comparison sites were not significantly different from one another in the majority of the analyses. Thus, provider screening and counseling rates within an individual site did not account for the significant effects of the intervention.

Discussion

This study evaluated an intervention to increase clinicians' delivery of preventive services to a wide age range of adolescent patients in a group-model HMO. The findings support the general hypothesis that a systems intervention, consisting of training and tools, resulted in higher rates of provider delivery of services in 6 targeted risk areas, compared with rates of delivery using the usual standard of care. A secondary set of hypotheses testing the additive effects of the 2 components of the system intervention was only partially supported: provider training resulted in significantly higher rates of clinician screening and counseling of adolescent patients across all of the targeted risk areas; however, the subsequent addition of a modified screening tool did not further significantly increase screening and counseling rates. Thus, although the full intervention of training and tools significantly increased clinician screening and counseling rates, most of this increase seems to be accounted for by the training component.

COMPONENT 1: TRAINING

The full-day provider training workshops that were conducted in the intervention sites were associated with large increases in rates of clinician screening and counseling (an average of 24%) across all targeted risk areas. The effect of this training is especially noteworthy as continuing medical education workshops alone have not been found to be an effective method of changing clinician behavior.[34] There are several reasons as to why this particular workshop might have been effective at changing clinician behavior. First, the training workshops, based on social cognitive theory,[33] addressed multiple barriers that impede implementation of preventive services for adolescents. The training focused on increasing knowledge, skills, and self-efficacy to deliver effectively preventive services to adolescents. Second, local opinion leaders were integrally involved in the intervention, a strategy that has been associated with improvements in professional practice.[24] The chief or assistant chief of pediatrics served as our MD champions in each of the intervention sites, and adolescent medicine specialists from within

the health care plan were involved in planning and conducting the training sessions. Third, the majority of clinicians, as well as the chief of pediatrics, attended the trainings together. This cohesive approach facilitated incorporating the screening and counseling methods not only into the practices of individual clinicians but also throughout the clinic system.

These findings support previous work on the effectiveness of skill-based training for clinicians.[28] However, these findings extend the previous work in several important ways. First, the inclusion of comparison sites further validates the efficacy of this skill-based training program. Second, this training focused on delivering preventive services to all adolescents. Consequently, adolescents who were screened and counseled ranged in age from 13 to 17 years. Earlier research had included only a cohort of 14-year-old patients. Third, the magnitude of the change in screening and counseling rates in this current study are considerably larger than reported in previous research. The larger increase in rates of screening and counseling may be because clinicians were encouraged to deliver preventive services to all adolescents who came to their clinic for a well visit. Although this may initially seem more difficult than delivering services to a subset of adolescents (eg, 14-year-olds), these findings suggest that delivering services systematically to all patients may make it easier to integrate new guidelines into practice.

FULL INTERVENTION: TRAINING AND MODIFIED SCREENING AND CHARTING TOOLS

Although studies have found that interventions that combine 2 or more modalities are more likely to improve clinical practice,[21,26,27] the subsequent addition of tools did not result in additional significant increases in screening and counseling rates in the intervention sites in relation to the comparison sites. Although rates of screening and counseling for helmet use increased between phases 2 and 3 in the intervention sites, once the full-model ANCOVA took into account any changes in the comparison sites and controlled for all covariates, this increase was not significant, relative to the comparison sites. Thus, although introducing the modified questionnaire had some impact on specific areas of screening and counseling, overall, it did not add significantly more than the initial training.

One likely explanation as to why the addition of tools may have had less impact than we expected is related to ceiling effects. After the training, adolescents reported being screened by their provider >80% of the time across all targeted areas, except for helmet use (at 70%). These are very high rates of screening across a wide age range of adolescent patients. It may be unrealistic to expect rates to increase greater than ~80% in a busy clinical practice when clinicians are attempting to screen all adolescents. After introducing the screening questionnaire, helmet use increased to approximately the same screening rate (81%) as the other risk areas. The consistent implementation of the adolescent screening questionnaire may have served to maintain the posttraining screening and counseling rates across all risk areas. The already high rates of screening posttraining may have led to the screening questionnaire's serving primarily as a maintenance tool.

It should also be noted that at baseline, before our intervention, all clinics were using a charting form that had previously been distributed by the HMO's Regional Health Education for use in adolescent well visits. We made only minor changes to this form for the purposes of this study. Because clinicians were already using the charting form during the baseline phase (when screening and counseling rates were lower), it is clear that distributing a charting form alone does not result in high rates of screening and counseling. However, because all clinicians had some tool to assist them before the intervention, the full-intervention tools phase was more of a modification/add-on phase than a pure tools phase. This also may have contributed to the addition of tools having less of an impact.

During the full intervention phase (posttools), clinicians screened adolescents across all targeted risk areas, on average, 81% of the time. Screening across all risk areas reached approximately the same level regardless of the differential in screening rates at baseline. Consistent with our previous research,[27] during the pretraining phase, clinicians

were most likely to screen adolescents for substance use and least likely to screen for seatbelt and helmet use. Thus, the greatest absolute increase in screening rates, as a result of the intervention, was in the areas of seatbelt and helmet use. This suggests that before our intervention, screening adolescents for seatbelt and helmet use was not focused on and/or viewed as important as other risk areas such as substance use. This is especially striking given that the majority of adolescent deaths are attributable to unintentional injuries,[1] screening for seatbelt and helmet use is relatively straightforward, and recent data suggest that clinician screening and counseling do have an effect on adolescent safety behavior.[35,36]

Although the findings of this intervention study are promising, a limitation of the study is that it was conducted within a group-model HMO that has distinct characteristics. For example, the ability to conduct a training that includes all primary care providers and is tailored to a particular clinic setting is not easily transferable to all health care settings. However, although the effect size may differ, the basic components of combining a provider skill-based training with tools that assist in enhancing or maintaining behavior change are generalizable to providers across a wide range of clinical settings.

Improving adolescent health is the ultimate goal of adolescent clinical preventive guidelines. However, an essential first step is to develop successful implementation models to facilitate prevention efforts.[37] This is the first study to propose a model to implement adolescent clinical preventive services into busy clinical practices within managed care, using a research design that includes intervention and comparison sites. It is now time for research to begin to assess the behavioral/health effects of adolescents who receive clinical preventive services.

This study offers strong support for an intervention to increase clinicians' delivery of preventive services to a wide age range of adolescent patients. The enhancement of screening and counseling across all 6 targeted risk behaviors, compared with delivery using the usual standard of care, indicates that it is possible to improve the delivery of preventive services in the context of outpatient pediatric visits. This is a key step toward fully using the context of the health care setting for promoting adolescent health.

Acknowledgments

This research was supported primarily by grant U18 HS11095 from the Agency for Healthcare Research and Quality. Additional support was provided through a cooperative agreement from the Centers for Disease Control and Prevention through the Association of American Medical Colleges (MM-0162-02/02); the Hellman Family Award for Early Career Faculty; and by the Maternal and Child Health Bureau (MCJ-000978), Health Resources and Services Administration, Department of Health and Human Services (T71MC00003, U45MC00002, and U45MC000023).

We thank Jan Babb, Martha Barbosa, Sherille Pedron, and Natalie Redmond for the exceptional job in data collection and Ilse Larson and Alison Goldberg for skillful work in organizing the trainings and helping with multiple aspects of this study. Sheila Husting has played an integral role in data management, and we thank Jeanne Tschann for consultation on data analysis. We also appreciate the assistance of Michael Berlin in the preparation of the manuscript. Finally, we are grateful to Charito Sico and Gail Udkow for support for this study as well as the clinicians and staff in the Kaiser Permanente Northern California clinics who participated in this study and demonstrated a commitment to delivering preventive health care to adolescents.

References

1. Ozer EM, Park MJ, Paul T, Brindis CD, Irwin CE Jr. *America's Adolescents: Are They Healthy?* San Francisco, CA: University of California, National Adolescent Health Information Center; 2003

2. Anderson RN. Deaths: leading causes for 2000 [serial online]. *Natl Vital Stat Rep.* 2002;50:1–85. Available at: www.cdc.gov/nchs/products/pubs/pubd/nvsr/50/50-16. htm. Accessed September 3, 2003

3. National Center for Injury Prevention and Control. Injury mortality reports 1999–2000 [database online]. Atlanta, GA: Centers for Disease Control and Prevention, National Center for Injury Prevention and Control; 2002. Available at: webapp.cdc.gov/sasweb/ncipc/ mortrate10.html. Accessed September 3, 2003

4. National Highway Traffic Safety Administration. *Traffic Safety Facts 2000: A Compilation of Motor Vehicle Crash Data From the Fatality Analysis Reporting System and the General Estimates System.* Washington, DC: National Highway Traffic Safety Administration, National Center for Statistics and Analysis, US Department of Transportation; 2001. Available at: www-fars.nhtsa.dot.gov/pubs/1.pdf. Accessed September 3, 2003

5. Mackay AP, Fingerhut LA, Duran CR. *Adolescent Health Chartbook. Health, United States, 2000.* Hyattsville, MD: National Center for Health Statistics. Available at: www.cdc.gov/nchs/products/pubs/pubd/hus/2010/ 2010.htm#hus00. Accessed September 3, 2003

6. Newacheck PW, Brindis CD, Cart CU, Marchi K, Irwin CE Jr. Adolescent health insurance coverage: recent changes and access to care. *Pediatrics.* 1999; 104(suppl):195–202

7. Elster AB, Kuznets N. *Guidelines for Adolescent Preventive Services (GAPS): Recommendations and Rationale.* Chicago, IL: American Medical Association; 1994

8. Green M, ed. *Bright Futures: Guidelines for Health Supervision of Infants, Children and Adolescents.* Arlington, VA: National Center for Education in Maternal and Child Health; 1994

9. Stein M, ed. *Health Supervision Guidelines.* 3rd ed. Elk Grove Village, IL: American Academy of Pediatrics; 1997

10. Department of Health and Human Services, Public Health Service, Office of Disease Prevention and Health Promotion. *The Clinician's Handbook of Preventive Services: Put Prevention Into Practice.* Alexandra, VA: International Medical Publishers; 1994

11. US Preventive Services Task Force. *Guide to Clinical Preventive Services.* 2nd ed. Baltimore, MD: Williams & Wilkins; 1996

12. Igra V, Millstein S. Current status and approaches to improving preventive services for adolescents. *JAMA.* 1993;269:1408–1412

13. Park MJ, Macdonald TM, Ozer EM, et al. *Investing in Clinical Preventive Health Services for Adolescents.* San Francisco, CA: University of California, Policy Information and Analysis Center for Middle Childhood and Adolescence, and National Adolescent Health Information Center; 2001

14. Franzgrote M, Ellen JM, Millstein SG, Irwin CE Jr. Screening for adolescent smoking among primary care physicians in California. *Am J Public Health.* 1997;87: 1341–1345

15. Halpern-Felsher BL, Ozer EM, Millstein SG, et al. Preventive services in a health maintenance organization: how well do pediatricians screen and educate adolescent patients? *Arch Pediatr Adolesc Med.* 2000;154:173–179

16. Ellen JM, Franzgrote M, Irwin CE Jr, Millstein SG. Primary care physicians' screening of adolescent patients: a survey of California physicians. *J Adolesc Health.* 1998; 22:433–438

17. Cabana MD, Rand CS, Powe NR, et al. Why don't physicians follow clinical practice guidelines? A framework for improvement. *JAMA.* 1999;282:1458–1465

18. Hallfors D, Van Dorn RA. Strengthening the role of two key institutions in the prevention of adolescent substance abuse. *J Adolesc Health.* 2002;30:17–28

19. Blum RW, Bearinger LH. Knowledge and attitudes of health professionals toward adolescent health care. *J Adolesc Health.* 1990;11:289–294

20. McPherson TL, Hersch RK. Brief substance use screening instruments for primary care settings: a review. *J Subst Abuse Treat.* 2000;18:193–202

21. Bero LA, Grilli R, Grimshaw JM, Harvey E, Oxman AD, Thomson MA. Closing the gap between research and practice: an overview of systematic reviews of interventions to promote the implementation of research findings. *BMJ.* 1998;317:465–468

22. Greco PJ, Eisenberg JM. Changing physicians' practices. *N Engl J Med.* 1993;329:1271–1273

23. Lomas J, Haynes RB. A taxonomy and critical review of tested strategies for the application of clinical practice recommendations: from "official" to "individual" clinical policy. *Am J Prev Med.* 1988;4(suppl 4):77–97

24. Oxman AD, Thomson MA, Davis DA, Haynes RB. No magic bullets: a systematic review of 102 trials of interventions to improve professional practice. *CMAJ.* 1995;153:1423–1431

25. Simpson L, Kamerow D, Fraser I. Pediatric guidelines and managed care: who is using what and what difference does it make? *Pediatr Ann.* 1998;27:234–240

26. Klein JD, Allan MJ, Elster AB, et al. Improving adolescent preventive care in community health centers. *Pediatrics.* 2001;107:318–327

27. Ozer EM, Adams SH, Lustig JL, et al. Can it be done? Implementing adolescent clinical preventive services. *Health Serv Res.* 2001;36(suppl):150–165

28. Lustig JL, Ozer EM, Adams SH, et al. Improving the delivery of adolescent clinical preventive services through skills-based training. *Pediatrics.* 2001;107:1100–1107

29. Green LW, Eriksen MP, Schor EL. Preventive practices by physicians: behavioral determinants and potential interventions. *Am J Prev Med.* 1988;4(suppl4):101–110

30. Lawrence RS. Diffusion of the U.S. preventive services task force recommendations into practice. *J Gen Intern Med.* 1990;5(suppl 5):S99–S103

31. Walsh JM, McPhee SJ. A systems model of clinical preventive care: an analysis of factors influencing patient and physician. *Health Educ Q.* 1992;19:157–175

32. Bandura A. *Social Foundations of Thought and Action: A Social Cognitive Theory.* Englewood Cliffs, NJ: Prentice Hall; 1986

33. Bandura A. *Self-efficacy: The Exercise of Control.* New York, NY: WH Freeman; 1997

34. Davis DA, Thompson MA, Oxman AD, Haynes RB. Changing physician performance. A systematic review of the effect of continuing medical education strategies. *JAMA.* 1995;274:700–705

35. Ozer EM, Adams SH, Lustig JL, et al. The effect of preventive services on adolescent behavior [abstract]. *Pediatr Res.* 2003;53(suppl 4):265A

36. Johnston BD, Rivara FP, Droesch RM, Dunn C, Copass MK. Behavior change counseling in the emergency department to reduce injury risk: a randomized, controlled trial. *Pediatrics.* 2002;110:267–274

37. Agency for Healthcare Research and Quality. *Translating Evidence Into Practice: Conference Summary.* Rockville, MD: Agency for Health Care Policy and Research; 1998. Available at: www.ahcpr.gov/clinic/trip1998. Accessed September 3, 2003

Management of Substance Abuse

Caroline J. Barangan, MD, * *Elizabeth M. Alderman, MD*†

Objectives

After completing this article, readers should be able to:

1. Characterize the degree of use of illicit substances among adolescents.
2. Describe the most important treatment of substance abuse among adolescents.
3. Discuss the process required to make a diagnosis of substance abuse.
4. Explain the appropriate use of laboratory tests in the management of substance abuse.
5. Delineate the conditions for referral for treatment of an adolescent who is abusing drugs.

Introduction

Substance abuse among adolescents continues to be a serious problem. It affects all age groups, including the newborn of the addicted mother, the preadolescent exposed to various forms of drug use through the media, and the adolescent who is experimenting or addicted. Pediatricians can make a difference in the lives of all who are affected by substance abuse. First, they have an important responsibility in the prevention, diagnosis, and treatment of substance abuse. This should be fulfilled at every routine office visit with the preadolescent and adolescent and at prenatal visits with expectant parent(s). Second, they are role models and sources of information and support to patients and their families. Third, they can be leaders in their communities by participating in prevention programs that provide education in the schools.

Some pediatricians may avoid dealing with this issue because they feel that they are not sufficiently knowledgeable. Many may be uncomfortable with this topic because they fear alienating the patient or the family. Some also may be in denial that substance abuse could be a problem in their patients. Because it is well known that the patterns of lifetime substance abuse are established during adolescence, the necessity of becoming educated in its management is apparent.

Epidemiology

To manage substance abuse properly in the individual patient, it is important to know about the epidemiology of cigarette, alcohol, and illicit drug use. Two national surveys often are cited in describing the statistics and trends of substance abuse in the preadolescent and adolescent populations. The University of Michigan has been conducting the *Monitoring the Future (MTF) Survey* annually since 1975. It surveys 8th-, 10th-, and 12th-grade students in public and private high schools. The *Youth Risk Behavior Surveillance System (YRBSS)*, established by the Centers for Disease Control and Prevention, has been reporting on health risk behaviors, including substance use, in samples of high school and college students biennially since 1991. These studies likely underestimate overall substance use in the preadolescent and adolescent populations because the samples are only school-based.

Tobacco use has serious long-term effects on health. Despite this awareness, preadolescents and young adolescents are particularly drawn to its use. According to the most recent MTF study, lifetime tobacco use has remained about the same (70%) over the past 8 years. One fourth of students had reported lifetime daily cigarette use (defined as at least one cigarette every day for 30 d) to the YRBSS. Both surveys have shown

Fellow, Division of Adolescent Medicine, Department of Pediatrics.

†*Associate Professor, Clinical Pediatrics, Albert Einstein College of Medicine/Montefiore Medical Center, New York, NY.*

that children initiate cigarette use generally before 13 years of age.

Alcohol, a central nervous system depressant, is the psychoactive substance used most commonly by adolescents. According to the MTF survey, lifetime alcohol use by adolescents has remained steady at 50% over the past 8 years. The same survey reported that 80% of students have consumed alcohol by the end of high school, and 52% have done so by the 8th grade. One third of students reported that they had their first drink of alcohol before age 13 years. One third of students reported riding in a car with a driver who had been drinking alcohol, and 13% of students reported driving after drinking alcohol at least once during the 30 days prior to the survey.

Marijuana is the most commonly used illicit drug among high school students. It is a euphoriant and a hallucinogen. It can be smoked in a cigarette (joint), cigar (blunt), or pipe or ingested when baked into foods. In the 1999 YRBSS, 47% of students had used it during their lifetime, 26.7% had used it at least once during the 30 days prior to the survey, and 11.3% had tried marijuana before they were 13 years old. The MTF survey showed that lifetime use has increased since 1991.

The epidemiology and risk factors associated with illicit drug use were covered in an article by Kaul and Coupey last month (*Pediatr Rev.* 2001;23:85–94). Fortunately, not all adolescents at risk develop a substance abuse problem. It is important for the pediatrician to identify protective factors that promote abstinence. Various studies report that healthy relationships and open communication with parents and family members, family rituals (meals, celebrations, holidays), involvement with extracurricular school activities, worship/religious beliefs, self-esteem, assertiveness, personal success at socialization and academics, and ability to set limits are associated with decreased drug use. Other studies have shown that despite poor home environments, certain adolescents develop traits such as self-reliance, appropriate supportive relationships outside the home, and personal achievement, which decrease their risk for substance

abuse. Traits that also contribute to resilience are insight, initiative, creativity, humor, and morality.

Clinical Aspects

The pediatrician must be skilled in identifying the patient who is at risk for substance abuse as well as the patient who is using those substances. Having a high index of suspicion is important. Collecting information from parents and the patient's school can be valuable. If the patient has had interaction with the police, obtaining information from these records, if possible, is also important. The interview and physical examination are the most important tools for making the diagnosis. Laboratory tests should be used only under specific circumstances.

The interview should be conducted confidentially and nonjudgmentally and should address various areas of the patient's life. The patient's past medical history and family history, specifically any substance abuse and mental illness, should be explored. The acronym **HEADSSS** (**H**ome, **E**ducation, **A**ctivities, **D**rugs, **S**afety, **S**exuality, **S**uicide/depression) may help prompt questions to obtain a comprehensive psychosocial history. Another tool to assess health risk behaviors quickly is the GAPS (Guidelines for Adolescent Preventive Services) questionnaire, which can be completed while the patient is in the waiting room. The goal is to identify problems that require intervention, including risk-taking behaviors such as substance use. It is important to note that risk-taking behaviors, including substance abuse, high-risk sexual activity, and delinquency, tend to exist in clusters. If one risk-taking behavior is uncovered, there is a good chance that others also exist.

If a history of substance use is confirmed, it is important to identify the drugs being used, the frequency of use, and the circumstances under which they are used. Any drug-related dysfunction, such as delinquency, poor school performance, mood swings/personality changes, depression, isolation from family and friends, changes in sleep or eating habits, or associated risk-taking behavior under the influence of drugs such as drinking and driving and promiscuous sexual activity, should be thoroughly investigated and discussed. When a patient admits to substance abuse, he or she may minimize or exaggerate use, with the former being more likely. When a patient denies use, inappropriate or inconsistent responses to questions should raise suspicions about that denial. The findings on physical examination will help in constructing the full picture of the patient's use.

Most teenagers who are involved with drugs do not present to the doctor's office in an acute state of intoxication. In most instances, these patients are managed in the emergency department. In the doctor's office, symptoms may be subtle or nonexistent. Other times, a seemingly common complaint, such as headache, chronic cough, rhinorrhea, or epistaxis, overlies a substance abuse problem. Specific physical findings (Table 1) can be attributed to various drugs.

The use of laboratory tests in the diagnosis of substance abuse should be considered only in specific circumstances to augment information obtained during the interview and physical examination of the patient; they should not be used as the sole method of diagnosing abuse. Pediatricians should become familiar with the American Academy of Pediatrics (AAP) statement regarding the testing for drugs of abuse in children and adolescents in anticipation of potential associated ethical issues regarding consent and confidentiality that frequently arise. Screening and diagnostic testing in the older, competent adolescent may be carried out, with few exceptions, only with the patient's consent. Parental permission is not sufficient for involuntary screening or testing in these patients. To ignore this is to place the therapeutic relationship between the patient and the physician in jeopardy, creating an adversarial relationship in which trust is lost. Consent may be waived when the patient's competency is in doubt or when findings from the interview and physical examination strongly suggest that the patient is at high risk for serious harm from substance use and that this harm could be avoided if the substance is identified. Other indications for drug screening include emergent presentations of altered mental status, acute injuries that may have been due to drug abuse, life-threatening symptoms that require a correct diagnosis to

provide appropriate treatment, monitoring for abstinence in drug rehabilitation centers, and court-ordered drug testing. Results of testing are not to be shared with anyone other than the patient unless the patient gives permission or if a substance is found to be the cause of an acute medical problem, and additional care and monitoring are required.

Table 1. Possible Findings on Physical Examination Indicating Substance Abuse

General Findings
- Altered mood
- Poor dress/hygiene
- Inappropriate or strange behavior

Chronic Substance Abusers
- Mood swings
- Depression
- Paranoia
- Anxiety
- Poor hygiene
- Bizarre behavior

Vital Signs
- Weight loss
- Hypertension (cocaine, amphetamine)
- Hypotension (heroin)
- Hyperthermia (cocaine, amphetamine)
- Hypothermia (heroin)
- Tachycardia (marijuana, cocaine, amphetamine)

Ear-Nose-Throat
- Red eyes (marijuana)
- Dilated pupils (marijuana, cocaine, amphetamine)
- Constricted pupils (heroin)
- Nasal irritation

Cardiac
- Arrhythmias (heroin, cocaine, amphetamine)

Abdomen
- Hepatomegaly

Skin
- Abscesses
- Tattoos
- Needle track marks

Neurologic
- Altered sensorium
- Poor coordination
- Ataxia (amphetamine)
- Nystagmus
- Hyporeflexia or hyperreflexia (marijuana, cocaine, amphetamine)

If laboratory tests are employed, pediatricians should become familiar with the screening panels used to evaluate asymptomatic patients and the diagnostic tests used to confirm positive screening test results or to evaluate patients whose physical examination or interview results are suggestive of substance use. The capabilities and certification of laboratories also should be examined. The sensitivity and specificity of each test should be considered when reviewing results because false-positive and false-negative results do occur. False-positive results are usually due to cross-reactivity with substances that have similar structures, such as poppy seeds for narcotics, pseudoephedrine for amphetamines, and diphenhydramine for phencyclidine. False-negative results are due to pharmacokinetic characteristics of the test, technological shortcomings, and intentional alterations of the specimen by the person being tested. Some examples of intentional alterations of a urine sample are substitution with another person's urine, dilution with another fluid, addition of substances such as golden seal tea, and drinking of excessive fluids or use of a diuretic before sample submission. Test results can only provide information about one moment in time; positive results cannot define frequency, duration, or severity of drug use.

Management

The best treatment for substance abuse is prevention during each health supervision visit. Prevention can begin as early as the prenatal visit, during which the parent(s)' family history of substance abuse and their own history can be reviewed and appropriate counseling undertaken. The dangers of environmental tobacco and risk of harm to the child by caregivers who are impaired by substance use should be discussed. In early childhood, parental modeling of and exposure to alcohol and tobacco use through the media can be discussed.

The school-age visits are appropriate venues to encourage parents to begin to talk with their children about substance abuse. One technique for parents is to initiate such conversations when tobacco and alcohol use are observed on television as advertising or by characters in sitcoms/movies. The parent can ask the child what he or she thinks about what is being shown, why the substance is being used, if any schoolmates smoke or drink alcohol, if he or she ever has been offered a cigarette or alcohol, and how he or she feels about cigarettes and alcohol use. This will provide the parent with a framework for discussing substance use: possible dangers associated with substance use, responsible ways of dealing with friends who drink alcohol (designated driver, not getting into a car with someone who has been drinking), and methods of dealing with peer pressure (role playing). This discussion can lead to subsequent conversations about other drugs, such as marijuana, inhalants, and "hard" drugs. Pediatricians can provide parents with advice, written information, and resources (eg, Web sites, Table 2). Such information also can be disseminated outside the office through talks to school, religious, and community groups.

Late childhood (middle and junior high school) usually is when children begin to experiment with drugs. The pediatrician should have direct and confidential discussions with the patient on the subject. If the patient denies any use, encouragement and support can be given along with education and counseling about the effects of different drugs on the body and the health and safety hazards involved with their use. This should be approached in an interactive (asking questions, attentive listening) and objective (knowing the facts about substance abuse,

Table 2. Web Site Resources for Patients, Parents, and Physicians

- www.tipsonteens.com
- www.parentingresources.ncjrs.org
- www.adolescenthealth.org
- www.aap.org
- www.teengrowth.com
- www.raisingtodaysteens.org
- www.ama-assn.org/adolhlth
- www.tobaccofreekids.org
- www.cdc.gov/tobacco/
- www.health.org
- www.caas.brown.edu/plndp
- www.samhsa.gov
- www.cdc.gov/nccdphp/dash/yrbs—Youth Risk Behavior Surveillance System
- www.monitoringthefuture.org—Monitoring the Future Survey

nonjudgmental) manner in an effort to prevent even experimental drug use.

Once an adolescent is identified as having had some experience with drug use, the extent of drug use should be determined. A helpful staging system is the Five Stages of Adolescent Substance Abuse described by Comerci in 1985 (Table 3). Stage 1 describes adolescents who have not had any personal experience with drugs but are at high risk for future drug use. Screening for risk factors for substance abuse, as discussed in the article by Kaul and Coupey, can identify adolescents in this stage. Stage 2 is the experimentation stage in which patients "learn the euphoria." They use drugs such as tobacco, alcohol, and marijuana with their friends. Experimentation with drugs is very common among adolescents, but it should not be condoned or trivialized because of the potential for further use and subsequent abuse. This is the basis for the concept that tobacco, alcohol, and marijuana are "gateway drugs," the

first substances commonly tried because of their accessibility and perceived safety relative to other drugs. It is believed that adolescents are at high risk for substance abuse and other substance use once they have experimented with the gateway drugs. Stage 3 is defined as regular use in which adolescents are "seeking the euphoria." There is use of more illicit drugs, such as LSD and stimulants, and use is more frequent and solitary. Stage 4 is defined as regular (daily) use, "preoccupation with the high." There is loss of control, risk-taking, and estrangement from family and friends. Stage 5 is defined as burnout. Drugs are used to feel "normal" at this stage. Polysubstance abuse, deterioration of physical and mental health, self-destructive behavior, withdrawal, and shame are characteristic.

The management of substance abuse by the pediatrician depends on the extent of the problem, which can be based on the staging system for substance abuse just described and the *DSM-IV* (*Diagnostic and Statistical Manual of Mental Disorders*, 4th ed.) criteria for substance abuse and substance dependence (Tables 4 and 5). The AAP Committee on Substance Abuse has

Table 3. Stages of Adolescent Substance Abuse*

Stage 1: Potential for Abuse
- Decreased impulse control
- Need for immediate gratification
- Availability of tobacco, drugs, alcohol, inhalants
- Need for peer acceptance

Stage 2: Experimentation: Learning the Euphoria
- Use of inhalants, tobacco, marijuana, and alcohol with friends
- Few, if any, consequences
- May increase to regular weekend use
- Little change in behavior

Stage 3: Regular Use: Seeking the Euphoria
- Use of other drugs (eg, stimulants, LSD, sedatives)
- Behavioral changes and some consequences
- Increased frequency of use; use alone
- Buying or stealing drugs

Stage 4: Regular Use: Preoccupation With the "High"
- Daily use of drugs
- Loss of control
- Multiple consequences and risk-taking
- Estrangement from family and "sober" friends

Stage 5: Burnout: Use of Drugs to Feel Normal
- Use of multiple substances; cross-addiction
- Guilt, withdrawal, shame, remorse, depression
- Physical and mental deterioration
- Increased risk-taking, self-destructive or suicidal behavior

*Adapted from Comerci

Table 4. *DSM-IV** Criteria for Substance Abuse

1. A maladaptive pattern of substance use leading to clinically significant impairment or distress, as manifested by 1 or more of the following, occurring within a 12-month period:
   a. recurrent substance use resulting in a failure to fulfill major role obligations at work, school, or home (ie, repeated absences or poor work performance related to substance use; substance-related absences, suspensions, or expulsions from school; neglect of children or household)
   b. recurrent substance use in situations in which it is physically hazardous (ie, driving an automobile or operating a machine when impaired by substance use)
   c. recurrent substance-related legal problems (ie, arrests for substance-related disorderly conduct)
   d. continued substance use despite having persistent or recurrent social or interpersonal problems caused or exacerbated by the effects of the substance (ie, arguments with spouse about consequences of intoxication, physical fights)
2. The symptoms have never met the criteria for substance dependence for this class of substance.

*Diagnostic and Statistical Manual of Mental Disorders. 4th ed.

Table 5. *DSM-IV** Criteria for Substance Dependence

A maladaptive pattern of substance use, leading to clinically significant impairment or distress, as manifested by 3 or more of the following, occurring at any time in the same 12-month period:

1. tolerance, as defined by either of the following:
   a. a need for markedly increased amounts of the substance to achieve intoxication or desired effect
   b. markedly diminished effect with continued use of the same amount of the substance
2. withdrawal, as manifested by either of the following:
   a. the characteristic withdrawal syndrome for the substance
   b. the same (or a closely related) substance is taken to relieve or avoid withdrawal symptoms
3. the substance is often taken in larger amounts or over a longer period than was intended
4. there is a persistent desire or unsuccessful efforts to cut down or control substance use
5. a great deal of time is spent in activities necessary to obtain the substance (ie, visiting multiple doctors or driving long distances), use the substance (ie, chain-smoking), or recover from its effects
6. important social, occupational, or recreational activities are given up or reduced because of substance use
7. the substance use is continued despite knowledge of having a persistent or recurrent physical or psychological problem that is likely to have been caused or exacerbated by the substance (ie, current cocaine use despite recognition of cocaine-induced depression or continued drinking despite recognition that an ulcer was made worse by alcohol consumption)

*Diagnostic and Statistical Manual of Mental Disorders. 4th ed.

developed guidelines for management, as have others. Once the severity of drug use is determined, a decision can be made about whether management can continue by the pediatrician in the office or requires referral for mental health or specialized substance abuse evaluation and possible treatment. It is very helpful to identify other health professionals in the community for consultation who have specific drug abuse expertise.

In the early stages of adolescent substance abuse (stages 1 and 2), there usually are no adverse consequences or disruption in the patient's life. Education and counseling in the office and in-office follow-up generally is sufficient. The primary treatment for adolescents in stage 1 is prevention. If the adolescent is in stage 2, and there are adverse consequences associated with the drug use (injuries, legal troubles, decline in performance and attendance in school, or negative effects on health), intervention at the discretion of the physician should be initiated. At this point, family members should become involved in the therapeutic process. In addition to counseling, self-help groups (eg, Alcoholics Anonymous and Narcotics Anonymous), therapy with a social worker or peer counselor, and family therapy may be recommended. A contract between the physician, the patient, and the family can be established to define rules about tobacco, alcohol, and drug use. Follow-up visits should be scheduled on a monthly basis initially to monitor for any continued drug use and associated dysfunction. These visits are opportunities for constructing smoking cessation plans, giving anticipatory guidance on safety (drinking and driving, designated drivers), discussing alternative drug-free activities, and providing positive reinforcement when efforts at drug abstinence are successful. It also is important to provide the patient and the family with resources (eg, Web sites) during these visits. There are no indications for the use of laboratory testing for drugs at stage 1 or 2.

According to AAP guidelines, if office management of adolescent substance abuse fails or if an adolescent meets the criteria for stage 3 to 5 or the *DSM-IV* criteria for substance abuse or dependence, he or she must be referred or admitted to a treatment program. It is important for pediatricians to seek out programs that view substance abuse as a disease, have a strict abstinence policy, and include strong integration of the family in the therapeutic process. Guidelines for where referred patients should be placed are being established by managed care organizations and have been defined by the American Society of Addiction Medicine (ASAM) based on various criteria or "dimensions" (Table 6). These six criteria describe conditions and complications (biomedical, emotional, behavioral, and environmental) that influence how safely and successfully an adolescent undergoing treatment would recover from substance abuse. For example, early intervention (level 0.5) is for adolescents who do not have withdrawal risk or coexisting unstable conditions

Table 6. Adolescent Substance Use: Criteria for Levels of Intervention*

Criteria Dimensions	Levels of Intervention				
	Level 0.5 Early Intervention	Level 1 Outpatient Treatment	Level 2 Intensive Outpatient Treatment	Level 3 Medically Monitored Intensive Inpatient Treatment	Level 4 Medically Managed Intensive Inpatient Treatment
1. Acute intoxication and/or withdrawal potential	No withdrawal risk	No withdrawal risk	Manifests no overt symptoms of withdrawal risk	Risk of withdrawal syndrome present but manageable in Level 3	Severe withdrawal risk
2. Biomedical conditions and complications	None or very stable	None or very stable	None, or if present, do not distract from addiction treatment; manageable at Level 2	Requires medical monitoring but not intensive treatment	Requires 24-hr medical and nursing care
3. Emotional/behavioral conditions and complications	None or very stable	None or manageable in an outpatient structured environment	Mild severity, with the potential to distract from recovery efforts	Moderate severity; requires 24-hr structured setting	Severe problems require 24-hr psychiatric care, with concomitant addiction treatment
4. Treatment acceptance/resistance	Willing to understand how current use may affect personal goals	Willing to cooperate, but needs motivating and monitoring strategies	Resistance high enough to require structured program, but not so high as to render outpatient treatment ineffective	Resistance high despite negative consequences; needs intensive motivating strategies in a 24-hr structured setting	Problems in this dimension do not qualify patient for Level 4 treatment
5. Relapse/continued use potential	Needs understanding of or skills to change current use pattern	Able to maintain abstinence and recovery goals with minimal support	Intensification of addiction symptoms; high likelihood of relapse without close monitoring and support	Unable to control use despite active participation in less intensive program; needs 24-hr structure	Problems in this dimension do not qualify patient for Level 4 treatment
6. Recovery environment	Social support system or significant others increase risk of personal conflict about alcohol/other drug use	Supportive recovery environment and/or patient has skills to cope	Environment unsupportive, but with structure or support, patient can cope	Environment dangerous for recovery, necessitating removal from the environment; logistical impediments to outpatient treatment	Problems in this dimension do not qualify patient for Level 4 treatment

* Approximate summary to illustrate the principal concepts and structure of the criteria.

Adapted from the American Society of Addiction Medicine.

(biomedical, emotional, or behavioral); are willing to receive treatment; want to make the change required to recover; and have a strong support systems inside and outside the home. In contrast, medically managed intensive inpatient treatment (level 4) is recommended for adolescents who are in severe withdrawal, have biomedical conditions that require 24-hour medical and nursing care, or have severe psychiatric problems that require 24-hour psychiatric care.

There are four levels of intervention in the treatment of adolescents who have substance abuse problems (Table 7). Early intervention programs and outpatient treatment involve a skilled counselor who has back-up resources and includes office management and self-help groups such as Alcoholics Anonymous and Narcotics Anonymous. Intensive outpatient treatment programs are managed by a multidisciplinary team and are located in hospitals or community-based health clinics. Examples of medically monitored intensive inpatient treatment

Table 7. Description of Interventions

Early Intervention and Outpatient Treatment
- Office management by pediatrician
- Skilled counselor with backup resources (eg, psychiatrist)
- Self-help groups (Alcoholics Anonymous, Narcotics Anonymous)

Intensive Outpatient Treatment
- Located in hospital-based outpatient clinics or community-based health clinics
- Methadone maintenance for narcotic addiction
- Multidisciplinary team, generally consisting of substance abuse counselors, psychiatrists, and social workers in consultation with the primary physician

Medically Monitored Intensive Inpatient Treatment
- Located in therapeutic communities, half-way homes, group homes
- Ideal for situations when environmental changes are needed
- For patients who have run away or those who do not respond to intensive outpatient treatment

Medically Managed Intensive Inpatient Treatment
- Hospital inpatient unit
- For patients undergoing withdrawal or who have suicidal ideation, deterioration of emotional and physical condition that threatens their life, or behavior that threatens the lives of their family and friends
- For patients who do not respond to all other treatments

programs are therapeutic communities, half-way houses, and group homes. These are ideal when environmental changes are required to facilitate recovery. Methadone maintenance programs are intensive outpatient treatments for those who are addicted to narcotics.

Candidates for inpatient treatment have significant psychiatric illnesses; are undergoing withdrawal; have suicidal ideation, runaway behavior, deterioration of their emotional and physical condition that threatens their lives, or behavior that threatens the lives of their family and friends; or have not responded to intensive outpatient treatment.

A high prevalence of psychiatric disorders, such as depression and psychoses, has been reported in substance abusers who receive inpatient treatment. It is unclear whether the psychiatric symptoms are due to the substance abuse or to the psychiatric diagnosis, which is why a comprehensive psychosocial evaluation and physical and mental status examinations are important. If a patient does not do well or fails treatment, there should be a high index of suspicion for a coexisting psychiatric diagnosis. Patients who have psychiatric symptoms require appropriate referral to a treatment program where a mental health specialist is available.

Prognosis

Recovering from substance abuse is a lifelong process. A high risk for relapse always exists and is an expected part of recovery. The pediatrician's role is to provide support and additional referral if relapse occurs. Pediatricians should maintain close follow-up during and after treatment regardless of whether the patient is referred or treated in the office.

Suggested Reading

American Academy of Pediatrics, Committee on Substance Abuse. Indications for management and referral of patients involved in substance abuse. *Pediatrics.* 2000;106:143–148

American Academy of Pediatrics, Committee on Substance Abuse. Role of the pediatrician in prevention and management of substance abuse. *Pediatrics.* 1993;91:1010–1013

American Academy of Pediatrics, Committee on Substance Abuse. Testing for drugs of abuse in children and adolescents. *Pediatrics.* 1996;98:305–307

American Academy of Pediatrics, Committee on Substance Abuse. Tobacco, alcohol, and other drugs. The role of the pediatrician in prevention and management of substance abuse. *Pediatrics.* 1998;101:125–128

American Psychiatric Association. *Diagnostic and Statistical Manual of Mental Disorders.* 4th ed. Washington, DC: American Psychiatric Association; 1994

Brown RT, Coupey SM. Illicit drugs of abuse. *Adolescent Medicine: State of the Art Reviews.* 1993;4:321–339

Comerci GD. Recognizing the 5 stages of substance abuse. *Contemp Pediatr.* 1985;2:57–68

Elster AB, Kuzsets N. *Guidelines for Adolescent Preventive Services (GAPS).* Baltimore, Md: Williams & Wilkins; 1993

Fuller PG, Cavanaugh RM. Basic assessment and screening for substance abuse in the pediatrician's office. *Pediatr Clin North Am.* 1995;42:295–307

Goldenring JM, Cohen E. Getting into adolescent heads. *Contemp Pediatr.* 1988;5:75–90

Heyman RB, Adger H. Office approach to drug abuse prevention. *Pediatr Clin North Am.* 1997;44:1447–1455

Johnston LD, O'Malley PM, Bachman JG. *The Monitoring the Future National Results on Adolescent Drug Use (Overview of Key Findings, 1999).* Washington, DC: The University of Michigan, Institute for Social Research; National Institute on Drug Abuse; United States Department of Health and Human Services; 2000

Kann L, Kinchen SA, Williams BI, et al. Youth risk behavior surveillance - United States, 1999. *MMWR: CDC Surveillance Summaries.* Atlanta, Ga: United States Department of Health and Human Services, Centers for Disease Control and Prevention; 2000

Mee-Lee D. *ASAM Patient Placement Criteria for the Treatment of Substance-Related Disorders.* 2nd ed. Chevy Chase, Md: The American Society of Addiction Medicine, Inc; 1996

Schwartz B, Alderman EM. Substances of abuse. *Pediatr Rev.* 1997;13:204–215

Office Management of Substance Use

by Sharon Levy, MD, MPH, FAAP, and John R. Knight, MD, FAAP

Substance use by adolescents is a problem commonly encountered in pediatric practice. This paper, which focuses on the screening, assessment, and management of adolescents at risk, opens with a brief review of the epidemiology and consequences of substance use.

Epidemiology

Substance use by adolescents is a major public health problem in the United States. Alcohol, tobacco, and marijuana are the drugs most commonly used by teens. One recent survey,[1] found that by the end of high school, 80% of teens have consumed alcohol (more than a few sips), 61% have tried cigarettes, and 49% have used marijuana. More than half (54%) have used an illicit drug before finishing high school, up from a low of 41% in 1992. There has been a dramatic increase in use of 3,4- methylenedioxymethamphetamine (MDMA or "Ecstasy") during recent years; 5.8% of high school seniors reported ever using Ecstasy in 1998, compared to 11.7% in 2001.

All adolescents, regardless of demographic, racial, or ethnic factors, are at risk for substance use and associated problems. There is little difference in drug use between urban and nonurban youth. African American youth have substantially lower rates of drug use than do white teens and rates among Hispanic youngsters generally fall in the middle. Males have higher rates of illicit drug use and heavy drinking than females. Teens with plans to attend college are considerably less likely to use illicit substances, drink heavily, or smoke than are those who are not college-bound.[1]

Consequences of Substance Use

Alcohol and other drug use are associated with the 3 leading causes of death among American

Learning Objectives

After reading this article, pediatricians will be better able to identify and intervene on behalf of adolescents who are engaged in problematic use of drugs or alcohol, and should be better prepared to:

- Discuss the epidemiology of adolescent substance use, including trends in the extent of use and common drugs of abuse
- Recognize the potential consequences of the misuse of alcohol and drugs
- Describe techniques for interviewing adolescents about their use of alcohol and drugs
- Discuss screening tests that may be employed in the office setting to identify adolescents at risk
- Explain the role of laboratory testing in the detection of adolescent substance use
- Employ brief intervention techniques for teens who are using drugs or alcohol and support continued abstinence for those who are not
- Recognize and counsel adolescents who require referral
- Manage parent/child conflicts concerning substance abuse, including requests by parents to have their adolescents' urine tested

Sharon Levy, MD, MPH, FAAP, is an instructor in pediatrics at the Harvard Medical School and an associate investigator at the Center for Adolescent Substance Abuse Research at Children's Hospital Boston (CHB). Dr Levy also serves as director of pediatrics for the Adolescent Substance Abuse Program at CHB. John R. Knight, MD, FAAP, is an assistant professor of pediatrics at the Harvard Medical School (HMS) and the associate director for medical education at the HMS Division on Addictions. Dr Knight is also director of the Center for Adolescent Substance Abuse Research at CHB.

teens: accidents, homicide, and suicide.[2] Mortality from unintentional vehicular injury is a particular concern because adolescents are novice drivers. In 2001, the U.S. Centers for Disease Control and Prevention (CDC) reported that greater than 1 in 3 motor vehicle fatalities among adolescents 15 to 20 years old were associated with the use of alcohol,[3] making driving under the influence of alcohol more dangerous for teens than for adults.[4] This number would certainly be higher if other drugs were included. Alcohol and drug use are also implicated in other types of fatal accidents and serious health risks (eg, weapon-carrying, truancy, and early sexual activity).[5-10]

Early experimentation with drugs and alcohol is associated with increased risk of long-term substance abuse and dependence in adulthood; the youngest adolescents are at greatest risk.[11] Adolescent substance use is particularly damaging, as the adolescent brain is not fully mature and the neuropsychological changes caused by some substances, such as MDMA, appear to be irreversible.[12] Therefore, some teens who use drugs may never achieve their full intellectual potential.

Screening

Given the high rates of alcohol and drug use by teens, adolescents should be asked about drug use at each yearly health maintenance visit.[13-15] However, a recent survey of pediatricians found that less than half screen all of their adolescent patients for drug use.[16] Perceived lack of time, reimbursement, screening tools, intervention strategies, and effective treatments are likely the most significant barriers to clinician screening.[17]

A number of valid and reliable self-administered screening questionnaires are available, including the Drug and Alcohol Problem Quickscreen,[18] the Problem Oriented Screening Instrument for Teenagers (POSIT)[19] and the Alcohol Use Disorders Identification Test (AUDIT).[20] However, questionnaires are not practical in all office settings and may pose a risk to adolescents' confidentiality when parents are present.

An alternative is to discuss sensitive issues such as alcohol and drug use privately (when parents have left the examination room). Not all adolescents will be completely truthful in responding to questions about substance use. A few simple techniques may increase the likelihood of getting honest answers. Physician and teen should review confidentiality provisions before these conversations take place.[21] Ask about substance use in a straightforward, nonthreatening way. Many pediatricians begin with a normalizing statement, such as "The next questions I'm going to ask are things that I ask *all* my patients about." Employ simple phrasing that leaves little room for interpretation. One approach is to begin with the following three questions:

1. Have you ever smoked a cigarette?
2. Have you ever had an alcoholic drink?
3. Have you ever used marijuana or any other drug to get high?

Including the word "ever" in each sentence yields a more clear and sensitive question than, for example, "Do you drink?" Some experienced clinicians prefer to begin the conversation with a discussion of drug use by peers and friends to break the ice. Even teens who do not report any drug use within their peer groups should be asked about personal use, as many teens have multiple circles of friends with varying drug use. Specifically screen all teens, including those who say that they have never used alcohol or drugs, for the risk of riding with an intoxicated driver.

Teens who answer "no" to all 3 of the above questions and are functioning well require little additional substance use assessment. Regardless of how patients answer these questions, however, the veracity of a response should be questioned if there are problems at school, difficulties at home, or conflicts with police. Also, if a parent presents with concerns regarding drug use the physician should probe further.

Further screening is recommended for adolescents who answer "yes" to any of the 3 initial questions. Our office employs the CRAFFT test (Figure 1), which consists of 6 orally administered questions that simultaneously screen for drug and alcohol problems. The CRAFFT test is brief, developmentally appropriate, easy to administer and score, and it has been well validated with adolescents.[22] Each "yes" answer scores one point, and

Figure 1. The CRAFFT questions

C_ Have you ever ridden in a **CAR** driven by someone (including yourself) who was 'high' or had been using alcohol or drugs?

R_ Do you ever use alcohol or drugs to **RELAX**, feel better about yourself, or fit in?

A_ Do you ever use alcohol or drugs while you are by yourself, **ALONE?**

F_ Do you ever **FORGET** things you did while using alcohol or drugs?

F_ Do your family or **FRIENDS** ever tell you that you should cut down on your drinking or drug use?

T_ Have you ever gotten into **TROUBLE** while you were using alcohol or drugs?

Copyright Children's Hospital Boston 1999. Reproduced with permission from the Center for Adolescent Substance Abuse Research (CeASAR) at Children's Hospital Boston.

a total score of 2 or more indicates high risk for a serious substance-related problem or disorder.

Assessment

Patients with a CRAFFT score of 2 or higher require additional assessment, either at follow-up or via referral to a mental health professional.

HISTORY

The first step in assessment is a complete substance use history. Ask what substances the teen is using. For each psychoactive substance, inquire about duration of use, how the pattern of use has changed over time, what the current pattern is, and whether he or she has ever tried to cut down or quit. Include questions about problems that have been associated with use of each substance (eg, trips to the emergency room after drinking alcohol, or arrests or school suspensions due to marijuana use). One useful question is "What's the worst thing that ever happened to you when you were drinking or using drugs?"

Once this history has been completed for each of the teen's "preferred" drugs, ask whether he or she has tried using other drugs to get high. Ask about inhalants, Ecstasy and other club drugs, stimulants, cocaine, opioids (eg, codeine, oxycodone, or dextromethorphan), benzodiazepines (eg, diazepam, clonazepam), phencyclidine (PCP), lysergic acid (LSD), over-the-counter medications, prescription drugs, or any other substance. Ask the patient when he or she last was intoxicated, and with which substance.

Teens who use drugs other than alcohol and marijuana tend to have more serious health and/or legal problems. Ask about illnesses (current, chronic, or recurrent), hospitalizations, surgeries, current medications, sexual experiences, and school functioning, with an emphasis on the potential impact of drug use on each of these areas. Finally, take a family history, including an extended family history of mental illness and substance use. Patients with a strong family history of substance abuse or dependence are more likely than their peers to abuse substances as teens and to have continued problems as adults.[23,24]

PHYSICAL EXAMINATION

A general screening physical is part of a thorough substance abuse assessment. Signs of acute intoxication, such as vital sign irregularities (brady- or tachycardia, hypertension), erythema of the conjunctivae, or pupil irregularities, are unusual in the primary care setting but of great diagnostic importance if present. Signs of chronic drug use are also unusual in teens, but may include inflammation or erosion of the nasal mucosa from insufflation of powdered drugs or skin lesions resulting from injection drug use. A careful assessment for wheezing should be performed on any adolescent who smokes tobacco, marijuana, or another drug. Hepatomegaly or right upper quadrant tenderness may be seen with chronic heavy drinking or hepatitis from infectious causes.

It may be of therapeutic educational value to tell the patient what you are checking for during each part of the physical examination. Any positive physical findings related to substance use should be discussed with the teen.

LABORATORY TESTING

Laboratory testing for alcohol and other drugs is generally not indicated as a screening procedure, but may be part of the assessment for a substance use disorder. Liver enzyme tests, such as carbohydrate-deficient transferrin (CDT) or gamma-glutamyl transpeptidase (GGT), may be elevated in some adolescents who engage in frequent heavy drinking, and this finding may be useful to motivate behavior change. Urine drug testing may have value in certain circumstances, but has limitations that few parents understand. (Please see the section on "Parent/Child Conflicts" on page 540 and "Consultant's Corner" in this edition of *AAP News* for further discussion.)

Intervention

Screening and assessment are necessary to identify the adolescent's stage of use, which indicates the needed level of intervention. Those who are abstinent should receive anticipatory guidance and positive feedback. Those reporting experimentation or nonproblematic use should receive brief advice aimed at risk reduction. Motivational interviewing and/or referral for more intensive treatment are indicated when there is problem use, abuse, or dependence.

ANTICIPATORY GUIDANCE

Teens who have never used drugs should be encouraged and supported. Ask these patients what strategies they have used or could imagine using to avoid drugs in the future. Ask those who have never been offered drugs whether they have a plan for such an eventuality, and what that plan would be. Reinforce patients' healthy choices and remind them that they can talk to you in confidence about drugs at any time.

Anticipatory guidance regarding substance use should be aimed at both children and parents. When parents ask how they can help their children avoid substance use problems, advise them to set a good example by drinking responsibly, never driving after drinking, avoiding illicit drugs, and establishing clear expectations that their children will not drink or use drugs. Consumption of small amounts of alcohol in religious or social settings with parental supervision are exceptions to this rule.

Not all parents understand that they should never permit their teens to get drunk or allow children's friends to drink in their home. Some parents believe that "supervised" teen drinking while a parent is at home is "safe." These are

situations that lead to tragedy, and parents may be held legally responsible.

RISK REDUCTION

Teens who answer "yes" to the first CRAFFT question, as well as those who report occasionally using alcohol and/or drugs, should be given brief advice regarding risks related to driving after drinking or using drugs. All teens should be reminded of the hazards of riding with an intoxicated driver. Some clinicians give patients a copy of the "Contract for Life," and urge them to discuss it with their parents, and sign it. The Contract for Life, created by Students Against Destructive Decisions (www.saddonline.com), establishes a written pact between teen and parents. The teen promises to do his or her best to remain alcohol- and drug-free. Both parents and teen agree that they will always wear a seatbelt and that they will neither drive after using drugs or alcohol nor ride in a car driven by someone who is impaired. The parents promise to provide a safe ride home, at any time and under any circumstances, if the teen calls for one. We suggest arranging a follow-up appointment with these teens to discuss whether or not they were able to contract with their parents and, if not, what other methods they might use to minimize future risk.

COMMITMENT TO ABSTAIN FROM DRUG USE

Teens who have used alcohol or drugs and who score 2 or higher on the CRAFFT test are often amenable to a time-limited trial of abstinence, which can be used as a diagnostic "challenge." In proposing this to the teen, give feedback about the risks of substance use, acknowledge that the teen is in control, offer clear advice to stop using, and then discuss making a commitment to abstain from all alcohol and drug use. Clarify misconceptions about drugs in a nonjudgmental fashion. In our clinic, we ask teens to sign a contract with specific provisions (no use of alcohol or any other drug, no riding in a car with a driver who has been drinking or using other drugs) for a given period of time, usually 1 to 3 months. We explain to teens that before the period is over we will plan a follow-up visit to discuss their success. We give positive reinforcement to teens who are

---

Case Study #1

Risk Reduction

The Patient:

Jimmy is a healthy 15-year-old boy who presents to your office for his annual physical. Neither he nor his mother have any particular concerns. After speaking briefly with Jimmy and his mother together, you interview him privately about alcohol and drug use. He says that he has been drunk 3 times in the past 2 months. He has never smoked tobacco or marijuana, nor has he tried other drugs. His CRAFFT score is 1. His relationships with family and friends are stable. He is doing well in school and has not experienced legal difficulties.

Feedback:

"Jimmy, I am glad that you have not yet had any problems related to alcohol, but I am worried about you because getting drunk is dangerous. Every year kids die in car crashes and other accidents related to drinking. This is a leading cause of death for kids your age."

Acknowledging the patient is in control and giving advice:

"Only you can decide whether or not you are going to drink. My recommendation is that you do not drink, at least until you are older. However, what I am most concerned about is your riding in a car with friends who have been drinking, because that can lead to tragedy. I recommend to all my patients that they make a promise to themselves to never ride in a car with someone who has been using alcohol or drugs."

(You present a copy of the "Teen Education Handout")

"Please look this over. It gives some ideas for ways to get home if you find yourself in trouble. Many parents are also willing to make an agreement that they will pick you up any time without asking questions until the next morning when you are ready to talk about it."

Issuing the Challenge:

"I can help you talk to your parents and arrange an agreement, without telling them any of the details of what we have discussed. Would you be willing to come back in a few weeks with your parents so that we can discuss it?"

Jimmy accepts the handout but doesn't comment on it. He agrees to make a follow-up visit in 1 month.

---

successful, and encourage them to continue to abstain from drug use. Patients who are not successful are more likely to have an alcohol or drug use disorder and should be referred for more intensive assessment and treatment. Patients who refuse to make a commitment not to use drugs or alcohol should be encouraged to reduce their use and counseled regarding risk reduction. Ask these patients to promise that, at the very least, they will not drive after using or ride with anyone who has, and try to persuade them to return for follow up within a few weeks.

MOTIVATIONAL INTERVIEWING

Motivational interviewing is a counseling style that encourages patients to change problem behaviors.[25] It is based on a core assumption that motivation is a product of interpersonal interaction and not an inherent character trait. The physician encourages the patient to change by exploring discrepancies between goals and current behavior. A second assumption is that ambivalence toward change is normal and acceptable. According to this view, adolescents who use alcohol and drugs are in constant conflict, simultaneously experiencing both positive and negative feelings about it. Their "decisional balance" can be viewed as an old-fashioned pan scale, with the pros and cons of substance use represented by the relative weights on the 2 sides. The role of the counselor is to tip the balance of the scale in favor of positive behavioral change.

Motivational interviewing employs four key strategies:

- *Empathize* — Offer unconditional positive regard for your patients, but not their behavior, and try to understand their point of view.
- *Develop discrepancy* — Explore discrepancies between your patient's words and actions, as well as between stated goals and current behaviors.
- *Roll with resistance* — Resistance is a natural response to confrontation; avoid arguing because it only increases resistance.
- *Support self-efficacy* — Patients will only attempt to change their behavior if they believe they can be successful. Encourage your patients by pointing out their strengths and expressing belief in their ability to change.

Although a full discussion of motivational interviewing is beyond the scope of this article, it is a concept worth pursuing (see Miller and Rollnick in resource list).

REFERRAL FOR TREATMENT

The first step in substance abuse treatment for any teen at risk of acute withdrawal from alcohol, opioids, or benzodiazepines, is hospital-based inpatient detoxification. Those with suspected psychiatric or psychological comorbidities who are not at risk of acute withdrawal should be referred to a mental health provider for further assessment and comprehensive treatment.

Teens with less serious problems who are unwilling or unable to change their behavior with the limited support available in a primary care office should be referred for more intensive treatment. This usually takes the form of individual or group therapy specifically targeted at substance abuse. Resources vary by locality. The Substance Abuse and Mental Health Services Administration (SAMHSA) provides a treatment locator on the Internet (http://www.findtreatment.samhsa.gov).

Parent/Child Conflicts

One of the most challenging situations in a primary care office is deciding what to do when a parent demands a drug test against the will of an adolescent. The physician must acknowledge and evaluate the concerns of the parents while maintaining the patient's trust. Speak briefly with the parent about why he or she would like a drug test.

Case Study #2

Commitment to Abstain from Alcohol and Drug Use

The Patient:

Betty is a 17-year-old girl who comes to your office for follow-up after an emergency room visit because of acute alcohol intoxication. She gives a history of drinking at parties on most weekends and smoking marijuana occasionally. She has also tried Ecstasy, cocaine, and "magic mushrooms." Her grades have fallen during the last quarter and she was dropped from the girls' basketball team as a result. Her parents took away her use of the car after the most recent incident and Betty is frustrated because this forces her to ride the school bus every morning. Betty does not think that alcohol or drugs are a problem for her, and tells you "I could stop if I wanted to, I just don't want to."

Feedback using motivational interviewing

"Betty I understand that you don't think that your drinking is a problem, but it certainly seems to be standing in the way of your parents returning your car privileges."

Advice and Issuing the Challenge

"You know, even teens with serious drug and alcohol problems often believe that they can stop, but it almost always turns out to be impossible for them. One way for us to find out if you have lost control or not, and an important first step for rebuilding trust with your parents, is to have you try not using for a while, let's say the next 60 days. Do you think you could do it?"

Betty agrees to give it a try. She also agrees to return to see you in the office in six weeks to discuss how it is going.

It may be best to have this conversation without the teen present. After clarifying the parents' specific questions, first validate their concerns. Explain the limits of laboratory testing and the possibility that it may compromise what is now a trusting physician/patient relationship. Advise that the information they have provided, coupled with a thorough, confidential history and physical, is the most sensitive and specific means of assessing drug use. Specify that information provided by the teen will be kept confidential unless there are concerns for the teen's safety.

The next step is to interview the adolescent privately, beginning with an explanation of confidentiality and its limits. A useful way to open further discussion is simply to ask "Why did your

---

Case Study #3

The Motivational Interview

The Patient:

Sara is a 16-year-old girl who comes to your office at her mother's insistence because of marijuana use. When interviewed privately, Sara admits to smoking marijuana for the past two years, but denies drinking alcohol, smoking tobacco, or using other drugs. Her CRAFFT score is 4. You take a substance use history and find that last year Sara smoked marijuana about once a month, but increased her use over the summer and is currently smoking 4 to 5 times a week. Sara's parents have grounded her on several occasions. Her grades have dropped at school, which she blames on a "bad geometry teacher and a history teacher who doesn't like me." She has not been suspended or arrested, though she once had to run from a party when the police came. Medical history is noncontributory. Family history is negative for emotional problems or substance use disorders. You note that when asked whether her 12-year-old sister has ever smoked marijuana Sara becomes defensive and says, "I would never let her try weed." Throughout the interview Sara insists that smoking marijuana is not a problem for her, and that she has no intention of changing. You decide to use motivational interviewing to encourage behavioral change.

Developing a Discrepancy:

"Sara, you told me several times that smoking marijuana does not cause problems, yet you also told me that since you started smoking you have been fighting more with your parents and your grades at school have fallen. Like your parents, I'm worried about you."

Sara replies that her grades were unrelated to marijuana use and that her parents were "worried about nothing." "Everyone in my school smokes, including some of the students on the Honor Roll," she insists. "Smoking has nothing to do with anything."

Rolling with Resistance:

"OK, then let's talk about something else. I'm curious about why you would want to keep your younger sister away from marijuana, since smoking doesn't cause any problems." Sara replies, "My sister is too young — she could get into trouble if she doesn't know what she is doing."

"So it sounds like marijuana can cause problems sometimes."

"Not really, not unless you are too young and don't know what your doing. Are we almost finished?"

Empathizing and Supporting Self Efficacy:

"I'm sorry if this conversation is difficult for you. It's just that I'm very worried about you. You really have some wonderful qualities, like the way you would like to protect your sister. I believe you have a lot of potential, but I'm afraid that continuing to use marijuana will stand in the way of your future. In some ways you really have thought a lot about marijuana. Would you agree to think about it some more and come back and talk to me again in a week or two? Also, in the meantime, would you at least agree to not ride in a car with a driver who has been using marijuana, alcohol, or any other drugs? I care about your health and just don't want to see you get injured."

Sara agrees to a follow-up appointment in two weeks and to not ride in a car with a driver who has been using alcohol or drugs.

parents feel you needed to see me today? Why do you think they want you to have a drug test?"

When there is a discrepancy between history obtained from a teen and that obtained from the parent, or when a parent remains suspicious despite a teen's denial of drug use, the physician may decide to give the teen the option to take a drug test. From a teen's perspective, the test can be done to support his or her denial of use. Both teen and parent should understand the reason for performing a test and the limits of testing. The physician should emphasize that a negative test indicates only that none of the substances in the test panel were detected in the urine. Since the half-life of most drugs is brief, a negative drug test generally indicates no use within the past 24 to 48 hours. Marijuana is a notable exception; urine tests can remain positive for weeks in chronic users. A single positive urine test for cannabis indicates that a teen has used marijuana, it does not confirm a diagnosis of a substance use disorder. Passive inhalation of marijuana will cause positive drug tests only when exposure has been significant. This may occur if a teen intentionally remains in a small, poorly ventilated space (such as a car) with many smokers; and should be considered a true positive. Please see "Consultant's Corner" for further information.

In some instances an adolescent will refuse to give a urine sample despite staunch denial of substance use. Although this raises concern that the adolescent may be using substances, *the American Academy of Pediatrics clearly states that testing against the will of a competent adolescent is not recommended.* In these cases we recommend close follow-up with child and parent. The true history will almost certainly become apparent with time.

Home drug testing kits have been on the market since 1995, and now parents can easily obtain them from the Internet. Given the complexity of drug testing and the difficulty of interpreting the results, we do not believe that home testing kits provide enough support for parents to get meaningful information from this procedure. Further, parents who drug test their children at home are at risk of damaging their relationship with their teens. *Therefore, we do not recommend that parents use home drug testing products under any circumstances.*

A second common dilemma that occurs in the pediatric office regarding substance use is the issue of when to breach confidentiality. It is helpful to set confidentiality rules prior to taking the history from an adolescent. We recommend telling the patient that confidentiality will be maintained unless acute safety concerns arise. Determining when a patient's safety is at risk is a

Confidentiality Tips

- As a general rule, the older the patient, the more confidentiality can be afforded.
- Physicians cannot maintain complete confidentiality for patients who need acute hospitalization or residential treatment.
- Confidentiality should be breached if a patient is at risk of harming him/herself or others.
- When confidentiality must be breached, the specific reasons and the information to be revealed should be discussed with the teen prior to the discussion with parents. The physician should limit revealing details and focus on the need for treatment.
- If parents request a copy of the written medical record, they should be discouraged and told that such a breach of confidentiality may damage the physician patient relationship and limit the potential for further therapeutic intervention. (Laws regulating such demands vary by state.)
- Physicians should include relevant information only in the chart (ie, only that information used to make the diagnosis or treatment plan). Specific details, such as who supplies drugs, who uses drugs with the patient, etc need not be recorded in the chart.
- Certain information (substance abuse treatment) in clinic records may be protected under special federal confidentiality rules (42 CFR, Part 2) and can only be released with specific signed consent; a general medical release form is not adequate for this purpose. These pages should be signaled in the chart, by placing a header on top of the note or by using a different color paper.

matter of clinical judgment. The box at left provides a set of guidelines to help physicians determine whether confidentiality should be breached.

Conclusion

Substance use is common among American teenagers. Primary care health supervision visits provide an opportunity for assessment, brief intervention, and treatment. All teens should be asked confidentially about substance use at each primary care visit. Those who have ever used substances should be further assessed using the CRAFFT questions. Pediatricians can give important risk reduction information to teens who have not had problems associated with substance use and provide brief interventions for those who have had problems related to alcohol or illicit drugs.

PRINT RESOURCES

American Academy of Pediatrics, Committee on Substance Abuse. Alcohol use and abuse: a pediatric concern. *Pediatrics.* 2001;108:185–189

American Academy of Pediatrics, Committee on Substance Abuse. Testing for drugs of abuse in children and adolescents. *Pediatrics.* 1996;98:305–307

American Academy of Pediatrics, Committee on Substance Abuse. *Testing Your Teen for Illicit Drugs: Information for Parents.* [Patient education brochure available from the Academy through the AAP Web site (www.aap.org) or by calling 888/227-1770]

American Academy of Pediatrics, Committee on Substance Abuse. Tobacco, alcohol, and other drugs: the role of the pediatrician in prevention and management of substance abuse. *Pediatrics.* 1998;101:125–128

American Academy of Pediatrics. *Substance Abuse: A Guide for Health Professionals.* 2nd ed. Elk Grove Village, IL: American Academy of Pediatrics; 2002

Miller WR, Rollnick S. *Motivational Interviewing: Preparing People for Change.* 2nd ed. New York, NY: Guilford Press; 2002

INTERNET RESOURCES

National Clearinghouse for Alcohol and Drug Information
http://www.health.org/

National Institute on Drug Abuse
http://www.nida.nih.gov/

National Institute on Alcohol Abuse and Alcoholism
http://www.niaaa.nih.gov/

Substance Abuse & Mental Health Services Administration
http://www.samhsa.gov/

Students Against Destructive Decisions
http://www.saddonline.com/

Acknowledgment

The editors would like to acknowledge technical review by Richard B. Heyman, MD, FAAP, for the AAP Section on Adolescent Health.

The authors would like to acknowledge support from grant R01 AA12165 from The National Institute on Alcohol Abuse and Alcoholism and The Substance Abuse and Mental Health Services Administration; grants 36126, 45222 and 40557 from The Robert Wood Johnson Foundation; and grant 5T20MC000-11-06 from the Maternal and Child Health Bureau.

References

1. Johnston LD, O'Malley PM, Bachman JG. *Monitoring the Future national results on adolescent drug use: overview of key findings, 2001.* (NIH publication No. 02-5105). Bethesda, MD: National Institute on Drug Abuse; 2002

2. Kann L, Kinchen SA, Williams BI, et al. Youth Risk Behavior Surveillance—United States, 1999. *J Sch Health.* 2000;70:271–285

3. U.S. Centers for Disease Control and Prevention. Alcohol involvement in fatal motor-vehicle crashes—United States, 1999–2000. *MMWR.* 2001;50:1064–1065

4. National Institute on Alcohol Abuse and Alcoholism. Alcohol and Transportation Safety. *Alcohol Alert.* 2001;52:1

5. Riggin O. Substance abuse as an antecedent to premature death in pre-adolescents and young adults. Paper presented at: Annual National Conference of the Association for Medical Education and Research in Substance Abuse; November 6, 1999; Alexandria, VA

6. DuRant RH, Krowchuk DP, Kreiter S, Sinal SH, Woods CR. Weapon carrying on school property among middle school students. *Arch Pediatr Adolesc Med.* 1999;153:21–26

7. DuRant RH, Smith JA, Kreiter SE, Krowchuk DP. The relationship between early age of onset of initial substance use and engaging in multiple health risk behaviors among young adolescents. *Arch Pediatr Adolesc Med.* 1999;153:286–291

8. Woods ER, Lin YG, Middleman A, Beckford P, Chase L, DuRant RH. The associations of suicide attempts in adolescents. *Pediatrics.* 1997;99:791–796

9. Jessor R, Jessor SL. *Problem Behavior and Psychosocial Development: A Longitudinal Study of Youth.* New York, NY: Academic Press; 1977

10. Jessor R, Turbin MS, Costa FM. Protective factors in adolescent health behavior. *J Pers Soc Psychol.* 1998; 75:788–800

11. Weinberg NZ, Rahdert E, Colliver JD, Glantz MD. Adolescent substance abuse: a review of the past 10 years. *J Am Acad Child and Adolesc Psychiatry.* 1998;37:252–261

12. Freese TE, Miotto K, Reback CJ. The effects and consequences of selected club drugs. *J Subst Abuse Treat.* 2002; 23:151–156

13. Elster AB, Kuznets NJ, eds. *AMA Guidelines for Adolescent Preventive Services (GAPS): Recommendations and Rationale.* Baltimore, MD: Williams & Wilkins; 1994

14. Green M, Palfrey J, eds. *Bright Futures: Guidelines for Health Supervision of Infants, Children, and Adolescents.* 2nd ed, rev. Arlington, VA: National Center for Education in Maternal and Child Health, Georgetown University; 2002

15. American Academy of Pediatrics Committee on Substance Abuse. Alcohol use and abuse: a pediatric concern. *Pediatrics.* 2001;108:185–189

16. American Academy of Pediatrics, Division of Child Health Research, Periodic Survey of Fellows No. 31. Practices and Attitudes Toward Adolescent Drug Screening; 1997

17. Knight JR. The role of the primary care provider in preventing and treating alcohol problems in adolescents. *Ambul Pediatr.* 2001;1:150–161

18. Schwartz RH, Wirtz PW. Potential substance abuse. Detection among adolescent patients using the Drug and Alcohol Problem (DAP) Quick Screen, a 30-item questionnaire. *Clin Pediatr.* 1990;29:38–43

19. Rahdert ER, ed. *Adolescent Assessment/Referral System Manual.* DHHS Publication No. (ADM) 91-1735. Rockville, MD: US Dept Health and Human Services, ADAMHA National Institute on Drug Abuse; 1991

20. Babor T, de la Fuente J, Saunders J, Grant M. *AUDIT, The Alcohol Use Disorders Identification Test: Guidelines For Use In Primary Care.* 2nd ed. Geneva Switzerland: World Health Organization; 2001

21. American Academy of Pediatrics Committee on Substance Abuse. Tobacco, alcohol, and other drugs: the role of the pediatrician in prevention and management of substance abuse. *Pediatrics.* 1998;101:125–128

22. Knight JR, Sherritt L, Shrier LA, Harris SK, Chang G. Validity of the CRAFFT substance abuse screening test among adolescent clinic patients. *Arch Pediatr Adolesc Med.* 2002;156:607–614

23. Keller MB, Lavori PW, Beardslee W, Wunder J, Drs DL, Hasin D. Clinical course and outcome of substance abuse disorders in adolescents. *J Subst Abuse Treat.* 1992;9:9–14

24. Webb JA, Baer PE, McKelvey RS. Development of a risk profile for intentions to use alcohol among fifth and sixth graders. *J Am Acad Child Adolesc Psychiatry.* 1995; 34:772–778

25. Miller WR, Rollnick S. *Motivational Interviewing: Preparing People For Change.* 2nd ed. New York, NY: Guilford Press; 2002

Frequently Asked Questions About Alcohol and Drugs — A Guide for Parents

Which drugs are kids using now?

The drugs most commonly used by kids are alcohol, tobacco, and marijuana.

Don't all kids try alcohol and drugs?

Not everyone tries drugs. By the end of high school 80% of kids have tried alcohol, which is to say that 20% of kids have not. Less than half of all teens try marijuana before graduating high school and very few kids have tried other drugs.

What can parents do to protect their children from drugs?

A few simple guidelines can help decrease the chances that your child will have a problem with drugs or alcohol:

● Set a good example. Use alcohol in moderation, never drive after drinking, and don't ever use illicit drugs.
● Always know where your child is and whom he or she is with.
● Set clear expectations for non-use. Make house rules against drinking alcohol with friends or using drugs.
● Never serve alcohol to your children's friends.
● Help your child organize alcohol-free celebrations for occasions like proms or graduation.

These suggestions are helpful but not foolproof. Encourage your child to speak openly with you about difficult topics, including drugs.

If my kids are going to drink anyway, isn't it better that they drink at home where I know they're safe?

No. Drinking is not safe, even at home with a parent present. When teens drink together they get drunk, and put themselves at risk of having an accident or overdosing on alcohol. Serious accidents associated with teen drinking do not always involve driving. Making sure that none of the teens will drive does not make teen drinking safe. Parents should never serve alcohol to their children's friends; it is dangerous and it sends the wrong message to teens. Parents are often held legally responsible when tragedy occurs.

What should I do if I think my son or daughter has a serious problem?

If you believe your child has a serious drug problem, consult a professional. Explain your concerns to your child, but then insist that he or she have a formal evaluation. If your child claims you are "overreacting," explain that you will feel much better after a physician or counselor has done an evaluation.

Shouldn't we get a drug test?

It is best to let a professional decide whether a drug test is warranted. In most cases a drug test is not necessary and demanding a drug test against your child's will can be counterproductive. Drug testing is complicated—both to perform and to interpret. Parents should not attempt to do drug testing at home.

This patient education sheet is distributed in conjunction with the July 2003 issue of Adolescent Health Update, *published by the American Academy of Pediatrics. The information in this publication should not be used as a substitute for the medical care and advice of your pediatrician. Pediatricians are encouraged to photocopy this page for distribution to patients and parents.*

Know What You Know and You'll Know What to Do: Advice for Teens

OK, you've heard about alcohol and drugs before. You've heard it from your parents, at school, at the doctor's office, even on TV. Do all of these people really expect that you will *never* drink or use drugs? Are alcohol and drugs really that dangerous? Maybe you should read Michelle's story:

> "I always knew that it was dangerous to drive after drinking or using drugs. That's why I always slept over at parties instead of looking for a ride home. One night I went to a party at Kim's house. I met a bunch of new people, who seemed pretty cool, and I had a great time. I felt safe because I knew I was sleeping over, so I just kept drinking. Some time later, after a lot of drinks, I guess I blacked out. I have no idea what I said or did, I only remember waking up with a guy I didn't know on top of me. You just don't know how gross that made me feel. I never thought something like that could happen to me. It made me realize that alcohol and drugs are dangerous in lots of ways. I don't want to drink any more, at least not for now." —Michelle

Top 5 strategies for saying "no" to alcohol and drugs

1. Plan ahead. If you are going to a party or concert, decide not to drink or use drugs BEFORE YOU LEAVE YOUR HOUSE.
2. Arrange to spend time with friends who don't use.
3. Think of ways to have fun without drugs. If you can't think of anything you may really have a big problem.
4. Tell your friends you are trying to avoid using. If they still push you to use, maybe you need to think about who your friends are.
5. Think of all that you can accomplish with your life. Then think about how alcohol

and drugs can get in the way. Is using really that important?

Don't go yet—read Evan's story before you put this paper down:

> "I've always known that drinking and driving is dangerous. But I'm smart; I promised my parents and myself that I would never get behind the wheel if I was drunk. I didn't drink that much anyway. Smoking weed was a lot more fun. I would light up with my friends and we didn't worry about that because we all knew we could drive better after smoking. It wasn't until after the accident that I learned how much marijuana can slow your reflexes and affect your judgment. That's probably why I didn't see the car coming down the street as I was pulling out of the driveway. My friend Billy got really messed up. Now we don't know if he'll even be able to walk again. Nothing will ever be the same now."—Evan

Top 5 strategies for saying "no" to a ride home with an impaired driver

1. Plan ahead. Have a ride home worked out BEFORE YOU LEAVE YOUR HOUSE.
2. Have a back-up plan in case something goes wrong. Be prepared to take a bus, call a taxi, sleep at a friend's house, or call your parents if your ride falls through.
3. If your ride has been drinking or using a drug, tell him that you "feel sick" and don't want to get in the car.
4. Don't try to decide if you or someone else is "all right" to drive. If you drank or used anything at all that night, DON'T DRIVE.
5. Sign the "Contract for Life" with your parents (provided on the Internet by Students Against Destructive Decisions at www.saddonline.com)

This patient education sheet is distributed in conjunction with the July 2003 issue of Adolescent Health Update, *published by the American Academy of Pediatrics. The information in this publication should not be used as a substitute for the medical care and advice of your pediatrician. Pediatricians are encouraged to photocopy this page for distribution to patients and parents.*

The Role of the Pediatrician in Youth Violence Prevention in Clinical Practice and at the Community Level

Task Force on Violence

ABSTRACT. Violence and violent injuries are a serious threat to the health of children and youth in the United States. It is crucial that pediatricians define their role and develop the appropriate skills to address this threat effectively. From a clinical perspective, pediatricians should incorporate into their practices preventive education, screening for risk, and linkages to necessary intervention and follow-up services. As advocates, pediatricians should become involved at the local and national levels to address key risk factors and assure adequacy of preventive and treatment programs. There are also educational and research needs central to the development of effective clinical strategies. This policy statement defines the emerging role of pediatricians in youth violence prevention and management. It reflects the importance of this issue in the strategic agenda of the American Academy of Pediatrics for promoting optimal child health and development.

ABBREVIATIONS. AAP, American Academy of Pediatrics; HELP, Handgun Epidemic Lowering Plan; TFOV, (AAP) Task Force on Violence; VIPP, Violence Intervention and Prevention Program.

Background

Violence has become increasingly prominent in the lives of children in the United States, which has the highest youth homicide and suicide rates among the 26 wealthiest nations in the world and one of the highest rates of homicide worldwide.[1-3] Homicide and suicide have become the second and third leading causes of death of teenagers; homicide is the leading cause of death of black youth.[3,4] Children and youth face serious short- and long-term physical and emotional consequences as victims, witnesses, and perpetrators of violence.[5,6] Furthermore, violence is an issue that crosses all geographic (urban to rural) and socioeconomic boundaries.

Homicide rates for males 15 to 19 years of age increased 113% between 1985 and 1995, surpassing rates for males of all other age groups except those 20 to 24 years of age, with firearm-related homicides accounting for almost all of this increase.[3] Teenagers are now more likely to die of gunshot wounds than all natural causes combined.[7,8]

Data on nonfatal violent injuries are less available and reliable than those on homicide, in part, because many victims do not seek medical attention. It is estimated that for every homicide, there may be as many as 100 nonfatal violent assaults that receive treatment in an emergency department.[9] In 1995, children and adolescents 17 years or younger had 517 000 hospital emergency department visits for assault-related injuries.[10] Health care workers in urban trauma centers have noted that assaultive trauma is recurrent, with hospital readmission rates for subsequent assaults noted to be as high as 44% and subsequent homicides as high as 20%.[11-15]

As youth homicide rates have continued to rise, so have permanent physical disabilities attributable to assaults. One estimate is that during the early 1990s, the number of severe nonfatal central nervous system injuries attributable to gunshot wounds in Los Angeles, California, was equal to the number of fatalities.[16] More than 15% of all spinal cord injuries are caused by intentional trauma,[17] and an unknown, but presumably substantial, number of traumatic brain injuries are the result of violence. The number, specific injury cause, and degree of long-term disability of the victims remain poorly described in the literature because no surveillance system has been established to document these conditions, despite their prevalence.

The situations in which fatal and nonfatal adolescent assault injuries occur are similar.[18] Violent injury and death result from altercations between family members and acquaintances far more often than from robberies or other criminal activity.[19] National surveys indicate that large numbers of youth, male and female, are involved in violent altercations.[20] Furthermore, the risk of involvement with violence has been associated with many issues relevant to pediatric practice including disciplinary methods (such as corporal punishment), television viewing (particularly violent programming), exposure to domestic violence and child abuse, and handgun ownership.[21-28]

A growing number of reports confirm that numerous children witness violence.[29-32] Although it is unclear how many children are exposed to domestic and other forms of violence, no doubt exists that children are harmed—cognitively, emotionally, and developmentally—when they witness violence.[6,31,33-37] Exposures to violence and victimization are also strongly associated with subsequent acts of violence by the victim.[38-40]

The Role of Pediatricians

Pediatricians have a long and admirable history of addressing the major health issues of children in the United States by: promoting access to health care and the prevention of unintentional injury; recognizing and treating institutional injuries and child abuse; providing preventive care, such as immunizations; and by fostering early care and education, such as quality child care and the Head Start program.

This statement outlines roles for pediatricians in the prevention and management of youth violence. It establishes an agenda for making this a routine part of pediatric practice in four major areas: clinical services, community advocacy, research, and education. This broad agenda builds on a still-evolving body of knowledge, but the urgency of youth violence prevention requires further and immediate action by pediatricians.

CLINICAL CARE

The epidemiology of violent injury identifies contributing factors affecting risk for involvement with violence, and the influences of violence on children (short- and long-term).[21-28] Many of these risk factors are in areas traditionally and

routinely addressed by pediatricians in their anticipatory guidance activities and so provide a familiar starting point for violence prevention efforts.[41]

Because many pediatricians encounter children and youth who are experiencing or are at risk for violence, pediatricians are well situated to intervene. Prevention of youth violence requires that pediatricians recognize violence-related risk factors and diagnose and treat violence-related problems at all stages of child development. See section on "Safety and Screening" on page 550.

The Academy encourages pediatricians to use a stepwise approach to promote a healthy nonviolent environment at all phases of child and adolescent development.

EARLY NURTURING

- *Infancy.* Children need loving and caring relationships early in life to develop skills for nonviolent behavior throughout life. Pediatricians can promote care and support systems for families to help them nurture children. Key elements include appropriate bonding and attachment between parents and the infant and identification of factors that threaten bonding and attachment (ie, postpartum and other family depression, family strife, and lack of support systems for parents).

- *Preschool.* During the preschool years, pediatricians can encourage parents to spend time with their children, read to them (starting in infancy), teach them positive social skills, and monitor and provide guidance for their television viewing. Pediatricians can educate parents on normal age-appropriate (see Table 1) behaviors and guide them in how to model nonviolent behavior and conflict resolution for their children.

- *School age.* During this time, children develop communication skills and problem-solving skills. Parents can teach and model nonviolent anger management and conflict resolution skills as well as foster appropriate empathy skills. Pediatricians should support and encourage parents in this process by identifying positive activities for children, such as

Table 1. Age-Appropriate Interventions*

Category	Infancy/Early Childhood (0–2 Years)	Preschool (3–5 Years)	School Age (6–12 Years)	Early Adolescence (13–16 Years)	Late Adolescence (16 Years and Older)

Early nurturing	Pregnancy planned?
	Assess support system
	Assess bonding and attachment
	Parent education:
	● bonding and attachment
	● reading to child
	Assess child care arrangements
	Assess sibling issues
		Ability to cope with stress
		Assess support system
		Assess bonding and attachment
		Parent education:
		● reading to child
		● teaching social skills
		● knowing normal age-appropriate behavior
		● modeling age-appropriate behavior
		● spending time with children
			Assess ability to cope with stress
			Assess support system
			Parent education: (same as preschool plus):
			● promote:
			  – communication skills
			  – empathy skills
			  – anger-management skills
			  – problem-solving skills
			  – opportunities for positive activities (eg, sports)
				Continued parental involvement
				Parent education: (same as school age)
					Continued parental involvement
					Foster safe separation
					Support growth and development:
					· education
					· recreation
					Educate about:
					· parenting
					· bonding and attachment

Limit setting	Promote parenting skills that emphasize positive reinforcement Avoid corporal punishment Promote age-appropriate disciplinary practices, including praise for positive behavior	Promote appropriate parenting skills Avoid corporal punishment Consistency in discipline Appropriate time-outs Develop family rules Praise for positive behavior	Promote appropriate parenting skills Avoid corporal punishment Consistency in discipline Appropriate time-outs Expand family rules Include responsibility ● school ● chores	Promote appropriate parenting skills Avoid corporal punishment Consistency in discipline Appropriate restrictions ● driving ● drugs ● curfews Establish boundaries for dating and relationship Establish conflict resolution techniques with friends and peers	Same as for early adolescence
Safety and screening	Assess family: ● child care ● parental stress ● treatment of mental illness or drug abuse ● support system ● gang involvement Assess disciplinary attitudes and practices Assess for domestic violence Assess conflict resolution at home Assess for guns in the home	Assess family: ● child care ● parental stress ● treatment of mental illness or drug abuse ● support system Assess disciplinary attitudes and practices Assess for domestic violence Assess conflict resolution at home Assess for guns in the home Assess exposure to violence: ● media ● community ● school	Assess family: ● child care ● parental stress ● treatment of mental illness or drug abuse ● support system (plus inquire about situations that threaten the child; assess whether the child is victimized) Assess disciplinary attitudes and practices Assess for domestic violence Assess conflict resolution at home Assess for gang involvement Assess exposure to violence: ● media ● community ● school Assess for substance abuse	Assess family: ● child care ● parental stress ● treatment of mental illness or drug abuse ● support system Assess disciplinary attitudes and practices Assess for domestic violence Assess conflict resolution at home Assess for gang involvement Assess exposure to violence: ● media ● community ● school Assess victimization risk factors Assess for substance abuse	Assess family: ● child care ● parental stress ● treatment of mental illness or drug abuse ● support system Assess disciplinary attitudes and practices Assess for domestic violence Assess conflict resolution at home Assess for guns in the home Assess exposure to violence: ● media ● community ● school Assess victimization risk factors (Use HEADS to further access risk factors) Assess for substance abuse
Treatment and referral	Make referrals for problems identified. Refer to: ● parenting programs ● services for domestic violence ● drug treatment program ● mental illness treatment Provide counseling on the dangers of guns in the home	Make referrals for problems identified. Refer to counseling if the child: ● witnesses violence ● is excessively aggressive ● has been victimized Provide counseling on the dangers of guns in the home Case management for high-risk youth	Make referrals for problems identified. Refer to counseling if the child: ● witnesses violence ● is excessively aggressive ● has been victimized Provide counseling on the dangers of guns in the home Case management for high-risk youth	Make referrals for problems identified. Refer to counseling if the child: ● witnesses violence ● is excessively aggressive ● has been victimized Provide counseling on the dangers of guns in the home Case management for high-risk youth	Make referrals for problems identified. Refer to counseling if the child: ● witnesses violence ● is excessively aggressive ● has been victimized Provide counseling on the dangers of guns in the home Case management for high-risk youth

supervised sports, music, theater, recreational, and community life projects that are both socially acceptable and that build useful skills.

● *Adolescence.* As children mature, the pediatrician can encourage parents to foster independence, educate their children about the responsibilities of adulthood, but also maintain their attachment to and involvement with their children during this process.

LIMIT SETTING

● *Infancy.* Limit setting during the infant's first year should center on educating parents about appropriate parenting and nurturing skills. Pediatricians can ask about parental views regarding spoiling and discipline. Parents must learn that corporal punishment is less effective than other limit-setting strategies.

● *Preschool.* Pediatricians can encourage the parents and other caregivers to avoid corporal punishment and use more effective nonviolent disciplinary restrictions to alter misbehavior such as natural and logical consequences and time-out strategies for specific behaviors.[43] Pediatricians can advise parents against disciplining a child for age-appropriate behavior, such as exploring their environment or spilling their milk. When children knowingly misbehave, parents and others must be as consistent as possible, and when children behave appropriately, they should be praised and encouraged. Pediatricians can provide advice on managing assertive and aggressive behaviors, as well as on supporting and reinforcing prosocial behaviors.

● *School age.* Pediatricians can help parents understand the child's need to assume greater responsibilities. They can help parents understand the importance of developing consistent, clearly articulated family rules and agreed-on consequences for breaking these rules. They can also encourage consistent discipline among different caregivers and nonviolent disciplinary strategies.

● *Adolescence.* Pediatricians can help parents establish family rules that address potential areas of conflict, such as driving privileges, curfews, substance abuse, and school and household responsibilities. Pediatricians can discuss with the adolescent what constitutes safe, appropriate dating and relationships, as well as strategies for avoiding or resolving interpersonal conflicts with friends and peers.

SAFETY AND SCREENING

Pediatricians need to identify the risk factors for violence among their patients. Violence-related assessment and screening should focus on the following areas:

● history of mental illness, previous domestic violence, or substance abuse in the parents or other family members;

● family stresses that could lead to violence (eg, unemployment, divorce, or death);

● appropriate supervision and care and support systems (eg, child care arrangements, the family and social network);

● disciplinary attitudes and practices of the parents or caregivers (particularly about corporal punishment and physical/emotional abuse);

● exposure to violence in the home (domestic violence[44] or child abuse), school, or community;

● degree of exposure to media violence;

● access to firearms (especially handguns) in their or a neighbor's home, or the community;

● gang involvement or gang exposure in family, school, or neighborhood;

● situations in which a child or adolescent experiences physical assault or sexual victimization from anyone;

● presence of signs of poor self-esteem, or depression; and

● other factors affecting risk, such as poor school performance and physical, emotional, or developmental disabilities.

TREATMENT AND REFERRAL

When pediatricians identify risk factors for violence or actual violence-related problems during the screening process, appropriate treatment or referral should occur. Some of the problems can be handled by the pediatrician through follow-up visits and office-based counseling, particularly when the issues are television viewing, removal of handguns, and nonurgent behavioral issues. The issue of gun ownership is a particularly frustrating and difficult one. Pediatricians should be prepared for resistance. Maintaining a focus specifically on the risks of handgun ownership can help keep the message clear and reduce controversy.

Some problems require referral for additional services to child welfare agencies (eg, for suspected child abuse), mental health services (eg, for victims of and witnesses to violence), emergency shelters and other domestic violence counseling and legal services, substance abuse treatment, or high-risk youth services. Repeated referral efforts may be required to achieve linkage to services.

ADVOCACY

Pediatricians should apply their proven professional influence to violence-prevention efforts. Pediatricians can advocate at patient, community, or broader public policy levels.

The first level of advocacy focuses on individual patients and families who present in the pediatrician's office. Individual advocacy might involve interventions and interactions with patients' insurance companies, schools, hospitals, mental health services, and other specific programs.

The second level of advocacy focuses on the community where pediatricians can partner with others to increase services, promote prevention activities, and influence community attitudes that affect risk and incidence of violence. Examples include reducing corporal punishment in schools and homes, participating in child death review teams, reducing or eliminating access to handguns, working with hospitals to develop protocols for treatment of victims and witnesses of violence (eg, using the American Academy of Pediatrics' [AAP] Adolescent Assault Victim statement[45]), and educating the local media.

The third level of advocacy focuses on public policy. Pediatrician involvement can influence legislation and regulation.[21] Laws and regulations pertinent to violence prevention include those that require safe gun storage, trigger locks, and other gun control measures, (particularly the reduction or elimination of handguns); prohibition of corporal punishment in schools; programs to provide home visitation for new parents, after-school care and recreational opportunities for youth, quality child care, and programs that educate parents and children.

Advocacy is an integral activity of the Academy, its state chapters, and other state medical societies. By working with the AAP individual pediatricians can achieve more than any single individual. Other organization collaborators include education groups (the state and local parent-teacher associations, state and local teacher associations, local chapters of the National Association for the Education of Young Children), youth service programs (Girl Scouts and Boy Scouts, girls and boys clubs, YMCA, YWCA), public health associations, community service organizations (Lions, Jaycees, Junior League), law enforcement agencies and organizations, religious institutions, organizations of child care providers, gun control organizations (eg, the Handgun Epidemic Lowering Plan [HELP] Network), and groups of local business leaders and associations. The AAP Department of Government Liaison and Division of State Government and Chapter Affairs can help pediatricians plan advocacy at the federal and state levels.

EDUCATION

Pediatricians need comfort and familiarity with the issues and the strategies related to violence prevention. Education on the issue should occur at all levels for trainees, from undergraduate to residency and fellowship programs, and for practicing clinicians through continuing medical education.

RESEARCH

Although the literature includes substantial data on risks and causes of violence, little published research addresses the effectiveness of prevention and treatment strategies.

Practicing pediatricians can be involved directly in violence-related research through practice-based research projects. Practicing pediatricians are crucial in this work because they bring direct clinical experience to choosing the right questions that will lead to useful interventions.

Pediatricians also need to advocate for resources to support research activities. Ongoing public health tracking of violent injuries should be a cornerstone for monitoring trends and characteristics of violence, as well as for measuring the effectiveness of prevention and intervention programs. To do this, the public and private sectors should invest in research on youth violence prevention. Investing in understanding youth violence and how to reduce it should match the level of concern about the issue. In particular, further research should explore what can be done early in the lives of children, given the research on early brain and child development.[46]

Recommendations

CLINICAL PRACTICE

Clinical practice guidelines for the prevention and management of youth violence need to be established that include:

- promoting a healthy environment for all children, in the family and in the community;
- assessing for high-risk situations and behaviors;
- responding to problems identified with appropriate treatment and referrals;
- violence-prevention counseling and screening as early as the pediatric prenatal visit and continuing into adulthood; and
- maintaining familiarity with the relevant and appropriate counseling and treatment services in communities.

ADVOCACY

Pediatricians should advocate for:

- provision of affordable, quality child care for all families who require it, as well as other family support programs, such as postnatal home visitation;
- elimination of corporal punishment as a recommended form of child discipline in all settings;
- reduction of violence and expanded reporting of healthful activities in the media;
- reduced availability or elimination of handguns in all communities through handgun regulation and public education;
- increased treatment resources and services for substance abuse and domestic violence in all communities; and

- increased recreational, therapeutic, and occupational services and programs for children and youth, particularly in low-income communities.

Pediatricians should work as a group to strengthen such efforts and should link with other disciplines and advocacy groups to maximize effectiveness in these efforts.

EDUCATION

Many pediatricians lack education to acquire the skills and comfort they need to participate effectively in violence prevention. To remedy this situation:

- Medical schools and pediatric residency programs should develop and institute appropriate curricula on prevention and management of youth violence.
- Practicing pediatricians should enhance their knowledge and comfort in violence prevention and management through continuing medical education.

RESEARCH

Pediatricians can contribute to needed research by:

- participating in violence-related practice-based research projects;
- advocating for resources to:
  - enhance the level of violent injury tracking activities;
  - enhance the level of public and private funding for violence prevention and management research.

TASK FORCE ON VIOLENCE, 1997–1998
Howard Spivak, MD, Chairperson
Katherine Kaufer Christoffel, MD, MPH
Herman B. Gray, Jr, MD
Maxine Hayes, MD
Renee Jenkins, MD
Luis Montes, MD
C. Damon Moore, MD

LIAISON REPRESENTATIVES
Stephanie Bryn, MPH
    Maternal and Child Health Bureau
Alex Crosby, MD
    Centers for Disease Control and Prevention

CONSULTANT
Carl Bell, MD
    Community Medical Health Center

References

1. Centers for Disease Control and Prevention. Rates of homicide, suicide, and firearm-related death among children: 26 industrialized countries. *MMWR Morb Mortal Wkly Rep.* 1997;46:101–105

2. Krug EG, Dahlberg LL, Powell KE. Childhood homicide, suicide, and firearm deaths: an international comparison. *World Health Stat Q.* 1996;49:230–235

3. Anderson RN, Kochanek KD, Murphy SL. Report of final mortality statistics: 1995. *Mon Vital Stat Rep.* 1997;45 (suppl 2):1–80

4. Centers for Disease Control and Prevention. Homicide among young black males: United States, 1978–1987. *MMWR Morb Mortal Wkly Rep.* 1990;39:869–873

5. Prothrow-Stith D. *Deadly Consequences.* New York, NY: HarperCollins; 1991

6. Osofsky JD, ed. *Children in a Violent Society.* New York, NY: Guilford Press; 1997

7. Centers for Disease Control and Prevention. Homicides among 15–19 year-old males: United States, 1963–1991. *MMWR Morb Mortal Wkly Rep.* 1994;43:725–727

8. Fingerhut LA, Kleinman JC, Godfrey E, Rosenberg H. Firearm mortality among children, youth and young adults, 1–34 years, trends and current status: United States, 1979–88. *Mon Vital Stat Rep.* 1991;39(suppl):1–16

9. Barancik JI, Chatterjee BF, Greene YC, Michenzi EM, Fife D. Northeastern Ohio trauma study, I: magnitude of the problem. *Am J Public Health.* 1983;73:746–751

10. Stussman BJ. *National Ambulatory Medical Care Survey: 1995 Emergency Department Summary.* Advance Data From Vital and Health Statistics, No. 285. Hyattsville, MD: National Center for Health Statistics; 1997

11. Sims DW, Bivins BA, Obeid FN, Horst HM, Sorensen VJ, Fath JJ. Urban trauma: a chronic recurrent disease. *J Trauma.* 1989;29:940–947

12. Poole GV, Griswold JA, Thaggard VK, Rhodes RS. Trauma is a recurrent disease. *Surgery.* 1993;113:608–611

13. Goins WA, Thompson J, Simpkins C. Recurrent intentional injury. *J Natl Med Assoc.* 1992;84:431–435

14. Morrissey TB, Byrd CR, Deitch EA. The incidence of recurrent penetrating trauma in an urban trauma center. *J Trauma.* 1991;31:1536–1538

15. Reiner DS, Pastena JA, Swan KG, Lindenthal JJ, Tischler CD. Trauma recidivism. *Am Surg.* 1990;56:556–560

16. Montes L. Physical morbidity. Presented at the Annual Meeting of the Handgun Epidemic Lowering Plan; October 18–19, 1993; Chicago, IL

17. Stover SL, Fine PR. *Spinal Cord Injury: The Facts and Figures.* Birmingham, AL: University of Alabama at Birmingham; 1986

18. Hausman AJ, Spivak H, Roeber JF, Prothrow-Stith D. Adolescent interpersonal assault injury admissions in an urban municipal hospital. *Pediatr Emerg Care.* 1989; 5:275–280

19. Federal Bureau of Investigation. *Crime in the United States, 1996: Uniform Crime Reports.* Washington, DC: Government Printing Office; 1997

20. Centers for Disease Control and Prevention. Behaviors related to unintentional and intentional injuries among high school students: United States, 1991. *MMWR Morb Mortal Wkly Rep.* 1992;41:760–762,771–772

21. Spivak H, Harvey B, eds. The role of the pediatrician in violence prevention: proceedings of a conference: Chantilly, Virginia, March 4–5, 1994. *Pediatrics.* 1994; 94:576–651

22. Kann L, Warren CW, Harris WA, et al. Youth risk behavior surveillance: United States, 1993. *MMWR CDC Surveill Summ.* 1995;44:1–56

23. DuRant RH, Cadenhead C, Pendergrast RA, Slavens G, Linda CW. Factors associated with the use of violence among urban black adolescents. *Am J Public Health.* 1994;84:612–617

24. Webster DW, Gainer PS, Champion HR. Weapon carrying among inner-city junior high school students: defensive behavior vs aggressive delinquency. *Am J Public Health.* 1993;83:1604–1608

25. Sosin DM, Koepsell TB, Rivara FP, Mercy JA. Fighting as a marker for multiple problem behaviors in adolescents. *J Adolesc Health.* 1995;16:209–215

26. Valois RF, McKeown RE, Garrison CZ, Vincent ML. Correlates of aggressive and violent behaviors among public high school adolescents. *J Adolesc Health.* 1995; 16:26–34

27. Callahan CM, Rivara FP. Urban high school youth and handguns: a school-based survey. *JAMA.* 1992;267: 3038–3042

28. Cotten NU, Resnick J, Browne DC, Martin SL, McCarraher DR, Woods J. Aggression and fighting behavior among African-American adolescents: individual and family factors. *Am J Public Health.* 1994;84:618–622

29. Hutson HR, Angling D, Pratts MJ Jr. Adolescents and children injured or killed in drive-by shootings in Los Angeles. *N Engl J Med.* 1994;330:324–327

30. Dowd MD, Knapp JF, Fitzmaurice LS. Pediatric firearm injuries, Kansas City, 1992: a population-based study. *Pediatrics.* 1994;94:867–873

31. Osofsky JD, Wewers S, Hann DM, Fick AC. Chronic community violence: what is happening to our children? *Psychiatry.* 1993;56:36–45

32. Pynoos RS, Eth S. Children traumatized by witnessing acts of personal violence: homicide, rape, or suicide behavior. In: Eth S, Pynoos RS, eds. *Post-Traumatic Stress Disorder in Children.* Washington, DC: American Psychiatric Press; 1985:19–43. Spiegel D, series ed. The Progress in Psychiatry Series

33. American Bar Association. *The Impact of Domestic Violence on Children: A Report to the President of the American Bar Association.* Chicago, IL: American Bar Association; 1994

34. Shakoor BH, Chalmers D. Co-victimization of African-American children who witness violence: effects on cognitive, emotional, and behavioral development. *J Natl Med Assoc.* 1991;83:233–238

35. Jenkins EJ, Bell CC. Violence among inner city high school students and post-traumatic stress disorder. In: Friedman S, ed. *Anxiety Disorders in African Americans.* New York, NY: Springer Publishing Co; 1994:76–88

36. Fitzpatrick KM, Boldizar JP. The prevalence and consequences of exposure to violence among African-American youth. *J Am Acad Child Adolesc Psychiatry.* 1993;32:424–430

37. Groves B. The child witness to violence project. *Discharge Plann Update.* 1994:14–18

38. Durant RH, Pendergrast RA, Cadenhead C. Exposure to violence and victimization and fighting behavior by urban black adolescents. *J Adolesc Health.* 1994;15:311–318

39. Widom CS. The cycle of violence. *Science.* 1989;244: 160–166

40. Miller TR, Cohen MA, Rossman SB. Victim costs of violent crime and resulting injuries. *Health Aff (Millwood).* 1993;12:186–197

41. Bass JL, Christoffel KK, Widome MD, et al. Childhood injury prevention counseling in primary care settings: a critical review of the literature. *Pediatrics.* 1993;92: 544–550

42. American Academy of Pediatrics. *Guidelines for Health Supervision III.* 3rd ed. 1997

43. American Academy of Pediatrics, Committee on Psychosocial Aspects of Child and Family Health. Guidelines for effective discipline. *Pediatrics.* 1998;101:723–728

44. American Academy of Pediatrics, Committee on Child Abuse and Neglect. The role of the pediatrician in recognizing and intervening on behalf of abused women. *Pediatrics.* 1998;101:1091–1092

45. American Academy of Pediatrics, Task Force on Adolescent Assault Victim Needs. Adolescent assault victim needs: a review of issues and a model protocol. *Pediatrics.* 1996;98:991–1001

46. Shore R. *Rethinking the Brain: New Insights Into Early Development.* New York, NY: Families and Work Institute; 1997

Report to the AAP Board of Directors From the Task Force on Violence

Introduction

Violence and violent injuries are a serious threat to the health of children and youth in the United States. It is crucial that pediatricians define their role and develop the appropriate skills to effectively address this threat. From a clinical perspective, pediatricians should incorporate into their practices: preventive education, screening for risk, and linkages to necessary intervention/follow-up services. As advocates, pediatricians should become involved at the local and national levels to address key risk factors and assure adequacy of preventive and treatment programs. There are also educational and research needs central to the development of effective clinical strategies.

Background

Violence has become increasingly prominent in the lives of children in the United States, which has the highest youth homicide and suicide rates among the 26 wealthiest nations in the world and one of the highest rates of homicide worldwide. Homicide and suicide have become the second and third leading causes of death of teenagers; homicide is the leading cause of death of black youth. Children and youth face serious short- and long-term physical and emotional consequences as victims, witnesses, and perpetrators of violence. Furthermore, violence is an issue that crosses all geographic (urban to rural) and socioeconomic boundaries.

Homicide rates for males 15 to 19 years of age increased 113% between 1985 and 1995, surpassing rates for males of all other age groups except those 20 to 24 years of ages, with firearm-related homicides accounting for almost all of this increase. Teenagers are now more likely to die of gunshot wounds than all natural causes combined. Data on nonfatal violent injuries are less available and reliable than those on homicide, in part, because many victims do not seek medical attention. It is estimated that for every homicide, there may be as many as 100 nonfatal violent assaults that receive treatment in an emergency department. In 1995, children and adolescents ages 17 years or younger had 517 000 hospital emergency department visits for assault-related injuries. Health care workers in urban trauma centers have noted that assaultive trauma is recurrent, with hospital readmission rates for subsequent assaults noted to be as high as 44% and subsequent homicides as high as 20%.

As youth homicide rates have continued to rise, so have permanent physical disabilities attributable to assaults. One estimate is that in the early 1990s, the number of severe central nervous system injuries from gunshots in Los Angeles was equal to the number of fatalities. Over 15% of all spinal cord injuries are caused by intentional trauma, and an unknown, but presumably significant, number of traumatic brain injuries are the result of violence. These victims remain poorly described in the literature—in terms of the number, specific injury cause, and degree of long-term disability—because no surveillance system has been established to document these conditions, despite their prevalence.

The situations in which fatal and nonfatal adolescent assault injuries occur are similar. Violent injury and death result from altercations between family members and acquaintances far more often than they are related to robberies or other criminal activity. National surveys indicate that large numbers of youth, male and female, are involved in violent altercations. Furthermore, risk of involvement with violence has been associated with many issues relevant to pediatric practice including disciplinary methods such as corporal punishment, television viewing (particularly violent programming), exposure to domestic violence and child abuse, and handgun ownership.

A growing number of reports confirm that numerous children witness violence. Although it is unclear how many children are exposed to domestic and other forms of violence, no doubt exists that children are harmed when they witness violence—cognitively, emotionally, and developmentally. Exposure to violence and victimization are also strongly associated with subsequent acts of violence by the victim.

History of the AAP Task Force on Violence

The Task Force on Violence (TFOV) was established in June 1996 and included seven members, two governmental agency liaison representatives, and a consultant from the field of community psychiatry. The Task Force held four meetings that primarily focused on the following activities:

a) the development of a policy statement on the role of the pediatrician in violence prevention that is broken down into the following categories: clinical care, advocacy, research, and education and training;

b) the development of a report to the Board of Directors recommending strategies and action steps for the organization to take related to violence prevention in each of the four categories listed above; and

c) consideration of goals/objectives for the possible convening of an interorganizational council on youth/peer violence including an assessment of more than 20 select health- and education-related national organizations to determine interest in participating on this council.

Other Highlights/Activities of the Task Force

● The Task Force worked very closely with staff from the Division of Child Health Research on the development and fielding of a Periodic Survey on violence and violence prevention. The survey is currently underway.

● The Task Force served as a reviewing body and resource for the development of an ACQIP exercise on violence/violence prevention that was distributed to ACQIP subscribers in January 1998.

● The Task Force developed questions on violence prevention for inclusion in a survey on managed care and children with special health care needs that was disseminated to major managed care organizations (by the Division of Physician Payment Systems); survey results have been analyzed by staff and will be written up for a possible article in *AAP News*.

- The Task Force submitted program proposal recommendations to the Committee on Scientific Meetings for consideration at the 1998 Spring Session (not approved) and the 1998 Annual Meeting (approved as a Plenary Session—Howard Spivak, MD, Faculty).
- Staff developed an AAP violence prevention resource compendium that is available in hard copy format and on the Academy's Website (Advocacy Page).
- The Task Force outlined ideas for the components to be included in a Violence Intervention and Prevention Program (VIPP) anticipatory guidance program if funding is secured for its development, implementation, and evaluation.
- The Task Force has encouraged other Academy committees to develop policy statements on specific areas of violence prevention that relate to issues that fall under their purview.
- The Task Force encouraged staff involvement throughout the process of the development of the policy statement, recommendations to the Board of Directors, and in educational issues.

Recommendations to the AAP Board

CLINICAL CARE

1. That the Academy undertake the development of a VIPP anticipatory guidance program.

Action Necessary:

- Identify resources for the development and evaluation of the program and subsequent training of pediatricians and other health professionals in its use.
- Inventory current Academy patient education materials to determine what might be repackaged to be utilized as part of the program.

2. That in its meetings with representatives of several of the major managed care organizations, the Academy leadership discuss violence prevention programs and initiatives as a priority issue especially as it relates to the impact on Medicaid managed care systems.

Action Necessary:

- Identify lead staff and AAP members to assist in the development of key messages to be shared with managed care organizations related to violence prevention.

ADVOCACY AND POLICY

1. That the Academy continue and intensify its focus on violence prevention in its goals and objectives.
- Action Necessary: That the Academy promote and enhance, where possible, its involvement in handgun regulatory activities.
- That the Academy promote and enhance, where possible, its involvement in child death investigations at the federal and state levels including working with the American Bar Association and others, and to promote the AAP model state legislation on this issue.
- That the Academy advocate for additional funding for research on the aforementioned topics.
- That the Committee on Adolescence and the Department of Government Liaison expedite and prioritize the development of Academy policy on juvenile justice issues.
- That the Department of Communications continue to emphasize messages regarding preventing media violence via the Academy's Media Matters campaign.
- That the Academy continue to prioritize its efforts in the area of media education specifically related to combatting media violence.
- That the Academy's leadership take a strong stand against corporal punishment in the home as they have done with respect to other settings such as schools.

2. That the Academy focus on the development of materials for use in education and training of pediatricians as advocates in the area of violence prevention.

Action Necessary:

- That a public speaking and media training session specifically focused on violence prevention be coordinated and facilitated by the Division of Public Relations.
- That the Division of Public Relations develop and promote speaking points and key media messages on violence prevention specifically focusing on positive images of youth in ways that emphasize nonviolence, resilience, and special accomplishments of youth.

- That the Division of Member Communications continue to prioritize articles on violence, and that a feature article be included in a future issue of *AAP News* that discusses the root causes of violence, encourages members to become involved in local/community-based coalitions and efforts related to violence prevention, and includes a section on additional resources.
- That the Violence Prevention Resources pages on the Academy's Website be promoted to the membership and others via *AAP News* and other publications.

3. That the Academy provide a nominal amount of funds to be used for the replication of the AAP violence prevention resource folder/packet so that an offer of the materials to the membership can be included in a future issue of *AAP News* as well as other Academy publications.

Action Necessary:

- That the Academy allocate funds for the production and distribution of the violence prevention resource folder/packet so that an offer of the materials can be made to the full Academy membership via *AAP News* and other publications.

4. That the Academy take the lead in convening an interorganizational council on youth/peer violence to enhance communication, collaboration, and public policy initiatives of several health and education organizations in an effort to coordinate clinical care messages, intervention and prevention strategies, and other activities.

Action Necessary:

- That the Academy allocate a nominal amount of funding for planning and convening a preliminary meeting of an interorganizational council on youth/peer violence. (Funds for AAP representatives' travel and expenses and for the council members' meals are being requested).
- That lead staff and AAP members be identified to coordinate and plan this activity.

RESEARCH

1. That the Academy identify opportunities to promote expanded attention to research in the area of violence prevention.

Action Necessary:

- That the Academy leadership promote violence prevention as a topic to be addressed by the soon-to-be established Child Health Research Center.
- That the Academy's Department of Research place emphasis on pediatric practice-based research projects on violence prevention via ongoing AAP research programs.

2. That the Academy via its Departments of Government Liaison and Research advocate for violence-related research funding from public and private sector sources.

Action Necessary:

- Work with appropriate staff from Centers for Disease Control and Prevention, the Department of Health and Human Services, the Maternal and Child Health Bureau, and the Department of Justice to identify opportunities to support violence prevention research in the budget process.

3. That the Academy, via the Councils on Pediatric Practice and Pediatric Research and the Department of Government Liaison, prioritize its advocacy efforts related to enhanced surveillance of violence-related injuries and deaths.

Action Necessary:

- Work with the Centers for Disease Control and Prevention to identify opportunities for funding of surveillance in the budget process.

4. That the results of the recently undertaken Periodic Survey on violence prevention be promoted earnestly to the membership and to other health care professionals and organizations in both the public and private sectors.

Action Necessary:

- Upon completion of the fielding of the Periodic Survey on violence prevention and tabulation of the results, the Division of Child Health Research will write up the results and submit an article(s) for publication in a peer-reviewed journal. Information about the results also will be published in *AAP News*.

EDUCATION AND TRAINING

1. That the Academy recommend the development of enhanced continuing medical education programming, enhanced undergraduate medical education, and enhanced medical school education in the area of violence prevention.

Action Necessary:

- That the Board of Directors encourage the Section and Committee on Injury and Poison Prevention to make efforts to submit program proposals on violence prevention to the Committee on Scientific Meetings for consideration.

- That the Section on Injury and Poison Prevention focus at least one session on this topic at each national meeting as part of its educational programming.

- That the Practical Pediatrics Course Workgroup include violence prevention training in their future program planning.

- That the Committee on Scientific Meetings include the topic of violence prevention as part of their curriculum.

- That the PREP Planning Group consider including one article per year on violence prevention in *Pediatrics in Review*.

That the Council on Pediatric Education discuss violence prevention at their next meeting and determine an appropriate course of action for future endeavors in pediatric education and training related to same.

Safety and Efficacy of the Nicotine Patch and Gum for the Treatment of Adolescent Tobacco Addiction

Eric T. Moolchan, MD; Miqun L. Robinson, MD, PhD; Monique Ernst, MD, PhD; Jean Lud Cadet, MD; Wallace B. Pickworth, PhD; Stephen J. Heishman, PhD; and Jennifer R. Schroeder, PhD

ABSTRACT. *Objectives.* To determine the safety and efficacy of the nicotine patch and gum for adolescents who want to quit smoking.

Design. Double-blind, double-dummy, randomized, 3-arm trial with a nicotine patch (21 mg), nicotine gum (2 and 4 mg), or a placebo patch and gum; all participants received cognitive-behavioral group therapy.

Setting. Inner-city, outpatient clinic on the East Coast.

Subjects. Thirteen- to 17-year-old adolescents who smoked ≥10 cigarettes per day (CPD), scored ≥5 on the Fagerström Test of Nicotine Dependence, and were motivated to quit smoking.

Intervention. Twelve weeks of nicotine patch or gum therapy with cognitive-behavioral therapy, with a follow-up visit at 6 months (3 months after the end of treatment).

Main Outcome Measures. Safety assessed on the basis of adverse event reports for all 3 groups, prolonged abstinence, assessed through self-report and verified with exhaled carbon monoxide (CO) levels of ≤6 ppm, in intent-to-treat analyses, and smoking reduction (CPD and thiocyanate concentrations) among trial completers.

Results. A total of 120 participants were randomized (72% white, 70% female; age: 15.2 ± 1.33 years; smoking: 18.8 ± 8.56 CPD; Fagerström Test of Nicotine Dependence score: 7.04 ± 1.29) from 1999 to 2003. Participants started smoking at 11.2 ± 1.98 years of age and had been smoking daily for 2.66 ± 1.56 years; 75% had at least 1 current psychiatric diagnosis. Mean compliance across groups was higher for the patch (mean: 78.4–82.8%) than for the gum (mean: 38.5–50.7%). Both the patch and gum were well tolerated, and adverse events were similar to those reported in adult trials. Changes in mean saliva cotinine concentrations throughout treatment were not statistically significant. Intent-to-treat analyses of all randomized participants showed CO-confirmed prolonged abstinence rates of 18% for the active-patch group, 6.5% for the active-gum group, and 2.5% for the placebo group; the difference between the active-patch and placebo arms was statistically significant. There was no significant effect of patch versus gum or gum versus placebo on cessation outcomes. Abstinence rates at the 3-month follow-up assessment were sustained but were not significantly associated with treatment group. Mean smoking rates, but not CO or thiocyanate concentrations, decreased significantly in all 3 arms but not as a function of treatment group.

Conclusions. Nicotine patch therapy combined with cognitive-behavioral intervention was effective, compared with placebo, for treatment of tobacco dependence among adolescent smokers. Decreases in the numbers of cigarettes smoked appeared to be offset by compensatory smoking. Additional study of nicotine gum, with enhanced instructional support, is needed to assess its efficacy among adolescent smokers. *Pediatrics* 2005; 115:e407–e414. URL: www.pediatrics.org/cgi/doi/ 10.1542/peds.2004-1894; *treatment, adolescent, tobacco, nicotine patch, nicotine gum, cessation, smoking reduction.*

ABBREVIATIONS. CPD, cigarettes per day; NRT, nicotine replacement therapy; FTND, Fagerström Test of Nicotine Dependence; CO, carbon monoxide; IDR, incidence density ratio; CI, confidence interval; OR, odds ratio.

After having peaked in the late 1990s, smoking prevalence among adolescents declined slightly, although remaining high. Percentages of eighth-, 10th-, and 12th-graders who reported having smoked in the past 30 days were 10.2%, 16.7%, and 24.4%, respectively, in 2003.[1] More importantly, tobacco addiction develops among adolescent smokers, and they experience withdrawal

From the Teen Tobacco Addiction Research Clinic, Clinical Pharmacology and Therapeutics Research Branch, National Institute on Drug Abuse, Baltimore, Maryland.

Accepted for publication Nov 9, 2004. doi:10.1542/peds.2004-1894

No conflict of interest declared.

Reprint requests to (E.T.M.) Teen Tobacco Addiction Research Clinic, Clinical Pharmacology and Therapeutics Research Branch, National Institute on Drug Abuse, Intramural Research Program, 5500 Nathan Shock Dr, Baltimore, MD 21224. E-mail: emoolcha@intra.nida.nih.gov

symptoms similar to those of adult smokers when they try to abstain from smoking.[2] A large proportion of adolescent smokers have tried unsuccessfully to stop smoking at least once, most frequently with acute abstinence ("cold turkey") methods,[3] and many desire treatment to help with cessation.[4] Most adolescents with established smoking habits continue to smoke as adults and incur both short-term and long-term health consequences, including premature death.[5] Therefore, safe and effective smoking cessation interventions for adolescent smokers are critically needed.

Although several informative reviews of the adolescent smoking-cessation literature have been published in recent years, one challenge remains, namely, how best to tailor the setting and modalities for cessation interventions for youths.[6-8] Various counseling and behavioral, classroom-based approaches have included infrequent and low-level smokers with more intense smokers, with some yielding encouraging short-term quit rates of 30 to 50%.[9,10] Although advocated by expert opinion in a clinical practice guideline,[11] very few pharmacologic interventions have been evaluated for treating dependent teenage smokers. In open-label trials of the nicotine patch in combination with group counseling support, abstinence rates remained very low (4.5–11.5%).[12,13] A small-sample (N = 16), open-label, bupropion study reported an abstinence rate of 31% after 4 weeks of treatment.[14] Two randomized, adolescent, patch trials have been reported. In the first, participants were randomized to the patch or placebo, in combination with intense cognitive-behavioral and contingency management therapies to reinforce tobacco abstinence. Cessation rates reached 18% at 3 months, but no significant treatment effect was observed.[15] In the other trial, teen smokers were assigned randomly to either patch plus bupropion or patch plus placebo, with weekly group skills training. Abstinence rates measured at weeks 10 and 26 were 23% and 8% for the patch plus bupropion group and 28% and 7% for the patch plus placebo group, respectively.[16] Although no treatment effect was observed, these cessation rates were encouraging.

Relatively low abstinence rates in previous treatment trials with addicted adolescent smokers prompted us to evaluate biochemically verified reduced smoking as a treatment outcome variable. Treatment-generated reductions in smoking rates among adults have been reported with pharmacologic methods[17-19] and demonstrate the potential for deferred quitting.[20,21] Despite limited effects on cessation in the open-label youth trials,[12,13] transdermal nicotine therapy was associated with significant self-reported decreases in cigarette consumption. This type of effect has been linked to a reduction of adolescents' smoking in the long term,[5] which might translate into health benefits on a population basis if accompanied by decreases in toxin exposure.[22] Moreover, in a longitudinal trial with Swiss youths, a reduction of 5 cigarettes per day (CPD) during adolescence doubled the chances of being abstinent 3 years later.[23] As suggested in a previous report, lower systemic support for quit attempts, and potentially less motivation, preparation, and success in achieving total cessation among adolescents, compared with adult smokers, might prompt the consideration of tobacco exposure reduction as an intermediate treatment goal for adolescent smokers.[24] Gradual reduction of smoking might also appeal to subgroups of teen smokers who smoke to self-medicate negative cognitive or affective states.[23,25]

On the basis of the clinical practice guideline[11] and the observation that youths do purchase and have access to nicotine replacement therapy (NRT),[1,26] we designed this pilot trial to determine the safety and preliminary efficacy of the nicotine gum and patch, used in combination with cognitive-behavioral group therapy,[27] to help young smokers achieve cessation. Because of the growing interest in therapies that might aid in reducing smoke exposure and the possibility that many addicted adolescent smokers might not be ready for complete cessation,[23,24] we were also interested in determining whether treatment could produce a substantial reduction in smoking rates among trial-completers.

Methods

SAMPLE

This study was approved by the National Institute on Drug Abuse institutional review board and was conducted in Baltimore, Maryland. Outreach and recruitment were performed from September 1999 to September 2003, through various media (print, audiovisual, and electronic) advertisements and through various community channels, such as schools and churches. Adolescent smokers desiring to quit were encouraged to call for a structured telephone interview, to determine their initial preeligibility. Callers who reported major physical health problems or untreated acute psychiatric problems were excluded. Only participants who were able to discuss their smoking with their parent/guardian, were motivated to quit (>5 on a 10-point integer scale), and were planning to remain in the area for the duration of the trial were invited for on-site screening.

Final eligibility was determined after an on-site history recording, physical examination, and basic laboratory screening. Adolescents 13 through 17 years of age who were in general good health, had smoked ≥10 CPD for ≥6 months, had a minimal score of 5 on the Fagerström Test of Nicotine Dependence (FTND), and were motivated to stop smoking were eligible to participate. Pregnancy, lactation, chronic skin conditions, use of other tobacco products, and current use (within the past 30 days) of medications for smoking cessation (eg, NRT or bupropion) were reasons for exclusion. Drug or alcohol dependence other than nicotine and current mania, psychosis, and acute depression, according to the Diagnostic Interview of Children and Adolescents,[28] which was based on the *Diagnostic and Statistical Manual of Mental Disorders, Fourth Edition,* were also exclusion criteria. However, candidates taking psychotropic medications not prescribed for smoking cessation were included in the trial.

PROCEDURES

Adolescents who qualified through a 10- to 15-minute telephone screening were invited, with a parent or guardian, to an orientation meeting in which an overview of the study and clinic functioning was presented. Signed informed assent and consent were obtained from all adolescents and their parents or legal guardians, respectively. A "universal" Fagerström questionnaire, which included the FTND and more youth-appropriate versions of the questionnaire, and other baseline sociodemographic assessments were completed. Expired-air carbon monoxide (CO) testing (Vitalograph, Lenexa, KS) was performed, blood was drawn, and saliva was collected for measurement of baseline (while the subjects were smoking their usual numbers of cigarettes) nicotine, cotinine, and thiocyanate concentrations. Female adolescents of childbearing potential were required to have a negative pregnancy test before being randomized. The target quit date was set 1 week after the 2 baseline clinic visits.

On the quit date, participants were instructed in the use of the 21-mg nicotine patch and gum (2 mg if smoking ≤24 CPD or 4 mg if smoking >24 CPD), according to Food and Drug Administration labeling, and were given self-help materials from the package insert used for the over-the-counter products. Participants weighing <100 pounds (45 kg) and smoking <20 CPD at baseline received the 14-mg patch. GlaxoSmithKline (Research Triangle Park, NC) provided study medication (Nicoderm, 21 mg and 14 mg; Nicorette, 2 mg and 4 mg) but did not participate in the study design, study performance, or data analysis. Participants were told to use the gum as needed, with the approximate goal of using one half their baseline reported CPD values in numbers of pieces of gum (eg, 10 pieces of gum for smokers smoking 1 pack per day, as a guideline) for the beginning of treatment. For this double-blind study, adolescents were randomized to 1 of 3 groups according to an algorithm held by the National Institute on Drug Abuse Pharmacy, with true replacement of trial-noncompleters. Because both the patch and gum are used commonly, the 3 groups included (1) active patch and placebo gum, (2) active gum and placebo patch, and (3) placebo gum and placebo patch. Adolescents were asked to complete a weekly questionnaire recording the number of cigarettes smoked, tobacco craving, and symptoms of tobacco withdrawal and depression.[29] Nurses recorded vital signs, including height and weight, and provided minimal individual counseling (3-4 minutes) to address possible medication side effects and proper use of the nicotine patch and gum. Trained study assistants aided in data collection. After the 2 baseline visits, participants attended 11 visits over a total of 12 weeks of treatment (Fig 1 illustrates the study timeline). At each visit, vital signs and exhaled CO were measured and saliva specimens were collected for later cotinine and thiocyanate assays. Assays were completed by Labstat, Inc (Kitchener, Ontario, Canada). Used and unused patches were collected, and a new supply was dispensed. Participants were queried regarding any adverse reactions and concomitant medication use since the last visit. Information on adverse events was elicited through open-ended questions (eg, "How have you been feeling since the last visit") and also through direct prompting of teens to indicate

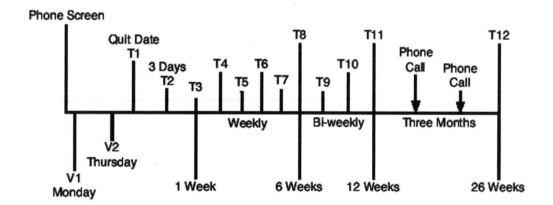

Fig 1. Study timeline.

whether specific side effects on a questionnaire had been experienced. A monthly urine pregnancy test was performed for female participants. Subjects returned at 6 months (3-month posttreatment follow-up visit) for assessment of self-reported smoking status and expired-air CO measurements; saliva samples were collected for quantification of cotinine and thiocyanate. Participants attended a 45-minute cognitive-behavioral group therapy session led by a trained social worker at the end of each treatment visit. The aim of the cognitive-behavioral therapy was to help participants identify and address specific factors that led either to smoking or to maintaining abstinence from smoking behavior and manage life stressors better by using effective, adaptive, coping skills.[27] Study participants were compensated with $90 for the baseline assessment and $135 after study completion for research activities other than treatment.

DATA ANALYSES

Given 3 study groups, for a power of .80 and an α level of .05, based on reported values for adult populations[30] and assuming a 70% reduction of smoke exposure in the active-medication groups, the approximate sample size needed to perform an analysis of variance for the main outcome variable (saliva thiocyanate concentrations) was estimated at 17 for each group. Given an anticipated attrition rate of 55%, 40 patients for each group were required to obtain a total of 51 completers. The sample of 53 completers slightly exceeded the 51 planned.

The other study end points were measures of cessation, ie, point prevalence abstinence and prolonged abstinence. For weekly point prevalence abstinence rates, subjects were considered abstinent from smoking if they self-reported not smoking during the 7 days before a visit and had an expired-air CO level of ≤6 ppm at that visit. Subjects missing visits for any reason were considered to be smoking at the time of the missed visits. Prolonged abstinence was defined as point prevalent abstinence maintained throughout the trial, after an initial 2-week grace period after the quit date.[31,32]

Self-reported smoking rates reported at each visit were summarized as mean CPD values and calculated as change from baseline. The data were summarized with weekly means for each of the 6 weeks of the medication phase and at the 12-week and 6-month follow-up visits.

The 3 treatment groups were compared with respect to demographic and smoking history variables with analysis of variance for continuous variables and χ^2 tests for categorical variables. Any variable found to be associated with treatment group assignment was considered a potential confounder and was included as a covariate in outcome analyses if also associated with the outcome measure. Nonparametric survival analysis techniques (log-rank and Wilcoxon tests) were used to determine whether treatment groups differed with respect to retention. Incidence density ratios (IDRs) were calculated to compare rates of adverse events in each active-treatment group with those in the placebo group; the IDR equals the adverse event count per person-weeks of follow-up monitoring for each active-medication group divided by the adverse event count per person-weeks of follow-up monitoring for the placebo group. When the rate of adverse events in either active-medication arm exceeded that in the placebo arm (ie, IDR > 1), a 1-sided hypothesis test was used to determine whether the excess was statistically significant ($P < .05$). The normal approximation to the binomial was used when warranted; otherwise, an exact binomial test was performed.

Fisher's exact tests, χ^2 tests, and logistic regression analyses were used to assess the effect of treatment group assignment on smoking cessation (both prolonged abstinence and point prevalence abstinence). Treatment groups were coded such that each active-medication arm was compared with placebo. Fisher's exact tests and χ^2 tests were performed to determine whether frequencies of participants achieving abstinence were associated with treatment group assignment, with contingency tables, and whether maximal likelihood parameter estimates from logistic regression models differed from 0; the treatment effect was considered statistically significant if the P value was <.05. Analysis of variance with planned contrasts (patch versus placebo and gum versus placebo) was used to determine whether continuous outcome measures (compliance rates, reductions in CPD values, CO levels, and saliva thiocyanate levels, and withdrawal symptoms) were associated with treatment group assignment. Compliance for the patch was defined as the number of patches used for the first 30 days of treatment divided by 30; compliance for the gum was defined as the number of reported pieces of gum used during the first 30 days divided by one half the baseline reported CPD value times 30. Paired t tests were used to determine the significance of changes observed in continuous measures of smoking during the trial (before/after differences in CPD values, CO levels, and saliva thiocyanate levels). For cessation end points, an intent-to-treat analysis was performed that included all participants randomized ($n = 120$); participants who dropped out were assumed to have been smoking. For all other end points, the analysis included participants for whom data were available.

Results

PARTICIPANT CHARACTERISTICS

Of 1347 adolescents who telephoned the clinic in response to advertisements, 329 were preeligible in telephone screenings and 159 presented for on-site screening, as described in a separate report.[33] Of the 159 adolescents who presented for enrollment, 39 (24.5%) were not randomized, after on-site evaluations indicated their ineligibility (Fig 2).

One hundred twenty participants were randomized to receive treatment; 53 completed the study. Overall, randomized subjects were 15.2 ± 1.33 years of age, 72.5% white, and 70.0% female. At the time of admission, they smoked an average of 18.8 ± 8.56 CPD and had a mean FTND score of 7.04 ± 1.29, indicating high dependence. Participants started smoking at 11.2 ± 1.98 years of age and had been smoking daily for 2.66 ± 1.56 years. Table 1 provides the characteristics according to treatment group. Only the age at which subjects started smoking was significantly associated with treatment group assignment [$F(2111) = 4.25, P = .017$]; participants assigned to receive the patch started smoking at a later age. The age at which subjects started smoking was significantly associated with prolonged abstinence and CPD reduction; therefore, this variable was used as a covariate in analyses of these outcomes.

Baseline psychiatric assessments revealed that 90 subjects (75%) had at least 1 current

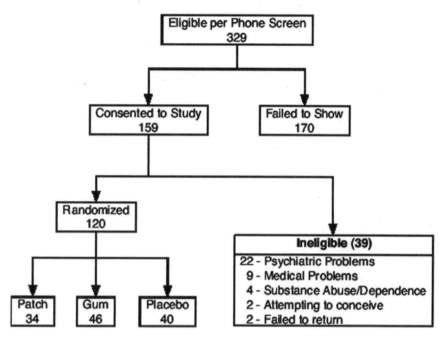

Fig 2. Participant enrollment flow chart.

psychiatric diagnosis, according to the Diagnostic Interview for Children and Adolescents.[28] The most frequently represented categories were oppositional defiant disorder (40%), conduct disorder (15%), attention-deficit/hyperactivity disorder (current: 7%; previous: 11%), and premenstrual dysphoric disorder (11%). The percentages of participants with at least 1 psychiatric diagnosis in each treatment group were as follows: patch, 64%; gum, 75%; placebo, 85%. Several applicants were enrolled in the trial while taking prescribed psychotropic medications, including (categories not mutually exclusive) sertraline (6 subjects), methylphenidate (4 subjects), paroxetine (4 subjects), fluoxetine (3 subjects), hydroxyzine (2 subjects), citalopram (2 subjects), trazodone (2 subjects), venlafaxine (2 subjects), risperidone (1 subject), and olanzapine (1 subject).

The proportions of randomized participants who completed the study were 41.3% (19 of 46 subjects) for the gum group, 52.9% (18 of 34 subjects) for the patch group, and 40.0% (16 of 40 subjects) for the placebo group; differences in study completion rates were not statistically significant (χ^2 test). Treatment group differences in retention times were not statistically significant ($P = .71$ with log-rank test and $P = .60$ with Wilcoxon test for homogeneity of survival curves).

SAFETY

Safety was assessed on the basis of all self-reported adverse events throughout the trial and nicotine and cotinine concentrations in saliva. Of 745 total adverse events documented during the trial, the frequencies of events, in descending

Table 1. Participant Characteristics (N = 120)

	Patch (n = 34)	Gum (n = 46)	Placebo (n = 40)
Age, y	15.4 ± 1.41	15.0 ± 1.31	15.2 ± 1.29
Female, %	61.8	69.6	77.5
White, %	79.4	65.2	75.0
FTND score	7.00 ± 1.11	7.09 ± 1.39	7.00 ± 1.32
CPD	17.7 ± 6.45	18.9 ± 8.96	19.6 ± 9.70
Age started smoking, y*	12.1 ± 1.87	11.0 ± 1.99	10.9 ± 1.91
Years smoked daily	2.57 ± 1.29	2.73 ± 1.88	2.66 ± 1.35

* $P < .05$.

order, were as follows: pruritus, 130 cases; erythema, 111 cases; headache, 86 cases; fatigue, 67 cases; viral infection, 63 cases; insomnia, 43 cases; cough, 32 cases; nausea, 31 cases; jaw pain, 30 cases; anxiety, 26 cases; sore throat, 24 cases; hiccup, 22 cases; dyspepsia, 22 cases; shoulder or arm pain, 18 cases; dizziness, 15 cases; congestion, 10 cases; edema, 10 cases; constipation, 3 cases; diarrhea, 2 cases; other, 18 cases. Active medication was associated with a statistically significant increase in adverse events for the following symptom categories: sore throat (gum versus placebo, $IDR = 4.79$, $P = .0007$), hiccups (gum versus placebo, $IDR = 2.79$, $P = .014$), shoulder/arm pain (patch versus placebo, $IDR = 4.63$, $P = .0011$), pruritus (patch versus placebo, $IDR = 1.63$, $P = .033$; gum versus placebo, $IDR = 1.95$, $P = .003$), and erythema (patch versus placebo, $IDR = 1.97$, $P = .0045$). Table 2 provides the frequency of adverse events according to treatment arm. Overall, the highest (mean ± SD) saliva cotinine concentrations were observed at the 2.5-month postquit visit (T10), but the increase over baseline was not significant in either treatment group (data not shown).

CESSATION

The proportions of participants who achieved prolonged abstinence (continuous abstinence as of 2 weeks after randomization) were as follows: patch group, 6 of 34 subjects (17.7%); gum group, 3 of 46 subjects (6.5%); placebo group, 1 of 40 subjects (2.5%) (Fig 3). For prolonged abstinence, a trend toward statistical significance was found for the overall effect of treatment (2-tailed Fisher's exact test, $P = .066$). Two-tailed Fisher's exact tests showed that the direct comparison between patch and placebo was statistically significant ($P = .043$), whereas the comparison between gum and placebo was not statistically significant ($P = .62$). Post hoc comparisons of the patch and gum groups revealed no statistically significant difference. The odds ratio (OR) of prolonged abstinence for the patch group, compared with the placebo group, was 8.36 (95% confidence interval [CI]: 0.95–73.3; $P = .055$) and that for the gum group, compared with the placebo group, was 2.72 (95% CI: 0.27–27.3; $P = .39$); adding the age at which the subjects started smoking as a covariate in the logistic regression model did not alter the results substantively.

Table 2. Adverse Events Among Randomized Participants ($N = 120$), Listed In Order of Decreasing Overall Frequency, According to Treatment Group

	Patch (476 person-wk)	Gum (552.1 person-wk)	Placebo (439.9 person-wk)	Elevated in Active-Medication Group, Compared with Placebo
Pruritus	44	61	25	Patch, $P = .033$; gum, $P = .003$
Erythema	49	39	23	Patch, $P = .0045$
Headache	24	26	36	
Fatigue	15	20	32	
Viral infection	14	30	19	
Insomnia	13	17	13	
Cough	9	15	8	
Nausea	10	10	11	
Jaw pain	10	12	8	
Anxiety	6	13	7	
Sore throat	3	18	3	Gum, $P = .0007$
Hiccups	4	14	4	Gum, $P = .014$
Dyspepsia	4	10	8	
Shoulder or arm pain	15	0	3	Patch, $P = .00011$
Dizziness	3	3	9	
Congestion	3	3	4	
Edema	4	2	4	
Constipation	3	0	0	
Diarrhea	0	0	2	

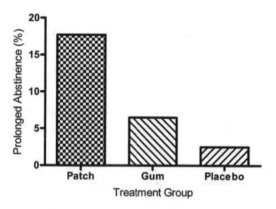

Fig 3. Prolonged abstinence at 3 months, according to intent-to-treat analysis.

In addition to prolonged abstinence, we examined point prevalence abstinence at 3 time points, ie, 1 week after the quit date, at the end of the study, and 3 months after study completion. At 1 week after the quit date, a time at which patient follow-up monitoring might begin in a standard medical practice, proportions of abstinent participants were as follows: patch group, 9 of 34 subjects (26.5%); gum group, 8 of 46 subjects (17.4%); placebo group, 2 of 40 subjects (5.0%). The OR of point prevalence abstinence for the patch group, compared with the placebo group, was 6.84 (95% CI: 1.36–34.33; $P = .02$) and that for the gum group, compared with the placebo group, was 4.00 (95% CI: 0.80–20.1; $P = .09$). Two-tailed Fisher's exact tests found the effect for patch versus placebo to be statistically significant ($P = .030$), whereas the effect for gum versus placebo was not ($P = .45$). Post hoc comparison of the patch and gum groups revealed no statistically significant difference in rates of point prevalence abstinence at 1 week after the quit date. The proportions of abstinent participants according to group did not change from study completion to 3 months after study completion:

patch, 20.6%; gum, 8.7%; placebo, 5%. Point prevalence abstinence results were highly concordant at the end of treatment (T11) and at the 3-month follow-up evaluation (T12). In the patch group, 1 participant was abstinent at T11 but not at T12 and another participant was abstinent at T12 but not at T11; the same was true for the gum group. For the placebo group, 2 participants were abstinent at T11 but not T12 and another 2 were abstinent at T12 but not T11. At study completion (T11) and 3 months after study completion (T12), logistic regression analyses showed a trend toward significance for the effect of the patch, compared with placebo (OR: 4.93; 95% CI: 0.95–25.6; $P = .058$), and no significance for the effect of gum (OR: 1.81; 95% CI: 0.31–10.4; $P = .51$). Figure 4 displays point prevalence abstinence, according to intent-to-treat analysis, at each visit throughout the study.

REDUCTION

Percent reduction was calculated with the following formula: % reduction = 100 ∞ [(follow-up value – baseline value)/baseline value]. Therefore, a negative sign indicates reduction and a positive sign denotes increase. Mean reductions in self-reported CPD values exceeding 80% were observed for all 3 treatment groups at the end of the treatment phase; these reductions were significantly different from 0 with paired t tests. However, analysis of variance with contrasts showed that these decreases were not associated with treatment group assignment (Table 3). Adding the age at which subjects started smoking as a covariate did not alter the findings. The mean changes in both expired CO and saliva thiocyanate levels did not differ from 0 and did not differ according to treatment group (Table 3).

Table 3. Percentage Reductions in Measures of Smoking Among Completers, According to Treatment Group ($N = 52$)

	Patch	Gum	Placebo
Change in CPD, T11 – V1, %	−80.4 ± 7.52 ($N = 18$)*	−85.1 ± 5.13 ($N = 18$)*	−89.6 ± 4.98 ($N = 16$)*
Change in CO level, T11 – V1, %	10.5 ± 19.7 ($N = 18$)	37.7 ± 30.5 ($N = 18$)	30.8 ± 33.2 ($N = 16$)
Change in saliva thiocyanate level, T11 – V1, %	1.69 ± 26.6 ($N = 13$)	17.7 ± 23.7 ($N = 12$)	9.90 ± 13.5 ($N = 9$)

* Percentage change significantly different from 0 ($P < .05$) by paired t test.

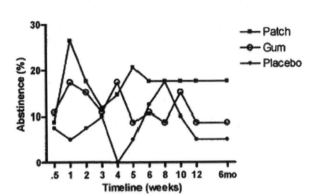

Fig 4. Point prevalence abstinence, according to intent-to-treat-analysis.

COMPLIANCE

Mean compliance rates based on daily use of the patch were 78.4% for the patch group, 82.8% for the gum group, and 80.9% for the placebo group. Analyses of variance showed no significant differences among treatment groups in the proportions of patches used.

Compliance rates for gum use during the first month of the trial (based on the recommended amount of use according to pretreatment CPD values) were 42.1% for the patch group, 38.5% for the gum group, and 50.7% for the placebo group. Analysis of variance with planned contrasts showed that compliance in the gum group differed significantly from that in the placebo group [$F(1100) = 5.59$, $P = .020$].

Discussion

The main finding from our study was that the nicotine patch was significantly more effective than placebo in helping dependent adolescent smokers receiving cognitive-behavioral therapy quit smoking (prolonged abstinence). Despite the absence of significant group differences in rates measured at the end of treatment, there was a trend toward higher point prevalence abstinence rates in the patch group, compared with the placebo group, that was sustained at the 3-month follow-up visit. The large effect size (OR: 8.36) for the comparison of the patch versus placebo for prolonged abstinence suggests a clinically significant effect; however, the wide CI (95% CI: 0.95–73.3) indicates a lack of statistical power. This is not surprising, because the study

was designed to have sufficient statistical power to detect a significant reduction but not a cessation effect. Future studies of NRT among adolescent smokers should be designed to detect group differences in abstinence rates.

Despite substantial psychiatric comorbidity in our recruited sample, cessation rates obtained in this study were comparable to those reported previously from youth studies[12,15,34] and slightly lower than those from adult studies (15–28% at 6 months) with NRT.[35–37] Unlike cessation, reductions in cigarette consumption were not significantly associated with treatment group assignment. Although the degree of reduction in smoking achieved by study participants (means exceeding 80% for all 3 groups) appeared encouraging, neither biomarker of smoke exposure (ie, expired CO or saliva thiocyanate levels) declined during the trial, perhaps because of compensatory smoking (eg, deeper inhalation), reducing the inference of any health benefit related to smoking reduction. Alternatively, teens might have reported their cigarette consumption inaccurately. These results are consistent with findings from 2 adult studies, in which reductions in the numbers of cigarettes smoked were not accompanied by reductions in CO or thiocyanate concentrations[34] or reductions smaller than corresponding reductions in cigarette consumption were observed.[21] Active medication did not affect withdrawal scores in the current study, contrary to a previous study in which the patch group experienced a significant decrease in withdrawal scores, compared with placebo (data not shown).[15]

The nicotine patch and gum were well tolerated in this study and appeared safe. For the patch, this was similar to previous studies with adolescents,[12,13,15,16] and the adverse event profile was consistent with that from previous studies with adults.[38] Although we were not able to obtain adverse event data from trial dropouts, our clinical impression was that adverse events did not affect retention substantially. This is also suggested by the superior cessation outcome for the patch group, which reported the highest rate of side effects. We did not find any previously reported controlled studies of the gum among adolescents. Although not considered an adverse event, our clinical perception was that the aversive taste of the gum might have reduced compliance in the active-gum arm. Cotinine concentrations remained within the range from other similar studies, which suggests that the patch and gum remained safe for adolescents who continued to smoke. Although our attrition rate of 54% was high, it had been anticipated and was comparable to the 61% dropout rate recently reported for adolescent participants who attended trial visits at a research office.[15] Clearly, creative strategies are needed to retain adolescents in future medication trials that aim to treat tobacco dependence.

Several limitations of this study warrant attention. Only a small percentage of applicants who inquired via telephone were enrolled, compared with a previous randomized trial.[15] Stringent consumption and dependence eligibility criteria for this trial seem to have offset our otherwise liberal inclusion of participants with psychiatric disorders and drug and alcohol use. Alternatively, differences in sociodemographic characteristics in our trial, compared with the trial by Hanson et al,[15] might have affected eligibility for study participation. One example of this is our previously reported inadvertent exclusion of some black adolescents because of the their lower FTND scores.[39,40] The enrollment/randomization of only a small percentage of initial applicants is regrettable; however, as a first step, important information for developing and implementing other youth cessation research was obtained.[33] This was a rather lengthy study (3 months), with trial-related research procedures (eg, group therapy and questionnaire completion) exceeding standard practice-based cessation procedures at each visit. We wanted to obtain practical information pertaining to the use of both available over-the-counter modalities of NRT (of which only 1 was active) simultaneously. The external validity of this approach was based on the observations that both the patch and the gum are used commonly, often in combination, for cessation or reduction attempts.[37,38] The high degree of psychiatric comorbidity in this sample might have reduced cessation success.[41,42] Overall, gum

compliance was suboptimal. Higher gum use in the placebo group might be attributable to increased use in a continued attempt to obtain an effect of the medication or, alternatively, less aversion for the placebo versus the active gum. Future studies with the nicotine gum among adolescents should test the recently available mint-flavored gum and provide increased, detailed, instructional support and rehearsal of gum use.

Because of the inclusion of highly addicted adolescents with substantial comorbidity, results from our sample can be extended to a broad range of settings in which adolescents might be seen for treatment of tobacco addiction and other clinical concerns. Although these results do not answer definitively the question of the efficacy of the patch or gum for treating adolescent smokers, the current findings lend empirical support to the US Public Health Service clinical practice guideline[11] for pediatricians, family practitioners, and other practitioners to prescribe or to recommend more consistently the nicotine patch, in addition to developmentally appropriate behavioral and counseling support, for adolescent smokers who are attempting to quit.

Acknowledgments

This work was supported by funds from the National Institute on Drug Abuse, Intramural Research Program.

We thank GlaxoSmithKline (Research Triangle Park, NC) for providing us with study medications (21- and 14-mg Nicoderm, 2- and 4-mg Nicorette, and placebo patch and gum). This trial would not have been possible without the support of the Teen Tobacco Addiction Treatment Research Clinic staff, including Alex Radzius, MHS, A. Thiri Aung, MD, Maria Gasior, MD, Frederick H. Franken, BS, Charles Collins, BA, Nelda Snidow, RN, and Debra Zimmerman, RN. We are grateful to Susan J. Ruckel, LCSW-C, and the staff of NOVA Research. Finally, we acknowledge the invaluable contributions of Drs Jack E. Henningfield, Edward J. Cone, and Marilyn A. Huestis.

References

1. Johnson KC, Klesges LM, Somes GW, Coday MC, DeBon M. Access of over-the-counter nicotine replacement therapy products to minors. *Arch Pediatr Adolesc Med.* 2004;158:212–216

2. Rojas NL, Killen JD, Haydel KF, Robinson TN. Nicotine dependence among adolescent smokers. *Arch Pediatr Adolesc Med.* 1998;152:151–156

3. Myers MG, MacPherson L. Smoking cessation efforts among substance abusing adolescents. *Drug Alcohol Depend.* 2004;73:209–213

4. Centers for Disease Control and Prevention. *Preventing Tobacco Use Among Young People: A Report of the Surgeon General.* Washington, DC: US Government Printing Office; 1994

5. Chassin L, Presson CC, Sherman SJ, Edwards DA. The natural history of cigarette smoking: predicting young-adult smoking outcomes from adolescent smoking patterns. *Health Psychol.* 1990;9:701–716

6. Backinger CL, McDonald P, Ossip-Klein DJ, et al. Improving the future of youth smoking cessation. *Am J Health Behav.* 2003;27(suppl 2):S170–S184

7. Sussman S. Effects of sixty six adolescent tobacco use cessation trials and seventeen prospective studies of self-initiated quitting. *Tob Induced Dis.* 2002;1(1):35–81

8. McDonald P, Colwell B, Backinger CL, Husten C, Maule CO. Better practices for youth tobacco cessation: evidence of review panel. *Am J Health Behav.* 2003;27 (suppl 2):S144–S158

9. Sussman S, Dent CW, Lichtman KL. Project EX: outcomes of a teen smoking cessation program. *Addict Behav.* 2001; 26:425–438

10. Adelman WP, Duggan AK, Hauptman P, Joffe A. Effectiveness of a high school smoking cessation program. *Pediatrics.* 2001;107(4). Available at: www.pediatrics.org/ cgi/content/full/107/4/e50

11. Fiore M, Bailey W, Cohen S. *Treating Tobacco Use and Dependence: Clinical Practice Guideline.* Rockville, MD: US Department of Health and Human Services; 2000

12. Smith TA, House RF Jr, Croghan IT, et al. Nicotine patch therapy in adolescent smokers. *Pediatrics.* 1996;98: 659–667

13. Hurt RD, Croghan GA, Beede SD, Wolter TD, Croghan IT, Patten CA. Nicotine patch therapy in 101 adolescent smokers: efficacy, withdrawal symptom relief, and carbon monoxide and plasma cotinine levels. *Arch Pediatr Adolesc Med.* 2000;154:31–37

14. Upadhyaya HP, Brady KT, Wang W. Bupropion SR in adolescents with comorbid ADHD and nicotine dependence: a pilot study. *J Am Acad Child Adolesc Psychiatry.* 2004;43:199–205

15. Hanson K, Allen S, Jensen S, Hatsukami D. Treatment of adolescent smokers with the nicotine patch. *Nicotine Tob Res.* 2003;5:515–526

16. Killen JD, Robinson TN, Ammerman S, et al. Randomized clinical trial of the efficacy of bupropion combined with nicotine patch in the treatment of adolescent smokers. *J Consult Clin Psychol.* 2004;72:729–735

17. Bolliger CT, Zellweger JP, Danielsson T, et al. Smoking reduction with oral nicotine inhalers: double blind, randomised clinical trial of efficacy and safety. *BMJ.* 2000;321:329–333

18. Etter JF, Laszlo E, Zellweger JP, Perrot C, Perneger TV. Nicotine replacement to reduce cigarette consumption in smokers who are unwilling to quit: a randomized trial. *J Clin Psychopharmacol.* 2002;22:487–495

19. Windsor RA, Li CQ, Boyd NR Jr, Hartmann KE. The use of significant reduction rates to evaluate health education methods for pregnant smokers: a new harm reduction behavioral indicator? *Health Educ Behav.* 1999;26:648–662

20. Eliasson B, Hjalmarson A, Kruse E, Landfeldt B, Westin A. Effect of smoking reduction and cessation on cardiovascular risk factors. *Nicotine Tob Res.* 2001;3:249–255

21. Wennike P, Danielsson T, Landfeldt B, Westin A, Tonnesen P. Smoking reduction promotes smoking cessation: results from a double blind, randomized, placebo-controlled trial of nicotine gum with 2-year follow-up. *Addiction.* 2003;98:1395–1402

22. Stratton K, Shetty P, Wallace R, Bondurant S. Clearing the smoke: the science base for tobacco harm reduction: executive summary. *Tob Control.* 2001;10:189–195

23. Schmid H. Predictors of cigarette smoking by young adults and readiness to change. *Subst Use Misuse.* 2001;36:1519–1542

24. Moolchan ET, Aung AT, Henningfield JE. Treatment of adolescent tobacco smokers: issues and opportunities for exposure reduction approaches. *Drug Alcohol Depend.* 2003;70:223–232

25. Windle M, Windle RC. Depressive symptoms and cigarette smoking among middle adolescents: prospective associations and intrapersonal and interpersonal influences. *J Consult Clin Psychol.* 2001;69:215–226

26. Klesges LM, Johnson KC, Somes G, Zbikowski S, Robinson L. Use of nicotine replacement therapy in adolescent smokers and nonsmokers. *Arch Pediatr Adolesc Med.* 2003;157:517–522

27. Moolchan E, Ruckel S. Tobacco cessation for adolescents: developing a group therapy approach. *J Child Adolesc Subst Abuse.* 2002;12:65–92

28. Reich W. Diagnostic Interview for Children and Adolescents (DICA). *J Am Acad Child Adolesc Psychiatry.* 2000; 39:59–66

29. Hughes JR, Hatsukami D. Signs and symptoms of tobacco withdrawal. *Arch Gen Psychiatry.* 1986;43:289–294

30. Jarvis MJ, Tunstall-Pedoe H, Feyerabend C, Vesey C, Saloojee Y. Comparison of tests used to distinguish smokers from nonsmokers. *Am J Public Health.* 1987; 77:1435–1438

31. Hughes JR, Keely JP, Niaura RS, Ossip-Klein DJ, Richmond RL, Swan GE. Measures of abstinence in clinical trials: issues and recommendations. *Nicotine Tob Res.* 2003;5:13–25

32. Mermelstein R, Colby SM, Patten C, et al. Methodological issues in measuring treatment outcome in adolescent smoking cessation studies. *Nicotine Tob Res.* 2002;4: 395–403

33. Moolchan ET, Robinson ML, Schroeder JR. Adolescent smokers screened for a smoking cessation treatment study: correlates of eligibility and enrollment. Presented at: 11th Annual Meeting and 7th Annual European Conference of the Society for Research on Nicotine and Tobacco; March 19–23, 2005; Prague, Czech Republic

34. Hurt RD, Croghan GA, Wolter TD, et al. Does smoking reduction result in reduction of biomarkers associated with harm? A pilot study using a nicotine inhaler. *Nicotine Tob Res.* 2000;2:327–336

35. Lerman C, Kaufmann V, Rukstalis M, et al. Individualizing nicotine replacement therapy for the treatment of tobacco dependence: a randomized trial. *Ann Intern Med.* 2004;140:426–433

36. Silagy C, Lancaster T, Stead L, Mant D, Fowler G. Nicotine replacement therapy for smoking cessation. *Cochrane Database Syst Rev.* 2004: CD000146

37. Bolliger CT. Practical experiences in smoking reduction and cessation. *Addiction.* 2000;95(suppl 1):S19–S24

38. Tonnesen P. Smoking cessation: nicotine replacement, gums and patches. *Monaldi Arch Chest Dis.* 1999;54: 489–494

39. Moolchan ET, Berlin I, Robinson ML, Cadet JL. African-American teen smokers: issues to consider for cessation treatment. *J Natl Med Assoc.* 2000;92:558–562

40. Moolchan ET, Berlin I, Robinson ML, Cadet JL. Characteristics of African American teenage smokers who request cessation treatment: implications for addressing health disparities. *Arch Pediatr Adolesc Med.* 2003;157:533–538

41. Brown RA, Lewinsohn PM, Seeley JR, Wagner EF. Cigarette smoking, major depression, and other psychiatric disorders among adolescents. *J Am Acad Child Adolesc Psychiatry.* 1996;35:1602–1610

42. Glassman AH, Helzer JE, Covey LS, et al. Smoking, smoking cessation, and major depression. *JAMA.* 1990; 264:1546–1549

Teen Reach: Outcomes From a Randomized, Controlled Trial of a Tobacco Reduction Program for Teens Seen in Primary Medical Care

Jack F. Hollis, PhD*; Michael R. Polen, PhD*; Evelyn P. Whitlock, MD, MPH*; Edward Lichtenstein, PhD‡;
John P. Mullooly, PhD*; Wayne F. Velicer, PhD§; and Colleen A. Redding, PhD§

ABSTRACT. *Objective.* **To test the long-term efficacy of brief counseling plus a computer-based tobacco intervention for teens being seen for routine medical care.**

Methods. **Both smoking and nonsmoking teens, 14 to 17 years of age, who were being seen for routine visits were eligible for this 2-arm controlled trial. Staff members approached teens in waiting rooms of 7 large pediatric and family practice departments within a group-practice health maintenance organization. Of 3747 teens invited at ≥1 visits, 2526 (67%) consented and were randomized to tobacco intervention or brief dietary advice. The tobacco intervention was individually tailored on the basis of smoking status and stage of change. It included a 30-second clinician advice message, a 10-minute interactive computer program, a 5-minute motivational interview, and up to two 10-minute telephone or in-person booster sessions. The control intervention was a 5-minute motivational intervention to promote increased consumption of fruits and vegetables. Follow-up smoking status was assessed after 1 and 2 years.**

Results. **Abstinence rates after 2 years were significantly higher for the tobacco intervention arm, relative to the control group, in the combined sample of baseline smokers and nonsmokers (odds ratio [OR]: 1.23; 95% confidence interval [CI]: 1.03–1.47). Treatment effects were particularly strong among baseline self-described smokers (OR: 2.42; 95% CI: 1.40–4.16) but were not significant for baseline nonsmokers (OR: 1.25; 95% CI: 0.97–1.61) or for those who had "experimented" in the past month at baseline (OR: 0.95; 95% CI: 0.45–1.98).**

Conclusions. **Brief, computer-assisted, tobacco intervention during routine medical care increased the smoking cessation rate among self-described smokers but was less effective in preventing smoking onset.** *Pediatrics* **2005;115:981–989;** *tobacco, adolescents, intervention, cessation, primary care.***

ABBREVIATIONS. OR, odds ratio; CI, confidence interval; GEE, generalized estimating equations; PTC, Pathways to Change.

Tobacco use remains the number 1 cause of preventable morbidity and death in the United States, each year resulting in >430 000 deaths,[1] >5 million years of potential life lost,[2] and $50 billion of direct medical expenditures related to smoking alone.[3] Among adults who have ever smoked daily, 82% first tried cigarettes and 53% smoked daily before age 18 years.[4] According to recent estimates, almost one half of current adolescent smokers who continue to smoke regularly will die from a smoking related disease.[5]

After several decades of decline, rates of smoking in the past month increased in the early 1990s for grades 9 through 12 and peaked in 1997 at 37% for grade 12. Smoking rates have since declined but remain unacceptably high at ~27% for 12th-graders.[6] Rates of adolescent smoking are higher among whites (40%) than among either Hispanics (34%) or blacks (23%).[5] Male and female adolescents have similar smoking rates, except among blacks (only 17% of high school girls smoke cigarettes, compared with 28% of boys).[5] For most adolescent subgroups, rates of tobacco use must be at least halved to meet Healthy People 2010 targets.[5]

Tobacco use can be reduced among youths by preventing (or delaying) initiation and promoting cessation. The large volume of research on smoking prevention in schools and communities has

From the *Center for Health Research, Kaiser Permanente, Portland, Oregon; ‡Oregon Research Institute, Eugene, Oregon; and §University of Rhode Island, Kingston, Rhode Island.*
Accepted for publication Sep 1, 2004. doi:10.1542/peds.2004-0981
Conflict of interest: Dr Velicer has received royalties from the University of Rhode Island from the licensing of smoking cessation programs.
Reprints requests to (J.F.H.) Center for Health Research, Kaiser Permanente, 3800 N Interstate Ave, Portland, OR 97227. E-mail:
jack.hollis@kpchr.org

been summarized in several government reports[4,7] and meta-analyses.[8] Although many interventions based on social influence or life skills training show significant short-term results, the effects dissipate over time. A comprehensive, long-term study by Peterson et al[9] showed no effects for a multiyear, school-based, prevention program, which provides sobering evidence of the limitations of school-based programs alone. A recent smoking prevention intervention among families enrolled in 2 managed care organizations similarly found no effect on smoking susceptibility or experimentation among preteens.[10] Comprehensive programs that include both school-based and community components show more durable effects.[11,12] The clinical care setting is a potentially important, unexplored contributor to youth tobacco use prevention and cessation efforts.

In contrast to prevention programs, few adolescent cessation programs have been evaluated rigorously.[13] School-based cessation programs, even when preceded by extensive formative research,[14] typically recruit few smokers in that setting, experience high attrition rates, and produce low cessation rates.[4] Very few studies have recruited adolescents in medical settings or used state-of-the-art approaches, such as computer-based expert systems.[15] To date, these studies have been limited by nonexperimental designs and/or short-term outcomes.

The Teen Reach (Research Approaches to Cancer in a Health Maintenance Organization) program was a randomized, controlled trial of the long-term efficacy of brief clinician advice, the Pathways to Change (PTC) interactive computer program,[15,16] and brief motivational counseling to reduce the prevalence of smoking among teens seen for routine medical care. This population-based, individually tailored intervention capitalized on the teachable moment present at the primary care physician visit and the attractiveness to teens of a multimedia, computer-based, interactive program. Other attributes of this strategy included (1) a focus on the whole population of adolescents (whether smoking at entry or not), (2) a stage-based, theory-driven intervention, (3) the ease and practicality of the intervention for clinicians, and (4) the relatively low cost of

delivering the intervention to teens during routine medical care.

Methods

SETTING

Participants were adolescent members of Kaiser Permanente Northwest, a health maintenance organization in the Portland, Oregon, and Vancouver, Washington, metropolitan areas that serves ~450 000 individuals. Pediatrics and family practice departments at 7 Kaiser Permanente Northwest medical centers participated in the study during a 23-month recruitment period, from October 1997 through August 1999.

PARTICIPANTS

Figure 1 shows the flow of participants through the study. Study staff members scanned electronic appointment records to identify age-eligible teens with appointments at participating medical centers. Staff members invited adolescent primary care patients waiting to see their physician or allied health care provider to participate in a study of "healthy lifestyles and changes in health habits." Eligibility criteria included age 14 through 17 years, willingness to stay after the visit for ~15 minutes, and no intention to leave the geographic area within 1 year. No incentives were offered. Subjects who agreed to participate signed consent forms and completed short, self-administered questionnaires. We assigned participants randomly to either a tobacco prevention/cessation intervention or a brief dietary intervention (both described below). Hollis et al[17] provided additional details about recruitment and characteristics of the study sample.

RANDOMIZATION

Random assignment to the smoking intervention group or diet intervention group was blocked over time and stratified according to medical center and 30-day cigarette smoking status (smoked or did not smoke) at study enrollment. Study staff members not involved in recruitment or randomization printed the stratified allocation assignments on index cards and concealed the cards in envelopes. Recruitment/intervention staff members opened the envelopes after gaining teens' written consent to participate in the study and determining the teens' smoking status from questionnaire responses. The Kaiser Permanente Northwest institutional review board approved and monitored this study.

TOBACCO INTERVENTION

We designed the tobacco intervention to reduce the prevalence of cigarette smoking by preventing smoking uptake among nonsmokers and increasing cessation among smokers. The intervention included 3 primary elements at the enrollment visit. (1) Staff members provided a written prompt (ie, a suggested 30–60-second advice message) to primary care clinicians to encourage teens to quit smoking or to not start. Clinicians were also asked to encourage the patient to talk briefly with a health counselor (study staff member) immediately after the visit. (2) Teens had a 10- to 12-minute session on a computer with the PTC expert system, which was developed by Prochaska, Velicer, and colleagues[16,18,19] for use with adolescent nonsmokers and smokers. This multimedia interactive version of the print-based system has been successful in trials with adult smokers.[20-23] The PTC program assessed the stage of readiness to begin smoking (for nonsmokers) or the stage of change to quit smoking (for smokers) and then delivered highly

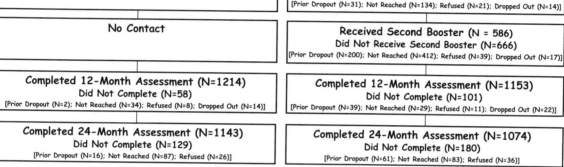

Fig 1. Flow of participants through the study.

individualized advice and encouragement tailored to the teen's reported readiness stage. The program included brief (5–10-second), stage-relevant, teen testimonial movies and graphics designed specifically to appeal to teens. (3) Teens had 3 to 5 minutes of post-PTC motivational counseling with bachelor's or master's degree-level health counselors trained in motivational interviewing techniques.[24] Handouts included a synopsis of the stage-relevant advice or encouragement generated by the PTC program, topic-specific information sheets generated by the computer program as requested by the participant, and small quit kits (eg, cinnamon sticks and Pez candy dispensers) to encourage nonsmoking.

In addition, we conducted 2 individual booster sessions with the PTC and health counselor during the next 11 months. Whenever possible, counselors met with teens at future visits within the intervention contact window to deliver the intended follow-up interventions. In practice, counselors conducted most follow-up intervention sessions via telephone, reading the text of the computer queries and advice messages to the teen and mailing the printed reports generated by the PTC program. Counselors made up to 25 contact attempts at a variety of day, evening, and weekend times, left up to 5 telephone messages, and sent up to 2 letters requesting callbacks.

DIET INTERVENTION

Teens allocated to the diet intervention served as attention control subjects. Health counselors provided 3 to 5 minutes of motivational counseling to promote increased consumption of fruits and vegetables. The recommendations followed the National Cancer Institute Five-a-Day campaign. Counselors provided teens with 2 nutritional information brochures and a small snack-packet of fruit leather. This intervention did not include a computer component. We assumed that some teens would also receive brief tobacco advice as a part of usual care, but we did not prompt clinicians.

INTERVENTION TRAINING AND QUALITY ASSURANCE

Counselors used motivational interviewing techniques[24] during the structured counseling sessions for both the tobacco and diet interventions. The lead health behavior interventionist, a master's degree-level counselor with substantial experience in adolescent health behavior changes, provided the initial counselor training and monitored quality and consistency over time. Interventionists conducted solo sessions only after completing training certification. In the field, interventionists documented components of intervention delivery, including whether they notified the clinician to deliver the brief advice message for the tobacco intervention group. These data were monitored to evaluate the quality of intervention delivery.

To assess the frequency of clinician tobacco cessation advice, research staff members asked participants in both study groups whether their clinician discussed any of the following topics during the visit: nutrition, sun exposure, tobacco use, and exercise. These questions were completed immediately after the consultation with the clinician and, for treatment subjects, just before receiving other intervention components (eg, the computer program).

FOLLOW-UP ASSESSMENTS

A combination of mailed questionnaires and telephone interviews (for those who did not respond to the mailing) provided outcome data after follow-up periods of 1 and 2 years. One month before each annual anniversary of the teen's enrollment, research staff members mailed a questionnaire and a cover letter to the teen. Two weeks later, we mailed a second questionnaire if the first had not been returned. Two weeks after the second mailing, if necessary, study staff members attempted contact via telephone. Blinded study personnel conducted all follow-up assessments. To enroll more participants, we extended the recruitment period beyond our original plans and thus reduced the calendar time available for the 2-year assessment. The second annual follow-up period was therefore truncated by 2 to 3 weeks for the last 140 participants enrolled in the study. The mean follow-up period from study enrollment was 12.4 months (SD: 0.84) for the first assessment and 24.4 months (SD: 0.80) for the second assessment. Follow-up assessments were completed by the end of September 2001.

MEASURES

Outcomes

The primary outcome of the study was the proportion of teens who reported no smoking in the 30 days before the 1- and 2-year follow-up assessments. We hypothesized that abstinence rates would be higher in the tobacco treatment group, compared with the diet control group. Our projected sample size of 2538 assumed a usual care smoking prevalence at follow-up evaluations of ~30% (actual value: 31.4%), α of .05, 0.85 power, a 2-tailed test for the difference in proportions, and a 20% reduction in smoking prevalence in the treatment group. We also used self-reported 30-day use of cigarettes, cigars, pipes, and chewing tobacco at follow-up evaluations to assess abstinence from all forms of tobacco.

Covariates

Table 1 lists additional sociodemographic, tobacco use, and health-habit measures. We briefly summarize these measures here; Hollis et al[17] described them in more detail. We based the depression screen on the 3 items recommended by Rost et al.[25] Stage of acquisition for smoking and stage of smoking cessation were based on the algorithms described by Pallonen et al.[26] Susceptibility to smoking in the next year was based on the algorithm described by Pierce et al.[27,28]

An index of 6 questions derived from the National Cancer Institute Five-a-Day campaign and used previously in dietary research[29,30] provided measures of consumption of servings of fruits, vegetables, and combined fruits and vegetables. French fries were excluded from this measure. A square root transformation was applied to improve normality, and we excluded the overall index scores if >2 items were missing.

Analyses

We compared characteristics of the study groups at baseline by examining percentage distributions of categorical variables and means of continuous variables. We used a generalized estimating equations (GEE) approach for repeated categorical measures to assess the effects of the tobacco intervention across the 2 follow-up years. In these models, treatment group-time interactions provided the tests of hypothesized treatment effects. The primary test of the tobacco intervention's efficacy was the overall difference in rates of abstinence from smoking at follow-up evaluations. Secondary questions of interest, however, were whether the tobacco intervention reduced smoking onset among baseline nonsmokers, promoted cessation among baseline smokers, or both. Consequently, we examined GEE models for cigarette nonsmokers and smokers (30-day use) at baseline and for subcategories within these groups on the basis of a question about self-described smoking status. Most analyses were conducted with SAS software,[31] although we used the Solas software package[32] for the multiple-imputation procedure described below.

Missing Data Imputation

Because of the current debate regarding how to handle missing data in tobacco trials, we examined study outcomes by using 6 alternative methods for handling missing smoking outcome data.[33,34] The first method used the available raw data (ie, "complete cases"), with no adjustments and no imputation for missing data. The second approach, propensity analysis, adjusted the intervention effect at each follow-up time for differences in participants' predicted propensity for being lost to follow-up monitoring. The propensity model was based on baseline age, gender, race/ethnicity, smoking status, stage of change, friends' smoking, smokers in the home, educational aspirations, BMI, exercise patterns, and depression. The third approach, the pattern-mixture method, adjusted the intervention effect for differences in the pattern of missing data (ie, no missing data, missing at either year 1 or year 2, or missing at both year 1 and year 2).

The last 3 methods imputed missing outcome data in various ways. Method 4 assigned the baseline value when follow-up smoking status was missing. Method 4 was equivalent to the traditional "intent-to-treat" procedure for baseline smokers, but baseline nonsmokers with missing outcomes were assumed to still be nonsmokers. Method 5, a single-imputation regression approach, used a combination of baseline variables (ie, same as for the propensity analysis) to predict and impute missing outcomes. Finally, a multiple-imputation regression approach used these same baseline predictor variables but created and then averaged 5 imputed values for each missing case. Multiple imputation provides a more accurate estimate of the variance for the intervention effect than does single imputation. Conclusions were largely consistent among the various missing-data procedures, and we therefore relied on the multiple-imputation procedure for our primary presentation of the main outcomes.

RESULTS

RECRUITMENT AND PATIENT CHARACTERISTICS

Figure 1 shows that 67% of teens (2526 of 3747 teens) approached ≥1 times in medical office waiting rooms consented to the study and were randomized. Table 1 presents baseline characteristics, smoking influences among family and friends, status on a depression screen, smoking status, stage of readiness for smoking acquisition or cessation, and smoking susceptibility. The tobacco and diet study arms were similar with respect to all items, with the exception of a small but significant difference in the proportions of subjects who screened positive for depressive symptoms.

INTERVENTION PROCESS MEASURES

Table 2 shows that a high percentage of clinicians in the tobacco arm received a written prompt to deliver brief tobacco advice. Immediately after the clinical encounter, patients in the tobacco arm were somewhat more likely than those in the diet arm to report that their clinician discussed the tobacco issue, although only 41% recalled such advice. As expected, reports of discussions

Table 1. Baseline Characteristics According to Study Group Characteristics

	Treatment		Control		Total	
	No.	%	No.	%	No.	%
No.	1254		1270		2524*	
Female	738	58.9	758	59.6	1496	59.2
Age						
14 y	345	27.5	329	25.9	674	26.7
15 y	316	25.2	334	26.3	650	25.7
16 y	321	25.6	316	24.8	637	25.2
17 y	272	21.7	293	23.0	565	22.4
Ethnicity						
Black	60	4.8	58	4.6	118	4.7
Asian/Pacific Islander	47	3.8	46	3.6	93	3.7
Hispanic/Latino	56	4.5	62	4.9	118	4.7
Native American/Alaskan Native	24	1.9	29	2.3	53	2.1
White	989	79.6	973	76.9	1962	78.2
Other	67	5.4	97	7.7	164	6.5
Highest level of schooling planned						
Less than high school graduate	16	1.3	13	1.0	29	1.2
High school	81	6.5	101	8.0	182	7.2
2-y college or technical school	211	16.9	199	15.7	410	16.3
4-y college or more	938	75.3	951	75.2	1889	75.3
Exercises for ≥30 min						
Once a week or less	305	24.4	312	24.6	617	24.5
More than once a week	947	75.6	958	75.4	1905	75.5
BMI (tertiles)						
Lower (<20.7)	390	31.1	400	31.5	790	31.3
Middle (20.7–23.7)	384	30.6	400	31.5	784	31.0
Higher (>23.7)	412	32.9	391	30.7	803	31.8
Unknown (missing height or weight)	68	5.4	81	6.4	149	5.9
Tried to lose weight in past year?	572	45.7	596	46.9	1168	46.3
How many friends smoke cigarettes?						
Few or none	743	59.4	737	58.1	1480	58.7
Up to approximately one half	266	21.3	288	22.7	554	22.0
More than one half	243	19.4	244	19.2	487	19.3
No. of smokers in home						
None	803	64.2	771	60.8	1574	62.5
≥1	448	35.8	498	39.3	946	37.6
Positive screen for depressive disorder	606	48.5	689	54.3	1295	51.4
Smoking acquisition stage						
Acquisition precontemplation	886	91.7	883	90.7	1769	91.2
Acquisition contemplation	48	4.9	49	5.0	97	5.0
Acquisition preparation	32	3.3	42	4.3	97	3.8
Smoking cessation stage						
Cessation precontemplation	52	18.5	53	18.7	105	18.6
Cessation contemplation	58	20.6	64	22.5	122	21.6
Cessation preparation	60	21.4	57	20.1	117	20.7
Cessation action	82	29.2	76	26.8	158	28.0
Cessation maintenance	29	10.3	34	12.0	63	11.1
Susceptible to smoke in 1 y	491	39.2	519	40.8	1010	40.0

All comparisons were nonsignificant at $P < .05$ except for depression screen results ($P < .01$).

* Subtotals vary slightly because of missing data, and 2 deceased subjects in the diet condition were excluded.

Table 2. Process Indicators of Intervention Delivery According to Study Group

Indicator/Measure	Study Group				
	Treatment (n = 1254)		Control (n = 1272)		P
	No.	%	No.	%	
Clinician prompted to give tobacco message	1012	80.8	NA	NA	NA
Teen recalls clinician discussion of*					
Tobacco	443	40.9	325	28.8	<.0001
Nutrition	210	19.4	208	18.5	NS
Ultraviolet radiation	56	5.2	45	4.0	NS
Exercise	326	30.1	332	29.5	NS
Teen completed intervention at†					
Baseline	1223	97.5	1132	89.0	
Booster 1	1054	84.0	NA	NA	
Booster 2	586	46.7	NA	NA	

NA indicates not applicable; NS, not significant.

* Denominators exclude 170 missing data in the tobacco intervention group and 145 missing data in the diet intervention group.

† Values exclude 52 missing data among those who received the baseline tobacco intervention and 64 missing data among those who received the baseline diet intervention.

of other lifestyle topics were similar in the 2 treatment groups.

Almost all participants (97.5%) in the tobacco arm received the baseline computer- and counselor-delivered intervention components (mean length: 15.9 minutes), most received at least 1 computer-assisted booster session (in person or via telephone), and approximately one half completed 2 booster sessions. Most (89%) in the diet arm received brief dietary counseling (mean length: 6.7 minutes) to increase consumption of fruits and vegetables. An index of the counselors' ratings of the participants' talkativeness, friendliness, interest, and cooperativeness showed similar levels of rapport in the tobacco and diet groups (15.2 vs 15.3; $P = .34$).

LOSS TO FOLLOW-UP MONITORING

Both annual assessments achieved high response rates, with 2367 of 2526 subjects (93.7%) completing the 1-year follow-up assessment (963 by mail and 1404 by telephone) and 2218 of 2526 (87.8%) completing the 2-year follow-up assessment (743 by mail and 1474 by telephone). Figure 1 shows the reasons for nonresponse at each assessment. Loss to follow-up monitoring at 2 years was significantly greater ($P < .001$) in the tobacco arm (181 of 1254 subjects, 14.3%), compared with the diet arm (128 of 1272 subjects, 10.1%), primarily because those in the tobacco arm had more contact with staff members and thus more opportunities to decline participation.

DIET TREATMENT OUTCOMES

Self-reported servings of fruits and vegetables combined did not differ for subjects in the diet control group and the tobacco arms at baseline (3.66 vs 3.63, $P > .78$), 1 year (3.59 vs 3.62, $P > .77$), or 2 years (3.61 vs 3.60, $P > .92$). Similarly, no treatment effects were seen for intake of fruits alone at 1 year (0.99 vs 1.02, $P > .40$) or 2 years (0.97 vs 0.95, $P > .80$) or intake of vegetables alone at 1 year (1.50 vs 1.49, $P > .92$) or 2 years (1.50 vs 1.46, $P > .48$).

TOBACCO TREATMENT OUTCOMES

Table 3 shows the proportions of participants who were smoke-free for ≥30 days at the 1- and 2-year assessments, with planned contrasts from a GEE analysis for treatment effects at each follow-up time, relative to baseline. We imputed missing values by using a baseline regression model with multiple imputations. The tobacco intervention, relative to the diet arm, increased significantly the

Table 3. Percent Smoke-Free and GEE ORs and CIs at 1 and 2 Years, According to Study Group and Baseline Smoking Status

Baseline Smoking Status	No.	Year 1 Assessment			Year 2 Assessment		
		Treatment, %	Control, %	OR (95% CI)	Treatment, %	Control, %	OR (95% CI)
All participants	2524*	77.2	72.8	1.27 (1.08–1.51)	72.8	68.6	1.23 (1.03–1.47)
Nonsmokers	1935*	90.8	87.9	1.37 (1.01–1.85)	85.8	83.1	1.25 (0.97–1.61)
Smoked in past 30 d	589†	32.5	23.1	1.55 (1.05–2.31)	29.7	20.9	1.55 (1.02–2.36)
Experimenters	140	46.4	50.0	0.80 (0.40–1.60)	49.7	48.7	0.95 (0.45–1.98)
Smokers	448‡	28.4	13.8	2.45 (1.43–4.20)	23.9	11.4	2.42 (1.40–4.16)

Smoke-free was defined as no cigarettes in the past 30 days, with multiple imputation for missing values at follow-up visits.

* Excludes 2 subjects who died before the first follow-up assessment.

† Includes both self-described experimenters and smokers and 1 teen who had smoked within 30 days but did not provide self-description data.

‡ Includes those who smoked in the past 30 days and who described themselves as either smokers or former smokers at baseline.

proportion of all participants (ie, both smokers and nonsmokers at baseline) who were smoke-free for 30 days at the 1-year assessment. This modest treatment effect diminished somewhat by the time of the 2-year assessment but remained statistically significant. Treatment effects did not vary according to (ie, interact with) facility. A similar pattern of results applied when the outcome was defined as no tobacco use (including pipes, cigars, and smokeless tobacco) (data not shown).

Among the nonsmokers at baseline (77%), the tobacco intervention significantly reduced smoking onset at the 1-year assessment, but this prevention effect was no longer significant by year 2. Among all those who had smoked ≥1 cigarettes in the past 30 days at baseline (ie, experimenters, smokers, and recent quitters), the tobacco intervention produced significant effects at both the 1- and 2-year assessments, although the intervention had no effect on the small subgroup ($n = 140$) of self-described experimenters at baseline. In contrast, the tobacco intervention had a strong cessation effect among those who considered themselves to be smokers at baseline (odds ratio [OR]: 2.4; 95% confidence interval [CI]: 1.40–4.16). Conclusions were similar when the outcome was defined as no tobacco in the past 30 days.

In separate posthoc analyses of baseline self-described smokers, the tobacco intervention produced a statistically significant effect among nonwhites (OR: 4.10; 95% CI: 1.01–16.71), despite the small sample size and large CI. The OR was nearly double that seen for whites (OR: 2.16; 95% CI: 1.14–4.08), although the CIs for whites and nonwhites overlapped. In process analyses for all participants in the tobacco treatment arm only, quit rates were higher among those who completed 1 (OR: 2.65; 95% CI: 1.89–3.73) or 2 (OR: 4.03; 95% CI: 2.87–5.65) booster calls, compared with those who completed none. The same was true for baseline nonsmokers who received 1 (OR: 2.72; 95% CI: 1.35–5.47) or 2 (OR: 2.89; 95% CI: 1.48–5.60) booster calls but not for the smaller group of baseline regular smokers (OR: 2.00; 95% CI: 0.83–4.90; and OR: 1.88; 95% CI: 0.73–4.83; respectively). Table 4 shows the ORs and CIs for treatment effects at the 2-year follow-up assessment with 6 alternate methods for handling missing data.[33,34] Results and conclusions were generally similar across methods. For baseline nonsmokers, the regression-based imputation yielded somewhat lower ORs than did imputing the baseline value (ie, assuming that baseline nonsmokers with missing data were still not smoking). For self-described smokers at baseline, the traditional intent-to-treat approach of imputing the baseline value (ie, imputing smoking for missing values) yielded smaller but still strongly significant differences in 30-day abstinence rates between the diet and

Table 4. Comparison of Effects of 6 Missing-Data Procedures on Intervention Results for Abstinence at 2 Years

Baseline Smoking Status	No.	OR (95% CI)					
		No Imputation			**Imputation**		
		No Adjustment	Propensity Model	Pattern Mixture	Baseline Value	Single Imputation	Multiple Imputation
All participants	2524*	1.26 (1.06–1.50)	1.43 (1.12–1.82)†	1.24 (1.03–1.48)	1.17 (1.00–1.36)	1.16 (0.98–1.36)	1.23 (1.03–1.47)
Nonsmokers	1935*	1.25 (0.96–1.63)	1.28 (0.98–1.68)	1.25 (0.96–1.64)	1.30 (0.99–1.69)	1.15 (0.91–1.46)	1.25 (0.97–1.61)
Smoked in past 30 d	589‡	1.67 (1.11–2.52)	1.76 (1.15–2.70)	1.68 (1.11–2.53)	1.29 (0.86–1.93)	1.68 (1.12–2.52)	1.55 (1.02–2.36)
Experimenters	140	1.05 (0.52–2.16)	1.03 (0.50–2.12)	1.05 (0.51–2.16)	0.85 (0.43–1.67)	1.16 (0.57–2.34)	0.95 (0.45–1.98)
Smokers	448§	2.43 (1.39–4.28)	2.55 (1.42–4.60)	2.45 (1.40–4.29)	1.86 (1.07–3.23)	2.43 (1.39–4.22)	2.42 (1.40–4.16)

* Excludes 2 subjects who died before the first follow-up assessment.

† Based on a 1- and 2-year repeated-measures GEE model including baseline smoking status as a covariate.

‡ Includes both self-described experimenters and smokers and 1 teen who had smoked within 30 days but did not provide self-description data.

§ Includes those who smoked in the past 30 days and who described themselves as either smokers or former smokers at baseline.

tobacco arms at 2 years (OR: 1.86; 95% CI: 1.07–3.23).

Discussion

In recruiting for this randomized trial of brief tobacco intervention for teens during routine medical care visits, we found that 67% of smoking and nonsmoking adolescents 14 to 17 years of age were willing to extend their visits to receive counseling about tobacco or diet. The tobacco intervention included clinician advice combined with an interactive, computer-based, expert system and brief counseling and was designed to capitalize on both the teachable moment created by the clinical encounter and the appeal of interactive, computer-based technology. Other key attributes of this strategy were a focus on the whole population of adolescents (whether smoking at entry or not) and a highly tailored, theory-driven intervention.

Among the entire sample of baseline smokers and nonsmokers, the computer-assisted tobacco intervention produced a significant, albeit modest, reduction in self-reported smoking prevalence at both the 1- and 2-year follow-up assessments. Intervention effects for self-described smokers at baseline were considerably stronger, however, and these effects were largely maintained over 2 years of follow-up monitoring. The 2-year quit rate of 24% among self-defined smokers was high for a relatively brief intervention. This result was, however, within the 22% to 25% cessation rate range reported for 4 adult smoking-cessation studies

that used a print-based version of the multimedia expert system intervention used in this study.[20-23] If this approach was implemented broadly and achieved similarly high recruitment and quit rates, then the expected impact on cessation at the population level would be striking.

Quit rates were relatively high (ie, 21% at 2 years) among control subjects who reported at least 1 cigarette in the past 30 days at baseline. This subgroup, however, included self-described experimenters, of whom almost one half (48%) in the control group reported abstinence 2 years later. Among self-described baseline smokers in the control group, the abstinence rate was much lower (11%). Clearly, the smoking patterns of many experimenters are in flux, which might argue for longer (eg, 2-year) follow-up intervals than are common in studies of adults (eg, 6–12 months).

As has been true for school-based, smoking prevention programs,[9] our intervention was less effective in preventing smoking onset among baseline nonsmokers. Treatment effects were significant, although modest, at 1 year and became nonsignificant at the 2-year follow-up assessment. Similarly, no effects were seen among the small group of self-described recent experimenters who did not view themselves as smokers at entry. Why might tobacco prevention programs have so little effect on preventing onset among nonsmokers and those who are early in the tobacco uptake process? One possibility is that those who are still in the experimentation or social smoking phase fail to appreciate just how addicting tobacco really is. Previously, we reported[17] that most of these experimenters at baseline (76.3%) had no intention to smoke in the future. Indeed, many intend to smoke just at parties, to smoke only for a while, or to quit well before any serious health effects would befall them. Unfortunately, many do become addicted and remain long-term smokers. Increasing awareness about the actual frequency of addiction and long-term smoking may be useful.

We found no evidence that our control condition, a 3- to 5-minute motivational intervention, increased intake of fruits and vegetables. The tobacco intervention, however, was well received by patients. In addition to the high recruitment rate, we found that 98% of those randomized to the tobacco arm used the computer program and received brief counseling. Although clinicians were prompted to advise treatment participants but not control subjects, treatment participants were only modestly more likely than control subjects (41% vs 28%) to report that their clinician discussed tobacco during the visit. It is possible that teens under-reported clinicians' tobacco advice, although teens' reports were given immediately after the visit and just before use of the computer program. Most participants (84%) completed 1 follow-up support call, and nearly one half completed 2 calls after extensive efforts to reach them. Other posthoc correlational analyses showed that those in the treatment arm who completed booster calls were more likely to be abstinent. This finding could reflect a true "dose-response effect" or perhaps could indicate simply that new and continuing smokers were less willing to take the calls. Although some teens were difficult to reach, it should be recalled that they were not volunteers who came to us for help with smoking. They were both smoking and nonsmoking patients with a wide range of interest in the tobacco issue who received a very brief intervention as a part of a routine visit.

Although the overall follow-up rates at 1 year (94%) and 2 years (88%) were high, loss to follow-up monitoring was somewhat greater in the treatment arm, compared with the control arm (14% vs 10%). We applied a variety of recommended methods to account for or impute missing data.[33,34] We found that the various methods had relatively little effect on the outcomes or conclusions about treatment effects. For baseline smokers, the traditional approach of imputing the baseline value (ie, assuming that smokers with missing values were still smoking) yielded a lower, although still clearly significant, OR. For nonsmokers at baseline, multiple imputation was more conservative than substituting the baseline value and assuming that they were still not smoking. An even more conservative approach would be to assume that all baseline nonsmokers with missing follow-up values had started smoking. This assumption is hard to justify, however, given that 83% to 86% of baseline nonsmokers with follow-up data were still abstinent. We view the multiple imputation method as the more reasonable and sophisticated approach for handling missing data for a population that includes both smokers and nonsmokers at baseline. It is reassuring that the various missing-data procedures had minimal impact on the overall study conclusions.

A limitation here is that our study sample was largely white (78%). Power was insufficient for specific race or ethnicity subgroup comparisons, but treatment effects for nonwhites were significant and at least as strong as those seen for whites. Another limitation is that our end points were based on self-reported smoking status, which might understate or bias actual smoking rates. Ideally, we would have confirmed biochemically the smoking status at both follow-up points, but current biochemical verification procedures are not well suited for detecting the light and/or occasional smoking patterns typical among adolescents. Because our aim was to conduct a real-life and highly externally valid study, we judged that limiting participation to only those adolescent patients willing to consent to come back for future face-to-face follow-up visits to provide saliva samples would not be feasible and would likely reduce substantially the participation rate and generalizability. The Society for Research on Nicotine and Tobacco Subcommittee on Biochemical Confirmation[35] also concluded that, in large-population, low-intensity, intervention trials, biochemical confirmation is often neither feasible nor desirable. Although self-report may inflate quit rates, the committee determined that the magnitude of such inflation is small and "rarely is differential across intervention conditions."[35] Verification is warranted for teens and/or adults where there is an incentive to deceive, such as in diversion programs or when outcomes are shared with parents or other authority figures. This study had minimal incentives to deceive, because all participants were assured that their data would not be shared with either their parents or their clinician. In this relatively low-intensity, low-demand setting, we expect that misreporting would be modest, similar across groups, and unlikely to have accounted for the large treatment effects seen 2 years after treatment. The baseline age-specific prevalence of reported smoking in this population was also similar to that seen in anonymous statewide surveys, which suggests that most patients were willing to report honestly. However, reporting bias cannot be ruled out completely as a possible explanation for the findings.

The clinical context of our study and the individualized attention from trained counselors might have contributed to the strong effects on quitting among the youth smokers. A European study[36] used an earlier version of the same computer program in a classroom setting, with no adjunct counseling or follow-up support, and found no prevention or cessation effects. That study suffered from having nonequivalent groups at baseline and a relatively short follow-up period. A follow-up report found that lack of engagement in the intervention was a predictor of subsequent smoking.[37] One possibility is that individual patients in a clinical setting might be more likely to engage in the intervention than students in a classroom, although we could not assess this directly.

Although our intervention protocol was designed as a prototype for a practical, office-based strategy, research staff members delivered all aspects of the intervention other than the clinician's brief advice. In real-world practice, office staff members would need to assess smoking status, introduce the teen to the computer program, provide brief motivational counseling, and complete follow-up support. Highly motivated clinicians and support staff members could reasonably offer a similar intervention, but these components would likely prove challenging to integrate into most practice settings. Realistically, health care delivery systems will likely need additional research evidence and a more easily managed approach before they invest significant resources. Future research should explore ways to take advantage of the power and opportunity of clinical encounters while minimizing the time and training demands on clinicians. For example, clinical staff members could provide the first 3 A's (ie, ask, advise, and assess interest) and then refer interested teens for centralized, multisession, proactive, telephone counseling, combined with an interactive website that teens could access conveniently and repeatedly from home. Although they are potentially more practical, the efficacy of more centralized approaches needs to be determined, and we are currently testing 1 such model. We recommend currently that clinicians follow the US Public Health Service recommendations[38] for adolescents and routinely ask about smoking, offer brief advice, assess smokers' interest in quitting, and provide brief assistance and follow-up monitoring as appropriate.

Conclusions

This study is the first large randomized trial to test a brief computer-assisted tobacco prevention and cessation intervention for adolescents in a medical setting. The high acceptance rate, combined with the strong effects on cessation among both white and nonwhite adolescents, shows that a relatively brief tobacco intervention during routine office visits can help teen smokers quit.

Acknowledgments

This research was supported by National Cancer Institute grant PO1 CA72085.

We thank the following contributors to this work: Unto Pallonen, PhD, for helping develop and implement the expert system intervention; Steven Berg-Smith, for developing the motivational counseling components of the tobacco and diet interventions; Christine Catlin, for assuming lead interventionist/recruiter responsibilities; Donna White, for lead follow-up interviewing; Xiuhai Yang, MA, for data analysis; Kristine Funk, MS, RD, for manuscript production; Jennifer Coury, MA, for editing; Center for Health Research recruitment and intervention staff members; Kaiser Permanente Northwest physicians and medical office staff members; and the volunteer teen participants who made this research possible.

References

1. McGinnis JM, Foege WH. Actual causes of death in the United States. *JAMA.* 1993;270:2207–2212

2. Centers for Disease Control and Prevention. Smoking-attributable mortality and years of potential life lost: United States, 1984. *MMWR Morb Mortal Wkly Rep.* 1997;46:444–451

3. Centers for Disease Control and Prevention. Medical-care expenditures attributable to cigarette smoking: United States, 1993. *MMWR Morb Mortal Wkly Rep.* 1994;43:469–472

4. US Department of Health and Human Services. *Preventing Tobacco Use Among Young People: A Report of the Surgeon General.* Atlanta, GA: US Department of Health and Human Services; 1994

5. US Department of Health and Human Services. *Healthy People 2010.* Washington, DC: US Department of Health and Human Services; 2000

6. Johnston LD, O'Malley PM, Bachman JG. *The Monitoring the Future National Survey Results on Adolescent Drug Use: Overview of Key Findings, 2002.* Bethesda, MD: National Institute on Drug Abuse; 2003

7. Lynch BS, Bonnie RS. *Growing Up Tobacco Free: Preventing Nicotine Addiction in Children and Youths.* Washington, DC: National Academy Press; 1994

8. Bruvold WH. A meta-analysis of adolescent smoking prevention programs. *Am J Public Health.* 1993;83:872–880

9. Peterson AV Jr, Kealey KA, Mann SL, Marek PM, Sarason IG. Hutchinson Smoking Prevention Project: long-term randomized trial in school-based tobacco use prevention: results on smoking. *J Natl Cancer Inst.* 2000;92:1979–1991

10. Curry SJ, Hollis J, Bush T, et al. A randomized trial of a family-based smoking prevention intervention in managed care. *Prev Med.* 2003;37:617–626

11. Perry CL, Kelder SH, Murray DM, Klepp KI. Community-wide smoking prevention: long-term outcomes of the Minnesota Heart Health Program and the Class of 1989 Study. *Am J Public Health.* 1992;82:1210–1216

12. Biglan A, Ary DV, Smolkowski K, Duncan T, Black C. A randomised controlled trial of a community intervention to prevent adolescent tobacco use. *Tob Control.* 2000;9:24–32

13. Sussman S, Lichtman K, Ritt A, Pallonen UE. Effects of thirty-four adolescent tobacco use cessation and prevention trials on regular users of tobacco products. *Subst Use Misuse.* 1999;34:1469–1503

14. Sussman S, Dent CW, Stacy AW, et al. Project towards no tobacco use: one-year behavior outcomes. *Am J Public Health.* 1993;83:1245–1250

15. Pallonen UE, Velicer WF, Prochaska JO, et al. Computer-based smoking cessation interventions in adolescents: description, feasibility, and six month follow-up findings. *Subst Use Misuse.* 1998;33:935–965

16. Velicer WF, Prochaska JO. An expert system intervention for smoking cessation. *Patient Educ Couns.* 1999;36:119–129

17. Hollis JF, Polen MR, Lichtenstein E, Whitlock EP. Tobacco use patterns and attitudes among teens being seen for routine primary care. *Am J Health Promot.* 2003;17:231–239

18. Redding CA, Prochaska JO, Pallonen UE, et al. Transtheoretical individualized multimedia expert systems targeting adolescents' health behaviors. *Cogn Behav Pract.* 1999;6:144–153

19. Velicer WF, Prochaska JO, Bellis JM, et al. An expert system intervention for smoking cessation. *Addict Behav.* 1993;18:269–290

20. Prochaska JO, DiClemente CC, Velicer WF, Rossi JS. Standardized, individualized, interactive, and personalized self-help programs for smoking cessation. *Health Psychol.* 1993;12:399–405

21. Velicer WF, Prochaska JO, Fava JL, Laforge RG, Rossi JS. Interactive versus non-interactive interventions and dose-response relationships for stage-matched smoking cessation programs in a managed care setting. *Health Psychol.* 1999;18:21–28

22. Prochaska JO, Velicer WF, Fava JL, et al. Counselor and stimulus control enhancements of a stage-matched expert system intervention for smokers in a managed care setting. *Prev Med.* 2001;32:23–32

23. Prochaska JO, Velicer WF, Fava JL, Rossi JS, Tsoh JY. Evaluating a population-based recruitment approach and a stage-based expert system intervention for smoking cessation. *Addict Behav.* 2001;26:583–602

24. Miller W, Rollnick S. *Motivational Interviewing.* New York, NY: Guilford Press; 1991

25. Rost K, Burnam MA, Smith GR. Development of screeners for depressive disorders and substance disorder history. *Med Care.* 1993;31:189–200

26. Pallonen UE, Prochaska JO, Velicer WF, Prokhorov AV, Smith NF. Stages of acquisition and cessation for adolescent smoking: an empirical integration. *Addict Behav.* 1998;23:303–324

27. Pierce JP, Farkas AJ, Evans N, Gilpin E. An improved surveillance measure for adolescent smoking? *Tob Control.* 1995;4(suppl 1):S47–S56

28. Pierce JP, Choi WS, Gilpin EA, Farkas AJ, Merritt RK. Validation of susceptibility as a predictor of which adolescents take up smoking in the United States. *Health Psychol.* 1996;15:355–361

29. Buller DB, Morrill C, Taren D, et al. Randomized trial testing the effect of peer education at increasing fruit and vegetable intake. *J Natl Cancer Inst.* 1999;91:1491–1500

30. Buller DB, Buller MK, Larkey L, et al. Implementing a 5-a-day peer health educator program for public sector labor and trades employees. *Health Educ Behav.* 2000; 27:232–240

31. SAS Institute. *SAS/STAT User's Guide, Version 8.* Cary, NC: SAS Institute; 2000

32. Statistical Solutions. *Solas v. 3.0.* Cork, Ireland: Statistical Solutions; 2001

33. Hall SM, Delucchi KL, Velicer WF, et al. Statistical analysis of randomized trials in tobacco treatment: longitudinal designs with dichotomous outcome. *Nicotine Tob Res.* 2001;3:193–202

34. Schafer JL, Graham JW. Missing data: our view of the state of the art. *Psychol Methods.* 2002;7:147–177

35. SRNT Subcommittee on Biochemical Verification. Biochemical verification of tobacco use and cessation. *Nicotine Tob Res.* 2002;4:149–159

36. Aveyard P, Cheng KK, Almond J, et al. Cluster randomised controlled trial of expert system based on the transtheoretical ("stages of change") model for smoking prevention and cessation in schools. *BMJ.* 1999;319:948–953

37. Aveyard P, Markham WA, Almond J, Lancashire E, Cheng KK. The risk of smoking in relation to engagement with a school-based smoking intervention. *Soc Sci Med.* 2003; 56:869–882

38. Fiore MC, Bailey WC, Cohen SJ, et al. *Treating Tobacco Use and Dependence: Clinical Practice Guideline.* Rockville, MD: US Department of Health and Human Services; 2000

Tobacco Prevention and Cessation in Pediatric Patients

Jonathan D. Klein, MD, MPH, Deepa R. Camenga**

Objectives

After completing this article, readers should be able to:

1. List the leading preventable cause of disease and death in the United States.
2. Describe the potential effects of environmental or passive smoke exposure in children.
3. Delineate when smoking usually begins.
4. Describe the roles of pediatricians in counseling patients and parents about tobacco use and smoke exposure.

Introduction

Tobacco use is the most preventable cause of disease and death in the United States. Despite major efforts to prevent and reduce smoking, initiation of tobacco use among children and adolescents remains high (Table 1). More than 2,000 young people become regular smokers every day, as many as one in three adolescents currently smokes, more than 15% of high school students report having smoked a cigar in 2001, and 8% of all teens report smokeless tobacco use. Additionally, many children are exposed to environmental or secondhand smoke.

Tobacco is the only legal substance that, when used as intended, causes death and disease. Although complex psychological and sensory factors contribute to smoking initiation, nicotine is a strong pharmacologically addictive substance. Maintenance of smoking is due in great part to the addictive nature of nicotine as well as to the continued effects of social influence.

Children are most vulnerable to secondhand smoke during the pre- and perinatal period and during the first 7 years of life, when most lung

Table 1. Findings from Youth Tobacco Surveillance—United States 2000

- 34.5% of high school students and 15.1% of middle school students currently use some form of tobacco.
- Cigarettes are the most used tobacco product, followed by cigars and smokeless tobacco.
- Exposure to secondhand smoke is very high among both middle school and high school students. During the week before the survey, approximately 9 of 10 current smokers and 50% of those who had never smoked were in the same room with someone who was smoking.
- Approximately 70% of middle school and 57% of high school students who currently smoke live in a home where someone smokes cigarettes.
- Among middle school students, male students (17.6%) were significantly more likely than female students (12.7%) to use tobacco. Among high school students, the gap between boys and girls widens, with 39.1% of males and 29.8% of females using tobacco.
- Among middle school students, white (14.3%), black (17.5%), and Hispanic (16.0%) students were significantly more likely than Asian (7.5%) students to use a tobacco product. Among high school students, whites (38.0%) were significantly more likely than blacks (26.5%), Hispanics (28.4%), or Asians (22.9%) to use tobacco currently.
- Approximately 11% of middle school and 16% of high school students who had never used tobacco would wear something with a tobacco company name or picture on it, a rate that increases to nearly 60% for current tobacco users.

Adapted from Youth Tobacco Surveillance—United States, 2000.
MMWR Morbid Mortal Wkly Rep. 2001;50(SS-04).

growth occurs. Most preschoolers recognize cigarettes, and 55% think that they will smoke as adults. Children and adolescents are most vulnerable to tobacco use during the second decade of life, when most smokers start using tobacco and become addicted to nicotine. One fifth of high

*Department of Pediatrics, Division of Adolescent Medicine, and the AAP Center for Child Health Research, University of Rochester, Rochester, NY.

Pediatrics in Review, *Vol 25, No. 1, January 2004*

school students report smoking their first cigarette before age 13 years. Significant nicotine dependence has been identified among adolescents, and recent reports suggest that addiction may occur very early, even after only a few cigarettes. Early addiction is the only way to produce new smokers.

Prevention of smoke exposure by children and prevention of smoking by youth is the first step in preventing tobacco-related deaths. Although the health risks associated with smoking typically do not become evident until mid-life, mild airway obstruction, slower lung growth, and increased respiratory symptoms are seen more in adolescent smokers than in nonsmokers.

This article reviews the initiation and maintenance of smoking and smokeless tobacco use and reviews strategies that have been developed by the United States Public Health Service (USPHS) and National Cancer Institute (NCI) to help clinicians prevent tobacco use by children and adolescents. Guidelines and resources for pediatricians and other primary care clinicians interested in providing smoking cessation counseling are also discussed.

Environmental Tobacco Exposure

The toxic effects of environmental smoke exposure have been well documented in reports from the NCI and the Environmental Protection Agency. Infants and children are exposed to environmental smoke from parents and from other caregivers. Environmental tobacco smoke (ETS), or secondhand smoke, is a complex mixture of tobacco product fumes and smoke exhaled by the smoker. ETS contains more than 4,000 chemicals, including hydrogen cyanide, sulfur dioxide, and many known mutagens and carcinogens.

Smoking during pregnancy is believed to contribute to 5% to 6% of perinatal deaths and to be the cause of 17% to 26% of low-birthweight births, 7% to 10% of preterm deliveries, and an increased risk of miscarriage and fetal growth retardation. Infants and young children exposed to ETS have increased rates of lower respiratory tract infections, including bronchitis and pneumonia. These children also have more otitis media, reduced rates of lung growth, and an increased risk of death from sudden infant

death syndrome. New cases of asthma, as well as worse chronic respiratory symptoms, also are associated with children who are exposed to parental smoking.

ETS is estimated to be responsible for an increased risk of death from lung cancer and 35,000 to 62,000 deaths among nonsmoking adults from heart disease in the United States each year. Cigarettes are believed to be responsible for 25% of deaths from fires. From 1995 to 1999, smoking caused more than $150 billion in annual health-related economic losses, including $75.5 billion in excess medical expenditures in 1998.

Prevention and Cessation in Primary Care

In the Surgeon General's 1994 report, "Preventing Tobacco Use Among Young People," interventions for the primary prevention of smoking were found to be most effective if they targeted the broad social environment, including countering the promotion of tobacco products. The Surgeon General also found that both primary and secondary prevention of smoking were important in primary care practice. Recent preventive service guidelines, American Academy of Pediatrics (AAP) guidelines, and all other primary care practice organizations' policies call for smoking prevention and cessation efforts as part of routine preventive care for youth. Although few studies have been conducted on smoking cessation approaches for adolescents, NCI guidelines and the most recent USPHS guidelines (Table 2) recommend brief counseling interventions modeled after interventions that have been demonstrated to be effective with adults. Most of those who have quit smoking have done so without formal, one-on-one intervention. Additionally, most smokers, including adolescent smokers, want to quit and are concerned about the personal consequences of their smoking.

Despite this consensus for counseling, surveys have found that only about one third of pediatricians consistently counsel patients or parents not to smoke, and fewer than two thirds of internists or family physicians routinely spend time counseling smokers, even at new patient visits. Even fewer clinicians use recommended strategies to

Table 2. Methods to Increase Effectiveness of Counseling Against Tobacco Use

Direct, face-to-face advice and suggestions
- Give a brief, unambiguous statement to stop using tobacco.
- Review the short- and long-term health, social, and economic benefits of quitting.
- Foster the tobacco user's belief in his or her ability to stop.
- If the patient is not contemplating cessation, try to motivate the patient again at the next visit.
- If the patient is contemplating stopping, try to gain agreement on a specific "quit date" and prepare the patient for withdrawal symptoms.

Reinforcement
- Schedule "support visits" or follow-up telephone calls, especially during the first 2 weeks.

Office reminders
- Use a register system or chart stickers for tobacco users to increase the probability of delivering an antitobacco message at each visit.

Self-help materials
- Provide materials in the waiting room and distribute them to patients to motivate and aid the majority of tobacco users, who quit on their own.

Community programs
- Suggest such programs to provide additional help in quitting.

Drug therapy
- Prescription of nicotine products as adjuncts to counseling may help cessation by relieving withdrawal symptoms. Persons using the nicotine patch or gum should stop all tobacco use and prevent accidental ingestion by children or pets.
- The nicotine patch is applied daily to clean, dry skin sites for 6 to 8 weeks, over which time the dosage of nicotine is weaned. Nicotine gum is chewed slowly and intermittently to allow absorption by the buccal mucosa. Nicotine gum is used for up to 3 months, then tapered over 3 months. Although the potential risks of nicotine adjuncts must be weighed against the known effects of tobacco, nicotine should not be used in persons who have cardiac disease or are pregnant and should be used with caution among those with ulcer disease, claudication, renal or hepatic insufficiency, or accelerated hypertension. Nicotine gum also is contraindicated in people who have temporomandibular joint disease.

Source: *Guide to Clinical Preventive Services.* 2nd ed. US Preventive Services Task Force; 1996.

help patients quit. Smoking cessation messages are most effective when they are presented through multiple routes, repeated over time, and received from various sources and in various settings. To be most effective, physicians must address the causes contributing to children's perceptions of cigarettes and motivations to smoke, including family and peer behavior and media messages. Cognitive developmental considerations among adolescents include challenging limits on their behavior and a belief in their own invulnerability, both of which make the risk of smoking high. The themes used in brand advertising not only sell cigarettes, they also sell the social acceptability of smoking. This often results in experimentation with tobacco and a subsequent addiction to nicotine. Learning and practicing resistance skills can help provide "social inoculation" and, thus, help youth to avoid these unhealthy behaviors.

How much of the focus of adolescent tobacco prevention efforts should be to prevent all experimental smoking or to target addicted, continued smoking by adolescents is controversial. Although social influence plays a significant role in the decision to experiment with smoking, recent evidence suggests that many adolescents quickly become addicted to nicotine. Thus, primary care prevention efforts are especially important, and pediatricians and other health care practitioners can help people quit through interventions directed at both psychological and physiologic effects of smoking. Formal training in smoking cessation techniques (and in delivery of more effective preventive services) has been demonstrated to improve the rates of smoking cessation counseling by physicians. However, just like the many people who stop smoking without the benefit of a formal course, physicians can incorporate effective smoking interventions into their practices without formal training. The USPHS practice guideline "Treating Tobacco Use and Dependence" provides guidance for primary care physicians. In addition, the NCI has developed a variety of materials for primary care clinicians to use to help their patients not smoke. (NCI resource materials are available free by calling 1-800-4CANCER.) The AAP, American Academy of Family Physicians, American Medical Association, and other groups have worked with the NCI to provide smoking cessation training continuing medical education programs for practitioners.

Effective Counseling Techniques: The 5As

The USPHS smoking cessation guideline contained in "Treating Tobacco Use and Dependence" is based on a mnemonic involving the 5As: Ask, Advise, Assess, Assist, and Arrange (Table 3). The goal is to ensure that every patient who uses tobacco is identified and offered treatment. This counseling technique is designed for the adult patient who is willing to quit smoking and is intended to be brief, requiring less than 3 minutes of direct clinician involvement.

EARLY CHILDHOOD (AGES 0 TO 5 YEARS): TARGET PARENTS AND OTHER ADULTS

Ask

Providers should ask about all possible exposures to smoking, including in child care settings and cars, as well as from parents at home.

Advise

The pediatrician should advise parents to maintain a smoke-free environment for the child. Advice should focus on the parents' own health,

the health effects of environmental smoking, and the importance of parents as role models for children.

Assess

The clinician should determine whether the smoking parent is ready to quit. Willingness to quit will help guide further motivational interviewing.

Assist

Assistance includes helping motivated quitters set a quit date, providing self-help material or referrals to the parents' own clinicians, and recommending nicotine replacement or other pharmacotherapy (Table 4). Although some clinicians may prefer not to recommend or prescribe medications to parents, nicotine replacement is available as an over-the-counter product for adults, and pediatricians should be familiar with pharmacotherapy options for adolescents and for the parents of their patients who smoke.

Arrange

Arranging for follow-up varies, depending on how pediatricians decide to provide assistance. Some may refer parents to community agencies, available over-the-counter nicotine replacement products, or telephone or Internet cessation adjuncts that support quitting attempts and provide information and motivational counseling. Pediatricians also may choose to refer parents to their own physicians for follow-up, especially for prescription nicotine replacement or other pharmacotherapy. Because nicotine replacement products are replacing other therapies already being used, pediatricians should feel comfortable prescribing replacement in conjunction with

Table 3. The 5As for Brief Intervention

Ask about tobacco use	Identify and document tobacco use status for every patient at every visit.
Advise to quit	In a clear, strong, and personalized manner, urge every tobacco user to quit.
Assess willingness to attempt quitting	Is the tobacco user willing to attempt quitting at this time?
Assist in quit attempt	For the patient who is willing to attempt quitting, use counseling and pharmacotherapy to help.
Arrange follow-up	Schedule follow-up contact, preferably within the first week of the quit date.

Source: Fiore MC, Bailey WC, Cohen SJ, et al. *Treating Tobacco Use and Dependence. Clinical Practice Guideline.* Rockville, MD: U.S. Department of Health and Human Services. Public Health Service; June 2000.

Table 4. Clinical Guidelines for Prescribing Pharmacotherapy for Smoking Cessation for Adults

Question	Guideline
Who should receive pharmacotherapy for smoking cessation?	All smokers trying to quit, except in the presence of special circumstances. Special consideration should be given before using pharmacotherapy with selected populations: those who have medical contraindications, those smoking fewer than 10 cigarettes per day, pregnant/breastfeeding women, and adolescent smokers.
What are the first-line pharmacotherapies recommended?	All five of the United States Food and Drug Administration-approved pharmacotherapies for smoking cessation are recommended, including bupropion SR, nicotine gum, nicotine inhaler, nicotine nasal spray, and the nicotine patch.
What factors should a clinician consider when choosing among the five first-line pharmacotherapies?	Because of the lack of sufficient data to rank order these five medications, choice of a specific first-line pharmacotherapy must be guided by factors such as clinician familiarity with the medications, contraindications for selected patients, patient preference, previous patient experience with a specific pharmacotherapy (positive or negative), and patient characteristics (eg, history of depression, concerns about weight gain).
Are pharmacotherapeutic treatments appropriate for lighter smokers (eg, 10 to 15 cigarettes per day)?	If pharmacotherapy is used with lighter smokers, clinicians should consider reducing the dose of first-line nicotine replacement therapy. No adjustments are necessary when using bupropion SR.
What second-line pharmacotherapies are recommended in this guideline?	Clonidine and nortriptyline.
When should second-line agents be used for treating tobacco dependence?	Consider prescribing second-line agents for patients who are unable to use first-line medications because of contraindications or for patients for whom first-line medications are not helpful. Monitor patients for the known adverse effects of second-line agents.
What pharmacotherapies should be considered for patients who are particularly concerned about weight gain?	Bupropion SR and nicotine replacement therapies, in particular nicotine gum, have been shown to delay, but not prevent, weight gain.
Are there pharmacotherapies that should be considered for patients who have a history of depression?	Bupropion SR and nortriptyline appear to be effective with this population.
Should nicotine replacement therapies be avoided in patients who have a history of cardiovascular disease?	No. The nicotine patch, in particular, is safe and has been shown not to cause adverse cardiovascular effects.
May tobacco dependence pharmacotherapies be used long term (eg, 6 months or more)?	Yes. This approach may be helpful for smokers who report persistent withdrawal symptoms during the course of pharmacotherapy or who desire long-term therapy. A minority of individuals who successfully quit smoking use ad libitum nicotine replacement therapy medications (gum, nasal spray, inhaler) long term. The long-term use of these medications does not present a known health risk. Additionally, the United States Food and Drug Administration has approved the use of bupropion SR for long-term maintenance.
May pharmacotherapies ever be combined?	Yes. There is evidence that combining the nicotine patch with either nicotine gum or nicotine nasal spray increases long-term abstinence rates over those produced by a single form of nicotine replacement therapy.

Source: Fiore MC, Bailey WC, Cohen SJ, et al. *Treating Tobacco Use and Dependence. Clinical Practice Guideline.* Rockville, Md: U.S. Department of Health and Human Services. Public Health Service; June 2000.

cessation counseling and follow-up visits (unless parents have cardiac illness or other chronic diseases). At follow-up visits, ask again, emphasize the importance of quitting smoking for the child's health, and monitor the progress of parents and others who still may be smoking.

SCHOOL-AGE CHILDREN (AGES 5 TO 12 YEARS)

Ask

Children should be asked if they think it is harmful to try smoking and if they think they will smoke as adults; these questions can help predict who is more at risk for future smoking. They also should be asked if they have tried smoking and if they, their friends, or adults in their lives (eg, parents, teachers, coaches) smoke.

Advise

Children who have tried tobacco or who are experimental smokers should be advised to stop. Advice for children should focus on the short-term effects of tobacco use, consistent with the concrete operational stage of cognitive development in school-age children. The facts that cigarettes smell bad; stain teeth, clothes, or fingers; decrease athletic performance; and are addicting are more salient to children than is the risk of heart or lung disease (unless they have a recent family history of these problems). Additionally, those who have not smoked should be praised and advised to be prepared to refuse offers to try tobacco.

Advice to parents should include discussion of their responsibility as role models and the continued risk of passive smoke exposure. Parents also should be encouraged to educate their children about the messages they receive from the media and from consumer products that promote smoking. Education and efforts to develop media literacy among children can help counter advertising's inappropriate messages about the social acceptability of smoking. These strategies include parents expressing disapproval of tobacco logo items and smoking-related play (eg, as exhibited with candy cigarettes).

Assess

School-age children at risk for nicotine addiction should have their risk assessed. Pediatricians also should determine whether smoking parents are ready to quit as well as whether parents perceive their child to be at risk.

Assist

Assisting children requires different resources from pediatricians, depending on the age and developmental stage of patients and families. Children at lower risk for becoming tobacco users and those who have never experimented with tobacco need praise and reinforcement of their healthy behaviors. Those at increased risk for smoking and those who are experimenting with tobacco need help in developing specific refusal skills to be able to "say no" to tobacco while maintaining their self-esteem with peers. Practicing these skills at first in the office and then at home is effective for helping children remain nonsmokers. Parents who smoke also should be assisted in smoking cessation.

Arrange

Clinicians need to follow-up with children who are experimenting with tobacco or who have ever smoked. Children who are at high risk for smoking based on their attitudes, behaviors, lack of motivation, or lack of confidence in their ability to resist also need follow-up and reinforcement of antismoking messages. For parents willing to quit, follow-up varies, depending on how pediatricians decide to address the Assist step.

ADOLESCENTS/YOUNG ADULTS (AGES 13 TO 20 YEARS): PREVENTION AND CESSATION AS SHORT-TERM GOALS

Ask

Although smoking is common among adolescents, the behavior seldom is volunteered unless providers ask confidentially. Asking about smoking by parents, friends, and siblings in addition to the adolescent's own behavior may facilitate disclosure and can help pediatricians assess the adolescent's risk and target preventive messages more precisely. It also is important to ask about patterns of use consistent with adolescent lifestyles because some adolescents only smoke on the weekends or when not participating on a sports team during the season. Smokeless tobacco use also is common at these ages, and specific questions should be asked about these products.

Screening or trigger questionnaires can help identify efficiently and effectively those youth in need of greater discussion during the face-to-face part of clinical encounters. A trigger questionnaire that is kept as a part of the chart serves several purposes: 1) It informs adolescents about topics that might be considered during their visits, 2) It provides an initial screen for risky behaviors (including smoking), 3) It reminds clinicians about the various topics to be covered during prevention care visits, and 4) It documents the content of care delivered.

Advise

As with younger children, emphasizing the immediate and short-term effects of smoking and smokeless tobacco use on health and athletic performance and discussing the short-term benefits of not smoking are more salient to youth than are the long-term health effects of tobacco use. All adolescents who are smoking should be advised to quit and offered help in making a cessation plan. Those who are nonsmokers should be praised again for their healthy behavioral choices and encouraged to remain nonsmokers.

Assess

Clinicians should determine whether the adolescent is motivated or willing to quit. For those who are willing, the Assist step provides specific tools for the clinician to use to help patients quit more effectively. For others, understanding the process of quitting can be helpful in providing assistance to adolescent and adult smokers. Prochaska and DiClemente's stages of change model for behavior can be useful in thinking about helping smokers quit. These stages—precontemplation, contemplation, preparing to act, action, and maintenance—are useful in determining the stage at which a smoker is with regard to quitting. They also help in setting intermediate goals along the continuum toward maintaining cessation (not smoking).

Adolescents (or parents) who are not willing to quit should receive some assistance, and the following techniques for adults may be used to improve the probability of quitting among adolescents. For the adult patient unwilling to quit, the USPHS guidelines have designed an intervention centered on the 5 Rs (Table 5). The patient should be encouraged to determine why quitting is personally *relevant* to his or her well-being. The pediatrician then should encourage the patient to identify the *risks* of smoking, and in the case of the adolescent, again emphasize the short-term negative consequences of tobacco use. The patient should recognize the potential benefits or *rewards* of quitting smoking, such as having better-smelling breath and saving money. Then, the patient should identify *roadblocks* to quitting, which may include weight gain or fear

Table 5. The 5Rs for Brief Intervention

Relevance	Encourage the patient to indicate why quitting is personally relevant, being as specific as possible.
Risks	Ask the patient to identify potential negative consequences of tobacco use and suggest those that seem most relevant to the patient.
Rewards	Ask the patient to identify potential benefits of stopping tobacco use.
Roadblocks	Ask the patient to identify barriers or impediments to quitting and note elements of treatment (problem solving, pharmacotherapy) that could address barriers.
Repetition	Repeat the motivational intervention every time an unmotivated patient visits the clinic. Tell tobacco users who have failed in previous attempts to quit that most people make repeated quit attempts before they are successful.

Source: Fiore MC, Bailey WC, Cohen SJ, et al. *Treating Tobacco Use and Dependence. Clinical Practice Guideline.* Rockville, Md: U.S. Department of Health and Human Services. Public Health Service; June 2000

of not being accepted by friends. Lastly, the pediatrician should provide *repetition* of these techniques every time the unmotivated patient visits the office.

Assist

Smokers can be given assistance by offering them age-appropriate self-help materials. For those who are ready and motivated to quit, it is especially important to set a quit date. Adolescents should identify potential challenges and determine how they will overcome them. It also is important to encourage youth to enlist social support from parents and friends and to work on strengthening their coping responses. Nonsmoking adolescents or those who are smoking experimentally should be encouraged to use their problem-solving skills to counter potential peer pressure influence and to help them say no effectively.

If symptoms of addiction are present, nicotine replacement may be offered to adolescent smokers. Nicotine replacement requires a prescription for adolescents, but many health insurance plans that include pharmaceutical coverage also provide coverage for nicotine replacement. In general, adults who smoke more than one half pack per day, who smoke within a short time after awakening, or who report withdrawal symptoms after quit attempts (anxiety, tension, irritability, and the craving for cigarettes) have been found to benefit from nicotine replacement or bupropion use. Nicotine replacement therapy has been found to be safe for adolescents; efficacy is currently under investigation.

Arrange

As with adults, adolescents who agree to a quit date should have follow-up contact within 1 to 2 weeks after their quit date and again within the first month to discuss progress and problems with quitting and to encourage another attempt for those who were unable to quit successfully. Most successful quitters have quit an average of seven times before attaining success. Thus, the possibility of relapse should be acknowledged. Clinicians should encourage patients to discuss why they relapsed and then brainstorm about

how they can prevent relapse during subsequent quitting attempts.

The Clinical Office Environment

In addition to smoking cessation counseling, school health education and community/public health strategies promote health and reinforce antitobacco and smoking cessation efforts. Reinforcement of cessation efforts in clinical practice can take many forms. The office environment and the staff must be involved. Consistent nonsmoking messages help counter the social influences that portray tobacco use as acceptable or the norm. Thus, the office should be smoke-free, and the waiting room should contain affirmative health messages (eg, posters, pamphlets, books). Health education content may be added to other patient communications (eg, letters, billing or encounter forms, or other patient reminders). Explicitly countering the tobacco advertisements in many magazines can help sensitize patients and their families to the pervasive and false nature of these messages.

Involving nurses and other office staff in counseling smokers increases the likelihood of counseling, reduces the burden on the physician, and significantly increases adult cessation rates compared with physician advice alone. A trigger questionnaire or other screening form completed by adolescents (or parents), chart sticker systems that identify smoking patients or parents, and a problem list or chart flow sheet that prompts or otherwise reminds both physicians and nursing staff about smoking (and other preventive services) are important parts of systematizing preventive counseling in clinical practice. To be most effective, implementation programs from USPHS and other preventive services recommend identifying a smoking cessation coordinator or an office or practice prevention coordinator. This person can assume responsibility for establishing systems to remind clinicians to deliver smoking cessation and prevention messages, make sure appropriate handouts are in place, and provide ongoing reinforcement and support to other staff within the practice.

Several preventive service guideline initiatives that incorporate effective preventive counseling techniques into their materials are listed in the Suggested Reading. In addition to the USPHS guidelines, the AMA "Guidelines for Adolescent Preventive Services Implementation Manual" and the Office of Disease Prevention and Health Promotion's "Put Prevention into Practice" contain specific recommendations for effective use of an office prevention coordinator.

Schools, Community Health, and Tobacco

As child health advocates, pediatricians have many opportunities to speak for effective use of community resources to prevent youth from smoking. The recent settlement between the State Attorneys General and the major tobacco companies has resulted in the availability of new resources in states and in many communities. There are new federal and state governmental initiatives as well as efforts supported by the American Legacy Foundation, the Robert Wood Johnson Foundation, and others. The NCI has funded a series of studies to improve the evidence and knowledge base for prevention and cessation, the AAP has been active in advocacy at the national level, and the AAP's Child Health Research Center has identified tobacco as one of its top priorities for improving children's health.

It is especially important for pediatricians to be advocates for appropriate school-based education. Tobacco use prevention in schools may be undertaken separately or can be part of a comprehensive health education curriculum. However, several sessions over at least 2 years is necessary for sustained program effects. Effective programs should include information about the social influences of tobacco, information about the short-term effects of tobacco on the body, and training in refusal skills, including modeling and practicing resistance.

The content of school programs is even more important. Curricula based on "social inoculation" that help youth rehearse cigarette refusal skills through role-playing and highlight the negative health effects of tobacco help to prevent smoking. In contrast, those based solely on "improving self-esteem" are unlikely to have effects. More importantly, pediatricians must be aware that smoking "prevention" curricula based on "delaying" the decision to smoke and emphasizing the adult nature of those decisions are harmful. These programs (some of which have been sponsored by the tobacco industry) do not mention the detrimental health effects of smoking and may, in fact, have a paradoxic effect by associating smoking with being more like an adult.

Previously, most smoking prevention activities have been aimed at protecting nonsmokers from the adverse effects of environmental tobacco smoke and reducing the demand for tobacco among young people through education. Activities that restrict the supply of tobacco to minors have progressed slowly because laws that restrict the availability of cigarettes often are not well enforced. However, recent data suggest that local coalitions, especially those active in clean indoor air ordinances and point-of-sale enforcement, have made a difference in smoking by youth. Physicians who choose to be active in antismoking legislation will find readily available information about a variety of initiatives, including banning smoking in and around schools or in other public places, banning all cigarette advertising (especially those targeting youth), and limiting teenagers' access to tobacco products (by enforcing laws that restrict sales to minors, eliminating vending machine sales, increasing cigarette prices, or limiting advertising).

Both enforcement of age-of-sale laws and taxation to maintain high prices have been effective in reducing cigarette acquisition among youth. However, continued advocacy by health professionals is important to counter the influence of the tobacco industry. Illegal sales to adolescents are believed to account for domestic tobacco sales of nearly 1 billion packs a year. Cigarette advertising undermines prevention and cessation efforts.

Advocacy by pediatricians and other clinicians, both as individuals and through organizations, can help prevent youth from starting smoking and make it easier for smokers to quit. In addition to providing clinical prevention and cessation services, clinicians can become aware of programs in schools, reinforce their messages with patients and parents, consult with schools, develop referral lists for tobacco cessation programs for youths, and advocate to maintain effective community programs.

Conclusion

With continued clinical and public health efforts, pediatricians can help reduce smoking and tobacco-related disease among children in the United States. The Centers for Disease Control and Prevention's National Center for Chronic Disease Prevention and Health Promotion Office on Smoking and Health has an extensive collection of resources, including the Surgeon General's reports, community and school prevention guidelines, clinical materials, and other public health materials, at http://www.cdc.gov/tobacco. The NCI also offers materials for patients and professionals, including "You Can Quit Smoking Consumer Guide" and "How to Treat Tobacco Use and Dependence." NCI Trainers can be identified for those interested in local training for groups of clinicians. Telephone services and some publications are available in Spanish. Telephone: 1-800-4CANCER, and ask for "How to Treat Tobacco Use and Dependence." NCI and PHS guidelines, as well as clinician, patient, and other resource materials, are available at http://www.surgeongeneral.gov/tobacco/.

Suggested Reading

Beyond smoking outside. *AAP Pediatric Update.* 2003;24(3):1–9

DiClemente CC, Prochaska JO, Fairhurst SK, Velicer WF, Velasquez MM, Rossi JS. The process of smoking cessation: an analysis of precontemplation, contemplation, and preparation stages of change. *J Consult Clin Psychol.* 1991;59:295–304

Elster AB, Kuznets NJ. *Guidelines for Adolescent Preventive Services.* Baltimore, Md: Williams and Wilkins; 1994

Fiore MC, Bailey WC, Cohen SJ, et al. *Treating Tobacco Use and Dependence. Clinical Practice Guideline.* Rockville, Md: U. S. Department of Health and Human Services. Public Health Service; June 2000

Institute of Medicine. *Growing Up Tobacco Free: Preventing Nicotine Addiction in Children and Youths.* Washington, DC: National Academy Press; 1994

The Maternal and Child Health Bureau, United States Public Health Service. *Bright Futures.* Washington, DC: 1994

U.S. Department of Health and Human Services. Preventing tobacco use among young people. A report of the Surgeon General. Executive summary. *MMWR Morbid Mortal Wkly Rep.* 1994;43:1–10

U.S. Preventive Services Task Force. *Guide to Clinical Preventive Services.* 2nd ed. 1996. Available online from the National Library of Medicine at http://text.nlm.nih.gov or through following the US Preventive Services links on the Agency for Health Care Research and Quality (AHRQ) Web site at www.ahrq.gov.

tobacco:
straight talk for teens

Most teens don't smoke

Did you know that about 80% of teens in the United States don't smoke? They've made a healthy choice.

But think about this:
- One third of all new smokers will eventually die of smoking-related diseases.
- And nearly 90% of all smokers started when they were teens.

This is what smoking does to your body

- Carbon monoxide in tobacco smoke takes oxygen from your body.
- Your lungs will turn gray and disgusting.
- Nicotine, a drug contained in tobacco, can cause your heart to beat faster and work less effectively.

Tobacco can kill

Each time you take a puff on a cigarette, you inhale **400 toxic chemicals like:**

- Nicotine (a drop of pure nicotine can **kill**)
- Cyanide (a deadly **poison**)
- Benzene (used in **making paints,** dyes, and plastics)
- Formaldehyde (used to **preserve dead bodies**)
- Acetylene (fuel used in **torches**)
- Ammonia (used in **fertilizers**)
- Carbon monoxide (**poisonous gas**)

Athletes who smoke can't run or swim as well as nonsmoking athletes because their bodies get less oxygen. This is why coaches tell athletes never to smoke.

Before you start smoking or if you're trying to quit...think about this:

It's a proven fact that the earlier a person starts smoking, the greater the risk of these diseases:
- Cancer
- Heart disease
- Chronic bronchitis—a serious disease of the airways to the lung
- Emphysema—a crippling lung disease

Smoking is addictive

Some of the chemicals in cigarettes cause people to become addicted very soon after they start smoking. If you are a smoker, you'll know you're addicted when
- You crave cigarettes.
- You feel nervous without cigarettes.
- You try to quit smoking and have trouble doing it.

Quitting can be hard, and it can take a long time. **The longer you smoke, the harder it is to stop.**

If you're already addicted, there's help available to you.

Smoking is ugly

- Smoking causes **bad breath** and **stained teeth.** Some teens say that kissing someone who smokes is like kissing an ashtray.
- Smoking often makes other people not want to be around you.
- Smoking stinks. If you smoke you may not smell smoke on you, but other people do.
- Studies show that most teens would rather date someone who doesn't smoke.

Smoking costs a lot of money

Do the math
One pack of cigarettes per day	$3
Multiplied by the days in a year	x 365
Yearly cost for cigarettes	**$1,095**

That's more than **$1,000 a year** that you could be spending on CDs, clothes, a car, or college.

Chewing tobacco and snuff ("dip") are just as bad for you.

If you use smokeless tobacco you are at increased risk for illnesses that hurt your mouth, such as cancer and gum disease. You could lose some teeth. Also, you probably won't be able to taste or smell things as well as before.

Tobacco companies are targeting YOU

Tobacco companies spend billions of dollars every year promoting their products on TV, in movies and magazines, on billboards, and at sporting events. Teens are the main targets of many of these ads.

Most ads falsely show smokers as healthy, energetic, sexy, and successful.

The tobacco companies and advertisers don't mention the bad effects of smoking, like cancer, heart disease, bad breath, and stained teeth.

The fact is, tobacco companies need 3,000 new smokers every day to make up for the 400,000 people who die each year from tobacco-related diseases.

Think about it.

Quitting

If you smoke, quitting is the best thing you can do for yourself, your friends, and your family.

Myth

Many teens think they are not at risk from smoking. They tell themselves, "I won't smoke forever," or "I can quit any time."

Fact

If you ignore the warning signs and continue to smoke, your body will change. It will get used to the smoke. You won't cough or feel sick every time you puff on a cigarette, yet the damage to your body will get worse each time you smoke.

Deciding to stop smoking is up to you. Once you make the commitment to stop, get support from friends and family. You can get help from your pediatrician or school health office as well.

If you don't succeed at quitting the first time, keep trying.

From your doctor

For more information, visit the Web site of the American Academy of Pediatrics at **www.aap.org** or contact any of the following organizations:

Campaign for Tobacco-Free Kids
800/803-7178
www.tobaccofreekids.org

The truth: A campaign developed by teens
www.thetruth.com

American Cancer Society
800/ACS-2345 (800/227-2345)
www.cancer.org

American Heart Association
800/242-8721
www.americanheart.org

American Lung Association
800/586-4872
www.lungusa.org

Please note: Listing of resources does not imply an endorsement by the American Academy of Pediatrics (AAP). The AAP is not responsible for the content of the resources mentioned in this brochure. Phone numbers and Web site addresses are as current as possible, but may change at any time.

The information contained in this publication should not be used as a substitute for the medical care and advice of your pediatrician. There may be variations in treatment that your pediatrician may recommend based on individual facts and circumstances.

American Academy of Pediatrics

DEDICATED TO THE HEALTH OF ALL CHILDREN™

The American Academy of Pediatrics is an organization of 60,000 primary care pediatricians, pediatric medical subspecialists, and pediatric surgical specialists dedicated to the health, safety, and well-being of infants, children, adolescents, and young adults.

American Academy of Pediatrics
PO Box 747
Elk Grove Village, IL 60009-0747
Web site — http://www.aap.org

Section V Further Reading

Comerci GD, Schwebel R. Substance abuse: an overview.
Adolesc Med. 2000;11:79–101

Morris RE. The health of youth in the juvenile justice system.
Adolesc Med. 2001;12:471–483

Reproductive Health

Adolescent Gynecomastia

Question

I have definitely noticed a changing clinical trend in my practice that I cannot explain. Twenty years ago, I only occasionally encountered an adolescent male who had gynecomastia. Recently, however, I seem to be seeing many adolescents who have "physiologic" gynecomastia, and many of these boys are earlier in adolescence than the ones I had seen previously. Have other pediatricians noticed this trend? The teens certainly are not happy about it!

Judy Fuschino, MD
Troy, NY

Answer

I am aware of no epidemiologic evidence to suggest that the prevalence of gynecomastia is increasing, but it would not be surprising if it were, and Dr Fuschino's observation may, in fact, be accurate.

Gynecomastia refers to the presence of true breast tissue (not adipose tissue) in males. It generally is caused by a relative imbalance of estrogen and androgen, which may prove to be either physiologic or pathologic. Transient gynecomastia occurs in 60% to 90% of newborns as a result of stimulation by maternal estrogen. Elderly men frequently develop gynecomastia too, often as a result of an age-related decrease in levels of bioavailable testosterone and frequently complicated by chronic cardiovascular, liver, or other disorders or by medications used in their treatment.

Up to two thirds of boys develop physiologic gynecomastia during puberty. Although these boys have similar levels of testosterone, estradiol, estrone, follicle-stimulating hormone (FSH), leutenizing hormone (LH), and prolactin as their peers, they also have been shown to have self-limited lower ratios of androgen to estrogens. Boys who have physiologic gynecomastia exhibit palpable, sometimes tender, subareolar breast tissue. Breast enlargement is often asymmetric; tissue may appear only unilaterally or may appear bilaterally, but at different times. Breast enlargement typically regresses spontaneously after several months, but it may persist for as long as 2 years. Gynecomastia that persists beyond 2 years is unlikely to resolve on its own.

There are many pathologic causes of gynecomastia (Table 1); most are uncommon. A wide range of prescribed, illicit, or accidentally ingested

Table 1. Causes of Gynecomastia in Pubertal Males

- **Physiologic gynecomastia**
- **Pseudogynecomastia (fatty enlargement of the breasts)**
- **Decreased androgen production**
  - Congenital abnormalities of testosterone production
  - Suppression of LH secretion due to hyperestrogenic states
  - Congenital anorchia
  - Syndromes of androgen resistance
  - Acquired testicular failure
    - ■ Viral orchitis
    - ■ Trauma
    - ■ Castration
    - ■ Granulomatous diseases
  - Renal disease
  - Drugs that decrease androgen production (see Table 2)
- **Increased estrogen activity**
  - Estrogen-producing tumors
  - Estrogenic drugs (see Table 2)
  - Conditions that increase activity of estrogen aromatase
    - ■ Adrenal disease
    - ■ Liver disease/cirrhosis
    - ■ Starvation
    - ■ Thyrotoxicosis
  - True hermaphroditism
- **Idiopathic gynecomastia**

drugs can cause gynecomastia (Table 2). Gabapentin, metoclopramide, omeprazole, and a variety of antipsychotic medications are all known to cause gynecomastia. Treatment with human growth hormone can cause gynecomastia, even prepubertally. Gynecomastia as a result of the surreptitious use of anabolic steroids or heavy use of marijuana also is well described. Herbal, "natural," or complementary medicine products that have estrogenic properties, as well as the accidental ingestion of estrogens, also should be considered.

Tumors that produce estrogen (eg, testicular Leydig cell tumors or adrenal tumors) can cause gynecomastia, as can any condition that increases the activity of extraglandular estrogen aromatase, predominantly in adipose tissue, the liver, or muscle. Congenital or acquired conditions associated with decreased synthesis of testosterone (eg, Klinefelter syndrome) also can cause gynecomastia. In Klinefelter syndrome, for example, plasma levels of testosterone are subnormal, LH and FSH levels are high, and about 50% of those affected develop gynecomastia.

The evaluation of a young man who has gynecomastia begins with the initial identification of the condition. Teenage males are generally reluctant patients and are even more reluctant to broach embarrassing issues such as breast enlargement. A complete physical examination, sometimes performed opportunistically as part of an acute illness visit or a preparticipation sports physical, allows the clinician to discover the finding and to respond, typically with reassurance—and a big sigh of relief from the patient. Pseudogynecomastia (fatty enlargement of the breasts) should be differentiated from true glandular enlargement. Similarly, gynecomastia should be distinguished from other breast masses, which can include benign tumors (lipomas, neurofibromas, dermoid cysts), or rarely, carcinomas.

The evaluation of a young male who has gynecomastia should include a careful history and physical examination. The history should specifically include a drug and exposure to drug history. The physical examination should seek signs of congenital endocrinopathies and should pay special attention to the liver and the testes.

Table 2. Drugs That Can Cause Gynecomastia

Drugs known to decrease androgen production
- Ketoconazole
- Spironolactone
- Metronidazole
- Cimetidine

Drugs known to act as estrogens
- Oral contraceptives and other hormonal agents
- Anabolic steroids
- Diethylstilbestrol
- Digitalis
- Estrogen-containing cosmetics
- Estrogen-contaminated foods

Drugs whose mechanisms are unknown
- Calcium channel blockers
- Tricyclic antidepressants
- Antipsychotics
- Metoclopromide
- Omeprazole
- Human growth hormone
- Antiretroviral drugs
- Gabapentin
- Marijuana
- Heroin

Laboratory evaluation is reserved for patients who have additional symptoms or if other findings suggest a pathologic cause for the gynecomastia. Patients who have macromastia (breast size greater than 4x4 cm) may be more likely to have an underlying pathologic explanation for their breast enlargement. The initial laboratory evaluation can be limited to liver function studies and measurement of serum testosterone, estradiol, LH, and dehydroepiandrosterone sulfate (DHEAS) (elevated in adrenal diseases). Further evaluation can be performed if any of these measurements is abnormal.

Most cases of gynecomastia are physiologic and can be managed with reassurance, follow-up, and the passage of time. Management of pathologic causes of gynecomastia is directed to the specific underlying conditions. Testosterone replacement can be helpful for patients who have androgen insufficiency. Antiestrogens and aromatase inhibitors also have been tried, but their use has not been validated in controlled trials. Pathologic gynecomastia, or gynecomastia that has persisted over a long period of time, often results in fibrosis and other changes that do not regress. For these patients, surgery is the usual treatment of choice, predominantly for cosmesis and to address psychological sequelae.

It is easy to speculate on reasons for a potential increasing prevalence of gynecomastia. The prevalence of obesity is rising, making more pseudogynecomastia likely. Use of psychotropic medications, a common cause of drug-induced gynecomastia, also is increasing, as is the use of unprescribed anabolic steroids and herbal and "natural" products. Finally, because of new guidelines suggesting annual health supervision visits for adolescents, we simply may be identifying more physiologic gynecomastia than before. Whether the prevalence of true gynecomastia has increased, the condition is sufficiently common that every pediatrician will encounter it frequently. Reassurance of the boy usually is sufficient, but a minority of patients require further investigation, and a few ultimately require surgical intervention.

David S. Rosen, MD, MPH
Editorial Board

Adolescent Sexual Behavior and Sexual Health

Renee E. Sieving, PhD, RNC,* Jennifer A. Oliphant, MPH,* Robert Wm. Blum, MD, PhD*

Objectives

After completing this article, readers should be able to:

1. Describe the trends related to adolescent sexual and reproductive health in the United States.
2. Explain the steps of becoming a sexually healthy adult in the United States.
3. Describe the continuum of sexual risk.
4. Delineate the best method of encouraging behavior change among adolescents.
5. Characterize how the law affects adolescents' access to reproductive health care.

Introduction

Adolescent sexual behavior is influenced by a complex set of interactions of biology and genetics, individual perceptions, personality characteristics, and sociocultural norms and values. This article addresses trends related to sexual and reproductive health of adolescents as well as clinical assessment and interventions designed to reduce sexual risk and promote sexual health of the adolescents in the United States.

Patterns and Trends in Adolescent Sexual Health

SEXUAL BEHAVIOR

Perhaps in no other single area has there been as dramatic a change in the past decade as in adolescent sexual and reproductive health. There has been a small but significant decline in the percentage of teens who report having had sexual intercourse today compared with a decade ago. Specifically, in 1988, 53% of teenage females and 60% of males reported ever having had sexual intercourse; a decade later it was 50% and 55%, respectively. However, there has been an even more dramatic trend toward early initiation of sex. In 1988, 11% of adolescent females 14 years of age and younger reported having had sexual intercourse; a decade later it was 19%.

Although we tend to think of youths who have initiated intercourse as being "sexually active," substantial data suggest otherwise. In fact, Terry and Manlove noted that in 1997, only 37% of females and 33% of males who reported ever having had sexual intercourse said that they had sex in the past 3 months. In 1995, the majority of sexually experienced high school teens (54% of males and 70% of females) had either no partners or one partner in the previous year.

SEXUAL ORIENTATION

Children engage in sexual play with same-gender friends as a normative part of development. During adolescence, engaging in sexual activity with boys and girls may be a way of testing one's own sexual feelings. Although sexual orientation is believed to be determined before adolescence, its expression may be postponed until early adulthood or indefinitely, making it difficult to estimate the prevalence of homosexuality and bisexuality among adolescents. Uncertainty about sexual orientation may diminish during the adolescent years, with corresponding increases in homosexual and heterosexual affiliation. Among

*Division of General Pediatrics and Adolescent Health, Department of Pediatrics, Medical School, University of Minnesota, Minneapolis, MN.

Preparation of this article was supported, in part, by grants from the Centers for Disease Control and Prevention, DHHS, to the National Teen Pregnancy Prevention Research Center (U48/CCU513331); and from the Maternal and Child Health Bureau, HRSA, DHHS, to the Leadership Education in Adolescent Health Program (MCJ279640A).

adults, sexual orientation prevalence estimates vary with the operational definition of homosexuality. Using a definition that included both homosexual behaviors and attractions, Sell and colleagues estimated the prevalence of homosexuality nationwide to be about 20.8% among adult males and 17.8% among adult females.

In part due to the social stigma surrounding homosexuality and the lack of socially sanctioned ways to explore their sexuality, gay and lesbian adolescents typically experience a period of identity confusion in their process of sexual identity development. Some young people deal with this confusion through sexual encounters with multiple same- and opposite-gender partners or by engaging in other high-risk behaviors. For example, research suggests that adolescent girls who report being bisexual or lesbian have pregnancy rates that are as high or higher than their heterosexual female peers.

CONTRACEPTION

Over the past 20 years, there has been a continuous rise in contraceptive use by America's teenagers. Specifically, according to data from the National Survey of Family Growth, 48% of young people ages 15 to 19 years used any contraception at first intercourse in 1982. This rose to 76% by 1995. Most of the increase reflected a nearly threefold increase in condom use during that 13-year period (Fig. 1).

Despite these positive trends, other indicators of contraceptive use among teenagers have decreased significantly. Specifically, although 43% of sexually active adolescent females said that they used oral contraceptives (OCPs) in 1988, the usage rate had decreased to 23% by 1995. Although the decline in OCP use was offset partly by increases in the use of injectable contraceptives, it was not offset by the use of other contraceptives at most recent intercourse, which remained stable (26% in 1998 compared with 28% in 1995).

PREGNANCY

Birth rates among 15- to 19- year-olds decreased dramatically during the 1990s, from a high of 62.1 per 1,000 in 1991 to 49.6 per 1,000 in 1999, which is the lowest rate since records were first collected in 1940. The 1999 rate represents a 20% decline for the decade. When the trends in pregnancy rates are analyzed by age, the greatest decline was seen among the youngest teens (<15 y), in which there was a decrease of 24% compared with declines of 17% among 15- to 17-year-olds and 12% among 18- to 19-year-olds. There was a 29% reduction in births over the same period for those younger than 15 years, 21% for 15- to 17-year-olds, and 13% for those 18 to 19 years old. Among ethnic groups, the birth rates for African-American teens dropped most dramatically (26%) compared with whites

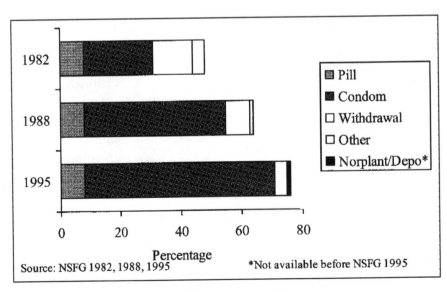

Source: NSFG 1982, 1988, 1995   *Not available before NSFG 1995

Figure 1. Trends in contraceptive use at first sex among females ages 15 to 19 years.

(19%), Asian/Pacific Islanders (16%), and Native Americans (15%). Concurrent with this downward trend has been a decline in abortions among adolescents, from 37.6 per 1,000 adolescent women ages 15 to 19 years in 1991 to 29.2 per 1,000 in 1996. Darroch and Singh attribute 75% of the decline in adolescent pregnancy rates to improved contraceptive use, with the remaining 25% attributable to abstinence. Although other authors have reached similar conclusions, key influences in the decline of teen pregnancy remain a hotly debated topic.

Adolescent Sexual Health: What Is It? How Do We Promote It?

A key developmental task of adolescence is to become a sexually healthy adult (Table 1). As clinicians, we can encourage development of sexual health among our adolescent patients by providing accurate information about sexuality, fostering responsible communication and decision-making skills, and offering guidance and support for young people to explore sexual attitudes and develop positive sexuality values. We also can encourage parents to communicate with their adolescent children in ways that promote sexual health and discourage risky sexual behavior. As members of individual communities and society at large, we can advocate for teenagers' access to comprehensive sexuality education; affordable, sensitive, and confidential reproductive health-care services; and high-quality education and employment.

Adolescents should be encouraged to delay sexual activity until they are physically, cognitively, and emotionally ready for mature sexual relationships and their consequences. They should receive education about intimacy, sexual limit-setting, resistance to negative sexual pressures, benefits of abstinence, prevention of sexually transmitted infections (STIs), contraception, and delay of pregnancy. Because many adolescents are or will be sexually active, they should receive support and guidance in developing skills to evaluate their readiness for responsible sexual relationships.

Research has shown that adolescents get their sexual health information from a variety of

Table 1. Adolescent Sexual Health

Includes:
- Sexual development
- Reproductive health

As well as the following abilities:
- Appreciation of one's own body
- Development and maintenance of meaningful interpersonal relationships
- Avoidance of exploitative or manipulative relationships
- Affirmation of one's own sexual orientation and respect for the sexual orientation of others
- Interaction with both genders in respectful and appropriate ways
- Expression of affection, love, and intimacy in accord with personal values
- Expression of one's sexuality while respecting the rights of others

Adapted from Sexuality Information and Education Council of the United States, 1996; 2000.

sources. In a recent survey, 412 tenth graders were asked about their major sources of sexual information. Similar to patterns in previous research, friends were mentioned most often, with 63% of respondents noting that they obtained information related to sexual health from their friends. Siblings and cousins, the Internet, and magazines tied as the second most common source (31% of respondents); parents and clinics/health-care practitioners also were common sources of sexual information (each noted by 29% of respondents). However, when these teens were asked about their most valued sources of information on birth control and safer sex, their four top endorsements included friends, parents, siblings and cousins, and clinics/health-care practitioners. Because teens value adults as sources of information, it is important for parents and health-care practitioners to initiate conversations and share timely, accurate information, lest adolescents obtain information only from other, perhaps less reliable, sources.

Interviewing Adolescents: Asking the Right Questions

Individuals face many risks related to sexual and reproductive health as they venture through the developmental stages of adolescence. However, as

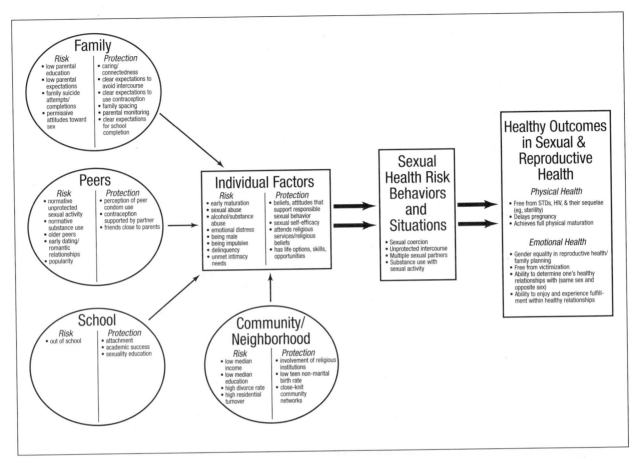

Figure 2. Predictors and protectors of sexual risk among adolescents. Adapted from a paper prepared for the World Health Organization by R. Blum, 2001.

noted in Figure 2, individual-level and environmental protective factors buffer many teens from these risks.

In the span of a brief office visit, how can health-care practitioners assess risk and protective factors in the life of a young person? The HEADSSS mnemonic (Home and family; Education and school; Activities and friends; Drugs, alcohol, and tobacco use; Sexuality and sexual activity; Safety, violence, and abuse; Suicide, depression, and emotional distress) provides an optimal strategy for clinical assessment. Assessment within these domains provides information that is pertinent to the health of adolescents.

Starting with general, open-ended questions from the HEADSSS assessment, followed by more specific sexual health questions, allows the clinician to assess risk and protective factors while gaining an adolescent patient's trust. Adolescents are most likely to respond honestly to opened-ended, nonjudgmental questions. Close-ended

or seemingly judgmental questions tend to elicit socially desirable (although not necessarily honest) responses. Before beginning a HEADSSS assessment, clinicians should explain briefly the routine nature of their questions and why they ask them (eg, "As I do with all the teens I see in clinic, I'm going to ask you several questions to give me a better sense of things that can affect your health."). This explanation may be especially important with new adolescent patients and with younger teens, who may be acutely aware or easily embarrassed by the physical, emotional, and social changes they are experiencing.

Although there are no "magic" questions, certain interviewing strategies result in more accurate understandings. Using HEADSSS as a guide, the clinician starts by asking questions about home, education, and activities and proceeds toward sexuality. Opening questions related to sexual health could include "With whom do you spend time?" or "Is there someone special in your life you consider to be your boyfriend or girlfriend?" These can be followed by more specific questions such as "What kinds of questions do you have about sex that you've never really had the chance to ask?" and "Is there anyone with whom you are having sex now. . .have had sex in the past. . .or are planning to have sex in the near future?" Screening questions regarding sexual attractions and behaviors should be phrased in ways that allow adolescents to discuss same- and opposite-sex attractions, behaviors, and affiliations.

Asking questions that define sexual intercourse help both the clinician and patient clarify what types of sexual risk the adolescent may be taking and allows discussion of abstinence. For example, a clinician might ask, "There are different kinds of sex—anal, oral, and vaginal sex. What kinds of sex are you having?" or "Now or in the past have you had sexual relations with males, females, or both?" Discussing types of sexual activity is important because involvement and understanding vary greatly among adolescents. Giving a range of choices may be surprising to some teens, but may elicit honest responses from others.

Counseling about contraception and pregnancy prevention is especially pertinent with an adolescent. Even those currently practicing abstinence need to learn about contraception for future consideration. A question such as "What are you doing to protect yourself from pregnancy?" or "What are you doing to protect yourself from sexually transmitted infections?" works for both males and females and for abstinent patients.

Finally, closing with a question inviting additional comments shows adolescents that the clinician cares about him or her and about a specific health concern, a characteristic that adolescents consistently remark they desire in health-care practitioners. For example, a clinician might ask, "Is there anything else that I need to know or that you want to ask me so I can provide you with good health care?" This type of question encourages adolescent patients to take control of their own health and provides them an opportunity to address health issues not previously discussed.

Assessing Adolescents' Level of Risk

Sexual risk behaviors, including early sexual debut, unprotected sexual intercourse, and multiple sexual partners, occur in a broader context. Table 2 provides guidelines for assessing adolescents' risk for negative outcomes associated with risky sexual behaviors. The intensity of involvement in sexual risk behavior ranges from no sexual relationship to unprotected sexual intercourse with multiple partners and prostitution. Although risky sexual behavior does not always indicate a high-risk lifestyle, sexual risk behaviors often cluster with other risk behaviors, including substance use, violence involvement, and poor school performance. Adolescents who engage in sexual intercourse at young ages are at higher risk for outcomes that can compromise their health. Finally, sexually active teens who exhibit few positive or prosocial behaviors, such as involvement in organized activities at school or in the community, are at higher risk for outcomes such as early sexual activity and pregnancy during their teenage years.

These guidelines help to differentiate high- from lower-risk clinical situations. High-risk situations are those in which there is serious and long-term involvement in an organized pattern of risk behaviors and few protective behaviors. Clinicians need to intervene whenever an adolescent's risk-taking behavior creates the potential for outcomes that can compromise health or when the behavior threatens the achievement of normal developmental tasks. The intensity of interventions must match

Table 2. Assessing an Adolescent's Level of Sexual Risk

● Intensity of involvement in sexual risk behavior from a level of experimentation to a level of commitment
● Number of different risk behaviors in which an adolescent is involved and degree to which behaviors constitute an organized pattern or lifestyle
● Age of onset of sexual risk behavior
● Degree of simultaneous involvement in protective behaviors

Adapted from R. Jessor, 1991

both the individual adolescent's level of involvement in risk behavior and his or her readiness to change behavior.

Impact of Clinician Values When Working With Youth

Values are an inherent aspect of sexuality. Patients and practitioners alike view sexuality through their own values "lenses." Sexual values are learned from home, school, religious organizations, media, and other social institutions. They are affected by exposure to life circumstances, values of one's peers, and one's own comfort with sexuality. It is important for clinicians to recognize their own values and be aware of situations in which these values have a positive or negative impact on the care being provided. Although it is not appropriate for clinicians to impose values on patients, it is appropriate to be a catalyst in helping adolescent patients explore and understand their own values. To be effective in working with adolescents, clinicians must first understand their own values.

Guidelines for Brief Office-based Interventions

Among the "best bets" in brief office-based interventions are those that: 1) focus on building protection and reducing risk, 2) help teens build motivation or skills necessary for behavior change, 3) counsel parents about adolescent sexuality in ways that protect the adolescent patients' rights to confidential services, and 4) are based on an understanding of the legal framework related to adolescents' sexuality-related health care.

A DUAL APPROACH: BUILDING PROTECTION WHILE REDUCING RISK

Some behaviors, perceptions, and social forces increase adolescents' risk; other social and individual factors act as protective buffers, reducing the likelihood that young people will engage in risky sexual behaviors. Resnick and others suggest that the most effective interventions for adolescents simultaneously build protection and address risks that are amenable to change. Protective and risk factors are present within social contexts in which teens live and work as well as in the perceptions, beliefs, and behaviors of individual teens.

BEHAVIOR CHANGE: UNDERSTANDING MOTIVATION AND SKILLS

Adopting healthy behaviors or giving up risky behaviors can be thought of as a process involving several distinct stages (Table 3). From this perspective, change is a "spiral" process in which people typically regress and cycle back through earlier stages several times before they succeed in maintaining healthy behaviors.

Early in the process of behavior change, people often lack the necessary motivation for change. In later stages, people tend to lack skills or confidence to bring about a behavior change. Assessing an adolescent's level of motivation and confidence to engage in or avoid a particular behavior gives clinicians a reference for initiating brief office-based counseling (Table 4).

Table 3. Stages of Behavior Change

Precontemplation
- Not intending to change behavior in the foreseeable future.

  Example: The sexually active adolescent who is not using condoms and has no intention to start doing so.

Contemplation
- Thinking about a change in behavior; considering the pros and cons of change.

  Example: The sexually active adolescent who is not using condoms, but is considering use because he or she is worried about sexually transmitted diseases.

Preparation
- Intending to take action in the near future.

  Example: The adolescent who has decided to talk with his or her partner tomorrow about using condoms when they have sex.

Action
- Actively modifying behavior, experiences, or environment to make a change.

  Example: The teen who uses a condom the first time he or she has sex with a partner.

Maintenance
- Working on continuing or reinforcing behaviors adopted during the action stage.

  Example: The teen who has been using condoms every time he or she has had sex with this partner over the past 6 months.

Table 4. Assessing Motivation and Confidence

● On a scale of 1 to 10, with 10 being really motivated, how motivated are you to _____ (eg, use birth control)?

What would it take to move you from a 3 to a 7 in terms of motivation?

● On a scale of 1 to 10, with 10 being really confident, how confident are you that you could start to _____ (eg, use birth control)?

What would it take to move your confidence from a 3 to a 7?

Depending on where an adolescent is in the process of change, different types of interviewing strategies are useful in promoting healthy decision-making and action.

"Typical Day" strategies are useful in opening discussions and assessing an adolescent's readiness to change behavior. For example, a clinician might open a conversation about relationships, sex, and contraception in the following way: "Tell me about a typical day for you and your boyfriend . . .What happens when you're together, how do you feel, when and how might you decide to have sex?"

"Good and Less Good Things" strategies are useful for exploring positive and negative perceptions teens may hold about an existing or new behavior. These strategies are useful with teens in early stages of behavior change. The goal is to help a teen identify and consider reasons that he or she might have for changing behavior. The following example illustrates a "good/less good" strategy: "For you, what are some of the good things about using a condom? And what are some of the less good things about using condoms?"

"So What?" strategies are useful in helping teens express concern about an issue. These strategies are useful with teens who are contemplating behavior change. The goal of these strategies is to have a teen voice a reason or reasons for change. The clinician might follow a discussion of good/less good things about an existing situation with a question such as: "What concerns you most about the way things are?"

"Now What?" skill-oriented strategies are most appropriate for teens in the preparation, action, and maintenance stages of behavior change. With these strategies, the goal is to help the teen plan and practice skills that allow him or her to take action in the direction of healthy behavior change.

Table 5 provides an additional set of guidelines to help adolescents develop and exercise decision-making skills. Rollnick and colleagues expand on office-based strategies that support healthy behavior change (see Suggested Reading).

COUNSELING PARENTS

Research clearly documents that parents have an influence on their adolescent childrens' sexual behaviors. Although parents cannot determine whether their children have sex, use contraception, or become pregnant, their values, parenting practices, and quality of their relationships with their children can make a difference.

Ideally, practitioners should set aside time during routine health supervision visits to talk privately with parents about issues related to parenting adolescents. Grounded in research on parental influence, the National Campaign to Prevent Teen Pregnancy articulated "Ten Tips" along with a list of resources for parents and other adults who work with young people for talking about love, sex, and relationships. These tips provide a useful guide for talking with parents around promoting sexual health and reducing sexual risk of their adolescent children.

Table 5. Help with Making Decisions

● Don't rush the teen into making a decision
● Present options for the future rather than a single course of action
● Describe what other teens have done when faced with similar situations
● Emphasize that "You are the best judge of what's best for you"
● Provide information in a neutral, nonpersonal manner
● Remember that failure to reach a decision is not a failed counseling session
● Resolutions to change often break down; make sure the adolescent understands this and doesn't avoid future contact with you if things change
● Acknowledge that commitment to change is likely to fluctuate; empathize with the teen

Be clear about your own sexual values and attitudes. Before communicating with teens about sex, love, and relationships, it is important to clarify your own values and attitudes around these topics as they relate to adolescence.

Talk early and often with your children about sex. Kids have lots of questions about sex, and they often say that they'd like to go to their parents for answers. Initiate an honest and respectful conversation, remembering that two-way conversations are often more effective than one-way lectures. Ask teens what *they* think and what they want to discuss so you can start at their point of interest. Research clearly shows that talking with children about sex does *not* encourage them to become sexually active.

Help your teenagers find options for their future that are more attractive than early pregnancy and parenthood. The chances that your children will delay sex and pregnancy are increased substantially if their futures appear bright. As parents, you can help your children reach toward the future by helping them set meaningful goals, talking to them about what it takes to make the future plans come true, and helping them reach their goals. In particular, by becoming involved in community service, adolescents learn job skills and come into contact with a group of committed and caring adults.

Let your teens know that you value education. Encourage your children to take school seriously and set high expectations for their school performance. Be attentive to your children's progress in school; intervene early if they are not doing well. Get to know your children's teachers, principals, coaches, and guidance counselors. Volunteer at school if possible.

Know what your kids are watching and reading and to what they are listening. The media is full of material sending the wrong messages: Sex rarely has meaning, unplanned pregnancy seldom happens, and few people having sex appear to be especially committed to each other. Is this consistent with your values? If not, it's important to talk with your children about what the media portray and what you think about it. Encourage your children to think critically, asking them what they think about the programs they watch and the music to which they listen.

Supervise and monitor your children. Establish rules, curfews, and standards for behavior, preferably through a process of respectful family communication.

Know your children's friends and their families. Friends have substantial influence on each other, so help your children to become friends with kids whose families share your values. Welcome your children's friends into your home and talk to them openly. Consider talking with parents of your children's friends to establish common rules and expectations.

Discourage early, frequent, and steady dating. Group activities among teenagers are important and fun, but allowing teens to begin steady, one-on-one dating much before age 16 years can lead to trouble. Let your children know your expectations about dating throughout childhood or they may think that you just don't like a particular person or invitation.

Build close, caring relationships with your children early in childhood. The previous tips work best when they occur in the context of caring, connected parent-child relationships. Strive for relationships that are warm, firm in discipline, rich in communication, and that emphasize mutual trust and respect.

For more information as well as resources for parents to talk with teens, visit the Campaign's website at http://www.teenpregnancy.org.

LEGAL CONSIDERATIONS

The legal precedent that many minors have the capacity and, indeed, the right to make important decisions about health care has been established in federal and state policy. At a minimum, the law must offer two different kinds of protection: 1) federal and state laws must allow an adolescent who is a minor to give his or her own consent for care, and 2) laws must ensure that information about care will not be disclosed without the young person's agreement, except in uncommon circumstances. To ensure these protections, experts recommend that the source of health-care funding accommodate provision of independent and confidential services to minors.

The necessity for the law to provide for and protect confidential access to reproductive and sexuality-related care is not inconsistent with the idea that parents play an important role in the care of their adolescent children's health-care needs. Practitioners, parents, and adolescents interact to different degrees around decisions related to health care, depending on the nature of medical issues, family dynamics, and the developmental maturity and legal status of the minor. Many adolescents voluntarily involve their parents in health-care decisions, and many parents are aware of health-care services that adolescents receive. However, some adolescents cannot or will not involve their parents when seeking care. For these young people, legal protection of the ability to give consent and to receive confidential services is necessary.

Many states specifically authorize minors to consent to contraceptive services, testing and treatment for human immunodeficiency virus infection and other STIs, prenatal care and delivery services, treatment for alcohol and other drug abuse, and outpatient mental health care. English and colleagues provide a state-by-state review of minor consent statutes (see Suggested Reading).

Conclusion

Office-based interventions are most likely to contribute to a reduction of risks and promotion of sexual health among young people if they occur in concert with other efforts in schools, communities, and families. Kirby describes key characteristics of successful multilevel efforts to prevent pregnancy and promote sexual health of adolescents. Building skills in effective office-based interventions is worth the effort because although adolescents frequently appear to dismiss our guidance, they listen actively to what clinicians have to say. Whether such interactions facilitate an adolescent's process of making behavior change depends on the accuracy of information provided and the clinician's skills in connecting with and understanding a particular young person's perspectives and readiness for change. Finally, because clinicians may be one of very few adult resources in the lives of some teens, they must be mindful of keeping "an open door" for ongoing conversation and support.

Suggested Reading

Abma J, Chandra A, Mosher W, Peterson L, Piccinino L. Fertility, family planning and women's health: new data from the 1995 National Survey of Family Growth. National Center for Health Statistics. *Vital Health Stat.* 1997;23(19)

Borzekowski D, Rickert V. Adolescent cybersurfing for health information. *Arch Pediatr Adolescent Med.* 2001;155:813–817

Darroch J, Singh S. *Why Is Teen Pregnancy Declining? The Roles of Abstinence, Sexual Activity and Contraceptive Use.* New York, NY: The Alan Guttmacher Institute; 1999

DiCenso A, Borthwick V, Busca C, et al. Completing the picture: adolescents talk about what's missing in sexual health services. *Can J Pub Health.* 2001;92:35–38

Dittus P, Jaccard J. Adolescents' perceptions of maternal disapproval of sex: relationship to sexual outcomes. *J Adolesc Health.* 2000;26:268–278

Emmons K, Rollnick S. Motivational interviewing in health care settings: opportunities and limitations. *Am J Prev Med.* 2001;20:68–74

English A, Simmons P. Legal issues in reproductive health care for adolescents. *Adolescent Medicine: State of the Art Reviews.* 1999;10:181–194

English A, et al. *State Minor Consent Statutes: A Summary.* 2nd ed. Chapel Hill, NC: Center for Adolescent Health & the Law; 2001

Goldenring J, Cohen E. Getting into adolescent heads. *Contemp Pediatr.* 1988;5:75–90

Jessor R. Risk behavior in adolescence: a psychosocial framework for understanding and action. *J Adolesc Health.* 1991;12:597–605

Kirby D. *Emerging Answers.* Washington, DC: National Campaign to Prevent Teen Pregnancy; 2001

Kirby D. *No Easy Answers.* Washington, DC: National Campaign to Prevent Teen Pregnancy; 1997

Meininger E, Cohen E, Neinstein L, Remafedi G. Gay, lesbian and bisexual adolescents. In: Neinstein L, ed. *Adolescent Health Care: A Practical Guide.* 4th ed. Baltimore, Md: Williams & Wilkins; 2002

Miller B. *Families Matter: A Research Synthesis of Family Influences on Adolescent Pregnancy.* Washington, DC: National Campaign to Prevent Teen Pregnancy; 1998

National Campaign to Prevent Teen Pregnancy. *Ten Tips For Parents To Help Their Children Avoid Teen Pregnancy.* Washington, DC: National Campaign to Prevent Teen Pregnancy; 1998

Paroski P. Health care delivery and the concerns of gay and lesbian adolescents. *J Adolesc Health Care.* 1987;8:188

Philliber S. In search of peer power: a review of research on peer-based interventions for teens. *Peer Potential: Making the Most of How Teens Influence Each Other.* Washington, DC: National Campaign to Prevent Teen Pregnancy; 1999

Remafedi G. Adolescent homosexuality: psychosocial and medical implications. *Pediatrics.* 1987;79:331

Remafedi G, Resnick M, Blum R, et al. Demography of sexual orientation in adolescents. *Pediatrics.* 1992;89:714–721

Resnick M. Protective factors, resiliency, and healthy youth development. *Adolescent Medicine: State of the Art Reviews.* 2000;11:157–164

Rollnick S, Mason P, Butler C. *Health Behavior Change: A Guide For Practitioners.* New York, NY: Churchill Livingstone; 1999

Saewyc E, Bearinger L, Blum R, et al. Sexual intercourse, abuse and pregnancy among adolescent women: does sexual orientation make a difference? *Fam Plan Perspect.* 1999;31:127

Sell R, Wells J, Wypij D. The prevalence of homosexual behavior and attraction in the United States, the United Kingdom and France: results of national population-based samples. *Arch Sexual Behav.* 1995;24:235–248

Sexuality Information and Education Council of the United States. *Annotated Bibliography: Adolescent Sexuality.* Available at: www.siecus.org/pubs/biblio/bibs0001.htm. Accessed April 2001

Sexuality Information and Education Council of the United States. *Guidelines for Comprehensive Sexuality Education: Kindergarten–12th Grade.* 2nd ed. Washington, DC: Sexuality Information and Education Council of the United States; 1996

Sieving R, Sucoff C, Blum R. Maternal expectations, mother-child connectedness, and adolescent sexual debut. *Arch Pediatr Adolesc Med.* 2000;154:809–816

Terry E, Manlove J. Trends in sexual activity in contraceptive use among teenagers. *Pregnancy Prevention for Youth (PPFY) Newsletter.* 2000:5

Troiden R. Homosexual identity development. *J Adolesc Health Care.* 1988;9:105

Adolescents and Human Immunodeficiency Virus Infection: The Role of the Pediatrician in Prevention and Intervention

Committee on Pediatric AIDS and Committee on Adolescence

ABSTRACT. Half of all new human immunodeficiency virus (HIV) infections in the United States occur among young people between the ages of 13 and 24. Sexual transmission accounts for most cases of HIV during adolescence. Pediatricians can play an important role in educating adolescents about HIV prevention, transmission, and testing, with an emphasis on risk reduction, and in advocating for the special needs of adolescents for access to information about HIV.

ABBREVIATIONS. HIV, human immunodeficiency virus; AIDS, acquired immunodeficiency syndrome.

Introduction and Background

Age-appropriate education concerning sexuality, drug use, and disease prevention is an important aspect of preadolescent and adolescent health care. The American Academy of Pediatrics has previously addressed important issues of adolescent sexuality and sexually transmitted diseases.[1-3] Specific information regarding sex and sexually transmitted diseases, including human immunodeficiency virus (HIV) infection and acquired immunodeficiency syndrome (AIDS), is an essential component of anticipatory guidance provided by pediatricians to their adolescent patients. Pediatricians play an important role together with parents in discussing the importance of postponing sexual activity, safer sex, and sexually transmitted diseases with adolescents. In addition, pediatricians can be advocates for school health education on HIV prevention. Educating adolescents about sex does not increase sexual activity.[4]

Half of all new HIV infections in the United States occur in young people between the ages of 13 and 24.[5] Thus, pediatricians and adolescents should be concerned and knowledgeable about HIV infection. The risk of exposure to HIV varies by prevalence of HIV infection in the community, sexual behaviors, and concurrent substance use. Sexual transmission accounts for most cases of HIV infection during adolescence. Females account for more than one half of all new cases in adolescents, and three quarters of new infections in adolescent females occur via heterosexual transmission. Among adolescent males, at least two thirds of HIV transmissions occur via male-to-male sex.[6] African American and Hispanic adolescents are at a disproportionately high risk of becoming infected with HIV.

Although abstinence from sexual intercourse (including oral sex) is the safest method of avoiding sexual exposure to HIV, it is impossible to predict which adolescents will remain abstinent. Therefore, education about safer sexual practices, including latex condom use, and other barrier methods should be provided so adolescents might opt to stop or alter their sexual behavior. Alternatives to sexual intercourse, such as masturbation and petting, should be discussed with adolescents. Adolescents should be educated about the potential consequences of sexually transmitted diseases, including deleterious effects on ultimate reproductive capacity (eg, infertility, ectopic pregnancy).

Addressing the consequences of drug use is an essential part of adolescent health care. Although injection drug use is not common among adolescents, any needle sharing, including that done in administration of anabolic steroids, carries a risk of transmission of HIV. In addition, the use of

PEDIATRICS (ISSN 0031 4005). Copyright © 2001 by the American Academy of Pediatrics.

noninjection drugs, including alcohol, marijuana, and cocaine, is associated with an increased risk of contracting HIV infection, because impaired judgment associated with intoxication may increase the likelihood of unsafe sexual practices. Fear of HIV infection may not be sufficient motivation for a young person to forgo substance use, but pediatricians nevertheless should include HIV on the list of risks inherent to such behavior.

Adolescents at risk for HIV because of treatment with blood or blood products should understand that heat treatment of factor VIII concentrates and testing of blood donors for HIV antibody since April 1985 has greatly reduced the risk of HIV transmission from transfusion of blood and blood products. Adolescents should be educated about precautions to reduce the risk of transmission of HIV or other bloodborne pathogens from contact with blood or open wounds (as in contact sports).[7]

Counseling

Counseling of adolescents should be directed at behaviors that place adolescents at risk. Adolescents should be informed of the risk of continued potential exposure to HIV and other sexually transmitted diseases so that they might opt to stop or alter their sexual behavior, use latex condoms, and engage in safer sex. Adolescents with a sexually transmitted disease, in particular ulcerative diseases such as herpes simplex or syphilis, should be informed about the association between these conditions and transmission of HIV. In addition to serving as a marker for unprotected sexual intercourse, these conditions increase the likelihood of HIV transmission.

Discussion of the dangers of sharing needles and methods for sterilizing needles may be appropriate for the adolescent who continues injection drug use despite efforts to interrupt this behavior.

Testing for HIV

Because it is estimated that more than half of all HIV-infected adolescents have not been tested and, thus, are unaware of their infection, discussion also should address availability and importance of testing for the presence of HIV. Testing is important for prevention of HIV transmission and for referral of HIV-infected adolescents to care. A negative HIV test result can allay anxiety resulting from a high-risk event or high-risk behaviors and is a good opportunity to counsel on, and to reduce future, high-risk behavior. Pediatricians should remember that HIV seropositivity may not appear for several months after infection (window period), so retesting after 6 months is advisable in the context of recent or ongoing high-risk behaviors. The risk reduction activities discussed previously should be reinforced. For adolescents with a positive HIV test result, it is important to provide support, address medical and psychosocial needs, and arrange referrals to appropriate care. Awareness of a positive HIV test result helps facilitate reasoned planning of future behavior, which can affect not only the welfare of HIV-infected adolescents but also that of as-yet uninfected partners or contacts. Results should be reported in a straightforward way, and adolescents should be given time to react before the meaning of the test result is discussed. Adolescents may be linked with a specialist in adolescents and HIV disease or an infectious diseases specialist. Pediatricians should recognize the stress of being informed of the presence of HIV infection and offer support and referral to appropriate counseling as needed. In addition, pediatricians are encouraged to arrange for follow-up and ensure that such adolescents enter appropriate care programs.

Advances in the treatment of HIV infection and AIDS include early use of combination regimens of antiretroviral medications, which can relieve HIV-related symptoms and prolong survival. An important benefit of knowledge of HIV seropositivity for adolescent females who become pregnant is the ability to reduce the risk of mother-to-child HIV transmission by intervening with antiretroviral therapy, including zidovudine. Zidovudine, started in the second trimester and given through delivery and then to the infant for 6 weeks, reduces the HIV vertical transmission rate by two thirds, from 25% to 8%.[8] Combination regimens of antiretroviral medications currently being studied and in widespread clinical use, may reduce the risk of HIV vertical transmission even further.

Adolescents who are infected with HIV may exhibit reluctance or refusal to inform sexual partners of their serostatus. In such cases, pediatricians should explore with their patients the reasons for refusal, which may include fear of rejection or even potential violence. Pediatricians should offer support and counseling as needed, and if helpful, provide the assistance of public health experts in partner notification, who will maintain the anonymity of the HIV infected individual. Pediatricians also may be able to offer assistance in informing the sexual partner(s) through role playing and/or providing a safe and supportive setting in which to make the disclosure.

Consent and Confidentiality

Laws concerning consent and confidentiality for HIV care and treatment vary from state to state, and pediatricians need to be familiar with the laws of the state in which they practice. In general, individuals 18 years or older may consent to their own medical care. Similarly, individuals younger than 18 years who are self-supporting, married, parents themselves, or members of the armed services may consent to their own health care without the need for parental involvement. In addition, public health statutes and legal precedents allow for medical evaluation and treatment of minors for certain categorical illnesses, in particular sexually transmitted diseases, without parental knowledge or consent. To date, however, not every state has explicitly defined HIV infection as a condition for which evaluation or treatment of a minor may proceed without parental consent.

Some adolescents may not wish to involve a parent in decisions relative to evaluation or treatment of HIV infection. Such reluctance may arise from a desire not to inform family members about HIV status or a reluctance to reveal behaviors that placed the adolescent at risk for infection. Although it is usually best to involve the family in the health care of adolescents, this is not always the case. Deference to parental wishes to be informed must not interfere with needed evaluation or treatment of adolescents. For adolescents who are able to understand the implications of testing and treatment and are capable of informed consent, and in the absence of local laws to the contrary, it is best to proceed on the basis of this consent alone rather than insisting on parental involvement. Similarly, an adolescent's consent should be obtained before release of any information concerning HIV status.

Generally, pediatricians should respect an adolescent's request for privacy. Nevertheless, questions about whether pediatricians may disclose or receive information about a patient's HIV status without the consent of the patient can arise in several contexts, including disclosure by obstetricians to pediatricians, mandated reporting to health departments, reporting to institutional authorities and employers, the care of accused or convicted sex offenders, instances of accidental needle sticks involving known HIV-infected patients, and issues of charting HIV status in the medical record. Although each of these contexts may at times involve an adolescent patient, they are not specific to young people. Accordingly, disclosure of the HIV status of an adolescent should be held to the same legal and ethical standards as disclosure of the HIV status of an adult. A concern most relevant to the care of HIV-infected adolescents is the limits of confidentiality as they would apply to sexual partners. A difficult question is whether to disclose HIV status to the sexual partner(s) of a patient known to be HIV positive and who persistently refuses to agree to such disclosure. There should be little debate about the desirability of using all reasonable means to persuade an infected person to inform his or her partner(s) on a voluntary basis.

Physicians who intend to disclose information about HIV infection status to sexual partners should consider their duty to inform adolescent patients before testing that results will be disclosed to partners and under what circumstances. Partner notification (without revealing the source of exposure) is available in many areas through local health departments. Maintaining confidentiality is important. Disclosure of HIV infection status is regulated by state laws. Disclosure of HIV infection status to school authorities without an adolescent's consent generally is not indicated.[9]

When desired by an adolescent, pediatricians can play an important role in disclosure and education of school authorities.

Conclusions and Recommendations

1. Information about HIV infection and AIDS and the availability of HIV testing should be regarded as an essential component of the anticipatory guidance provided by pediatricians to all adolescent patients. This guidance should include information about HIV prevention and transmission and implications of infection.

2. Prevention guidance should include helping adolescents understand the responsibilities of becoming sexually active. Information should be provided on abstinence from sexual activity and use of safer sexual practices to reduce the risk of unplanned pregnancy and sexually transmitted diseases, including HIV. All adolescents should be counseled about the correct and consistent use of latex condoms to reduce risk of infection.

3. Availability of HIV testing should be discussed with all adolescents and should be encouraged with consent for those who are sexually active or substance users.

4. Although parental involvement in adolescent health care is a desirable goal, consent of an adolescent alone should be sufficient to provide evaluation and treatment for suspected or confirmed HIV infection.

5. A negative HIV test result can allay anxiety resulting from a high-risk event or high-risk behaviors and is a good opportunity to counsel on reducing high-risk behaviors to reduce future risk.

6. For adolescents with a positive HIV test result, it is important to provide support, address medical and psychosocial needs, and arrange linkages to appropriate care.

7. Pediatricians should help adolescents with HIV infection to understand the importance of informing their sexual partners of their potential exposure to HIV. Pediatricians can provide this help directly or via referral to a state or local health department's partner referral program.

8. Pediatricians should advocate for the special needs of adolescents for information about HIV, access to HIV testing and counseling, and HIV treatment.

COMMITTEE ON PEDIATRIC AIDS, 2000–2001
Mark W. Kline, MD, Chairperson
Robert J. Boyle, MD
Donna Futterman, MD
Peter L. Havens, MD
Susan King, MD
Lynne M. Mofenson, MD
Gwendolyn B. Scott, MD
Diane W. Wara, MD
Patricia N. Whitley-Williams, MD

LIAISON
Mary Lou Lindegren, MD
    Centers for Disease Control and Prevention

STAFF
Eileen Casey, MS

COMMITTEE ON ADOLESCENCE, 2000–2001
David W. Kaplan, MD, MPH, Chairperson
Ronald A. Feinstein, MD
Martin M. Fisher, MD
Jonathan D. Klein, MD, MPH
Luis F. Olmedo, MD
Ellen S. Rome, MD, MPH
W. Samuel Yancy, MD

LIAISONS
Paula J. Adams Hillard, MD
    American College of Obstetricians
    and Gynecologists
Glen Pearson, MD
    American Academy of Child and
    Adolescent Psychiatry
Diane Sacks, MD
    Canadian Paediatric Society

SECTION LIAISON
Barbara L. Frankowski, MD, MPH
    Section on School Health

STAFF
Tammy Piazza Hurley

REFERENCES

1. American Academy of Pediatrics, Committee on Adolescence. Condom availability for youth. *Pediatrics.* 1995;95:281–285

2. American Academy of Pediatrics, Committee on Adolescence. Contraception and adolescents. *Pediatrics.* 1999;104:1161–1166

3. American Academy of Pediatrics, Committee on Adolescence. Sexually transmitted diseases. *Pediatrics.* 1994;94:568–572

4. Kirby D, Short L, Collins J, et al. School-based programs to reduce sexual risk behaviors: a review of effectiveness. *Public Health Rep.* 1994;109:339–360

5. Futterman D, Chabon B, Hoffman ND. HIV and AIDS in adolescents. *Pediatr Clin North Am.* 2000;47:171–188

6. US Department of Health and Human Services, Public Health Service. *HIV/AIDS Surveillance Report.* Atlanta, GA: Centers for Disease Control and Prevention; 1999; 11:1–42

7. American Academy of Pediatrics, Committee on Sports Medicine and Fitness. Human immunodeficiency virus and other blood-borne viral pathogens in the athletic setting. *Pediatrics.* 1999;104:1400–1403

8. Centers for Disease Control and Prevention. Public Health Service Task Force recommendations for the use of antiretroviral drugs in pregnant women infected with HIV-1 for maternal health and reducing perinatal HIV-1 transmission in the United States. *MMWR Morb Mortal Wkly Rep.* 1998;47(RR-2):1–30. Updates available at: http://www.hivatis.org

9. American Academy of Pediatrics, Committee on Pediatric AIDS. Education of children with human immunodeficiency virus infection. *Pediatrics.* 2000;105:1358–1360

Availability of Adolescent Health Services and Confidentiality in Primary Care Practices

Lara J. Akinbami, MD*; Hiren Gandhi, MD‡; and Tina L. Cheng, MD, MPH§

ABSTRACT. *Background.* Little is known about availability of services and confidential care for adolescents in primary care practices or how availability among pediatric practices compares to that among other primary care practices. The objective of this study was to assess self-reported availability of services for medically emancipated conditions and confidential care in primary care practices, to compare physician responses to those from office staff who answer appointment lines, and to compare availability in pediatric practices to other primary care practice types.

Methods. We conducted a telephone survey of randomly selected practices from the Washington, DC, metropolitan area in pediatrics (Peds), internal medicine (IM), and family medicine (FM). We asked staff who answer appointment lines about availability of services for medically emancipated conditions and confidential appointments for adolescents. Physicians received the same questions via a mail survey. Responses from office staff and physicians in the same practice were linked for comparison.

Results. Of 434 practices contacted by telephone, 372 (86%) responded. Of the 615 physicians surveyed from these 372 practices, 264 (43%) from 170 practices responded to the mail survey. Peds practices were less likely than FM and IM practices to offer services for medically emancipated conditions and were less likely than FM practices to offer confidential services to adolescents. Office staff and physicians from FM and IM had higher agreement compared with Peds about availability of services for medically emancipated conditions. Agreement between office staff and physicians about provision of confidential appointments to adolescents was low among all practice types. However, having a written office policy on adolescent confidentiality was significantly associated with agreement between office staff and physicians about availability of confidential services.

Conclusions. Care for medically emancipated conditions and confidential services for adolescents are limited among primary care practices, especially among pediatric practices. All primary care practice types had significant disagreement between office staff and physicians about availability of confidential services to adolescents. Adolescents who call appointment lines are likely to receive inaccurate information about confidentiality policies. Establishing written office policies on adolescent confidentiality may help to improve access to confidential care for adolescents. *Pediatrics* 2003;111: 394–401; *adolescent health services, confidentiality, primary health care.*

ABBREVIATIONS. STD, sexually transmitted disease; Peds, pediatric medicine; FM, family medicine; IM, internal medicine; AOR, adjusted odds ratio; CI, confidence interval.

Adolescents have identified lack of confidentially as a barrier to seeking health care; they are more willing to seek care from and communicate with physicians who assure confidentiality[1-3] and may forgo health care to prevent their parents from finding out.[3-5] Each state in the United States legally entitles adolescents to consent to treatment for medically emancipated conditions that may include contraception, pregnancy, diagnosis and treatment of sexually transmitted diseases (STDs), human immunodeficiency virus or other reportable diseases, treatment of substance abuse problems, and mental health.[6-9] Having the legal right to consent to care is closely related to being guaranteed confidentiality—adolescents who are considered cognitively mature enough to give consent

From the *Infant and Child Health Studies Branch, National Center for Health Statistics, Centers for Disease Control and Prevention, Hyattsville, Maryland; ‡Mt Washington Pediatrics Hospital, Cheverly, Maryland; and §Division of General Pediatrics and Adolescent Medicine, Johns Hopkins Children's Center, Johns Hopkins University, Baltimore, Maryland. At the time this work was started, the authors were affiliated with Children's National Medical Center, George Washington University, Washington, DC.

Received for publication May 7, 2002; accepted Sep 4, 2002.

Address correspondence to Lara J. Akinbami, National Center for Health Statistics, 6525 Belcrest Rd, Rm 790, Hyattsville, MD 20782. E-mail: lakinbami@cdc.gov

are also granted the right to patient confidentiality.[6] However, the availability of confidential care for medically emancipated conditions among primary care practices is not well-characterized.

Although pediatricians recognize adolescents as their patients, studies have found that a high proportion feel uncomfortable with providing services for medically emancipated conditions and/or providing confidential care.[10-14] Despite the 1978 recommendations by the Task Force on Pediatric Education to improve training for adolescent health care,[15] there is evidence that pediatricians still lack confidence in their ability to address adolescent issues and remain uncommitted to providing comprehensive care to adolescents.[10,16] Furthermore, it is unclear how service and confidentiality for adolescents in pediatric practices compares to that in other types of primary care practices.

We conducted a survey in the Washington, DC, metropolitan area to assess availability of services for emancipated conditions to adolescents, the ability of an adolescent to receive care on a confidential basis, and differences among primary care practice types. Because agreement of the entire office staff about confidentiality policies is essential to ensure confidentiality,[13] we surveyed both physicians and office staff who answer appointment lines. Obtaining responses from office staff and physicians in the same practice allows comparison of actual physician policy to information that patients receive when they call appointment lines. We asked about services for pelvic examinations, contraception, and STD testing. The jurisdictions in the metropolitan areas included in this study (Virginia, Maryland, and Washington, DC) all have statutes that allow minors to consent for these services.[9]

Methods

Physician offices that provide primary care within a 25-mile radius of Washington, DC, were identified through listings in the *Washington Physicians Directory*.[17] The listings in this private publication are compiled from medical society rosters, the yellow pages, and requests from practitioners for inclusion. Only physicians in primary care specialties were surveyed. A medical practice was defined as any number of practitioners operating at a single site. The list of practices was divided into pediatric and adolescent medicine (Peds; 270 practices), family medicine (FM; 305 practices), and internal medicine (IM; 442 practices), depending on the specialty of the practitioners. Practices with physicians

from multiple primary care specialties were excluded because of their small number (17 practices).

The telephone survey was conducted with office staff who answered appointment lines between February and July 1998. To determine the necessary sample size to attain an 80% power in discerning differences among practice types in responses about available services, we performed a pilot telephone survey of a randomly chosen subgroup of 50 practices. The final study sample comprised 481 practices. Each practice was called until a response or refusal was obtained or until it was determined that the practice was ineligible (47 were retired physicians or not a clinical practice). Identifying information was stripped from responses after participation, and each practice was assigned a study number.

For the mail survey, conducted between November 1998 and February 1999, all physicians from practices that completed the telephone survey were mailed questions identical to those in the telephone survey. The mail survey was pilot-tested among 20 physicians at our institution to ensure good comprehension. Three successive mailings were undertaken to maximize response rates. Physician responses were anonymous and identified only by the study number assigned to their practice. Using the study number, we linked responses from the telephone and mail surveys so that the practice became the unit of analysis. A total of 170 practices participated in both the telephone and mail surveys. Analysis was conducted with data from the 137 practices that had at least 1 physician who reported seeing adolescent patients (defined as at least up to 18 years of age) and with no missing office staff or physician responses to questions about service provision. To measure agreement between office staff and physician responses, we scanned all physician responses for each practice to determine whether any physician responded that he or she provided the service. When any physician responded "yes," the physician response for that practice was categorized as "yes." We assessed agreement between office staff and physician responses for each practice type by calculating percentage agreement "yes," percentage agreement "no," and percentage of discordant responses. To assess differences among practice types in rates of agreement, we used the Breslow-Day test for homogeneity of odds ratios and reported whether the P value was <.05.

Respondent characteristics were determined from survey questions and from information printed in the *Washington Physicians Directory* (medical school graduation date and board certification status). We calculated the mean number of decades since medical school graduation and the proportion of board-certified physicians for all physicians in each participating practice regardless of whether all physicians in that practice had participated in the mail survey.

We constructed logistic regression models to assess the association between availability of services and practice characteristics. In 5 separate models, availability of service to adolescents (for pelvic examination, contraception, STD testing, confidential contraception, and confidential STD testing) was the dichotomous dependent variable. The following independent variables were included on the basis of findings in previous studies[10,12,14,16,18,19] and entered simultaneously: >50% of physicians in the practice were board certified (dichotomous), mean number of decades since physician graduation from medical school, whether the practice typically saw >5 adolescent per week (dichotomous), existence of a specific office policy on adolescent confidentiality (dichotomous), 4 dummy variables combining solo practitioner status and presence of at least 1 female physician in the practice, and 3 dummy variables for primary care practice type. We also used logistic regression models to assess the association between practice characteristics and agreement between office staff and physicians about availability of confidential services. Agreement between office staff and physicians in the same practice about confidential contraception and confidential STD testing was the dichotomous dependent variable (both "yes" or both "no" responses versus discordant responses) in each of 2 models. The independent variables were the same as above. For each model, the Hosmer and Lemeshow goodness-of-fit χ^2 test was used and confirmed the null hypothesis that the data fit the model in each case. The Children's National Medical Center Institutional Review Board approved the study.

Results

The response rate for the telephone survey of office staff was 86%. The response rate for the mail survey of physicians from the 372 practices that responded to the telephone survey was 43%, ranging from 30% among IM physicians to 68% among pediatricians (Table 1). A total of 170 practices had both office staff and physician responses that could be compared. Table 2 shows respondent characteristics for each practice type. For the telephone survey, IM practices were less likely than Peds and FM practices to see adolescent patients ($P <.0001$). Overall, 88% of respondents were nonphysician office staff. FM practices were significantly more likely to have a medical assistant or physician answer the telephone survey ($P =.006$). We did not exclude practices for which physicians answered the telephone survey because it was likely that physicians regularly answered appointment lines in those practices. IM practices were more likely to have physicians who graduated from medical school 2 decades ago or less ($P =.03$). Among physicians who responded to the mail survey, IM physicians were least likely to see adolescent patients ($P =.02$). Pediatricians and FM physicians were significantly more likely to see greater numbers of adolescent patients per week ($P <.0001$).

The remainder of the analysis included the 137 practices in which at least 1 physician saw adolescent patients and for which there were no missing responses for questions about provision of services. When asked about services available, office staff and physicians from FM and IM practices were more likely than those from Peds practices to say that pelvic examinations, contraceptive services, and STD testing were available to adolescents (Table 3). For example, 97% of FM physicians and 79% of IM physicians provided pelvic examinations to adolescents compared with 50% of pediatricians. Differences among practice types for both office staff and physicians were statistically significant. When physician and office staff responses from the same practice were compared for all services, 16% to 39% of practices gave discordant responses. The highest level of disagreement was between pediatricians and their office staff about whether STD testing was available to adolescents at their practice.

Next we analyzed confidential services among the 92 practices whose physicians offered services for medically emancipated conditions (Table 4). Although office staff and physicians from IM practices were the least likely to say that confidential services were available, the difference among practice types did not reach statistical significance. Disagreement between office staff and physicians about providing confidential services (Table 4) was substantially higher among all practice types than for provision of services (Table 3). Between 45% and 63% of practices had discordant responses between office staff and physicians about provision of contraceptive and STD services to adolescents without parental knowledge.

When the overall proportion of practices providing confidential services for medically emancipated conditions is compared among practice types, the greatest proportion of FM practices offered such services (data not shown). Compared with 16% of all Peds practices and 6%

Table 1. Response Rates: Telephone Survey and Mail Survey

	Office Staff (Telephone Survey) (Response Rate % [n])	Physicians (Mail Survey) (Response Rate % [n])	Practices With Both Telephone and (Response Rate % [n])
Total	86% (372/434)	43% (264/615)	170
Peds	83% (100/121)	68% (135/200)	71
FM	93% (116/125)	32% (63/194)	43
IM	83% (156/188)	30% (66/221)	56
P value	.76	<.0001	

Table 2. Respondent Characteristics: Office Staff (Telephone Survey) and Physicians (Mail Survey)

Characteristics	Peds	FM	IM	P Value
Telephone survey (office staff/practice) ($n = 170$)				
Practice sees adolescent patients	100%	93%	57%	<.0001
Receptionist/office manager/RN respondent (versus medical assistant/MD)	93%	75%	96%	.006
Physicians in practice w/mean medical school graduation ≤2 decades ago	28%	38%	52%	.03
Practices with >50% board-certified physicians	85%	93%	80%	.2
Mail survey (physician) ($n = 264$)				
Sees adolescent patients	99%	98%	86%	.002
Male gender	53%	65%	70%	.06
Solo practice	24%	40%	24%	.06
>5 adolescents seen per wk	83%	82%	9%	<.0001

RN indicates registered nurse.

of IM practices, 29% of FM practices had office staff and physicians who agreed that contraceptive services were available at their practice and that an adolescent could make an appointment for contraception without parental knowledge ($P = .02$). The differences among practice types for confidential STD testing were not statistically significant: 23% of Peds and 17% of IM practices versus 31% of FM practices had office staff

and physicians who agreed that STD testing was available and that an adolescent could make an appointment for testing without parental knowledge ($P = .28$).

To assess the association between provision of services to adolescents and practice characteristics, we used logistic regression models for each of 5 services asked about in the survey: pelvic examination, contraceptive services, STD testing,

Table 3. Services Provided to Adolescents for Medically Emancipated Conditions and Agreement Between Office Staff and Physicians

	"Yes" Response		Agreement Between Office Staff (Telephone) and Physician (Mail) Responses[†]		
	Office Staff (Telephone)	Physician* (Mail)	Agreement "Yes"	Agreement "No"	Discordant Responses
Pelvic exam available?					
Peds ($n = 70$)	43%	50%	39%	46%	16%
FM ($n = 39$)	85%	97%	82%	0%	18%
IM ($n = 28$)	86%	79%	71%	7%	21%
P value	<.0001	<.0001			
Contraceptive services available?					
Peds ($n = 70$)	43%	59%	40%	39%	21%
FM ($n = 39$)	77%	97%	77%	3%	21%
IM ($n = 28$)	86%	71%	64%	7%	29%
P value	<.0001	<.0001			
STD testing available?					
Peds ($n = 69$)	52%	80%	46%	15%	39%
FM ($n = 39$)	85%	95%	79%	0%	21%
IM ($n = 27$)	85%	96%	81%	0%	19%
P value	.0002	.02			

*All physician responses for each practice were scanned. When <u>any</u> physician responded that he or she provided the service, the physician response for that practice was categorized as "yes."

[†]Differences among practice types in agreement rates were assessed with Breslow-Day test for homogeneity of odds ratios. For all services in this table, agreement rates were not significantly different among practice types, ie, all P values were >.05.

Table 4. Services Provided Confidentially to Adolescents and Agreement Between Office Staff and Physicians, Among Practices

	"Yes" Response		Agreement Between Office Staff (Telephone) and Physician (Mail) Responses[†]		
	Office Staff (Telephone)	Physician* (Mail)	Agreement "Yes"	Agreement "No"	Discordant Responses
Contraceptive services available without parental knowledge?					
Peds (n = 29)	38%	83%	38%	17%	45%
FM (n = 33)	39%	85%	36%	12%	52%
IM (n = 19)	32%	63%	16%	21%	63%
P value	.84	.15			
STD testing available without parental knowledge?					
Peds (n = 35)	49%	91%	46%	6%	49%
FM (n = 34)	41%	88%	38%	9%	53%
IM (n = 23)	39%	78%	35%	17%	48%
P value	.73	.33			

* All physician responses for each practice were scanned. When any physician responded that he or she provided the service, the physician response for that practice was categorized as "yes."

† Differences among practice types in agreement rates were assessed with Breslow-Day test for homogeneity of odds ratios. For all services in this table, agreement rates were not significantly different among practice types, ie, all P values were >.05.

confidential contraceptive services, and confidential STD testing (Table 5). The adjusted odds ratios (AORs) for which the 95% confidence interval (CI) excludes the value of 1.0 are shown in bold type. Three factors were associated with providing services for medically emancipated conditions and providing confidential service. First, practice type had the strongest association with providing pelvic examinations, contraception, and STD testing to adolescents. Physicians in FM practices were at significantly higher odds than those in Peds practices to offer all of the services about which we asked and to provide them confidentially. Physicians in IM practices were at significantly higher odds than those in Peds practices to offer pelvic examinations and STD testing and to offer STD testing confidentially. Second, practices that usually saw >5 adolescents per week were at significantly higher odds of providing STD testing and confidential STD testing to adolescents than practices with a lower volume of adolescent patient visits. Having >50% board-certified physicians in a practice was also associated with providing services to adolescents but only significantly with confidential contraceptive services. Third, when solo practitioner status and practitioner gender were considered, group practices with at least 1 female physician (referent group) were at higher odds of providing all 5 services than solo practices with either a male or a female physician and group practices with no female physicians, although the 95% CI of the AOR included 1.0 in some cases.

We also analyzed the association between practice characteristics and agreement between office staff and physicians in the same practice about availability of confidential services. For both models, only having >50% board-certified physicians and having a written office policy on adolescent confidentiality were significantly associated with agreement about confidential services. For agreement about whether adolescents could get contraceptive services without parental knowledge, having >50% board-certified physicians was negatively associated with an AOR of 0.1 (0.02–0.8) and having an office policy positively associated with an AOR of 3.5 (1.2–10.6). For agreement about confidential STD testing for adolescents, having >50% board-certified physicians had an AOR of 0.1 (0.01–0.7) and having an office policy had an AOR of 4.5 (1.5–13.6).

Table 5. Logistic Regression Results: Association Between Practice Characteristics With Physician Response That Service Was Available*

Independent Variables	Pelvic Exam	Contraception	STD Testing	Confidential Contraception	Confidential STD Testing
Practice type					
FM	**77.6 (8.8–688.3)**	**42.1 (5.0–352.7)**	**6.9 (1.3–37.3)**	**8.2 (2.6–25.5)**	**4.1 (1.3–12.8)**
IM	**13.6 (2.6–72.7)**	2.8 (0.7–12.0)	**21.6 (3.0–158.1)**	2.7 (0.7–11.0)	**6.9 (1.6–29.6)**
Peds	ref	ref	ref	ref	ref
Practice characteristics					
>50% board-certified physicians in practice	2.1 (0.7–6.3)	2.8 (0.9–8.5)	2.1 (0.5–8.5)	**3.2 (1.1–9.9)**	2.2 (0.7–6.4)
Decades since medical school graduation (practice mean)†	0.8 (0.5–2.0)	0.8 (0.5–1.2)	1.5 (0.8–2.9)	1.2 (0.8–1.8)	1.3 (0.8–2.1)
Practice sees >5 adolescents per week‡	1.7 (0.5–6.4)	0.7 (0.2–2.3)	**4.7 (1.2–18.5)**	1.6 (0.5–5.0)	**4.2 (1.4–13.2)**
Office has written policy on adolescent confidentiality	1.2 (0.4–3.4)	0.7 (0.2–1.9)	0.9 (0.3–3.0)	1.3 (0.5–3.3)	1.3 (0.5–3.5)
Presence of female physicians in solo/group practice					
Solo practice, male physician	0.4 (0.1–1.5)	0.3 (0.1–1.3)	0.4 (0.1–2.0)	**0.1 (0.03–0.4)**	**0.2 (0.04–0.6)**
Solo practice, female physician	0.5 (0.1–2.0)	**0.2 (0.1–0.8)**	0.8 (0.1–4.6)	**0.2 (0.1–0.8)**	**0.2 (0.1–0.9)**
Group practice, no female physician	**0.1 (0.03–0.5)**	**0.1 (0.03–0.4)**	0.2 (0.1–1.2)	**0.1 (0.03–0.3)**	**0.2 (0.1–0.7)**
Group practice, at least 1 female physician	ref	ref	ref	ref	ref

* All physician responses for each practice were scanned. When <u>any</u> physician responded that he or she provided the service, the physician response for that practice was categorized as "yes."

† The odds ratio represents the risk for each additional decade since graduation from medical school for the practice mean.

‡ For solo practices, the response of the solo practitioner was used. For group practices, when any physician said that the practice saw >5 adolescents per week, that group practice was considered to see >5 adolescents per week.

Respondents were also asked about other aspects of providing services that may improve access for adolescents (Table 6). Respondents from IM practices were least likely and those from Peds practices most likely to say that same-day urgent appointments were available. Peds practices had the lowest disagreement between office staff and physicians about availability of same-day appointments. A low percentage of office staff and physicians from all practice types said that the fee required at the time of service for adolescents without health insurance was lower than $50 or that their practice offered a sliding-scale fee schedule based on ability to pay. In general, FM practices seemed to have lower up-front fees for adolescents without insurance, although the differences among practice types was not always statistically significant. There was also a high level of disagreement between office staff and physicians

about amount of payment required for uninsured patients and whether a sliding-scale fee schedule was available: discordance rates ranged from 32% to 56%. Finally, when asked whether the practice had a specific office policy on adolescent confidentiality, respondents from Peds practices were most likely to say yes. IM respondents were more likely to say no but had the lowest percentage of discordant responses.

Table 7 shows reasons given by pediatricians for not providing pelvic examinations or contraceptive services to adolescents. The most common reasons for not providing pelvic examinations were lack of equipment and expertise, low patient demand for this service, and inadequate staffing. Pediatricians who did not provide contraceptive services were most likely to respond that they did not provide pelvic examinations (and therefore could not provide the medical surveillance

Table 6. Comparison of "Adolescent-Friendly" Policies Among Primary Care Practice Types and Agreement Between Office Staff and Physicians

	"Yes" Response		Agreement Between Office Staff (Telephone) and Physician (Mail) Responses[†]		
	Office Staff (Telephone)	Physician* (Mail)	Agreement "Yes"	Agreement "No"	Discordant Responses
Same-day urgent appointment available?					
Peds (n = 70)	91%	97%	91%	3%	6%
FM (n = 40)	88%	90%	78%	0%	23%
IM (n = 27)	70%	89%	59%	0%	41%
P value	.03	.20			
If no insurance, required fee up front <$50?					
Peds (n = 59)	20%	42%	10%	47%	42%
FM (n = 36)	25%	53%	11%	33%	56%
IM (n = 23)	9%	52%	4%	43%	52%
P value	.30	.54			
Sliding-fee scale based on ability to pay?					
Peds (n = 63)	35%	27%	11%	49%	40%
FM (n = 38)	61%	50%	29%	18%	53%
IM (n = 19)	47%	37%	26%	42%	32%
P value	.04	.06			
Adolescent confidentiality policy?					
Peds (n = 56)	70%	77%	52%	5%	43%
FM (n = 32)	50%	69%	34%	16%	50%
IM (n = 26)	12%	42%	8%	54%	38%
P value	<.0001	.008			

* All physician responses for each practice were scanned. When <u>any</u> physician responded that he or she provided the service, the physician response for that practice was categorized as "yes."

† Differences among practice types in agreement rates were assessed with Breslow-Day test for homogeneity of odds ratios. For all services in this table, agreement rates were significantly different among practice types only for availability of same-day urgent appointment (P <.05).

necessary for contraceptive services), that they lacked expertise, and that patient demand for contraception was low.

Discussion

Providing confidential care to adolescents is challenging. The Society for Adolescent Medicine[6] has called for health providers to inform patients and families about the requirements of confidential care and to strike the difficult balance between respecting an adolescent's wishes about sharing information and involving responsible adults when necessary. The tumultuous nature of adolescence and the varied stages of autonomy among adolescents pose challenges. In addition, practitioners face barriers such as limited time for office visits; lack of training in adolescent issues; difficulties in keeping billing and medical

records confidential; and private, public and political debates about confidential health care for adolescents.[6]

Our results show that care for medically emancipated conditions for adolescents is not universally available in primary care practices in metropolitan Washington, DC, and that confidential care is even less accessible to adolescents. This is especially true in Peds practices, a finding supported by previous studies.[14,20] The most common reasons given by pediatricians in our study for not providing pelvic examinations and contraceptive services are lack of expertise and equipment and low patient demand. Given the high rates of sexual activity, pregnancy, and STDs among adolescents,[21] the perception of low patient demand is probably attributable to the fact that adolescent patients perceive that pediatricians are

Table 7. Reasons Given by Pediatricians for Not Providing Pelvic Exams and Contraceptive Services Among Pediatricians Who Do Not Offer These Services* (Responses From Mail Survey Only)

	% Citing Reason for Not Providing Pelvic Exams (n=67)	% Citing Reason for Not Providing Contraceptive Services (n=59)
Do not provide pelvic exams	NA	78%
Lack equipment	61%	NA
Lack expertise	58%	47%
No patient demand for service	40%	27%
Lack adequate staff	33%	NA
Family negotiations difficult	NA	10%
Uncomfortable/prefer not to see adolescents	6%	7%
Refer to obstetrics/gynecology (more appropriate specialty)	6%	5%
Religious reasons	NA	2%
Lack of time	4%	2%
Inadequate reimbursement	1%	0%

NA indicates not applicable.

* Respondents were able to give >1 response; sum of percentages therefore exceeds 100%.

unable or unwilling to provide the needed services and seek these services elsewhere.[20,22] It may be that pediatric training in gynecologic skills remains insufficient, that pediatricians have less opportunity to use these skills in practice, or both. Few pediatricians cited being uncomfortable with the family negotiations involved or being reluctant to see adolescent patients as found in previous work.[12] Because pediatricians are positioned to guide patients and families through the sensitive issues that arise in adolescence, they should enter practice well-prepared to exercise the spectrum of skills necessary for this role. Past work has shown that training in adolescent medicine during and after residency is associated with physicians seeing more adolescent patients and that continuing medical education was associated with increased provision of services for medically emancipated conditions.[14] Our study reinforces the need to provide both adolescent medicine training in

pediatric residency and continuing medical education in treating adolescents.

The multivariate analysis revealed that primary care practice type had the strongest association with provision of services and with provision of confidential care. Other work has shown that a high percentage of FM physicians deliver reproductive preventive services: >70% reported asking adolescent patients about contraceptive use, condom use, and sexual relationships and regularly discussing confidentiality with their adolescent patients.[18] We also found that seeing >5 adolescents per week was associated with providing STD services and providing confidential STD testing. Belonging to a group practice of male practitioners or being a solo practitioner (regardless of gender of practitioner) was negatively associated with providing services and providing confidential services. This pattern may indicate that other barriers exist to increasing access to care for adolescents. For example, solo practitioners may face a larger opportunity cost than group practitioners of spending nonreimbursed time to counsel parents and patients about providing confidential care to adolescents. Practitioner gender may pose a barrier for female patients who may be apprehensive about being examined by a male physician, or, as shown in previous studies,[10,14,16] male physicians may feel less confident in providing pelvic examinations and contraceptive counseling. The mean number of decades since medical school graduation for all physicians in a practice had no significant association with provision of services, although our measure was crude. Another concerning finding is the large degree of disagreement between office staff who answer appointment lines and physicians in the same practice about the availability of confidential care for medically emancipated conditions to adolescents. Other studies have shown that a substantial proportion of adolescents wish to be seen without their parent's knowledge.[3-5] Information that they receive about confidentiality when trying to schedule an appointment may be a deciding factor in whether to seek health care. To ensure that adolescents receive needed care, office staff should be fully informed of services available and the office policy on adolescent confidentiality[13] and also have specific referral information if the services that adolescent patients seek are not available at the practice. Our results suggest that having a written office policy on adolescent confidentiality is an important way to ensure consistency within a practice. Ideally, such a policy should establish that providers inform adolescents and their parents about the process of developing a provider-patient relationship as the adolescent gains ability to make independent decisions. Providers should also discuss the conditions under which information will be shared with others, such as suspected physical or sexual abuse or when the adolescent poses a severe risk of harm to her- or himself or to others. The adolescent's wishes on how the information will be shared should be respected.[6] Ongoing education about laws and regulations about adolescent confidentiality should be included in the policy.

The responses to our questions about fees required up front and sliding-scale fee schedules suggest that payment may pose additional barriers both to obtaining care and to keeping the care received confidential. Adolescents who seek care without insurance or outside their parent's insurance plan may face high payments up front; uninsured adolescents report missing care because of high cost.[4] Although statutes may authorize adolescents to consent to their own care, provisions are rarely made for making services financially accessible for adolescents. Agreements about payment for services among practitioners and adolescents and their parents are important in increasing access to confidential care.[6]

LIMITATIONS

The generalizability of our study is limited by a number of factors. First, the survey was limited to the Washington, DC, metropolitan area. There may be large regional variation in availability of confidential services based on state law, the supply of primary care providers, availability of alternative sites for health care, and local attitudes toward providing confidential services to adolescents. Second, the response rate of physicians to the mail survey was low, particularly for FM and IM physicians. Also, because of limited physician participation, sample sizes for each practice type

were low for analyses of confidential services. The power of our study is therefore limited. Third, a large health maintenance organization in the Washington, DC, area declined to respond to our survey. Thus, a large provider of primary care was not represented in the study. We cannot compare the sample population to the physician population of the area as a whole because we did not collect information on nonresponding physicians. However, among the 86% of sampled practices that responded to the telephone survey, we compared characteristics of those with responding and nonresponding physicians. Practices with responding ($n = 170$) versus nonresponding ($n = 202$) physicians had the same percentage of physicians with 2 or fewer decades since graduation (38%). However, practices with nonresponding physicians were less likely to see adolescent patients (73% vs 84%) and less likely to have >50% of its physicians board certified (73% vs 85%). These differences may have biased our findings, but we surmise that access for adolescents in the practices with nonresponding physicians may have been even more restricted than in practices with responding physicians. Fourth, because clinics such as school-based health clinics and family planning clinics are not included in the *Washington Physicians Directory*, it is not possible to use the survey results to assess overall availability of confidential care in the Washington, DC, area. Finally, another limitation is possible bias as a result of social desirability in survey response. This bias would likely result in overestimation of service availability and may account for some of the discordance between the telephone and mail surveys.

Conclusion

It has long been clear that clinical services are an important component in health-promotion and disease-prevention efforts required to address STDs, unintended pregnancies, and other health problems among adolescents.[23] Confidentiality is essential to providing such services to adolescents.[6] Ongoing changes may be required in pediatric residency training and continuing medical education to improve health care for adolescents and to ensure that pediatricians feel confident in treating adolescents. Pediatric practices that are unable or unwilling to provide these services must be able to screen for health risk behaviors and to offer adolescents a referral to a specific practice or specialist who is proficient in providing the needed care. Establishing an office policy and ensuring that all office staff are knowledgeable about the policy may help to ensure greater access for adolescents to these services.

Acknowledgments

We thank Kanti Patel, PhD, for statistical assistance and Larry D'Angelo, MD, MPH, Julia Rhodes, PhD, and Ken Schoendorf, MD, MPH, for critical review.

References

1. Ford CA, Millstein SG, Halpern-Felsher BL, Irwin CE. Influence of physician confidentiality assurances on adolescents' willingness to disclose information and seek future health care. *JAMA*. 1997;278:1029–1034

2. Lane MA, McCright J, Garrett K, Millstein SG, Bolan G, Ellen JM. Features of sexually transmitted disease services important to African American adolescents. *Arch Pediatr Adolesc Med*. 1999;153:829–833

3. Thrall JS, McCloskey L, Ettner SL, Rothman E, Tighe JE, Emans SJ. Confidentiality and adolescents' use of providers for health information and for pelvic examinations. *Arch Pediatr Adolesc Med*. 2000;154:885–892

4. Klein JD, Wilson KM, McNulty M, Kapphahn C, Scott Collins K. Access to medical care for adolescents: results from the 1997 Commonwealth Fund Survey of the Health of Adolescent Girls. *J Adolesc Health*. 1999;25:120–130

5. Cheng TL, Savageau JA, Sattler AL, DeWitt TG. Confidentiality in health care: a survey of knowledge, perceptions, and attitudes among high school students. *JAMA*. 1993;269:1404–1407

6. Sigman G, Silber TJ, English A, Gans Epner JE. Confidential health care for adolescents: position paper for the Society of Adolescent Medicine. *J Adolesc Health*. 1997;21:408–415

7. English A. Treating adolescents: legal and ethical considerations. *Adolesc Med*. 1990;74:1097–1112

8. English A. Reproductive health services for adolescents: critical legal issues. *Obstet Gynecol Clin North Am*. 2000;27:195–211

9. Boonstra H, Nash E. Minors and the right to consent to health care. The Guttmacher Report on Public Policy, August 2000. Available at: www.agi-usa.org/pubs/ib_minors_00.pdf

10. Fisher M, Golden NH, Bergeson R, et al. Update on adolescent health care in pediatric practice. *J Adolesc Health*. 1996;19:394–400

11. Marks A, Fisher M, Lasker S. Adolescent medicine in pediatric practice. *J Adolesc Health Care*. 1990;11:149–153

12. Neinstein LS, Shapiro JR. Pediatrician's self-evaluation of adolescent health care training, skills, and interest. *J Adolesc Health Care*. 1986;7:18–21

13. Acquavella AP, Braverman P. Adolescent gynecology in the office setting. *Pediatr Clin North Am*. 1999;46:489–503

14. Key JD, Marsh LD, Darden PM. Adolescent medicine in pediatric practice: a survey of practice and training. *Am J Med Sci*. 1995;309:83–87

15. American Academy of Pediatrics, Task Force on Pediatric Education. *The Future of Pediatric Education*. Evanston, IL: American Academy of Pediatrics; 1978

16. Chastain DO, Sanders JM, DuRant RH. Recommended changes in pediatric education: the impact on pediatrician involvement in health care delivery to adolescents. *Pediatrics*. 1988;82(suppl):469–476

17. *The Washington Physicians Directory*. Silver Spring, MD: National Directories, Inc; 1997

18. Kelts EAS, Allan MJ, Klein JD. Where are we on teen sex? Delivery of reproductive health services to adolescents by family physicians. *Fam Med*. 2001;33:376–381

19. Fleming GV, O'Connor KG, Sanders JM. Pediatricians' view of access to health services for adolescents. *J Adolesc Health*. 1994;15:473–478

20. Chamie M, Eisman S, Forrest JD, Orr MT, Torres A. Factors affecting adolescents' use of family planning clinics. *Fam Plann Perspect*. 1982;14:126–127, 131–139

21. MacKay AP, Fingerhut LA, Duran CR. *Adolescent Health Chartbook. Health, United States, 2000*. Hyattsville, MD: National Center for Health Statistics; 2000

22. Klein JD, McNulty M, Flatau CN. Adolescents' access to care: teenagers' self-reported use of services and perceived access to confidential care. *Arch Pediatr Adolesc Med*. 1998;152:676–682

23. United States Congress, Office of Technology Assessment. *Adolescent Health: Summary and Policy Options, I*. Washington, DC: US Government Printing Office; 1991. Publ. No. OTA-H-468

Care of the Adolescent Sexual Assault Victim

Committee on Adolescence

ABSTRACT. Sexual assault is a broad-based term that encompasses a wide range of sexual victimizations, including rape. Since the American Academy of Pediatrics published its last policy statement on this topic in 1994, additional information and data have emerged about sexual assault and rape in adolescents, the adolescent's perception of sexual assault, and the treatment and management of the adolescent who has been a victim of sexual assault. This new information mandates an updated knowledge base for pediatricians who care for adolescent patients. This statement provides that update, focusing on sexual assault and rape in the adolescent population.

ABBREVIATIONS. STDs, sexually transmitted diseases; HBV, hepatitis B virus; HIV, human immunodeficiency virus.

Definitions

Understanding the definitions of the terms sexual assault, rape, acquaintance rape, date rape, molestation, and statutory rape are important in the identification, treatment, and management of the adolescent victim. *Sexual assault* is a comprehensive term that includes multiple types of forced or inappropriate sexual activity. Sexual assault includes situations in which there is sexual contact with or without penetration that occurs because of physical force or psychologic coercion. This includes touching of a person's "sexual or intimate parts or the intentional touching of the clothing covering those intimate parts."[1]

The term *molestation* is applied when there is noncoital sexual activity between a child and an adolescent or adult. Molestation can include viewing of sexual materials, genital or breast fondling, or oral-genital contact.[1]

From legal and clinical perspectives, *rape* is defined as "forced sexual intercourse" that occurs because of physical force or psychologic coercion. Rape involves vaginal, anal, or oral penetration by the offender. This definition also includes incidents in which penetration is with a foreign object, such as a bottle, or situations in which the victim is unable to give consent because of intoxication or developmental disability.[1,2] The terms *acquaintance rape* and *date rape* are applied to those situations in which the assailant and victim know each other.

Statutory rape involves sexual penetration by a person 18 years or older of a person under the age of consent.[1] Statutory rape laws are based on the premise that, until a person reaches a certain age, he or she is legally incapable of consenting to sexual intercourse. The age of consent varies from state to state. In some states, there are new statutory rape laws mandating that sexual intercourse and sexual contact must now be reported if certain age differences exist between a minor (usually defined as younger than 18 or 21 years) and his or her sex partner (whether minor or adult), even if the sexual act was voluntary and consensual. There is concern that the new laws and mandated reporting statutes can have a significant impact on the interaction between the health care provider and the patient. Adolescents and health care providers may have concerns regarding medical or social history, access to care, and confidentiality, and some adolescents may refuse to seek care or refuse to disclose personal risk information because of possible reporting of sexual partners.[3-5]

PEDIATRICS (ISSN 0031 4005). Copyright © 2001 by the American Academy of Pediatrics.

Epidemiology

National data show that adolescents continue to have the highest rates of rape and other sexual assaults of any age group. Annual rates of sexual assault per 1000 persons (males and females) were reported in 1998 by the US Department of Justice to be 3.5 for ages 12 through 15 years, 5.0 for ages 16 through 19 years, 4.6 for ages 20 through 24 years, and 1.7 for ages 24 through 29 years.[6] There are significant gender differences in adolescent rape and sexual assault, with female victims exceeding males by a ratio of 13.5:1.[6] National Crime Victimization Survey statistics reported 308 569 rapes and sexual assaults in females 12 years or older and 21 519 rapes and sexual assaults in males 12 years or older in 1998.[6] This represents a decrease from peak rates of rape and sexual assault reported in 1992.[6,7] The US Department of Justice reported that more than half of all rape and sexual assault victims in 1998 were females younger than 25 years.[6]

Studies have demonstrated that two thirds to three quarters of all adolescent rapes and sexual assaults are perpetrated by an acquaintance or relative of the adolescent.[8-11] Older adolescents are most commonly the victims during social encounters with the assailants (eg, a date). With younger adolescent victims, the assailant is more likely to be a member of the adolescent's extended family. Adolescents with developmental disabilities, especially those in the mildly retarded range, are at particular risk for acquaintance and date rape.[12]

Adolescent rape victims are more likely than adult victims to have used alcohol or drugs and are less likely to be physically injured during a rape, as the assailants in adolescent rape tend to use weapons less frequently.[8,9] Adolescent female victims are also more likely to delay seeking medical care after rape and sexual assault and are less likely to press charges than adult women.[8,9]

Male victims are less likely to report a sexual assault than are female victims.[13,14] Studies of sexual assault of males have demonstrated that up to 90% of perpetrators are male. Sexual assault of males by females is more commonly reported by older adolescents or young adults, compared with children or young adolescents.[12] Male perpetrators of male sexual assault more commonly identify themselves as heterosexual than homosexual, and there is lack of clarity in the literature whether adolescent and young adult victims are more commonly heterosexual or homosexual.[13-14] The rate of perpetration by an acquaintance of the victim is similar for male and female victims, but multiple assailants, use of a weapon, and forced oral assaults are more common in assault of males than females.[14]

Alcohol or drug use immediately before a sexual assault has been reported by more than 40% of adolescent victims and adolescent assailants.[15] The recent increase in the rate of adolescent acquaintance rape has been associated with the illegal availability of flunitrazepam (Rohypnol, manufactured by Roche Pharmaceuticals Inc, outside of the United States). This so-called "date rape drug" is a benzodiazepine sedative/hypnotic. The effects of flunitrazepam begin 30 minutes after ingestion, peak within 2 hours, and can persist for up to 8 to 12 hours. Drug effects include somnolence, decreased anxiety, muscular relaxation, and profound sedation. There may also be amnesia for the time that the drug exerts its action. This drug can go undetected if added to any drink, thus increasing the risk of sexual assault, especially in the adolescent population.[16-19]

Adolescents' Perceptions and Attitudes Regarding Sexual Assault and Rape

Exploring the perceptions and attitudes of adolescents regarding rape and other forced or unwanted sexual encounters is important. The acquaintance rape phenomenon raises issues of victim credibility, because there may have been voluntary participation until the assault occurred. Aggressive behavior on the part of a male perpetrator may be seen by some adolescents as normative in this context.[20-23] One study demonstrated that male and female adolescents who viewed a vignette of unwanted sexual intercourse accompanied by a photograph of the victim dressed in provocative clothing were more likely to indicate that the victim was responsible for the assailant's behavior, more likely to view the male's behavior as justified, and less likely to judge the act as rape.[24]

Exploration of unwanted sexual experiences and rape from the adolescent's perspective can lead to additional insight into health behaviors and outcomes.[21,22,25,26] A large survey of unwanted sexual experiences among middle and high school students indicated that 18% of females and 12% of males reported having had an unwanted sexual experience.[26] In 1 study, this led to unexpected gender-reversed patterns of behavior, including the internalizing behavior, bulimia, in males and externalizing behaviors, such as fighting, in females.[27] Other studies of female adolescents have found rape during childhood or adolescence to be associated with younger age of first voluntary intercourse, lower internal locus of control, higher depression scores, increased seeking and receipt of psychologic services, increased rate of pregnancy, and greater amounts of illegal drug use as well as evidence of physical abuse and negative mental health states.[28,29]

Treatment and Management

The pediatrician who is involved in the management of adolescents who are the victims of sexual assault should be trained in the forensic procedures required for documentation and collection of evidence or should refer to an emergency department or rape crisis center where there are personnel experienced with adolescent rape victims. New colposcopic procedures allow examiners to better document genital trauma, including microtrauma, seen in rape cases, with a growing body of literature demonstrating the patterns of genital injury in sexual assault victims.[30-32]

It is essential that the forensic examination be performed by a person who can ensure an unbroken chain of evidence and accurate documentation of findings.[1,33-38] Details of the required examination and documentation are presented in a handbook by the American College of Emergency Physicians, *Evaluation and Management of the Sexually Assaulted or Sexually Abused Patient*.[39] Pediatricians who treat sexually abused or assaulted patients need to be aware of the legal requirements, including completion of appropriate forms and reporting to appropriate authorities, specific to their locale. Pediatricians should also

be aware that the availability of DNA amplification technology now used to more accurately identify assailants allows for performance of a forensic examination beyond the 72-hour period that was previously considered the cutoff for such examinations.[36,40-41]

The diagnosis and management of sexually transmitted diseases (STDs) is an important component of treatment of the assault victim.[42] Blood and tissue specimens should be obtained from appropriate sites (as identified in the history) to detect *Neisseria gonorrhea* and *Chlamydia trachomatis*. Vaginal secretions should be microscopically examined for *Trichomonas* species. Specimens should be tested for herpes virus if there is a clinical indication (eg, vesicles). Serum samples should be obtained to test for syphilis, hepatitis B virus (HBV), and human immunodeficiency virus (HIV). These tests serve as a baseline indicating the presence of any STDs in the victim before the assault but are considered controversial by some authorities who prefer performing the initial STD tests 2 weeks after the assault. All authorities agree that the syphilis and HBV tests should be repeated in 6 weeks and that the HIV test should be repeated in 3 to 6 months.[1,36-39,42]

Pregnancy prevention and postcoital contraception should be addressed with every adolescent female rape and sexual assault victim. This discussion should include risks of failure and options for pregnancy management. A baseline urine pregnancy test should be performed. This is important because the adolescent could be pregnant from sexual activity that occurred before the assault.[1,36-39]

Current recommendations are to provide prophylactic treatment for *Chlamydia* infection and gonorrhea to adolescent sexual assault victims and to provide prophylaxis for pregnancy prevention.[1,36-39,42] HIV prophylaxis is not universally recommended but should be considered when there is mucosal exposure (oral, vaginal, or anal). Factors to consider include the risks and benefits of the medical regimen, whether there was repeated abuse or multiple perpetrators, if the perpetrator is known to be HIV-positive, or if there is a high prevalence of HIV in the geographic area where the sexual assault occurred.[1,36-39,43] HBV vaccination is recommended for those who have not received a complete HBV series or who have a negative surface antibody despite previous vaccination.[36-39]

Adolescent Reactions to Rape

Posttraumatic stress disorder occurs in up to 80% of rape victims.[44] Rape trauma syndrome is described as consisting of an initial phase lasting days to weeks during which the victim experiences disbelief, anxiety, fear, emotional lability, and guilt followed by a reorganization phase lasting months to years during which the victim goes through periods of adjustment, integration, and recovery.[37,45] Counseling designed to specifically address these issues as well as additional psychologic trauma that results from date or acquaintance rape should be available. Psychotropic medications may be required in some instances. The pediatrician should be knowledgeable about services available in the community to address these issues and should provide initial psychologic support.

Other victim reactions to rape can include the feeling that his or her trust has been violated, increased self-blame, less positive self-concept, anxiety, alcohol abuse, and effects on sexual activity (including younger age at first voluntary sexual activity, poor use of contraception, greater number of abortions and pregnancies, STDs, victimization by older partners, and sexual dissatisfaction).[28,34,46-49] Adolescent victims may feel that their actions contributed to the act of rape and have confusion as to whether the incident was forced or consensual.[50-52]

Because responses to rape can vary, it is important for pediatricians to not only manage the physical needs of the victim but also be sensitive to the psychologic needs of the adolescent. Pediatricians should be aware that self-blame, humiliation, and naiveté may prevent the adolescent from seeking medical care. Effective screening, referral, and follow-up allow for support of the adolescent rape victim and appropriate delivery of health care services. Because patients treated in emergency departments often do not return for follow-up care,[53] it is important that the emergency treatment team refer the assaulted adolescent back to his or her medical home. Thus, pediatricians should be prepared to provide such services as follow-up STD testing, completion of the HBV vaccination series, treatment of injuries, screening for mental health problems, and management of substance use issues.

Sexual Assault and Rape Prevention Strategies

Adolescent rape exists in a sociocultural context in which issues of male dominance, appropriate gender behaviors, female victimization, and power imbalances in relationships are highly visible. Prevention messages for adolescents need to be designed for males and females.[33,34,54-56] Adolescents need to be able to identify high-risk situations and should be encouraged to seek medical care after a rape. Factors that may increase the likelihood of assault (eg, late night use of drugs or alcohol) and strategies to prevent rape should be discussed, and associated educational materials should be distributed.[33,34,54-56]

Screening of adolescents for sexual victimization should be part of a routine history. Adolescents should be asked direct questions regarding their past sexual experiences. These questions should include those that explore age of first sexual experience, unwanted voluntary or forced sexual acts, and a description of events. Exploration of gender roles and relationship parameters (eg, exploitative, nonconsensual vs healthy) are critical. The patient needs the opportunity to describe the experience in his or her own words.[30-34]

RECOMMENDATIONS

1. Pediatricians should be knowledgeable about the epidemiology of sexual assault in adolescence.
2. Pediatricians should be knowledgeable about the current reporting requirements for sexual assault in their communities.
3. Pediatricians should be knowledgeable about sexual assault and rape evaluation services available in their communities and when to refer adolescents for a forensic examination.

4. Pediatricians should screen adolescents for a history of sexual assault and potential sequelae.

5. Pediatricians should be prepared to offer psychologic support or referral for counseling and should be aware of the services in the community that provide management, examination, and counseling for the adolescent patient who has been sexually assaulted.

6. Pediatricians should provide preventive counseling to their adolescent patients regarding avoidance of high-risk situations that could lead to sexual assault.

COMMITTEE ON ADOLESCENCE, 2000–2001
David W. Kaplan, MD, MPH, Chairperson
Ronald A. Feinstein, MD
Martin M. Fisher, MD
Jonathan D. Klein, MD, MPH
Luis F. Olmedo, MD
Ellen S. Rome, MD, MPH
W. Samuel Yancy, MD

LIAISONS
Paula J. Adams Hillard, MD
    American College of Obstetricians
    and Gynecologists
Diane Sacks, MD
    Canadian Paediatric Society
Glen Pearson, MD
    American Academy of Child and
    Adolescent Psychiatry

SECTION LIAISON
Barbara L. Frankowski, MD, MPH
    Section on School Health

STAFF
Tammy Piazza Hurley

References

1. American Academy of Pediatrics, Committee on Adolescence. Sexual assault and the adolescent. *Pediatrics.* 1994;94:761–765

2. Perkins C, Klaus P. *Criminal Victimization 1994: National Crime Victimization Survey.* Washington, DC: Bureau of Justice Statistics; 1996. Available at: http://www.ojp.usdoj.gov/bjs/abstract/cv94.htm. Accessed November 6, 2000

3. Teare C, English A. An analysis of Assembly Bill 327: New California Child Abuse Reporting Requirements for Family Planning Providers. San Francisco, CA: National Center for Youth Law for the California Health Council Inc; 1998. Available at: http://www.youth.law.org/ab327.pdf. Accessed November 6, 2000

4. Ford CA, Millstein SG. Delivery of confidentiality assurances to adolescents by primary care physicians. *Arch Pediatr Adolesc Med.* 1997;151:505–509

5. Donovan P. Can statutory rape laws be effective in preventing adolescent pregnancy? *Fam Plann Perspect.* 1997;29:30–34, 40

6. Rennison CM. *Criminal Victimization 1998: Changes 1997-1998 With Trends 1993-1998.* Washington, DC: Bureau of Justice Statistics; 1999. Available at: http://www.ojp.usdoj.gov/bjs/abstract/cv98.htm. Accessed November 6, 2000

7. Greenfield LA. *Sex Offenses and Offenders: An Analysis of Data on Rape and Sexual Assault.* Washington, DC: Bureau of Justice Statistics; 1997. Available at: http://www.ojp.usdoj.gov/bjs/pub/pdf/soo.pdf. Accessed November 6, 2000

8. Muram D, Hostetler BR, Jones CE, Speck PM. Adolescent victims of sexual assault. *J Adolesc Health.* 1995;17:372–375

9. Peipert JF, Domagalski LR. Epidemiology of adolescent sexual assault. *Obstet Gynecol.* 1994;84:867–871

10. National Victim Center. *Rape in America: A Report to the Nation.* Arlington, VA: National Victim Center; 1992

11. Heise LL. Reproductive freedom and violence against women: where are the intersections? *J Law Med Ethics.* 1993;21:206–216

12. Quint EH. Gynecological health care for adolescents with developmental disabilities. *Adolesc Med.* 1999;10:221–229

13. Holmes WC, Slap GB. Sexual abuse of boys: definition, prevalence, correlates, sequelae, and management. *JAMA.* 1998;280:1855–1862

14. Lacy HB, Roberts R. Sexual assault on men. *Int J STD AIDS.* 1991;2:258–260

15. Seifert SA. Substance use and sexual assault. *Subst Use Misuse.* 1999;34:935–945

16. Schwartz RH, Weaver AB. Rohypnol: the date rape drug. *Clin Pediatr (Phila).* 1998;37:321

17. Simmons MM, Cupp MJ. Use and abuse of flunitrazepam. *Ann Pharmacother.* 1998;32:117–119

18. Rickert VI, Weimann CM. Date rape: office-based solutions. *Contemp Ob/Gyn.* March 1998:133–153

19. Anglin D, Spears KL, Hutson HR. Flunitrazepam and its involvement in date or acquaintance rape. *Acad Emerg Med.* 1997;4:323–326

20. Parrot A. Acquaintance rape among adolescents: identifying risk groups and intervention strategies. *J Soc Work Hum Sex.* 1989;8:47–61

21. Small SA, Kerns D. Unwanted sexual activity among peers during early and middle adolescence, incidence and risk factors. *J Marriage Fam.* 1993;55:941–952

22. Kershner R. Adolescent attitudes about rape. *Adolescence.* 1996;31:29–33

23. Boxley J, Lawrance L, Gruchow H. A preliminary study of eighth grade students' attitudes toward rape myths and women's roles. *J Sch Health.* 1995;65:96–100

24. Cassidy L, Hurrell RM. The influence of victim's attire on adolescent's judgments of date rape. *Adolescence.* 1995;30: 319–323

25. Kellogg ND, Hoffman TJ. Unwanted and illegal sexual experiences in childhood and adolescence. *Child Abuse Negl.* 1995;19:1457–1468

26. Erickson PI, Rapkin AJ. Unwanted sexual experiences among middle and high school youth. *J Adolesc Health.* 1991;12:319–325

27. Shrier LA, Pierce JD, Emans SJ, DuRant RH. Gender differences in risk behaviors associated with forced or pressured sex. *Arch Pediatr Adolesc Med.* 1998;152:57–63

28. Miller BC, Monson BH, Norton MC. The effects of forced sexual intercourse on white female adolescents. *Child Abuse Negl.* 1995;19:1289–1301

29. Nagy S, DiClemente R, Adcock AG. Adverse factors associated with forced sex among southern adolescent girls. *Pediatrics.* 1995;96:944–946

30. Slaughter L, Brown CR, Crowly S, Peck R. Patterns of genital injury in female sexual assault victims. *Am J Obstet Gynecol.* 1997;176:609–616

31. Lenahan LC, Ernst A, Johnson B. Colposcopy in evaluation of the adult sexual assault victim. *Am J Emerg Med.* 1998;16:183–184

32. Biggs M, Stermac LE, Divinsky M. Genital injuries following sexual assault of women with and without prior sexual intercourse experience. *Can Med Assoc J.* 1998;159: 33–37

33. American College Obstetricians and Gynecologists. Sexual assault. *ACOG Educ Bull.* 1997;242:1–4

34. American College Obstetricians and Gynecologists. Adolescent victims of sexual assault. *ACOG Educ Bull.* 1998;252:1–5

35. Campbell R, Bybee D. Emergency medical services for rape victims: detecting the cracks in service delivery. *Womens Health.* 1997;3:75–101

36. Hampton HL. Care of the woman who has been raped. *N Engl J Med.* 1995;332:234–237

37. Petter LM, Whitehill DL. Management of female sexual assault. *Am Fam Physician.* 1998;58:920–926, 929–930

38. Linden JA. Sexual assault. *Emerg Med Clin North Am.* 1999;17:685–697

39. American College of Emergency Physicians. *Evaluation and Management of the Sexually Assaulted or Sexually Abused Patient.* Dallas, TX: American College of Emergency Physicians; 1999. Available at: http://www.acep.org/library/index.cfm/id/2101. Accessed November 6, 2000

40. Chakraborty R, Kidd KK. The utility of DNA typing in forensic work. *Science.* 1991;254:1735–1739

41. Ledray LE, Netzel L. DNA evidence collection. *J Emerg Nurs.* 1997;23:156–158

42. Reynolds MW, Peipert JF, Collins B. Epidemiologic issues of sexually transmitted diseases in sexual assault victims. *Obstet Gynecol Surv.* 2000;55:51–57

43. Bamberger JD, Waldo CR, Gerberding JL, Katz MH. Postexposure prophylaxis for human immunodeficiency virus (HIV) infection following sexual assault. *Am J Med.* 1999;106:323–326

44. Pynoos RS, Nader K. Post traumatic stress disorder. In: McAnarney ER, Kreipe RE, Orr DP, Comerci GD, eds. *Textbook of Adolescent Medicine.* Philadelphia, PA: WB Saunders Co; 1992:1003–1009

45. Beebe DK. Sexual assault: the physician's role in prevention and treatment. *J Miss State Med Assoc.* 1998;39: 366–369

46. Boyer D, Fine D. Sexual abuse as a factor in adolescent pregnancy and child maltreatment. *Fam Plann Perspect.* 1992;24:4–11,19

47. Moore KA, Nord CW, Petterson JL. Nonvoluntary sexual activity among adolescents. *Fam Plann Perspect.* 1989;21: 110–114

48. Smith MD, Besharov DT, Gardiner KN, Hoff T. *Early Sexual Experiences: How Voluntary? How Violent?* Menlo Park, CA: Henry J. Kaiser Family Foundation; 1996

49. Taylor D, Chavez G, Chabra A, Boggess J. Risk factors for adult paternity in births to adolescents. *Obstet Gynecol.* 1997;89:199–205

50. American Medical Association. *Strategies for the Treatment and Prevention of Sexual Assault.* Chicago, IL: American Medical Association; 1995

51. Louis Harris and Associates. *In Their Own Words: Adolescent Girls Discuss Health and Healthcare Issues.* New York, NY: The Commonwealth Fund; 1997

52. Koval JE. Violence in dating relationships. *J Pediatr Health Care.* 1989;3:298–304

53. Holmes MM, Resnick HS, Frampton D. Follow-up of sexual assault victims. *Am J Obstet Gynecol.* 1998;179: 336–342

54. Holmes MM. The primary health care provider's role in sexual assault prevention. *Womens Health Issues.* 1995;5: 224–232

55. Vickio CJ, Hoffman BA, Yarris E. Combating sexual offenses on the college campus: keys to success. *J Am Coll Health.* 1999;47:283–286

56. Scarce M. Same-sex rape of male college students. *J Am Coll Health.* 1997;45:171–173

Condom Use by Adolescents

Committee on Adolescence

ABSTRACT. The use of condoms as part of the prevention of unintended pregnancies and sexually transmitted diseases (STDs) in adolescents is evaluated in this policy statement. Sexual activity and pregnancies decreased slightly among adolescents in the 1990s, reversing trends that were present in the 1970s and 1980s, while condom use among adolescents increased significantly. These trends likely reflect initial success of primary and secondary prevention messages aimed at adolescents. Rates of acquisition of STDs and human immunodeficiency virus (HIV) among adolescents remain unacceptably high, highlighting the need for continued prevention efforts and reflecting the fact that improved condom use can decrease, but never eliminate, the risk of acquisition of STDs and HIV as well as unintended pregnancies. While many condom education and availability programs have been shown to have modest effects on condom use, there is no evidence that these programs contribute to increased sexual activity among adolescents. These trends highlight the progress that has been made and the large amount that still needs to be accomplished.

ABBREVIATIONS. STD, sexually transmitted disease; HIV, human immunodeficiency virus; CDC, Centers for Disease Control and Prevention.

Introduction

The medical and social consequences of adolescent sexual activity are a national health concern highlighted by unintended pregnancies and the acquisition of sexually transmitted diseases (STDs), including human immunodeficiency virus (HIV). How to best decrease pregnancy and STD rates among adolescents is the focus of much debate, with particular controversy surrounding the roles of sexuality education and condom availability for youth. From a public health perspective, primary prevention of unintended pregnancy and STDs in adolescents involves a delay in the initiation of sexual activity until psychosocial maturity or marriage, depending on the religious or cultural perspective. Secondary prevention in adolescents involves the use of safer sex practices by those who are sexually active and who do not plan on abstaining from sexual activity.

In this policy statement, the use of condoms as part of the secondary prevention of unintended pregnancies and STDs in adolescents is evaluated. The statement reviews current pregnancy, STD, and HIV infection rates; recent changes in condom use by adolescents and factors affecting condom use; the types of condoms, their proper use, and their breakage rates; the effectiveness of condoms in pregnancy, STD, and HIV prevention; and the roles that schools are playing in condom education and availability for youth. This statement updates a previous statement published in 1995[1] and refers only to the male condom; information on the female condom, which is newer and not currently used by many adolescents, may be obtained from other sources.[2]

Trends in Adolescent Sexual Activity

Although recent data have shown encouraging signs that primary and secondary prevention efforts may be starting to have an effect, current rates of sexual activity, pregnancy, and STDs among adolescents remain a public health concern. An evaluation of data available for female and male adolescents demonstrates the changes that have taken place throughout time and ongoing reasons for concern.

Data from a series of studies demonstrated that sexual intercourse among 15- to 19-year-old adolescent females living in metropolitan areas increased significantly in the 1970s, from 37%

PEDIATRICS (ISSN 0031 4005). Copyright © 2001 by the American Academy of Pediatrics.

reporting being sexually active in 1971, to 43% in 1976, to 50% in 1979.[3] Smaller changes took place during the 1980s, with a series of national studies demonstrating an increase in the number of 15- to 19-year-old adolescent females who were sexually active, from 47% in 1982% to 53% in 1988.[4] Rates decreased slightly in the 1990s, with the Centers for Disease Control and Prevention (CDC) reporting in its Youth Risk Behavior Surveys that 50% of females in grades 9 through 12 were sexually active in 1991, with an increase to 52% in 1995 and a decrease to 48% in 1999.[5,6] As the 1990s ended, the rate of sexual activity among adolescent females in high school had remained between 47% and 53% for 2 decades.

Changes in sexual activity among adolescent males have been somewhat more dramatic. The rate of 17- to 19-year-old males living in metropolitan areas who reported having sexual intercourse in a series of national studies increased from 66% in 1979 to 76% in 1988.[7] This was followed, however, by a second series of studies that demonstrated a decrease in the number of males 15 to 19 years old who reported having sexual intercourse, from 60% in 1988 to 55% in 1995.[8] The CDC data demonstrate a decrease among males in grades 9 through 12 who report being sexually active, from 57% in 1991, to 54% in 1995, to 49% in 1997.[5] The data demonstrate that, although adolescent males have had higher rates than adolescent females throughout most of the past 2 decades, approximately 50% of high school students of both sexes now report having sexual intercourse.

With approximately half of all adolescents being sexually active, rates of adolescent pregnancies and STDs remain a significant concern. Approximately 900 000 adolescents become pregnant each year, with up to two thirds of these pregnancies occurring in women 18 to 19 years old and one third in women 17 years or younger.[9] Approximately 51% of adolescent pregnancies result in a live birth, 35% end with an abortion, and 14% end with a miscarriage or stillbirth.[9,10] Among adolescent women who are sexually active, approximately 9% of 14-year-olds, 18% of 15- to 17-year-olds, and 22% of 18- to 19-year-olds become pregnant each year, with most pregnancies

described as unintended.[11,12] The birth rate to adolescents increased 24% from 1986 to 1991 (from 50.1 to 62.1 births per 1000 females 15–19 years old) but then decreased 12% from 1991 to 1996 (from 62.1 to 54.7 births per 1000).[12-13] The abortion rate among adolescents increased significantly from 1975 to 1980 but has decreased steadily since then (from 42.8 per 1000 females 15–19 years old in 1980 to 25 per 1000 in 1993).[12-14] Despite these decreases, the United States continues to have the highest adolescent birth rate among all developed countries, even compared with countries that have similar or higher rates of sexual activity. Mixed messages concerning sexuality that are delivered in this country are believed to be a primary cause of this discrepancy.

Rates of STD acquisition by adolescents also remain high, and the Institute of Medicine recently recommended that "a major part of a national strategy to prevent STDs should focus on adolescents."[15] The CDC estimates that approximately 3 million adolescents acquire an STD each year, representing 25% of all new STD cases annually, and that two thirds of all individuals who acquire STDs are younger than 25 years.[15] Data from published studies indicate that up to 30% of sexually active adolescent females test positive for infection with *Chlamydia* organisms; as many as 30% to 50% of sexually active adolescents have been infected with the human papillomavirus; sexually active adolescents between 15 and 19 years old have higher rates of gonorrhea than any other age group; rates of genital herpes infections are estimated to have increased more than 50%; and up to 25% of newly acquired HIV infections are estimated to occur among those who are 22 years or younger.[11,15-20] In total, rates of adolescent sexual activity, unintended pregnancy, and acquisition of STDs remain an area of major concern.

Condom Use

RECENT TRENDS IN ADOLESCENT USE

Survey data from male and female adolescents indicate a significant increase in condom use by adolescents during the past 2 decades. Among sexually active adolescent males 17 to 19 years old living in metropolitan areas, reported condom use at last intercourse increased from 21% in 1979 to 58% in 1988.[7] Reported condom use at first intercourse among adolescent women 15 to 19 years old increased from 23% in 1982 to 47% in 1988.[4] Data from the 1988 and 1995 National Surveys of Adolescent Males indicate that these increases have continued, with reported condom use at last intercourse among 15- to 19-yearolds increasing from 57% in 1988 to 67% in 1995.[8] The CDC data indicate increases in reported condom use at last intercourse from 38% to 51% among females and from 56% to 63% among males for those in grades 9 through 12 between 1991 and 1997.[5]

Despite noted improvements in condom use, significant problems still remain. Condom use by one half to two thirds of adolescents is not sufficient to significantly decrease rates of unintended pregnancy and acquisition of STDs. Furthermore, the data show that only 45% of adolescent males report condom use for every act of intercourse and that condom use actually decreases with age when comparing males 15 to 17 years old with males 18 to 19 years old.[7,8] Also, females report less frequent use of condoms during intercourse than males, presumably because many adolescent females are sexually active with older partners.[5] For these reasons, rates of pregnancies and STDs in females are unlikely to decrease beyond current levels unless condom use by adolescents and young adults continues to increase significantly in the years ahead.

FACTORS THAT INFLUENCE USE

Demographic, attitudinal, and educational factors have all been associated with increased condom use by adolescents, although studies on each of these factors are far from clear. As noted earlier, younger age has been associated with condom use in a national study of males; in that same study, black adolescents, adolescents who had more educated parents, and adolescents who were older at first intercourse also had greater condom use.[7] A study of females demonstrated that being from an intact family and having a mother with higher educational achievement were associated with greater condom use at first intercourse,[21]

and studies have shown that increased communication with parents is also associated with increased condom use.[22] Attitudes associated with increased condom use among males include having a strong belief in male contraceptive responsibility, being more worried about acquisition of HIV, believing that a partner would appreciate condom use, believing that a partner could be infected with HIV, and being less embarrassed about discussing condom use and purchasing a condom.[23-37] Other factors associated with condom use include receiving sexuality education, accessibility of condoms for use, believing that condoms can prevent STDs and HIV infection, being able to communicate with partners about STDs and HIV, perceiving peer norms as supportive of condom use, and availability of a physician with whom to discuss condom use.[23-37]

Effectiveness of Condom Use

The effectiveness of condoms in preventing unintended pregnancy and acquisition of STDs depends on consistent and proper use and avoidance of breakage, slippage, or leakage. Despite recent trends toward increased use by adolescents, consistent condom use (ie, for all episodes of vaginal or anal intercourse) is reported by less than half of all sexually active adolescents.[7,8] In addition, data demonstrate that effectiveness increases with experience, leaving those adolescents with the least experience at greatest risk for improper use.

Most condoms used in the United States are made of latex.[23,38] Natural condoms (made of lamb intestine) may be permeable to microorganisms (possibly including HIV). Polyurethane condoms also have recently become available for use.[39-40] As summarized by a CDC report, proper use of a condom requires: 1) using a new condom for each act of vaginal, oral, and anal intercourse; 2) putting the condom on correctly before any genital contact; 3) withdrawing while the penis is still erect and holding the condom firmly to keep it from slipping off; and 4) using only water-based lubricants, not those that are petroleum based (because condoms can be damaged by petroleum jelly, mineral oil, vegetable oil, cold creams, body lotions, and several antifungal medications).[23,38,41-42] The most important errors that lead to clinical failure are breakage, slippage, and failure to use throughout intercourse.[43-45] Other errors that can lead to condom failure include tearing or nicking the condom as the package is opened, unrolling the condom before placing it on the penis, failing to squeeze the tip of the condom as it is rolled onto the penis, delaying use of the condom until after intercourse starts, removing the condom too early (before ejaculation), and failing to hold the condom on the penis during withdrawal.[23]

Problems with condom use include latex allergy, which can be decreased by using a polyurethane condom, and decreased glans sensitivity, which can partly be overcome by use of textured, ribbed, ultrathin, or lubricated condoms.[23,38,41,42] The female condom, which is made of polyurethane, can be used as an alternative by those with latex allergy but cannot be used together with the male condom because they adhere to each other.[2] Breakage and slippage rates of the male condom have each been estimated to be less than 2%, although rates vary by study and with user experience.[42-46] Leakage attributable to faulty manufacturing is not currently considered to be a problem in the United States—efforts by the Food and Drug Administration have resulted in improved production and increased inspection in this country—but condoms imported from other countries may still be a cause for concern.[42-46] Condoms should be stored in cool, dark places, because heat, including body heat, can cause condoms to weaken.

Problems with inconsistent use, incorrect use, breakage, and leakage clearly indicate that condoms cannot be 100% effective in preventing pregnancy, STDs, and HIV infection. The data on pregnancy prevention are relatively clear, with theoretical annual failure rates (ie, pregnancy occurring during a year of use when the condom is used consistently and correctly) estimated to be 2%.[47] Actual failure rates range from 5% to 20%, depending on the age of the users.[47] Although failure rates are higher for adolescents than for older women, highest failure rates are reported to occur in women 20 to 24 years old; frequency of use and levels of fertility may play a role in these

findings.[38] One study reported first-year failure rates as low as 2% to 4% in adolescents, demonstrating that proper use can be attained in some populations of adolescents.[48]

Determining the efficacy of condom use in preventing transmission of STDs and HIV is much more complicated, because each STD must be considered individually. Several articles have reviewed the literature on this topic, with additional studies examining the effects of condom use on transmission of HIV and specific STDs.[49-60] The literature findings can be summarized as follows:

1. Condom use appears to decrease the rate of, but does not fully eliminate, transmission of most, and possibly all, STDs to males. Protection rates of one half to three quarters (ie, relative risk ratios of one half to two thirds) have been found in several studies of *Neisseria gonorrhoeae* and *Ureaplasma urealyticum* transmission, with 2 studies demonstrating 100% protection with short-term, consistent use.[49] Less clear is the demonstration of protection against *Chlamydia trachomatis* and *Treponema pallidum* in males, and there are no definitive studies to date on protection against herpes simplex and human papillomavirus, 2 organisms that can be transmitted by skin-to-skin contact for which the condom may offer less protection.[49-55]

2. Because a female is more likely to acquire an STD from an infected male partner than a male is from a female partner, condom use offers less protection from STD acquisition for females than for males. Studies of gonorrhea and *Trichomonas* infection demonstrate protection rates with condom use of only one third to one eighth (ie, relative risk ratios of 0.66-0.87).[49] Although some studies show no protection, others demonstrate some protection for women against infection with human papillomavirus and *C trachomatis* and bacterial vaginosis and decreased rates of infertility and hospitalizations for pelvic inflammatory disease among those who use condoms for contraception compared with those who use no protection.[49]

3. Condom use decreases the rate of acquisition of HIV by those who engage in high-risk sexual activity or whose partners are seropositive for HIV, with relative risk ratios generally in the range of 0.04 to 0.4 (ie, 60%–96% protective).[49,56-60] In 1 study of serodiscordant partners, consistent condom use decreased the rate of HIV conversion by the negative partner to 1%, compared with 7% in those who did not use condoms.[56] A recent meta-analysis of condom use in HIV-discordant couples yielded a consistent HIV infection incidence of 0.9 per 100 persons per year in those who always used condoms.[61]

In general, the data indicate that condom use is less protective against transmission of STDs and HIV than it is for pregnancy when used correctly and consistently ("theoretical effectiveness") and in real-life use ("actual effectiveness"). The fact that any single act of intercourse is more likely to result in transmission of disease from an infected partner than in pregnancy may partially account for this difference.[49] From a public health perspective, condoms, especially if used consistently and correctly, can be expected to decrease the rates of unintended pregnancy and STD and HIV acquisition among those who are sexually active, including adolescents. For the individual, however, condom use, even if consistent and correct, does not ensure prevention of unintended pregnancy or acquisition of an STD or HIV. It is for this reason that abstinence remains the major focus of primary prevention in efforts to decrease adolescent pregnancy, STDs, and HIV infection, whereas condom use is the main focus of secondary prevention for those who are already sexually active and plan to remain so.

Use of Condoms and Other Methods

Use of spermicides, especially those containing nonoxynol-9, had previously been recommended by some as a means of increasing the efficacy of condom use in prevention of pregnancy and STDs.[38,47,49] Several considerations were taken into account in making this recommendation. In favor of spermicide use were findings that spermicides kill or inactivate not only sperm but also *N gonorrhea*, HIV, *Trichomonas vaginalis,* herpes simplex, *T pallidum, U urealyticum,* and possibly *C trachomatis.*[49] Of concern, however, were the following facts: 1) no studies ever definitively demonstrated a beneficial effect of spermicides on STD or HIV transmission with condom use; 2) spermicide use may have adverse effects (although earlier concerns about birth defects and possible urinary tract colonization have not been confirmed)[62,63]; and 3) spermicides have been shown to cause vaginal irritation in some studies, leading to an increased risk of genital ulcers and a potentially increased risk of HIV infection.[49,64] This last concern has now been confirmed in a study performed in Africa by the Joint United Nations Program on AIDS, which found in a controlled study of more than 1000 women that those who used a condom and a spermicide with nonoxynol-9 became infected with HIV at about a 50% higher rate than those who used a condom and a placebo gel.[65] The CDC therefore issued a letter in August 2000 recommending against the use of nonoxynol-9 as a means of preventing STDs and HIV infection.[66]

More recently, use of condoms together with hormonal contraception (the "belt and suspenders" approach) has been advocated as the optimal approach to preventing unintended pregnancy, STDs, and HIV infection in those who are sexually active. Data indicate that some, but not many, adolescents use this approach. In a 1995 study, 8% of adolescent females in the United States reported using a condom and the birth control pill at last intercourse, and 21% of those using the pill reported that they also used a condom.[16,67-68] Clearly, this is less than the 37% reporting condom use overall in the same study, indicating that additional efforts are required to remind those who use birth control pills or other methods of hormonal contraception that condom use is also required for STD and HIV prevention.

Efforts Aimed at Increasing Condom Use

Efforts aimed at increasing condom use by adolescents have taken place in clinical, community, and school settings. Several organizations have provided official guidelines for clinicians who have adolescents patients. These include the American Academy of Pediatrics,[69] American Medical Association,[70] Maternal and Child Health Bureau of the Health Resources and Services Administration,[71] American Academy of Family Physicians,[72] and US Department of Health and Human Services.[73] Each of these guidelines recommends that counseling about the use of contraceptives, including the condom, be offered to sexually active adolescents as part of preventive health care in clinical settings. There have been multiple studies, however, which have shown that clinicians are inconsistent in following these recommendations.[74]

In community settings, youth development programs incorporate condom use into messages being transmitted to high-risk adolescents, but there have been no specific studies of the efficacy of this approach.[16] Community-based HIV prevention programs have also incorporated condom use into their messages, with some evidence of significant but generally small effects.[16] A direct mailing to adolescent males about condom use also had a small but significant effect.[75] Condom sales have responded to social marketing internationally, and studies showed increased condom sales in the United States after the release of the US Surgeon General's Report on AIDS in 1987.[76] Condom advertising remains taboo on national network television in the United States, however, despite some studies that have shown that most adults would approve of airing ads for contraceptives.[77]

By far the most common, most effective, and best studied efforts aimed at increasing condom use among adolescents, as well as the most controversial, have taken place in school settings. These efforts fall into 2 main categories: education about condom use as part of sex education and HIV prevention programs and direct condom availability programs.

School-based sex education programs during the past few years have generally been of 3 types: 1) abstinence-only programs, which generally do not include information on condoms or other contraceptive methods (except their failure rates); 2) pregnancy prevention programs, which focus on the use of contraception, including the condom, for those who are sexually active; and 3) HIV

prevention programs, which focus on condom use as a major component of the incorporation of safer sex strategies.[16]

Multiple studies evaluating the effects of these programs on sexual activity and contraceptive use have been performed during the past few years. These studies have failed to show a delay in the initiation of intercourse, a decrease in frequency of intercourse, or a decrease in the number of sexual partners for abstinence-only programs, when used alone.[16] Studies have shown beneficial effects of some pregnancy and HIV prevention programs, and no studies have shown an increase in intercourse (by hastening onset, increasing frequency, or increasing number of partners) for any of the programs.[16,78] Increased contraceptive use, including increased use of condoms, has been reported in the evaluation of some pregnancy and HIV prevention programs, with HIV prevention programs having the greatest influence on condom use.[16,78] It is not yet clear whether this important difference is attributable to the different messages delivered by the programs, the greater impact of HIV infection as opposed to pregnancy for males, better funding or evaluation methods for more recent HIV prevention programs, or other as yet unknown factors.[16,78]

Despite the controversy that surrounds them, it is becoming clear that sexuality education programs (ie, pregnancy prevention and especially HIV prevention programs) can have some effect on delaying the onset of intercourse, reducing sexual activity, and increasing the use of contraception, including condom use. Unfortunately, the magnitude of these effects is relatively small, in keeping with the known limitations of the effects that education can have on complex social and sexual behaviors.[78]

Because of these limitations, the concept of increasing condom availability through the schools has been implemented with the hope that providing increased access in addition to education can have a beneficial effect. It is estimated that more than 400 high schools in the United States, including many in the largest cities, have instituted condom availability programs during the past decade.[79] Many of the programs were begun amid great controversy, with many parents strongly in favor and many parents vehemently opposed.[80] Some programs include parental consent, whereas others do not; some involve school-based health centers, whereas others assign the job of condom distribution to a school nurse or specific faculty members; some include educational components, whereas others make condoms available solely through vending machines, baskets, or drawers.[79,81]

Several recent studies have evaluated the effectiveness of school-based condom availability programs. One study demonstrated that 93% of respondents in a high school were aware of their school's condom distribution program, 26% of respondents had received condoms, and 67% of respondents who had received condoms used them.[82] A Seattle study demonstrated that, although students took large numbers of condoms, neither sexual activity nor condom use were reported to have increased.[83] A Philadelphia study showed an insignificant increase in condom use, from 52% to 58% at last intercourse.[84] In a study in Santa Monica, California, 34% of students who had used a condom at last intercourse reported obtaining the condom from the school-based availability program, total sexual activity was not increased, and the program was strongly accepted among students.[85,86] In a study comparing New York City schools that have condom availability programs with Chicago schools that do not have such programs, New York students reported equal rates of sexual activity but higher rates of condom use (with an overall odds ratio of 1.36:1).[87,88] Similar to results achieved by educational programs, data from condom availability programs demonstrate no increases in sexual activity, with modest increases in condom use after introduction of the programs into school-based settings.

Recommendations

1. Abstaining from intercourse should be encouraged for adolescents, because it is the surest way to prevent STDs, including HIV infection, and pregnancy. Adolescents who have been sexually active previously should also be counseled regarding the benefits of postponing future sexual relationships.

2. Pediatricians are urged to actively support and encourage the correct and consistent use of reliable contraception and condoms by adolescents who are sexually active or contemplating sexual activity. The responsibility of males as well as females in preventing unwanted pregnancies and STDs should be emphasized. Pediatricians need to be actively involved in community programs directed toward this goal.

3. In the interest of public health, restrictions and barriers to condom availability should be removed.

4. Schools should be considered appropriate sites for the availability of condoms, because they contain large adolescent populations and may potentially provide a comprehensive array of related educational and health care resources.

5. To be most effective, condom availability programs should be developed through a collaborative community process and accompanied by comprehensive sequential sexuality education, which is ideally part of a K-12 health education program, with parental involvement, counseling, and positive peer support.

6. Pediatricians can actively help raise awareness among parents and communities that making condoms available to adolescents does not increase the rate of adolescent sexual activity and that condoms, despite their limitations, can decrease rates of unintended pregnancy and acquisition of STDs and HIV infection.

7. Research is encouraged to identify methods to increase correct and consistent condom use by sexually active adolescents and to evaluate effectiveness of strategies to promote condom use, including condom education and availability programs in schools.

COMMITTEE ON ADOLESCENCE, 2000–2001
David W. Kaplan, MD, MPH, Chairperson
Ronald A. Feinstein, MD
Martin M. Fisher, MD
Jonathan D. Klein, MD, MPH
Luis F. Olmedo, MD
Ellen S. Rome, MD, MPH
W. Samuel Yancy, MD

Liaisons

Paula J. Adams Hillard, MD
American College of Obstetricians
and Gynecologists

Diane Sacks, MD
Canadian Paediatric Society

Glen Pearson, MD
American Academy of Child and
Adolescent Psychiatry

Section Liaison

Barbara L. Frankowski, MD, MPH
Section on School Health

Staff

Tammy Piazza Hurley

References

1. American Academy of Pediatrics, Committee on Adolescence. Condom availability for youth. *Pediatrics.* 1995;95:281–285

2. McCabe E, Golub S, Lee AC. Making the female condom a "reality" for adolescents. *J Pediatr Adolesc Gynecol.* 1997;10:115–123

3. Zelnik M, Kantner JF. Sexual activity, contraceptive use, and pregnancy among metropolitan-area teenagers: 1971–1979. *Fam Plann Perspect.* 1980;12:230–237

4. Forrest JD, Singh S. The sexual and reproductive behavior of American women, 1982–1988. *Fam Plann Perspect.* 1990;22:206–214

5. Centers for Disease Control and Prevention. Trends in sexual risk behaviors among high school students—United States, 1991–1997. *MMWR Morb Mortal Wkly Rep.* 1998;47:749–752

6. Centers for Disease Control and Prevention. Youth risk behavior surveillance—United States, 1999. *MMWR Morb Mortal Wkly Rep.* 2000;49:1–94

7. Sonenstein FL, Pleck JH, Ku LC. Sexual activity, condom use and AIDS awareness among adolescent males. *Fam Plann Perspect.* 1989;21:152–158

8. Sonenstein FL, Ku LC, Lindberg LD, Turner CF, Pleck JH. Changes in sexual behavior and condom use among teenage males: 1988 to 1995. *Am J Public Health.* 1998;88:956–959

9. American Academy of Pediatrics, Committee on Adolescence. Adolescent pregnancy—current trends and issues: 1998. *Pediatrics.* 1999;103:516–520

10. Ventura SJ, Mosher WD, Curtin SC, Abma JC, Henshaw S. Trends in pregnancies and pregnancy rates by outcome: estimates for the United States, 1976-96. *Vital Health Stat 21.* 2000;56:1–47

11. The Alan Guttmacher Institute. *Sex and America's Teenagers.* New York, NY: The Alan Guttmacher Institute; 1994

12. Flinn MA, Hauser D. Teenage pregnancy: the case for prevention. Washington, DC: Advocates for Youth; 1998

13. Centers for Disease Control and Prevention. State-specific birth rates for teenagers—United States, 1990-1996. *MMWR Morb Mortal Wkly Rep.* 1997;46:837–842

14. Koonin LM, Smith JC, Ramick M, Strauss LT, Hopkins FW. Abortion surveillance—United States, 1993 and 1994. *MMWR Morb Mortal Wkly Rep.* 1997;46:37–98

15. Institute of Medicine, Committee on Prevention and Control of Sexually Transmitted Diseases. *The Hidden Epidemic.* Eng TR, Butler WT, eds. Washington, DC: National Academy Press; 1997

16. Santelli JS, DiClemente RJ, Miller KS, Kirby D. Sexually transmitted diseases, unintended pregnancy, and adolescent health promotion. *Adolesc Med.* 1999;10:87–108

17. Fleming DT, Quillan GM, Johnson RE, et al. Herpes simplex virus type 2 in the United States, 1976 to 1994. *N Engl J Med.* 1997;337:1105–1111

18. Office of National AIDS Policy. *Youth and HIV/AIDS: An American Agenda.* Washington, DC: Office of National AIDS Policy; 1996

19. Reddy SP, Yeturu SR, Slupik R. Chlamydia trachomatis in adolescents: a review. *J Pediatr Adolesc Gynecol.* 1997; 10:59–72

20. Gutman LT. Human papillomavirus infections of the genital tract in adolescents. *Adolesc Med.* 1995;6:115–128

21. Kahn JR, Rindfuss RR, Guilkey DK. Adolescent contraceptive method choices. *Demography.* 1990;27:323–335

22. Miller KS, Levin ML, Whitaker DJ, Xu X. Patterns of condom use among adolescents: the impact of mother-adolescent communication. *Am J Public Health.* 1998; 88:1542–1544

23. Joffe A. Adolescents and condom use. *Am J Dis Child.* 1993;147:746–754

24. Pleck JH, Sonenstein FL, Ku LC. Adolescent males' condom use: relationships between perceived cost-benefits and consistency. *J Marriage Fam.* 1991;53:733–745

25. Pleck JH, Sonenstein FL, Ku L. Changes in adolescent males' use of and attitudes toward condoms, 1988-1991. *Fam Plann Perspect.* 1993;25:106–110,117

26. Kegeles SM, Adler NE, Irwin CE. Adolescents and condoms: associations of beliefs with intentions to use. *Am J Dis Child.* 1989;143:911–915

27. Hingson RW, Strunin L, Berlin BM, Heeren T. Beliefs about AIDS, use of alcohol and drugs, and unprotected sex among Massachusetts adolescents. *Am J Public Health.* 1990;80:295–299

28. Hingson R, Strunin L, Berlin B. Acquired immunodeficiency syndrome transmission: changes in knowledge and behaviors among teenagers, Massachusetts statewide surveys, 1986 to 1988. *Pediatrics.* 1990;85:24–29

29. DiClemente RJ, Durbin M, Siegel D, Krasnovsky F, Lazarus N, Comacho T. Determinants of condom use among junior high school students in a minority, inner-city school district. *Pediatrics.* 1992;89:197–202

30. Murphy JJ, Boggess S. Increased condom use among teenage males, 1988–1995: the role of attitudes. *Fam Plann Perspect.* 1998;30:276–280,303

31. Weisman CS, Plichta S, Nathanson CA, Ensminger M, Robinson JC. Consistency of condom use for disease prevention among adolescent users of oral contraceptives. *Fam Plann Perspect.* 1991;23:71–74

32. Valdiserri RO, Arena VC, Proctor D, Bonati FA. The relationship between women's attitudes about condoms and their use: implications for condom promotion programs. *Am J Public Health.* 1989;79:499–501

33. Pendergast RA Jr, Durant RH, Gaillard GL. Attitudinal and behavioral correlates of condom use in urban adolescent males. *J Adolesc Health.* 1992;13:133–139

34. Adler NE, Kegeler SM, Irwin CE Jr, Wibbelsman C. Adolescent contraceptive behavior: an assessment of decision processes. *J Pediatr.* 1990;116:463–471

35. Shafer MA, Boyer CB. Psychosocial and behavioral factors associated with risk of sexually transmitted diseases, including human immunodeficiency virus infection, among urban high school students. *J Pediatr.* 1991; 119:826–833

36. Orr DP, Langefeld CD. Factors associated with condom use by sexually active male adolescents at risk for sexually transmitted diseases. *Pediatrics.* 1993;91:873–879

37. Plichta SB, Weisman CS, Nathanson CA, Ensminger ME, Robinson JC. Partner-specific condom use among adolescent women clients of a family planning clinic. *J Adolesc Health.* 1992;13:506–511

38. Sikand A, Fisher M. The role of barrier contraceptives in prevention of pregnancy and disease in adolescents. *Adolesc Med.* 1992;3:223–240

39. Frezieres RG, Walsh TL, Nelson AL, Clark VA, Coulson AH. Evaluation of the efficacy of a polyurethane condom: a randomized, controlled clinical trial. *Fam Plann Perspect.* 1999;31:81–87

40. Rosenberg MJ, Waugh MS, Solomon HM, Lyszkowski AD. The male polyurethane condom: a review of current knowledge. *Contraception.* 1996;53:141–146

41. Centers for Disease Control and Prevention. Update: barrier protection against HIV infection and other sexually transmitted diseases. *MMWR Morb Mortal Wkly Rep.* 1993;42:589–591,597

42. Anderson FWJ. Condoms: a technical guide. *Female Patient.* 1993;18:16,21

43. Albert AE, Warner DL, Hatcher RA, Trussell J, Bennett C. Condom use among female commercial sex workers in Nevada's legal brothels. *Am J Public Health.* 1995;85:1514–1520

44. Spruyt A, Steiner MJ, Joanis C, et al. Identifying condom users at risk for breakage and slippage: findings from three international sites. *Am J Public Health.* 1998; 88:239–244

45. Warner L, Clay-Warner J, Boles J, Williamson J. Assessing condom use practices: implications for evaluating method and user effectiveness. *Sex Transm Dis.* 1998;25:273–277

46. Consumer's Union. Can you rely on condoms? *Consumer Reports.* 1989;54:135–141

47. Hatcher RA, Trussell J, Stewart F, et al. *Contraceptive Technology.* 17th ed. New York, NY: Ardent Media; 1998

48. Goldman JA, Dicker D, Feldberg D, Samuel N, Resnik R. Barrier contraception in the teenager: a comparison of four methods in adolescent girls. *Pediatr Adolesc Gynecol.* 1985;3:59–76

49. Cates W Jr, Stone KM. Family planning, sexually transmitted diseases and contraceptive choice: a literature update—Part I. *Fam Plann Perspect.* 1992;24:75–84

50. Morris BA. How safe are "safes"? Efficacy and effectiveness of condoms in preventing STDs. *Can Fam Phys.* 1993;39:819–822,827

51. d'Oro LC, Parazzini F, Naldi L, La Vecchia C. Barrier methods of contraception, spermicides, and sexually transmitted diseases: a review. *Genitourin Med.* 1994; 70:410–417

52. Zenilman JM, Weisman CS, Rompalo AM, et al. Condom use to prevent incident STDs: the validity of self-reported condom use. *Sex Transm Dis.* 1995;22:15–21

53. Jamison JH, Kaplan DW, Hamman R, Eagar R, Beach R, Douglas JM Jr. Spectrum of genital human papillomavirus infection in a female adolescent population. *Sex Transm Dis.* 1995;22:236–243

54. Kreiss JK, Kiviat NB, Plummer FA, et al. Human immunodeficiency virus, human papillomavirus, and cervical intraepithelial neoplasia in Nairobi prostitutes. *Sex Transm Dis.* 1992;19:54–59

55. Hippelainen MI, Hippelainen M, Saarikoski S, Syrjanen K. Clinical course and prognostic factors of human papillomavirus infection in men. *Sex Transm Dis.* 1994;21: 272–279

56. Saracco A, Musicco M, Nicolosi A, et al. Man-to-woman sexual transmission of HIV: longitudinal study of 343 steady partners of infected men. *J Acquir Immune Defic Syndr.* 1993;6:497–502

57. Weller SC. A meta-analysis of condom effectiveness in reducing sexually transmitted HIV. *Soc Sci Med.* 1993; 36:1635–1644

58. de Vincenzi I. A longitudinal study of human immunodeficiency virus transmission by heterosexual partners. *N Engl J Med.* 1994;331:341–346

59. Guimaraes MD, Munoz A, Boschi-Pinto C, Castilho EA. HIV infection among female partners of seropositive men in Brazil. *Am J Epidemiol.* 1995;142:538–547

60. Deschamps MM, Pape JW, Hafner A, Johnson WD Jr. Heterosexual transmission of HIV in Haiti. *Ann Intern Med.* 1996;125:324–330

61. Davis KR, Weller SC. The effectiveness of condoms in reducing heterosexual transmission of HIV. *Fam Plann Perspect.* 1999;31:272–279

62. Louik C, Mitchell AA, Werler MM, Hanson JW, Shapiro S. Maternal exposure to spermicides in relation to certain birth defects. *N Engl J Med.* 1987;317:474–478

63. Shapiro S, Sloane D, Heinonen OP, et al. Birth defects and vaginal spermicides. *JAMA*. 1982;247:2381-2384

64. Hira SK, Feldblum PJ, Kamanga J, Mukelebai G, Weir SS, Thomas JC. Condoms and nonoxynol-9 use and the incidence of HIV infection in serodiscordant couples in Zambia. *Int J STD AIDS*. 1997;8:243-250

65. van Damme L. Advances in topical microbicides. Paper presented at: XIII International AIDS Conference; July 9-14, 2000; Durban, South Africa

66. Gayle HD. Nonoxynol-9 trial the implications [letter]. Atlanta, GA: Centers for Disease Control and Prevention, Public Health Service, US Department of Health and Human Services; August 4, 2000. Available at: http://www.cdc.gov/hiv/pubs/mmwr/mmwr11aug00.htm. Accessed November 6, 2000

67. Abma JC, Chandra CA, Mosher WD, Peterson LS, Piccinino LJ. Fertility, family planning, and women's health: new data from the 1995 National Survey of Family Growth. *Vital Health Stat*. 1997;23:1-114

68. Santelli JS, Warren CW, Lowry R, et al. The use of condoms with other contraceptive methods among young men and women. *Fam Plann Perspect*. 1997;29:261-267

69. American Academy of Pediatrics, Committee on Practice and Ambulatory Medicine. Recommendations for preventive pediatric health care. *Pediatrics*. 1995;96:373-374

70. Elster AB, Kuznets NJ. *AMA Guidelines for Adolescent Preventive Services (GAPS): Recommendations and Rationale*. Baltimore, MD: Williams & Wilkins; 1992

71. Green M, ed. *Bright Futures: Guidelines for Health Supervision of Infants, Children and Adolescents*. Arlington, VA: National Center for Education in Maternal and Child Health; 1994

72. American Academy of Family Physicians. *Age Charts for Periodic Health Examinations*. Kansas City, MO: American Academy of Family Physicians; 1995

73. US Preventive Services Task Force. *Guide to Clinical Preventive Services*. 2nd ed. Baltimore, MD: Williams & Wilkins; 1996

74. Fisher M. Adolescent health assessment and promotion in office and school settings. *Adolesc Med*. 1999;10:71-86

75. Kirby D, Harvey PD, Claussenius D, Novar M. A direct mailing to teenage males about condom use: its impact on knowledge, attitudes and sexual behavior. *Fam Plann Perspect*. 1989;21:12-18

76. Moran JS, Janes HR, Peterman TA, Stone KM. Increase in condom sales following AIDS education and publicity, United States. *Am J Public Health*. 1990;80:607-608

77. Strasburger VC. Children, adolescents and the media: five crucial issues. *Adolesc Med*. 1993;4:479-493

78. Kirby D. Reducing adolescent pregnancy: approaches that work. *Contemp Pediatr*. 1999;16:83-94

79. Kirby DS, Brown NL. Condom availability programs in US schools. *Fam Plann Perspect*. 1996;28:196-202

80. Rafferty Y, Radosh A. Attitudes about AIDS education and condom availability among parents of high school students in New York City: a focus group approach. *AIDS Educ Prev*. 1997;9:14-30

81. Fortenberry JD. Condom availability in high schools. *Adolesc Med*. 1997;8:449-454

82. Wolk LI, Rosenbaum R. The benefits of school-based condom availability: cross-sectional analysis of a comprehensive high school-based program. *J Adolesc Health*. 1995;17:184-188

83. Kirby D, Brener ND, Brown NL, Peterfreund N, Hillard P, Harrist R. The impact of condom availability in Seattle schools on sexual behavior and condom use. *Am J Public Health*. 1999;89:182-187

84. Furstenberg FF Jr, Geitz LM, Teitler JO, Weiss CC. Does condom availability make a difference? An evaluation of Philadelphia's health resource centers. *Fam Plann Perspect*. 1997;29:123-127

85. Schuster MA, Bell RM, Berry SH, Kanouse DE. Students' acquisition and use of school condoms in a high school condom availability program. *Pediatrics*. 1997;100:689-694

86. Schuster MA, Bell RM, Berry SH, Kanouse DE. Impact of a high school condom availability program on sexual attitudes and behaviors. *Fam Plann Perspect*. 1998;30:67-72,88

87. Guttmacher S, Lieberman L, Ward D, Freudenberg N, Radosh A, Des-Jarlais D. Condom availability and New York City public high schools: relationships to condom use and sexual behavior. *Am J Public Health*. 1997;87:1427-1433

88. Guttmacher S, Lieberman L, Wai HC, et al. Gender differences in attitudes and use of condom availability programs among sexually active students in New York City public high schools. *J Am Med Womens Assoc*. 1995;50:99-102

Contraception and Adolescents

Committee on Adolescence

ABSTRACT. The risks and negative consequences of adolescent sexual intercourse are of national concern, and promoting sexual abstinence is an important goal of the American Academy of Pediatrics. In previous publications, the American Academy of Pediatrics has addressed important issues of adolescent sexuality, pregnancy, sexually transmitted diseases, and contraception.[1-3] The development of new contraceptive technologies mandates a revision of this policy statement, which provides the pediatrician with an updated review of adolescent sexuality and use of contraception by adolescents and presents current guidelines for counseling adolescents on sexual activity and contraceptive methods.

ABBREVIATIONS. STDs, sexually transmitted diseases; IM, intramuscular; IUD, intrauterine device; ECPs, emergency contraceptive pills.

Pediatricians have an important role in adolescent reproductive health care. Because pediatricians have long-term relationships with their patients and families, this continuity of care provides opportunities to promote healthy behavior and to reduce the potential negative consequences of high-risk adolescent sexual activity. Pediatricians have an active role in reducing the risk of unintended pregnancies and sexually transmitted diseases (STDs) in their adolescent patients.

Adolescent Sexual Behavior and Use of Contraception

An adolescent's decision to initiate or delay sexual activity is complex.[4-10] Evidence exists that consensual sexual intercourse may serve a variety of psychosocial needs in the adolescent, including mastery of psychosocial development, rebellion, peer group identification and validation, and as a way of coping with frustration and failure.[4,5] The factors that determine if adolescent sexual activity begins earlier or later are listed in Table 1.[6-10]

During the past 3 decades the level of sexual activity in adolescents in the United States has increased. The majority of US adolescents begin having sexual intercourse by mid- to late adolescence, with an average age of first intercourse between 15 and 17 years.[11] The results of the National Youth Risk Behavior Study of the Centers for Disease Control and Prevention disclosed that at least half of all high school students have had sexual intercourse, with 36.9% of 9th graders and 66.4% of 12th graders reporting coital experience.[12,13]

There is no evidence that refusal to provide contraception to an adolescent results in abstinence or postponement of sexual activity. In fact, if adolescents perceive obstacles to obtaining contraception and condoms, they are more likely

Table 1. Factors Associated With Early and Later Initiation of Sexual Intercourse

Early initiation
    Early onset of puberty
    Sexual abuse
    Absence of a nurturing or supportive parent
    Poor academic achievement
    Poverty
    Participation in other high-risk activities
    Mental illness
Later initiation
    Emphasis on abstinence
    Parental consistency and firmness in discipline
    Goal orientation
    High academic achievement
    Regular attendance at a place of worship

PEDIATRICS (ISSN 0031 4005). Copyright © 1999 by the American Academy of Pediatrics.

to have negative outcomes to sexual activity.[16] In addition, no evidence exists that provision of information to adolescents about contraception results in increased rates of sexual activity, earlier age of first intercourse, or a greater number of partners. Two school-based controlled studies that demonstrated a delay of onset of sexual intercourse in the intervention group used a comprehensive approach that included a discussion of contraception.[17-19] Availability of contraception is not causally related to sexual experimentation.[19,20]

An adolescent's decision about whether to use contraception is complex. Although trends have improved, with more adolescents reporting current use of contraception, more use of contraception at first intercourse, and more frequently with continuing sexual intercourse, the consistent use of any contraception remains a challenge for most adolescents. About 35% of female adolescents do not use contraception at the time of first intercourse[7,21]; the approximate time between an adolescent female becoming sexually active and seeking medical services for contraception is 12 months.[7,22,23] Approximately half of all adolescent pregnancies occur within the first 6 months after the adolescent becomes sexually active, and one fifth of pregnancies occur within the first month.[24]

Individual methods of contraception used by adolescents vary according to such factors as race, ethnicity, age, marital status, education, income, and fertility intentions. Trends in methods of contraception used during 1982–1995 show a decrease in pill use among adolescents 15 to 19 years old and increased male condom use.[25] Reported male condom use has steadily increased among adolescents since 1970; use tripled between 1982 and 1992.[15,26-28] The increase in male condom use occurred faster among black and Hispanic adolescents, increasing from 13% in 1982 to 38% in 1995 in the 15- to 19-year-old age group, while their white adolescent counterparts increased their use from 23% in 1992 to 36% in 1995.[14] The most recent Youth Risk Behavior Study data confirmed 58% of sexually active adolescents aged 14 to 17 years used a condom at last intercourse, and 78% of all sexually active adolescents reported use of a reliable method of contraception at last intercourse. However, use of a contraceptive method during each sexual encounter was inconsistent and sporadic.[14,15,27]

Adolescents who incorrectly or inconsistently use (are poor users of) contraception include younger adolescents who may be less likely to be involved in a stable, long-term relationship and youth who are involved in casual relationships. In addition, more than one fourth of female adolescents who have had their first intercourse at 14 years or younger report that their participation was involuntary.[7] Contraception clearly is problematic for these young women. Other factors that contribute to lack of contraceptive use include adolescent developmental issues such as reluctance to acknowledge one's sexual activity, a sense of invincibility (belief that they are immune from the problems or issues surrounding sexual intercourse or pregnancy), and denial of the possibility of pregnancy and misconceptions regarding use or appropriateness of contraception. However, an adolescent's level of knowledge about how to use contraception effectively does not necessarily correlate with consistent use. Some of the reasons given by adolescents for the delay in using contraception are fear that their parents will find out, ambivalence, and the perception that birth control is dangerous.[5,22]

The Role of the Pediatrician

Pediatricians should be able to encourage abstinence and provide appropriate counseling about sexual behaviors. Counseling should include discussion about the prevention of STDs, education on contraceptive methods, and family planning services for the sexually active patient. When these services are provided in the pediatrician's office, policies and procedures for the provision of such services should be developed.[20]

COUNSELING ADOLESCENTS ABOUT CONTRACEPTION

Comprehensive health care of adolescents should include a sexual history that should be obtained in a safe, nonthreatening environment through open, honest, and nonjudgmental communication, with assurances of confidentiality.[3,20] During the preadolescent years the pediatrician can provide anticipatory guidance by discussing puberty and offering health education materials to the youth and family. With the onset of puberty, the patient's history should include information regarding attitudes and knowledge about sexual behavior, degree of involvement in sexual activity, and use of contraception. At the onset of puberty, private, confidential interviews with the adolescent should be part of a health maintenance visit.

CONFIDENTIALITY AND CONSENT

The primary reason adolescent's hesitate or delay obtaining family planning or contraceptive services is concern about confidentiality.[29] It is important for pediatricians to develop office policies that assure confidentiality. State requirements and standards of practice should be reviewed and the development of clear, concise, and standardized office protocols for confidentiality should be developed for staff, patients, and parents.[30] These policies should include information regarding when confidentiality must be waived, guidelines for reimbursement for services, medical record access, appointment scheduling, and office policy regarding information disclosure.

SEXUAL RESPONSIBILITY

The promotion of healthy and responsible sexual decision-making is one of the goals of counseling adolescents about contraception. Pediatricians can help adolescents identify their own goals for safe and responsible sexual behavior, including abstinence. Issues of health concerns and individual risk assessments may lead to appropriate discussions between the adolescent and pediatrician. Successful counseling requires the pediatrician to be supportive and nonjudgmental. The teaching of responsible sexual decision-making requires effective dialogue, skillful history taking, careful listening, and repeated simple messages that contain essential information.[20]

SEXUAL DECISION MAKING

Adolescents should be strongly encouraged to postpone the initiation of sexual intercourse. For patients already engaged in sexual intercourse or who are contemplating having sexual intercourse,

a discussion of contraceptive methods and prevention of STDs (including acquired immunodeficiency syndrome/human immunodeficiency virus), is essential. Discussions should address and explore, in a nonjudgmental way, the adolescent's reasons for becoming sexually active and the impact that sexual intercourse may have on relationships with peers, parents, and significant others.

For sexually active adolescents who are using contraception, the role of the caregiver is to support compliance, manage side effects, change the method of contraception as circumstances require, and provide referrals and frequent follow-up with periodic screening for STDs.

METHODS OF CONTRACEPTION

Numerous current reviews and protocols for prescribing and managing contraception are available.[31,34] The following comments focus on the appropriateness of the various contraceptive methods for adolescents. The pediatrician should emphasize the need for prevention of STDs as well as contraception with each patient.[20,35]

ABSTINENCE

Abstinence is the most effective means of birth control. Abstinence education generally focuses on delaying the initiation of adolescent sexual activity until adulthood. Many schools have adopted abstinence-dominant or abstinence-only education programs for school sexuality curricula. To date, the evidence regarding the efficacy of such interventions in the reduction of sexual behaviors remains controversial.[36] Recent studies have demonstrated the importance of youth, parent, physician, and education partnerships in the prevention of health risk behaviors such as early initiation of sexual intercourse.[37,38] There is some consensus that abstinence-based education and intervention is most effective when targeted toward younger adolescents and before their becoming sexually active.[39-41] However, abstinence may be difficult for adolescents. About 26% of adolescent couples trying to abstain from intercourse will become pregnant within 1 year.[42] Teenage couples who choose to abstain from sexual intercourse should be encouraged and supported by their parents, peers, and society (including the media) and especially by their pediatrician. But they need to know about other contraceptive options BEFORE or IF they decide to have intercourse.

CONDOMS

The male condom is a mechanical barrier method of contraception. Its effectiveness is enhanced by use of a spermicide. Latex condoms significantly reduce the transmission of STDs and should therefore be used by all sexually active adolescents regardless of whether an additional method of contraception is being used. Adolescents must understand that the use of a condom is not optional and that a new condom must be used each time they have sexual intercourse. They must also be instructed in the correct use of a condom. Adolescents need to understand that no other contraception method provides the same protection from STDs.[4,27,33,34,43] Male condoms have several other advantages. They allow for males to share in the responsibility for contraception, they are easily accessible and available, they can be obtained without prescription, they are inexpensive, and they can be legally purchased by minors.[3,33,44,45]

The female condom is also a barrier method of contraception. Available data suggest it may be effective in the prevention of STDs and as effective as the diaphragm in preventing pregnancy. Acceptability in the adolescent population is unknown, but may be limited by the high cost, lack of availability, and the difficulty of insertion.[20,31,46,47]

SPERMICIDES AND CONDOMS

Spermicides have a relatively high contraceptive failure rate when used alone and must be applied with each act of intercourse to be effective. If used consistently with male condoms, the birth control effectiveness approaches that of oral contraceptives. Spermicides consist of 2 agents: nonoxynol 9 and octoxynol 9, applied intravaginally through a variety of forms (gel, foam suppository, and film). The combination of spermicide and condoms is a very effective means of contraception

for adolescents because it provides effective prevention of pregnancy and STDs, is available without a prescription, and is inexpensive.[7,20,31,44,45]

ORAL CONTRACEPTIVES

Oral contraceptives are reliable and effective for the prevention of pregnancy, are available by prescription, and are the most popular method of contraception among adolescents.[25] Currently 3 forms of oral contraceptive pills are available: the fixed-dose combination (each tablet contains the same dose of estrogen and progestin), the phasic dose (the triphasic and biphasic packs containing varying doses of estrogen and progestin), and the mini-pill (progestin only). The newest generation of birth control pills have a low dose of estrogen (20 to 35 mm), and new forms of progestin. The standard 28-day pack of pills (21 days of hormone and 7 days of placebo) continues to be widely and successfully used by adolescents[2,25,33,43,48] and should be encouraged over the 21-day pack for promoting daily compliance.

Benefits of the use of combination oral contraceptives are listed in Table 2. Breakthrough bleeding is the most common side effect and usually resolves within 3 months. Weight gain, nausea, and headaches are infrequent.[33,39,43,49-51]

The failure rate of oral contraceptives when used correctly is <1%.[50] However, the failure rate among adolescents may be as high as

Table 2. Benefits of Oral Contraceptives

Protection against
  Ovarian and endometrial cancer
  Ectopic pregnancy
  Ovarian cysts
  Iron deficiency anemia
  Benign breast disease

Possible decreased risks of bacterial STDs progressing to pelvic inflammatory disease

Therapy for dysmenorrhea

Other noncontraceptive uses:
  Regulation of menses
  Treatment of dysfunctional uterine bleeding
  Decreased risk of osteoporosis
  Treatment of acne

15% because of inconsistent use.[52,53] One study suggests that adolescents miss an average of 3 pills per month.[54]

Adolescent compliance with oral contraceptive use may be enhanced by appropriate patient education and problem-solving techniques. This includes careful instruction regarding the use of oral contraceptives, anticipatory guidance about side effects and their management, a discussion of correct pill usage (including when the first pill should be taken during the menstrual cycle or what to do if a pill is missed), and frequent follow-up and monitoring.[34,43,51]

Oral contraceptives are best for adolescent females who desire regular menses and are organized and motivated to take a pill every day; additionally, a condom must be used in conjunction with oral contraceptives to give protection against STDs. Ideally, adolescents should receive a complete gynecological examination by the pediatrician before taking oral contraceptives. In some circumstances (such as when a patient shows anxiety), the pelvic examination may be deferred and oral contraceptives prescribed if the patient is healthy, not pregnant, and has no contraindications to taking the pills. Therefore, oral contraceptives can be prescribed by the pediatrician and the adolescent can be referred for an examination and Papanicolaou smear within the next 3 months.

MEDROXYPROGESTERONE ACETATE INJECTION (DEPO-PROVERA)

Medroxyprogesterone acetate is a long-acting progestin given every 12 weeks as a single 150-mg intramuscular (IM) dose. For adolescents, this contraceptive method has many benefits, including effective pregnancy prevention, convenience (requires no daily drug regimen, no need for planning before intercourse), lack of estrogen-related side effects, and protection against endometrial cancer and iron deficiency anemia. The major disadvantages of this contraceptive method for adolescents are menstrual cycle irregularities (present for nearly all patients originally), the need for IM administration, and the side effects (weight gain, headaches, bloating, depression, and mood changes). Medroxyprogesterone acetate is also associated with a delayed return to fertility and possibly a reversible osteopenia.[34,43,44,55,56]

This contraceptive method may be safely recommended for adolescents who have chronic illnesses (ie, seizures, sickle cell disease), are lactating, or are at risk for complications with estrogen. Medroxyprogesterone acetate injection is the best type of contraception for adolescents who do not remember to take daily medication. Pediatricians need to be sure to discuss the potential side effects and to ensure that the patient is not pregnant at the time of each injection. Condoms must be used in conjunction with medroxyprogesterone acetate for protection from STDs.

LEVONORGESTREL IMPLANTS (NORPLANT SYSTEM)

Levonorgestrel implants are a highly effective long-acting progestin contraceptive that provides pregnancy prevention for up to 5 years. It requires insertion and removal of subcutaneous Silastic capsules by a trained health care professional.[34,43]

For some adolescents levonorgestrel implants have proven to be a long-term effective method of contraception.[43,56-60] This contraception may be indicated in adolescents who desire long-term spacing between births, want an extended length of protection, have a history of problems with oral contraceptives, or are already mothers.[33,34,56,61] The major disadvantages for use in the adolescent population include high initial cost, the potential side effects (breakthrough bleeding, headaches), and the need to have an experienced health care professional remove the implant.

Adolescents using subdermal implants have experiences similar to adults, particularly when appropriate counseling is provided.[61] They have the same concerns or problems but may be more likely to have the implants removed than would an adult.[62,63] Although most pediatricians do not insert or remove the implants, they should be aware of the resources in the community that can serve as referral sources for their patients. Condoms must be used in conjunction with levonorgestrel implants for protection from STDs.

INTRAUTERINE DEVICES (IUDS)

When used appropriately, IUDs are safe, effective methods of contraception. IUDs should be reserved for adolescent females who cannot use other contraceptive methods and whose sexual behavior does not put them at risk for STDs. Some controversy exists as to whether IUDs are an appropriate method of contraception for adolescents.[35] Condoms must be used in conjunction with IUDs for protection against STDs.

DIAPHRAGM AND CERVICAL CAP

The diaphragm and cervical cap are effective barrier methods of contraception that require use of spermicides and condoms. These contraceptive methods have limited usefulness in adolescents as they require a prescription, a visit with a health care professional for a fitting, and a motivated adolescent who is comfortable and skilled with insertion. Consistent, correct use is critical.

RHYTHM AND OTHER PERIODIC ABSTINENCE METHODS

Rhythm and other methods of periodic abstinence require sophistication, awareness of fertility, motivation, and timing of intercourse that may be too complicated for most adolescents. However, pediatricians should be prepared to teach adolescents about the menstrual cycle and the times of increased fertility as an educational tool. The rhythm method provides little or no protection against STDs.

WITHDRAWAL

Withdrawal, which involves the male partner's attempt to withdraw the penis before ejaculation, is still widely used by adolescents in sexual relationships. Adolescents should receive counseling that discusses the high failure rate of withdrawal for pregnancy prevention. In addition, counseling should stress that this method provides little or no protection against STDs.

EMERGENCY CONTRACEPTIVE PILLS (ECPs)

There are many prescribed methods of emergency postcoital contraception. The most commonly prescribed method consists of 2 doses of combined estrogen and progestin contraceptive pills taken within 72 hours of unprotected intercourse followed by 2 pills 12 hours later.[64] For this method of ECPs, the dose depends on the oral contraceptive agent used (Table 3). The US Food and Drug Administration has indicated that the use of ECPs is safe and effective. Nausea is a likely side effect that may be relieved by the use of antiemetics. Pediatricians should inform adolescents that ECP is available in cases of emergency but should not be considered a substitute for ongoing contraception.

The ECP has an efficacy of approximately 75% in the prevention of conception.[64] It is contraindicated in adolescents who are unable to use oral contraceptives and if more than 72 hours have transpired since intercourse. A pregnancy test should be done before administration of the pills and 3 weeks after administration to detect any treatment failures.

COMPLIANCE AND FOLLOW-UP

Frequent follow-up is important to maximize compliance for all methods of contraception, to promote and reinforce healthy decision-making, and to screen periodically for risk-taking behaviors and STDs. Follow-up visits should include: periodic reassessment for contraception method, STD surveillance, and cervical cytology (Papanicolaou smear). The timing and frequency of reassessment will vary depending on the contraceptive method. In general, adolescents should have an annual Papanicolaou smear and a screen for STDs every 6 months, and a quarterly contraceptive reassessment to discuss issues such as utilization, compliance, and complications. Each adolescent should receive ongoing support, personal guidance, and reinforcement to enhance effective and consistent contraceptive use; parental support (if possible); and couples counseling or the opportunity

Table 3. Emergency Contraception Choices

	Tablets Within 72 Hours	Tablets 12 Hours Later
Ovral	2	2
Lo/Ovral; Nordette; Levlen	4	4
Triphasil or Tri-Levlen (yellow tablets only)	4	4

for couples interaction with the health care professional. In addition, condom use needs to be advised and reinforced at every visit.

SPECIAL CONSIDERATIONS

The issue of contraception in adolescents with chronic illness or disability is often forgotten. An estimated 10% to 20% of children and adolescents experience a disability or chronic illness by age 20 years.[65] Pediatricians should be aware that extensive information regarding contraception choices and decisions for adolescents with chronic illness or disability are available in references and texts on adolescent medicine.

Recommendations

1. Pediatricians should encourage and promote sexual abstinence to their adolescent patients at every appropriate opportunity.
2. Pediatricians should be prepared to provide nonjudgmental education and preventive counseling about sexuality to their adolescent patients.
3. Pediatricians need to counsel their sexually active patients about the consequences of sexual activity, including pregnancy and STDs.
4. Pediatricians may wish to provide basic contraceptive services for their patients in their offices, providing an environment that is conducive to trust and confidentiality, or they may wish to refer their patients to another appropriate site for these services while still maintaining primary care of the adolescent.
5. Pediatricians who wish to provide basic contraceptive services for their patients should update their skills and information about adolescent sexuality and gynecology. This may require specific training.
6. Pediatricians should be aware that it is acceptable to prescribe oral contraceptives up to 3 months before the first pelvic examination.
7. Pediatricians who offer contraceptive services to adolescents should provide appropriate follow-up to ensure compliance. Time needs to be allocated for counseling, education, problem solving, and periodic reassessment of the adolescent's contraceptive needs.

COMMITTEE ON ADOLESCENCE, 1998–1999
Marianne E. Felice, MD, Chairperson
Ronald A. Feinstein, MD
Martin Fisher, MD
David W. Kaplan, MD, MPH
Luis F. Olmedo, MD
Ellen S. Rome, MD, MPH
Barbara C. Staggers, MD

LIAISON REPRESENTATIVES
Paula Hillard, MD
    American College of Obstetricians
    and Gynecologists
Glen Pearson, MD
    American Academy of Child and
    Adolescent Psychiatry
Diane Sacks, MD
    Canadian Paediatric Society

SECTION LIAISON
Samuel Leavitt, MD
    Section on School Health

References

1. American Academy of Pediatrics, Committee on Adolescence. Adolescent pregnancy—current trends and issues: 1998. *Pediatrics.* 1999;103:516–520
2. American Academy of Pediatrics, Committee on Adolescence. Sexually transmitted diseases. *Pediatrics.* 1994;94:568–572
3. American Academy of Pediatrics, Committee on Adolescence. Contraception and adolescents. *Pediatrics.* 1990;86:134–138
4. Boyer CB. Psychosocial, behavioral, and educational factors in preventing sexually transmitted diseases. *Adolesc Med State Art Rev.* 1990;1:597–613
5. Brooks-Gunn J, Furstenburg FF. Adolescent sexual behavior. *Am Psychol.* 1989;10:249–257
6. Jaskiewicz JA, McAnarney ER. Pregnancy during adolescence. *Pediatr Rev.* 1994;15:32–38
7. Allan Guttmacher Institute. *Sex and America's Teenagers.* New York, NY: The Allan Guttmacher Institute; 1994
8. Hollerth S, Hayes C, eds. Contraceptive decision-making among adolescents. In: *Risking the Future: Adolescent Sexuality, Pregnancy, and Childbearing, II.* Washington, DC: National Academy Press; 1987
9. Jaccard J, Dittus PJ, Gordon VV. Maternal correlates of adolescent sexual and contraceptive behavior. *Fam Plann Perspect.* 1996;28:159–165
10. Jaccard J, Dittus P. Parent-Teen Communication. *Toward the Prevention of Unintended Pregnancy.* New York, NY: Springer-Verlag; 1991

11. Smith CA. Factors associated with early sexual activity among urban adolescents. *Soc Work*. 1997;42:334–346

12. Leigh BC, Morrison DM, Trocki K, Temple MT. Sexual behavior in American adolescents: results from a US national survey. *J Adolesc Health*. 1994;15:117–125

13. Goldfarb AF. Adolescent sexuality. *Ann N Y Acad Sci*. 1997;816:395–403

14. Centers for Disease Control and Prevention. Youth risk behavior surveillance—United States, 1995. *MMWR CDC Surveill Summ*. 1996;45:1–84

15. Kann L, Warren CW, Harris WA, et al. Youth risk behavior surveillance—United States, 1993. *MMWR CDC Surveill Summ*. 1995;44:1–56

16. Guttmacher S, Lieberman L, Ward D, Freudenberg M, Radosh A, Jarlais D. Condom availability in New York City schools: relationships to condom use and sexual behavior. *Am J Public Health*. 1997;87:1427–1433

17. Kirby D, Barth RP, Leland N, Fetro JV. Reducing the risk: impact of a new curriculum on sexual risk-taking. *Fam Plann Perspect*. 1991;23:253–263

18. Zabin LS, Hirsch MB, Smith EA, Streett R, Hardy J. Evaluation of a pregnancy prevention program for urban teenagers. *Fam Plann Perspect*. 1986;18:119–126

19. Howard M, Mitchell M. Preventing teenage pregnancy. *Pediatr Ann*. 1993;22:109–111

20. Beach RK. Contraception for adolescents: part 1. *Adolescent Health Update*. 1994;7:1

21. Zelnik M, Shah FK. First intercourse among young Americans. *Fam Plann Perspect*. 1983;15:64–70

22. Zabin LS, Stark HA, Emerson MR. Reasons for delay in contraceptive clinic utilization: adolescent clinic and nonclinic populations compared. *J Adolesc Health*. 1991;12:225–232

23. Leslie-Harwit M, Meheus A. Sexually transmitted disease in young people: the importance of health education. *Sex Trans Dis*. 1989;16:15–20

24. Zabin LS, Kanter JF, Zelnik M. The risk of adolescent pregnancy in the first months of intercourse. *Fam Plann Perspect*. 1979;11:215–222

25. Piccinino L, Mosher W. Trends in contraception in the United States—1982–1985. *Fam Plann Perspect*. 1998;30:4–10,46

26. Centers for Disease Control and Prevention. Sexual behavior among high school students—1990. *MMWR Morbid Mortal Wkly Rep*. 1992;40:885–888

27. Forrest JD, Fordyce RR. US women's contraceptive attitudes and practices: how have they changed in the 1980s? *Fam Plann Perspect*. 1988;20:112–118

28. Sonenstein FL, Pleck JH, Ku LC. Sexual activity, condom use, and AIDS awareness among adolescent males. *Fam Plann Perspect*. 1989;21:152–158

29. American Medical Association, Council on Scientific Affairs. Confidential health services for adolescents. *JAMA*. 1993;269:1420–1424

30. Wildel L, ed. *State Minor Consent Statutes: A Summary*. Cincinnati, OH: Center for Continuing Education in Adolescence; 1995

31. Emans SJH, Lauter MR, Goldstein DP. *Pediatric and Adolescent Gynecology*. ed 4. Boston, MA: Little, Brown and Co; 1998

32. Greydanus DE, Lonchamp D. Contraception in the adolescent: preparation for the 1990s. *Med Clin North Am*. 1990;74:1205–1224

33. Beach RK. Contraception for adolescents: part 2. *Adolescent Health Update*. 1995;7:2

34. Grimes DA, ed. Contraception and adolescents: highlights from the NASPAG conference. *The Contraception Report*. 1995;6(3):4–11

35. Rauh JL. The pediatrician's role in assisting teenagers to avoid the consequences of adolescent pregnancy. *Pediatr Ann*. 1993;22:90–91

36. Kirby D. *No Easy Answers: Research Findings on Programs to Reduce Teen Pregnancy*. Washington, DC: The National Campaign to Prevent Teen Pregnancy; 1999

37. Alan Guttmacher Institute. School-based sexuality education: the issues and challengers. *Fam Plann Perspect*. 1998;30:188–193

38. Hawkins JD, Catalano RF, Kosterman R, Abbott R, Hill KG. Preventing adolescent health risk behaviors by strengthening protection during childhood. *Arch Pediatr Adolesc Med*. 1999;153:226–234

39. Jemmott JB III, Jemmott LS, Fong GT. Abstinence and safer-sex HIV risk-reduction interventions for African American adolescents: a randomized control trial. *JAMA*. 1998;279:1529–1536

40. Kirby D, Korpi M, Barth RP, Cagampang HH. The impact of postponing sexual involvement curriculum among youth in California. *Fam Plann Perspect*. 1997;29:100–108

41. Haignere CS, Gold R, McDaniel HJ. Adolescence abstinence and condom use, are we sure we are really teaching what is safe? *Health Ed Behav*. 1999;26:43–54

42. Hatcher RA, Trussell J, Stewart F, et al. *Contraceptive Technology*. New York, NY: Irvington Publishers, Inc; 1994

43. Hatcher RA. *Contraceptive Technology*. ed 17. New York, NY: Ardent Media, Inc; 1998

44. Greydanus DA. Contraception in adolescence: an overview for the pediatrician. *Pediatr Ann*. 1980;9:111–118

45. Sikand A, Fisher M. The role of barrier contraception in the prevention of pregnancy and disease in adolescents. *Adolesc Med State Art Rev*. 1992;3:223–240

46. Grimes DA, ed. ARHP meeting highlights: the female condom. *The Contraception Report*. 1995;5(6):4–17

47. Trussell J, Sturgen K, Strickler J, Dominik R. Comparative contraception efficacy of the female condom and other barrier methods. *Fam Plann Perspect*. 1994;26:66–72

48. Forrest JD, Singh S. The sexual and reproductive behavior of American women, 1982–1988. *Fam Plann Perspect*. 1990;22:206–214

49. Grace E, Emans SJ, Havens KK, Merola JL, Woods ER. Contraceptive compliance with a triphasic and monophasic norethindrone-containing oral contraceptive pill in a private adolescent practice. *Adolesc Pediatr Gynecol.* 1994;7:29-33

50. ACOG Committee Opinion. *Safety of Oral Contraceptives for Teenagers.* 1991 (No. 90)

51. Grimes DA, ed. Highlights from the 1992 AAFP symposium. *The Contraception Report—Special Edition.* 1993;3(6):4-12

52. Trussell J, Hatcher RA, Cates W Jr, Stewart FH, Kost K. Contraceptive failure in the United States: an update. *Stud Fam Plann.* 1990;21:51-54

53. Jones EF, Forrest JD. Contraceptive failure rates based on the 1988 NSFG. *Fam Plann Perspect.* 1992;24:12-19

54. Blassone ML. Risk of contraceptive discontinuation among adolescents. *J Adolesc Health Care.* 1989; 10:527-533

55. Cromer BA. DEPO-PROVERA—wherefore art thou? *Adolesc Pediatr Gynecol.* 1992;5:155-162

56. Hatcher RA, Stewart F, Kowal D, Grant F, Stewart GK, Cates W. *Contraceptive Technology, 1990-1992.* New York, NY: Irvington Publishers; 1990

57. Rosenthal SL, Biro FM, Kollar LM, Hillard PJ, Rauh JL. Experience with side effects and health risks associated with Norplant implant use in adolescents. *Contraception.* 1995;52:283-285

58. Blumenthal PD, Wilson LE, Remsburg RE, Cullins VE, Huggins GR. Contraceptive outcomes among postpartum and post-abortal adolescents. *Contraception.* 1994;50:451-460

59. Berenson AB, Wiemann CM. Use of levonorgestrel implants versus oral contraceptives in adolescence: a case-control study. *Am J Obstet Gynecol.* 1995;172:1128-1135

60. Polaneckzy M, Slap G, Forke C, Rappaport A, Sondheimer S. The use of levonorgestrel implants (Norplant) for contraception in adolescent mothers. *N Engl J Med.* 1994;331:1201-1206

61. Berenson AP, Wiemann CM. Patient satisfaction and side effects with levonorgestrel implant (Norplant) use in adolescents 18 years of age or younger. *Pediatrics.* 1993;92:257-260

62. Cullins VE, Remsburg RE, Blumenthal PD, Huggins GR. Comparison of adolescent and adult experiences with Norplant levonorgestrel contraceptive implants. *Obstet Gynecol.* 1994;83:1026-1032

63. Levine A, Holmes M, Haselden C, et al. *Norplant Continuation Rates in Adolescents and Adults in a Family Planning Clinic.* Presented at NASPAG Ninth Annual Meeting; April 22-28, 1995; Toronto, Canada

64. Trussel J, Stewart F. The effectiveness of postcoital hormonal contraception. *Fam Plann Perspect.* 1992; 24:262-264

65. Blum RW. Sexual health needs of adolescents with chronic conditions. *Arch Pediatr Adolesc Med.* 1997; 15:290-297

Counseling the Adolescent About Pregnancy Options

Committee on Adolescence

ABSTRACT. When consulted by a pregnant adolescent, pediatricians should be able to make a timely diagnosis and to help the adolescent understand her options and act on her decision to continue or terminate her pregnancy. Pediatricians may not impose their values on the decision-making process and should be prepared to support the adolescent in her decision or refer her to a physician who can.

ABBREVIATIONS. β-hCG, β-subunit human chorionic gonadotropin; hCG, human chorionic gonadotropin.

Pediatricians are likely to encounter adolescent patients who become pregnant and need counseling on the options available to them. The American Academy of Pediatrics continues to endorse the principles published in its statement on this topic in 1989,[1] namely:

1. The statement represents an objective guide for pediatricians assisting patients and their families in making decisions about adolescent pregnancy.

2. None of the options offered is necessarily ideal or universally preferred by physicians or their patients.

3. The pediatrician, the adolescent patient, and other concerned persons must be given complete information on all available options to help the adolescent make an informed decision.

More than 1 million individuals <20 years old become pregnant annually.[2-4] Slightly >50% of adolescent pregnancies result in a birth.[2,4] The basic approach to effective ethical counseling has not changed since the 1989 statement; however, medical, sociological, and technological advances warrant an update of earlier information.

Premarital sex, pregnancy, and abortion engender strong personal and individual feelings. Pediatricians and other health professionals should not allow their personal beliefs and values to interfere with optimal patient health care. The physician needs to respect the adolescent's personal decision and her legal right to continue or to terminate her pregnancy and not impose barriers to health services from another provider. Should a pediatrician choose not to counsel the adolescent patient about sexual matters such as pregnancy and abortion, the patient should be referred to other experienced professionals.

Identification

All pregnancy options benefit from an early diagnosis. Some adolescents will seek medical care with characteristic signs and symptoms of pregnancy or as the result of a positive home pregnancy test. However, pregnancy symptoms may also be vague and nonspecific, particularly in the younger adolescent. The pediatrician cannot always rely on the menstrual and sexual history of the patient to diagnose pregnancy. Psychological denial may exist to such an extent that the adolescent may not consider pregnancy to be the cause of her symptoms, even when it is evident to others.

Laboratory test results for pregnancy are likely to become positive before the appearance of clinical symptoms or signs on physical examination. A serum β-subunit human chorionic gonadotropin (β-hCG) assay may show positive results as early as 1 week after conception. Most pregnancies are diagnosed by monoclonal human chorionic gonadotropin (hCG) urine pregnancy

This statement has been approved by the Council on Child and Adolescent Health.

The recommendations in this statement do not indicate an exclusive course of treatment or serve as a standard of medical care. Variations, taking into account individual circumstances, may be appropriate.

tests, which are rapid, cost-effective, specific to hCG, and almost as sensitive as the serum hCG assays. These urine tests will also demonstrate positive results within 7 to 10 days after conception, before the first missed menstrual period. Office personnel can be educated to perform these tests. When there is clinical suspicion of pregnancy, a negative test result suggests the need to repeat the test in 1 to 2 weeks. The pediatrician should use the negative result of the pregnancy test as an opportunity for further counseling.

The physical diagnosis of a normal intrauterine pregnancy can usually be made by 6 weeks from the last menstrual period with the finding of an enlarged softened uterus during a pelvic examination. The fetal heart tones may be detected as early as 10 weeks' gestation by Doppler fetoscopy. The observation or notice of fetal movement occurs at about 20 weeks in women experiencing their first pregnancy. If questions remain about uterine size or the confirmation of pregnancy, obstetric consultation or ultrasonography should be arranged. Ultrasonography can confirm an intrauterine pregnancy, with cardiac activity demonstrable at approximately 6 weeks from the last menstrual period. Concurrent with pregnancy evaluation, appropriate testing for sexually transmitted diseases should be performed.[4,5] Early first trimester complications include ectopic pregnancy and spontaneous abortion, and these problems should be considered if abdominal pain or vaginal bleeding develops. An ectopic pregnancy should also be considered in a patient with a positive pregnancy test in the absence of expected uterine enlargement.

Communication

While waiting for the results of a urine pregnancy test, the pediatrician has the opportunity to discuss the adolescent's expectations and feelings about her possible pregnancy. The pediatrician should convey the results of the pregnancy test to the adolescent alone in a private setting.

Minors have legal rights protecting their privacy about the diagnosis and treatment of pregnancy. Pediatricians should be familiar with local confidentiality laws being aware that they vary

from state to state. In considering confidentiality, the pediatrician should assess the adolescent's ability to understand the diagnosis of pregnancy and appreciate the implications of that diagnosis. The diagnosis should not be conveyed to others, including parents, until the patient's consent is obtained, except when there are concerns about suicide, homicide, or abuse. The pediatrician should be sensitive to the possibility of sexual abuse or incest in the young or developmentally delayed pregnant adolescent. In those cases, the pediatrician should inform child protective services as required by the law in most jurisdictions.

Reactions to the diagnosis of pregnancy vary. Some adolescents may be pleased, while others may be upset or confused. Some may have already discussed potential options with their family or sexual partner. The pediatrician needs to be sensitive to family, social, and cultural issues that may influence the adolescent and her decisions about pregnancy.[5,6] Adolescents should be encouraged to include their parents in a full discussion of their options. The pediatrician should explain how parental involvement can be helpful and that parents generally are supportive. If parental support is not possible, minors should be urged to seek the advice and counsel of adults in whom they have confidence, including other relatives, counselors, teachers, or clergy. This is especially true for younger adolescents, age 12 to 15 years.

Management

The duration of the pregnancy should be assessed and documented because options depend on this assessment. Usually, the adolescent has the following options available:

1. Carrying her pregnancy to delivery and raising the baby.
2. Carrying her pregnancy to delivery and placing the baby for adoption.
3. Terminating her pregnancy.

The pediatrician should discuss with or counsel the adolescent about all three options or refer the adolescent to a health care professional who will discuss all three options.

Financial status should not deprive a person of her options for management of the pregnancy. The pediatrician should be knowledgeable about local funding resources for continuing or terminating her pregnancy. The patient should be counseled to consider all options, encouraged to return for as many visits as needed, and helped to understand the need to make a timely decision. She should be encouraged to include her parents and the father of the baby in these counseling sessions. If the adolescent is reluctant to reveal the identity of the father, the pediatrician should consider the possibility of sexual abuse, sexual assault, or incest. Pediatricians should be aware of state laws about reporting suspected abuse or statutory rape and take appropriate action.

The pediatrician should address any coexisting medical conditions—chronic medical illness, physical disability, or psychiatric illness—that could affect the decision to continue or terminate the pregnancy. If there is a question of the adolescent's mental competence to make an informed decision about the pregnancy, the pediatrician should be aware of state law and procedures necessary to make this determination.

If the adolescent decides to continue the pregnancy, the pediatrician should refer her for timely and appropriate prenatal care. Adolescents receiving prenatal care in comprehensive adolescent pregnancy programs generally have had better outcomes than adolescents not in such programs, and pediatricians may choose to refer preferentially to such programs, when available.[7] Family and social support systems are essential for optimal outcomes for young adolescent parents and their infants.[8]

Adoption is an important option for the pediatrician to discuss with the adolescent. To make appropriate referrals, the pediatrician should be familiar with the available medical, legal, counseling, and social service resources that facilitate adoption. Throughout the pregnancy, the adolescent should have the opportunity to discuss the possibility of adoption with the pediatrician or other health care professionals.

If the adolescent decides to terminate her pregnancy, the pediatrician should be knowledgeable about community resources, considering the stage of pregnancy and any coexisting medical conditions. The pediatrician should also consider the adolescent's financial resources and should be aware of local or federal law affecting the availability of services, parental notification, or consent.[9] With the anticipated US Food and Drug Administration approval of pharmacologic agents, such as mifepristone, and the availability of prostaglandin analogues and methotrexate to induce abortion nonsurgically, pediatricians need to become aware of the nature and availability of these methods and have a clear understanding of their role in the counseling, provision of care, or referral for these methods.

Whatever the adolescent's decision, the pediatrician should follow up with the patient to ensure that there has been a successful referral and that appropriate social support is in place and to discuss the prevention of future unintended pregnancies. If the adolescent chooses to continue her pregnancy, the pediatrician should remain available for further discussion during the pregnancy should later events require reconsideration of decisions made at the time of the initial confirmation of pregnancy. If the adolescent chooses to place the child for adoption or to terminate her pregnancy, the pediatrician should be available to provide for her subsequent health care and emotional support. In either case, the pediatrician should encourage the adolescent to continue her education and be available to help her identify appropriate community scholastic programs.

The diagnosis of pregnancy is a sensitive and emotional time for the adolescent, her family, and her sexual partner. A warm and accepting environment in which the adolescent feels sufficiently secure to explore her own feelings about pregnancy is essential. Becoming a parent, placing a child for adoption, or having an abortion may have significant personal and long-term consequences for adolescents. It is important to ensure continuing help and support, regardless of the adolescent's decisions about her pregnancy. Ideally, the pediatrician has the counseling expertise, an understanding of adolescent developmental and medical issues, and, often, a longstanding relationship with the patient, and, therefore, is the appropriate person to review these issues with her.

References

1. American Academy of Pediatrics, Committee on Adolescence. Counseling the adolescent about pregnancy options. *Pediatrics*. 1989;83:135–137

2. Alan Guttmacher Institute. *Sex and America's Teenagers.* New York, NY: The Alan Guttmacher Institute; 1994

3. *Facts at a Glance.* Washington, DC: Child Trends Inc; January 1996

4. Alan Guttmacher Institute. *Contraception Counts: State-by-State Information.* New York, NY: The Alan Guttmacher Institute; 1997

5. American Academy of Pediatrics, Committee on Adolescence. Sexually transmitted diseases. *Pediatrics*. 1994;94:568–572

6. Davis BJ, Voegtle KH. *Culturally Competent Health Care for Adolescents: A Guide for Primary Care Providers.* Chicago, IL: American Medical Association; 1994

7. Klerman LV, Horowitz SM. Reducing the adverse consequences of adolescent pregnancy and parenting: the role of service programs. *Adolesc Med State Art Rev.* 1992;3:2:299–316

8. American Academy of Pediatrics, Committee on Adolescence. Care of adolescent parents and their children. *Pediatrics*. 1989;83:138–140

9. American Academy of Pediatrics, Committee on Adolescence. The adolescent's right to confidential care when considering abortion. *Pediatrics*. 1996;97:746–751

Diagnosis and Management of Sexually Transmitted Disease Pathogens Among Adolescents

Gale R. Burstein, MD, MPH,* Pamela J. Murray, MD, MPH†

Objectives

After completing this article, readers should be able to:

1. List the possible clinical presentations and sequelae of *Neisseria gonorrhoeae* and *Chlamydia trachomatis* genital infections in males and females.
2. Describe the various types of licensed *N gonorrhoeae* and *C trachomatis* laboratory tests as well as their advantages and disadvantages.
3. List the Amsel criteria and available laboratory tests for diagnosis of bacterial vaginosis.
4. Describe the various treatments for vulvovaginal candidiasis.
5. Describe patient, partner, and practitioner barriers to implementing effective partner notification.

Introduction

Sexually transmitted diseases (STDs) have been labeled a "hidden epidemic" among adolescents, with adolescent females experiencing some of the highest rates of most STDs. Most adolescent STDs, regardless of pathogen, are asymptomatic. A primary care visit presents the perfect window of opportunity to screen for STDs. Clinical preventive care guidelines, such as the Guidelines for Adolescent Preventive Services (GAPS), Bright Futures, and the American Academy of Pediatrics Recommendations for Preventive Pediatric Health Care, recommend screening adolescents for sexual risk behaviors and offering STD diagnostic tests to all sexually active adolescents. The National Committee for Quality Assurance adopted chlamydia screening of sexually active females ages 15 to 25 years as a new Health Plan Employer Data and Information Set (HEDIS) performance measure for managed care organizations in 2000. New nucleic acid amplification diagnostic technology allows for a widening scope of STD screening without performing an invasive genital examination.

This article reviews the epidemiology and clinical presentation of common curable STDs acquired by adolescents and provides information on new diagnostic technologies and treatments for these STDs. Screening and treating STDs can be offered readily as part of routine adolescent health services.

Chlamydia and Gonorrhea Infection

EPIDEMIOLOGY

Chlamydia trachomatis and *Neisseria gonorrhoeae* are the sexually transmitted genital pathogens reported most commonly among adolescents. Both infections frequently are asymptomatic in males and females. A large multisite, randomized, controlled trial found that 62% of chlamydial infections in both males and females and 28% of male and 51% of female gonorrheal infections were asymptomatic. Most sexually active adolescents are unaware of their risk for these infections. Typically, chlamydial infections in adolescents are diagnosed by screening asymptomatic females. Adolescent males are not screened routinely for STDs. Undetected and, therefore, untreated chlamydial infections among

*Centers for Disease Control and Prevention, Atlanta, GA.

†Children's Hospital, Pittsburgh, PA.

The authors gratefully acknowledge Dr. Kimberly Workowski for her manuscript review.

Use of trademark names is for identification purposes only and does not constitute endorsement by the federal government.

Pediatrics in Review, *Vol 24, No. 3, March 2003*

males contribute to the high rates of infection among adolescent females.

Although often asymptomatic, chlamydial and gonorrheal infections can present as various STD syndromes, depending on the site of infection. Both males and females may develop urethritis, proctitis, or pharyngitis. Females may develop cervicitis. Neither infection causes vaginitis.

Sequelae of uncomplicated gonorrheal and chlamydial infection can be devastating for females. Infection can ascend into the pelvis, causing pelvic inflammatory disease (PID). Many PID cases are "silent," with no symptoms or atypical symptoms that are not perceived as infection. Females who have a history of PID are at high risk for an ectopic pregnancy, chronic pelvic pain, and tubal factor infertility. Chlamydial screening and treatment of adolescent females reduces the incidence of PID.

Sequelae of chlamydial and gonorrheal infections are rare among males. The incidence of epidydimitis among males is much lower than the prevalence of PID among females. Evidence for a causal association between chlamydial and gonorrheal urethritis and male infertility is lacking.

Although uncommon, both males and females are at risk for developing disseminated gonococcal infection and reactive arthritis (Reiter syndrome). Exudative STDs, such as chlamydia and gonorrhea, may facilitate human immunodeficiency virus (HIV) transmission and infection.

DIAGNOSIS

Nucleic acid amplification tests (NAATs) are a new class of highly sensitive and specific diagnostic tests for C trachomatis and N gonorrhoeae infections. Four NAATs are licensed for both gonorrhea and Chlamydia testing, and some only require a single specimen for both tests (Table 1). These tests can detect as few as 10 strands of chlamydial DNA or RNA in a specimen by replicating strands up to 10 million-fold. Advantages over older methods of testing include superior sensitivity, ability to test urine specimens, and practical convenience (Tables 2 and 3). NAATs have made chlamydia and gonorrhea testing more acceptable for asymptomatic patients by eliminating the need for an invasive genital examination.

Symptomatic adolescents, especially females, also require a full genital examination to evaluate for PID and other infections that cause vaginal or urethral discharge (eg, trichomoniasis, bacterial vaginosis, and vulvovaginal candidiasis).

MANAGEMENT

Uncomplicated genital chlamydial and gonorrheal infections can be treated with a single dose of cefixime*, ciprofloxacin, ceftriaxone, ofloxacin, or levofloxacin (Table 4). Because adolescents infected with N gonorrhoeae often are coinfected with C trachomatis, the Centers for Disease Control and Prevention (CDC) recommend

Table 1. Licensed Amplification Tests for *Chlamydia trachomatis* and *Neisseria gonorrhoeae*

Test	Manufacturer	Specimen	Clinical Utility
Polymerase Chain Reaction	Roche Molecular System (Branchburg, NJ)	Cervical, urethral, first-void urine	N gonorrhoeae,* C trachomatis, combination N gonorrhoeae and C trachomatis
Ligase Chain Reaction[†]	Abbott Laboratories (Abbott Park, IL)	Cervical, urethral, first-void urine	N gonorrhoeae, C trachomatis, combination N gonorrhoeae and C trachomatis
Transcription-Mediated Amplification	Gen-Probe (San Diego, CA)	Cervical, urethral, first-void urine	C trachomatis, combination N gonorrhoeae and C trachomatis
Strand Displacement Amplification	Becton Dickinson (Sparks, MD)	Cervical, urethral, first-void urine	N gonorrhoeae, C trachomatis, combination N gonorrhoeae and C trachomatis
Hybrid Capture II System	Digene (Beltsville, MD)	Cervical	N gonorrhoeae, C trachomatis, combination N gonorrhoeae and C trachomatis

*Polymerase chain reaction is not approved for N gonorrhoeae testing with female urine or asymptomatic male urethral swabs.

[†]Abbott Laboratories will discontinue this product June 30, 2003.

*In July 2002, Wyeth Pharmaceuticals (Collegeville, PA) discontinued manufacturing cefixime in the United States. No other pharmaceutical company manufactures or sells cefixime tablets in the United States.

Table 2. Advantages and Disadvantages of Specific Laboratory Tests for *Chlamydia trachomatis*

Test	Advantages	Disadvantages
Culture	Specificity nearly 100%	Expensive Technically demanding Time-consuming Labor-intensive Sensitivity of about 80% Requires cervical or urethral specimens
EIA	Inexpensive Technically straightforward	Sensitivity of about 60% Requires cervical or urethral specimens
DNA Probe	Inexpensive Easier transport	Sensitivity of about 65% Requires cervical or urethral specimens
Nucleic Acid Amplification	Sensitivity of 85% Specificity of 97% to 99% Can perform on urine specimens	Expensive

Table 3. Advantages and Disadvantages of Specific Laboratory Tests for *Neisseria gonorrhoeae*

Test	Advantages	Disadvantages
Culture	Sensitivity of approximately 85% Specificity of nearly 100% Inexpensive Low labor demands Technically straightforward Rectal specimens Can determine antimicrobial susceptibility	Transport in CO_2 medium Requires cervical or urethral specimens
DNA Probe	Sensitivity of about 85% Inexpensive Easy transport	Requires cervical or urethral specimens
Gram Stain	Inexpensive Easy transport Rectal specimens Sensitivity of 85% for urethral specimens	Requires cervical or urethral specimens Sensitivity of 55% for cervical specimens
Nucleic Acid Amplification	Sensitivity of 80% to 90% Specificity of 97% to 99% Can be performed on urine specimens	Expensive

Table 4. The Centers for Disease Control and Prevention Recommended Treatment for Uncomplicated Genital *Chlamydia trachomatis* and *Neisseria gonorrhoeae* Infections*

Pathogen	Treatment
C trachomatis	Azithromycin 1 g orally in a single dose OR Doxycycline 100 mg orally twice daily for 7 days
N gonorrhoeae	Cefixime[†] 400 mg orally in a single dose OR Ciprofloxacin 500 mg orally in a single dose OR Ofloxacin 400 mg orally in a single dose OR Levofloxacin 250 mg orally in a single dose OR Ceftriaxone 125 mg IM in a single dose AND Treatment for C trachomatis[††]

*Adapted from the Centers for Disease Control and Prevention. 2002 guidelines for treatment of sexually transmitted disease. *Morbid Mortal Weekly Rep MMWR.* 2002;51(No. RR-6):32–42.

[†]In July 2002, Wyeth Pharmaceuticals (Collegeville, PA) discontinued manufacturing cefixime in the United States. No other pharmaceutical company manufactures or sells cefixime tablets in the United States.

[††]The Centers for Disease Control and Prevention recommends treating persons who have a positive gonorrhea test result for both gonorrhea and chlamydial infection unless a negative result has been obtained with a sensitive nucleic acid amplification chlamydia test.

treating persons who have a positive gonorrhea test result for both gonorrheal and chlamydial infection unless a negative result has been obtained with a sensitive chlamydia test. Abstinence should be recommended for at least 7 days after initiation of therapy for both infected patients and their sex partners to decrease the risk of reinfection.

Although once considered an infection responsive to a wide spectrum of antibiotics, treatments for gonorrhea now are limited. In response to the progressive rise in *N gonorrhoeae* resistance to penicillin and tetracycline caused by plasmid-producing beta-lactamase and other antibiotic-resistant mediators, the CDC advises against use of these antibiotic classes for treatment of gonorrhea infection. Although it is an effective treatment for *C trachomatis* infection, a single 1-g azithromycin dose is associated with suboptimal gonorrhea cure rates. A single 2-g dose provides adequate therapy, but a high frequency of gastrointestinal adverse effects and high cost prohibit its practical use. Accordingly, single-dose azithromycin should not be used as monotherapy for both gonorrheal and chlamydial genital infection.

Fluoroquinolones have not been recommended for persons younger than 18 years of age because they damage articular cartilage in juvenile animal models. However, no joint damage attributable to therapy has been observed among children treated with flouroquinolones. Currently, quinolones should not be used to treat gonorrheal infections acquired in Asia, the Pacific, California, or Hawaii, due to documented resistance in those areas.

FOLLOW-UP

A "test of cure" is not recommended routinely following treatment of adolescent gonorrheal or chlamydial infection. However, clinicians should advise all females to be rescreened 3 to 4 months after treatment. Some experts recommend chlamydial testing for all females every 6 months because the risk of infection is high.

Bacterial Vaginosis

EPIDEMIOLOGY

Bacterial vaginosis (BV) is a sexually associated noninflammatory disturbance of the normal vaginal ecosystem. It is characterized by an overgrowth of several anaerobic bacterial species usually found in the vagina, including *Mobiluncus* sp, *Prevotella* sp, *Gardnerella vaginalis,* and *Mycoplasma hominis,* and a decrease in H_2O_2-producing *Lactobacillus* sp. It occurs more frequently among sexually active than sexually inexperienced females. BV is not an infection and is not accompanied by local vaginal inflammation visible on clinical examination or by microscopy. However, it has been associated with an increase in preterm labor, perinatal morbidity, PID, and risk of HIV infection, suggesting that BV may play an important role in several major women's reproductive health problems.

DIAGNOSIS

BV is diagnosed by the presence of a gray-white, homogenous, nonviscous vaginal discharge. It is not associated with the usual signs or symptoms of inflammation (eg, itching, abdominal pain, or dysuria). BV is diagnosed clinically by the presence of at least three of the four criteria listed in Table 5.

New commercial tests are available for the diagnosis of BV. These tests can be used to document pH, a positive "whiff" test, and microscopy. The FemExam® pH and Amines Test Card™

Table 5. Amsel Criteria for Diagnosis of Bacterial Vaginosis

- Vaginal discharge: thin, homogenous, white, uniformly adherent
- Vaginal pH >4.5
- Positive "whiff" test: fishy odor after mixing discharge with 10% KOH
- >20% "clue" cells on microscopic examination: bacteria-coated squamous epithelial cells in which both the periphery (cell membrane) and cytoplasm have a granular, irregular "moth-eaten" appearance

(Quidel® Corp, San Diego, CA) can detect an elevated vaginal pH and the presence of trimethylamine. The FemExam® PIP Activity Test Card™ (Quidel® Corp, San Diego, CA) can identify an enzyme expressed by *G vaginalis*. The Affirm VP III Microbial Identification Test® (Becton Dickinson, Sparks, MD) is a DNA probe for the etiologic diagnosis of vaginitis: BV, candidiasis, and trichomoniasis. Correlation with clinical symptoms and elevated vaginal pH is recommended with this test. Ordinary cultures are neither recommended nor clinically helpful in diagnosing BV.

MANAGEMENT

The goal of treatment is to decrease symptoms and signs and to eliminate excess reproductive risks. Treatment is recommended for symptomatic nonpregnant and all pregnant patients. Options for treatment include oral and vaginal regimens (Table 6). Abstinence from alcohol during treatment with metronidazole and for 24 hours afterward should be stressed because of the disulfiramlike effect of that drug. Clindamycin cream and ovules are oil-based and should not be used by women who use latex barrier contraceptives, such as condoms and diaphragms.

The same treatments are used in HIV-positive individuals. Follow-up and tests of cure are not indicated for nonpregnant patients. No treatment of partners is indicated. Possible future developments include prevention or treatment of BV by restoration of vaginal ecology with H_2O_2-producing lactobacilli in vaginal suppositories.

Trichomoniasis

EPIDEMIOLOGY

Trichomoniasis is a sexually transmitted infection of squamous epithelial tissues that is caused by a pathogenic, flagellated, single-celled, parasitic protozoan, *Trichomonas vaginalis*. It causes an impressive inflammatory response in females and infects the urethra, exocervix, and periurethral glands as well as the vagina.

Trichomoniasis classically presents in a postpubertal female with an irritating, profuse, yellow-green vaginal discharge accompanied by vulvovaginal itching and discomfort. Pelvic

Table 6. Recommended Bacterial Vaginosis Treatment Regimens*

Nonpregnant Females
- Metronidazole 500 mg orally twice daily for 7 days
  OR
- Metronidazole gel, 0.75%, one full applicator (5 g) intravaginally once a day for 5 days
  OR
- Clindamycin cream, 2%, one full applicator (5 g) intravaginally once a day for 5 days

Pregnant Females
- Metronidazole 250 mg orally three times daily for 7 days
  OR
- Clindamycin 300 mg orally twice daily for 7 days
  OR
- Clindamycin ovules 100 g intravaginally at bedtime for 3 days

*Adapted from the Centers for Disease Control and Prevention. 2002 guidelines for treatment of sexually transmitted diseases. *Morbid Mortal Weekly Rep MMWR.* 2002;51(No RR-6):42–44

discomfort occurs in about 15% of infected individuals. Trichomoniasis may cause vaginitis, urethritis, and cervicitis and, thus, may present with abnormal vaginal or postcoital bleeding or dysuria. Skene and Bartholin glands also may harbor infection. The vulva may be edematous, excoriated, and erythematous. Discharge often is visible at the introitus. Similarly, the vagina may appear red and inflamed. The cervix may be red and swollen, with punctate hemorrhagic ulcerations looking like a "strawberry," a finding that is highly specific for trichomoniasis and can be seen with a colposcope in 50% of infected females. In males, trichomoniasis usually is asymptomatic, with fewer organisms and less inflammation. However, it is increasingly recognized and identified as a cause of urethritis that is not responsive to the usual antibiotic regimens for nonspecific urethritis.

DIAGNOSIS

Trichomoniasis is diagnosed by microscopic visualization of the organism on a wet preparation that is identified by the characteristic erratic twirling motion caused by the flagellae. Phase-contrast microscopy is helpful, but at best, microscopy is 50% to 70% sensitive. Staining does not improve the detection rate. The vaginal pH usually is high (pH ≥6.0). The inflammatory response may be so overwhelming that large numbers of white blood cells (WBCs) surround and obscure the trichomonads. In this case, dilution of the saline preparation with nonbacteriostatic saline and warming of the solution to body temperature may improve identification of motile organisms.

More sensitive diagnostic alternatives include laboratory culture with Diamond modified media, which establishes the "gold standard" for identification. InPouch TV Culture® (BioMed Diagnostics, San Jose, CA) is a United States Food and Drug Administration (FDA)-approved self-contained culture medium-filled bag that can be inoculated and incubated with a vaginal fluid specimen from females or a first-void urine specimen from males in the office and viewed under the microscope for up to 5 subsequent days. The Affirm VP III Microbial Identification Test® (Becton Dickinson, Sparks, MD) also tests for trichomoniasis. A positive test may be obtained with at least $5 \infty 10^3$ trichomonads. For men, the maximum yield from cultures may combine specimens from the urethra and spun urine. Reports of trichomonads on Papanicolaou smears have high false-positive and false-negative rates that preclude their use for diagnosis.

MANAGEMENT

Trichomoniasis is treated easily in about 85% to 95% of infected patients with a single 2-g dose of metronidazole accompanied by concurrent partner treatment with the same regimen regardless of the partner's clinical picture. To avoid reinfection, abstinence is recommended until both partners have taken their medication and are asymptomatic. Abstinence from alcohol for 24 hours should be stressed because of the disulfiramlike effect of metronidazole. Topical treatments are not effective because the anatomic extent of the infection in many individuals includes the urethra and periurethral glands. Nonresponders should be retreated with a 7-day course of 500 mg metronidazole twice daily. If this regimen fails, an alternative is 2 g metronidazole daily for 3 to 5 days. However, nonadherence to partner treatment or abstinence always

should be explored because these behaviors commonly cause reinfections. For patients who have laboratory-documented infection, do not respond to the 3- to 5-day treatment regimen, and in whom reinfection has been excluded, determination of *T vaginalis* susceptibility and consultation with an expert should be sought. (Consultation is available from the CDC at 404-639-8363.)

HIV-infected individuals should receive the same regimens. Metronidazole treatment is complicated by an unpleasant metallic taste and nausea in approximately 10% of patients taking the single-dose regimen. Because no teratogenic effects have been demonstrated, treatment with a single 2-g metronidazole dose is recommended during pregnancy.

Candida Vulvovaginitis

EPIDEMIOLOGY

Candidiasis or yeast vaginitis is an infection that develops in the estrogenized, low pH, vaginal environment. It is not transmitted sexually and rarely is acquired from a colonized partner.

Candidiasis presents commonly with acute vulval pruritis and vaginal discharge of varying character and consistency. Other signs and symptoms include "external" dysuria, vaginal soreness and irritation, vulvar burning, and painful intercourse. The physical examination may demonstrate redness and swelling of the vagina and vulva. Sometimes, papular satellite lesions are apparent. Symptoms often escalate before the menses. Only some patients have a classic vaginal thrush, characterized by clumps of adherent thick white discharge. Local adenopathy may be present. Self-diagnosis based on vaginal complaints has been shown to be unreliable in many studies.

DIAGNOSIS

Microscopic evaluation of vaginal discharge may support the diagnosis of candidiasis, but simultaneous evaluation for other causes of vaginal discharge is necessary. Vaginal pH usually is normal (4 to 4.5), germinated yeast (pseudohyphae) can be identified in the saline or KOH preparations, and a modest increase in WBCs may be noted. Large numbers of WBCs suggest other causes or concomitant infection. Yeast and pseudohyphae may be seen under low or high power, but direct microscopy may miss as many as 50% of infections. Rapid tests are probably no better than microscopy and are more expensive. After microbiologic cure, 20% to 25% of women are reinfected with the same strain 30 days posttreatment.

MANAGEMENT

Candidiasis is treated with many topical azole preparations that have as their active agent clotrimazole, miconazole, butoconazole, terconazole, or tioconazole. Most regimens result in clinical and microbiologic cure rates of 80% to 90%. Oral fluconazole in a 150-mg single dose is as effective as the topical treatments. Local relief may be delayed with oral treatments. Local irritation may occur from the topical agents, although this complaint may be difficult to differentiate from the disease. Effective over-the-counter vaginal agents are available, and "azoles" are more effective than nystatin. Topical antifungal preparations may weaken latex barrier contraceptives, such as condoms and diaphragms. Single-dose treatments are prepared in vehicles that keep the antifungal agent active in the vagina for several days, but they may be less effective in the treatment of recurrent infections. All topical azoles can be used in pregnancy. A longer duration of treatment (10 to 14 d) may be needed in pregnancy and for severe and recurrent infections. Treatment of acute vulvovaginal candidiasis in the HIV-positive patient employs the same recommended treatment regimens.

Partner Notification

Sexual partners of adolescents infected with chlamydia, gonorrhea, or trichomoniasis must be notified and treated; otherwise, the patient is likely to become reinfected. Partners are usually asymptomatic and unlikely to seek screening and treatment without notification. Because many health departments do not have resources to support partner notification (PN) services, the responsibility often falls on the clinician and patient.

Various clinician PN strategies have varying success rates and challenges. Patients directly advising their partners to be evaluated and treated for an STD has some advantages, although both patient and partner barriers often render this an ineffective strategy. Patient barriers include poor self-efficacy, denial, and fear of partner violence. Partner barriers to evaluation and treatment include their health-seeking behaviors and clinicians failing to offer partner treatment. Scheduling the partner to be seen in the practitioner's clinic is one option, but reimbursement issues, especially in a managed care setting, present a challenge. Some advocate providing patients with prescriptions for their partners to fill. However, in some states, prescribing medications to patients never examined can result in legal sanctions. Low-cost clinical settings, such as STD clinics, offer options for STD care of sex partners. Although family planning and Planned Parenthood® clinics traditionally have limited their services to only females, some have begun offering clinical services for male partners of infected females.

Despite the challenges, treating asymptomatic partners who otherwise would never receive treatment reduces the risk of reinfection for the patient. Pediatricians can significantly contribute to STD control in their communities by ensuring PN and treatment.

Conclusion

Fifty percent of United States high school students are sexually experienced. The simple question, "Have you ever had sexual intercourse?" can identify many of the adolescent patients in need of reproductive health services. Assumptions of sexual activity status among adolescent patients could result in devastating sequelae from untreated STDs. Technology has simplified the procedures for STD diagnosis and treatment. Pediatricians have the opportunity to maintain good reproductive health and prevent chronic disease for their patients by providing these services at the adolescent preventive care visit. Suggested resources for patients and clinicians are listed in Table 7.

Table 7. Resources*

Health Care Clinician Information

- Centers for Disease Control and Prevention, Division of STD Prevention
  - http://www.cdc.gov/nchstp/dstd/dstdp.html
- Holmes KK, Sparling PF, March PA, et al, eds. *Sexually Transmitted Diseases.* 3rd ed. New York, NY: McGraw Hill; 1999
- Neinstein LS, ed. *Adolescent Health Care.* 5th ed. Baltimore, Md: Williams & Wilkins; 2002

Patient Information

- American Social Health Association (ASHA) for patient information brochures, STD and AIDS Hotline telephone number, and online STD and HIV information
- 800-783-9877
- http://www.ashastd.org

Adolescent-appropriate STD Information Web Sites

- http://www.iwannaknow.org
- http://www.itsyoursexlife.com
- http://www.teenwire.com
- http://www.kidshealth.org

*The authors and publishers take no responsibility for the content of the Web sites mentioned in this article. These sites are recommended on the basis of their content at time of manuscript preparation. This list of sites is not inclusive.

Suggested Reading

American Academy of Pediatrics, Committee on Practice and Ambulatory Medicine. Recommendations for preventive pediatric health care. *Pediatrics.* 2000;105:pullout

Burstein GR, Gaydos CA, Diener-West M, Howell MR, Zenilman JM, Quinn TC. Incident. *C. trachomatis* infections among inner city adolescent females. *JAMA.* 1998;280: 521–526

Centers for Disease Control and Prevention. 2001 guidelines for treatment of sexually transmitted diseases. *Morbid Mortal Wkly Rep MMWR.* 2002;51(No. RR-6):1–80

Elster A, Kuznets N. *AMA Guidelines for Adolescent Preventive Services (GAPS): Recommendations and Rationale.* Baltimore, Md: Williams & Wilkins; 1994

Eng TR, Butler WT, eds. *The Hidden Epidemic: Confronting Sexually Transmitted Diseases.* Washington, DC: National Academy Press; 1997

Green M, ed. *Bright Futures: Guidelines For Health Supervision of Infants, Children, and Adolescents.* Arlington, Va: National Center for Education in Maternal and Child Health; 1994: 195–258

Kamb ML, Newman D, Peterman TA, et al. Most bacterial STDs are asymptomatic. Presented at Sexually Transmitted Infections at the Millennium Conference, Baltimore, Md; May 3–7, 2000

Kann L, Kinchen SA, Williams BI, et al. Youth risk behavior surveillance — United States, 1999. *Morbid Mortal Weekly Rep MMWR.* 2000;49(SS05):19

Scholes D, Stergachis A, Heidrich FE, Andrilla H, Holmes KK, Stamm WE. Prevention of pelvic inflammatory disease by screening for cervical chlamydial infection. *N Engl J Med.* 1996;334:1362–1366

Dysfunctional Uterine Bleeding

Mary E. Rimsza, MD*

Objectives

After completing this article, readers should be able to:

1. Identify the primary cause of dysfunctional uterine bleeding (DUB).
2. Characterize the management of DUB.
3. Explain how coagulation disorders can cause menorrhagia.
4. Describe methods of reducing menstrual blood loss.
5. Delineate the most common ovarian cause of DUB.

Introduction

The normal menstrual cycle is defined as having a mean interval of 28±7 days, with a mean duration of 4±3 days. The amount of blood loss averages 30 mL per cycle but may be as high as 80 mL. Although abnormal endometrial bleeding occurs in women of all ages, it is particularly common in adolescence. Dysfunctional uterine bleeding (DUB) is defined as abnormal endometrial bleeding in the absence of pelvic pathology. Approximately 95% of the abnormal endometrial bleeding in adolescence is DUB due to anovulation. Patterns of abnormal endometrial bleeding include menorrhagia (prolonged bleeding occurring at regular intervals), metrorrhagia (uterine bleeding occurring at irregular intervals), and menometrorrhagia (uterine bleeding that is prolonged, excessive, and occurring at irregular intervals).

Epidemiology

DUB is most common during the first 2 years after menarche, when approximately 55% to 82% of menstrual cycles are anovulatory. Even after 5 years of menstruation, 20% of cycles remain anovulatory. The earlier the onset of menarche, the shorter the duration of anovulatory cycles. If menarche occurs before 12 years of age, 50% of cycles are ovulatory after 1 year, whereas if menarche occurs after 13 years of age, it may be 4.5 years until 50% of cycles are ovulatory. In the United States, the mean age of menarche is 12.88 years for Caucasian and 12.16 years for African-American girls. Approximately 90% of adolescents reach menarche by the time their breast and pubic hair development has reached sexual maturity rating (SMR) stage 4. Thelarche (onset of breast development) usually occurs 2 years before menarche.

Normal Menstrual Cycle

Ovulation leads to normal repetitive menstrual bleeding. The first phase of the ovulatory menstrual cycle is the follicular phase during which pulsatile release of gonadotropin-releasing hormone (GnRH) from the hypothalamus stimulates the pituitary gland to secrete luteinizing hormone (LH) and follicle-stimulating hormone (FSH), which stimulates ovarian follicular growth (Fig. 1). The growing follicle predominantly secretes estrogen, which induces proliferation of the endometrium. The second phase of the menstrual cycle is the ovulatory phase. In this phase, the pituitary gland releases increased amounts of LH, and ovulation occurs within 12 hours of this midcycle surge in LH.

The third phase of the ovulatory cycle is the luteal phase, which follows ovulation. In this phase, the corpus luteum that is formed by luteinization of the follicular cells begins

*Director of Health, Arizona State University, Professor of Pediatrics, Mayo Graduate School of Medicine and University of Arizona College of Medicine, Tempe, AZ.

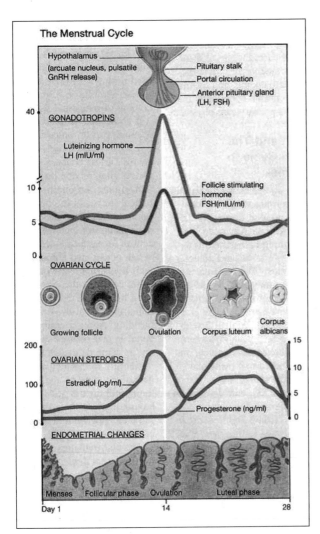

Figure 1. The ovulatory menstrual cycle.

producing progesterone, which counteracts the effects of estrogen on the endometrium. Progesterone inhibits proliferation of the endometrium and produces glandular changes that make the endometrium receptive to implantation by a fertilized ovum. Without fertilization and the production of human chorionic gonadotropin, the corpus luteum cannot survive. As the corpus luteum regresses, estrogen and progesterone levels fall, triggering the synchronous sloughing of the endometrial lining (menstruation) approximately 14 days after ovulation.

Anovulatory Menstrual Cycle

When anovulatory cycles occur, the endometrium experiences continued estrogen stimulation that is unopposed by progesterone. Growth of the vascular and glandular elements of the endometrium

that are stimulated by estrogen are not accompanied by the stromal support that usually is provided by progesterone. For most adolescents who are anovulatory, increasing levels of estrogen cause a negative feedback on the hypothalamic-pituitary axis. This feedback causes a decrease in estrogen levels, which results in endometrial bleeding that mimics an ovulatory cycle. Adolescents who develop DUB seem to have impairments in this negative feedback system. Thus, increasing levels of estrogen do not cause a decrease in FSH secretion with subsequent suppression of estrogen secretion. In these girls, many different follicles are stimulated, none becomes dominant, and progesterone levels remain low. The endometrium becomes excessively thickened and unstable. Eventually, the endometrial lining begins to break down asynchronously and irregularly. Thus, endometrial bleeding in the absence of ovulation becomes prolonged, irregular, and sometimes profuse. The more prolonged an adolescent's anovulation, the greater the risk for DUB because even an occasional ovulatory cycle stabilizes and coordinates sloughing of the endometrium.

Although immaturity of the hypothalamic-pituitary-ovarian axis is the most common cause of anovulation in adolescence, there are many other causes. Almost any systemic illness, especially if the illness is prolonged or associated with excessive weight loss, can cause anovulation. For example, poorly controlled diabetes mellitus, inflammatory bowel disease, and cystic fibrosis are associated with anovulation. Poor nutritional status as well as emotional distress can cause anovulation. Girls who have anorexia nervosa frequently have anovulatory cycles due to both of these factors. In contrast, bulimia generally is not associated with menstrual irregularities, perhaps because the bulimic adolescent usually maintains a normal weight. It is hypothesized that 17% total body fat is needed to initiate menses and that 22% total body fat is needed for regular ovulatory cycles. Aromatization of androgen precursors in fat provides another source of estrogen; it is theorized that this additional estrogen is necessary for hypothalamic pituitary regulation and the onset and maintenance of vaginal bleeding. If this hypothesis is correct, any medical or psychological disorder that results in a decrease in total body fat potentially can cause anovulation. Thus, it is important to obtain both a dietary and weight history in the evaluation of the adolescent who has DUB.

Other causes of anovulation include endocrine disorders and primary ovarian dysfunction. The most common endocrine disorder associated with anovulation and DUB is hypothyroidism. In a recent study, approximately 25% of women who had hypothyroidism had DUB. Hyperprolactinemia due to a pituitary tumor also is a rare cause of anovulation. Adrenal causes of anovulation include Cushing syndrome (Fig. 2), Addison disease, and congenital adrenal hyperplasia (Fig. 3).

The most common primary ovarian cause of anovulation is polycystic ovarian syndrome (PCOS), which affects 5% to 10% of women. PCOS is associated with irregular menses, usually from the time of menarche, and physical signs

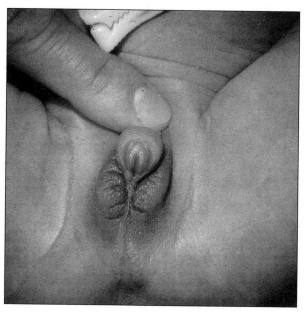

Figure 3. Clitoromegaly in a child who has congenital adrenal hyperplasia.

of hyperandrogenism. The classic findings on ultrasonography are multiple 2 to 8 mm follicles arranged in a peripheral pattern and associated with increased stroma relative to follicles ("string of pearls"). However, many adolescents have normal-appearing ovaries on ultrasonography because the prevalence of "polycystic ovaries" increases with increasing gynecologic age (years since menarche). Small follicular cysts are consistent with the diagnosis of PCOS, but they are nonspecific findings because other conditions that cause anovulation also may be associated with multiple ovarian cysts. Indeed, young adolescents who are anovulatory due to immature hypothalamic-pituitary-ovarian axis often have multiple ovarian cysts on ultrasonography due to continued FSH secretion. Signs of hyperandrogenism in the adolescent who has PCOS include hirsutism, acne (Fig. 4), and rarely clitoromegaly. Obesity occurs in 50% of patients and often is associated with other metabolic abnormalities, including insulin resistance, glucose intolerance, and lipid abnormalities. On physical examination, acanthosis nigrans, a thickening and increased pigmentation of the skin, frequently is noted on the nape of the neck, axilla, and intertriginous areas (Fig. 5).

Anovulatory menstrual cycles usually are painless. Thus, questioning the adolescent about

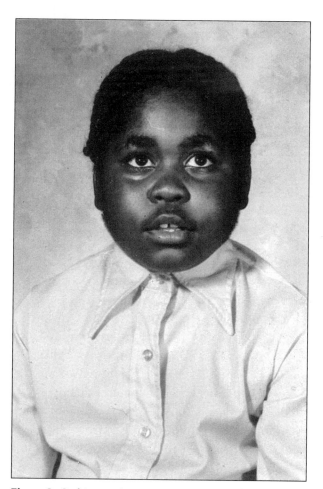

Figure 2. Cushing syndrome.

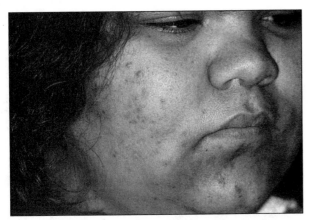

Figure 4. Facial acne in an adolescent who has polycystic ovarian syndrome.

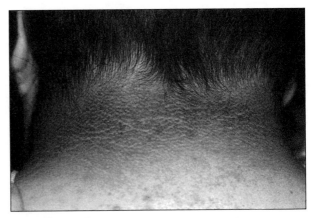

Figure 5. Acanthosis nigrans.

symptoms of dysmenorrhea can help the physician determine the cause of abnormal endometrial bleeding. In adolescence, the most common causes of painful uterine bleeding are primary dysmenorrhea, pregnancy complications (eg, ectopic pregnancy, missed abortion), and infection (eg, endometritis, pelvic inflammatory disease). Other less common causes include trauma and gynecologic tumors.

Abnormal uterine bleeding sometimes is the initial presentation of a blood dyscrasia. Indeed, in one study of adolescent females, 20% of the girls who had menorrhagia were found to have a blood dyscrasia. These disorders are most likely to present as regular but heavy menses. An underlying coagulation disorder should be considered especially if menorrhagia is severe or presents at the time of menarche. In one study of young adolescent Canadian girls, 25% of adolescents who had hemoglobin measurements less than 10 g/dL (100 g/L) and 50% of adolescents who presented with menorrhagia at menarche were found to have a coagulation disorder. Because platelets and fibrin are directly involved in the hemostasis achieved in a bleeding menstrual endometrium, thrombocytopenia and disorders associated with platelet dysfunction (eg, platelet storage pool diseases, von Willebrand disease) are some of the most common blood dyscrasias associated with menorrhagia.

Evaluation

The evaluation of the adolescent who has abnormal endometrial bleeding should begin with a detailed menstrual history, including age of menarche, frequency and amount of menstruation, and character and duration of flow. If the menstrual pattern has changed, it is important to ask about other events that may have coincided with the change, including weight change, family or personal stress, and illness. One should also seek a history of unusual nonmenstrual bleeding, including easy bruisability or prolonged bleeding after minor cuts or dental surgery. A sexual history is critical because the differential diagnosis of abnormal bleeding in the sexually active girl includes sexually transmitted diseases (eg, pelvic inflammatory disease) and gestational events (eg, ectopic pregnancy, missed abortion). A comprehensive general medical history and review of systems also is important because many chronic illnesses are associated with anovulation. Pertinent aspects of the family history include bleeding disorders, infertility, menstrual disorders, and thyroid disease.

The physical examination should begin with vital signs. Postural changes in heart rate and blood pressure may provide objective evidence of hypovolemia. The complete physical examination should focus particular attention on evidence of nongenital bleeding, thyroid examination, and signs of PCOS (eg, hirsutism, acne, obesity, acanthosis nigrans). The breast examination is important not only to assess sexual maturity, but to determine if galactorrhea is present.

Funduscopic examination and visual field testing may provide evidence of a pituitary lesion. An abdominal examination may reveal an ovarian or uterine mass.

An external genital examination always is indicated. Sexual maturity rating, clitoral size, and hymenal characteristics should be assessed. An internal genital examination is mandatory if the adolescent is sexually active or has painful bleeding. The goals of the internal bimanual genital examination are assessment of adnexal and uterine size; determination of abdominal, ovarian, or cervical motion tenderness; and presence of any lower abdominal or pelvic mass. A speculum examination also allows assessment of the vagina and cervix. A bluish coloration of the cervix may be a sign of early pregnancy, and a widened cervical os in association with active endometrial bleeding may indicate a spontaneous abortion. The amount and character of the bleeding should be noted. The presence of large clots may suggest a spontaneous abortion, but this also can occur with severe primary dysmenorrhea. In the sexually active adolescent, cervical swabs should be obtained for determining the presence of *Neisseria gonorrhoeae* and *Chlamydia trachomatis*. A Papanicolau smear should be obtained if there is no active bleeding at the time of the examination. If there is active bleeding, it is best to defer the Papanicolau test until the bleeding has stopped. It usually is possible to perform an internal bimanual examination in a virginal adolescent, but a speculum examination may be more difficult. In some situations, a rectal examination may be helpful in assessing uterine size. Pelvic ultrasonography can aid in the assessment of the virginal adolescent when the bimanual examination is not possible.

Laboratory testing should be guided by findings of the history and physical examination. For the patient who is actively bleeding, the most important tests to obtain are those that will assist in determining the best treatment for the bleeding. At a minimum, all patients should have a hemoglobin and complete blood count (CBC) done. Beta-human chorionic gonadotropin testing usually is indicated to rule out pregnancy. Coagulation studies, including, at a minimum, platelet count, prothombin time (PT), and partial thromboplastin time (PTT), also generally are indicated. These studies always should be performed if the adolescent has a family history of bleeding disorders and a personal history of excessive nonmenstrual bleeding or anemia. It is important to remember that the CBC, PT, and PTT results may be normal in patients who have von Willebrand disease, especially when there is active bleeding. Thus, if this disorder is suspected, a von Willebrand screen or referral to a hematologist should be considered.

Additional laboratory tests often can be deferred until the bleeding is controlled to minimize further blood loss due to testing. If galactorrhea is present, serum prolactin should be measured. If there are signs of PCOS, measurement of FSH, LH, and testosterone levels will be helpful. Thyroid screening should be considered, even in patients who do not have clinical signs or symptoms of hypothyroidism.

Abdominal and pelvic ultrasonography may be helpful in assessing the patient and always are indicated for patients who are suspected of having an ectopic pregnancy or who have a palpable pelvic or abdominal mass.

Treatment

If the history, physical examination, and laboratory test results are consistent with the diagnosis of DUB, treatment can be guided by the severity of the bleeding and the need for contraception. For the young virginal adolescent who is not anemic and is in her first or second gynecologic year, a conservative approach is warranted if the history and physical examination findings are normal. The cause of the DUB should be discussed with the patient and her parent. A menstrual calendar and follow-up visit in 3 to 6 months should be scheduled. Appropriate iron supplementation should be provided to prevent anemia. If the irregular menses are bothersome, hormonal treatment can be considered, but this rarely is necessary.

For the adolescent who is anemic, hormonal and iron therapy are indicated. Both estrogen and progesterone should be used to stop the bleeding. Estrogen provides hemostasis, and progesterone stabilizes the endometrial lining. Combined oral contraceptive pills (OCPs) containing both hormones are the most convenient method of administering these hormones. If the adolescent is not actively bleeding, OCPs can be given in a once-daily regimen. Pills containing at least 30 mcg of ethinyl estradiol should be prescribed. If there is active bleeding, the OCPs should be given in a daily multiple-pill regimen that is followed by a tapering dosage. The regimen begins with four pills every 6 hours until the bleeding has stopped for at least 24 hours. An antiemetic may be needed to control any nausea. For most patients, bleeding will cease within 48 hours. If the bleeding persists for more than 2 days, additional evaluation and consultation should be considered because patients who have persistent bleeding despite high-dose OCPs often have an underlying bleeding disorder or pelvic pathology. After the bleeding has stopped, the dosage of OCPs is decreased to three pills per day for the next 3 days, followed by two pills per day for 3 days. The patient then is maintained on a once-a-day regimen. If bleeding recurs during tapering, the dosage can be increased to the lowest effective dose necessary to control bleeding. If the hemoglobin is less than 10 mg/dL (100 g/L), the OCPs can be administered continuously without placebos for 6 to 9 weeks. The patient should be instructed to take only the first 21 pills of each pack. This regimen delays withdrawal menses until the hemoglobin concentration has increased. When withdrawal bleeding does occur, the patient should be advised that the menstrual flow might be heavier and more prolonged than normal because the OCPs have been taken continuously for more than 1 month. After tapering the dosage of OCPs, the patient continues cycling on OCPs for 3 to 6 months. Generally, no further treatment is needed for the young adolescent who has had DUB due to anovulatory cycles. However, many adolescents wish to continue the OCPs if they are sexually active. It is important to talk to the adolescent privately about the need for contraception.

If estrogen is contraindicated or not tolerated by the patient, cyclic progesterone therapy can be substituted for the daily OCP regimen. Progesterone induces stromal stability that is followed by withdrawal menstrual flow, but this regimen is not as effective as OCPs because estrogen improves hemostasis by increasing platelet aggregation and levels of fibrinogen and factors V and IX. Medroxyprogesterone acetate 10 mg daily can be administered for 10 days per month. The therapy should be continued for 3 to 6 months.

If the hemoglobin level is very low (<10 mg/dL [100 g/L]) or there is hemodynamic instability, intravenous conjugated estrogen can be used to stop the bleeding rapidly. Usually one to three intravenous doses of 25 mg conjugated estrogen administered at 4- to 6-hour intervals will stop the bleeding. If bleeding does not stop within 24 hours, a gynecologic surgical consultation is indicated. Blood transfusions are rarely needed, even in patients who have hemoglobin levels as low as 6 mg/dL (60 g/L). Dilatation and curettage is used as a last resort and seldom is needed in adolescents.

Systematic reviews of randomized control trials have shown that nonsteroidal anti-inflammatory drugs (NSAIDs) reduce menstrual blood loss. When administered during menses, blood loss may be reduced by 30% to 50%. The NSAIDs should be started at the onset of menstruation and continued until the end of menses. These drugs are a helpful adjunct to hormonal therapy for adolescents who have DUB and may be especially useful in the adolescent who has menorrhagia. In one systematic review of NSAIDs versus placebo, mefenamic acid, naproxen, meclofenamic acid, and diclofenac reduced menstrual blood loss by 23 to 74 mL. Ibuprofen may be less effective than mefenamic acid or naproxen in reducing blood loss.

Other drugs that have been used to control menstrual blood loss in adult women include desmopressin, antifibrinolytic drugs (eg, tranexamic acid, aminocaproic acid), danazol, and GnRH agonists. There is little experience with any of these drugs in adolescents, however. Desmopressin may help in the management of the adolescent who has von Willebrand disease or hemophilia A. Antifibrinolytic therapies may reduce blood loss by up to 50%, but adverse effects are frequent and include nausea, diarrhea, headaches, and abdominal pain. In addition, systemic thrombosis has been reported. Administration of GnRH agonists suppresses gonadotropin secretion and, thus, estradiol levels, resulting in amenorrhea. Long-term use is associated with osteoporosis similar to that seen in ovarian failure. However, GnRH agonists have been used as a short-term therapy for the adolescent who has severe but transitory thrombocytopenia associated with chemotherapy if there is a poor response to hormonal medications. Danazol is an androgen derivative that induces amenorrhea. Anabolic and androgenic adverse effects, such as weight gain, acne, and hirsutism, are very common.

The long-term prognosis for the adolescent who has abnormal uterine bleeding depends on the underlying cause. For the young adolescent who has anovulatory cycles due to immaturity of the hypothalamic-pituitary-ovarian axis, the prognosis is excellent. In contrast, adolescents who have PCOS often continue to have abnormal uterine bleeding, and retrospective studies suggest that they are at increased risk for adverse cardiovascular events. Recent research suggests that increased insulin resistance may be one of the key pathophysiologic factors in the development of PCOS. Use of insulin-sensitizing agents (eg, metformin, troglitazone) recently has been shown to decrease hyperandrogenism and induce ovulation, thus causing a return of regular menses. The use of these agents for the long-term management of adolescents is under investigation. Adolescents who have a blood dyscrasia often continue to have menorrhagia and require therapy throughout their reproductive years.

Suggested Reading

Gordon CM. Menstrual disorders in adolescents. Excess androgens and the polycystic ovary syndrome. *Pediatr Clin North Am.* 1999;46:519–543

Iglesia EA, Coupey SM. Menstrual cycle abnormalities: diagnosis and management. *Adolescent Medicine: State of the Art Reviews.* 1999;10:255–274

Mitan LAP, Slap GB. Adolescent menstrual disorders update. *Med Clin North Am.* 2000;84:851–868

Sanfilippo JS, Hertweck SP. Physiology of menstruation and menstrual disorders. In: Friedman SB, Fisher MM, Schonberg SK, Alderman AM, eds. *Comprehensive Adolescent Health Care.* 2nd ed. St. Louis, Mo: Mosby; 1998:990–1017

Shwayder JM. Contemporary management of abnormal uterine bleeding. Pathophysiology of abnormal uterine bleeding. *Obstet Gynecol Clin North Am.* 2000;27:219–234

Early Detection of Imperforate Hymen Prevents Morbidity From Delays in Diagnosis

Jill C. Posner, MD, MSCE, and Philip R. Spandorfer, MD, MSCE

ABSTRACT. *Objective.* Although it is detectable at all ages through inspection of the external genitalia, imperforate hymen (IH) is a diagnosis that is missed commonly. We hypothesized that children with late diagnoses (predefined as ≥8 years of age, chosen to reflect the timing of normal menarche) would be more likely to be symptomatic, undergo more diagnostic testing, and lack appropriate documentation in their medical records, compared with children with earlier diagnoses (ie, <8 years of age).

Methods. All patients with IH were identified through searches of 3 hospital databases with *International Classification of Diseases, Ninth Revision,* codes. The medical records of eligible subjects were reviewed by a single, blinded researcher. Comparisons were made between children diagnosed at younger versus older ages.

Results. A bimodal distribution of age at diagnosis was demonstrated; 43% (*n* = 10) of girls were diagnosed at <8 years of age, and 57% (*n* = 13) were diagnosed at ≥8 years of age. Among older girls, 100% were symptomatic (abdominal pain and/or urinary symptoms; duration of symptoms: 1–120 days), whereas 90% of cases in the younger group were detected incidentally. Documentation was lacking for breast development (77%), pubic hair development (69%), and menstrual history (46%) among the older girls. Older children were more likely to present symptomatically (odds ratio: 42.0; 95% confidence interval: 3.1–1965.7) and to undergo ancillary testing (odds ratio: 20.3; 95% confidence interval: 1.6–983.1).

Conclusions. Two distinct populations of girls with IH exist, ie, those diagnosed without symptoms at a young age and those not diagnosed until >8 years of age. By incorporating an examination of the external genitalia into their routine practice, clinicians caring for children can prevent the significant delays in diagnosis, misdiagnosis, and morbidity associated with the latter group. *Pediatrics* 2005;115:1008–1012; *imperforate*

hymen, hydrocolpos, hydrometrocolpos, hematocolpos, hematometrocolpos.

ABBREVIATION. IH, imperforate hymen.

Imperforate hymen (IH) is a rare congenital anomaly in which the hymenal membrane occludes outflow from the female genital tract. This obstruction results in an accumulation of uterine and vaginal secretions. Large amounts of retained fluid have been reported.[1,2] The presentations of patients with IH can be variable. There are reports of cases detected incidentally[1,3,4] or with symptoms of abdominal[1,5-9] or back[10-12] pain, constipation,[13,14] dysuria or acute urinary retention,[14-20] peritonitis,[21,22] or primary amenorrhea,[23] as well as a report of acquired IH associated with sexual abuse.[24]

Menarche is a relatively late event in the pubertal process, and most girls have attained Tanner stage 3 at the time of menarche. A discrepancy between a teen's advanced stage of pubertal development and the absence of menarche is a key clinical clue to the possibility of IH. Despite the ease of diagnosis at all ages with simple inspection of the external genitalia, the detection of IH can be delayed or missed, resulting in preventable morbidity and unnecessary diagnostic testing.

Previous works regarding IH consisted of case reports or small case series and therefore were limited in the ability to allow definitive

From the Division of Emergency Medicine, Department of Pediatrics, Children's Hospital of Philadelphia, University of Pennsylvania School of Medicine, Philadelphia, Pennsylvania.

Accepted for publication Sep 1, 2004. doi:10.1542/peds.2004-0183

This work was presented in part at the Ambulatory Pediatrics Association Regional Conference; March 5, 2002; Philadelphia, PA.

No conflict of interest declared.

Address correspondence to Jill C. Posner, MD, MSCE, Division of Emergency Medicine, Children's Hospital of Philadelphia, 34th Street and Civic Center Boulevard, Philadelphia, PA 19104. E-mail: posner@email.chop.edu

conclusions. To our knowledge, no previous work systematically investigated a population of children with IH. The objective of this study was to describe a population of patients with IH who were treated at a large, tertiary care, referral children's hospital. Specifically, we aimed to characterize the presenting features and diagnostic evaluations performed and to assess the frequency with which the menstrual history, pubertal staging, and hymenal examination results were documented in the medical evaluation. We hypothesized that children with late diagnoses (predefined as ≥8 years of age, chosen to reflect the timing of normal menarche) would be more likely to be symptomatic, undergo more diagnostic testing, and lack appropriate documentation in their medical records, compared with children with earlier diagnoses (ie, <8 years of age).

Methods

We conducted a retrospective, case-series study of all patients who were diagnosed with and treated for IH at a large, tertiary care, children's hospital during a 13-year period (January 1, 1987, through December 31, 2000). Eligible patients were identified through a search of the hospital's health information management (ie, medical records) database with *International Classification of Diseases, Ninth Revision*, codes for IH and related terms (hydrocolpos, hydrometrocolpos, hematocolpos, and hematometrocolpos). Additional searches of the urologic procedures database and the operative anesthesia database were performed to supplement the primary search. We used this strategy to optimize the identification of patients with IH. These databases were not mutually exclusive. Because we aimed to describe the presentation of uncomplicated IH, patients with genetic syndromes or coexistent genital anomalies were excluded. The medical records of identified subjects were abstracted for data pertaining to the presentation and diagnostic evaluation. All available components of the hospital medical records were subject to review, including emergency department records, preoperative evaluation findings, operative reports, and inpatient records. Demographic features, presenting symptoms, documentation of Tanner stage, hymenal examination results, menstrual history, preliminary diagnosis, ancillary test findings, operative procedure, and final diagnosis were recorded on a standardized data collection sheet by a single researcher, who was blinded with respect to the study hypothesis.

The sample size was based on identification of all eligible patients. Statistical analyses were conducted with Stata 7.0 software (Stata Corp, College Station, TX). The sample was described with means, SDs, medians, and ranges for continuous variables and frequencies for categorical variables. Between-group comparisons (ie, older versus younger girls) were performed with exact χ^2 tests.

This study received institutional review board approval. After chart abstraction had been completed, all data were deidentified.

Results

Computerized searches of the databases resulted in the identification of 95 girls. Fourteen patients were excluded because of multiple congenital anomalies or genetic syndromes associated with IH. Of the remaining 81 patients, 58 were excluded because of diagnoses other than IH, most commonly dysfunctional uterine bleeding. There were 23 patients in the final study sample, 74% ($n = 17$) white, 22% ($n = 5$) black, and 4% ($n = 1$) Asian (Table 1). The distribution of age at diagnosis demonstrated a clear bimodal distribution that was even more dramatic than results with the predefined cutoff point of 8 years (Fig 1); 43% of patients ($n = 10$) were diagnosed at <4 years of age (median age: 1.2 years; range: 9 days to 3.7 years), and the remaining 57% ($n = 13$) were diagnosed at >10 years of age (median age: 12.3 years; range: 10.9–14.2 years).

In the older group, 100% of patients ($n = 13$) were symptomatic at the time of diagnosis. In the younger group, almost all patients (90%, $n = 9$) were asymptomatic. One girl in the younger group was diagnosed during an evaluation because of dysuria at 3 years of age. Although it was unclear whether the presence of an IH predisposed this patient to develop dysuria, we considered this patient to be symptomatic for the purposes of analysis.

In the group of older girls, all presented with abdominal pain ($n = 6$), urinary symptoms ($n = 2$), or both abdominal pain and urinary symptoms ($n = 5$). In the same group, the median duration of symptoms before diagnosis was 15 days (range: 1–120 days). Almost one half of the older girls (46%, $n = 6$) were given preliminary diagnoses other than IH, including urinary tract infection ($n = 2$), appendicitis ($n = 2$), nephrolithiasis ($n = 1$), and abdominal tumor ($n = 1$). In the older group, the medical records lacked documentation of breast development in 77% of cases ($n = 10$), pubic hair development in 69% ($n = 9$), and menstrual history in 46% ($n = 6$). Most of the older girls (85%, $n = 11$) underwent ancillary testing before definitive diagnosis, including blood analyses ($n = 10$),

Table 1. Characteristics of the Patients With IH

Patient No.	Age at Evaluation*	Race	Symptoms at Diagnosis	Imaging Performed	Additional Comments
1	9 d	White	None	Confirmatory US	Detected as a pelvic cyst on prenatal US at 7 mo
2	22 d	White	None	Confirmatory US	Diagnosed in routine newborn examination
3	3 mo	White	None	None	Repaired at 9 y of age
4	4 mo	White	None	None	Repaired at 8 mo of age; younger sister of patient 8
5	7 mo	White	None	Confirmatory US	Diagnosed in routine examination
6	21 mo	White	None	Renal US and VCUG as part of previous UTI evaluation	Detected during evaluation for recurrent UTIs beginning at 6 wk
7	2.0 y	Asian	None	None	Surgical repair at 13 y of age
8	2.1 y	White	None	None	Older sister of patient 4
9	2.1 y	White	None	None	
10	3.7 y	White	Dysuria	None	
11	10.9 y	Black	Vomiting, right lower abd pain	Diagnostic US	US was obtained in an evaluation for appendicitis and was diagnostic of IH; no appendicitis
12	11.3 y	Black	Abd pain, dysuria	Confirmatory US	Referred for evaluation of an abd mass
13	11.5 y	Black	1 mo of abd and back pain	Abd CT and diagnostic US	Preliminary diagnosis of nephrolithiasis
14	11.7 y	Black	Dysuria, abd pain	Diagnostic US	Treated for UTI 1 mo previously
15	12.2 y	White	1 wk of dysuria	None	Diagnosed through physical examination
16	12.2 y	White	2 wk of abd pain	Diagnostic US	Preliminary diagnosis of UTI
17	12.3 y	White	1 d of inability to void	Confirmatory US	Diagnosed through physical examination
18	13.3 y	White	2 mo of lower abd pain	Diagnostic US	
19	13.3 y	White	2 mo of urinary retention, back pain, and abd pain	Diagnostic US	
20	13.6 y	White	4 mo of cyclic abd pain and dysuria	Confirmatory US	
21	13.8 y	Black	3 mo of abd pain	Confirmatory US	Sister had IH
22	13.9 y	White	2 wk of intermittent abd pain, 1 d of dysuria	Diagnostic US	
23	14.2 y	White	2 d of abd pain	Diagnostic US	Preliminary diagnosis of appendicitis

US indicates ultrasound; CT, computed tomography; VCUG, voiding cystourethrogram; UTI, urinary tract infection; abd, abdominal.

*The age of the patient at the first evaluation at the Children's Hospital of Philadelphia.

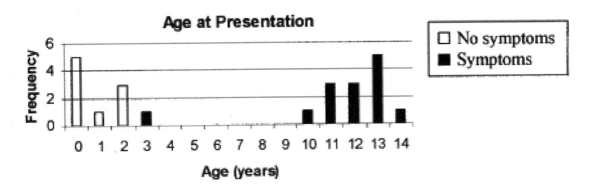

Fig 1. Age and presence of symptoms at the diagnosis of IH.

urinalyses ($n = 9$), and abdominal plain radiographic evaluations ($n = 4$). In comparison, the only patient in the younger group to undergo diagnostic testing before definitive diagnosis was the child diagnosed as having vesiculoureteral reflux after a previous urinary tract infection.

Ultrasonographic imaging was performed for 15 of the 23 patients. Interestingly, all 3 of the ultrasonographic evaluations performed in the younger group were to confirm diagnoses of IH that were made first through physical examination; however, 8 of the 12 ultrasonographic evaluations performed in the older group were part of diagnostic evaluations that led to the eventual diagnosis of IH. Of note, there was no documentation of any clinical suspicion of sexual abuse in either of the groups.

Compared with the younger children, the older children were more likely to present symptomatically (odds ratio: 42.0; 95% confidence interval: 3.1–1965.7; $P < .001$) and undergo laboratory or plain radiographic testing (odds ratio: 20.3; 95% confidence interval: 1.6–983.1; $P < .001$). All children underwent hymenectomy at or near the time of diagnosis, with the notable exception of 2 young children for whom surgery was delayed for several years.

Discussion

In this study, the first large case series of patients with IH exclusively, we demonstrated that 2 distinct subpopulations of girls with IH exist, on the basis of the age at diagnosis and the presenting

clinical features. One group was composed of younger girls, nearly all of whom were asymptomatic and were diagnosed incidentally through physical examination alone. The other group consisted of older girls, all of whom presented symptomatically. Although we planned in our analyses to compare girls ≥8 years of age with those <8 years of age (coinciding with the lower limit of normal puberty), a more striking dichotomy in age was observed. All patients in the younger group were <4 years of age, whereas the older group consisted of girls ≥10 years of age. This finding is consistent with the age distribution reported in a case series that aimed to describe the utility of laparoscopy in the evaluation of vaginal malformations.[25]

Girls in the older group commonly experienced protracted symptoms before being diagnosed as having IH. Although this might be attributable, in part, to a delay in seeking care by the girl and/or her family, our results indicate that the medical evaluation might also be contributory. Nearly one half of the older girls were assigned an incorrect preliminary diagnosis. In addition, this group was significantly more likely to undergo unnecessary laboratory and radiographic studies, further delaying the eventual diagnosis. Furthermore, we found that a substantial proportion of the older girls had incompletely documented histories and physical examination results and frequently lacked appropriate pubertal evaluations. Specifically, no genital examination was performed for two thirds of the older patients, and there was no breast examination for three fourths. Almost one half of the older patients were not asked about menstrual history.

The diagnosis of IH can be made from a physical examination alone, eliminating the need for expensive laboratory testing or radiographic evaluations. Observation of the hymen and viewing into the vaginal vault are best accomplished by applying gentle labial traction with the child in the supine frog-leg or knee-chest position.[26] An uncomfortable speculum examination is not indicated, because mere observation of a bulging mass at the vaginal introitus for an older patient (Fig 2) or, ideally, of a membrane obstructing the view into the vaginal vault for an infant or young child establishes the diagnosis. Our results indicate, however, that some patients with IH experience delays in diagnosis, misdiagnosis, and additional diagnostic evaluations. It can be surmised that, if each older girl had undergone a complete examination of the external genitalia as part of a routine well-child visit early in her life, then none would have had to endure the symptoms and diagnostic evaluations associated with late diagnosis. It is our recommendation, therefore, that the hymenal examination be emphasized as a routine part of newborn and infant health maintenance evaluations. In addition, routine periodic hymenal

reexaminations should be performed to document the hymenal changes that may occur with normal development.[27,28]

Treatment of IH consists of surgical hymenectomy, releasing the obstructing hymenal tissue. The majority of patients in our study were treated surgically at or near the time of diagnosis, although there were 2 notable exceptions of patients who underwent delayed treatment. The optimal timing for this procedure is unclear. However, it is possible that patients with IH may be at higher risk of endometriosis.[25] Therefore, treating physicians must weigh the risks of anesthesia for young children against the potential risks resulting from delayed correction.

There are limitations to this study that should be considered in interpreting our results. First, as with all retrospectively conducted investigations, there is a potential for information bias. It is possible that key components of the history and physical examination were actually performed but were not documented in the medical record. This could have led to an overestimation of incomplete pubertal evaluations for older girls. However, the fact that older girls experienced significant delays in diagnosis and underwent additional testing supports the validity of our results. Second, ascertainment bias might have occurred, resulting in incomplete identification of all eligible patients. However, we minimized the potential for this bias by using 3 hospital databases (not mutually exclusive) to ensure inclusion of all patients diagnosed with IH during the study period. Third, although this study of IH is the largest to date, the small sample size led to wide confidence intervals around the odds ratios. Finally, this study was undertaken at a tertiary children's hospital; therefore, the results might not be reflective of all children with IH.

Clinicians caring for children and teens should incorporate inspection of the female genitalia into their routine practices. If clinicians detect IH among young children, they can prevent the morbidity associated with delays in diagnosis, including the development of symptoms and additional diagnostic testing. For older girls presenting with abdominal or urinary symptoms, the complete

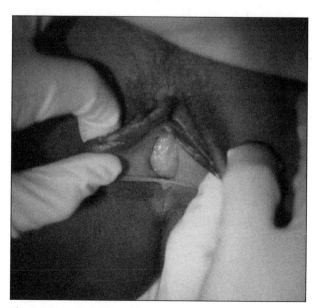

Fig 2. IH in an adolescent female patient.

medical evaluation must include a review of the menstrual history and an examination of the breasts and external genitalia. A high index of suspicion for IH should be maintained, especially if a discrepancy is noted between the Tanner stage of pubertal development and a reported lack of menarche.

Acknowledgment

We thank Gina Ruggierio for her assistance with data management.

References

1. Bogen DL, Gehris RP, Bellinger MF. Picture of the month. *Arch Pediatr Adolesc Med.* 2000;154:959–960

2. Loscalzo IL, Catapano M, Loscalzo J, Sama A. Imperforate hymen with bilateral hydronephrosis: an unusual emergency department diagnosis. *J Emerg Med.* 1995; 13:337–339

3. Henderson KC. Hydrometrocolpos in a newborn. *Am J Dis Child.* 1975;129:1190–1191

4. Kahn R, Duncan B, Bowes W. Spontaneous opening of congenital imperforate hymen. *J Pediatr.* 1975;87:768–770

5. Ward A, Maher P. Hematocolpos: an unusual presentation. *Br J Clin Pract.* 1979;33:83–84

6. Dickson CA, Saad S, Tesar JD. Imperforate hymen with hematocolpos. *Ann Emerg Med.* 1985;14:467–469

7. Maffeo DA, Santagata P, Santagata M. Hematocopos by imperforated hymen: case report. *Clin Exp Obstet Gynecol.* 1999;26:230–231

8. Schneider K, Hong J, Fong J, Sanders CG. Hematocolpos as an easily overlooked diagnosis. *Curr Opin Pediatr.* 1999;11:249–252

9. McIvor RA. Haematocolpos, once-in-a-lifetime cause of recurrent abdominal pain. *Arch Emerg Med.* 1990;7:51–57

10. London NJ, Sefton GK. Hematocolpos: an unusual cause of sciatica in an adolescent girl. *Spine.* 1996;21: 1381–1382

11. Buick RG, Chowdhary SK. Backache: a rare diagnosis and unusual complication. *Pediatr Surg Int.* 1999;15:586–587

12. Letts M, Haasbeek J. Hematocolpos as a cause of back pain in premenarchal adolescents. *J Pediatr Orthop.* 1990; 10:731–732

13. Isenhour JL, Hanley M, Marx JA. Hematocolpometra manifesting as constipation in the young female. *Acad Emerg Med.* 1999;7:752–753

14. Kitapci F, Avsar AG, Senses DA. A girl with constipation and acute urinary retention. *Eur J Pediatr.* 1999;158: 337–338

15. Hall DJ. An unusual case of urinary retention due to imperforate hymen. *J Accid Emerg Med.* 1999;16:232–233

16. Peterson-Sweeney KL, Stevens J. 13-year-old female with imperforate hymen. *Nurse Pract.* 1996;21:90–94

17. Nisanian AC. Hematocolpometra presenting as urinary retention: a case report. *J Reprod Med.* 1993;38:57–64

18. Wort SJ, Heman-Ackah C, Davies A. Acute urinary retention in the young female. *Br J Urol.* 1995;76:659–670

19. Yu T, Lin M. Acute urinary retention in two patients with imperforate hymen. *Scand J Urol Nephrol.* 1993; 27:543–544

20. Hammond Y. Haematocolpos. *Nurs Times.* 1970;66: 1131–1132

21. Bakos O, Berglund L. Imperforate hymen and ruptured hematosalpinx: a case report with a review of the literature. *J Adolesc Health.* 1999;24:226–228

22. Gazit E, Frand M, Mashiah S, Rotem Y. Imperforate hymen causing pyocolpos in an infant. *Clin Pediatr.* 1975;14:414–415

23. Siegberg R, Tenhunen A, Ylostalo P. Diagnosis of mucocolpos and hematocolpos by ultrasound: two case reports. *J Clin Ultrasound.* 1985;13:421–423

24. Botash AS, Jean-Louis F. Imperforate hymen: congenital or acquired from sexual abuse. *Pediatrics.* 2001;108(3). Available at: www.pediatrics.org/cgi/content/full/ 108/3/e53

25. Philbois O, Guye E, Richard O, et al. Role of laparoscopy in vaginal malformation. *Surg Endosc.* 2004;18:87–91

26. Christian C, Decker JM. Prepubertal genital examination. In: Henretig FM, King C, eds. *Textbook of Pediatric Emergency Procedures.* Philadelphia, PA: Lippincott Williams & Wilkins; 1997:961–970

27. Berenson AB, Grady J. A longitudinal study of hymenal development from 3 to 9 years of age. *Pediatrics.* 2002; 140:600–607

28. Berenson AB. A longitudinal study of hymenal morphology in the first three years of life. *Pediatrics.* 1995;95: 490–496

Oral Contraceptives: Part 1

by Margaret Polaneczky, MD, FACOG

This issue begins a two-part series that will enhance the pediatrician's knowledge and skill in providing oral contraception to adolescent patients. Part 1 will focus on the basics of prescribing oral contraceptives (formulations, risks, benefits, contraindications, drug interactions, and use of pills in certain medical conditions), and will also review emergency contraception. Part 2 will address the practical aspects of providing oral contraceptives to adolescents (patient selection, choosing and initiating pill use, confidentiality, and counseling) and will briefly address the newer long-acting alternatives to oral contraceptives.

While discussion of barrier contraceptives is beyond the scope of this article, educating patients about protection against sexually transmitted diseases is well within the scope of the pediatrician's responsibilities. Readers are referred to the October 2001 issue of *Adolescent Health Update,* which can be accessed on the members-only channel of the AAP Web site (www.aap.org.)

Overview

The combination oral contraceptive pill (OCP) is the most popular contraceptive among adolescents. The most recent data (1995) show that 44% of the 2.7 million teens using contraception rely on the pill. Thirty-seven percent use condoms, and 20% use either injectables or the contraceptive implant.[1] Although condom use has increased and new methods have been introduced in recent years, for many teens, the words "birth control" still mean "the pill."

Oral contraceptive pills are a safe and effective form of birth control. When taken properly, pregnancy rates are less than 1%. Noncompliance results in somewhat higher pregnancy rates among adolescent pill users; some studies suggest that less than 41% of adolescent pill users take their pill every day.[2] Discontinuation rates among adolescent pill users are also high. This is attributed to concerns about minor side effects and the sporadic nature of adolescent sexual activity, which leads some teens to believe that they have only an intermittent need for protection against pregnancy.

Prescribing birth control pills is not as simple as writing a prescription and sending the adolescent on her way. The myriad of pills available can make pill choice confusing to the clinician and patient alike. Myths and misperceptions persist about the use and safety of oral contraceptives. Managing side effects can be time consuming. However, birth control pills are an important contraceptive method, and the more clinicians

---

Learning Objectives

After reading this article, pediatricians will be better prepared to:
- Describe the various formulations of oral contraceptives
- Describe the noncontraceptive benefits of oral contraceptives
- List contraindications to oral contraceptive use
- Discuss considerations in prescribing oral contraceptives for adolescents with underlying medical conditions
- Describe important drug interactions with oral contraceptives
- Explain emergency contraception

Margaret Polaneczky, MD, FACOG is an associate professor of clinical obstetrics and gynecology, Weill Medical College of Cornell University, New York, NY

know about prescribing OCPs, the better their patients will use them.

Composition and Mechanism of Action

Oral contraceptives are either combination pills, containing estrogen and progestin, or progestin-only pills (POPs). (For the purposes of this review, "OCP" will refer to combination pills.) The majority of adolescents who take oral contraceptives use combination pills. OCPs may be classified as monophasic (ie, the hormone concentrations remain fixed throughout the cycle), biphasic, or triphasic (ie hormone concentrations vary in 2 or 3 phases throughout the cycle).

Oral contraceptives prevent pregnancy primarily by preventing ovulation (estrogen and progestin effect) and causing thickening of the cervical mucus (progestin effect). Secondary effects of oral contraceptives, such as thinning and deciduation of the endometrium and impairment of tubal motility, are likely to be less important in pregnancy prevention.

ESTROGEN COMPONENT

All currently marketed combination pills contain either ethinyl estradiol (EE) or mestranol as the estrogen component, in doses ranging from 20–50 µg. "Low dose" pills refers to monophasic combination oral contraceptives containing 20–35 µg of EE and triphasic pills containing 30–40 µg EE. "High dose" pills contain 50 µg EE or 50 µg mestranol. High dose OCPs are reserved for treatment of dysfunctional or breakthrough bleeding, for use in emergency contraception, and for special populations needing higher estrogen doses due to interaction of OCPs with other medications.

PROGESTIN COMPONENT

Progestins can be classified by "generations" (the order in which they were introduced into the marketplace), by steroid backbone (gonane or estrane), or according to in-vitro binding affinity for androgen receptors (androgenicity). (See Table 1)

Table 1. Progestins Used in Selected Low-Dose Oral Contraceptives

Progestin Grouping	Progestin	Relative Androgenicity*	Proprietary Names†
First generation (estrane)	norethindrone	++	Ortho-Novum 1/35, Ortho-Novum 7/7/7, Ovcon-35, Loestrin 1/20, Loestrin 1.5/30, Estrostep, Norinyl, Tri-Norinyl, Genora 0.5/35, Genora 1/35, Modicon, Jenest, Demulen 1/35
	ethynodiol diacetate	++	Micronor (POP)‡
Second generation (gonane)	levonorgestrel	+++	Nordette, Levlen, Alesse, Triphasil, Tri-Levlen, Levora, Levlite
	norgestrel	+++	Lo/Ovral, Ovrette (POP)
Third generation (gonane)	desogestrel	+	Desogen, Ortho-Cept, Cyclessa, Mircette
	norgestimate	+	Ortho-Cyclen, Ortho Tri-Cyclen
Other	drospirenone	–§	Yasmin

* Refers to the relative androgenicity of the progestin component alone and in-vitro, with + being less androgenic than +++. Androgenicity refers to the relative binding affinity of a progestin for testosterone receptors in in-vitro assays. It does not describe the overall androgenicity of pills containing that progestin, and does not take into account differences in progestin doses between pills.

† Here and elsewhere in the text, proprietary names illustrate products most often prescribed and with which pediatricians are likely to be familiar. This does not imply AAP endorsement. Equivalent products may be substituted. For a more complete listing, see Hatcher RA, Trussell J, Stewart F, et al. *Contraceptive Technology.* 17th rev. ed. New York, NY: Ardent Media; 1998:430–432

‡ POP: Progestin-only preparation

§ Drospirenone has additional anti-androgenic activity. See text.

Progestin-only pills (POPs) differ somewhat from estrogen-containing oral contraceptives. The failure rate of POPs, when taken correctly, is about 0.5% (compared with 0.1% for combination pills). POPs are taken continuously, with no placebos or pill-free days. Breakthrough bleeding is more frequent with progestin-only pills than combination pills, although the majority of POP users still have regular menses. Because overall hormonal doses are lower, back-up contraception is recommended if even one pill is missed or taken late. Despite these disadvantages, POPs are a good alternative for pill users unable to use estrogen-containing OCPs. There are almost no contraindications to POP use.

Benefits of OCP Use

For the healthy adolescent, the benefits of OCP use far outweigh associated risks. Younger postmenarchal adolescents can safely use oral contraception without adverse effects on growth or maturation of the hypothalamic-pituitary-ovarian axis. Unfortunately, the well-documented benefits of OCPs are not well known to the public. A 1996 survey by the Kaiser Family Foundation found that nearly two-thirds of women believe the pill is unsafe. Thirty percent think it causes cancer and heart disease, and most are unaware that OCPs benefit bone health. The time required to inform patients about the benefits of oral contraceptive use is a wise investment in compliance.

IMPROVEMENT OF DYSMENORRHEA

Dysmenorrhea is a common menstrual complaint among adolescents. In a survey of 70,000 adolescents, 60% reported dysmenorrhea and 14% had missed school due to cramps.[3] OCP use decreases menstrual pain in most women by inhibiting ovulation and decreasing endometrial prostaglandin production. OCPs are also used to treat pelvic pain associated with endometriosis. For severe dysmenorrhea, monophasic pills can be taken continuously (without placebos) and menstrual bleeding avoided altogether.

SHORTER, LIGHTER MENSTRUAL FLOW

OCPs reduce menstrual flow, benefiting teens who have anovulatory cycles, menorrhagia, or anemia. Patients should understand that lighter flow may take 2–3 cycles to become evident.

IMPROVEMENT IN ACNE AND HIRSUTISM

All combination oral contraceptive pills have the potential to improve acne and decrease unwanted (eg, facial) hair growth by causing a decrease in testosterone levels. Testosterone in the female is derived in large part from ovarian testosterone secretion and from peripheral conversion of androstenedione produced in the ovaries and the adrenals. OCPs suppress ovarian testosterone and androstenedione production, leading to decreased total testosterone levels. In addition, the estrogen component of OCPs induces an increase in hepatic production of sex hormone-binding globulin, in turn reducing free testosterone. The end result is improvement in acne and hirsutism. It is unclear to what extent, if any, the inherent androgenicity (ie, androgen receptor binding affinity) of the progestin component of a given pill modulates that pill's overall antiandrogenic effect.

Although some manufacturers have submitted data to the FDA on the anti-acne benefits of their pill and have permission to advertise this indication directly to patients, any combination OCP may be expected to achieve this benefit. In theory, third-generation pills with less androgenic progestins may be more beneficial to patients with acne and hirsutism, but few comparative studies have been performed. Yasmin has an added theoretical benefit in that its progestin, drospirenone, has direct antiandrogenic activity similar to spironolactone, from which it is derived. Spironolactone, a potassium-sparing diuretic, inhibits 5 α-reductase, which converts testosterone to its active metabolite, dihydrotestosterone, in the skin. Spironolactone also has a small and variable inhibitory effect on androgen production in the ovaries and adrenals.[4] Yasmin's drospirenone dose is equivalent to 25 mg spironolactone. Given that usual treatment doses of spironolactone for hirsutism are 200 mg, it is unclear if the lower equivalent dose in Yasmin has significant clinical impact.

PREVENTION OF FUNCTIONAL OVARIAN CYSTS

Oral contraceptives suppress ovulation, leading to a decrease in the incidence of functional cysts, especially symptomatic hemorrhagic corpus luteal cysts. Ovarian activity can occur during placebo weeks, however. For patients with particularly resistant ovarian cyst recurrences, changing to a pill with a higher estrogen dose (up to 50 µg) or using the pill continuously (omitting placebos) may be helpful. Oral contraceptive use will not resolve a preexisting functional cyst any faster than observation alone.

MITTELSCHMERZ

By preventing ovulation, combination pills can prevent the pain some women experience at ovulation.

PREVENTION OF OVARIAN AND ENDOMETRIAL CANCER

No other medication can claim such a well-documented benefit in cancer reduction. The risk reduction in ovarian cancer is 30% for 4 years of pill use, 60% for 5 to 11 years, and 80% after 12 or more years. For endometrial cancer, the risk reduction is 40% at 2 years and 60% with 4 years or more.[5]

PROTECTION AGAINST OSTEOPOROSIS

Multiple retrospective and cross-sectional studies in adult (primarily menopausal) women have demonstrated a link between OCP use and higher bone mass, a benefit that increases with duration of OCP use. This is thought to result from estrogen's prevention of age-related bone loss and possibly its therapeutic effects in individuals with estrogen-deficient states. A recent evidence-based review found 8 of 14 studies supporting a benefit to OCP use on bone mass.[6] In a recent 8-year prospective study, oral contraceptive use during adolescence had no adverse effects on bone mass achieved by age 20.[7] Low peak bone mass and osteoporosis at young ages may occur in adolescents who are hypoestrogenic due to athletics, eating disorders, or hypothalamic amenorrhea. Unfortunately, OCPs appear to be ineffective in preventing bone loss in anorexic patients unless

weight is normalized. Use of OCPs in normal-weight individuals and athletes with hypothalamic amenorrhea has not been as well studied. However, the absence of significant risk makes use of OCPs reasonable in these young women.

Risks and Contraindications

HYPERCOAGULABILITY

The only significant risk of combined oral contraceptives in the otherwise healthy, low-risk adolescent pill user is thromboembolic disease, primarily deep venous thrombosis (DVT). The risk in combination OCP users under age 35 is around 15 per 100,000. These risks are higher among smokers and carriers of inherited thrombophilic disorders, the most common being the factor V Leiden mutation. Presence of these disorders is an absolute contraindication to estrogen-containing oral contraceptives. Consider screening for hereditary thrombophilias prior to combination OCP prescription if family history reveals a blood clot or stroke at a young age in a first-degree relative, particularly if the event occurred in pregnancy or postpartum.

Teens who carry the methylenetetrahydrofolate reductase (MTHFR) mutation may safely use estrogen-containing pills if they are assured adequate folic acid intake. This mutation leads to elevated homocysteine levels, a risk factor for both arterial and venous thrombosis. Treatment with folic acid supplementation stabilizes the mutated enzyme, resulting in a normal homocysteine level and eliminating the excess risk for thrombosis. The dosage of folic acid used varies from 1 to 5 mg daily.

Pill users should be advised to notify their physician immediately if they have chest pain, shortness of breath, new-onset headache, or leg pain associated with swelling, redness, or heat, which may indicate presence of a clot. Many pediatricians teach their patients the ACHES acronym to remember signs of clots (A=abdominal pain, C=chest pain, H=severe, crushing headache, E=eye or visual loss, S=severe leg pain or swelling).

It may be worthwhile to warn all pill users against prolonged immobilization on long plane flights, which increases thrombotic risk. Common-sense strategies for long flights include drinking adequate water, avoiding caffeine and alcohol (which cause dehydration), moving about the plane hourly, and deplaning during layovers.

Recent meta-analysis suggests that pills containing the third generation progestins desogestrel (eg, Desogen, Ortho-Cept, Mircette and Cyclessa) and gestodene (not available in the US) may be associated with DVT risk twice that of pills containing the second-generation progestins, norethindrone and levonorgestrel. Multiple reanalyses of the data have failed to result in a unifying expert opinion on the matter. Most US experts agree that *if* there is an increased risk, its magnitude is not large enough to justify any change in prescribing practices. Suffice it to say that adolescents known to be at increased risk for thrombosis should not take an estrogen-containing contraceptive, regardless of the progestin used.

No increased risk for thrombosis has been reported in users of progestin-only contraceptive pills or other progestin-only methods. Despite statements to the contrary on package labeling, contraceptive experts agree that progestin-only methods are safe in women with a risk for thrombosis.

BREAST CANCER

Multiple studies, including several meta-analyses, have failed to show a consistent relationship between oral contraceptive use and breast cancer risk. Although there may be a small increase in breast cancer diagnoses among women under age 35 in the first 5 years of pill use, the lifetime risk of breast cancer is not elevated in pill users, even those with a family history.

Use of Oral Contraceptives in Adolescents with Special Medical Conditions

With careful evaluation and close monitoring, oral contraceptives are safe in most adolescents with chronic medical conditions. Specific considerations apply:

- **Diabetes:** OCP use is safe for patients whose diabetes is well controlled, who have no evidence of end organ or vascular involvement, or who have had diabetes for less than 20 years.
- **Post partum:** Avoid estrogen-containing pills in first 2–3 weeks post partum, since this period is associated with increased risk of thrombosis. Consider POPs.
- **Breast-feeding:** Consider progestin-only pills, which are lactogenic. After breast-feeding is well established, combination pills can be used.
- **Hypertension:** If hypertension is well controlled, OCPs are appropriate with careful monitoring. If hypertension occurs with pill use, consider POPs or other progestin-only methods.
- **Migraine headache:** Use a monophasic pill. Avoid OCP use if focal neurologic symptoms accompany migraines. For patients without neurologic symptoms, monitor headaches with pill use and discontinue if headaches increase in frequency or intensity. Headaches occurring in the pill-free interval may respond to continuous OCP use without placebo, since the migraine trigger may be estrogen withdrawal in these patients. Alternatively, a low dose estradiol patch can be prescribed for use in the pill-free interval.

- **Hyperlipidemia:** Consider a third-generation OCP (potentially less effect on lipids). Monitor closely.
- **Biliary tract disease:** Active disease contraindicates estrogen-containing OCPs. Prior cholecystectomy does not.
- **Hepatitis:** Active disease contraindicates OCP use. OCPs are safe in chronic hepatitis B or C carriers with normal liver enzymes.
- **Sickle cell anemia:** OCPs are safe in patients with sickle cell disease; any formulation can be used. Ischemia in sickle cell anemia is not related to abnormalities in the thrombotic cascade. Consider Depo-Provera because it has been shown to stabilize the red cell membrane and lead to decreased frequency of sickle crises. This effect has not been shown with other progestins.
- **Seizure disorders:** Adolescents with seizure disorders can safely use estrogen-containing OCPs. However, interaction between antiseizure medications and oral contraceptives must be considered (see drug interactions). Depo Provera may be a better choice for these patients.

CERVICAL CANCER

Multiple studies have raised concerns about increased risk of cervical cancer in OCP users. However, when confounding factors (eg, smoking, number of sexual partners, barrier use, and Pap smear frequency) are controlled, no consistent association is found, except for the very rare adenocarcinoma of the cervix. One recent study suggests an increased risk of cervical carcinoma in HPV-positive women who used the pill for longer than 5 years.[8] How this information translates to adolescent pill users who may transiently acquire HPV is unclear. Consistent condom use, limiting numbers of sexual partners, and getting annual Pap smears are currently the most important recommendations for preventing cervical cancer.

CHLAMYDIA AND PID RISKS IN OCP USERS

Research has shown lower rates of symptomatic pelvic inflammatory disease (PID) among oral contraceptive users. This may be due to thickening of cervical mucus and reduced menstrual flow. However, given the high rates of silent PID caused by chlamydia, rates of *symptomatic* PID may not be a reliable indicator of actual upper-tract infections in pill users. The risk of chlamydia cervicitis may actually be increased among users of OCPs, due to cervical ectopy. The importance of consistent condom use for STD prevention cannot be stressed enough.

OTHER RISKS

Other risks associated with OCP use are confined to certain population subgroups. For example, there is an increase in the incidence of myocardial infarction in OCP users over 35 who smoke or have cardiac risk factors such as hypertriglyceridemia. OCP-induced cholestasis may exacerbate or reveal underlying gallbladder disease. Benign liver tumors were associated with older high-dose OCPs, but not with currently used low-dose (35 µg or lower) pills. Preexisting benign liver tumors remain a contraindication to combined oral contraceptive use. Pseudotumor cerebri, common in reproductive-age women and in pregnancy, can occur in association with most hormonal contraceptives, including progestin-only methods. Oral contraceptives should be discontinued if pseudotumor cerebri is diagnosed.

CONTRAINDICATIONS TO COMBINED ORAL CONTRACEPTIVES

Most contraindications to oral contraceptives relate to the estrogen component of the pill, and are summarized in Table 2. Most relative contraindications relate to use of OCPs in individuals with underlying medical conditions. Recommendations for pill use in these adolescents are summarized in the box on page 685.

Drug Interactions With Oral Contraceptives

Drug interactions with OCPs fall into two categories: those drugs that affect oral contraceptive efficacy, and those drugs whose metabolism is affected by oral contraceptives. Most drugs that interact with OCPs induce hepatic cytochrome P450 enzymes, causing increased metabolism of

---

Table 2. Contraindications to Estrogen-Containing Oral Contraceptives*

- History of active thromboembolic disease or hypercoagulable state[†]
- Cerebrovascular or coronary artery disease[†]
- Known or suspected carcinoma of the breast
- Carcinoma of the endometrium or other known or suspected estrogen-dependent neoplasia
- Undiagnosed abnormal genital bleeding
- Cholestatic jaundice of pregnancy or jaundice with prior pill use
- Hepatic adenomas or carcinomas; active liver disease
- Known or suspected pregnancy

---

* For additional information about medical eligibility for OCP use, refer to Hatcher et al, *Contraceptive Technology* (see resource list), or visit the World Health Organization Web site for a downloadable copy of *WHO Medical Eligibility Criteria 2000* (go to http://www.who.int/ and search on medical eligibility)

† May consider POPs

the estrogen and/or progestin component of the pill, leading to lower hormonal blood levels and decreased efficacy. Other drugs alter gastrointestinal absorption or affect serum protein binding, changing free hormone levels.

ANTICONVULSANTS

Phenobarbital, phenytoin, primidone, carbamazepine, topiramate, and ethosuximide induce liver enzymes and lower hormone levels. Consider prescribing a high-dose (50 μg EE) oral contraceptive in adolescents taking these medications, reducing the pill-free interval to 3 or 4 days, or eliminating the placebo interval entirely. If breakthrough bleeding occurs on high-dose pills, efficacy is likely to be compromised and an alternative method should be used. Consider using Depo-Provera, as its metabolism is not affected by anticonvulsants. In addition, Depo-Provera itself is antiexcitatory in the central nervous system, and can actually lower seizure frequency. (*Note:* valproic acid does NOT affect oral contraceptive metabolism or efficacy.)

ANTIBIOTICS

The theory behind this interaction is that antibiotic-induced alterations in intestinal flora impair enterohepatic recirculation, leading to lower hormonal levels. Numerous case reports and uncontrolled retrospective studies have implicated antibiotics, most often ampicillin and tetracyclines, in reducing oral contraceptive efficacy. No pharmacokinetic data exist to support these claims for any antibiotic other than rifampin (a known cytochrome P450 inducer) and griseofulvin (probably hepatic enzyme induction). However, certain individuals may be at risk due to a combination of low bioavailability of EE, large enterohepatic recirculation, and/or susceptible intestinal flora. Current opinion is that short-term antibiotic use does not reduce oral contraceptive efficacy. If breakthrough bleeding or diarrhea occurs, barrier contraception can be used short term. Adolescents using antibiotics long term can preferentially use 30–35 μg pills; if breakthrough bleeding occurs, a higher dose (50 μg) pill may be prescribed.

ST JOHN'S WORT

Herbal and dietary supplement use, unregulated by the FDA, is widespread and increasing. St John's Wort is a particularly popular herb, usually taken as a pill or capsule, but also added to juices, soups, and even potato chips. St. John's Wort has been shown to induce hepatic cytochrome P450. The FDA issued a warning to physicians and patients about potential interactions between St. John's Wort and medications utilizing this pathway, including oral contraceptives. Reports of pregnancies and irregular bleeding in OCP users taking St. John's Wort are beginning to surface. Until more data are available, oral contraceptive users should be advised against using St. John's Wort.

VITAMIN C

Although the data are contradictory, several studies have shown that high doses of vitamin C (1 gm or more daily) may increase hormonal levels as much as 50% in OCP users by impairing hormonal metabolism. Although this would not impact efficacy, it could lead to heavier or erratic withdrawal bleeding. Vitamin C dosages should not exceed 500 mg daily.

THEOPHYLLINE

Oral contraceptives reduce clearance of theophylline by as much as 50%. Theophylline doses should be lowered accordingly. The same effect is noted with caffeine.

ANALGESICS AND CORTICOSTEROIDS

Oral contraceptive use appears to lower aspirin levels. Chronic acetaminophen use can lead to increased ethinyl estradiol levels in OCP users. Oral contraceptive use may lead to decreased clearance and prolonged elimination of certain corticosteroids, notably hydrocortisone, prednisone, and prednisolone.

BENZODIAZEPINES

Oral contraceptives can decrease clearance of benzodiazepines such as diazepam, alprazolam, nitrazepam, and chlordiazepoxide.

ANTIRETROVIRALS

Most of the antiretrovirals used to treat HIV infection have interactions with medications metabolized by the cytochrome P450 system. Ritonavir decreases ethinyl estradiol levels by as much as 40%, and alternative contraception is recommended. Nevirapine and nelfinavir are presumed to act similarly. Indinavir can raise ethinyl estradiol levels, which could increase side effects.

Emergency Contraceptive Pills (ECPs)

Emergency contraceptive pills, or ECPs, are high doses of estrogen and/or progestin given within a short period of time after unprotected intercourse in an attempt to prevent pregnancy. It is estimated that emergency contraception could prevent up to half of the 3 million unintended pregnancies in the United States annually. Despite this, only 1%–2% of women in the United States have ever used emergency contraception. Only 24% of pediatricians have ever prescribed ECPs and only 17% routinely discuss the method with their patients.[9-11]

ECPs are theorized to work in several possible ways: preventing or delaying ovulation, impairing corpus luteum function, or causing endometrial changes unfavorable to implantation. The efficacy of ECPs ranges from 75% to 89%, reducing the risk of pregnancy from a single act of unprotected intercourse from an average of 8% to 1%–2%. The sooner ECPs are taken after unprotected intercourse, the more effective they are. Although a 72-hour limit has been customary, newer data suggest that this time limit can be safely extended to 4 to 5 days after unprotected intercourse. However, efficacy diminishes with time. ECPs will not interrupt an implanted pregnancy

The only contraindications to ECPs are known or suspected pregnancy, hypersensitivity to the product's components, or undiagnosed genital bleeding. Pregnancies conceived despite ECP use have no increase in congenital anomalies or adverse outcomes. There is growing consensus that ECPs are safe enough to be available over the counter. In Washington state and California, ECPs are available in pharmacies through collaborative agreements in which a physician delegates authority to prescribe ECPs to a pharmacist who has undergone extensive training for this purpose. A survey of adolescents who used this pharmacy service showed that if the service were unavailable, almost half would not have known what to do or would have done nothing, despite the fact that the majority had a private physician. Adolescents were satisfied with the pharmacy service; 94% said they would recommend it to a friend.[12]

Adolescents requesting ECPs do not need a special examination; a health history will suffice, along with pregnancy testing if preexisting pregnancy is suspected. It is appropriate (and encouraged) to give prescriptions over the phone for established patients. Several ECP regimens are currently available. It is wise to become familiar with more than one regimen and to check pharmacy availability before prescribing a given regimen.

It is reasonable to provide all adolescents using barrier methods with an anticipatory prescription or packet of ECPs along with instructions for their use. Three large studies have shown that patients who have ECPs on hand at home are significantly more likely to use them than those given education alone, and do not abuse the method or use it repeatedly.[13-15] However, young women who request or use emergency contraception are at high risk for pregnancy in the year following ECP use.[16] They should be advised to call the office after ECP use to arrange for follow-up and contraceptive counseling.

Adolescents using ECPs should be advised that their next menses may be early (if ECP is taken in the follicular phase), or delayed (if taken in the luteal phase). Half will have a normally timed menses, and most will bleed normally. Almost all (98%) will menstruate within 21 days; if not, pregnancy is a concern.[17]

ECP REGIMENS

The Yuzpe regimen: The Yuzpe regimen is the oldest and most widely used method, and can be given using one of 7 different OCP formulations or a prepackaged product (Preven). (See Table 3). The most common side effects are nausea

Table 3.* Emergency Contraceptive Pill Regimens†

ECP	Dosing
Yuzpe Regimen	
Preven	2 pills Q 12 H ∞ 2 doses
Ovral, Ogestrel	2 white pills Q 12 H ∞ 2 doses
Alesse, Levlite	5 pink pills Q 12 H ∞ 2 doses
Aviane	5 orange pills Q 12 H ∞ 2 doses
Nordette, Levlen	4 light-orange pills Q 12 H ∞ 2 doses
Levora, Lo/Ovral, Low-Ogestrel	4 white pills Q 12 H ∞ 2 doses
Triphasil, Tri-Levlen	4 yellow pills Q 12 H ∞ 2 doses
Trivora	4 pink pills Q 12 H ∞ 2 doses
Progestin-only Method	
Ovrette	20 yellow pills Q 12 H ∞ 2 doses‡
Plan B	1 pill Q 12 H ∞ 2 doses

* Here and elsewhere in the text, proprietary names illustrate products most often prescribed and with which pediatricians are likely to be familiar. This does not imply AAP endorsement. Equivalent products may be substituted. For more information, providers and patients might access the Emergency Contraception Hotline (1-888-not-2-late) and website (http://ec.princeton.edu).

† Examples in the table reflect packaging of products available in the US at this writing. Other prepackaged regimens and OCPs available for use outside the United States may vary somewhat from those above.

‡ Patient can crush pills and take in applesauce or yogurt.

(3%–50%) and vomiting (12%–22%). Consider prescribing an antiemetic along with the Yuzpe regimen. Other minor temporary side effects include breast tenderness, headache, cramping, fatigue, and dizziness.

Progestin-only method: The advantage to using progestin alone for emergency contraception is twofold. It is more effective (89% reduction in pregnancy risk), and it has much lower rates of associated nausea (23%), vomiting (6%), dizziness, and fatigue than the Yuzpe regimen. Two progestin-only methods are available: one utilizes progestin-only pills; the other (Plan B) is prepackaged.

An excellent ECP resource for both patients and providers is the Emergency Contraception Hotline (1-888-not-2-late) and Web site (http://ec.princeton.edu).

Summary

Oral contraceptives are a safe and effective contraceptive method with relatively few contraindications, and important noncontraceptive benefits. OCPs are suitable for any healthy, sexually active female desiring pregnancy prevention. In Part 2 of this two-part series we will address the more practical aspects of initiating OCPs and managing the adolescent oral contraceptive user, and briefly review the new long-acting hormonal alternatives to oral contraceptives.

Acknowledgement

The editors would like to acknowledge technical review by Melanie A. Gold, DO, FAAP, FACOP, for the AAP Section on Adolescent Health.

REFERENCES

1. Alan Guttmacher Institute. *Facts in Brief: Contraceptive Use.* New York, NY: The Alan Guttmacher Institute; 2000
2. Rosenberg MJ, Burnhill MS, Waugh MS, Grimes DA, Hillard PJ. Compliance and oral contraceptives: a review. *Contraception.* 1995;52:137–141
3. Klein JR, Litt IF. Epidemiology of adolescent dysmenorrhea. *Pediatrics.* 1981;68:661–664
4. Speroff L, Glass RH, Kase NG. *Clincal Gynecologic Endocrinology and Infertility.* 6th ed. Baltimore, MD: Lippincott Williams & Wilkins; 1999:546
5. Hatcher RA, Trussell J, Stewart F, et al. *Contraceptive Technology.* 17th rev. ed. New York, NY: Ardent Media; 1998:410 (New edition scheduled for release September 2002)
6. Kuohung W, Borgatta L, Stubblefield P. Low-dose oral contraceptives and bone mineral density: an evidence-based analysis. *Contraception.* 2000;61:77–82
7. Lloyd T, Taylor DS, Lin HM, Matthews AE, Eggli DF, Legro RS. Oral contraceptive use by teenage women does not affect peak bone mass: a longitudinal study. *Fertil Steril.* 2000;74:734–738

8. Moreno V, et al, and International Agency for Research on Cancer (IARC) Multicentric Cervical Cancer Study Group. Effect of oral contraceptives on risk of cervical cancer in women with human papillomavirus infection: the IARC multicentric case-control study. *Lancet.* 2002; 359(9312):1085–1092

9. Kaiser Family Foundation. 1997 Kaiser Family Foundation Survey of Americans on Emergency Contraception. http://www.kff.org/content/archive/1352/methodol.pdf (accessed May 3, 2002)

10. Sills MR, Chamberlain JM, Teach SJ. The associations among pediatricians' knowledge, attitudes, and practices regarding emergency contraception. *Pediatrics.* 2000; 105:954–956

11. Golden NH, Seigel WM, Fisher M, Schneider M, et al. Emergency contraception: Pediatricians' knowledge, attitudes, and opinions. *Pediatrics.* 2001;107:287–292

12. Sucato GS, Gardner JS, Koepsell TD. Adolescents' use of emergency contraception provided by Washington State pharmacists. *J Pediatr Adolesc Gynecol.* 2001;14:163–169

13. Ellertson C, Ambardekar S, Hedley A, Coyaji K, Trussell J, Blanchard K. Emergency contraception: Randomized comparison of advance provision and information only. *Obstet Gynecol.* 2001;98:570–575

14. Raine T, Harper C, Leon K, Darney P. Emergency contraception: Advance provision in a young, high-risk clinic population. *Obstet Gynecol.* 2000;96:1–7

15. Glasier A, Baird D. The effects of self-administering emergency contraception. *N Engl J Med.* 1998;339:1–4

16. Falk G, Falk L, Hanson U, Milsom I. Young women requesting emergency contraception are, despite contraceptive counseling, a high risk group for new unintended pregnancies. *Contraception.* 2001;64:23–27

17. American College of Obstetrics and Gynecology. Emergency Oral Contraception. ACOG Practice Bulletin No. 25. Washington, DC: American College of Obstetrics and Gynecology; 2001

Birth Control Pills: Learn the Facts

Patient Education Sheet

MYTH	FACT
What your friends may say...	**What to say to your friends...**
"The pill doesn't work very well."	"If I take my pill correctly, my chance of getting pregnant is less than 1 in 100. Those are pretty good odds, wouldn't you say?"
"Birth control pills make you fat."	"What makes you gain weight is taking in more calories than you need and not exercising, whether you're taking the pill or not. Want to join me for a run tomorrow?"
"Birth control pills make you sterile."	"That's an old one. Women who take pills have the same fertility as those who never took pills. Stopping my pill puts me at risk for having a child I'm not ready to have."
"You need a break from the pill."	"There is no medical benefit in taking a break from the pill. Stopping and starting means getting my body used to the pill all over again. Plus, if I stop, my period will be heavier and more painful, like it was before I started the pill. And if I take a break, I could end up pregnant."
"Those pills will give you cancer."	"Actually, it's an anti-cancer pill. I'm lowering my risk for cancer of the ovary and uterus by taking birth control pills."
"You only need to take your pill on the day you have sex."	"Wrong! I need to take it every day. Otherwise, I could get pregnant."
"The pill is dangerous."	"Taking birth control pills is safer than driving a car, and definitely safer than being pregnant."
	"And by the way, did you know that taking the pill can lessen menstrual cramps, lighten menstrual blood flow, prevent ovarian cysts, and even treat acne?"
"The pill will give you a heart attack or a stroke."	"Not true. In healthy young women, there is no increase in these risks while using pills. There is a very small risk of blood clots, about 1 in 15,000. The chances of developing a blood clot would be greater if I were to get pregnant."
"You smoke—you can't take the pill."	"Not true. In healthy women under 35 who smoke, the pill is safe. But smoking is not safe—I think I'm ready to quit. Shall we quit together?"
"The pill causes birth defects."	"Not true. The children born to women who take the pill have no increase in abnormalities."

Who started these myths?

● Most of these myths come from misunderstanding and fears. The media rely on scare stories to keep the public interested, and until recently, rarely said anything positive about oral contraceptives.

● Some concerns arose years ago, when oral contraceptives contained much higher hormone doses and were not as safe as they are today. Sadly, some groups don't believe women should use birth control of any kind. They spread rumors and misinformation about birth control in order to discourage women from using it.

If you hear or read something that concerns you, ask your doctor before stopping your pills. Odds are it's another rumor!

Pediatricians are encouraged to photocopy this page for distribution to patients and parents.

This patient education sheet is distributed in conjunction with the July 2002 issue of Adolescent Health Update, *published by the American Academy of Pediatrics. The information in this publication should not be used as a substitute for the medical care and advice of your pediatrician.*

Oral Contraceptives: Part 2

by Margaret Polaneczky, MD, FACOG

In part 1 of this two-part series (*AHU* 14:3, 2002), we discussed the basics of oral contraceptive pills (OCPs). Part 2 will focus on the practical aspects of prescribing oral contraceptives in an adolescent practice, including management of side effects, timing of the pelvic exam, patient confidentiality and parental issues, and counseling to increase compliance. A brief overview of newer long-acting hormonal contraceptives is also included.

Initial Considerations

Any healthy, sexually active adolescent female is a candidate for oral contraception. Younger postmenarchal adolescents can safely use oral contraception without adverse effects on growth or maturation of the hypothalamic-pituitary-ovarian axis. Many adolescents with chronic medical conditions can also safely use OCPs. (See Part 1)

Before prescribing OCPs, counseling is important to determine whether the pill is the best choice for your patient and whether she can use it effectively. Some issues to address in the counseling session are summarized in Table 1. Good counseling takes time. Preprinted pamphlets, Web-based resources, and ancillary staff can be helpful in this regard.

The best adolescent candidate for OCPs is a responsible, mature, healthy female who can reliably take a pill daily, or one who has taken the pill or any other daily medication successfully in the past. Adolescents who have had problems with pills (eg, trouble swallowing pills or difficulty remembering to take them) may be better served with an injectable long-acting method, or by the newer vaginal ring or contraceptive patch.

INITIATING ORAL CONTRACEPTIVES

A complete history and physical examination, including a breast and pelvic examination, Pap smear, and (usually) screening for sexually transmitted diseases, have been the traditional prerequisites for initiation of OCPs in the United States. As the dose of hormone in the pill has lowered, and the safety of oral contraceptives has increased, this requirement has been challenged as an unnecessary barrier to contraceptive access.[1] While breast and pelvic examination are unlikely to reveal any conditions that contraindicate OCP use, a detailed medical and family history and blood pressure measurement should detect (or raise suspicion for) any that exist. Several international and US professional organizations recognize that while breast and pelvic examination and Pap smear screening are important elements of routine care, *they should not necessarily be tied*

Learning Objectives

After reading part 2, pediatricians will be better prepared to:
- Initiate and monitor oral contraceptive use
- Encourage long-term compliance
- Discuss principles underlying selection of an appropriate oral contraceptive
- Manage common side effects of oral contraceptives
- Use oral contraceptives to manage the menstrual cycle
- Understand how oral contraceptives compare with longer-acting hormonal contraceptive methods

---

Margaret Polaneczky, MD, FACOG is an associate professor of clinical obstetrics and gynecology, Weill Medical College of Cornell University, New York, NY

Adolescent Health Update, Vol 15, No. 1, October 2002

Table 1. Is Your Patient an Appropriate Candidate for Oral Contraception? Some Questions to Ask:

- Has she had previous experience with the pill? If so, what was it and how will this pill be different (or not)?
- Does she have a plan for remembering to take a pill every day?
- Where does she plan to keep her pills?
- Does she have fears or concerns about the pill?
- What have her friends told her and what has she heard in the media?
- Does she understand how the pill works?
- Does she know how to take the pill, and what to do if she misses a pill?
- Is she prepared to handle breakthrough bleeding in the first few cycles?
- Does her partner know about and support her pill use?
- Does she know about the noncontraceptive benefits of the pill?
- Does she acknowledge the need for barrier methods for STD prevention?

to the provision of oral contraceptives. In addition, the FDA has changed pill labeling to state: "A periodic history and physical examination is appropriate for all women, including women using oral contraceptives. The physical examination, however, may be deferred until after initiation of oral contraceptives if requested by the woman and judged appropriate by the clinician."

When adolescents are given the option to delay the pelvic examination, only a minority choose to do so; of these, close to 80% return for the examination within 6 months.[2,3] In one study, teens who delayed the exam had lower pregnancy rates and similar STD rates to those who did not delay.[4]

What should the pill-start visit include? A detailed medical and family history should be taken. Breast exam and pelvic examination with Pap smear and STD testing can then be performed. If there are no contraindications and the patient prefers it, the examination can be deferred for a later time. This allows more time to counsel the adolescent about safety and use of her pill, provide anticipatory guidance for minor side effects, and address any concerns and questions. Urine-based testing for gonorrhea and chlamydia can be done if the pelvic exam is deferred and STDs are a concern. Urine pregnancy testing is useful, especially if the teen has been having unprotected sex.

There are two typical options for starting OCPs: same-day start (day 1 of the menses) and Sunday-start (first Sunday of the menstrual cycle).

- If the pill is begun on the first day of menses, it will be effective immediately (although efficacy in the first few days is more likely due to the cycle phase than the contraceptive itself). There are two advantages to starting on day 1 of menses: the cycle is a good reminder, and back-up contraception is not needed in the first week of use.
- With a Sunday start, the adolescent takes her first pill on the Sunday after her next menses (or the day her menses begin if they begin on a Sunday). Back-up contraception should be used for the first week of pill use. Sunday starts usually mean menses-free weekends, which many teens see as an advantage. However, Sunday-start patients can become confused when menses begin on a Sunday and wait a week to begin their pills; these teens may be at risk for pregnancy.

Patient initiation of the pill is tied to the menses to assure a nonpregnant state. However, if the menstrual period is abnormal in any way (eg, lighter than usual, late in timing), advise the teen to come in for pregnancy testing prior to starting the pill.

Give a prescription for a year's supply of pills (either 1 per month or 3 per quarter, depending on the insurance plan requirements). A follow-up visit at 1 to 3 months may enhance compliance and provide an opportunity to address side effects. Due to the incidence of STDs in this age group, STD screening can be done twice yearly; Pap smear is annual. If continued compliance or high-risk sexual activity is a concern, more frequent office visits or telephone follow-up may be advisable. Do not require an office visit for a prescription refill, however; this increases the risk of pregnancy. Adolescent pill users should be advised to continue to use condoms for STD protection; this should be reinforced at each encounter.

CHOOSING A PILL

For the otherwise healthy adolescent without specific concerns or prior side effects from hormonal contraception, the pill of choice is any low dose (20–35 μg) combination pill that she can afford and obtain easily (and ideally one that you have in your sample cabinet so that you can show her the pack and familiarize her with its use). If she requests a certain pill and has no contraindications to its use, give her that pill. If she has used a pill successfully before, give her that pill again. A more detailed approach that takes into account patient-specific issues that might influence choice of pill is summarized in Table 2.

Remember that not all pill-choice issues can be resolved by switching formulations. Sometimes a different hormonal contraceptive or a barrier method would be more appropriate. Don't get stuck in the "pill-only" habit. Inform your patients about these new methods. The more options a teen has, the better the odds she will find a method that works well for her.

BODY WEIGHT AND OCP CHOICE

A recent study has raised concern that oral contraceptive efficacy may be lower in women who are overweight. This retrospective analysis used data collected from over 600 women in a study of ovarian cysts, and found that women currently over 155 pounds were more likely to report that they had become pregnant in the past while taking birth control pills. Estimated failure rates in this weight group ranged from 5.2 per 100 person-years of use for 30 μg pills, to 6.8 per 100 person-years for 20 μg pills. Researchers did not collect information about compliance or weight at the time of OCP use, and relied on patient recall for pill identification.

At this point, the data are insufficient to recommend any changes in OCP prescribing practices. There are no data to suggest that properly-taken low-dose OCPs have lower efficacy than higher dose pills in heavier women. However, typical OCP use usually implies 1 or more missed pills per cycle, and it is conceivable that lower dose pill regimens may be less "forgiving" of missed pills in higher-weight women.

It is important to remember that oral contraceptives remain superior to barrier methods in preventing pregnancy in teens of any weight, and that, ultimately, compliance that will have the biggest impact on pregnancy rates. However, until better data are available, there is no harm in instructing overweight teens to use a back-up method whenever they miss a pill.

Managing Side Effects

It is the minor, or nuisance, side effects that will most affect long-term compliance. It is important to discuss side effects and to have a

Table 2. Choosing a Pill

Issue	Pill of Choice*
Contraindication to estrogen	Progesterone-only pill
Concern/history of estrogen-related side effects (nausea, breast tenderness)	20 μg pill (Alesse, Mircette, Levlite, Loestrin 1/20)
Migraine headaches	20 μg monophasic pill (Alesse, Mircette, Levlite, Loestrin 1/20)
Menstrual migraines (worsening of migraine headaches at the time of menses)	Mircette. Any other 20 μg monophasic pill (Alesse, Levlite, Loestrin 1/20), either continuously (no days off) or with the estrogen patch on pill-free days
Acne, hirsutism, polycystic ovary syndrome	Any pill. If a less androgenic progestin is desired, (norgestimate, desogestrel, or drospirenone), try Ortho Tri-Cyclen, Ortho-Cyclen, Ortho-Cept, Desogen, or Yasmin. The least androgenic first generation pill is Ovcon-35
Breakthrough bleeding	Monophasic or triphasic 30-35 μg pill. If bleeding occurred on a 20 μg pill, choose a 30-35 μg pill. If on a triphasic pill, choose a monophasic preparation.

*Here and elsewhere in the text, proprietary names are used to illustrate products that are most often prescribed and with which pediatricians are likely to be familiar. This does not imply AAP endorsement. Equivalent products may be substituted. For a more complete listing of available oral contraceptives, see Hatcher RA, Trussell J, Stewart F, et al. *Contraceptive Technology.* 17th rev. ed. New York, NY: Ardent Media; 1998:430–432

plan for dealing with the more common ones that may prompt the adolescent patient to stop taking her pills. Although serious adverse effects (discussed in Part 1 of this series) are uncommon, your patient needs to know which symptoms warrant an immediate call to your office (see patient information sheet).

BREAKTHROUGH BLEEDING

Irregular bleeding or spotting is common in the first few cycles of pill use. Bleeding rates are higher in pills with 20 µg ethinyl estradiol than in those with 30 to 35 µg. If breakthrough bleeding begins or persists beyond the first few cycles, take a careful pill history—it is likely the adolescent is missing pills. Explore possible interacting medications, herbs, or vitamins (see Part 1). Screen for chlamydia, gonorrhea, and trichomonas infection, and for cervical dysplasia. If the patient is taking a triphasic pill, change her to a monophasic formulation. Increase the estrogen dose if she is on a 20 µg pill, or try a pill containing a different progestin or a higher dose of the same progestin. Most breakthrough bleeding will resolve over time, especially if noncompliance is the cause. If compliance continues to be a concern, consider a longer-acting hormonal method.

Breakthrough bleeding that persists despite these measures warrants sonogram and referral to a gynecologist for further evaluation.

Amenorrhea

Prolonged use of any oral contraceptive can lead to amenorrhea, although this side effect is more common in the 20 µg pills. The incidence is about 6%. Once pregnancy is ruled out, the patient can be reassured. If the patient desires regular menses, a higher dose pill can be prescribed, or a short course of estrogen (6 weeks) can be given to supplement the current pill. Stopping the pill for a cycle or two usually resolves the problem, but is not advised because it could lead to pregnancy in the intervening months.

WEIGHT GAIN

Weight gain is usually not a direct side effect of oral contraceptives. Studies of modern low-dose pills have failed to show significant weight changes in pill users when compared to those on placebo or using nonhormonal methods. Adolescent weight change can occur as a normal part of pubertal growth or as a result of changes in diet and exercise patterns. Because the weight gain may be perceived rather than real, obtaining a weight is critical. It is best to focus on diet, exercise, and lifestyle issues, and to be sure the adolescent's expectations of body weight are realistic. Changing to a pill with a different progestin or a lower estrogen dose may help the adolescent who gains weight due to fluid retention or who experiences undesired increase in breast size or appetite.

HEADACHE

Headaches are a common health complaint. Rather than assuming an adolescent's headaches are from the pill, rule out other causes before discontinuing necessary contraception. One exception is worsening or new-onset migraine with neurologic or visual symptoms; these patients are at increased risk for stroke. OCPs should be discontinued immediately and evaluation made.

It is important to note the timing of headaches in the pill cycle. Typical migraines or migraines in the pill-free interval may be due to estrogen withdrawal. Changing to a 20 µg monophasic pill, shortening the placebo interval, going to continuous OCP without placebos, or using a low-dose estradiol patch in the placebo week are all acceptable strategies for dealing with estrogen-withdrawal headaches. Mircette has a shortened placebo interval, although it has not been specifically studied for headache relief.

NAUSEA

Like most estrogen-related side effects, this problem usually resolves after the first few cycles. Taking pills with food and never in the morning on an empty stomach may be all that is needed to resolve the problem. If this is unsuccessful, change to a 20 µg pill. To be sure the problem is related to the pill and not a sign of gastrointestinal or biliary disease, ask about nausea in the pill-free week—it should resolve at that time. If nausea only occurs at the beginning of each new pack, consider trying Mircette (see headache), or using OCPs continuously without placebos. Adolescents who cannot take combination pills due to nausea are ideal candidates for progestin-only methods, or lower dose combination methods such as Lunelle.

BREAST TENDERNESS (MASTALGIA)

This is a relatively common complaint, usually confined to the first few cycles of pill use. Assuming it is bilateral and not associated with breast pathology, changing to a 20 µg pill can help. Use of a supportive bra and elimination or decrease in caffeine may help. Evening primrose oil, 1000 mg daily, has been shown to decrease mastalgia in placebo-controlled trials.

DEPRESSION OR MOOD CHANGES

Oral contraceptives have been reported to improve as well as worsen mood. A careful history will determine if symptoms are related to the pill or are preexisting. A symptom diary may reveal premenstrual syndrome (PMS), which can be treated without discontinuing pill use. Changing progestin dose or type, or switching to a lower estrogen dose or to a monophasic preparation may help. Yasmin, a new OCP, has been shown to decrease PMS symptoms as well as bloating, and may be worth trying.

Sometimes a pill-free interval is necessary to answer the question as to whether the pill is the problem or not. One cycle should be enough to know. During the trial, recommend abstinence and remind the patient that condom use for STD protection will also reduce risk of pregnancy.

CHLOASMA

Chloasma is an estrogen-related brown skin pigmentation that is harmless, and may be prevented with sunscreen or treated with skin-lightening agents. Changing to a progestin-only method may resolve the problem.

Negotiating the Teen-Parent Relationship

Caring for sexually active adolescents can become complicated when parents and teen disagree about contraceptive use, or when the teen desires confidential care despite parental presence or involvement. It is important to be clear with both teens and their parents on how you handle such situations.

No state specifically requires parental consent for the provision of contraceptive services to adolescents at this writing. However, Texas and Utah do restrict the use of state funds to provide contraception to minors without parental consent. By law, all Title X funded clinics are required to provide services regardless of age, sex, or income. Because restrictions can change at any time, it is important to stay current with state and federal laws.

It is best to establish the "ground rules" of your relationship with the adolescent patient. Explain to parents that you will provide confidential sexuality counseling, including the option of abstinence, contraception, STD treatment (and pregnancy-related care where permitted) to their daughter, all the while encouraging dialogue and openness between parent and child. A brochure can be helpful in relaying this information to parents.

It is best to see adolescents alone in the examining room, explaining to the parents that this encourages adolescents to take responsibility for their health. If you are uncomfortable about providing contraception in a confidential manner when requested, refer adolescents elsewhere.

In many situations, the noncontraceptive benefits of oral contraception provide legitimate reasons for their use in a sexually active young woman, allowing for parental knowledge and support of their use.

Certain situations may require parental involvement, such as chronic medical conditions or medication use that can be affected by a contraceptive. In these situations, it is important to explain to the patient why parental involvement is important to her health and to obtain her agreement before involving a parent in the discussion.

The need for long-delayed parent-child dialogue often becomes apparent when the issue of contraception is brought up. If both mother and daughter ask you privately about contraception, it's time to encourage a dialogue. Don't be afraid to step into the fray and get these individuals talking to one another.

Make sure your office staff is clear regarding confidentiality policies and that there is a plan for dealing with reimbursement issues related to office visits and laboratory tests. Establish a clear policy regarding responses to parents who ask to see confidential medical records.

Managing the Menstrual Cycle Using OCPs

One advantage of OCPs is that users can plan their cycles around travel, exams, proms, or other activities by taking consecutive pills without days off, reserving placebo use (and their menses) for a better time in their schedule. There are no known health risks to manipulating menses in this way. In fact, there can be significant benefits in having less frequent menses, particularly in teens who experience dysmenorrhea, menstrual migraines, or menorrhagia. This approach is probably most successful using a monophasic 30–35 μg pill.

Prolonged exposure of the endometrium to hormones in the pill without permitting withdrawal bleeding can lead to spotting in continuous oral contraceptive users, possibly due to down-regulation of estrogen receptors in the endometrium. While this is harmless, going to placebos for a week and then restarting usually resolves the problem. Most users find they will need to allow a withdrawal bleed every 2-6 months to avoid spotting.

Oral Contraceptives and Sexual Activity

There are no data to support the notion that providing contraception to adolescents encourages sexual activity, or conversely, that denying contraception prevents or delays sexual activity. Data from school-based clinics show that providing referral for contraceptive services does not increase rates of sexual activity among students in those schools.

One of the most important protective factors against teen pregnancy is a high quality parent-child relationship. Teens who report good relationships with their parents are far more likely to delay sexual activity, and are more likely to use contraception when they do become sexually active.

Hormonal Contraception: It's Not Just the Pill Anymore

The oral contraceptive pill has been the mainstay of pregnancy prevention in the United States for decades, and is still the most popular form of birth control used by adolescents. However, the pill has some drawbacks, most notably, the need to take it every day.

Enter the long-acting hormonal contraceptives. These methods are formulations of progestins, alone or combined with estrogen, designed to circumvent the need for daily compliance. All have efficacy rates very close to 100%, and like oral contraceptive pills, are extremely safe. For adolescents who have problems remembering to take a pill every day, or who desire the convenience of a long-acting method, these new methods provide a welcome alternative to the pill. In 1995, 20% of adolescents reported using either injectables or implants, a testimony to just how popular these methods may become. If you prescribe contraception in your practice, it is important to become well versed in all the viable options available to your patients.

DEPOT MEDROXYPROGESTERONE ACETATE (DEPO-PROVERA)

Depo-Provera is 150 mg of the progestin depot medroxyprogesterone acetate, given as an intramuscular injection once every 12 weeks in either the deltoid or gluteal muscle. The method is extremely effective, safe, and well tolerated. Side effects are typical for a progestin-only method, with menstrual alterations predominating. In this case, amenorrhea is the predominant bleeding pattern, with 70% of users amenorrheic by 2 years of use. However, for some, irregular bleeding can be problematic. Although the majority of adolescent Depo-Provera users maintain or lose weight, Depo-Provera users are more likely than oral contraceptive users to gain weight (25% vs 7% in one study), with weight gain possibly higher in teens who are overweight to begin with.[5,6]

Depo-Provera suppresses ovarian follicular development, and estradiol levels are suppressed to early follicular phase levels. There are concerns that this could affect long-term peak bone mass in younger adolescents. Although some experts advise against Depo-Provera use until after age 15, when the majority of bone has been laid down, the risk for pregnancy may outweigh this concern in those adolescents who cannot use other methods well.[7]

Advantages of Depo-Provera include long-acting effectiveness, lack of estrogen, few drug interactions, and induction of amenorrhea in patients with endometriosis, dysmenorrhea, or menorrhagia. Although Depo-Provera does not adversely affect fertility, return of ovulation may be delayed due to the long-acting nature of the drug. In adolescents, this may be seen as an advantage. The method is also private.

MONTHLY COMBINATION INJECTABLE (LUNELLE)

Lunelle is depot medroxyprogesterone acetate 25 mg/estradiol cypionate 5 mg in aqueous solution given as an intramuscular injection once a month. The small amount of estrogen in Lunelle minimizes irregular bleeding and other side effects associated with Depo-Provera use. In studies of adults, 75% of Lunelle users had regular menses. Rates of amenorrhea and breakthrough bleeding were about 15% and 10% respectively in any given cycle. The use of estrogen also addresses bone loss concerns associated with use of depot medroxyprogesterone acetate alone, although no clinical studies have confirmed this protective effect.

Like Depo-Provera, Lunelle was associated with some weight gain in clinical trials with adults (5.7% of users). Efficacy is high (99.7%) and return to fertility after discontinuation is rapid (2 to 4 months).

Contraindications for Lunelle are similar to those for estrogen-containing oral contraceptives. The lower dose of estrogen in Lunelle compared

---

Resources*

For providers

- Hatcher RA, Trussell J, Stewart F, et al. *Contraceptive Technology.* 17th rev. ed. New York, NY: Ardent Media; 1998. (New edition expected fall 2002; 1-800/218-1535.)
- Hatcher RA, Zieman M, Watt A, et al. *A Pocket Guide to Managing Contraception.* Tiger, GA: Bridging the Gap Foundation; 1999. Also online at http://www.managingcontraception.com/
- Contraception Online. An online resource sponsored by Baylor College of Medicine. Includes sample patient education materials and online access to the *Contraception Report.* http://www.contraceptiononline.org

For adolescents

- TeenGrowth.com. Physician-directed interactive site where adolescents can find sound information on a variety of health topics. http://www.teengrowth.com/
- The Center for Young Women's Health. Sponsored by Children's Hospital, Boston. Resources for adolescents, families, and health professionals. http://www.youngwomenshealth.org/
- I Wanna' Know. Information from the American Social Health Association on puberty, sexuality, and STDs. http://www.iwannaknow.org/

For parents

- The Facts of Life: A Guide for Teens and Their Families. Facts about contraception, abortion, STDs, and teen pregnancy from the Planned Parenthood Foundation. Extensive resource links. http://www.plannedparenthood.org/teens/teentalk1.html

These resources are included as sources of general information only. Their content has not been reviewed or endorsed by the American Academy of Pediatrics.

with oral contraceptives may make this method a good choice for teens who experience nausea or breast tenderness on oral contraceptives.

TRANSDERMAL PATCH (ORTHO EVRA)

Ortho Evra contains norelgestromin, a primary metabolite of norgestimate, and ethinyl estradiol in a 4.5 cm square polyester patch. The patch is applied to the lower abdomen, buttocks, upper outer arm, or upper torso (not the breast). Estrogen doses are similar to a 20 μg pill. The patch is changed once a week for 3 weeks, followed by a patch-free week to allow for menses.

Pregnancy rates with the patch were 1.2 per 100 person-years of use, compared with 2.2 pregnancies in oral contraceptive users in a large multicenter adult clinical trial.[8] Decreased contraceptive efficacy was suggested in women over 196 lbs.

About 20% of patch users experienced breakthrough bleeding in the first cycle, although this decreased over time to less than 10%. Compliance with the patch was significantly better than pills. The patch was well tolerated, with safety and side effect profiles similar to oral contraceptives. Exceptions were breast tenderness, which was slightly higher in the patch group, and patch site reactions. Application site reactions led to discontinuation of the patch in 3% of users. Visibility of the patch could be problematic for adolescents who need confidentiality. Contraindications are the same as for the combination oral contraceptives.

CONTRACEPTIVE VAGINAL RING (NUVARING)

The contraceptive vaginal ring is a soft, flexible, nonbiodegradable transparent ring approximately 2 inches in diameter. The ring is worn for 3 weeks (21 days), during which time it releases on average 0.12 mg of etonogestrel and 0.015 mg of ethinyl estradiol per day. The ring is then removed for 7 days to allow for menses. A new ring is then inserted for the next cycle.

The ring is inserted by the user within 5 days of the onset of menses. It can be worn during menstrual bleeding and during intercourse. Among adults, user satisfaction is high. The ring does not have to be fitted, and its exact positioning within the vagina is not critical for efficacy, so it cannot be incorrectly inserted within the vagina. There is no increase in vaginal infections during ring use.

The ring inhibits ovulation in a manner similar to oral contraceptives, with failure rates of 0.65 pregnancies per 100 woman years. Breakthrough bleeding rates are very low (less than 10%) and close to 100% of users have regular withdrawal bleeding, a profile better than that seen with oral contraceptive users in comparison studies. Greater than 90% of cycles were completely compliant.[9,10]

The safety profile and contraindications for the ring are similar to those of combination oral contraceptives. For teens who are comfortable with inserting and removing a vaginal device, the vaginal ring is a safe, effective, and private option for contraception.

THE LEVONORGESTREL IMPLANT (NORPLANT)

Norplant is six silastic capsules containing the progestin levonorgestrel that are placed under the skin on the inner surface of the arm, providing contraception for 5 years. Studies have shown Norplant to be safe and highly effective in preventing adolescent pregnancies. However, due to limitations in product component supply, it will no longer be manufactured. Current users remain protected against pregnancy for the 5-year duration of use.

Conclusion

The components of effective oral contraception provision include (1) identifying appropriate candidates for the pill, (2) choosing an appropriate formulation both for contraception and other beneficial effects, (3) counseling to maximize compliance and minimize unnecessary patient concerns, (4) management of side effects that can lead to method discontinuation, and (5) knowing the alternative methods available for adolescents who cannot or should not use the pill.

Although new contraceptive methods are becoming more popular, oral contraceptives remain a mainstay of pregnancy prevention for adolescents. Their long record of safety and efficacy, as well as numerous noncontraceptive benefits, make them an ideal contraceptive choice for many young women.

Acknowledgment

The editors would like to acknowledge technical review by Melanie A. Gold, DO, FAAP, FACOP, for the AAP Section on Adolescent Health.

References

1. Stewart FH, Harper CC, Ellerston CE, Grimes DA, Sawaya GF, Trussel J. Clinical breast and pelvic examination requirements for hormonal contraception: Current practice vs. evidence. *JAMA.* 2001;285:2232–2239

2. Armstrong KA, Stover MA. SMART START: An option for adolescents to delay the pelvic examination and blood work in family planning clinics. *J Adolesc Health.* 1994;15:389–395

3. Harper C, Balistreri L, Boggess J, Leon K, Darney P. Provision of hormonal contraceptives without a mandatory pelvic examination: The First Stop demonstration project. *Fam Plann Perspect.* 2001;33:13–18

4. Sawaya GF, Harper C, Balistreri E, Boggess J, Darney P. Cervical neoplasia risk in women provided hormonal contraception without a Pap smear. *Contraception.* 2001;63:57–60

5. Risser WL, Gefter LR, Barratt MS, Risser JM. Weight change in adolescents who used hormonal contraception. *J Adolesc Health.* 1999;24:433–436

6. Mangan SA, Larsen PG, Hudson S. Overweight teens at increased risk for weight gain while using depot medroxyprogesterone acetate. *J Pediatr Adolesc Gynecol.* 2002;15:79–82

7. Cromer BA, Blair JM, Mahan JD, Zibners L, Naumovski Z. A prospective comparison of bone density in adolescent girls receiving depot medroxyprogesterone acetate (Depo-Provera), levonorgestrel (Norplant), or oral contraceptives. *J Pediatr.* 1996;129:671–676

8. Audet MC, Moreau M, Koltun WD, et al. Evaluation of contraceptive efficacy and cycle control of a transdermal contraceptive patch vs an oral contraceptive: A randomized controlled trial. *JAMA.* 2001;285:2347–2354

9. Roumen FJ, Apter D, Mulders TM, Dieben TO. Efficacy, tolerability and acceptability of a novel contraceptive vaginal ring releasing etonogestrel and ethinyl oestradiol. *Hum Reprod.* 2001;16:469–475

10. Bjarnadottir RI, Tuppurainen M, Killick SR. Comparison of cycle control with a combined contraceptive vaginal ring and oral levonorgestrel/ethinyl estradiol. *Am J Obstet Gynecol.* 2002;186:389–395

Taking oral contraceptives

HOW THEY WORK

The hormones in your birth control pill prevent pregnancy primarily by:

- Preventing the ovary from releasing an egg
- Thickening the mucus at the entrance to the uterus, blocking the sperm from getting in

When birth control pills are taken properly, the chance of becoming pregnant is less than 1 in 100.

TAKING YOUR PILL

Take one pill every day, preferably at the same time each day. The pill only works if taken every day, even if you don't have sex very often.

When to start your first pack of pills:

You and your health care provider will decide one of two schedules to start your pills after discussing the benefits and drawbacks of each:

1. *Start your pills on the first day of your next period.* You will be protected from pregnancy right from the start.

   or

2. *Start your pills the first Sunday after the first day of your next period, or the first day of your period if your menses begin on a Sunday.* The pill will become effective after you take it for 7 days. Although using a condom for disease protection decreases your pregnancy risk, the safest thing to do is abstain from sex until you've taken a full week of pills.

   Your pill pack has two kinds of pills: "active" pills with hormone, and "placebo" pills without hormone. You need to take all the active pills to prevent pregnancy. Taking the placebos is the trigger for your period. Take the placebo pills unless your health care provider tells you otherwise. There is no sugar in the placebo pills.

IF YOU BLEED BETWEEN YOUR PERIODS

Breakthrough bleeding is common and expected in the first 3 months of pill use. It can be as light as spotting or as heavy as a period. DO NOT skip or stop your pills. DO call your health care provider if you are concerned.

WHAT TO DO IF YOU MISS AN "ACTIVE" PILL:

- *If you are late taking a pill,* take it as soon as you remember it.
- *If you miss taking a pill for one day,* take it as soon as you remember it the next day. Take that day's pill at the regular time. If this means taking 2 pills at once, that's ok.

- *If you miss two pills,* take 2 pills a day for the next two days, then finish your pack of pills as usual. You are at risk for getting pregnant in the 7 days after missing pills. Although using a condom for disease protection decreases your pregnancy risk, the safest thing to do is abstain from sex until you've taken a full week of pills again.
- *If you miss more than 2 pills,* throw out the pack of pills and start a new pack that day. You are at risk for getting pregnant in the 7 days after missing pills. Although using a condom for disease protection decreases your pregnancy risk, the safest thing to do is abstain from sex until you've taken a full week of pills again.

Call your doctor right away if you have:

- Severe stomach or chest pain
- Trouble breathing
- Unusual, severe or worsening headaches
- Difficulty seeing
- Leg pain or swelling

OTHER BENEFITS

Taking oral contraceptives may have certain additional benefits:

- Lighter, less painful, and more regular periods
- Decreased acne and less unwanted hair growth
- Fewer ovarian cysts
- Fewer benign (harmless) breast lumps
- Fewer pelvic infections
- Lower risk of ovarian and uterine cancer
- Stronger bones

WHAT ARE THE RISKS?

Women taking the pills have a small increased risk for getting a blood clot of the leg or lung. This risk is very low: about 1 in 15,000 women.

If you have any of the following conditions, you should not take the pill: breast or uterine cancer, unexplained vaginal bleeding, heart disease, blood clot or stroke, or liver disease. If you take any other medications or herbal supplements, discuss this with your health care provider.

The birth control pill does not protect against HIV (AIDS) or other sexually transmitted diseases. Regardless of contraceptive method, always use a condom!

This patient education sheet is distributed in conjunction with the October 2002 issue of Adolescent Health Update, *published by the American Academy of Pediatrics. The information in this publication should not be used as a substitute for the medical care and advice of your pediatrician.*

Pediatricians are encouraged to photocopy this page for distribution to patients and parents.

Oral Versus Vaginal Sex Among Adolescents: Perceptions, Attitudes, and Behavior

Bonnie L. Halpern-Felsher, PhD*; Jodi L. Cornell, MSW, MA*; Rhonda Y. Kropp, BScN, MPH*; and Jeanne M. Tschann, PhD‡

ABSTRACT. *Objective.* **Despite studies indicating that a significant proportion of adolescents are having oral sex, the focus of most empirical studies and intervention efforts concerning adolescent sexuality have focused on vaginal intercourse. This narrow focus has created a void in our understanding of adolescents' perceptions of oral sex. This study is the first to investigate adolescents' perceptions of the health, social, and emotional consequences associated with having oral sex as compared with vaginal sex, as well as whether adolescents view oral sex as more acceptable and more prevalent than vaginal sex.**

Methods. **Participants were 580 ethnically diverse ninth-grade adolescents (mean age: 14.54; 58% female) who participated in a longitudinal study on the relationship between risk and benefit perceptions and sexual activity. Participants completed a self-administered questionnaire that inquired about their sexual experiences and percent chance of experiencing outcomes from, attitudes toward, and perceived prevalence of oral versus vaginal sex among adolescents.**

Results. **More study participants reported having had oral sex (19.6%) than vaginal sex (13.5%), and more participants intended to have oral sex in the next 6 months (31.5%) than vaginal sex (26.3%). Adolescents evaluated oral sex as significantly less risky than vaginal sex on health, social, and emotional consequences. Adolescents also believed that oral sex is more acceptable than vaginal sex for adolescents their own age in both dating and nondating situations, oral sex is less of a threat to their values and beliefs, and more of their peers will have oral sex than vaginal sex in the near future.**

Conclusions. **Given that adolescents perceive oral sex as less risky, more prevalent, and more acceptable than vaginal sex, it stands to reason that adolescents are more likely to engage in oral sex. It is important that health care providers and others who work with youths recognize adolescents' views about oral sex and broaden their clinical preventive services to include screening, counseling, and education about oral sex.** *Pediatrics* **2005;115:**
845–851; *adolescent sexual behavior, risk perception, STDs, oral sex.*

ABBREVIATIONS. STI, sexually transmitted infection; ANOVA, analysis of variance.

Although the past several decades have produced a host of research on adolescent sexuality as well as numerous prevention and intervention efforts aimed at reducing adolescents' engagement in risky sexual behaviors, the majority of these efforts have focused solely on vaginal intercourse. This concentration has occurred despite studies indicating that a significant proportion of adolescents are engaging in noncoital sexual activities, including oral sex.[1-5] Studies indicate that between 14% and 50% of adolescents have had oral sex before their first experience with sexual intercourse,[3,5-8] that more adolescents have had oral sex than vaginal sex,[5,8,9] and that few adolescents who engage in oral sex are using barrier protection.[1,6,9] The emphasis on vaginal sex has resulted in intervention efforts providing limited education and guidance about oral sex, including the potential risk of sexually transmitted infections (STIs), including HIV.[1,10] Most clinical preventive service guidelines provide specific guidelines concerning only screening or education about vaginal sex or sex in more general terms.[11-14] To the extent that adolescents perceive oral sex as less risky and more acceptable and that these perceptions influence their decisions to engage in oral sex, it is critical that health care

From the *Division of Adolescent Medicine, Department of Pediatrics, University of California, San Francisco, California; and ‡Department of Psychiatry, University of California, San Francisco, California.

Accepted for publication Dec 3, 2004. doi:10.1542/peds.2004-2108

No conflict of interest declared.

Address correspondence to Bonnie L. Halpern-Felsher, PhD, Division of Adolescent Medicine, Department of Pediatrics, University of California, 3333 California St, Suite 245, Box 0503, San Francisco, CA 94118. E-mail: yafa@itsa.ucsf.edu

providers include screening and education about oral sex into their practice.

Although it is true that oral sex negates the risk of pregnancy and entails significantly less risk of STI transmission, various studies and case reports suggest that oral sex is still a potential transmission route for oral, respiratory, and genital pathogens,[6,15-18] including STIs such as herpes, hepatitis, gonorrhea, chlamydia, syphilis, and HIV.[15] Although HIV transmission rates are lower for oral sex than vaginal and anal sex,[17] HIV and STI transmission is still possible through oral sex,[6,16-18] with 1 estimate for HIV transmission through oral sex of 0.04% compared with 0.06% for anal sex,[17] and another estimate of 1% (range: 0.85–2.3%) for oral sex with a single partner, as compared with 10% (range: 4.2–12%) for anal sex.[18] There is a concern about the potential for a rise in STI transmission rates from oral sex as a result of a general misperception that oral sex entails no risk at all or very little risk as compared with vaginal or anal sex, and therefore it is engaged in more frequently and with no use of barrier protection.[1,6,10,15,16] Such concern has resulted in the need for research on why adolescents are engaging in oral sex and how they view oral sex.[1,4,6,8,15,16,18,19] Nevertheless, surprisingly few empirical studies have assessed adolescents' attitudes toward or perceptions of oral sex, especially as compared with vaginal sex. Only 1 study[6] has investigated adolescent oral sex experience and risk perceptions, finding that although 96% of the sample acknowledged HIV transmission risk for vaginal and anal sex, significantly fewer (68%) acknowledged the risk for oral sex. That study was limited in that it asked only about HIV risk and not other risks, such as other STIs or social and emotional risks that are pertinent to adolescent decision making, and it did not analyze the potential effect that experience with oral sex may have on the perceptions of risk. Furthermore, although there is evidence that adolescents are more likely to have vaginal intercourse if they believe that they will benefit from the experience,[20,21] no study has extended this research to oral sex.

Adolescents' perceptions of the extent to which peers are engaging in oral sex are also important, because studies have shown that adolescents are more likely to have vaginal sex when they perceive that it is more prevalent among their peers.[22-25] One study[9] investigated the influence of adolescent perceptions of best friends' oral sex behavior on engagement in oral sex, finding that perceptions of friends' behavior were significantly associated with engagement in oral but not vaginal sex. Although these results provide support for the relationship between perceptions of best friends' behavior and adolescents' own behavior, previous studies have not investigated perceived prevalence of oral sex among adolescents' peer group in general.

The goals of this study were to fill these gaps in our understanding of adolescents' engagement in oral sex by determining whether adolescents perceive oral sex as less risky, more beneficial, more acceptable, and more prevalent among peers than vaginal sex. In so doing, we tested the following hypotheses with young adolescents in ninth grade: (1) adolescents are more likely to have engaged in oral than vaginal sex, (2) adolescents will perceive oral sex as less likely to result in health risks (eg, STIs) and social risks (eg, getting into trouble) than vaginal sex, (3) adolescents will have more favorable attitudes about participating in oral sex than vaginal sex, and (4) adolescents will perceive the prevalence rates of oral sex among similar-aged youths to be greater than vaginal sex.

Methods

PARTICIPANTS

Participants were 580 adolescents (mean age: 14.54; SD: .56; 58% female, 42% male) who participated in a longitudinal study on the relationship between risk and benefit perceptions and sexual activity. In this longitudinal study, participants were surveyed every 6 months; however, all of the data included in the current study come from the second wave of data collection. Participants were ethnically diverse, with 40.0% describing themselves as white/non-Hispanic, 23.9% as Latino, 17.3% as Asian, 7.3% as Pacific Islander, 3.1% as African American, 0.2% as American Indian/Alaskan Native, and 8.3% as mixed or other. According to participants' reports, 9% of their mothers had a professional degree, 2.4% had some education after college, 16.4% had a 4-year college degree, 28.8% had at least some college education, 18.6% of the mothers had a high school degree, 12.5% did not graduate from high school, and 12.0% of the participants reported that they did not know their mother's educational level.

PROCEDURES

Participants were recruited from mandatory ninth-grade classes in 2 California public high schools. Researchers came to each class, introduced the study to the students, and invited all ninth-grade students to participate. Students received study information and consent forms during class time and were asked to bring the materials home to share with their parents. Interested participants signed the adolescent assent form, and parents signed the parental consent form. Of the 1180 students who received consent packets, 665 (56.36%) returned completed consent forms. Of these, 637 (95.79%) completed the first survey, for an overall participation rate of 53.98%. The 580 participants included in this study completed the second wave of data collection, representing 91% of the original 637 participants. Participants did not significantly differ from the overall population of students in their schools on ethnicity or socioeconomic status.

Participants completed the self-administered questionnaire during regular class periods at their school. Before beginning the survey, the researchers explained the instructions for completing the surveys and remained available to answer questions that arose during the survey. Refreshments were provided for all participants. In addition, schools were reimbursed for their assistance. This money was used for school supplies for the students. The Institutional Review Board at the University of California, San Francisco, approved the study.

MEASURES

Demographics

Participants provided information about their age, grade, gender, ethnicity, and mother's level of education.

Engagement in and Intentions to Have Oral and Vaginal Sex

Participants were asked about the number of times they had had oral sex and vaginal sex in their entire life, with the following 6 response choices: never, 1 time, 2 times, 3 times, 4 times, and 5 or more times. Participants were also asked whether they intended to have vaginal sex and oral sex in the next 6 months, with responses provided on a 5-point scale ranging from "definitely will not" (1) to "definitely will" (5) (Table 1). Vaginal sex was defined as "regular" sex, or "going all the way" (in which the boy's penis is inserted into the girl's vagina). This was also specified as consensual sex, whereby both partners choose to have sex and neither was forced.

Chance Estimates of Experiencing Risks and Benefits From Oral and Vaginal Sex

Participants read 2 scenarios concerning sexual behavior. The scenarios were identical except for the specification of having vaginal sex versus having oral sex (ie, "Imagine that you have been dating Tanya for 3 months. You both have had sex with 2 other people but not with each other. Tonight you and Tanya have sex (oral sex) 1 time. You do not use a condom or other safer sex method."). After reading this scenario, participants estimated the chance that they would personally experience 12 sex-related risks and benefits (see Tables 2 and 3 for the list of risks and benefits).

Participants' chance estimates were provided using any percentage between 0% and 100%. The quantitative response scale (0%–100%) was chosen over scales that use lexical probability terms (eg, "likely," "probably") to estimate risk due to the great variability in meaning ascribed to these terms by adolescents.[26-28]

Attitudes Toward Engagement in Oral and Vaginal Sex

Participants responded to 5 items concerning their attitudes and acceptability of vaginal sex and oral sex (see Table 4 for items). Participants responded to each item on a 5-point scale, ranging from "strongly agree" (5) to "strongly disagree" (1).

Perceived Peer Engagement in and Intentions to Have Oral and Vaginal Sex

For both vaginal and oral sex separately, participants indicated the number of teens their age, out of 100, whom they think have had sex, intend to have sex in the next 6 months, and will not have sex in the next 6 months (see Table 5 for more details).

Results

All analyses were conducted using the statistical software SPSS, Version 10.

EXPERIENCE WITH AND INTENTIONS TO HAVE ORAL AND VAGINAL SEX

Table 1 presents the number of participants overall and by gender who reported having had oral sex and vaginal sex and who intend to have oral and vaginal sex in the next 6 months. In this

Table 1. Participants' Engagement in and Intentions to Have Oral and Vaginal Sex

	Total, % (n)	Male, % (n)	Female, % (n)
Have had oral sex	19.60 (112)	18.20 (43)	20.80 (69)
Have had vaginal sex	13.50 (78)	14.00 (34)	13.10 (44)
Have had oral and vaginal sex	10.53 (60)	11.44 (27)	9.94 (33)
Intend to have oral sex in the next 6 mo	31.50 (178)	34.50 (80)	29.40 (98)
Intend to have vaginal sex in the next 6 mo	26.20 (148)	29.00 (67)	24.10 (80)

group of ninth graders, a significantly greater number of participants have had oral sex (19.6%) than vaginal sex (13.5%; $\chi^2 = 191.48$, df =1, $P < .000$), and more participants intended to have oral sex in the next 6 months (31.5%) than vaginal sex (26.3%; $\chi^2 = 216.18$, df = 1, $P = .000$). There were no gender differences in adolescents' sexual experiences or intentions.

PERCEIVED RISKS AND BENEFITS ASSOCIATED WITH ORAL AND VAGINAL SEX

A within-subjects, repeated measures analysis of variance (ANOVA) compared participants' chance estimates of experiencing positive and negative outcomes associated with having either oral sex or vaginal sex. Potential interaction effects of gender and oral sex experience (dichotomously scored) were also explored in this model. As shown in Table 2, results supported our hypotheses for 9 of the 12 outcomes. Adolescents correctly perceived the chance of experiencing health-related negative outcomes, including chlamydia, HIV, and pregnancy, as significantly less likely to occur from oral than vaginal sex. Concerning, however, was the greater number of participants who estimated absolutely zero chance of contracting chlamydia and HIV from oral sex (14% and 13%) versus vaginal sex (1% and 2%).

Adolescents also evaluated a number of social and emotional risks as less likely to occur for oral sex than for vaginal sex (Table 2). More specific, participants believed that it is less likely that their relationship with their partner will get worse, that they will get a bad reputation, that they will get into trouble, that they will feel bad about themselves, or that they will feel guilty from having oral sex compared with vaginal sex. Adolescents did believe that they were more likely to experience pleasure from vaginal sex than from oral sex. No significant differences were found between oral and vaginal sex regarding potential social or emotional benefits, including feeling good about oneself, being more popular, or relationship getting better.

Significant interactions between gender and outcome estimates were found for 2 outcomes: male adolescents believed that one's relationship is more likely to get better from having vaginal than oral sex (means: 50.33 and 46.97 for vaginal and oral sex, respectively) than did female adolescents (means: 38.06 and 39.96; F = 4.04, $P < .05$). Female adolescents believed that pleasure was more likely to occur from vaginal sex than oral sex (means: 68.66 and 51.88) than male adolescents (means: 85.24 and 81.48; F = 17.68, $P < .001$).

Table 2. Adolescents' Chance Estimates of Experiencing Positive and Negative Outcomes for Vaginal Compared With Oral Sex

	Vaginal Sex, Mean % (SD)	Oral Sex, Mean % (SD)	F Value	P Value
Risks				
Get chlamydia	52.98 (25.40)	37.55 (28.86)	105.69	.000
Get HIV	49.92 (26.77)	37.64 (30.06)	77.01	.000
Become pregnant	67.63 (23.41)	16.71 (29.31)	824.86	.000
Relationship gets worse	42.13 (26.86)	35.61 (26.41)	37.47	.000
Bad reputation	41.46 (28.60)	37.58 (28.54)	10.54	.001
Get into trouble	71.71 (31.86)	63.16 (35.56)	64.77	.000
Feel bad about self	54.81 (34.11)	45.90 (34.91)	31.70	.000
Feel guilty	55.42 (33.85)	48.19 (35.43)	46.95	.000
Benefits				
Experience pleasure	72.03 (30.44)	59.19 (36.41)	43.93	.000
Feel good about self	40.01 (32.58)	40.26 (33.75)	.000	.999
Be more popular	27.13 (26.76)	26.85 (26.94)	.066	.797
Relationship gets better	41.29 (25.29)	39.71 (26.53)	.310	.578

Significant within-subject interactions between adolescents' own experience with oral sex and their perceived chance of a risk resulting from having oral versus vaginal sex were found. Specifically, adolescents who have had oral sex reported a greater difference in risk estimates for oral versus vaginal sex than did adolescents without oral sex experience for the following 4 outcomes: pregnancy (means for adolescents with oral sex experience were 67.32 and 9.31 for getting pregnant if they have had vaginal and oral sex, respectively, compared with 67.69 and 18.54 for adolescents without oral sex experience; $F = 5.65$, $P < .05$), getting into trouble (means: 59.26 and 45.14 vs 73.13 and 65.83, respectively; $F = 6.56$, $P < .01$), having their relationship get worse (means: 38.49 and 27.80 vs 42.54 and 37.48, respectively; $F = 5.32$, $P < .05$), or feeling guilty (means: 38.49 and 25.24 vs 57.65 and 51.84, respectively; $F = 7.16$, $P < .01$). Nevertheless, for all 4 of these outcomes, adolescents with and without oral sex experience estimated the risks as less likely to happen from having oral sex than vaginal sex.

We also conducted a within-subjects, repeated measures ANOVA to determine whether participants' chance estimates of experiencing positive and negative outcomes associated with having either oral sex or vaginal sex varied by participants' intentions to have oral sex in the near future. As shown in Table 3, significant interactions were found for 6 of the 8 risks and none of the benefits. A close look at the means presented in Table 3 indicates that adolescents with intentions to have oral sex in the next 6 months perceived an even greater difference in their perceptions of experiencing a negative outcome from having oral than vaginal sex than did adolescents without intentions to have oral sex in the near future. Nevertheless, the pattern of results for differences in chance estimates for oral versus vaginal sex remained invariant across oral sex intentions. Specifically, for all outcomes, adolescents with and without oral sex intentions estimated the risks as less likely to happen from having oral sex than vaginal sex.

ADOLESCENTS' ATTITUDES ABOUT PARTICIPATING IN ORAL VERSUS VAGINAL SEX

A within-subjects, repeated measures ANOVA compared participants' attitudes toward oral sex versus vaginal sex (Table 4). As expected, adolescents believed that having oral sex is more acceptable for their age group than vaginal sex. Specifically, participants reported more acceptance of having oral sex with someone they are dating and with someone they are not dating than vaginal sex. Participants also agreed more that teens

Table 3. Adolescents' Chance Estimates of Experiencing Positive and Negative Outcomes for Vaginal Versus Oral Sex, for Adolescents With and Without Oral Sex Intentions

	Intentions		No Intentions		F Value	P Value
	Oral Sex, Mean % (SD)	Vaginal Sex Mean % (SD)	Oral Sex, Mean % (SD)	Vaginal Sex Mean % (SD)		
Risks						
Get chlamydia	30.93 (2.16)	51.87 (1.93)	40.91 (1.48)	54.24 (1.32)	8.94	.003
Get HIV	31.99 (2.26)	49.07 (2.03)	40.54 (1.54)	51.31 (1.39)	6.54	.011
Become pregnant	10.48 (2.17)	67.60 (1.76)	19.68 (1.50)	67.78 (1.22)	8.33	.004
Relationship gets worse	25.86 (1.94)	36.98 (2.04)	39.90 (1.32)	44.46 (1.39)	8.68	.003
Bad reputation	28.77 (2.10)	35.54 (2.14)	41.69 (1.45)	44.40 (1.47)	3.53	.061
Get into trouble	44.64 (2.51)	59.93 (2.33)	71.99 (1.71)	77.60 (1.59)	19.51	.000
Feel bad about self	28.86 (2.49)	40.07 (2.46)	54.01 (1.71)	61.76 (1.69)	1.83	.177
Feel guilty	25.12 (2.40)	40.41 (2.43)	59.31 (1.64)	62.71 (1.67)	27.52	.000
Benefits						
Experience pleasure	73.81 (2.64)	83.69 (2.22)	51.76 (1.83)	66.23 (1.54)	3.02	.083
Feel good about self	55.63 (2.43)	52.39 (2.40)	33.32 (1.66)	34.46 (1.64)	2.53	.112
Be more popular	32.44 (2.00)	33.13 (2.02)	23.97 (1.37)	24.84 (1.38)	.008	.928
Relationship gets better	48.79 (1.96)	48.86 (1.87)	35.72 (1.34)	37.61 (1.28)	.695	.405

Table 4. Adolescents' Attitudes Toward Engagement in Vaginal Sex Versus Oral Sex*

	Vaginal Sex, Mean (SD)	Oral Sex, Mean (SD)	*F* Value	*P* Value
It is okay for teens my age to have (vaginal/oral) sex with someone they are dating.	2.62 (1.19)	2.87 (1.25)	21.889	.000
Teens my age are too young to have (vaginal/oral) sex.	3.51 (1.23)	3.34 (1.27)	6.37	.012
It is okay for teens my age to have (vaginal/oral) sex with someone they are not dating.	1.96 (1.10)	2.17 (1.14)	27.36	.000
It is okay for teens my age to have (vaginal/oral) sex with someone they are in love with.	3.02 (1.30)	3.05 (1.32)	1.39	.239
Having (vaginal/oral) sex at my age is against my moral/ethical/religious beliefs.	3.08 (1.41)	2.93 (1.34)	4.62	.032

* Responses made on a 5-point scale, ranging from strongly agree (5) to strongly disagree (1).

their age were too young to have vaginal sex, compared with oral sex. In addition, participants believed that vaginal sex was more against their moral, ethical, or religious beliefs, compared with oral sex. Participants did not demonstrate a significant difference in attitudes between having oral or vaginal sex with someone with whom they are in love. Interaction effects of gender and oral sex experience (dichotomously scored) were also conducted for each attitude variable. No significant interactions were found for oral sex experience. There was 1 significant gender interaction ($F = 5.23$, $P < .05$), in which female adolescents agreed that vaginal sex at their age is against their ethical beliefs more than is oral sex (means: 3.08 for vaginal sex and 2.86 for oral sex), whereas male adolescents on average reported no difference in such beliefs between vaginal or oral sex (means: 2.60 for both sex types).

PERCEIVED PEER ENGAGEMENT IN AND INTENTIONS TO HAVE ORAL AND VAGINAL SEX

Results from a within-subjects ANOVA indicated that adolescents in this study believed that a greater number of adolescents their age have had and intend to have oral sex in the near future compared with vaginal sex. The adolescents also perceived that more teens will choose to abstain from vaginal sex in the near future and will wait to have vaginal sex until marriage, as compared with oral sex (Table 5).

Significant within-subject interactions between adolescents' own experience with oral sex and perceptions of peer engagement were noted for

2 outcomes. Adolescents who have had oral sex reported a greater difference in the number of their peers who have had oral sex than vaginal sex (means: 56.42 for oral sex and 47.38 for vaginal sex) than adolescents without oral sex experience (means: 43.41 and 38.41; $F = 4.36$, $P < .05$). Similarly, adolescents with oral sex experience reported a greater difference in the number of their peers who intend on having oral sex as compared with vaginal sex in the next 6 months (means: 47.68 and 37.82, respectively) than adolescents without oral sex experience (means: 36.26 and 32.66, respectively; $F = 14.18$, $P < .001$). For both of these outcomes, adolescents with and without oral sex experience perceived that more adolescents are having and intend on having oral sex than vaginal sex.

Discussion

Most studies of adolescent sexuality have focused on vaginal intercourse, thus failing to consider how adolescents perceive the risks, benefits, and prevalence rates of oral sex as compared with vaginal sex and the extent to which adolescents view oral sex as more acceptable than vaginal sex. The results from this study provide important insight into how young adolescents perceive oral sex as compared with vaginal sex, with critical implications for health care providers.

We found that more adolescents have had and intend to have oral sex than vaginal sex. Although the health risks associated with having oral sex are less than that of vaginal sex, oral sex does carry a risk for STI transmission, including

Table 5. Adolescents' Perceived Peer Engagement in Vaginal Versus Oral Sex

Out of 100 Teens Your Age, How Many...	Vaginal Sex, Mean (SD)	Oral Sex, Mean (SD)	F Value	P Value
Have had (vaginal/oral) sex?	40.87 (25.22)	46.72 (25.13)	49.39	.000
Will choose not to have (vaginal/oral) sex in the next 6 mo?	44.81 (26.01)	41.65 (25.45)	13.27	.000
Will have (vaginal/oral) sex in the next 6 mo?	34.27 (23.79)	39.02 (24.37)	65.52	.000
Will wait to have (vaginal/oral) sex until they are married?	31.29 (24.66)	26.80 (24.44)	33.08	.000

HIV. In this study, the majority of adolescents acknowledged that oral sex could result in chlamydia and HIV, and they correctly evaluated oral sex as resulting in these health risks significantly less often than vaginal sex. However, of concern is the finding that a small but important percentage of adolescents believed that there is no chance of contracting chlamydia or HIV from oral sex. Although there is limited information on the actual rates of STI and HIV transmission from oral sex, it is clear that the risk is not zero.[15-18] That so many adolescents are having oral sex and view it as safe, perceiving little or no risk resulting from engaging in oral sex, stresses the importance of needing more research on oral sex transmissibility rates and increased health education about oral sex.

In addition to fewer health risks, the adolescents in this study perceived fewer social and emotional risks for oral sex compared with vaginal sex. In particular, the adolescents in this study believed that they are less likely to get a bad reputation, get into trouble, feel bad about themselves, or feel guilty from having oral as compared with vaginal sex. Furthermore, they believed that having oral sex is less of a threat to one's relationship with their partner. Adolescents also believed that oral sex is more acceptable than vaginal sex for adolescents their own age in both dating and nondating situations, and less of a threat to their values and beliefs, and that more of their peers will have oral sex than vaginal sex in the near future. These results, coupled with the finding that adolescents' own experience with and intentions to have oral sex seem to confirm their perceptions of less risk, may help to explain statistics showing that a far greater number of adolescents are engaging in oral sex than vaginal sex and at younger ages.[1-9] Although limited research has not found evidence for oral sex predicting coitus in the future,[29] some researchers have suggested that noncoital behaviors could be predictors for engaging in intercourse.[7] Limited evidence also suggests a relationship between oral sex and intercourse, although it does not specify a predictive order.[30] Clearly, the dearth of information about the relationship and timing of oral sex in relation to coitus and other sexual activity, especially with longitudinal data, should be addressed to gain a better understanding of adolescent sexual behavior and its progression over time.

It is interesting that the adolescents in this study did not perceive any differences in social or emotional benefits between having oral sex or vaginal sex, suggesting that although adolescents believe that they will feel less guilty and bad about themselves if they have oral sex, they are no more likely to have positive emotions resulting from either type of sexual behavior. It is also interesting that the adolescents had similar attitudes toward having oral sex and vaginal sex with someone with whom they are in love. This finding is consistent with the literature showing a correlation between a committed relationship and more favorable attitudes toward and less risk associated with sexual activity as compared with casual sex relationships.[31-33]

To the extent that adolescents perceive oral sex as less risky, more beneficial, more prevalent, and more acceptable than vaginal sex, it stands to reason that adolescents are more likely to engage in oral than vaginal sex. These findings are important from a public health perspective and have critical implications for health practitioners. It is important that health care providers recognize the diversity of adolescent sexual experiences and that discussions regarding oral sex be included in clinical risk assessments and sexual health education.

Given the suggestion that adolescents do not view oral sex as sex and see oral sex as a way of preserving their virginity while still gaining intimacy and sexual pleasure,[2,4,10] they are likely to interpret sexual health messages as referring to vaginal sex. Unfortunately, most of the guidelines for clinical preventive services do not suggest specific education or guidance for any noncoital sexual activities. Although these guidelines do recommend talking to adolescents about their involvement in sexual behaviors and educating adolescents on ways to reduce their risk for STIs, they do not specifically address sexual risk assessment or education regarding oral sex. Instead, the guidelines typically use terms such as "sexually active" or "sexual behavior" or provide guidelines concerning only sexual intercourse.[11-14] It thus is imperative that health care providers specifically discuss oral sex and other noncoital sexual behaviors with adolescents, providing information and guidance about potential health risks and risk-reducing strategies such as barrier protection (eg, condoms, dental dams), as well as stressing the importance of talking to one's sexual partners about their sexual history, including noncoital experiences. The results from this study also highlight the importance of discussing not only health risks with adolescents but also the social and emotional risks and benefits associated with oral sex. Furthermore, the fact that adolescents are having oral sex early in adolescence suggests that such education should begin prior to the high school years.

There are limitations to this study that must be noted. First, the generalizability of our findings is limited. Although our study sample is reasonably representative of the ethnic and socioeconomic groups of the larger school population from which we sampled, we do not have additional demographic and sexual experience information about the nonparticipants. In addition, the sensitive nature of the topic of study and that parental consent was required for participation may factor into reasons for our low participation rate. Nonparticipants could have chosen not to participate based on fears of their sexual experience being revealed to adults and thus getting into trouble or being stigmatized. Furthermore,

our sample is limited to young adolescent ninth graders. Thus, our findings should be interpreted with caution because it is conceivable that they could be limited to young adolescents with relatively low levels of sexual experience. Clearly, more research is needed on older adolescents to investigate how risk perceptions change as adolescents mature and gain more exposure to and have more experience with oral as compared with vaginal sex. Second, although vaginal sex was defined explicitly on the survey, oral sex was not well defined and thus we cannot be sure which behaviors were included in participants' understanding of oral sex. This limits the interpretation of the findings because it is possible that participants included other behaviors, such as French kissing, in their interpretation of the term "oral sex." Similarly, we did not assess the extent to which the adolescents in this study have given or received oral sex. This information is important because some studies have shown gender differences in the extent to which adolescents perform and receive oral sex.[3,5-8] For example, Newcomer and Udry[5] found that girls were more likely to have received oral sex than to have given it and that fellatio was less common than vaginal sex or cunnilingus in their overall sample. These results, however, are in contrast to other studies that have not found significant gender differences.[3,6] Third, although a number of risks were assessed, the health risks queried about were limited to pregnancy, chlamydia, and HIV. Future studies that examine adolescents' perceptions of oral sex should include a wider range of STIs and other negative health outcomes. Finally, this study was not longitudinal and therefore cannot address the extent to which adolescents' perceptions and attitudes are motivating their engagement in oral sex or are instead reflective of their own experiences.

Despite these limitations, this is 1 of the first studies to provide a more comprehensive understanding of adolescents' perceptions of oral sex. The results clearly indicate that adolescents perceive oral sex as less risky, more beneficial, more prevalent, and more acceptable than vaginal sex. These findings stress the importance of understanding the beliefs and attitudes underlying the breadth of adolescents' sexual experiences and that adolescents are engaging in a broad range of sexual behaviors that include oral sex. To help adolescents make informed sexual decisions, parents, health care providers, and other educators must broaden their clinical and educational efforts to include screening, counseling, and education about oral sex, including discussion of the potential health, emotional, and social consequences and methods to prevent negative outcomes for all sexual activities, including non-coital behaviors such as oral sex.

Acknowledgments

This research was supported in part by grants awarded to Dr Halpern-Felsher from the National Institute of Child Health and Human Development (R01 HD41349) and the William T. Grant Foundation (2363).

We gratefully acknowledge Eric Peterson, Tricia M. Michels, and Tina Paul for assistance on the manuscript, as well as the participation of the adolescents and school administrators.

References

1. Conard LA, Blythe MJ. Sexual function, sexual abuse and sexually transmitted diseases in adolescence. *Best Pract Res Clin Obstet Gynaecol.* 2003;17:103–116

2. Remez L. Oral sex among adolescents: is it sex or is it abstinence? *Fam Plann Perspect.* 2000;32:298–304

3. Schwartz IM. Sexual activity prior to coital initiation: a comparison between males and females. *Arch Sex Behav.* 1999;28:63–69

4. Sanders SA, Reinisch JM. Would you say you "had sex" if? *JAMA.* 1999;281:275–277

5. Newcomer SF, Udry JR. Oral sex in an adolescent population. *Arch Sex Behav.* 1985;14:41–46

6. Boekeloo BO, Howard DE. Oral sexual experience among young adolescents receiving general health examinations. *Am J Health Behav.* 2002;26:306–314

7. Gates GJ, Sonenstein FL. Heterosexual genital sexual activity among adolescent males: 1988 and 1995. *Fam Plann Perspect.* 2000;32:295–297, 304

8. Schuster MA, Bell RM, Kanouse DE. The sexual practices of adolescent virgins: genital sexual activities of high school students who have never had vaginal intercourse. *Am J Public Health.* 1996;86:1570–1576

9. Prinstein MJ, Meade CS, Cohen GL. Adolescent oral sex, peer popularity, and perceptions of best friends' sexual behavior. *J Pediatr Psychol.* 2003;28:243–249

10. Gerbert B, Herzig K, Volberding P, Stansell J. Perceptions of health care professionals and patients about the risk of HIV transmission through oral sex: a qualitative study. *Patient Educ Couns.* 1999;38:49–60

11. Elster AB, Kuznets NJ. American Medical Association. *AMA Guidelines for Adolescent Preventive Services (GAPS): Recommendations and Rationale.* Baltimore, MD: Williams & Wilkins; 1994:191

12. Green ME, Palfrey JS. *Bright Futures: Guidelines for Health Supervision of Infants, Children, and Adolescents.* 2nd ed. Arlington, VA: National Center for Education in Maternal and Child Health; 2000

13. Stein ME. *Health Supervision Guidelines.* 3rd ed. Elk Grove Village, IL: American Academy of Pediatrics; 1997

14. US Public Health Service. *Clinician's Handbook of Preventive Services: Put Prevention Into Practice.* 2nd ed. Alexandria, VA: International Medical Publishing; 1998

15. Edwards S, Carne C. Oral sex and transmission of non-viral STIs. *Sex Transm Infect.* 1998;74:95–100

16. Hawkins DA. Oral sex and HIV transmission. *Sex Transm Infect.* 2001;77:307–308

17. Vittinghoff E, Douglas J, Judson F, McKirnan D, MacQueen K, Buchbinder SP. Per-contact risk of human immunodeficiency virus transmission between male sexual partners. *Am J Epidemiol.* 1999;150:306–311

18. Rothenberg RB, Scarlett M, del Rio C, Reznik D, O'Daniels C. Oral transmission of HIV. *AIDS.* 1998;12:2095–2105

19. O'Donnell BL, O'Donnell CR, Stueve A. Early sexual initiation and subsequent sex-related risks among urban minority youth: the reach for health study. *Fam Plann Perspect.* 2001;33:268–275

20. Gebhardt WA, Kuyper L, Greunsven G. Need for intimacy in relationships and motives for sex as determinants of adolescent condom use. *J Adolesc Health.* 2003;33:154–164

21. Michels TM, Kropp RY, Eyre SL, Halpern-Felsher BL. Initiating sexual experiences: how do young adolescents make decisions regarding early sexual activity? *J Res Adolesc.* In press

22. Kinsman SB, Romer D, Furstenberg FF, Schwarz DF. Early sexual initiation: the role of peer norms. *Pediatrics.* 1998;102:1185–1192

23. O'Donnell L, Myint-U A, O'Donnell CR, Stueve A. Long-term influence of sexual norms and attitudes on timing of sexual initiation among urban minority youth. *J Sch Health.* 2003;73:68–75

24. Basen-Engquist K, Parcel GS. Attitudes, norms, and self-efficacy: a model of adolescents' HIV-related sexual risk behavior. *Health Educ Q.* 1992;19:263–277

25. Selvan MS, Ross MW, Kapadia AS, Mathai R, Hira S. Study of perceived norms, beliefs and intended sexual behaviour among higher secondary school students in India. *AIDS Care.* 2001;13:779–788

26. Biehl M, Halpern-Felsher BL. Adolescents' and adults' understanding of probability expressions. *J Adolesc Health.* 2001;28:30–35

27. Cohn LD, Schydlower M, Foley J, Copeland RL. Adolescent's misinterpretation of health risks probability expressions. *Pediatrics.* 1995;95:713–716

28. Fischhoff B, Bostrom A, Jacobs-Quadrel M. Risk perception and communication. *Annu Rev Public Health.* 1993;14:183–203

29. Smith EA, Udry JR. Coital and non-coital sexual behaviors of white and black adolescents. *Am J Public Health.* 1985;75:1200–1203

30. Herold ES, Way L. Oral-genital sexual behavior in a sample of university females. *J Sex Res.* 1983;19:327–338

31. Ellen JM, Cahn S, Eyre SL, Boyer CB. Types of adolescent sexual relationships and associated perceptions about condom use. *J Adolesc Health.* 1996;18:471–421

32. Plichta SB, Weisman CS, Nathanson CA, Ensminger ME, Robinson JC. Partner-specific condom use among adolescent women clients of a family planning clinic. *J Adolesc Health.* 1992;13:506–511

33. Reisen CA, Poppen PJ. Partner-specific risk perception: a new conceptualization of perceived vulnerability to STDs. *J Appl Soc Psychol.* 1999;29:667–684

What's New with Emergency Contraception: Questions and Answers

By Melanie A. Gold, DO, FAAP
Section on Adolescent Health Executive Committee Member

WHAT IS THE HISTORY OF EMERGENCY CONTRACEPTION (EC) AND WHAT IS HAPPENING NOW?

In 1997, the FDA announced in the Federal Register that certain oral contraceptive pills (OCs) were effective and could be used for EC (1). In the late 1990's, the FDA approved two pre-packaged EC products: Preven® (a combination OC for EC) in 1998 and Plan B® (a high dose levonorgestrel for EC) in 1999. Since that time, EC has become a standard of care for preventing pregnancy after unprotected sex resulting from sexual assault, contraceptive method failure or no method use. On April 21, 2003, Women's Capitol Corporation, the makers of Plan B, submitted an application to the FDA for Plan B to switch from prescription-only to over-the-counter (OTC) status. On December 16, 2003, two FDA committees voted 23:4 in favor of Plan B® going over OTC. However, on May 6, 2004, the FDA rejected the OTC application—claiming there was insufficient information about how adolescents under 16 would use EC if available OTC. During this time, Barr laboratories acquired Plan B from Women's Capitol Corporation. On July 22, 2004, Barr Laboratories submitted an application to the FDA for dual prescribing status for Plan B®. This unique and unprecedented dual prescribing status would allow Plan B® to go OTC for women ages 16 and older but it would remain a prescription-only product for women 15 and younger. By January 21, 2005, the FDA was supposed to give their final response to the dual prescribing status application. However, as of Jan 22nd 2005 when this article was submitted, the FDA had delayed the decision with no clear time frame as to when a final decision would be made.

WHAT CRITERIA DOES THE FDA USE TO DETERMINE IF A PRESCRIPTION MEDICATION, LIKE PLAN B, CAN SWITCH TO OTC STATUS?

A medication must meet three criteria:
1) It cannot be addictive;
2) It must be safe for use OTC (in case of user error it cannot be dangerous to an individual's health);
3) The consumer needs to be able to self-determine when the medication is needed and be able to understand how to follow the OTC package instructions without professional guidance.

Plan B® meets these three criteria:
1) Levonorgestrel is a steroidal hormone that is not addictive;
2) If Plan B were taken in error (e.g. if it was taken when it was not needed or if a woman is already pregnant when it is taken) it does not cause a miscarriage or birth defects. There are few side effects associated with its use and if taken when not needed, no harm would result.
3) It is the woman, rather than her health care provider, who usually can best determine if she needs the medication (she knows if she has had unprotected sex) and studies have shown that adult and adolescent women are able to understand the product package instructions.

WHY DID THE FDA REJECT THE OTC APPLICATION FOR PLAN B AND IGNORE THEIR OWN TWO COMMITTEES' RECOMMENDATIONS TO APPROVE THE OTC STATUS?

Although Plan B met the above three criteria, the FDA claimed there was insufficient information about how adolescents under the age of 16 would use Plan B if it was available OTC. The concerns were not specifically about safety in terms of health related to taking Plan B inappropriately but rather what type of behavioral impact making Plan B might have on younger adolescents' sexual and contraceptive risk taking. This is one of the first medications for which the FDA has restricted OTC status because of concerns about behavioral impact rather than direct health impact from the medication itself. Many believe that the FDA is making decisions about Plan B based on politics rather than science (2,3).

WHAT IS THE SCIENTIFIC EVIDENCE TO SUPPORT THE FDA'S CONCERNS ABOUT THE IMPACT OF INCREASING ACCESS TO EC?

To date there have been numerous studies that demonstrate giving adolescent and adult women easier access to EC (through either advance provision or through pharmacy access to EC) does not have negative behavioral impact (4–12). Women with advance provision of EC do not have more unprotected sex or more sexual partners. They do not use condom less or have higher rates of sexually transmitted diseases. Most studies demonstrate that women with easier access to EC do not discontinue use of more effective contraceptive methods. However, women provided EC in advance are more likely to use EC when it is needed compared to women in control groups and they use it sooner after unprotected intercourse when it is more likely to be effective at preventing pregnancy. Research to date supports increasing access to EC and demonstrates that increased access does not have detrimental behavioral effects.

Other Common Questions About EC

WHY IS PREVEN® NO LONGER AVAILABLE?

Preven®, the first pre-packed method of EC, was FDA approved in 1998. It was composed of the standard Yuzpe regimen of 200 mcg of ethiny estradiol and 2.0 mg of norgestrel that was split into two doses given 12 hours apart. Preven® was the only pre-package combination method of EC available in the US until 2004. Gynetics, the company that made Preven®, sold the rights to Barr Laboratories, the company that now makes Plan B®. Barr decided that since Plan B® is a superior

product with higher efficacy and less side effects that it was best to take Preven® off the market.

THE TRADITIONAL YUZPE REGIMEN, USING COMBINATION ESTROGEN-PROGESTIN BIRTH CONTROL PILLS FOR EC, ONLY INCLUDES PILLS WITH THE PROGESTINS LEVONORGESTREL OR NORGESTREL. CAN PILLS WITH OTHER PROGESTINS BE USED?

Yes. One study found that combination pills with norethindrone given in high doses were as effective for EC as the standard Yuzpe regimen (13). This same study also found that giving half the Yuzpe regimen (giving the first dose without the second dose of the two standard dose regimen) was also effective at preventing pregnancy after unprotected sex and produced significantly less nausea than the standard Yuzpe regimen or the modified regimen with norethindrone.

WHAT DOES THE SOCIETY FOR ADOLESCENT MEDICINE RECOMMEND REGARDING EMERGENCY CONTRACEPTION?

The *Journal of Adolescents Health* published the Society for Adolescent Medicine (SAM) position statement recommendations for EC in the spring of 2004 (14). In the statement, SAM strongly supports changing the status of EC from prescription-only to over-the-counter without an age restriction.

In addition, the statement makes the following ten recommendations:

1. Counsel all adolescents about EC during visits for acute and routine health care visits
2. Counsel about EC and offer a complete course of medication to all female adolescents being treated for sexual assault
3. Inquire routinely about when an adolescent last experienced unprotected sex and offer EC up to 120 hours after unprotected intercourse. Do not restrict provision to 72 hours after unprotected sex since current data supports effectiveness up to 120 hours (15,16).
4. Do not restrict access to EC by requiring adolescents to get a pregnancy test, pelvic exams, STD or pap smear testing prior to prescribing EC.

5. Progestin-only EC (Plan B®) is the regimen of choice because of higher efficacy and lower side effects (17). Rather than splitting the dose (the FDA approved instructions), it is now recommended to instruct adolescents to take the two tablets of Plan B® at the same time (18) and as soon as possible after unprotected intercourse. If the Yuzpe regimen is the only EC available, continue to give in two separate doses divided 12 hours apart and offer an anti-nauseant.

6. Maintain the same degree of confidentiality when providing EC as with other aspects of adolescent reproductive health care

7. Offer all female adolescents an advance prescription or advance supply of EC to have at home for future use and put multiple refills on the prescription.

8. Establish written protocols that prevent barriers to EC access that might result from individual health care provider's or pharmacist's personal attitudes and beliefs

9. Develop and disseminate medically accurate, age-appropriate materials about EC

10. Advocate for parity of insurance coverage for all contraceptive methods including EC

Resources for Learning More About EC

BOOK CHAPTERS

Stewart F, Trussell J, Van Look PF. Emergency contraception. In: Hatcher RA, Trussell J, Stewart F, et al, eds. *Contraceptive Technology.* New York: Ardent Media; 2004 pp. 279–303.

Hatcher RA, Zieman M, Cwiak C, et al. *A Pocket Guide to Managing Contraception.* Tiger, Georgia: Bridging the Gap Foundation; 2004.

WEB SITES

http://www.managingcontraception.com
http://www.NOT-2-LATE.com
http://www.backupyourbirthcontrol.org

TELEPHONE RESOURCES

1-888-NOT-2-LATE

References

1. Prescription drug products; certain combined oral contraceptives for use as postcoital emergency contraception. *Federal Register.* 1997;62(37):8609–8612.
2. Drazen JM, Greene MF, Wood AJJ. The FDA, Politics and Plan B. *NEJM.* 2004;350(15):1561–1562.
3. Steinbrook R. Waiting for Plan B—The FDA and nonprescription use of emergency contraception. *NEJM.* 2004;350(23):2327–2329.
4. Glasier A, Baird D. The effects of self-administering emergency contraception. *N Engl J Med.* 1998;339(1):1–4.
5. Lovvorn A, Nerquaye-Tetteh J, Glover EK, Amankwah-Poku A, Hays M, Raymond E. Provision of emergency contraceptive pills to spermicide users in Ghana. *Contraception.* 2000;61:287–293.
6. Ellertson C, Ambardekar S, Hedley A, Coyaji K, Trussell J, Blanchard K. Emergency contraception: randomized comparison of advance provision and information only. *Obstet Gynecol.* 2001;98(4):570–575.
7. Jackson RA, Schwarz EB, Freedman L, Darney P. Advance supply of emergency contraception: effect on use and usual contraception—a randomized trial. *Obstet Gynecol.* 2003;102(1):8–16.
8. Lo SST, Fan SYS, Ho PC, Glasier AF. Effect of advanced provision of emergency contraception on women's contraceptive behaviour: a randomized controlled trial. *Hum Reprod.* 2004;19(10):2404–2410.
9. Raine T, Harper C, Leon K, Karney P. Emergency contraception: advance provision in a young, high-risk clinic population. *Obstet Gynecol.* 2000;96:1–7.
10. Gold MA, Wolford JE, Smith KA et al. The effects of advance provision of emergency contraception on adolescent women's sexual and contraceptive behaviors. *J Pediatr Adolesc Gynecol.* 2004;17:87–96.
11. Walker DM, Torres P, Gutierrez JP, et al. Emergency contraception use is correlated with increased condom use among adolescents: Results from Mexico. *J Adolesc Health.* 2004;35:329–334.
12. Raine TR, Harper CC, Rocca CH, Fischer R, Padian N, Klausner JD, Darney PD. Direct access to emergency contraception through pharmacies and effect on unintended pregnancy and STIs: a randomized controlled trial. *JAMA.* 2005;293:54–62.
13. Ellertson C, Webb A, Blanchard K et al. Modifying the Yuzpe regimen of emergency contraception: a multicenter randomized controlled trial. *Obstet Gynecol.* 2003;101(6):1160–1167.
14. Gold MA, Sucato G, Conard LE, Hillard P. Provision of emergency contraception to adolescents: A Position Paper of the Society for Adolescent Medicine. *J Adolesc Health.* 2004;35:66–70.
15. Ellertson C, Evans M, Ferden S, et al. Extending the time limit for starting the Yuzpe regimen of emergency contraception to 120 hours. *Obstet Gynecol.* 2003;101(6):1168–1171.

16. Rodrigues I, Grou F, Joly J. Effectiveness of emergency contraceptive pills between 72 and 120 hours after unprotected sexual intercourse. *Am J Obstet Gynecol.* 2001;184:531–537.

17. Task Force on Postovulatory Methods of Fertility Regulation. Randomised controlled trial of levonorgestrel versus the Yuzpe regimen of combined oral contraceptives for emergency contraception. *Lancet.* 1998;352:428–433.

18. von Hertzen H, Piaggio G, Ding J, et al. Low dose mifepristone and two regimens of levonorgestrel for emergency contraception: a WHO multicentre randomized trial. *Lancet.* 2002;360:1803–1810.

Breast Self-Exam

Once a month, right after your period, you should examine your breasts. Although breast cancer is rare in young women, it usually can be cured if found early, and a breast self-exam is the best way to find it.

Do the following to examine your breasts:

1. Stand in front of your mirror with your arms at your sides and see if there are any changes in the size or shape of your breasts. Look for any puckers or dimples, and press each nipple to see if any fluid comes out. Raise your arm above your head and look for changes in your breasts from this position.

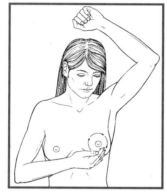

2. Lie down and place a towel or pillow under your right shoulder. Place your right hand under your head. Hold your left hand flat and feel your right breast with little, pressing circles. Think of each breast as a pie divided into 4 pieces. Feel each piece and then feel the center of the "pie" (the nipple area).

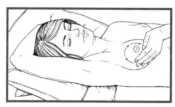

3. Now put your right arm down at your side, and do the same thing on the outside of the breast, starting under the armpit.
4. Repeat steps 2 and 3 for the other breast.

Most women have some lumpiness or texture to their breasts; breasts are not just soft tissue. Get to know your breasts, then be alert for any lumps or other changes should they ever appear. Remember, most lumps and changes are not cancerous. However, if you think you have found a lump or notice any other changes, don't press or squeeze it; see your pediatrician.

The information contained in this publication should not be used as a substitute for the medical care and advice of your pediatrician. There may be variations in treatment that your pediatrician may recommend based on individual facts and circumstances.

Illustrations by Lauren Shavell

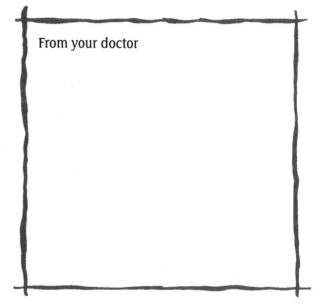

From your doctor

American Academy of Pediatrics

DEDICATED TO THE HEALTH OF ALL CHILDREN™

The American Academy of Pediatrics is an organization of 60,000 primary care pediatricians, pediatric medical subspecialists, and pediatric surgical specialists dedicated to the health, safety, and well-being of infants, children, adolescents, and young adults.

American Academy of Pediatrics
Web site — www.aap.org

Copyright ©1999
American Academy of Pediatrics

The Correct Use of Condoms
A Message to Teens

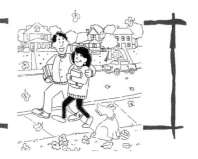

As a teen, you are faced with many challenges and decisions that will affect the rest of your life. Deciding when to begin having sex is one of the most important decisions you will ever make. It is perfectly normal not to have sex until marriage.

Sexually transmitted diseases (STDs) and unplanned pregnancies are at all-time highs for people your age. Not having sex (abstinence) is the only sure way to prevent pregnancy and STDs. It's also the only way to avoid getting sexually transmitted HIV, the AIDS virus. However, if you do decide to have sex, correct use of latex condoms will help you protect yourself and your partner against these risks. The American Academy of Pediatrics has designed this brochure to help you understand the importance of always using latex condoms and how to use them correctly.

Why use condoms?

A condom acts like a barrier or wall to keep semen, fluid from the vagina, and blood from passing from one person to the other during sex. These fluids can carry germs. If no condom is used, the germs can pass from the infected person to the uninfected person. Use of a condom also prevents unwanted pregnancies by keeping sperm out of the vagina.

Other good reasons to use condoms:
- They are cheap.
- They are easy to get (you don't need a prescription to buy them).
- They rarely have side effects.
- They are easy to use.

Some people have excuses for not using condoms, such as they are not comfortable, they lessen their enjoyment of sex, or they are unnatural. However, using a condom can make sex more enjoyable becauseboth partners are more relaxed and secure. Besides, the risks involved with **not** using condoms make any excuses seem pretty weak.

How to buy condoms

When buying condoms, be sure the ones you choose:
- are latex—some condoms are made of natural membranes (lambskin) and not latex. Only *latex* condoms have been proved to work against STDs because they prevent the passage of harmful germs.
- have a reservoir (nipple) at the tip to catch semen.
- are lubricated with *nonoxynol-9*, which is a spermicide (chemical) that has been proved to give additionalprotection against STDs, including the AIDS virus.

Condoms come in different colors, textures, and sometimes sizes. A good-quality condom is the most important feature for safer sex. Other points to keep in mind when buying condoms:
- Be sure to check the expiration date on the package. Do not buy or use them if they have expired.

- Condoms should be stored in a cool, dry place. You can carry a condom with you at all times, but do not store them where they will get hot (like in the glove box of a car). Heat can damage the condom. Also, carrying them in a purse or wallet is okay as long as it is not for long periods of time—this shortens their life.

Try not to feel embarrassed about buying condoms. By using condoms, you are proving that you are being responsible and there is nothing embarrassing about that.

How to put condoms on

Condoms are easy to use. However, they only work it they are used correctly. Follow these easy steps to make sure you are using them the right way (see illustration):

1. Carefully remove the condom from the package.
2. Put the condom on the end of the penis when the penis is *erect* ("hard").
3. Hold the condom by the tip and carefully roll the condom all the way to the base of the penis.
4. Leave extra space (1/4 to 1/2 inch) at tip of the condom to catch the semen.

If you do not have much experience with condoms, you should practice putting a condom on and taking it off **by yourself**, before you use it for sex with another person.

Be sure to put the condom on when an erection first occurs. Do not wait until you are ready to have sex—it may be too late. Drops of semen may leak from the uncovered penis. These small drops are enough to pass STDs to the other person or to cause a woman to get pregnant.

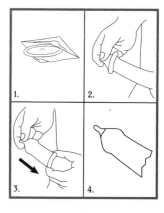

For added protection against STDs and pregnancy, use a spermicidal foam, cream, or jelly **along with** the condom. Make sure the spermicide you use contains nonoxynol-9.
- Before unrolling the condom, place a small amount of the spermicidal foam, cream, or jelly inside its tip.
- After unrolling the condom over the erect penis, place some more of the foam, cream, or jelly on the outside of the condom. Females can also use the spermicide inside the vagina for extra protection in case the condom breaks. Follow the directions on the spermicide package.

How to take condoms off

Withdraw the penis from the vagina right after ejaculation, while it is still erect or "hard." Hold on to the condom at the rim while the penis is withdrawn. Be careful as you slide it off the penis. Do not tug to pull condom off—it may tear. Throw away used condoms immediately. Never use a condom more than once. Be sure to keep used condoms away from your partner's genitals and other areas of the body as well. This will prevent semen from getting on hands or other body parts. If this happens, wash any areas of the body that have been touched by the semen.

Always insist that a condom be used *every* time you have sex. It is the only way to be sure that you are protected from infection. You should say **NO** to sex if you don't have a condom or if your partner refuses to use one.

Special points to remember

- Whenever possible, buy lubricated condoms.
- If you buy condoms that are not lubricated, you also may need a lubricant to help prevent the condom from breaking. Lubricants may also prevent irritation, which could increase the chances of infection.Use only **water-based** lubricants (like K-Y jelly). Do not use oil-based lubricants such as petroleum jelly (like Vaseline), hand or body lotions, or vegetable oil with latex condoms, since they can damage the condom.
- Other forms of birth control like the pill, diaphragm, or IUD **do not** prevent the spread of STDs—only condoms do. If another form of birth control is being used, a latex condom must also be used to make sure both partners are protected from STDs.

Why should I use a condom?

To prevent the spread of AIDS and other diseases
To prevent pregnancy

When should I use a condom?

Every time you have sex

How do I use a condom?

- Roll the condom all the way to the base of the erect penis.
- Leave space at the tip.
- After intercourse, carefully withdraw the penis and then slide the—condom off.
- Throw away the used condom - condoms can only be used once.

- If you have had sex and you did not use a latex condom, you could have an infection and not know it. Some STDs take several months to show symptoms and some have no symptoms. See your pediatrician if you or your partner have any of the following:
  - discharge from the vagina, penis, or rectum
  - pain or burning during urination or sex
  - pain in the abdomen, testes, buttocks, and legs
  - blisters, open sores, warts, rash, or swelling in the genital area or mouth
  - flu-like symptoms, including fever, headache, aching muscles, or swollen glands
  - miss a period and think you might be pregnant

Condoms do not make sex 100% safe, but if used properly, they will reduce the risk of STDs, including AIDS. Know the facts so that you can protect yourself and others from getting infected. Not having sex is the safest. However, if you are having sex, be sure to always use a latex condom. It is the best way for you and your partner to stay healthy. For more information about condoms and how to prevent STDs and pregnancy, talk with your pediatrician.

From your doctor

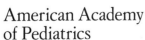

American Academy of Pediatrics

DEDICATED TO THE HEALTH OF ALL CHILDREN™

The American Academy of Pediatrics is an organization of 60,000 primary care pediatricians, pediatric medical subspecialists, and pediatric surgical specialists dedicated to the health, safety, and well-being of infants, children, adolescents, and young adults.

American Academy of Pediatrics
Web site—www.aap.org

Copyright © 1996
American Academy of Pediatrics

deciding to wait

No matter what you've heard, read, or seen, **not everyone your age is having sex,** including oral sex and intercourse. In fact, more than half of all teens choose to wait until they're older to have sex. If you have already had sex but are unsure if you should again, then wait before having sex again.

New feelings

Being physically attracted to another person and trying to figure out how to deal with these feelings is perfectly normal. Kissing and hugging are often accompanied by really intense sexual feelings. These feelings may tempt you to "go all the way."

Before things go too far, **try asking yourself the following questions:**

- Do I really want to have sex?
- Is this person pressuring me to have sex?
- Am I ready to have sex?
- What will happen after I have sex with this person?

Remember, you can **show how you feel** about someone **without having sex** (being abstinent) with him or her.

Can you be **sexual without having** sex?

Yes. Being sexual can mean

- Spending romantic time together
- Holding hands, kissing, or cuddling

Are you **ready?**

Ask yourself the following questions:

- **How do you feel** when you are with this person?
- Is this person kind and caring?
- Does this person *respect* you and your opinions?
- Have you **talked together** about whether to have sex?
- Have you talked together about condoms and other **birth control?**
- Will you stay together even if one of you does not want to have sex?
- Do you know if your partner has *ever had sex with other people?*
- **Do you feel pressured** to have sex just to please your partner?

If you and your partner find it hard to talk about sex, it might be a sign that **you are not ready to have sex.** Open and honest communication is important in any relationship, especially one that involves sex.

Know **the risks**

It's normal for teens to be curious about sex, but deciding to have sex is a big step.

Sex does increase your chances of becoming pregnant, becoming a teen parent, and getting a sexually transmitted disease (STD), and it may affect the way you feel about yourself or how others feel about you.

Some things to think about before you have sex are

- What would *your parents* say if you had sex?
- Are you **ready to be a parent?**
- Could you handle being told that you have an STD?
- Do you know where to go for **birth control methods?**
- How would you feel if your partner tells you *it's over after you have sex?*
- How would you feel if your partner tells people at school the two of you had sex?
- How would you handle feeling guilty, scared, or sad because you had sex?

Set your limits

If you don't want to have sex, set **limits** before things get too serious. Never let anyone talk you into doing something you don't want to do. Boys and girls need to understand that **forcing someone to have sex is wrong.**

Stick by your decision

If you don't know what to say, here are some suggestions

- "I like you a lot, but I'm just not ready to have sex."
- "You're really fun to be with, and I wouldn't want to ruin our relationship with sex."
- "You're a great person, but sex isn't how I prove I like someone."
- "I'd like to wait until I'm older before I make the decision to have sex."

Remember, **"no" means "no"**—no matter how far you go. If you feel things are going too far sexually, tell your partner to stop.

Better safe than sorry

If you choose to wait to have sex, try to avoid

- **Being alone with your date too often.** Spending time with your other friends is important too.
- Giving your date the wrong idea. Stick to your limits. It's also not a good idea for you and your date to "make out" or go too far sexually if you don't really want to have sex.
- Using alcohol or drugs. Both of these **affect your judgment**, which may make it hard to stick to your decision not to have sex.
- **Giving in to the pressure.** It may be tempting to keep up with the crowd, but keep in mind that they may not be telling the truth.

Why wait?

People who **wait** until they are older to have sex usually find out that it's

- More **special**
- More satisfying
- **Less risky** to their health
- **Easier** to act responsibly and take precautions to avoid infections and pregnancy
- More accepted by others

Be patient. At some point, you will be ready for sex. **Move at your own pace, not someone else's.**

From your doctor

American Academy of Pediatrics

DEDICATED TO THE HEALTH OF ALL CHILDREN™

The American Academy of Pediatrics is an organization of 60,000 primary care pediatricians, pediatric medical subspecialists, and pediatric surgical specialists dedicated to the health, safety, and well-being of infants, children, adolescents, and young adults.

American Academy of Pediatrics
Web site — www.aap.org

Copyright © 2005
American Academy of Pediatrics

making healthy decisions about sex

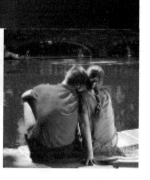

Are you thinking about having sex?

Is anyone trying to talk you into having sex? Does it seem like all your friends are having sex?

Before you make any decisions, or even if you have had sex but are unsure if you should again, read on for some **important information** about how to **stay healthy.** (And remember, if anyone has ever forced you to have sex, this is **WRONG** and not your fault! Tell someone you trust as soon as possible.)

It's OK to say NO Way!

Not everyone is having sex. **Half of all teens say "no" to sex.** There's nothing wrong if you decide to wait; in fact, it's a great idea. If you decide to wait, **stick with your decision.** Plan ahead how you are going to say "no" so that you are clearly understood. Stay away from situations that can lead to sex. Too many young people have sex without meaning to when they drink alcohol or use drugs. Not using alcohol and drugs will help you make clearer choices about sex. Whether you decide to have sex, it's important that you **know the facts** about birth control, diseases, and emotions.

Why wait?

- **Sex can lead to pregnancy. Are you ready** to be pregnant or a teen parent? *It's an awesome responsibility*—will your baby have food, clothes, and a safe place to live?

- **Sex has health risks.** You could become infected with one or more **sexually transmitted diseases (STDs)** like herpes, *Trichomonas,* or human immunodeficiency virus (HIV) (the virus that causes acquired immunodeficiency syndrome [AIDS]). One type of disease called human papillomavirus (HPV) may cause **cancer.**

- You may feel sad or angry if you let someone pressure you into having sex when you're not really ready.

- You also may feel sad or angry if you chose to have sex and then your partner leaves you. He may even tell other people that you had sex with him. **Can you handle that?**

If you don't want to **get an STD,** use condoms

If you're going to have sexual intercourse, using **condoms** is the best way to avoid getting STDs. Remember that **nothing will ever be 100% effective** in preventing diseases except abstinence (no sex). Use a **latex** condom every time you have sex—no matter what other type of birth control you and your partner also might use. To **protect** against getting a disease from having oral sex, use a condom, a dental dam, or non-microwavable plastic wrap. Your pediatrician can explain all these things to you. To make sure

you **stay healthy,** get regular medical checkups, urine testing for STDs, and a pelvic exam (if you're female).

Condoms are easy to use. They work best when you use them the right way. Here is **what you need to know.**

- **Use only latex or polyurethane condoms.** You also have a choice between a male condom or female condom. Never use these 2 types of condoms at the same time; they might tear. When buying male condoms, get the kind with a reservoir (nipple) at the tip to catch semen.

- **Follow the instructions** on the package to make sure you are using them the right way. Also, **check** the expiration date on the package. Don't buy or use expired condoms.

- **You can carry condoms with you at all times,** but do not store them where they will get hot (like in the glove compartment of a car). Heat can damage the condom. Also, you can carry them in a purse or wallet, but not for too long—this shortens their life.

If you don't want to get pregnant…

You need a **reliable form of birth control!**

- **Condoms** used the right way have a 90% chance of preventing pregnancy.

- "The pill" is the most popular type of birth control used by women. There are many brands of **the birth control pill.** For the pill to work, a woman must take it *every day.* When used correctly, the pill is 99% effective at preventing pregnancy.

- The birth control **patch** is similar to the pill and looks like an adhesive strip. The patch is placed on the skin and changed every week for 3 weeks. Side effects are similar to the pill.

- Depo-Provera is a **shot** that you get every 3 months. It is a popular choice for women who have trouble remembering to take the pill.

There may be **minor side effects** when using the pill, patch, or Depo-Provera like mild irregular bleeding, nausea, sore breasts, or weight gain. Your pediatrician will talk to you in detail about what to expect.

Other types of birth control

The following are **NOT recommended** for young people:

- **Withdrawal** (when the male "pulls out" of the female before he ejaculates or "cums") does not prevent pregnancy. If even a small amount of sperm enters a woman, pregnancy can occur.

- **Norplant.** It's no longer approved.

- **Diaphragms and spermicides.** These require some planning. The teen pregnancy rate using these methods is very high.
- The **"rhythm method."** This is when you avoid having sex during certain times of your monthly cycle. This method is not very effective at preventing pregnancy.
- The **intrauterine device (IUD)**, unless you have had a baby and are at a low risk for STDs.

The choice to become sexually active is **your choice.**

Choosing not to have sex is the **only** way to avoid all STDs and getting pregnant.

It's your choice!

Talk with your pediatrician about birth control—how safe and effective these methods are, what side effects they can cause, and how much they cost.

Note: Products are mentioned for informational purposes only and do not imply an endorsement by the American Academy of Pediatrics.

The information contained in this publication should not be used as a substitute for the medical care and advice of your pediatrician. There may be variations in treatment that your pediatrician may recommend based on individual facts and circumstances.

From your doctor

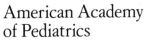

American Academy
of Pediatrics

DEDICATED TO THE HEALTH OF ALL CHILDREN™

The American Academy of Pediatrics is an organization of 60,000 primary care pediatricians, pediatric medical subspecialists, and pediatric surgical specialists dedicated to the health, safety, and well-being of infants, children, adolescents, and young adults.

American Academy of Pediatrics
Web site — www.aap.org

Copyright © 2005
American Academy of Pediatrics

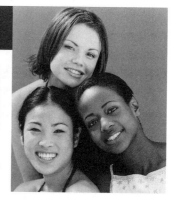

the pelvic exam

Pelvic exams are an important way to take care of your health. You should **get a pelvic exam** if you have ever had sex (even one time) or are having any problems with your periods.

Most women have questions and concerns about their first pelvic exam, but knowing what to expect can help you to feel more at ease. The pelvic exam only **takes about 5 minutes,** and your pediatrician will talk you through it and answer any questions you may have.

Why do I need a pelvic exam?

"Is a pelvic exam right for me now? If not now, when?" These are good questions to ask your pediatrician.

Basically, a pelvic exam is the best way for your pediatrician to **check** your reproductive system, which includes your vulva, vagina, cervix, ovaries, fallopian tubes, and uterus. The exam also includes **lab tests** that can check for problems like diseases that are easily treated if found early. Sometimes the pelvic exam includes tests for sexually transmitted diseases (STDs). However, for many patients with no symptoms a simple urine test can determine if you have 2 common STDs: chlamydia or gonorrhea.

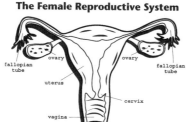

The Female Reproductive System

ovary · ovary · fallopian tube · fallopian tube · uterus · cervix · vagina

It's also a **great time to talk** with your pediatrician about things you may be thinking about, such as

- **Changes** in your body
- Your breasts
- Your **periods** (menstruation)
- **Sex**
- Pregnancy and birth control
- STDs
- Vaginal discharge
- Anything that hurts or bothers you

First a **mini-checkup**

Before the exam, your pediatrician may check your height, weight, blood pressure, lungs, heart, breasts, and stomach. You may be asked to give a small sample of urine and to empty your bladder so the pelvic exam is more comfortable.

There are **2 main parts** of your exam: the interview and the pelvic exam.

Part 1— The interview

Before the pelvic exam, your pediatrician will **ask you questions** about your **health** and your periods. So don't be surprised if you're asked questions like

- When did you get your first period?
- When was your last period?
- Do you have your periods regularly? How often?
- How long do they last?
- Do you have any pain, cramps, headaches, or mood swings with your periods?
- Do you use tampons, pads, or both?
- Have you ever had vaginal itching, discharge, or problems urinating?
- Do you douche? If yes, how often?

Don't be surprised if your pediatrician asks you about **sex.** You may be embarrassed or feel like your sex life is nobody else's business, but your pediatrician needs to know these things to help you protect your health. So be honest! And don't forget, whatever you say to your pediatrician is **confidential** and won't be discussed with anyone else without your permission (unless it's something life threatening, of course). These questions may include

Have you ever had any type of sexual intercourse (oral, anal, or vaginal)? **If yes,**

- When was the first time you had sex?
- Did you want to have sex, or were you forced to have sex?
- Have you had sex with more than 1 person? If yes, how many people?
- Have you had sex with men, women, or both men and women?
- How old were the people you had sex with?
- Do you use condoms or other types of birth control?

Remember, you can ask questions too. In fact, this is a great time to ask any questions you may have about your period, tampon use, sex, and other stuff. **Your pediatrician has lots of good information** and can give you advice on making good decisions, the benefits of not having sex (abstinence), and preventing pregnancy and diseases. **So don't be afraid to ask!**

Part 2— The pelvic exam

OK, so now it's time for the pelvic exam. You'll be left alone to undress and put on a gown. There will also be an extra sheet that you can use to cover yourself. Remember, **the entire exam only takes about 5 minutes.** Some girls think that having a pelvic exam will mean they are no longer virgins, but that's not true. The pelvic exam **doesn't change whether you are a virgin.** It's also not true that the pelvic exam is a "test" to see if you are a virgin. The exam can be done even if you have never had sexual intercourse, because the opening to your vagina is large enough to allow for the exam.

3 simple steps

Your pediatrician will describe each step of the exam. If you have any questions or feel uncomfortable, let your pediatrician know. Your pediatrician will have a nurse or assistant in the room during the exam. You can ask your mom, sister, or friend to join you if it makes you more at ease—it's up to you.

Step 1: The vulva (outside of your vagina and surrounding areas)
Your pediatrician will begin by looking at the outside of your vagina and surrounding areas to make sure everything looks normal.

Step 2: Inside your vagina
Then your pediatrician will use an instrument called a *speculum* to look inside your vagina. Specula are about the size of a tampon, made of disposable plastic or sterilized metal, and have no sharp edges.

- The speculum will be gently inserted into your vagina. You will feel some pressure, but it shouldn't hurt. Take **deep breaths** and try to **relax.** This will help relax your vaginal muscles and make this part of the test easier.
- Once the speculum is inside the vagina, it is opened so that your pediatrician can see your cervix.
- Then your pediatrician will use a cotton-tipped swab or a plastic brush to take a small sample of cells from your cervix. Samples are sent for tests, such as the **Pap smear,** which tests for abnormalities of the cervix. You may also be checked for diseases like gonorrhea and chlamydia with a second cotton swab.
- Once everything is collected, the speculum is gently removed. It's normal to have a little bit of spotting after the Pap smear.

Step 3: Uterus and ovaries

The last step of the exam checks your uterus and ovaries. Your pediatrician will gently insert 1 or 2 gloved fingers into your vagina and press on the outside of your abdomen with the other hand. It's quick and may feel a little funny, but shouldn't hurt.

That's it! Most women are surprised when their pelvic exam is over because it really is that quick.

Your sexual health

The following are 4 important things concerning your sexual health:

- **Having sexual feelings is normal.** Whether you decide to have sex is your choice. Talk with your partner about how you feel.
- **Not everyone your age is having sex,** including oral sex and intercourse. More than half of all teens **choose to wait** until they're older to have sex. Abstinence (not having sex, including oral, anal, and vaginal sex) means you won't become pregnant, become a teen parent, or get an STD.
- If you're going to have sex, using condoms is the best way to avoid getting STDs or becoming pregnant.
- To make sure you stay healthy, get regular medical checkups, urine testing for STDs, and a pelvic exam.

If your pediatrician finds a disease or any other problem, you may be referred to an OB/GYN (obstetrician/gynecologist). This type of doctor specializes in women's reproductive health.

Remember, the pelvic exam is an important part of taking care of your health. Ask your pediatrician if it's right for you.

The information contained in this publication should not be used as a substitute for the medical care and advice of your pediatrician. There may be variations in treatment that your pediatrician may recommend based on individual facts and circumstances.

From your doctor

American Academy of Pediatrics
DEDICATED TO THE HEALTH OF ALL CHILDREN™

The American Academy of Pediatrics is an organization of 60,000 primary care pediatricians, pediatric medical subspecialists, and pediatric surgical specialists dedicated to the health, safety, and well-being of infants, children, adolescents, and young adults.

American Academy of Pediatrics
Web site — www.aap.org

Copyright © 2005
American Academy of Pediatrics

puberty—ready or not
expect some big changes

Puberty is the time in your life when your body starts changing from that of a child to that of an adult. At times you may feel like your body is totally out of control! Your arms, legs, hands, and feet may grow faster than the rest of your body. You may feel a little clumsier than usual.

Compared to your friends you may feel too tall, too short, too fat, or too skinny. You may feel self-conscious about these changes, but many of your friends probably do too.

Everyone goes through puberty, but not always at the same time or exactly in the same way. In general, here's what you can expect.

When?

There's no "right" time for puberty to begin. **But girls start a little earlier than boys**—usually between 8 and 13 years of age. Puberty for boys usually starts at about 10 to 14 years of age.

What's happening?

Chemicals called hormones will cause many changes in your body.

Breasts!

Girls. The first sign of puberty in most girls is breast development—small, tender lumps under one or both nipples. The soreness goes away as your breasts grow. Don't worry if one breast grows a little faster than the other. By the time your breasts are fully developed, they usually end up being the same size.

When your breasts get larger, you may want to **start wearing a bra.** Some girls are excited about this. Other girls may feel embarrassed, especially if they are the first of their friends to need a bra. Do what is comfortable for you.

Boys. During puberty, boys may have swelling under their nipples too. If this happens to you, you may worry that you're growing breasts. **Don't worry—you're not.** This swelling is very common and only temporary. But if you're worried, talk with your pediatrician.

Hair, where?!

Girls & Boys. During puberty, soft **hair starts to grow** in the pubic area (the area between your legs and around your genitals—vagina or penis). This hair will become thick and very curly. You may also notice hair under your arms and on your legs. Boys might get hair on their faces or chests. Shaving is a personal choice. If you shave, remember to use your own clean razor or electric shaver.

Zits!

Girls & Boys. Another change that happens during puberty is that your skin gets **oilier** and you may start to sweat more. This is because your glands are growing too. It's important to wash every day to keep your skin clean. Most people use a deodorant or antiperspirant to keep odor and wetness under control. **Don't be surprised,** even if you wash your face every day, that you still get pimples. This is called acne, and it's normal during this time when your hormone levels are high. Almost **all teens** *get acne* at one time or another. Whether your case is mild or severe, **there are things you can do to keep it under control.** For more information on controlling acne, talk with your pediatrician.

Curves and muscles

Girls. As you go through puberty, you'll get taller, your hips will get wider, and your waist will get smaller. Your body also begins to build up fat in your belly, bottom, and legs. This is normal and gives your body the curvier shape of a woman.

Boys. As you go through puberty, you'll get taller, your shoulders will get broader, and as your muscles get bigger, your weight will increase.

Sometimes the weight gain of puberty causes girls and boys to feel so uncomfortable with how they look that they try to lose weight by throwing up, not eating, or taking medicines. This is not a healthy way to lose weight and may make you very sick. If you feel this way, or have tried any of these ways to lose weight, please talk with your parents or your pediatrician.

Does size matter?

Boys. During puberty, the penis and testes get larger. There's also an increase in *sex hormones.* You may notice you get erections (when the penis gets stiff and hard) more often than before. This is normal. Even though you may feel **embarrassed,** try to remember that unless you draw attention to it, most people won't even notice your erection. **Also, remember that** the size of your penis has nothing to do with manliness or sexual functioning.

Wet dreams

Boys. During puberty, your testes begin to produce sperm. This means that during an erection, you may also ejaculate. This is when semen (made up of sperm and other fluids) is released through the penis. This could happen while you are sleeping. You might wake up to find your sheets or pajamas are wet. This is called a nocturnal emission or "wet dream." This is normal and will stop as you get older.

Periods

Girls. Your *menstrual cycle,* or "period," starts during puberty. Most girls get their periods 2 to 2½ years after their breasts start to grow (between 10–16 years of age). During puberty, your ovaries begin to release eggs. If an egg connects with sperm from a man's penis (fertilization), it will grow inside your uterus and develop into a baby. To prepare for this, a thick layer of tissue and blood cells builds up in your uterus. If the egg doesn't connect with a sperm, the body does not need these tissues and cells. They turn into a blood-like fluid and flow out of your vagina. Your period is the monthly discharge of this fluid out of the body. A girl who has **started having periods is able to get pregnant,** even if she doesn't have a period every month.

You will need to wear some kind of sanitary pad and/or tampon to absorb this fluid and keep it from getting on your clothes. Most periods last from 3 to 7 days. Having your period does not mean you have to avoid any of your normal activities like swimming, horseback riding, or gym class. Exercise can even help get rid of cramps and other discomforts that you may feel during your period.

Voice cracking?

Boys. Your **voice** will get deeper, but it doesn't happen all at once. It usually starts with your voice cracking. As you keep growing, the cracking will stop and your voice will stay at the lower range.

New feelings

In addition to all the physical changes you will go through during puberty, there are many **emotional changes** as well. For example, you may start to care more about what other people think about you because you want to be accepted and liked. Your relationships with others may begin to change. Some become more important and some less so. You'll start to *separate more from your parents* and identify with others your age. You may begin to **make decisions** that could affect the rest of your life.

At times you may not like the attention of your parents and other adults, but they too are trying to adjust to the changes that you're going through. Many teens feel that their parents don't understand them—**this is a normal feeling.** It's usually best to let them know (politely) how you feel and then talk things out together. Also, it's normal to lose your temper more easily and to feel that nobody cares about you. **Talk about your feelings** with your parents, another trusted adult, or your pediatrician. You may be surprised at how much better you will feel.

Sex and sexuality

During this time, many young people also become more aware of their **feminine** and **masculine** sides. A look, a touch, or just thinking about someone may make *your heart beat faster* and produce a warm, tingling feeling all over. Talking with your parents or pediatrician is a good way to get information and to help you think about how these changes affect you.

You may ask yourself...

- When should I start dating?
- When is it OK to kiss?
- Is it OK to masturbate (stimulate your genitals for sexual pleasure)?
- How far would I go sexually?
- When will I be ready to have sexual intercourse?
- Will having sex help my relationship?
- Is oral sex really sex?

Some answers...

Masturbation is normal and won't harm you. Many boys and girls masturbate, many don't. Deciding to become sexually active, however, can be **very confusing.** On the one hand, you hear so many warnings and dangers about having sex. On the other hand, movies, TV, magazines, even the lyrics in songs all seem to be telling you that having sex is OK.

The fact is, sex is a part of life and, like many parts of life, **it can be good or bad.** It all depends on you and the choices you make. Take dating, for example. If you and a friend feel ready to start dating and it's OK with your parents, that's fine. You may find yourself in a more serious relationship. But if one of you wants to stop *dating,* try not to hurt the other person's feelings—just be honest with each other. After a breakup both partners may be sad or angry, but keeping on with normal activities and talking it over with a trusted adult is usually helpful.

Getting close to someone you like is OK too. Holding hands, hugging, and kissing may happen, but they *don't have to lead to having sex.* Deciding whether to have sex is one of the most important decisions you will ever make. Some good advice is in a brochure called *Deciding to Wait* that your pediatrician can give you. Why not **take your time** and think it through? Talk with your parents about your family's values. Waiting to have sex until you are older, in a serious relationship, and able to **accept the responsibilities** that come along with it is a great idea! And you can avoid becoming pregnant, getting someone pregnant, or getting deadly diseases. There is only one way to avoid pregnancy and infections related to sex, and **that is by not having sex.** And remember that oral sex is sex. You don't have to worry about pregnancy with oral sex, but you do have to worry about infections like herpes, gonorrhea, and HIV (the virus that causes AIDS).

However, if you decide to have sex, talk with your pediatrician about which type of birth control is best for you and how to **protect yourself** against sexually transmitted diseases.

Taking care of yourself

As you get older, there will be many decisions that you will need to make to ensure that you **stay healthy.** Eating right, exercising, and **getting enough rest** are important during puberty because your body is going through many changes. It's also important to feel good about yourself and the decisions you make. Whenever you have questions about your health or your feelings, don't be afraid to share them with your parents and pediatrician.

From your doctor

American Academy
of Pediatrics

DEDICATED TO THE HEALTH OF ALL CHILDREN™

The American Academy of Pediatrics is an organization of 60,000 primary care pediatricians, pediatric medical subspecialists, and pediatric surgical specialists dedicated to the health, safety, and well-being of infants, children, adolescents, and young adults.

American Academy of Pediatrics
Web site — www.aap.org

Copyright © 2005
American Academy of Pediatrics

Testicular Self-Exam

Most people think that cancer is a disease that only old people get. Cancer of the testicles — the male reproductive glands — is different. It is one of the most common types of cancer in men 15 to 34 years old.

Most testicular cancers are found by young men themselves. By doing a regular exam of your testicles, you greatly increase your chance of finding testicular cancer early if it does occur. It takes only 3 minutes a month to do a simple check for lumps on your testicles.

Here's How:

1. Do the exam once a month, after a warm bath or shower when the scrotal skin is most relaxed.
2. Roll each testicle gently between the thumb and first two fingers of both hands. The testicles should be smooth, with the consistency of a hard-boiled egg without the shell.

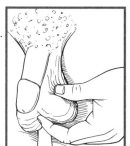

3. Feel for the small, comma-shaped cord, about the size of a pea, that is attached at the back of each testicle. This is a natural part of your testicles, and is called the epididymis. Learn what it feels like, so you will not confuse it with an abnormal lump.

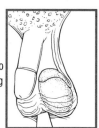

4. Check each testicle for lumps. If you find a lump, tell your doctor about it right away. Not all lumps are cancerous, but only your doctor will be able to tell the difference. Don't let fear keep you from getting the medical help you need.

What Is Normal?

- Testicles hang in the scrotum, and are about the same size.
- The left testicle usually hangs down a little more in the scrotum than the right testicle.
- A rope-like structure called the spermatic cord runs from your scrotum up into your groin.

What Are Possible Signs of Cancer?

- A lump on one of the testicles, which usually doesn't hurt.
- One testicle that gets larger than the other.
- A dull ache in your groin that doesn't go away.
- Your testicles feel heavy, like they are dragging.

The information contained in this publication should not be used as a substitute for the medical care and advice of your pediatrician. There may be variations in treatment that your pediatrician may recommend based on individual facts and circumstances.

Illustrations by Lauren Shavell

From your doctor

American Academy of Pediatrics

DEDICATED TO THE HEALTH OF ALL CHILDREN™

The American Academy of Pediatrics is an organization of 60,000 primary care pediatricians, pediatric medical subspecialists, and pediatric surgical specialists dedicated to the health, safety, and well-being of infants, children, adolescents, and young adults.

American Academy of Pediatrics
Web site — www.aap.org

Copyright © 1999
American Academy of Pediatrics

Section VI Further Reading

Blythe MJ. Common menstrual problems of adolescence. *Adolesc Med.* 1997;8:87–109

Economy KE, Laufer MR. Pelvic pain. *Adolesc Med.* 1999;10: 291–304

Iglesias EA, Coupey SM. Menstrual cycle abnormalities: diagnosis and management. *Adolesc Med.* 1999;10:255–273

Kahn JA, Gordon CM. Polycystic ovary syndrome. *Adolesc Med.* 1999;10:321–336

Perlman SE. Pap smears: screening, interpretation, treatment. *Adolesc Med.* 1999;10:243–254

Rome ES. Sexually transmitted diseases: testing and treating. *Adolesc Med.* 1999;10:231–241

Orthopedics and Sports Medicine

Correlates of Stress Fractures Among Preadolescent and Adolescent Girls

Keith J. Loud, MDCM, MSc*‡; Catherine M. Gordon, MD, MSc*; Lyle J. Micheli, MD‡; and Alison E. Field, ScD*§

ABSTRACT. *Objective.* Although stress fractures are a source of significant morbidity in active populations, particularly among young female athletes, the causes of stress fractures have not been explored among females <17 years of age or in the general population. The purpose of this study was to examine correlates of stress fractures in a large, population-based, national, cohort study of preadolescent and adolescent girls.

Methods. A cross-sectional analysis of data from 5461 girls, 11 to 17 years of age, in the Growing Up Today Study, an ongoing longitudinal study of the children of registered female nurses participating in Nurses' Health Study II, was performed. Mothers self-reported information regarding their children's histories of stress fractures on their 1998 annual questionnaire. Growing Up Today Study participants self-reported their weight and height, menarcheal status, physical activity, dietary intake, and disordered eating habits on annual surveys.

Results. In 1998, the mean age of the participants was 13.9 years. Approximately 2.7% of the girls had a history of stress fracture, 3% engaged in disordered eating (using fasting, diet pills, laxatives, or vomiting to control weight), and 16% participated in ≥16 hours per week of moderate to vigorous activity. Age at menarche, z score of BMI in 1998, calcium intake, vitamin D intake, and daily dairy intake were all unrelated to stress fractures after controlling for age. Independent of age and BMI, girls who participated in ≥16 hours per week of activity in 1998 had 1.88 greater odds of a history of stress fracture than did girls who participated in <4 hours per week (95% confidence interval [CI]: 1.18–3.30). Girls who participated in ≥16 hours per week of activity were also more likely than their peers to engage in disordered eating (4.6% vs 2.8%); however, disordered eating did not have an independent association with stress fractures (odds ratio [OR]: 1.33; 95% CI: 0.61–2.89). Independent of age and BMI, each hour per week of high-impact activity significantly increased the risk of stress fracture (OR: 1.05; 95% CI: 1.02–1.09). Among the high-impact physical activities, only running (OR: 1.13; 95% CI: 1.05–1.22) and cheerleading/gymnastics (OR: 1.10; 95% CI: 1.01–1.21) were independently associated with greater odds of stress fracture.

Conclusions. These findings suggest that, although activity can be beneficial for bone health, there is a threshold over which the risk of stress fracture increases significantly among adolescent girls. High-impact activities, particularly running, cheerleading, and gymnastics, appear to be higher risk than other activities. Prospective studies are needed to explore the directionality of these relationships, as well as the role of menstrual history. In the meantime, clinicians should remain vigilant in identifying and treating disordered eating and menstrual irregularities among their highly active, young, female patients. *Pediatrics* 2005; 115:e399–e406. URL: www.pediatrics.org/cgi/doi/10.1542/peds.2004-1868; *epidemiology, female, adolescents, stress fracture, activity.*

Abbreviations. GUTS, Growing Up Today Study; BMD, bone mineral density; OR, odds ratio; CI, confidence interval.

Stress fractures can be defined as skeletal defects that result from the repeated application of stress lower than that required to fracture a bone in a single loading.[1] Often called fatigue or insufficiency fractures, they are relatively uncommon in general but are a source of significant morbidity in active populations, with annual incidence rates ranging as high as 20% in prospective studies of young female athletes and military recruits.[2] In some cases, a stress fracture may be an indicator of inadequate bone mass.[3,4] These fractures would

From the *Division of Adolescent/Young Adult Medicine, Department of Medicine, and the ‡Division of Sports Medicine, Department of Orthopedic Surgery, Children's Hospital Boston and Harvard Medical School, Boston, Massachusetts; and §Channing Laboratory, Department of Medicine, Brigham and Women's Hospital and Harvard Medical School, Boston, Massachusetts.

Accepted for publication Nov 8, 2004. doi:10.1542/peds.2004-1868

No conflict of interest declared.

Reprint requests to (A.E.F.) Division of Adolescent/Young Adult Medicine, Children's Hospital Boston, 300 Longwood Ave, Boston, MA 02115. E-mail: alison.field@childrens.harvard.edu

be particularly important findings if noted during adolescence, a critical period for bone mass acquisition. More than one half of adult bone calcium is acquired during the teenage years and a woman's peak bone mineral density (BMD), a major determinant of her long-term risk of osteoporosis,[5,6] is thought to be achieved in early adulthood.[7,8] Weight-bearing exercise is a major stimulus for skeletal remodeling, increased bone mineralization, and thus increased BMD.[9,10] Therefore, maximization of peak BMD through participation in athletic activities during adolescence could assist in the prevention of osteoporosis later in these young women's lives.[11] Paradoxically, very high levels of activity may impair bone health. In addition, some female athletes who participate in high levels of activity resort to patterns of unhealthy eating,[12] which may lead to irregular menstrual cycles and an ensuing state of low serum estrogen levels that can counteract the beneficial effects of exercise on BMD.[13-15] This constellation of disordered eating, amenorrhea, and osteoporosis has come to be known as the "female athlete triad," a term coined by the American College of Sports Medicine in 1993.[16,17]

To begin to assess which stress fractures may be markers of compromised bone health, one must understand the epidemiology and causes of these injuries. Although stress fractures cause considerable impairment,[2] unfortunately little is known about the prevalence of or risk factors for stress fractures among young women. In a case-control study that included 38 adult female athletes, lower dietary calcium intake, current menstrual irregularity, lower use of oral contraceptives, and decreased bone density were identified as risk factors for stress fractures.[4] A large, cross-sectional survey of 2312 female active duty soldiers showed that a history of amenorrhea, smoking, white race, and a family history of osteoporosis were associated with a history of stress fracture.[18] In a case-control study, 27 female military recruits with stress fractures reported significantly higher levels of exercise and demonstrated lower femoral neck BMD than did 158 female subjects without fractures.[19]

Few studies have been conducted with samples of adolescent athletes, and none have examined factors related to stress fractures among girls <17 years of age. Therefore, the prevalence of stress fractures among children and adolescents is essentially unknown. In addition, the results from studies of older adolescent girls have not been consistent with those from studies of adult women.[20-25] Bennell et al[22] conducted a retrospective study of 53 Australian, female, track and field athletes 17 to 26 years of age and found that menstrual irregularities and restrictive eating behaviors were risk factors for stress fractures but low BMD was unrelated to fractures; however, in a prospective follow-up study of the same cohort, Bennell et al[23] found that lower bone density and a history of menstrual disturbances were significant predictors of stress fractures. A similar prospective study of 50 US, collegiate, track and field athletes found that a history of stress fracture and low BMD were significant predictors of stress fractures but menstrual history was not.[25] Hormonal status, serum calcium and vitamin D levels, nutritional history, and white ethnicity were not identified as significant predictors of stress fractures. The inconsistencies among earlier studies and more recent investigations may be accounted for by differences between military and nonmilitary populations[23] and differences in sample size, with some of the studies being underpowered to detect significant differences in the proposed predictors of stress fractures. Moreover, those investigators studied exclusively athletes whose primary sport involved running, thus precluding conclusions about correlates of stress fractures in the wider population of older adolescent females, the majority of whom are neither runners nor particularly athletic. To assess the prevalence and correlates of stress fractures among adolescent girls in general, we examined cross-sectional data for 5461 participants in an ongoing national cohort study.

Methods

OVERVIEW

The Growing Up Today Study (GUTS) was established by recruiting the children of women participating in Nurses' Health Study II who were 9 to 14 years of age in 1996. With the use of Nurses' Health Study II data, a detailed letter was sent to identified mothers who had children between the ages of 9 and 14 years. The purposes of GUTS were explained, and the mothers were asked to provide parental consent for their children to enroll. Additional details were reported previously.[26] Approximately 68% of the girls ($N = 9039$) and 58% of the boys ($N = 7843$) returned completed questionnaires, thereby assenting to participate in the cohort. The project was approved by the Human Subjects Committee at Brigham and Women's Hospital; this study was approved by that committee and by the Committee on Clinical Investigation at Children's Hospital Boston.

MEASURES

Self-reported physical activity, dietary intake, weight control behaviors, Tanner stage of development, weight, and height were assessed annually from 1996 through 1998. We calculated BMI values from self-reported weight and height information (weight [in kilograms]/height [in meters] squared) and calculated z scores on the basis of the Centers for Disease Control and Prevention growth charts (www.cdc.gov/growthcharts), which are age and gender specific. BMI values >3 SDs above the mean were excluded as outliers. In addition, BMI values of <12 for preadolescents or <12.5 for adolescents were excluded as being biologically implausible. Overweight was defined as a BMI ≥85th percentile for age and gender, whereas underweight was defined as a BMI <10th percentile. Drawings of the 5 Tanner stages of development of pubic hair were used for assessment of pubertal development.

Weight control methods (dieting, exercise, self-induced vomiting, diet pills, and laxatives) were assessed with questions adapted from the Youth Risk Behavior Surveillance System questionnaire.[27] Girls who reported using any of these methods to control their weight during the past year were requested to state the frequency of the behavior ("less than once a month," "1–3 times a month," "once a week," "2–6 times per week," or "every day"). Purging was defined as using laxatives or vomiting at least monthly to control weight in 1995–1996, 1997–1998, or 1998–1999. Disordered eating was defined as using vomiting, laxatives, fasting, or diet pills at least monthly to control weight in 1995–1996, 1996–1997, 1997–1998, or 1998–1999.

Dietary intake was assessed with the Youth/Adolescent Questionnaire, a validated, self-administered, semiquantitative, food frequency questionnaire assessing intake over the past year.[28] The questionnaire asked participants how often, on average, they consumed each of the 131 foods listed. Response categories for foods ranged from less than once per month to ≥4 times per day. Nutrient intake was computed by multiplying the frequency of consumption of the foods by their nutrient content, as estimated from standard food composition sources.

Physical activity was assessed with 18 questions on the hours per week, within each of the 4 seasons, that a participant engaged in a specific activity (eg, volleyball or soccer). Hours per week of moderate or vigorous activity were computed as the sum of the average hours per week engaged in basketball, baseball, biking, dance/aerobics, hockey, running, swimming, skating, skateboarding, soccer, tennis, cheerleading/gymnastics, lifting weights, volleyball, or karate. Reports of an average of >40 hours per week were considered implausible and were therefore set to missing and not used in the analysis. High-impact activity was computed as the sum of the average hours per week engaged in basketball, running, soccer, tennis, cheerleading, or volleyball. Medium-impact activity was computed as the sum of the average hours per week engaged in baseball, dance/aerobics, hockey, or karate. Nonimpact activity was computed as the sum of the average hours per week engaged in biking, swimming, skating, skateboarding, or lifting weights.

Menstrual status was assessed annually from 1996 through 1998. Girls were asked whether their menstrual periods had started. Girls who marked "yes" were asked the age when periods began (age at menarche).

The primary outcome measure was a history of a stress fracture. The 1999 questionnaire to the mothers asked the question, "Has a doctor ever said that this child had any of the following conditions?" The orthopedic conditions were tendonitis, stress fracture, Osgood-Schlatter syndrome, and anterior cruciate ligament tear.

SAMPLE

Participants included 7864 girls who completed the 1998 questionnaire. Those who completed the abbreviated questionnaire sent to participants who did not return the more complete questionnaire ($n = 973$), were <9 or >14 years of age at baseline (1996) ($n = 99$), did not provide plausible information or were missing information on physical activity ($n = 122$) or weight or height in 1998 ($n = 133$), or whose mother did not complete the mother's questionnaire ($n = 1076$) were excluded. After these exclusions, 5461 girls, 11 to 17 years of age in 1998, remained for analysis.

DATA ANALYSES

All analyses were conducted with the SAS statistical software package.[29] Generalized estimating equations (SAS proc genmod) were used for all multivariate analyses, to account for correlations between siblings. All statistical models assessing associations with a history of stress fracture controlled for age.

Hours per week of moderate or vigorous activity were initially divided into 8 groups, ie, <1, 1 to 3.9, 4 to 7.9, 8 to 11.9, 12 to 15.9, 16 to 19.9, 20 to 24.9, and ≥25 hours per week. Because of small group sizes, the top 3 categories were collapsed into 1 group for analyses, for a total of 6 groups. For multivariate analyses, the bottom 2 categories were also collapsed, making a total of 5 groups (<4, 4–7.9, 8–11.9, 12–15.9, and ≥16 hours per week). Participants who reported <4 hours per week of moderate or vigorous activity were used as the reference group. The Tanner stage of development was not included in the analysis because the majority of girls were in Tanner stage 4 or 5 (33% of girls were in Tanner stage 4 and 44% were in Tanner stage 5) and only 9% were in Tanner stage 1 or 2. All P values were 2-sided, with $P < .05$ being considered statistically significant.

Results

In 1998, the mean age of the girls was 13.9 years and 67.9% of the girls had achieved menarche. The mean BMI of the girls was 20.1 kg/m²; 7% of the girls were underweight and 15% were overweight. In addition, 3% of the girls engaged in disordered eating. Approximately 94% of the girls were white. Most girls participated in physical activity. Ninety-six percent of the girls engaged in ≥1 hour per week of moderate or vigorous activity, and 16% of the girls participated in ≥16 hours per week of activity (Table 1).

Approximately 2.7% of the girls (149 of 5461 girls) had a history of stress fracture. Age exhibited a J-shaped relationship with a history of stress fracture (Fig 1). Slightly more than 2% of 11- and 12-year-old subjects had a history of stress fracture, whereas 3.9% of 15-year-old subjects and 4.6% of 16-year-old subjects had a history of stress fracture. Stress fracture prevalence increased markedly at the highest levels of moderate or vigorous activity (Fig 2). The prevalence of stress fracture was approximately 2% to 3% for all categories of activity at <16 hours per week; however, 5% of girls who participated in ≥16 hours per week had a history of stress fracture.

In a bivariate analysis, being overweight appeared protective against stress fracture (1.7% of overweight girls and 2.9% of normal-weight girls had a stress fracture, $P = .056$). After adjustment for age, being overweight had an inverse but nonsignificant association with stress fracture (overweight versus normal-weight odds ratio [OR]: 0.62; 95% confidence interval [CI]: 0.36–1.07). Being underweight was unrelated to a history of fracture (underweight versus normal-weight OR: 0.76; 95% CI: 0.36–1.59). Girls who participated in ≥16 hours per week of activity were more likely than their peers (4.2% vs 2.8%, $P < .03$) to engage in disordered eating (using fasting, diet pills, laxatives, or vomiting to control weight); however, neither disordered eating (age-adjusted OR: 1.33; 95% CI: 0.61–2.89) nor purging (ie, using vomiting or laxatives to control weight) (age-adjusted OR: 0.63; 95% CI: 0.09–4.34) had an independent association with a history of stress fracture. Age at menarche (age-adjusted OR: 0.99; 95% CI: 0.84–1.17), quartile of calcium intake (age-adjusted OR: 1.06; 95% CI: 0.91–1.24), quartile of vitamin D intake (age-adjusted OR: 1.00; 95% CI: 0.86–1.16), and servings per day of dairy products (age-adjusted OR: 1.00; 95% CI: 0.87–1.15) were also unrelated to stress fracture.

Table 1. Age, Maturational Stage, Dietary Intake, and Activity of 5461 Girls in GUTS in 1998

Mean (SD) age, y	13.9 (1.6)
Mean (SD) BMI, kg/m^2	20.1 (3.3)
Mean (SD) BMI z score	0.1 (0.9)
Mean (SD) age at menarche, y	12.0 (1.1)
% Postmenarcheal	67.8 ($n = 3638$)
% Underweight	7.1 ($n = 386$)
% Overweight	14.9 ($n = 814$)
% Disordered eating	3.1 ($n = 172$)
Mean (SD) calcium intake, mg/d	1121 (491)
Mean (SD) vitamin D intake, IU/d	314 (218)
Mean (SD) daily servings of dairy	1.8 (1.2)
% with moderate or vigorous activity of *	
<1 h/wk	3.7 ($n = 204$)
1–3.9 h/wk	17.5 ($n = 957$)
4–7.9 h/wk	27.5 ($n = 1503$)
8–11.9 h/wk	21.2 ($n = 1156$)
12–15.9 h/wk	14.3 ($n = 782$)
16–19.9 h/wk	7.9 ($n = 430$)
20–24.9 h/wk	5.0 ($n = 274$)
≥25 h/wk	2.8 ($n = 155$)
Mean (SD) time of nonimpact activity, h/wk	3.6 (3.3)
Mean (SD) time of intermediate-impact activity, h/wk	1.7 (2.3)
Mean (SD) time of high-impact activity,† h/wk	4.2 (4.2)

*Sum of basketball, baseball, biking, dance/aerobics, hockey, running, swimming, skating, skateboarding, soccer, tennis, cheerleading, lifting weights, volleyball, and karate.

†Sum of basketball, running, soccer, tennis, cheerleading, and volleyball.

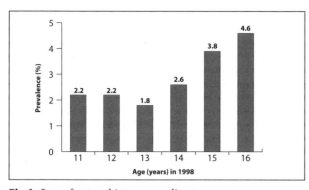

Fig 1. Stress fracture history according to age.

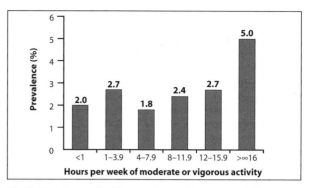

Fig 2. Prevalence of a history of stress fracture according to hours per week of moderate or vigorous activity.

The age of the participants was strongly associated with a history of stress fracture in all multivariate models tested (Tables 2–4), with a 27% to 29% increase in the odds of stress fracture for every year over 11 years of age in 1998. The BMI z score was not associated with stress fracture (age-adjusted OR: 0.91; 95% CI: 0.78–1.07), and inclusion of it in the multivariate models did not change substantially the effect estimates for other covariates (Table 2); therefore, the BMI z score was not included in the final statistical models. Being postmenarcheal in 1998 appeared to confer protection against stress fracture (age-adjusted OR: 0.61; 95% CI: 0.40–0.95) and remained significant in most models (Tables 2–4).

The association between the quantity of moderate or vigorous activity and stress fracture was complex. Compared with girls participating

in 4 hours per week of moderate or vigorous activity, girls participating in ≥16 hours per week had a significantly higher risk of stress fracture (OR: 1.88; 95% CI: 1.18–3.03) (Table 2). There was no evidence that girls participating in 8 to 11.9 hours per week or 12 to 15.9 hours per week of activity had any increase in the risk of stress fracture.

High-impact physical activity (basketball, running, soccer, tennis, cheerleading, or volleyball) was associated with a small but significantly increased odds of stress fracture (OR per hour of activity: 1.06; 95% CI: 1.03–1.10) (Table 3). Among the high-impact physical activities, only running (OR: 1.13; 95% CI: 1.05–1.22) and cheerleading/gymnastics (OR: 1.10; 95% CI: 1.01–1.21) were associated independently with greater odds of stress fracture (Table 4).

Table 2. Associations of Age, BMI, Menarcheal Status, and Activity With a History of Stress Fracture Among the Girls in GUTS

	OR, Adjusted for Age (95% CI)	OR, Adjusted for All Covariates in Model (95% CI)
Age		1.28 (1.12–1.46)
BMI z score	0.91 (0.78–1.07)	0.97 (0.81–1.16)
Postmenarcheal	0.61 (0.40–0.95)	0.62 (0.38–0.99)
<4 h/wk of activity*	1.00 (referent)	1.00 (referent)
4–7.9 h/wk of activity	0.71 (0.41–1.21)	0.66 (0.39–1.14)
8–11.9 h/wk of activity	0.94 (0.55–1.60)	0.90 (0.53–1.52)
12–15.9 h/wk of activity	0.94 (0.53–1.70)	0.89 (0.50–1.60)
≥16 h/wk of activity	1.86 (1.16–3.00)	1.88 (1.18–3.03)

There were 146 cases among 5219 girls with complete data. The ORs are from a generalized estimating equation model that adjusted for the covariates listed in the table. Information on correlates came from the 1998 GUTS questionnaire.

*Sum of basketball, baseball, biking, dance/aerobics, hockey, running, swimming, skating, skateboarding, soccer, tennis, cheerleading, lifting weights, volleyball, and karate.

Table 3. Association of Age, Menarcheal Status, and Type of Impact Activity With a History of Stress Fracture Among the Girls in GUTS

	OR, Adjusted for Age (95% CI)	OR, Adjusted for All Covariates in Model (95% CI)
Age		1.29 (1.14–1.47)
Postmenarcheal in 1998	0.61 (0.40–0.95)	0.61 (0.39–0.93)
Nonimpact activity, h/wk	1.03 (0.98–1.08)	1.03 (0.98–1.08)
Medium-impact activity, h/wk	1.00 (0.93–1.09)	1.00 (0.92–1.08)
High-impact activity, h/wk*	1.06 (1.02–1.10)	1.06 (1.03–1.10)

There were 146 cases among 5206 girls with complete data. The ORs were from a generalized estimating equation model that adjusted for the covariates listed in the table. Information on correlates came from the 1998 GUTS questionnaire.

*Sum of basketball, running, soccer, tennis, cheerleading, and volleyball.

Table 4. Association of Age, Menarcheal Status, and Type of Activity With a History of Stress Fracture Among the Girls in GUTS

	OR, Adjusted for Age (95% CI)	OR, Adjusted for All Covariates in Model (95% CI)
Age		1.27 (1.11–1.45)
Postmenarcheal in 1998	0.61 (0.40–0.95)	0.64 (0.41–1.01)
Nonimpact activity, h/wk	1.03 (0.98–1.08)	1.02 (0.97–1.07)
Medium-impact activity, h/wk	1.00 (0.93–1.09)	0.00 (0.92–1.08)
Running, h/wk	1.14 (1.06–1.21)	1.13 (1.05–1.22)
Basketball, h/wk	1.01 (0.91–1.11)	1.02 (0.92–1.12)
Soccer, h/wk	1.03 (0.94–1.14)	1.04 (0.94–1.15)
Cheerleading or gymnastics, h/wk	1.11 (1.03–1.21)	1.10 (1.01–1.21)
Tennis, h/wk	0.84 (0.62–1.14)	0.83 (0.61–1.13)
Volleyball, h/wk	1.05 (0.93–1.18)	1.05 (0.94–1.18)

There were 135 cases among 4954 girls with complete data. The ORs were from a generalized estimating equation model that adjusted for the covariates listed in the table. Information on correlates came from the 1998 GUTS questionnaire.

Discussion

This study is the first of which we are aware to report a lifetime prevalence of stress fracture (2.7%) among a large, general-population sample of adolescent girls living throughout the United States. Because this is the first general-population sample study, it is difficult to compare our results with estimates from other studies. Studies of collegiate athletes estimated that the annual incidence of stress fractures among late adolescent and young adult female athletes is between 2.7% and 6.9%.[30-32] The largest cohort studies of stress fracture have been among women in the US military and observed incidence rates among adult female recruits during basic training to be between 1.1% and 3.4%.[33,34] Although the mothers of the

GUTS participants were registered nurses and thereby potentially more accurate than lay persons in providing information regarding medical conditions, relying on maternal recollections of stress fracture diagnoses still might have resulted in an underestimate of the true prevalence of stress fractures in our sample. Alternatively, children of nurses might have greater access to medical care than other children and thus might be more likely to be diagnosed as having a stress fracture. Therefore, the prevalence of stress fractures in our sample might be higher than it would have been had we chosen to study a group of girls with less access to medical care. However, our results are consistent with those from other published studies that used medical records,[30,31] direct monitoring,[32-34] and radiographic confirmation of stress fractures.[20]

The age of the participants was the most consistent correlate of stress fractures in this sample. This is most likely because age might be a proxy for exposure time; the older an adolescent girl is, the longer she might have been participating in risk-associated activities and the greater the chance that she has sustained a stress fracture. Alternatively, it could be that the older girls had begun to participate in high school sports or other higher levels of competition, in which the intensity of the training sessions (a variable not assessed in the GUTS) is greater than the intensity of training sessions for girls at younger ages.

Menarche (the onset of menstrual periods) occurs near the end of the pubertal growth spurt, which is accompanied by rapid increases in bone mass and BMD.[6] BMD is one of the main determinants of a bone's ability to withstand loading.[2,6] Girls in this study who had achieved menses had decreased odds of stress fracture, which was possibly related to increased bone mass, although BMD was not measured in this cohort. Because menarche had not occurred for a nontrivial percentage of this sample, we must interpret associations of age at menarche with stress fracture that appear nonsignificant very cautiously. In a cohort of older adolescent, Australian, track and field athletes, age at menarche was an independent risk factor for stress fracture, with younger ages providing significant protection.[23] Other studies have not replicated this finding consistently, although none has suggested an inverse relationship between age at menarche and risk of stress fracture.[35] Numerous small studies also suggested consistently that stress fractures are less common among athletes with regular menses,[35] although the studies were not large enough to have adequate statistical power to allow firm conclusions. The presumed mechanism through which regular menses would offer protection against stress fracture is the improved BMD associated with an endogenous euestrogenic state.

Although clinicians and public health officials also target disordered eating, low calcium intake, low vitamin D intake, and fewer servings per day of dairy products as behaviors that can potentially be changed to improve bone mass and prevent future osteoporosis, none of these factors was significantly associated with a history of stress fracture in our sample. Because 50% to 85% of the variability in BMD is attributable to genetic factors,[6] any negative effects of these modifiable correlates on BMD might not have been large enough to affect stress fracture risk.

Identification of a threshold quantity of activity at which the risk of stress fracture increases would be valuable for clinicians, athletic trainers, coaches, and others guiding athletes in their training regimens. Because stress fractures result from repetitive stress loading,[1] training volume (ie, amount of exercise), which is related directly to the number of repeated applications (or "strain cycles"), is a key component in the pathophysiologic development of stress fractures.[2] Our finding of increased odds of stress fractures with ≥16 hours per week of moderate or vigorous activity requires additional refinement to define the "breakpoint" for increased odds of stress fracture, because higher strata of weekly exercise amounts contained too few participants with a history of stress fracture to allow meaningful associations. Prospective studies that can establish temporal directionality are also needed. Because this study was cross-sectional, it is impossible to identify whether the reported activity preceded the stress fractures. Because the activity reports were from 1998 and the mothers' questionnaire reported any stress fracture diagnosis up to 1999, it is possible that some of the activity assessments reflected a period after the stress fracture diagnosis had been made. It is likely that participants would have moderated their training volumes after a stress fracture diagnosis. Therefore, our effect estimate for the association between hours per week of activity and the risk of stress fracture might have underestimated the true association. The true breakpoint might have occurred at a volume of >16 hours per week, reflecting preinjury activity levels.

Similarly, it is unknown whether girls with stress fractures might have changed activity types after their diagnoses. Girls with stress fractures or even their precursors, ie, symptomatic stress reactions, might have chosen to switch to lower-impact activities; therefore, our results might underestimate the true effects of high-impact activities. The increased odds of stress fracture with running in this study were consistent with the results of other reports that showed high incidence rates for stress fractures among collegiate female runners.[30] Sample sizes for gymnastics in other studies were too small to allow comparisons. It is biologically plausible that these activities are most strongly associated with stress fractures, because the load applied to bone can equal 2 to 5 times body weight for jogging or running[36] and up to 12 times body weight for jumping and landing,[37] which are repetitive maneuvers in cheerleading and gymnastics.

Finally, recent evidence[38] reemphasized the observation that stress fractures result from an imbalance between the microfractures caused by repeated loading cycles and the bone's own responses to remodel the damaged region.[39,40] Because remodeling is a constant dynamic process, it may be inadequate acceleration of this process that results in stress fractures. Therefore, the more relevant activity parameter is likely to be the rate of increase in exercise volume, not the total volume itself. Our inability to date the stress fractures in this study precluded us from investigating this issue.

A limitation of this study was that the cohort was >90% white and was thus not representative of the US adolescent population. This limitation is mitigated because whites are a group at increased risk of stress fractures.[33] Therefore, the GUTS cohort represents an enriched sample in which to study this particular injury. Because the participants were children of registered nurses, the sample might underestimate female subjects of low socioeconomic status, potentially limiting the generalizability to female subjects of middle and upper socioeconomic status. Moreover, the high levels of physical activity demonstrated in this cohort contrast with the consistent findings of low and declining levels of physical activity among adolescent girls in other national surveys.[41] Therefore, the estimated levels of activity we observed might not be generalizable to a general

sample of adolescent female subjects. The strength of the association between the activity level and the risk of stress fracture should be generalizable, but other studies might observe lower rates of stress fractures because of having fewer girls who are highly active.

Although BMI and age- and gender-specific BMI percentile are used widely as proxy measures of weight status and body fatness, it is important to remember that highly active people who have substantial muscle mass may weigh slightly more than the standard for their height, despite having low body fat levels. Therefore, some girls might have been overweight according to the Centers for Disease Control and Prevention pediatric cutoff values but not overfat. Although the correlations between BMI, BMI percentile, and body fat are very high,[42-44] BMI is not a direct measure of body fatness; therefore, there is some misclassification when weight status is based on BMI alone, because BMI does not take into account lean body mass. The result of this misclassification might have been underestimation of the true association between weight status and risk of stress fracture. Another limitation was the lack of radiographic confirmation of stress fractures in this study, which could have resulted in overestimation of the prevalence of true stress fractures because of the difficulty of distinguishing them from stress reactions or other overuse injuries on the basis of clinical findings alone. If possible, future studies should define the outcome, namely, stress fracture, on the basis of objective findings and should specify the body part injured. Most importantly, the temporal relationship between stress fracture and activity should be clarified by assessing when the injury occurred and assessing the exposures before the diagnosis of stress fracture.

It is disturbing that highly active girls were more likely than their less-active peers to engage in disordered eating practices. This association may be attributable to girls using physical activity, as well as disordered eating, as a means to achieve a certain ideal body image. Although we did not observe an association between stress fractures and disordered eating, it is possible that the lack of association was attributable to a lack of statistical power rather than a true lack of association.

Therefore, clinicians should be advised to maintain their vigilance in screening their athletic and apparently healthy young female patients.

Given the significant gaps in knowledge about risk factors for stress fractures among active adolescent girls across a range of impact-loading sports, the results of this study provide critical information regarding the roles that amount and type of exercise play in the development of stress fractures in this population. The results provide preliminary information on how much exercise may be deleterious to skeletal health. Future studies should identify when the stress fracture occurred, so that only activity levels before the fracture are used in analyses trying to establish the point at which activity levels start to increase the risk of fracture. Moreover, future studies that examine more closely the amounts and types of weekly exercise, the types of training surfaces, and the menstrual history associated with stress fractures should help determine whether these injuries can be prevented and help identify whether some stress fractures should be considered markers of low bone mass and subsequent increased risk of long-term osteoporosis.

Acknowledgments

The analysis was supported by the Maternal and Child Health Bureau Leadership Education in Adolescent Health (grant 5T71 MC00009-12 0), the Glaser Pediatric Research Network, the Boston Obesity Nutrition Research Center (grant DK46200), and research grants (grants DK46834 and DK59570) from the National Institutes of Health.

References

1. Martin AD, McCulloch RG. Bone dynamics: stress, strain and fracture. *J Sports Sci.* 1987;5:155–163
2. Brukner P, Bennell K, Matheson G. *Stress Fractures.* Victoria, Australia: Blackwell Science; 1999
3. Marx RG, Saint-Phard D, Callahan LR, Chu J, Hannafin JA. Stress fracture sites related to underlying bone health in athletic females. *Clin J Sport Med.* 2001;11:73–76
4. Myburgh KH, Hutchins J, Fataar AB, Hough SF, Noakes TD. Low bone density is an etiologic factor for stress fractures in athletes. *Ann Intern Med.* 1990;113:754–759
5. Kanis JA. Assessment of fracture risk: who should be screened? In: Favus MJ, ed. *Primer on the Metabolic Bone Diseases and Disorders of Mineral Metabolism.* 5th ed. Washington, DC: American Society for Bone and Mineral Research; 2003:316–323
6. Eastell R. Pathogenesis of postmenopausal osteoporosis. In: Favus MJ, ed. *Primer on the Metabolic Bone Diseases and Disorders of Mineral Metabolism.* 5th ed. Washington, DC: American Society for Bone and Mineral Research; 2003:314–316
7. Bonjour JP, Theintz G, Buchs B, Slosman D, Rizzoli R. Critical years and stages of puberty for spinal and femoral bone mass accumulation during adolescence. *J Clin Endocrinol Metab.* 1991;73:555–563
8. Theintz G, Buchs B, Rizzoli R, et al. Longitudinal monitoring of bone mass accumulation in healthy adolescents: evidence for a marked reduction after 16 years of age at the levels of lumbar spine and femoral neck in female subjects. *J Clin Endocrinol Metab.* 1992;75:1060–1065
9. Wolman RL, Clark P, McNally E, Harries M, Reeve J. Menstrual state and exercise as determinants of spinal trabecular bone density in female athletes. *BMJ.* 1990;301:516–518
10. Lloyd T, Chinchilli VM, Johnson-Rollings N, Kieselhorst K, Eggli DF, Marcus R. Adult female hip bone density reflects teenage sports-exercise patterns but not teenage calcium intake. *Pediatrics.* 2000;106:40–44
11. Etherington J, Harris PA, Nandra D, et al. The effect of weight-bearing exercise on bone mineral density: a study of female ex-elite athletes and the general population. *J Bone Miner Res.* 1996;11:1333–1338
12. Rosen LW, McKeag DB. Pathogenic weight-control behavior in female athletes. *Phys Sports Med.* 1986; 14:79–84
13. Mansfield MJ, Emans SJ. Anorexia nervosa, athletics, and amenorrhea. *Pediatr Clin North Am.* 1989;36:533–549
14. Marcus R, Cann C, Madvig P, et al. Menstrual function and bone mass in elite women distance runners: endocrine and metabolic features. *Ann Intern Med.* 1985; 102:158–163
15. Rencken ML, Chesnut CH III, Drinkwater BL. Bone density at multiple skeletal sites in amenorrheic athletes. *JAMA.* 1996;276:238–240
16. Yeager KK, Agostini R, Nattiv A, Drinkwater B. The female athlete triad: disordered eating, amenorrhea, osteoporosis. *Med Sci Sports Exerc.* 1993;25:775–777
17. Otis CL, Drinkwater B, Johnson M, Loucks A, Wilmore J. American College of Sports Medicine position stand: the female athlete triad. *Med Sci Sports Exerc.* 1997;29:i–ix
18. Friedl KE, Nuovo JA, Patience TH, Dettori JR. Factors associated with stress fracture in young Army women: indications for further research. *Milit Med.* 1992; 157:334–338

19. Lauder TD, Dixit S, Pezzin LE, Williams MV, Campbell CS, Davis GD. The relation between stress fractures and bone mineral density: evidence from active-duty Army women. *Arch Phys Med Rehabil.* 2000;81:73–79

20. Bennell KL, Brukner PD. Epidemiology and site specificity of stress fractures. *Clin Sports Med.* 1997;16:179–196

21. Bennell KL, Malcolm SA, Brukner PD, et al. A 12-month prospective study of the relationship between stress fractures and bone turnover in athletes. *Calcif Tissue Int.* 1998;63:80–85

22. Bennell KL, Malcolm SA, Thomas SA, et al. Risk factors for stress fractures in female track-and-field athletes: a retrospective analysis. *Clin J Sport Med.* 1995;5:229–235

23. Bennell KL, Malcolm SA, Thomas SA, et al. Risk factors for stress fractures in track and field athletes: a twelve-month prospective study. *Am J Sports Med.* 1996; 24:810–818

24. Bennell KL, Malcolm SA, Thomas SA, Wark JD, Brukner PD. The incidence and distribution of stress fractures in competitive track and field athletes: a twelve-month prospective study. *Am J Sports Med.* 1996;24:211–217

25. Nattiv A. Stress fractures and bone health in track and field athletes. *J Sci Med Sport.* 2000;3:268–279

26. Field AE, Camargo CA Jr, Taylor CB, Berkey CS, Roberts SB, Colditz GA. Peer, parent, and media influences on the development of weight concerns and frequent dieting among preadolescent and adolescent girls and boys. *Pediatrics.* 2001;107:54–60

27. Kann L, Warren CW, Harris WA, et al. Youth Risk Behavior Surveillance: United States, 1995. *MMWR Surveill Summ.* 1996;45:1–84

28. Rockett HR, Breitenbach M, Frazier AL, et al. Validation of a youth/adolescent food frequency questionnaire. *Prev Med.* 1997;26:808–816

29. SAS Institute. *SAS User's Guide: Statistics, Version 6.* 4th ed. Cary, NC: SAS Institute; 1990

30. Lloyd T, Triantafyllou SJ, Baker ER, et al. Women athletes with menstrual irregularity have increased musculoskeletal injuries. *Med Sci Sports Exerc.* 1986;18:374–379

31. Goldberg B, Pecora C. Stress fractures: a risk of increased training in freshmen. *Phys Sports Med.* 1994;22:68–78

32. Johnson AW, Weiss CB Jr, Wheeler DL. Stress fractures of the femoral shaft in athletes: more common than expected: a new clinical test. *Am J Sports Med.* 1994; 22:248–256

33. Brudvig TJ, Gudger TD, Obermeyer L. Stress fractures in 295 trainees: a one-year study of incidence as related to age, sex, and race. *Milit Med.* 1983;148:666–667

34. Pester S, Smith PC. Stress fractures in the lower extremities of soldiers in basic training. *Orthop Rev.* 1992; 21:297–303

35. Bennell K, Matheson G, Meeuwisse W, Brukner P. Risk factors for stress fractures. *Sports Med.* 1999;28:91–122

36. Cavanagh PR, Lafortune MA. Ground reaction forces in distance running. *J Biomech.* 1980;13:397–406

37. McNitt-Gray JL. Kinetics of the lower extremities during drop landings from three heights. *J Biomech.* 1993;26: 1037–1046

38. Bennell K, Crossley K, Jayarajan J, et al. Ground reaction forces and bone parameters in females with tibial stress fracture. *Med Sci Sports Exerc.* 2004;36:397–404

39. Romani WA, Gieck JH, Perrin DA, Saliba EN, Kahler DM. Mechanisms and management of stress fractures in physically active persons. *J Athl Train.* 2002;37:306–314

40. Bennell KL, Malcolm SA, Wark JD, Brukner PD. Models for the pathogenesis of stress fractures in athletes. *Br J Sports Med.* 1996;30:200–204

41. Neumark-Sztainer D, Story M, Hannan PJ, Tharp T, Rex J. Factors associated with changes in physical activity: a cohort study of inactive adolescent girls. *Arch Pediatr Adolesc Med.* 2003;157:803–810

42. Field AE, Laird N, Steinberg E, Fallon E, Semega-Janneh M, Yanovski JA. Which metric of relative weight best captures body fatness in children? *Obes Res.* 2003;11: 1345–1352

43. Daniels SR, Khoury PR, Morrison JA. The utility of body mass index as a measure of body fatness in children and adolescents: differences by race and gender. *Pediatrics.* 1997;99:804–807

44. Goulding A, Gold E, Cannan R, Taylor RW, Williams S, Lewis-Barned NJ. DEXA supports the use of BMI as a measure of fatness in young girls. *Int J Obes Relat Metab Disord.* 1996;20:1014–1021

Dietary Supplements as Ergogenic Aids

by Joseph N. Chorley, MD, FAAP

An ergogenic aid can be any substance, treatment, or strategy employed to improve physical performance or appearance beyond the effects of training. Ergogenic aids include pharmacologic agents, hormones, nutritional supplements, relaxation techniques, improved equipment (shoes, poles, etc), and blood doping. ("Blood doping" refers to the use of erythropoietin or transfusion of previously donated blood to increase oxygen-carrying capacity.)

Dietary supplements are among the most commonly used ergogenic aids. In 1999, Americans spent $12.7 billion on dietary supplements. This represented a 250% increase over what was spent in 1993, the year before the Dietary Supplement Health and Education Act (DSHEA) became federal law.

The DSHEA significantly liberalized the definition of a dietary supplement in the United States. For regulatory purposes, dietary supplements now include not only essential vitamins and nutrients, but also herbs or other botanicals, amino acids, and dietary substances for use by man to supplement the diet. Substances categorized as dietary supplements are not subject to the stringent premarket safety evaluations that apply to other food ingredients.

The growth of the supplement industry cannot be attributed solely to deregulation. American society places a premium on youthful appearance and athletic achievement. Coupled with an increased acceptance of alternative medicine and a win-at-all-costs mentality in sports, supplements have found a fertile market.

The most prominent claims for dietary supplements assert that they will improve muscular strength, increase lean muscle mass, increase fat loss, decrease fatigue, and improve muscle repair. Adolescents are especially vulnerable to these claims at a time when they are searching for acceptance and accomplishment while experiencing pubertal body changes. Sports achievement and success during this life stage are extremely important.

While there are numerous ergogenic aids, this article will concentrate on the dietary supplements that are most commonly used and readily available. Discussion will consider what sound scientific research has and has not demonstrated, and how pediatricians can use this information to identify, counsel, and treat those adolescents who are taking nutritional supplements, or are thinking about it.

Epidemiology

In one cross-sectional study of nutritional supplement use among students in grades 7 through 12,

---

Learning Objectives

After reading this article, pediatricians will understand their role in counseling adolescents who use or are considering using dietary supplements as ergogenic aids. They will be able to:

- Describe the types of ergogenic aids likely to be used by adolescents
- Discuss the potential risks and benefits of ergogenic aids
- Present strategies to enhance performance or appearance through diet and training

---

Joseph N. Chorley, MD, FAAP, is an assistant professor of pediatrics in the Section of Adolescent Medicine and Sports Medicine, Baylor College of Medicine. Dr. Chorley, who is board certified in both pediatrics and sports medicine, is team physician for Texas Southern University as well as three high schools in the Houston area.

researchers found that males were more likely to use supplements than females. Males most often found out about supplements from their friends, while females were more likely to ask their parents. Rural schools had a higher prevalence of supplement use than urban and suburban schools. Only 5% of adolescents surveyed said that their parents did not know about their use.

Supplements are marketed to those who are trying to look better or get stronger. Body image dissatisfaction is present in both athletes and nonathletes. Although national data are not available, at least one study has countered the notion that "only the big jocks are using supplements," by demonstrating that the prevalence of steroid and supplement use among a group of high school males was highest among those with a body mass index (BMI) in the lowest 15th percentile.

Because anabolic/androgenic steroids are not dietary supplements, a discussion of their risks and benefits is beyond the scope of this paper. Brief mention is appropriate, however, because steroids continue to be used by adolescents. According to the 1999 National Institute on Drug Abuse Monitoring the Future Study, 2.7% of 8th and 10th graders, and 2.9% of 12th graders reported that they had taken anabolic steroids at least once in their lives. The 1999 levels represent a statistically significant increase from 1991, the first year that data on steroid use were collected. Survey results also showed that the proportion of 12th graders who perceived steroid use to be a health risk declined from 68% to 62% between 1998 and 1999.

Social and Political Context

While a drug manufacturer must first prove safety before marketing a product, manufacturers of dietary supplements are free to market their products without regulatory preapproval. Supplement manufacturers do not have to prove the purity of their products or document the amount of ingredients they contain. In fact, one study of 16 different brands of DHEA demonstrated that fewer than 50% contained the amount stated on the label. Supplement manufacturers also do not have to study how those products interact with other medications, demonstrate short- or long-term safety, or formulate a therapeutic dose. (The FDA does monitor for adverse reactions. If a consumer complaint prompts an FDA investigation, and if alleged negative side effects are proven, the FDA can restrict distribution.)

Manufacturers cannot claim that dietary supplements are useful to diagnose, treat, or cure any disease, but they can claim to maintain health. For example, while they cannot claim that a supplement is an effective treatment for osteoporosis, they can say that it will enhance bone health. Manufacturers will often include a disclaimer (eg, "some supplements do not accomplish their intended function as well as alleged," or words to that effect).

Although deaths have been reported in relation to their use, supplements are not subject to the same regulatory requirements as medications. The Federal Trade Commission, which regulates the sales and advertising practices of the industry, has sanctioned companies that implied that their supplements did not have side effects. While the companies that were sanctioned had to put warning labels on their supplements and advertisements, other companies not named in the suit selling similar products do not.

Claims regarding certain dietary supplements, such as creatine, DHEA, and androstenedione, are similar to those made for testosterone (eg, increased strength, muscle repair and recovery, and lean muscle mass). Deregulation made it possible to obtain these supplements without a prescription. While legal, the use of these supplements is ethically questionable and may be associated with many of the same health risks that have been seen with steroid use.

Selected Ergogenic Aids

New dietary supplements are continually introduced; it is not possible to present a comprehensive list. Figure 1 and Table 1 provide an overview. Some of the most commonly employed agents are discussed next.

Table 1. Supplements With Documented Usefulness

Supplement	Claims	Strength of Research
Alcohol	Decreases hand tremors in low doses	Limited
Alkaline salts	Buffer lactic acidosis	Strong
Antioxidants	Improve muscle tissue damage prevention	Limited
Aspartates	Preferentially accesses fat stores to protect muscle and liver glycogen during prolonged exercise	Limited
Caffeine	Neuromuscular stimulant. Preferentially accesses fat stores to protect muscle and liver glycogen during prolonged exercise	Strong
Carbohydrates	Provide energy substrate needed for prolonged exercise Increase glycogen stores for endurance competition	Strong
Choline	Related to maintenance of normal levels of the neurotransmitter acetylcholine	Limited
Creatine	Increases intacellular creatine kinase so that ATP can be resynthesized from ADP more efficiently	Mixed
Water	Maintains fluid balance during exercise to optimize hemodynamic performance and heat regulation	Strong
Glycerol	Allows the body to hyperhydrate	Limited
Phosphates	Uncertain, but may be related to ATP, intracellular buffering system, or increased level of 2,3 DPG and increased O_2 delivery to the muscle	Limited
Vitamin E	Antioxidant. Maintains optimal O_2 delivery at high altitudes	Limited

CREATINE

Creatine is a popular supplement with over $100 million per year in sales in the United States. Its widespread use has prompted increased research, although there is only one study involving adolescents. Creatine is synthesized in the liver and kidney from arginine and glycine, and is present in foods such as fish and red meat. There is no recommended daily allowance, but in the average adult, approximately 2 g are needed to replace the creatine excreted daily by the kidney in the form of creatinine.

Nearly 100% of oral creatine is absorbed by the GI tract and transported to muscle cells. A sodium-dependent transporter will selectively move creatine into the muscle cell depending on intracellular creatine concentration. This process may be augmented by exercise or by ingestion of 100 grams of simple carbohydrate. Excess creatine that is not incorporated into the muscle is excreted in the urine. There appear to be "responders and nonresponders" to creatine supplementation; persons with low intracellular creatine seem to be more likely to respond with increased strength and muscle mass. At this time, there is no screening test to predict responder status.

Creatine's effect at the muscular level is hypothesized to be related to its presence in the phosphorylated form, phosphocreatine. Phosphocreatine in the muscle can rephosphorylate low-energy ADP to the high-energy ATP, which is the energy source for short duration, high intensity exercise. Other proposed mechanisms of action include improved intracellular phosphate diffusion, acid buffering effects, and activation of glycogenolysis pathways. Initially, increased lean muscle mass is secondary to increased intracellular water accompanying the increased intracellular creatine concentration, rather than true muscular hypertrophy. With continued use, strength training has been shown to be more effective with creatine and can result in muscular hypertrophy. However, only one study (Grindstaff, et al) has included adolescents, and it did not include strength training.

Amino acids:
- Arginine, ornithine, lysine
- Branched-chain (leucine, isoleucine, valine)
- Glutamine
- Glycine
- Tryptophan

Bee pollen
Carnitine (L-carnitine)
Ciwujia
Coenzyme Q10 (ubiquinone)
Conjugated linoleic acid (CLA)
Dehydroepiandrosterone (DHEA)
Ephedrine, ephedra (Ma Huang)
Fructose 1,6-diphosphate
Gamma oryzanol (ferulic acid, FRAC)
Ginkgo biloba
Ginseng
Inosine
Medium chain triglycerides (MCTs)

Minerals
- Boron
- Chromium
- Iron
- Selenium
- Vanadium

Octacosanol

Omega-3 fatty acids
Polylactate
Protein
Smilax officianalis

Vitamins
- B-complex
  - Thiamin (B1)
  - Riboflavin (B2)
  - Niacin
  - Pyridoxine (B6)
  - Cyanocobalamin (B12)
  - Folacin
  - Pantothenic acid
- Antioxidants
  - Beta carotene
  - Vitamin C

Vitamin B15
Wheat germ oil
Yohimbine (yohimbe)

Based upon information extracted from: Williams MH. Nutritional ergogenics and sports performance. Table 1: Efficacy of some purported nutritional ergogenics. *The President's Council on Physical Fitness and Sports Research Digest.* 1998;3:2

Figure 1. Supplements promoted as ergogenic aids whose efficacy has not been established.

Although controversial, there is some reason to believe that creatine may benefit athletes engaged in short duration, high intensity, repetitive exercise. There is some evidence that creatine use has benefits for adults in activities which are predominantly anaerobic, such as high-intensity sprints (running, swimming, or cycling), and resistance weight training. Athletes involved in aerobic sports do not seem to benefit from creatine supplementation.

There have been no studies that demonstrate long-term safety with the use of creatine. Reported side effects of creatine have been anecdotal and not definitively linked to its use. Creatine's side effects have been minimal at doses ≤20 grams/ day. There are reports of gastrointestinal distress (nausea and vomiting), heat illness, muscle cramps and strains, and hypertension. Since creatinine is a direct metabolite of creatine, there

may be an elevated serum creatinine concentration; however, serum levels are generally normal. There have been two cases of renal disease in individuals using creatine that resolved following cessation of supplementation. (In one case, a patient developed interstitial nephritis. In the second, the patient developed focal segmental glomerular sclerosis and marked reduction in the glomerular filtration rate.) Those adults who have or are at risk for renal disease (eg, patients with hypertension, diabetes, or a family history of renal disease) should be medically monitored.

Creatine is usually taken in 4- to 12-week cycles, beginning with a loading dose of 20 g per day for 1 week, followed by a maintenance dose of 2 g to 5 g per day. Once the muscles have been "loaded," 2 grams per day will replace the normal turnover of creatine in the body. Higher doses will be excreted. The usual cost for this program ranges between $15 and $30 per month, depending on whether the supplement includes carbohydrate.

The limited understanding of how creatine affects adolescents makes it impossible to formulate a risk/benefit ratio regarding its use. The lack of scientific research about efficacy, need for long- and short-term safety profiles, concerns about the effect on growing bodies, and worry about adulterating substances that might be present in supplements that contain creatine, add to the apprehension about its use. While creatine is not listed as a banned substance, a recent American College of Sports Medicine roundtable stated clearly that "creatine supplementation is not advised for the pediatric population (ie, <18 years of age)."

DHEA AND ANDROSTENEDIONE

DHEA and androstenedione are two closely related steroid precursors marketed as testosterone "prohormones." They are both produced in the adrenal glands and testes, and are converted to testosterone, dihydrotestosterone, and estrogens. Their popularity has increased in recent years. Androstenedione is not illegal in major league baseball, although it has been banned by the National Collegiate Athletic Association, National Football League, National Hockey League, and at Olympic levels of competition. The FDA has stated that there are no medical indications for DHEA, and in 1996, it was banned from medical use. It is now available without a prescription.

Oral DHEA has been hypothesized to increase circulating testosterone as well as anabolic insulin-like growth factors (I-L GF). Androstenedione in doses of 300 mg daily has been shown to increase serum concentration of estrone, estradiol, and testosterone when compared with 100 mg daily and with placebo controls. The "recommended" daily dose of DHEA varies from 50 to 100 mg to as high as 1600 mg per day and for androstenedione is 100 to 300 mg per day. Unfortunately, athletes believe that more is better and will often take 5 to 10 times the amount used in the research studies.

Significant androgenic side effects associated with the use of these agents include breast enlargement, testicular atrophy, and infertility in males, and increased facial and body hair, voice deepening, and clitoral enlargement in females. Higher doses may increase these risks. Warning labels for these products caution that they should not be used by persons at risk for prostate or breast cancer. Liver toxicity was noted in animal studies with DHEA. Premature closure of epiphyses and irreversible shorter stature could result from prolonged use of higher doses of DHEA and androstenedione. Athletes who have not completed puberty should not use these substances. These side effects are similar to those of anabolic steroids.

GHB, GBL AND BD

Gamma hydroxybutyric acid (GHB), and its metabolites gamma butyrolactone (GBL) and 1,4 butanediol (BD) cause decreased mental status, altered sensorium, decreased respiratory drive, and coma. Although these drugs are taken primarily for recreational purposes, they have been used in some sports supplements. Recently, GHB, GBL, and BD have been linked to 122 serious illnesses and 3 deaths. Health authorities believe that manufacturers are renaming their products and substituting BD for GBL. However, the potential adverse effects associated with BD ingestion are as great as those of GHB and GBL.

Office Assessment

Pediatricians should assess for use of ergogenic aids by adolescents. Adult data show that most of those taking supplements do not voluntarily tell their primary care provider. Positive responses to screening questions should be pursued in a nonjudgmental way. One approach might be: "I hear that there are a lot of athletes taking supplements to get stronger. Are any athletes on your team taking them? Has anyone ever offered them to you? Did you take them? How much and for how long?"

Whether the context is a preparticipation sports evaluation or a health maintenance visit, a questionnaire may be useful. Questions with reference to sports participation and body weight and image are important screening tools. For example:

- Have you gained or lost weight in the past 6 months?
- Are you taking any medications, vitamins, or supplements?
- Are you trying to lose or gain weight?
- In what sports will you be participating this year?

Although the physical examination is of limited usefulness in this regard, some findings are associated with use of some ergogenic aids. Vital signs can be helpful in identifying patients with hypertension (stimulants) or profound weight gain (anabolic/androgenic steroids, creatine, DHEA).

Anabolic/androgenic steroids and androstenedione may cause skin changes, including jaundice, acne, coarsening, and male pattern baldness, as well as needle marks and bruising at the injection site. Steroids also may cause testicular atrophy and gynecomastia in males, and deepening of the voice, decrease in breast fat tissue, and clitoromegaly in females. Some of these changes are irreversible. Laboratory evaluation is not routine, but may show an altered lipid profile, elevated liver function tests, elevated serum creatinine, and altered serum and urine hormone concentrations.

Educating Patients About Fundamentals

Strength training and proper nutrition are the most important ergogenic methods to increase muscle mass in the adolescent athlete. These are the prime safe and effective alternatives to the use of anabolic steroids and supplements. It is important to emphasize that the use of dietary supplements in adolescents is largely unstudied, so that short and long term safety cannot be guaranteed. Other supplements initially thought to be safe in the past were later shown to have serious consequences (eg, eosinophilic myalgia syndrome linked to use of tryptophan or phenylalanine has been a documented cause of death in at least 38 cases). It is extremely difficult to keep up with the wide array of supplements that

are on the market; there is a new one every few months that "everyone is trying," despite very little solid information about its risks and benefits.

In counseling patients who may be taking or considering supplements, it is useful to present what is known about them, observe that there is much we do not know about them, and emphasize the solid scientific evidence showing that proper nutrition and strength training are safe and effective methods to achieve their goals.

NUTRITION

Areas for nutrition education include adequate fluids, calories, carbohydrates, and proteins.

Fluids

A body water deficit of as little as 1% can impair exercise performance and increase the probability of developing heat injury. Proper hydration includes drinking before, during, and after exercise. Some of the recommendations for fluids include:

- *Before*—It is recommended that individuals drink about 500 mL (about 17 ounces) of fluid about 2 hours before exercise to promote adequate hydration and allow time for excretion of excess ingested water.
- *During*—Athletes should start drinking early and at regular intervals (every 15–20 minutes) in an attempt to consume fluids at a rate sufficient to replace all the water lost through sweating, or consume the maximum amount that can be tolerated. Addition of proper amounts of carbohydrates and/or electrolytes to a fluid replacement solution is recommended for exercise events of duration greater than 1 hour. This rate of carbohydrate intake can be achieved without compromising fluid delivery by drinking 600 to 1200 mL per hour of solutions containing 4% to 8% carbohydrate (4 to 8 g/100cc) and sodium (0.5 to 0.7 g/L of water).
- *After*—If adequately hydrated during the workout, the postworkout weight should equal the preworkout weight. For every pound of weight lost, an athlete must consume 16 ounces or one-half liter of sports drink to replace fluid

lost. This will help to prevent increased risk of heat injury that may occur with cumulative dehydration over a number of days.

Carbohydrate

About 60% to 65% of daily calories should come from carbohydrate (6 to 10 g/kg of body weight). There are several ways to use carbohydrates as ergogenic aids. Carbohydrate loading may be employed by any athlete to augment performance in prolonged duration events (eg, marathons, 100-mile bike rides, and 2- to 3-day tournaments). It increases muscle glycogen concentration. Improved glycogen storage offers protection against "hitting the wall" or operating at a glycogen deficit.

Carbohydrate loading is begun 8 days before the anticipated event.

- *On the first day:* moderately long nonexhaustive workout with normal diet
- *The next 3 days:* 5 grams carbohydrate/kg/day with long, moderate-intensity exercise
- *The last 3 days:* 10 grams carbohydrate/kg/day with short duration, low-intensity exercise

Carbohydrates are also employed before and during aerobic and anaerobic events. In aerobic events, there is convincing evidence that such use benefits those athletes exercising for more than 60 minutes (there is little or no benefit in events lasting less than 60 minutes). Whether or not carbohydrate will improve performance in athletes in prolonged, intermittent, high-energy exercise (eg, soccer, hockey, and football) remains controversial.

It is important for athletes to practice consuming carbohydrate (eg, food, sports drink, sports bars, or gel) before and during exercise, because there is considerable difference between individuals' tolerance of carbohydrate ingestion.

Sources of Medically Sound Information

In addition to those discussed in this article, a plethora of supplements are available over the Internet, by mail, and in health food and grocery stores. Every few months, there is a new, "hot" supplement that is being talked about in the gym and written up in the muscle magazines. It is very difficult to keep up with the literature on the subject, most of which is scientifically flawed.

Listed below are several resources for current information, which can be employed to evaluate consumer literature.

Publications

Clark N. *Nancy Clark's Sports Nutrition Guidebook.* 2nd ed. Champaign, IL: Human Kinetics Publishers, Inc; 1997

Proceedings of the Gatorade Sports Science Institute Conference on Nutritional Ergogenic Aids, November 1994. *International Journal of Sport Nutrition & Exercise Metabolism.* 1995; 5 (suppl)

Fuentes RJ, Rosenberg JM, eds. *Athletic Drug Reference '99.* Durham, NC: Clean Data, Inc; 1999

Williams MH. *The Ergogenics Edge: Pushing the Limits of Sports Performance.* Champaign, IL: Human Kinetics Publishers, Inc; 1998

Web Sites

Office of Dietary Supplements, National Institutes of Health: http://odp.od.nih.gov/ods/site.html

International Bibliographic Information on Dietary Supplements (IBIDS) Database, National Agricultural Library Food & Nutrition Education Center, US Department of Agriculture: www.nal.usda.gov/fnic/IBIDS

Food and Drug Administration Center for Food Safety and Applied Nutrition: http://vm.cfsan.fda.gov/~dms/supplmnt.html

National Institute on Drug Abuse Web page on steroid abuse: www.steroidabuse.org

The President's Council on Physical Fitness and Sports: www.indiana.edu/~preschal/council.html. (Follow "health" link to *The President's Council on Physical Fitness and Sports Research Digest.*)

The quantity of pre-exercise carbohydrate depends on body size and time before competition.

- *4 hours before competition:* 4 g/kg body weight (eg, for a 60 kg athlete, this would translate to 3 cups of pasta, 1 cup sauce, 1 dinner roll, or 16 ounces juice)
- *1 hour before competition:* 1 g/kg body weight (eg, for a 60 kg athlete, 2 cups cereal, or 8 ounces skim milk)
- *10 minutes before competition:* 0.5 g/kg body weight (eg, for a 60 kg athlete, one small bagel)

During competition, 30 to 60 grams of carbohydrate should be ingested per hour. Sports drinks with fructose or carbohydrate concentrations greater than 8% should be avoided in order to minimize gastrointestinal side effects.

The body is most efficient at replacing glycogen stores when carbohydrate is consumed during the first hour after exercise. The athlete should consume 1.5 g/kg of carbohydrate and 0.5 g/kg protein during the first 15 minutes after exercise, and the same amount again in 2 hours. This can be achieved by drinking milk, or eating bananas, cereal, or a plain sandwich with 2 ounces of meat.

A number of carbohydrate products with and without protein have been marketed to athletes and are available in powder, bar, and gel forms. These products provide energy in a convenient form for active individuals, but offer no physiologic advantage over food sources. Many of the "energy bars" contain 35 to 40 g of carbohydrate and 10 g of protein, which can be obtained by eating a cereal bar and 8 ounces of skim milk. Convenience comes at a price; energy bars are often 2 to 3 times more expensive than the food equivalents.

Protein

The recommended daily allowance of protein for adolescents is 0.4 to 1.0 g/kg/day, and the average US diet contains 1.4 g/kg/day. Therefore, most adolescents consume adequate amounts. Because muscle contains a high percentage of protein, however, protein intake has been the focus of many strength-building programs in young athletes. The recommended intake levels of protein for adults, as published by the National Science Council are:

- *athletes:* 0.8 g/kg/day
- *strength athletes:* 1.2 to 1.7 g/kg/day
- *endurance athletes:* 1.2 to 1.4 g/kg/day

Protein powder supplements are not needed for the majority of athletes. Adolescents who do not get adequate dietary protein, such as those who restrict calories (especially females who may have the female athlete triad of disordered eating, amenorrhea, and osteopenia), vegetarians, or those who do not consume sufficient carbohydrates, may benefit from protein supplements. For those who consume insufficient carbohydrates, protein serves as another source of calories, and when taken with carbohydrates, protein slows their absorption so that there is a more sustained glucose elevation. In those with adequate caloric intake, excess protein is either burned as energy or stored as fat. Protein powder is more expensive than protein in food. Protein powder costs approximately 10 cents per gram of protein while egg whites cost about 1 to 2 cents per gram of protein. A practical way to augment protein-deficient diets is to add nonfat dry milk powder to milk (1/2 cup per gallon), or to mashed potatoes, grits, or hamburgers (1 tablespoon per serving of each food). This will give an additional 4 to 5 grams protein per serving. Three ounces of chicken, fish or meat contain the same amount of protein as one-third cup of powder at about one-third the cost.

About 20% to 25% of daily calories should be from protein sources. If there is inadequate caloric intake, endogenous protein will be broken down by gluconeogenesis; when this happens, the athlete's sweat smells a bit like ammonia. In order to gain 1 pound of muscle, an athlete must consume an additional 100 grams of protein and also strength train.

Strength Training

Strength training refers to conditioning programs to build strength. A properly supervised strength training program has shown increased strength for both male and female athletes, both before and after puberty. Muscle hypertrophy with weight training does not occur until puberty.

Although weightlifting is one of the essential elements, strength training includes exercises that use machines, weights, and the athlete's body weight to provide a training load. Olympic weightlifting, power lifting, and single-repetition maximum lift should be reserved for those athletes who have previous strength training experience, are skeletally mature, and have good balance and technique.

Equipment used for weight training (eg, isokinetic, circuit training, or variable resistance exercise machines), must be the correct size for the adolescent athlete. Each body part should be exercised twice weekly with at least 24 to 36 hours of rest between workouts of the same body part. A balanced workout regimen emphasizes opposite sides of the body (eg, quads and hamstrings, biceps and triceps). If each side is not exercised equally, there is potential for muscular imbalance and injury. The desired results dictate the number of repetitions. While strength athletes lift more weight fewer times (6 to 8 repetitions per set), endurance athletes lift less weight more times (12 to 15 repetitions per set). Increased muscular strength and muscular hypertrophy have been demonstrated in studies covering as little as 6 to 8 weeks. Aerobic training can supplement strength training in order to engage in a complete program.

Summary

The dietary supplement industry is growing rapidly. Unfortunately, the efficacy, safety, and proper dosing of these supplements have not been studied in adolescents. Pediatricians should identify and counsel athletes about potential risks, side effects, and costs of supplements. Adolescents may be advised that proper nutrition and appropriate strength training will allow them to achieve many of their athletic goals.

Bibliography

American Academy of Pediatrics Committee on Sports Medicine. Strength training, weight and power lifting, and body building by children and adolescents (RE9196). *Pediatrics.* 1990;86:801–803

American College of Sports Medicine. Position Stand: Exercise and fluid replacement. *Med Sci Sports Exerc.* 1996;28:i–vii

American College of Sports Medicine Roundtable on the Physiological and Health Effects of Oral Creatine Supplementation. *Med Sci Sports Exerc.* 2000;32:706–717

Bhasin S, Storer T, Berman N, et al. The effects of supraphysiologic doses of testosterone on muscle size and strength in normal men. *N Engl J Med.* 1996;335:1–7

Goldberg L, MacKinnon D, Elliot D, et al. The Adolescent Training and Learning to Avoid Steroids Program: Preventing drug use and promoting health behaviors. *Arch Pediatr Adolesc Med.* 2000;154:332–338

Grindstaff PD, et al. Effects of creatine supplementation on repetitive sprint performance and body composition in competitive swimmers. *Intl J Sport Nut Exerc Met.* 1997;7:330–346

Lawson MA, Fortenberry JD, Kraft D. Characteristics and frequency of use of nutritional supplements in adolescent athletes [abstract]. *J Adolesc Health.* 1999;24:85

Leder BZ, Longcope C, Catlin DH, Ahrens B, Schoenfeld DA, Finkelstein JS. Oral androstenedione administration and serum testosterone concentrations in young men. *JAMA.* 2000;283:779–782

Middleman AB, Faulkner AH, Woods ER, Emans SJ, DuRant RH. High-risk behaviors among high school students in Massachusetts who use anabolic steroids. *Pediatrics.* 1995;96:268–272

Neumark-Sztainer D, Story M, Falkner NH, Beuhring T, Resnick MD. Sociodemographic and personal characteristics of adolescents engaged in weight loss and weight/muscle gain behaviors: Who is doing what? *Prev Med.* 1999;28:40–50

Wang MQ, Yesalis CE, Fitzhugh EC, et al. Desire for weight gain and potential risks of adolescent males using anabolic steroids. *Percept Mot Skills.* 1994;78:267–274

Williams MH. *The Ergogenics Edge: Pushing the Limits of Sports Performance.* Champaign, IL: Human Kinetics Publishers, Inc; 1997:156–165,178–184,247–251

Williams M. Nutritional ergogenics and sports performance. *The President's Council on Physical Fitness and Sports Research Digest.* 1998;3:1–8

Acknowledgment

The editors would like to acknowledge technical review by Steven J. Anderson, MD, chair, AAP Committee on Sports Medicine and Fitness.

Improving Sports Performance: Tips for Patients

Dietary supplements have been promoted as tools to improve appearance, strength, and athletic performance, but not all supplements on the market have been proven safe and effective. Properly supervised nutrition and exercise programs have a solid track record. They can help you look and feel healthy and strong, now and in the future.

Many athletes feel compelled to excel, and many more feel pressure from coaches, friends, and parents to "do whatever it takes to win." Some athletes believe that dietary supplements will improve performance more effectively than a properly supervised routine of exercise and nutrition. This is not realistic.

This is a brief guide to safe and effective ways to build strength and stamina.

Supplements

SAFETY—Unlike medicines, supplements are not tested for safety, the correct dose, or for interactions with drugs. Serious illnesses and deaths have been associated with the use of some supplements. For example, androstenedione and DHEA can cause acne, baldness and decreased height. When males take these supplements, breasts can develop and testicles can shrink.

EFFECTIVENESS—Claims made on labels may be exaggerated. Very few scientific studies have addressed the safety and effectiveness of supplements when taken by adults. Even fewer studies have been done with athletes, and almost none with teenage athletes.

CONTENT—The amount of a supplement in the bottle may be much less than what is written on the label.

COST—It can cost 3 to 10 times as much to get the same amount of carbohydrate and protein in powders, bars, and gels instead of from food.

Resources

For more information about strength training, nutrition, and supplements, look to these resources.

BOOKS:

The Ergogenics Edge: Pushing the Limits of Sports Performance by Melvin Williams. Human Kinetics Publishers, Inc., Champaign, IL, 1997

Nancy Clark's Sports Nutrition Guidebook by Nancy Clark. Human Kinetics Publishers, Inc., 2nd ed., Champaign, IL, 1997

WEBSITES:

Sports Nutrition
www.sportsparents.com/nutrition/

National Institute on Drug Abuse Web page on steroid abuse
www.steriodabuse.org

The President's Council on Physical Fitness and Sports
www.fitness.gov

National Strength and Conditioning Association
www.nsca-lift.org/menu.asp

Strength Training

Strength training improves strength in males and females. If done correctly, strength training is safe for teenagers. Remember: Proper technique is important for a safe and effective workout.

● The equipment used must be well maintained and the proper size for the athlete.

● In order for muscles to get stronger, they must have time to recover between workouts; otherwise they just break down. At least 48 hours' rest is essential before working out the same muscle group again.

● It is very important to work both sides (front and back) of your body equally, otherwise an imbalance in strength and flexibility may result in injury.

Nutrition

Good nutrition gives the body the building blocks it needs to recover after you have worked out.

DON'T SKIP BREAKFAST—It really is the most important meal of the day. Athletes who work out early in the morning can try a liquid breakfast or sports drink, or have a snack before bed.

EAT SNACKS—Your muscles restock energy stores most efficiently if you eat a healthy snack within 1 hour after practice or workout.

EAT A WELL-BALANCED DIET—If you are trying to gain muscle be sure to take in adequate carbohydrates to give you enough energy and an extra serving (3 oz.) of meat, peanut butter, or a milk shake.

Performance-enhancing Substances and Their Use Among Adolescent Athletes

*Jason J. Koch, MD**

Objectives

After completing this article, readers should be able to:
1. List the names and actions of performance-enhancing substances.
2. Describe the signs and symptoms of anabolic steroid use.
3. Describe the signs and symptoms of growth hormone use.
4. Characterize the adverse effects of anabolic steroids and other performance-enhancing substances.
5. Describe the clinical changes seen in patients using anabolic steroids and growth hormone.

Introduction

Pediatricians see many adolescent patients who present for sports physical examinations, camp physical examinations, or immunizations. One area of concern in the health of these patients should be the use of performance-enhancing substances (PES), which may be better known as ergogenic aids or performance-enhancing drugs. The use of these agents has grown significantly among athletes to help performance and among nonathletes to improve appearance. Use of substances such as anabolic steroids, creatine, and dietary supplements is widespread among adolescents and is related to numerous pressures to excel in academics, at home, and on the athletic field.

To be prepared to discuss PES with our patients, we should know the names of the substances, how they are believed to work, and problems associated with their use. We should be aware of the current epidemiology, prevalence, and popular attitudes. We also should know the

clinical aspects of PES, including symptoms and signs of use and abuse as well as the science behind the chemicals and the studies that have been published. Finally, we should understand our role in the management of patients using these substances and how we can act as educators, spokespersons, and advocates for child athletes.

History and Definitions

PES have been present as long as there has been human competition. Aztec athletes and warriors ate human hearts to give them strength in battle and competition. Ancient Greek Olympians used special mushrooms they believed gave them added power. In the 1800s, European cyclists used heroin, cocaine, and ether-soaked tablets to enhance their performance. In 1904, the winner of the men's Olympic marathon used strychnine and brandy to help his performance. In 1920, the Olympic 100-meter dash champion drank sherry and ate raw eggs to augment his ability.

In the 1940s, testosterone was administered to racehorses to increase top speeds and endurance. In the 1950s, former Soviet Union power lifters began using anabolic steroids, and by 1964, anabolic steroid use was common among American, Soviet, and German weight lifters. In 1967, the International Olympic Committee (IOC) began to test competing athletes for substance use, but it did not begin testing for steroid compounds until 1976. Testing has escalated a sophisticated conflict between athletes and officials. At the 2000 Olympic Games in Sydney, Australia, reports were prevalent in the popular media about athletes who had been removed from competition and even had their awards confiscated due to positive tests for illegal or banned substances.

*Southdale Pediatrics, Edina, MN.

Table 1. Classification of Purported Performance-enhancing Substances

Supplements	Prescription Drugs	Illicit or Banned Substances
● Androstenedione	● Anabolic steroids	● Amphetamines
● Antioxidants	● Beta blockers	● Anabolic steroids
● Caffeine	● Beta$_2$ agonists	● Blood doping
● Creatine	● Diuretics	(Erythropoietin)
● Ephedra alkaloids (Ma Juang)	● Human growth hormone	● Cocaine
● Vitamins (B, C, E, Folate)	● Human chorionic	● Dihydroepiandrostenedione
● Minerals (Boron, Calcium, Chromium, Iron, Magne-	gonadotropin	(DHEA)
sium, Phosphates, Selenium, Sodium Bicarbonate,	● Corticotrophin (ACTH)	● Gamma-hydroxy butyrate
Vanadium, Zinc)	● Local anesthetics	● Human growth hormone
● Amino Acids (Arginine, Ornithine, Lysine, Aspartate,	● Theophylline	● Narcotics
Glutamine, Leucine, Tryptophan, Carnitine)		

In the present era of competition, the names of the substances have changed, but their presence has not. These substances can be divided into several classifications, including supplements, prescription drugs, and banned or illicit substances (Table 1). The distinction among these classes is not always clear, and several substances may fit into one or more categories.

Many of the PES available to young athletes today are considered to be supplements and are produced under the Dietary Supplement Health and Education Act. Under these guidelines, any substance can be packaged and sold as a beneficial supplement if it is not called a drug and is not purported to cure or to treat illness. This leaves the burden of proof regarding safety and efficacy on the United States Food and Drug Administration (FDA) and the federal government.

PES that may be classified as prescription drugs generally are obtained from physicians. These substances show medical effect in specific uses, but also may show an ergogenic advantage when used at higher doses or by healthy subjects.

PES that may be classified as illicit or banned substances have been made illegal by law or banned by governing boards of athletic competition. Some of these may be prescription drugs or even may be classified currently as dietary supplements.

Athletes and teens who are active in the culture of PES use often suggest that studies published in the medical and scientific literature have not been performed on athletes or active weight lifters, but rather on random, paid subjects such as medical students or college students "who are looking for money." Because their perception is that there is a paucity of well-performed studies, anecdotal evidence gains power. Teenagers and young athletes harbor significant skepticism toward the medical establishment, and educational programs that use scare tactics often fail in their goals, driving a larger wedge between the science and the target audience.

The American Academy of Pediatrics specifically condemns the use of anabolic and androgenic steroids, but has no specific position on the use of other dietary supplements, including creatine. The American College of Sports Medicine drafted a position statement in March 2000 concerning the physiologic and health effects of oral creatine supplementation. It stated that data on potential and real adverse effects in the pediatric (<18 y) population are grossly inadequate for formulating valid conclusions about the risk/benefit ratio of creatine supplementation. It suggested that there may be a potential enhancement of exercise performance, but supplementation is not advised in this age group.

Other governing boards, including the IOC and the National Collegiate Athletic Association (NCAA), have well-defined policies regarding the use of substances, banning several from use among participants.

Epidemiology and Prevalence

The prevalence of PES has grown to a striking level. In 1997, the legal supplement industry in the United States was conservatively estimated to bring in $1.26 to $3 billion per year, with expectations that the industry would be valued at $30 billion in 2000.

More than 90% of professional body builders admit to the use of substances during their career, and professional sports teams routinely supply PES to athletes in the training rooms. In a 1997 report, 98% of United States Olympians admitted they would take substances if they were guaranteed not to get caught. An anonymous descriptive survey at a major university showed almost 50% of male intercollegiate athletes using creatine, with a substantial number beginning their use during high school. One survey of collegiate athletes showed that 29% of football, 21% of men's track, and 16% of women's track athletes voluntarily admitted to some use of PES. Recent reports show that 8.2% of high school athletes used creatine, with up to one third admitting to daily use. In another study of high school students, 11% admitted to using androgenic and anabolic steroids. Although the majority of steroids are obtained by questionable means, 10% to 15% are obtained by prescription and likely distributed on a secondary market.

Physician influence and education regarding PES use among patients has been deficient. Fewer than 20% of school-age children reported that a physician had educated them on the dangers of steroid use or other performance-enhancing agents.

The importance of PES use by competitive athletes can be expressed in a frame of reference for physicians and scientists. Although a difference of 1 inch, 1 second, or 1% may not be statistically significant to a scientist, it may be the difference between victory and defeat to an athlete. Looking for the 5% difference to make research statistically significant is inconsequential compared with the minimal edge that high-level athletes and adolescents require to raise themselves above their competitors. It is this mindset that clinicians need to understand for meaningful discussions and recommendations.

Clinical Aspects

SUPPLEMENTS

Dietary supplements comprise the majority of PES used by teenagers. The presence of these compounds in health food stores and fitness centers allows for easy access. The lack of proven effect as well as safety allows their classification as supplements and, thus, lack of control on volume and distribution.

Creatine

Creatine received much attention in the popular press during the Major League Baseball home run race in the summer of 1998. More than 30% of American professional sports teams, including teams from professional football (NFL), basketball (NBA), hockey (NHL), and baseball (MLB) admitted voluntarily to supplying their players with creatine. Although this substance has no indication for use by the FDA, its use is not regulated, and it currently is not considered a banned substance by the MLB, IOC, or NCAA.

The first recorded use of creatine as a PES was in 1992 by British Olympic track athletes, and over the following year, widespread prevalence was documented among body builders. It has been reported to be used by more than 90% of current competing body builders at some point during their training.

Creatine is found naturally in the body, most notably in skeletal muscle. It is a tripeptide consisting of arginine, glycine, and methionine. As a normal part of a balanced diet, the average intake is less than 2 g daily. The daily requirement is slightly more than 2 g; the remainder is synthesized by the body in the liver, pancreas, and kidney to make up for any dietary deficiency.

Creatine exerts its physiologic activity through its conversion to phosphocreatine. The ability of the body to regenerate ATP depends on the supply of creatine and phosphocreatine, with phosphocreatine donating a phosphate group to convert ADP into ATP, bypassing the need for glycolysis for production of more ATP. Supplementation of creatine increases the phosphocreatine pool for rapid ATP synthesis and resynthesis in anaerobic exercise. Following vigorous and intense energy expenditures, the normal phosphocreatine stores are depleted in approximately 10 seconds, requiring other mechanisms for energy production. Having more creatine in the body enables an increase in the rate at which energy is supplied to muscle and prolongs the time before anaerobic production of ATP is needed.

Athletes use supplemental creatine in hopes of prolonging the time to anaerobic metabolism. Supplementation commonly is instituted with an initial loading dose of 20 to 40 g/d for 5 to 7 days in four to six divided daily doses and followed by maintenance dosing of 5 to 20 g/d divided in two to four doses. Kinetic studies reported by manufacturers suggest that peak levels are reached 60 to 90 minutes after oral ingestion. To maximize anabolic effects, ingestion pre- and postworkout is recommended.

Creatine has been shown to increase myofibrillar protein synthesis; these increases in whole body nitrogen retention, protein synthesis, and water retention allow muscle cells to become larger and heavier. Athletes and weightlifters undergo tremendous muscle breakdown in anaerobic exercise, and the addition of creatine presumably helps achieve zero or positive nitrogen balance. Athletes supplementing with creatine have lower body ammonia levels, which suggests less protein degradation.

Creatine cannot work without strength training; those who do not lift weights do not achieve the measured benefits compared with those who do lift. Creatine does not increase strength; rather, it increases an athlete's ability to train. Its greatest benefit seems to be in repetitive, short-burst sports (anaerobic) such as power lifting and wrestling rather than swimming and long-distance running (aerobic).

Creatine supplementation has been reported to give users more muscle strength earlier in their training compared with those not using the supplement. The psychological effect also is measurable in that those taking creatine truly believe that it works. Creatine has been reported to be ergogenic in repeated cycling sprints, to improve power output, and to prolong time of maximal output. Significant increases have been reported in strength, weight, and lean mass as well as an enhancing ability to maintain power in short maximal exercise. In one study, creatine supplementation increased performance capacity 7% to 13% in short-burst exercise. Creatine has been shown to improve body mass, strength, and endurance among college football players, and those in season were shown to have increased strength and maximal output.

The immediate and long-term safety of creatine is not known. No studies have been performed that meet the specific standards of protocol of pharmacology and toxicity as appears in Phase I trials of FDA-approved substances. Anecdotal and case report evidence exists on both sides of the safety argument. Muscle cramping and intestinal discomfort, likely due to the osmotic load presented to the body, are the most common adverse effects. Manufacturer-reported adverse effects include rash, dyspnea, vomiting, diarrhea, anxiety, fatigue, myopathy, seizure, and arrhythmia.

Kidney dysfunction, defined by increased creatinine and decreased glomerular filtration rate, is the most medically significant adverse effect reported in the medical literature. However, because creatinine is a major breakdown product of creatine, both anecdotal reports and published case reports have shown resolution of kidney function and normal creatinine levels following the removal of supplementation. This may suggest a simple increase in production of creatinine, rather than decreased or impaired excretion. In 1997, reports circulated that the deaths of three collegiate wrestlers were related to creatine use, but the FDA later found these claims to be unsubstantiated.

A major limitation of existing studies is that they have not tested the commonly used doses of 20 to 30 g/d, but rather the manufacturer's "recommended" doses of 5 g/d. A retrospective study showed that adverse effects, including muscle cramping and gastrointestinal upset, occurred in 38 of 52 athletes (73%) using creatine, but 87% said that they would continue to take the supplement. There are no studies in the current medical literature of the long- or short-term adverse effects on healthy men.

Androstenedione

Androstenedione has been available for many years. Following the revelation that Mark McGwire of the St. Louis Cardinals Baseball Club was using this product in 1998, sales increased 500% within months. Androstenedione is believed to work as a precursor to testosterone, but it is not considered a Schedule III medication like testosterone because of the lack of studies proving its efficacy.

Androstenedione has little activity, but theoretically acts as a precursor to increase blood testosterone levels. A recent study suggested that androstenedione use can result in a statistically significant increase in serum testosterone in healthy subjects for a transient period of time, even though most other studies have shown no increase. No proven effect on muscle mass has been shown in scientific studies, but the doses used in the studies are 25% to 50% of the manufacturer's recommended dose. No data exist on the adverse effects of androstenedione, and there is no evidence that it alters or modifies hypothalamic-pituitary function.

In the face of recent studies suggesting an associated increase in testosterone levels, the use of androstenedione becomes as significant as the use of other anabolic steroids. Androstenedione use in prepubertal or pubertal males theoretically could induce premature puberty or induce the premature closure of epiphyseal growth plates as well as cause the other adverse effects attributed to anabolic steroid use.

The rebuttal from the trade press and on the Internet suggests that the lack of measured effect lies in the limitations of scientific studies. Proponents of androstenedione use claim that reported results are false due to use of a different form of the compound, the use of nonathlete subjects, and selective reporting by the media. The anecdotal testimony and peer exposure continues to be overwhelmingly positive, and the pressures on teen athletes to use androstenedione remain intense.

Other Nutritional Additives

A significant number of other nutritional additives are used in hopes of deriving ergogenic and appearance-enhancing benefits. Carbohydrate loading and amino acid supplements are used to achieve positive nitrogen balance. This allows for an increase in weight, but does not lead directly to the muscle definition desired by athletes. The popular "Zone Diet," comprised of 40% carbohydrates, 30% fats, and 30% protein, is purported to alter the body's composition of fats and muscle. Antioxidant supplements, including vitamins B and E, are used for their protective and regenerative properties.

Many other substances are used in smaller numbers and in sport-specific instances for their perceived desirable effects and adverse effects. Chromium acts as an insulin cofactor, helping facilitate the anabolic effects of insulin, and vanadium acts as an insulin-like agent. Boron has been shown to increase testosterone levels in elderly women. L-carnitine acts as a transporter of fats and energy into skeletal muscle. Sodium bicarbonate acts as a buffer, decreasing muscle damage and breakdown and allowing more effort to go into anabolism, rather than repairing damage from the exercise.

PRESCRIPTION DRUGS

Prescription drugs are not used as widely as PES, although use is prevalent in certain populations and specific sports. The desired effect may be direct, as in sympathetic control, or an adverse effect, as in indirect lipolysis.

Beta-agonists are considered by the IOC to be both anabolic and stimulating and have been banned in competition without medical indication. Of interest, 15% of Olympic athletes had a diagnosis of exercise-induced asthma in 1984, but by the 1996 Olympic Games, nearly 60% had that same diagnosis, suggesting a possible way to allow for the presence of these substances. Beta-agonists stimulate lipolysis, not necessarily increasing strength, but adding definition to muscle and muscle groups.

Narcotics are used to decrease pain and increase ability and exertion. Beta-blockers, used in accuracy sports such as archery or biathalon, are used to control anxiety. Diuretics are used to shed weight, define muscle mass, and alter the composition of urine in athletes who may be undergoing testing. Insulin-like growth factor is used for its in vivo effects associated with growth hormone. It stimulates protein synthesis and increases uptake of glucose and amino acids while decreasing catabolism of protein and enhancing lipolysis. It is not detectable at this time by standard testing. The adverse effects are much like those of growth hormone, including acromegaly and organomegaly.

BANNED OR ILLICIT SUBSTANCES

The vast majority of banned substances are anabolic steroids and their derivatives. In addition, athletes and adolescents use other hormones, analogs, and releasing agents.

Anabolic Steroids

Anabolic steroids were synthesized initially in hopes of separating the anabolic effects from the virilization effects of known androgenic steroids. Steroids continue to be used widely and are the most common cause for a positive test for a banned substance in competitive athletes. Steroid use has increased among adolescent athletes, particularly weight lifters and gymnasts, in whom they increase strength and stunt growth. Among high school males, 5% to 11% admitted using anabolic and androgenic steroids by the time they finished high school, and one study reported that 2.7% had tried or used anabolic steroids by middle school.

Steroids have two broad effects: anabolic and anticatabolic. Through the androgen receptor, steroids increase protein synthesis, which results in gains in muscle strength and size. Studies have suggested that the concomitant use of testosterone with resistance training resulted in an increase in body weight, lean fat-free mass, nitrogen retention, total muscle mass, and overall strength. The anticatabolic effect essentially blocks the effects of cortisol, which is released in higher amounts during exercise and stress, causing muscle breakdown. Women seem to receive a greater anabolic effect from androgens,

Table 2. Side Effects of Steroid Use

- Acne
- Hirsuitism
- Hypertension
- Liver tumors
- Psychosis and aggression
- Emotional lability
- Increases in low-density lipoprotein (LDL)-cholesterol
- Decrease in high-density lipoprotein (HDL)-cholesterol
- Virilization (females)
- Premature closure of epiphyseal growth plates
- Dysplasia of collagen, resulting in tendon rupture
- Decreased sexual function and desire
- Testicular failure
- Gynecomastia

likely related to the relative balance of androgens and estrogens in the body.

The safety profile of anabolic and androgenic steroids is well known. Several of the adverse effects are listed in Table 2. Of further concern, the use of anabolic steroids among adolescents has been linked to other substance abuse, including intravenous drugs.

Anabolic steroids are used either orally or via injection, with most users taking 5 to 10 times what medical science has determined to be a safe physiologic dose. Different usage methods and schedules are common. "Cycling" involves taking steroid supplementation for several weeks, followed by several weeks off of the agents. "Stacking" involves use of several types of androgens or anabolic agents simultaneously. "Pyramiding" involves increasing the dose over a period of time.

The complexity of the supplement industry is on pace with the medical establishment. Antiestrogens, including tamoxifen, human chorionic gonadotropin, saw palmetto, indole-3, carbinol, and chrysin, are used commonly among those using androgenic and anabolic agents. These chemicals help block the conversion of androgens to estrogens, push estrogens to inactivation, and increase endogenous levels of androgens. Because the current test for the presence of androgens uses the testosterone/epitestosterone ratio, artificially increasing luteinizing hormone production as well as epitestosterone levels may help an athlete who is using anabolic steroids to evade an undesired positive test.

Dihydroepiandrostenedione (DHEA) is another androgenic compound in wide use. The FDA banned it in 1996 for proven androgenic effects and adverse effects. DHEA is a precursor to androgenic compounds and is used for the same theoretical value as androgens, but with the hope of fewer adverse effects. There has been no documented efficacy in men, although it does seem to increase androgen levels in women.

Human Growth Hormone

The use of HGH and its analogs and releasing agents has not yet been reported in the medical literature among adolescents. However, its use among competitive bodybuilders and higher level athletes is prevalent. HGH is used as an injectable anabolic compound. It was used initially in the 1980s as athletes began to search for substances that would have anabolic effects but would not show up in available tests. HGH acts in all body tissues. Its theoretical athletic benefit is to increase protein anabolism and lipolysis. Unlike exercise, it works by increasing the translation of existing mRNA. It is proposed to result in increased muscle definition and protein deposition as well as significant fat-free weight gain. Studies of HGH in normal subjects show no benefit, and although there is increased mass, it does not appear to be muscle mass.

Adverse effects of HGH can easily be observed in the clinical setting and are consistent with acromegaly (Table 3). Potential health problems include impurity of individual lots and possible infectious complications with cadaveric-obtained chemical or related to the injectable vehicle. Many athletes who use HGH refute the presence of such adverse effects, but it is not known if they are using fraudulent product or true HGH.

Athletes using HGH or HGH analogs employ dosages up to 20 times the maximum recommended physiologic doses. The cost can be $3,000 to $5,000/mo, which does not seem to be exclusionary among serious lifting athletes. Although HGH can be detected easily by gas chromatography, there is no reliable test to identify individuals using HGH as an anabolic agent. The 2000

Table 3. Growth Hormone Adverse Effects

- Behavioral changes
- Coarsening of facial features
- Growth of facial bones
- Enlargement in thickness of fingers and toes
- Increase in skull circumference
- Broadening of the nose
- Enlargement of the tongue
- Growth of the mandible
- Increased separation of the teeth
- Cardiovascular disease
- Diabetes
- Hypertension
- Peripheral neuropathy

Summer Olympics did not test athletes for HGH, although a tremendous amount of effort and money went into the development of such tests. Natural and theoretical HGH-releasing analogs are used, including arginine, ornithine, and tryptophan, in an attempt to increase endogenous HGH.

Other Illicit or Banned Substances

Gammahydroxy butyrate (GHB) has received increased exposure in the popular media, including reports of an NBA star being hospitalized after known use of GHB and a member of the NFL being arrested for possession of the substance. It has been available as a dietary supplement, either as a liquid or a powder, and was sold under several names, including "Liquid Ecstasy" and "Organic Quaalude." Possession became illegal in 1990, and it became a schedule I substance in March 2000, although it was widely available via international distribution sources. Its use increased in the mid to late 1990s as a "club drug" and among adolescents. GHB is available in single doses that mimic or augment the effects of alcohol for a cost of $5 to $10 per dose.

GHB depresses the central nervous system (CNS) by increasing CNS dopamine levels and also through the endogenous opioid system. Its use has been popular among bodybuilders and athletes who hold the belief that it facilitates the release of endogenous HGH by inducing the sleep patterns under which GH has its maximal release. It was developed initially as an anesthetic, but its use was discontinued due to unwanted adverse effects.

Gamma-butyrl lactone (GBL) and 1,4 butanediol (BD) can be converted easily to GHB both in vivo and in vitro. In January 1999, the FDA requested that products containing GBL be recalled, and some states, including California, have notified retailers that sale of these products is illegal. BD is still available in the United States as a solvent, but not as a supplement or nutritional additive.

Stimulants are used to mask fatigue in endurance athletes, to alter fuel utilization, and to increase fatty acid breakdown. Results are not statistically significant, although some trend of effects has been seen in swimmers, runners, and weight throwers as well as elite-trained athletes. Caffeine is a stimulant that has ergogenic properties at high doses. It stimulates the CNS and increases perception, allowing for longer exercise and increased endurance running. Ephedrine and other ephedra alkaloids, including the herbal Ma Juang, are widely available and have similar effects. Recent studies have been conducted to examine the use and dangers of ephedra alkaloids. A significant increase in the occurrence of hemorrhagic stroke was reported in one recently published case-control study. A case report also documented the occurrence of myocardial infarction in a healthy 19-year-old bodybuilder. Even though several ephedrine derivatives have been removed voluntarily from the market, herbal and "supplemental" forms remain widely available.

"Blood doping," which was banned by the IOC in 1990, refers to either transfusion of red blood cells or use of injected erythropoietin. This process exerts its ergogenic effects of improving the ability to perform in a submaximal and endurance exercise by increasing red blood cell mass and improving oxygen delivery to skeletal muscle. During the 2000 Olympic Games in Sydney, the IOC revealed the development of a new test to identify athletes using either natural or recombinant erythropoietin. Adverse effects and dangers of this increased red blood cell mass include increased viscosity and resultant vascular occlusions.

Management and Prognosis

Among the subculture of elite athletes and bodybuilders, supplements are widely available, and anecdotal evidence predominates. Even adolescents hoping to improve their appearance are beginning to use supplements at an alarming rate. Trade publications are filled with advertisements and selected studies that are unavailable or of questionable scientific basis. The Internet has allowed almost unregulated access to these chemicals and provides unproven information regarding their safety and efficacy. Many PES, including injectable anabolic steroids and narcotics, have easily defined and obvious deleterious adverse effects. Others, most notably creatine, seem to show beneficial effects with a minimal adverse effect profile.

Although random and directed drug testing is appropriate at the collegiate and Olympic levels, there is little use among adolescents and high school athletes. The most prevalent substances are not identified easily on basic screens available to most general practitioners. Clinical examination and history should be the first screening tools used to raise suspicion or identify use and abuse among patients.

We must be able to approach our patients with well-directed questions to elicit the information that we need without being judgmental. Simply asking patients if they or their friends are using anything to improve their appearance or performance is a good starting point (Table 4).

Our job as pediatricians is to educate patients to make sound medical decisions that will affect their current and future health. We need to notice clues of PES use in children in our practices. We

Table 4. Questions to Ask Regarding Substance Use

- Do you (or your friends/teammates) use anything to help you in sports or competition?
- Do you take any herbs, vitamins, or other natural medicines?
- Do you use anything to help improve your workouts?
- Do you take any supplements to help your appearance?

need to be honest with our patients, letting them know the medical data and their limitations. We need to let them know the health consequences and possible adverse effects. The pervasive influence of professional athletics and popular culture means that PES will continue to be available to adolescents, either by honest or dishonest means. We need to open communication with patients in an attempt to educate and influence them to make healthy and knowledgeable choices.

Suggested Reading

Anderson S, Bolduc S, Coryllos E, et al. Adolescents and anabolic steroids: a subject review. *Pediatrics.* 1997;99:904–908

Clarkson P, Thompson H. Drugs and sport—research findings and limitations. *Sports Med.* 1997;24:366–384

DuRant R, Escobedo L, Heath G. Anabolic steroid use, strength training, and multiple drug use among adolescents in the United States. *Pediatrics.* 1995;96:23–28

DuRant R, Rickert VI, Ashworth CS, Newman C, Slavens G. Use of multiple drugs among adolescents who use anabolic steroids. *N Engl J Med.* 1993;328:922–926

Eichner E. Ergogenic aids: what athletes are using—and why. *Physician Sports Med.* 1997;25:25

Faigenbaum A, Zaichkowsky LD, Gardner DE, Micheli LJ. Anabolic steroid use by male and female middle school students. *Pediatrics.* 1998;101:e6. Available at: www.pediatrics.org/cgi/content/full/101/5/e6

Leder BZ, Longcope C, Catlin DH, Ahrens B, Schoenfeld DA, Finkelstein JS. Oral androstenedione administration and serum testosterone concentrations in young men. *JAMA.* 2000;283: 779–782

NCAA Policy on Banned Substances. Available at: www.ncaa.org/sportssciences/drugtesting/introduction.html

Smith J, Dahm D. Creatine use among a select population of high school athletes. *Mayo Clin Proc.* 2000;75:1257–1263

Sturmi J, Diorio D. Anabolic agents. *Clin Sports Med.* 1998;17: 261–279

Tanner S, Miller D, Alongi C. Anabolic steroid use by adolescents: prevalence, motives, and knowledge of risks. *Clin J Sport Med.* 1995;5:108–115

Poortmans J, Francaux M. Long-term oral creatine supplementation does not impair renal function in healthy athletes. *Med Sci Sports Exercise.* 1999;31:1108–1110

Preparticipation Examination of the Adolescent Athlete: Part 1

Jordan D. Metzl, MD*

Objectives

After completing this article, readers should be able to:

1. Discuss the importance of preparticipation screening of young athletes.
2. Delineate the importance of the sports grading system.
3. List key points in the medical and family history that can affect sports performance and sports safety.

This series of two articles for Pediatrics in Review *addresses the preparticipation examination (PPE) as a method of screening adolescents for athletic participation. The first article addresses implementing the PPE as a screening tool and the important issues in the medical and family history portion of the examination. The second article, to be published next month, covers the medical and orthopedic examination portions of the PPE. Together, these two articles delineate a comprehensive approach to the safe and effective screening of the adolescent athlete. A sample PPE form is included at the end of the second article.*

Introduction

The number of adolescent athletes participating in organized sports continues to increase yearly in the United States, now totaling more than 14 million. Sports involvement is important for teenagers, teaching lessons such as leadership skills and group dynamics that are important for success in later life. Sports participation also encourages a dedication to physical fitness, which is especially important in the United States, where the incidence of pediatric and adolescent obesity has more than doubled over the past 30 years. Pediatricians, concerned with the healthy development of their teenage patients, should view the trend toward increasing sports involvement extremely favorably.

The pediatrician traditionally has provided medical clearance for young athletes involved in organized sports prior to the beginning of each sports season. In past years, this process was limited in scope and effectiveness, often addressing issues of general health such as cardiac and pulmonary disease, but offering minimal input about musculoskeletal pathology. Pediatric training programs, most of which offer fewer than 6 hours of sports medicine or orthopedic training to residents during the entire postgraduate education program, historically have contributed to this limited role by not emphasizing the importance of musculoskeletal evaluation skills.

Increasingly, the families of young athletes, who are involved in high-level sports as early as 6 years of age, are demanding more of their health-care practitioners. Pediatricians are being asked to evaluate sports-related injury more frequently and to provide helpful injury prevention strategies. The age-old, previously accepted mantra of "just stay off it until it feels better" no longer is accepted by patients and their families, who are eager for a safe and quick return to athletic competition.

For young and otherwise healthy adolescent athletes, many of whom do not see their physicians for annual health supervision visits, the preparticipation examination (PPE) is the most frequent interaction with a clinician during the teenage years. Used fully, the PPE offers an important opportunity to provide preventive care for young athletes.

*Medical Director, The Sports Medicine Institute for Young Athletes; Assistant Attending Physician, Sports Medicine Service, Hospital for Special Surgery, New York, NY.

The History of the PPE

The PPE was created approximately 25 years ago to provide medical clearance for athletes, screening primarily for congenital heart disease in an attempt to "hold" athletes who might be at risk for significant morbidity from increased exertion. Initially required by several states, the PPE has grown in both scope and popularity and now is mandated in 49 of 50 states. In most areas, the present-day PPE investigates family and medical history and includes a screening medical and musculoskeletal examination.

As the number of adolescent athletes increases, so does the number of PPEs being performed each year. In high school alone, the number of athletes being screened has increased by almost 50% in the past 10 years, due mostly to the increasing number of female athletes playing on school-sponsored sports teams. The trends in high school sports participation are shown in the Figure.

Unfortunately, the quality of the examination varies tremendously. In 21 of 50 states, nurses or physician assistants can complete the PPE; 11 states allow chiropractors to clear young athletes for competition. Most importantly, there is no standardized form for the PPE. Because of this lack of standardization, the content of the PPE varies considerably from state to state and even from school district to school district. Certain schools and districts have incomplete forms that offer little opportunity for meaningful prevention; other schools and districts have extensive forms that frustrate the pediatrician in a busy pediatric office.

Is the PPE a Waste of Time?

Some have argued that the PPE is a waste of time and money because of the lack of "positives" that result in disqualification from sports. A recent study found that only 1.9% of 2,729 high school athletes screened during the PPE were disqualified from sports participation. Seizing on this and similar data, insurance companies are increasingly hesitant to reimburse for the PPE, citing it as a superfluous procedure. For pediatricians, this often means completing multiple PPE forms, with a low chance of finding significant pathology, and receiving poor monetary reimbursement.

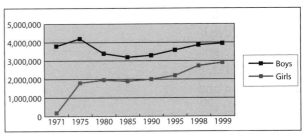

Figure. Trends in high school sport participation, 1972 through 1999. Based on data from the National Federation of State High Schools participation data, Kansas City, Missouri.

The overwhelming merits of the PPE, however, outweigh the limitations. The PPE remains the most common reason for healthy adolescents to visit their pediatricians and, therefore, should be viewed as an excellent and rare opportunity for health prevention in teenage patients. It can facilitate dialogue between adolescent patient and clinician and is an important method of preventing sports-related injury, much of which recurrs from season to season.

The PPE often discloses issues that require additional medical attention. In the study cited previously, although only 1.9% of athletes were disqualified from sports participation, 11.9% required follow-up, including physical therapy, nutritional counseling, and referral for previously undiagnosed hypertension. In many cases, positive findings on the PPE represent previous injuries and injury patterns that can be prevented in the future with effective preventive conditioning programs.

Making the PPE rewarding relies on the examiner's ability to focus the examination on the sport for which the athlete is being screened through a directed review of the medical and family history before starting the physical examination.

Examination Specifics: Where, When, and How

The PPE is performed best 4 to 6 weeks before the start of the sports season, which provides sufficient time for effective implementation of injury prevention programs. Practically, most young athletes receive their PPE forms before the start of the school year. Athletes should be encouraged to schedule screening visits earlier in the summer rather than waiting until the day before practice begins.

There are several formats for the screening of young athletes, including the station-based school examination and the traditional examination in the pediatric office. Both venues have merit, and if possible, both should be encouraged. Because healthy adolescents rarely interact with the medical system, the station-based examination at school should not replace the office-based PPE; rather, it should serve as a supplement.

The station-based examination at school is an excellent opportunity to compare athletes of similar ages and sports. For example, if a team of 12- to 15-year-old soccer players is screened in unison, comparing the ankle examinations allows for a better assessment of which ankles have significant ligamentous laxity or muscular weakness that would predispose a player to repeated inversion injuries. Comparing athletes of a specific age group and team identifies musculoskeletal pathology more easily. Furthermore, prevention programs implemented during the school-based format more easily can be made sport-specific. For example, the entire swim team can work on a rotator cuff strengthening program that is implemented during the school-based examination.

The office-based examination is important for two primary reasons. First, it promotes the physician-patient relationship. It offers an opportunity to address issues related directly to sports, such as developing a preventive ankle strengthening program for an athlete who has a history of ankle injuries, and issues not directly related to sports, such as "at-risk" behaviors (eg, drug and alcohol use, unsafe sexual practice). Second, office-based evaluation facilitates the exploration of more sensitive medical issues, such as the female athlete triad (anorexia, osteoporosis, amenorrhea), which frequently are poorly addressed in larger station-based examinations. The office-based examination allows for sport-specific screening, but more importantly, is an opportunity to implement general preventive health measures for adolescents.

A final issue that must be considered is the sport for which the athlete is being screened. Sports are graded, based on the level of contact, as high, moderate, and low (Table 1).

Table 1. Sports Grading Scale by Contact Level

High Contact/ Collision	Moderate, Limited Contact	Low, Noncontact
Basketball	Baseball	Archery
Boxing	Bicycling	Badminton
Diving	Canoeing/kayaking	Body Building
Field Hockey	Cheerleading	Bowling
Football	Fencing	Crew
Ice Hockey	Floor Hockey	Curling
Lacrosse	Gymnastics	Discus
Martial Arts	Handball	Golf
Rodeo	High Jump	Javelin
Rugby	Racquetball	Orienteering
Ski Jumping	Skating	Pole Vault
Soccer	Skiing	Race Walking
Team Handball	Softball	Riflery
Water Polo	Squash	Rope Jumping
Wrestling	Volleyball	Running
		Shot Put
		Strength Training
		Swimming
		Tennis
		Track

Generally, an injury pattern is associated with the contact grade of the sport. Macrotraumatic or acute traumatic injury results from one-time, kinetic energy force applied to the body and is common in high-contact sports such as soccer, football, and lacrosse. Therefore, for these sports, the examiner should focus on the previous history of macrotraumatic injury, such as concussion, fracture, or ligament injury. Microtraumatic or overuse injury is seen frequently in repetitive use sports, such as running or swimming, and is more common in the moderate- and low-contact sport categories. For example, a history of "terrible shin splints" should raise the suspicion of an undiagnosed tibial stress fracture during the previous year. In this scenario, the examiner should pay careful attention to the potential causes of stress fracture, including activity patterns, foot biomechanics, and potential medical problems that might cause osteopenia and increase the risk of stress fracture, such as hypoestrogenism or poor dietary calcium intake.

Objectives of the Examination

As a screening tool, the PPE should identify medical and musculoskeletal conditions that might affect the adolescent, both from a general health perspective and with sports-specific considerations. The examination, at minimum, should meet the following objectives:

1. Identify medical and musculoskeletal conditions that could make sports participation unsafe, with specific consideration of the sport for which the athlete is being cleared.
2. Screen for underlying illness through a medical and family history, review of systems, and physical examination.
3. Recognize pre-existing injury patterns from previous sports season(s) and devise rehabilitation programs to prevent recurrence.

Medical History

The PPE should start with a review of the medical history. The following considerations are important and should be considered based on the sport(s) in which the athlete is competing:

SUBJECTIVE FEELING OF FAINTNESS, WEAKNESS, OR FRANK SYNCOPE DURING EXERCISE

The report of syncope or alteration of consciousness during exercise is a "red flag" in the PPE. These concerns are especially noteworthy because cardiac deaths comprise the majority of sport-related fatalities in the United States (roughly 5 to 15 children per 1,000,000 participants). Asthma, hypoglycemia, and seizures can cause similar symptoms. Because the purpose of the examination is to screen for conditions that might require further evaluation, athletes who have symptoms of syncope or near-syncope should be evaluated by a pediatric cardiologist prior to participating in sports.

WHEEZING DURING SPORTS

Asthma is the most common chronic illness among adolescents. Of those affected, 85% have exercise-induced bronchospasm (EIB). The overall incidence of EIB is believed to be 10% to 35% of athletes and probably is underdiagnosed. The

diagnosis of EIB should be entertained in any athlete who has a history of wheezing during sports. Peak flow meter testing for baseline peak flow values is a valuable tool to establish baseline pulmonary function in affected athletes that is obtained easily during the PPE. Baseline values can be compared with initial readings later in the season if necessary. A decrease of 10% to 15% from baseline values is suggestive of EIB.

CONCUSSION

Recent data suggesting the long-term implications of concussion continue to raise awareness about the importance of identifying athletes who are predisposed to concussion. At present, there are no specific recommendations regarding the number of concussions suffered by an athlete and referral to a neurologist. In the adolescent athlete, however, a more conservative approach is warranted. Most sports medicine specialists consider a history of two or three concussions without the loss of consciousness (grade I) or one to two concussions with the loss of consciousness (grade II or III) as grounds for referral to a neurologist. Increasingly, this type of referral consists of neuropsychologic testing to establish a baseline level of neurologic function in addition to imaging studies. A history of concussion is especially important to consider when clearing an athlete for high- or moderate-contact sports.

At least 23 scales currently are used to assess the severity of concussion. Examiners should be familiar with at least one grading scale to assist with evaluation and treatment of the concussed athlete. The Cantu scale (Table 2) tends to be the most user-friendly.

RECENT MONONUCLEOSIS

Mononucleosis-induced splenomegaly can predispose an athlete involved in high- and moderate-contact sports to splenic rupture. Any adolescent who has had mononucleosis within 1 month of the onset of contact sports should be considered at risk for splenomegaly because spleen size peaks within 3 to 4 weeks of the onset of systemic signs of illness. Splenic rupture is the leading cause of death from mononucleosis and usually occurs

Table 2. Cantu Grading Scale for Assessment of Concussion

Grade	Symptoms	Treatment
Grade I (Mild)	No LOC. Complaints may include ringing, headache, dizziness, memory loss	Observation May not return to competition until symptom-free upon exertion
Grade II (Moderate)	LOC <5 min OR Post-traumatic amnesia >30 min	Observation May not return to competition for 1 wk from time of resolution of symptoms upon exertion
Grade III (Severe)	LOC >5 min OR Post-traumatic amnesia >24 hr	Admission to hospital Eventual referral to neurologist prior to resumption of contact sports

LOC = loss of consciousness. Reprinted with permission from Cantu RC. Head and spine injuries in youth sports. *Clin Sports Med.* 1995;14:517–532

within the first 3 weeks of illness. If physical examination findings are at all suspicious for a palpable spleen, ultrasonography or computed tomography can be used to assist in the evaluation of splenic size.

UNILATERAL ORGAN

Athletes who have unilateral organs, including kidneys and testicles, warrant special consideration prior to clearance for athletics. A single kidney is a contraindication to high-contact sports based on the recommendation of the American Academy of Pediatrics (AAP), and athletes wishing to play moderate-contact sports require a protective "flak" jacket. An athlete who has a single testicle requires mandatory protective cup use for all sports.

CURRENT MEDICATIONS

Prescription drugs such as beta-agonists (albuterol), methylxanthines (theophylline), tricyclic antidepressants (imipramine), macrolide antibiotics (erythromycin), nonprescription drugs such as decongestants (pseudoephrine), and illicit drugs (eg, cocaine, amphetamines) have been linked to arrhythmias. Therefore, it is important to document current drug use in the PPE.

MENSTRUAL HISTORY

Female athletes should be screened for amenorrhea during the medical history portion of the PPE. Primary amenorrhea (absence of menses by age 16) or secondary amenorrhea (absence of menses for more than three cycles) should

prompt further consideration of the female athlete triad (anorexia, amenorrhea, osteoporosis). If all three entities are present, bone density studies via dual-energy radiograph absorptiometry (DEXA) are being used increasingly to evaluate baseline bone density values. DEXA can be used to obtain baseline bone density measurements that can be compared with values obtained in subsequent years to assess bone health.

SEIZURE DISORDER

The history of a seizure disorder is not a direct contraindication to sports participation if the seizures are well controlled. However, athletes who experience ongoing epileptic activity, particularly if they are involved in aquatic sports, warrant careful review before clearance. The history of a seizure within the past 6 months should raise concern prior to clearance, particularly in those engaging in water sports.

PAST HISTORY OF INJURY

Included in this category are injuries that have caused a loss of playing time during the prior athletic season. Attempts should be made to devise rehabilitation protocols to prevent injuries such as chronic ankle sprains from recurring in the ensuing season.

ERGOGENIC AIDS

Unlike college or professional athletes, who are tested routinely, there currently is no authorized testing policy for ergogenic aid use in high school athletes. With an anabolic steroid user rate of 9%

reported in high school athletes and 3% in junior high athletes, the issues of steroid use are addressed best in the medical history section of the PPE.

The issue of nutritional supplement use is also of concern to adolescent athletes. None of the so-called "nutritional supplements" such as creatine or androstenedione ever has been tested in adolescents. Although the exact user rate of these substances in adolescents remains unknown, the incidence appears to be increasing.

The best method of approaching the subject of ergogenic aid use is with the question, "Have you ever taken a substance to enhance your athletic performance?"

Family History

A positive family history of these items in particular should prompt further consideration:

CARDIAC-RELATED DEATH IN A FIRST-DEGREE RELATIVE YOUNGER THAN 50 YEARS OF AGE

As the most common cause of sudden death in athletes, cardiac-related death deserves primary attention and consideration. This is especially important in young athletes because 90% of cardiac deaths in school-age athletes occur between the hours of 3 and 9 PM, during or just after sports participation. Congenital heart disease, arrhythmia, prolonged QT syndromes, hypertrophic cardiomyopathy, and Marfan syndrome are all inheritable cardiac diseases that should prompt suspicion if present in a first-degree relative.

FAMILY HISTORY OF CHRONIC DISEASE

Asthma, diabetes, epilepsy, and bleeding disorders are only several of the inherited chronic diseases commonly seen in childhood and adolescence. In many pediatric patients, these illnesses do not manifest until adolescence. A family history of any of these chronic diseases should alert the examiner for additional signs of chronic illness.

Suggested Reading

American Academy of Pediatrics Committee on Sports Medicine and Fitness. Athletic participation by children and adolescents who have systemic hypertension. Policy statement, RE9715, American Academy of Pediatrics. *Pediatrics.* 1997;99:637–638

American Academy of Pediatrics Committee on Sports Medicine and Fitness. Atlantoaxial instability in Down syndrome: subject review. *Pediatrics.* 1995;96:151–154

American Academy of Pediatrics Committee on Sports Medicine and Fitness. Medical conditions affecting sports participation. Policy statement, RE9432, American Academy of Pediatrics. *Pediatrics.* 1994;94:757–760

American Academy of Pediatrics Committee on Sports Medicine and Fitness. Strength training, weight and power lifting, and body building by children and adolescents. Policy statement, RE9196, American Academy of Pediatrics. *Pediatrics.* 1990;86:801–803

Anderson SJ. Soccer: a case-based approach to ankle and knee injuries. *Pediatr Ann.* 2000;29:177–188

Bernhardt DT. Football: a case-based approach to mild traumatic brain injury. *Pediatr Ann.* 2000;29:172–176

Callahan LR. The evolution of the female athlete, progress and problems. *Pediatr Ann.* 2000;29:149–153

Cantu RC. Functional cervical stenosis: a contraindication to participation in contact sports. *Med Sci Sports Exerc.* 1995;25:1082–1084

Collins MW, Grindel SH, Lovell MR, et al. Relationship between concussion and neuropsychological performance in college football players. *JAMA.* 1999;282:964–970

Corrardo D, Basso C, Schiavon M, et al. Screening for hypertrophic cardiomyopathy in young athletes. *N Engl J Med.* 1998;339:364–369

Luke A, Micheli L. Sports injuries: emergency assessment and field-side care. *Pediatr Rev.* 1999;20:291–301

Metzl JD. Strength training and nutritional supplement use in adolescent athletes. *Current Opin Pediatr.* 1999;11:292–296

Nattiv A, Agostini R, Drinkwater B, Yaeger K. The female athlete triad: the inter-relatedness of disordered eating, amenorrhea, and osteoporosis. *Clin Sports Med.* 1994;13:405–418

Rifat SF, Ruffin MT, Gorenflo DW. Disqualifying criteria in a preparticipation sports evaluation. *J Fam Pract.* 1995;41:42–50

Risser WL, Hoffman HM, Bellah GG Jr, et al. A cost-benefit analysis of preparticipation sports examinations of adolescent athletes. *J School Health.* 1985;55:270–273

Smith J, Lakowski ER. The preparticipation physical examination: Mayo clinic experience with 2,729 examinations. *Mayo Clin Proc.* 1998;73:419–429

Preparticipation Examination of the Adolescent Athlete: Part 2

Jordan D. Metzl, MD*

Objectives

After completing this article, readers should be able to:

1. Perform a sport-specific medical and musculoskeletal examination.
2. Explain why it is important to define pre-existing injury patterns.
3. Characterize preventive conditioning and rehabilitation programs for young athletes.

This is the second of two articles dedicated to the preparticipation examination of the adolescent athlete. The first article addressed the medical and family history, and this article discusses the medical and orthopedic portions of the examination.

Medical Examination

The medical examination portion of the preparticipation examination (PPE) should serve both as a follow-up for concerns raised in the medical and family history portion of the examination and as a screening for any medical conditions that might limit safe sports participation.

The medical examination begins with measurement of the vital signs, height, weight, blood pressure, heart rate, pulse, and respiratory rate. Blood pressure in the adolescent patient is an important marker for the presence of underlying, silent pathology, including primary hypertension or hypertension due to renal, endocrinologic, cardiac, or central nervous system causes. Secondary hypertension also can result from anabolic steroid use.

Blood pressure should be measured with the bladder encircling at least two thirds of the arm. The most common cause for an abnormal value is improper cuff sizing. If the initial value is elevated, two subsequent readings should be obtained before diagnosing hypertension. The guidelines regarding adolescent hypertension are listed in the Table. Of note, grade III hypertension requires removal from athletics until control is achieved, and grade IV hypertension is a contraindication to sports participation.

Once vital signs are established, the general medical examination should focus on sports-readiness. General markers for health are important, particularly excessive thinness or obesity and phenotypic manifestations of multisystem illnesses such as Marfan syndrome. Contagious skin conditions, including impetigo, molluscum contagiosum, and herpes gladiotorum, must be discovered prior to clearance for contact sports such as wrestling. Important aspects of the eye, ear, and nose examination include visual acuity, which needs to be 20/40 for clearance for competition, documentation of equal pupillary size, and a brief examination of the patient's dentition.

Table. Values for Adolescent Hypertension

Age	Mild (I)	Moderate (II)	Severe (III)	Very Severe (IV)
13 to 15 y	135 to 139 mm Hg	140 to 149 mm Hg	150 to 159 mm Hg	>160 mm Hg
	85 to 89 mm Hg	90 to 94 mm Hg	95 to 99 mm Hg	>100 mm Hg
16 to 18 y	140 to 149 mm Hg	150 to 159 mm Hg	160 to 169 mm Hg	>180 mm Hg
	90 to 94 mm Hg	95 to 99 mm Hg	100 to 109 mm Hg	>110 mm Hg

*Medical Director, The Sports Medicine Institute for Young Athletes; Assistant Attending Physician, Sports Medicine Service, Hospital for Special Surgery, New York, NY.

Cardiac examination is of paramount importance in the PPE and should include history, review of symptoms, measurement of vital signs, and auscultation. A recent study found that the three elements of cardiac screening—history of symptoms such as dizziness or chest pain with exercise, history of heart murmur or hypertension, and a family history of early cardiac death—were obtained in only 17.2% of high schools nationwide during the PPE. The overwhelming majority of adolescent patients who suffer cardiac death are previously asymptomatic.

Those in whom cardiac symptoms even are suggested need to be recognized. In the United States, more than 50% of cardiac-related deaths are due to hypertrophic cardiomyopathy (HCM), an autosomal dominant disorder characterized by cardiac muscle hypertrophy and eventual myocardial dysfunction upon exertion. An Italian study in 1998 suggested that the more stringent cardiac screening methods in Italy, which include preparticipation electrocardiography (ECG), recognized most cases of HCM. Only 2% of all cases of cardiac death in the Italian screened population that was studied were due to HCM compared with more than 50% in the United States. Currently, ECG is not recommended as a screening tool for HCM and is not recommended as part of the PPE in the United States. However, athletes who have a history of cardiac symptoms with exertion should be referred to a cardiologist prior to clearance for athletic competition. Often this referral will include baseline and stress ECGs to rule out electrophysiologic abnormalities and echocardiography to rule out structural cardiac defects.

The pulmonary examination offers an opportunity to screen for asthma in particular and to obtain a history that might suggest exercise-induced bronchospasm (EIB). It is important to determine that athletic patients who have asthma have a proper understanding of EIB and are aware of the timing of proper inhaler use prior to athletic competition. In addition, it is important to communicate with the school trainer during the school-based examination and to determine that the training bag has an adequate supply of metered dose inhalers containing beta-agonist medication to treat asthmatic

patients who might become symptomatic during athletic competition. Increasingly, preventive asthma medications such as leukotriene inhibitors and mast cell stabilizers are being used, and these products often are useful for athletes in conjunction with more symptomatic treatment such as beta-agonist therapy.

In addition to organomegaly caused by infectious etiologies such as hepatitis and mononucleosis, specific issues (eg, having a unilateral kidney) occasionally are raised with the abdominal examination. Medium- and low-contact sports are allowed in the case of a solitary kidney with proper protective gear.

Common points raised during the genitourinary portion of the examination include evaluation for hernia, especially for soccer players, and testicular protection in appropriate sports. The examiner should stress to both the athlete and his or her family that sexual maturity, based on secondary sexual development, rather than physical size, correlates with skeletal maturity. The large offensive lineman who might be at Sexual Maturity Rating stage 3 is at higher risk for suffering a physeal (growth plate) fracture than are his less developed or more developed peers; the muscular force exerted by testosterone-rich muscles across cartilaginous physes predisposes developing teens to physeal injury. The Sexual Maturity Rating best assesses the stage of sexual development.

Musculoskeletal Examination

The musculoskeletal portion of the PPE is the source of most sports-related pathology. It is especially useful to time the PPE approximately 4 to 6 weeks prior to the onset of a specific sports season so that findings that are amenable to rehabilitation can be addressed appropriately.

Conditions such as previous cervical spine injuries, especially those that have caused neurologic symptoms in the arms, hands, or legs, should prompt the clinician to obtain screening cervical radiographs that include flexion and extension views. Any concern about cervical stenosis also should prompt magnetic resonance imaging (MRI) of the cervical spine prior to clearance for high- and medium-contact sports.

Pediatric and adolescent athletes who have Down syndrome also warrant screening cervical radiographs, including flexion, extension, and odontoid views, prior to participation in sports that carry a risk of head injury to rule out atlantoaxial instability. The Special Olympics mandates such examinations prior to participation in sanctioned events, but the American Academy of Pediatrics has withdrawn this recommendation unless the athlete has been symptomatic.

Common adolescent spine problems such as Scheurmann kyphosis in the thoracic spine and scoliosis in all three portions of the spine should be evaluated visually. Spondylolysis and spondylolisthesis should be suspected in adolescents who have particular histories of pain upon extension. Discogenic back pain can account for low back pain in adolescents, although it is much less common than in adults. Rapid adolescent growth can cause muscle imbalance and lead to general muscle pain in the paraspinous musculature. Finally, a suspicion for neoplasm must be maintained in any adolescent who has unexplained back pain because this is a common site of primary and metastatic disease in this age group.

Examination of the back should focus on visual inspection, looking for abnormal curvature such as scoliosis, which is more common in adolescent females than males, and kyphosis, which is more common in adolescent males than females. The back should be palpated to identify any areas of tenderness, which often are present in patients who have muscular spasm. Functional movement, including flexion, rotation, and extension, should be performed to assess function of the spine. In general, pain with flexion, especially if a radicular component is involved, suggests discogenic pain; pain with extension suggests posterior element overuse such as spondylolysis. Rotational pain (pain that worsens with trunk rotation) often suggests paraspinous muscle pain. Finally, reflexes in the patellar and Achilles tendons should be assessed to evaluate neurologic function.

Shoulder problems represent common issues for adolescent athletes, particularly in "overhead" sports. In sports such as swimming, baseball, and tennis, adolescent athletes frequently develop rotator cuff overuse. Such overuse injuries tend

to recur and are treated best by preseason conditioning programs. Shoulder instability is another common adolescent problem and should be evaluated appropriately prior to sports participation. Effective preseason conditioning can greatly reduce the incidence and severity of many types of shoulder pathology in adolescent athletes. The details of preventive shoulder programs are discussed later in this article.

The history and examination of the knee should focus on the history of knee pain rather than the presence of knee instability. Both knees of all athletes should be screened for ligamentous instability prior to competition. Any patient who has a history of the knee "giving way" with activity warrants special attention. Anterior cruciate ligament (ACL) injury is increasingly common among young athletes and occurs three to four times more frequently in females than males. ACL injury is evaluated best with the Lachman test, and ligament injury is well visualized by MRI (Fig. 1).

For those adolescents who have a history of persistent knee pain with flexion as well as swelling, consideration should be given to obtaining a four-view knee series to rule out osteochondritis dessicans (Fig. 2) of the femoral condyle.

The ankle is the most commonly affected joint in sports injury, and chronic ankle problems are

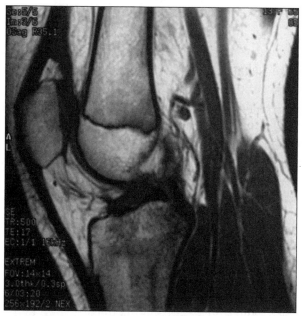

Figure 1. Sagittal MRI of knee showing a torn ACL.

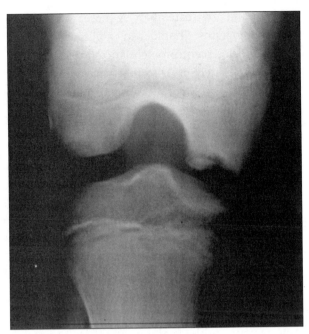

Figure 2. Tunnel view radiograph of the knee showing an osteochondritis dessicans lesion in the femur.

related primarily to repetitive sprains and subsequent instability. Preventive strengthening programs are effective in supporting the ankle and should be encouraged. The details of preventive ankle strengthening programs are discussed later in this article.

Preventive Conditioning Programs

Preventive conditioning programs can help to reduce the rate of injury before the sports season begins. General programs can be implemented for all athletes, and focused programs can be undertaken for athletes who have a history of specific injury patterns.

General prevention programs include both weight training and aerobic conditioning. Weight training, if supervised properly, can be tremendously helpful in improving sports performance, increasing bone density, and reducing injury. Safely designed programs can be implemented in both preadolescents and adolescents. Weight training programs, especially in preadolescents, should focus on high repetition and low resistance. Such programs are especially important for young athletes who are skeletally less mature than their peers and are attempting to participate in high- or medium-contact sports. Baseline strength

can be improved by 30% to 40% through preadolescent strengthening programs and can reduce the strength gap between underdeveloped athletes and their more physically mature peers.

When prescribing a strength training program for a prepubertal adolescent, it is especially important to stress the difference between power lifting and strength training. Power lifting, which uses maximum force for several repetitions, never should be undertaken by a preadolescent because of the potential risk of apophyseal avulsion fracture. Strength training, which involves high repetition training to increase baseline strength through increased recruitment of muscle fiber, is safe in preadolescents if a proper program is designed and implemented with supervision. General conditioning programs also should involve an aerobic component, with 3 to 4 days of aerobic fitness per week.

Focused prevention programs can prevent the recurrence of chronic injury patterns during the upcoming season. Athletes such as soccer players who have a history of ankle sprains during the past few seasons or swimmers who have a history of shoulder pain when swimming increasing yardage are commonly patients in the pediatric office. These repetitive injury patterns require prevention strategies. Preventive sport-specific and joint-specific programs can be instituted during the PPE. Ankle and shoulder injuries deserve special mention because these two sites are especially amenable to office-based conditioning programs.

ANKLE INJURY

A common scenario for ankle injury found during the PPE is the athlete who has a history of recurrent sprains, most often from repeated inversion injury. During the medical history, the athlete often describes multiple episodes of "rolling over" on the ankle during the previous sports season. If the athlete is not yet skeletally mature, it is important to distinguish a history of physeal (growth plate) injury from ligament injury. During the physical examination, the ankle that has a history of chronic sprain often shows residual swelling in the area of the anterior talofibular ligament (ATFL) (Fig. 3), the most commonly sprained ligament in the body, as well as laxity

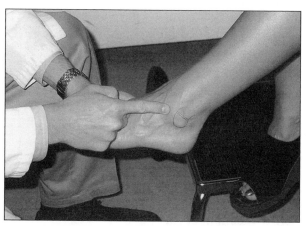

Figure 3. Examiner pointing to the anterior talofibular ligament (ATFL), with the distal fibular physis drawn as a line across the distal fibula. The same inversion injury likely will injure the physis in a skeletally immature athlete and the ATFL if the physis is closed.

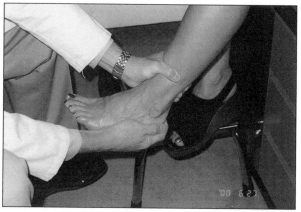

Figure 4. Anterior drawer test for lateral ankle stability. The force is applied anteriorly to gauge laxity in the ATFL.

during the anterior drawer test. In this test, the ankle is flexed to 90 degrees from the tibia (neutral position), and an anterior force is applied to the heel, producing an anterior translation force in the talofibular joint (Fig. 4). If the ATFL has been injured previously, the anterior drawer test will produce anterior laxity. The examiner should compare the noninjured side to the injured side to establish a control.

Once the patient has been shown to have ligamentous laxity, the next important step is to grade the strength in the ankle, particularly in the peroneal muscle group, the major lateral muscular stabilizer of the ankle. Athletes who have a history of chronic inversion injury often demonstrate associated peroneal weakness in addition to

underlying ligamentous laxity. This further contributes to lateral ankle instability and the chronic ankle sprain pattern. Strength grading is accomplished best by having the patient evert the foot against the examiner's hand at 90 degrees of flexion (neutral) (Fig. 5) and using the noninjured ankle as a control.

A strengthening program designed to improve lateral ankle stability can have very favorable results, especially in child and adolescent athletes. An easily implemented ankle strengthening program is three sets of 15 repetitions daily using resisted inversion and eversion with an ace bandage (Figs. 6 and 7). As strength in the ankle improves, the risk of continued inversion injury diminishes. The school trainer can be an invaluable resource for such strengthening programs.

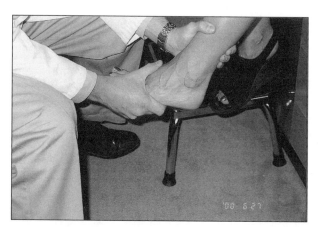

Figure 5. Examiner testing strength in the peroneal muscle group through resisted eversion of the foot.

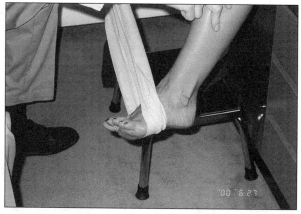

Figure 6. Peroneal muscle strengthening program that can improve lateral ankle stability and decrease the recurrence of inversion injury.

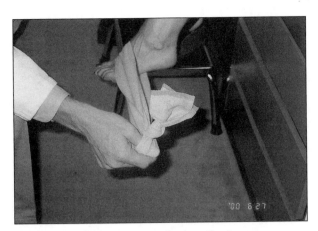

Figure 7. Tibialis posterior muscle strengthening program can aid in improving lateral ankle stability.

SHOULDER INJURY

Common adolescent shoulder injury patterns found during the PPE include shoulder instability and rotator cuff overuse. Athletes who report a slipping sensation in the shoulder, often with a throwing motion, are describing glenohumeral instability, a graded phenomenon from subluxation (slipping) to dislocation. In adolescent patients, recognition of subluxation and aggressive institution of a shoulder stabilization program often represent the best chance of avoiding dislocation and eventual surgical fixation.

Rotator cuff muscle overuse is common in overhead sports such as swimming and tennis and often is described in the medical history as shoulder pain during the previous season that worsened with overhead activity, such as a freestyle swimming stroke or repetitive serving of tennis balls. Instead of the slipping sensation

described in glenohumeral instability, patients who have rotator cuff muscle overuse often describe a pain that "pinches" in the shoulder, generally without the sensation of the shoulder "giving out" that suggests ligamentous injury.

Examination of the shoulder during the PPE should focus on the nature of the complaint. The four major joints of the shoulder, the acromioclavicular, glenohumeral, sternoclavicular, and scapulothoracic joints, can be potential causes of shoulder pain in the adolescent. Furthermore, soft-tissue injury, including muscle, tendon, ligament, or labrum cartilage injury, can cause shoulder pain. Referred pain, especially from the neck among athletes playing contact sports such as football, always should be considered in those complaining of a "shooting" pain down the arm. Of these problems, glenohumeral instability and rotator cuff overuse are common among teenage athletes.

Examination of the shoulder should commence with the testing of the range of motion, including abduction, internal rotation, and external rotation (Figs. 8, 9, and 10). Results of an examination of an affected shoulder always should be compared with the opposite side.

Rotator cuff muscle testing follows range of motion evaluation. The rotator cuff, a group of four small-size muscles (supraspinatus, infraspinatus, teres minor, subscapularis) is responsible for providing dynamic stabilization of the glenohumeral joint. For example, the rotator cuff preserves the normal glenohumeral anatomic relationship by keeping the humeral head centered in

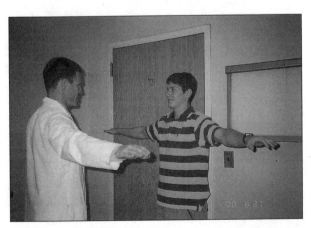

Figure 8. Testing of shoulder abduction. Normal values generally are 0 to 180 degrees.

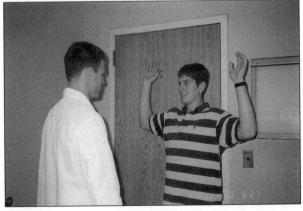

Figure 9. Testing of external rotation. Normal values generally are 0 to 90 degrees.

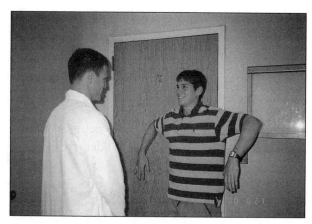

Figure 10. Testing of internal rotation. Normal values generally are 0 to 90 degrees.

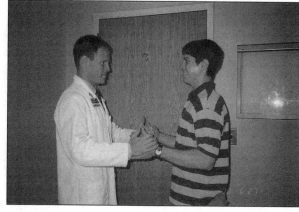

Figure 11. Testing external rotation against resistance to evaluate teres minor and infraspinatus strength.

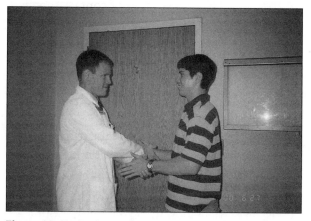

Figure 12. Testing internal rotation against resistance to evaluate subscapularis strength.

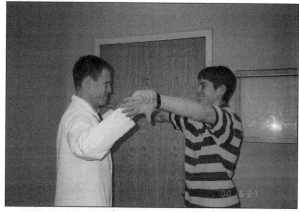

Figure 13. Testing for supraspinatus weakness. In this test, the patient's thumbs are pointed downward, the arms are extended to 45 degrees, and an upward force is exerted against the examiner.

the glenohumeral joint in a pitcher who throws repeatedly, using the larger muscle groups, such as the deltoid and pectoralis muscles, to generate arm velocity and throw the ball. Underlying laxity in the glenohumeral capsule and ligament complex is common among overhead sport athletes, and this creates a greater degree of baseline laxity in the glenohumeral joint, putting an even greater stress on the dynamic muscular stabilizers. If the rotator cuff is excessively weak, the shoulder often becomes "sore" with overuse; the muscles are not strong enough to function properly. The same scenario occurs in swimming where the larger muscle groups can overpower a weaker rotator cuff group, producing excessive glenohumeral motion and shoulder pain due to rotator cuff overuse. Testing the strength of the rotator cuff group before the

sports season begins is essential to evaluate baseline dynamic stability.

Rotator cuff muscle strength is evaluated by testing the major functions, external rotation (teres minor, infraspinatus), and internal rotation (subscapularis) and using the supraspinatus test to evaluate for supraspinatus weakness (Figs. 11, 12, and 13). Side to side comparisons are very helpful in determining specific rotator cuff weakness.

Ligamentous stability must be determined in patients in whom a history of glenohumeral instability is elicited during the medical history of the PPE prior to clearance for high- and medium-contact sports participation. These patients might present with a history of shoulder dislocation or subluxation or a "slipping shoulder" during the past season. In adolescents, glenohumeral instability

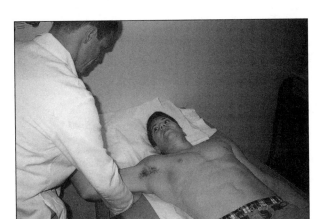

Figure 14. Anterior apprehension test for glenohumeral laxity.

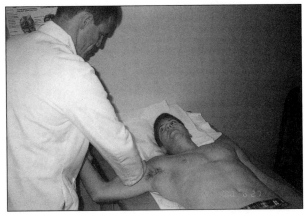

Figure 15. Anterior relocation test to confirm the presence of anterior glenohumeral laxity.

can occur anteriorly, posteriorly, or inferiorly. Instability that occurs in two or more directions is termed multidirectional.

When attempting to determine the type of glenohumeral instability, the examiner should focus on which maneuver appears to elicit the sensation of instability. Athletes most often show signs of anterior instability for two reasons. First, the humeral head sits in an anterior position in the glenohumeral joint, predisposing it to anterior instability. Second, the anterior portion of the glenohumeral ligament is the weakest, reducing the anterior structural support in the joint. It is most important for the examiner to find athletes who have glenohumeral instability, evaluate the degree of ligamentous laxity, and design a muscle strengthening program to help stabilize the joint and prevent further episodes. Cases of previous glenohumeral dislocation should be referred to a specialist.

Anterior glenohumeral laxity is evaluated by using the apprehension-relocation test (Figs. 14 and 15). With the arm abducted to 90 degrees and rotated externally, the anterior portion of the glenohumeral ligament is maximally stressed. In this position, a sense of apprehension indicates a positive test for anterior glenohumeral laxity. In the same position, a posterior force applied to the humeral component of the glenohumeral joint without a sensation of apprehension indicates a positive relocation test.

Two common patterns of shoulder pain in the young athlete are rotator cuff muscle overuse and glenohumeral instability. Early recognition of these problems and effective rehabilitation for 4 to 6 weeks prior to the commencement of the sports season can decrease the risk of recurrent shoulder problems significantly during the ensuing sports season.

Conclusion

As sports participation increases among young athletes, so too does the need for effective and efficient preparticipation clearance. In most cases, this responsibility falls on the pediatrician. Because many injury patterns are sports-specific, consideration of the sport for which an athlete is being cleared is the first step of the PPE. Attention to the pertinent family history; investigation of the medical problems that can affect sports safety and sports performance, such as asthma or concussion; and a specific focus on recurrent musculoskeletal problems from the previous sports season are important considerations. The Appendix features a sample preparticipation examination form. With a focused, sports-specific approach, the PPE can be an extremely rewarding experience for both the athlete and the pediatrician that can enhance the safety and enjoyment of sports participation by young athletes.

Suggested Reading

American Academy of Pediatrics Committee on Sports Medicine and Fitness. Athletic participation by children and adolescents who have systemic hypertension. Policy statement RE9715, American Academy of Pediatrics. *Pediatrics.* 1997; 99:637–638

American Academy of Pediatrics Committee on Sports Medicine and Fitness. Atlantoaxial instability in Down syndrome: subject review. *Pediatrics.* 1995;96:151–154

American Academy of Pediatrics Committee on Sports Medicine and Fitness. Medical conditions affecting sports participation. Policy statement RE9432, American Academy of Pediatrics. *Pediatrics.* 1994;94:757–760

American Academy of Pediatrics Committee on Sports Medicine and Fitness. Strength training, weight and power lifting, and body building by children and adolescents, RE9196, American Academy of Pediatrics. *Pediatrics.* 1990;86:801–803

Anderson SJ. Soccer: a case-based approach to ankle and knee injuries. *Pediatr Ann.* 2000;29:177–188

Bernhardt DT. Football: a case-based approach to mild traumatic brain injury. *Pediatr Ann.* 2000;29:172–176

Callahan LR. The evolution of the female athlete—progress and problems. *Pediatr Ann.* 2000;29:149–153

Cantu RC. Functional cervical stenosis: a contraindication to participation in contact sports. *Med Sci Sports Exerc.* 1995; 25:1082–1084

Collins MW, Grindel SH, Lovell MR, et al. Relationship between concussion and neuropsychological performance in college football players. *JAMA.* 1999;282:964–970

Corrardo D, Basso C, Schiavon M, et al. Screening for hypertrophic cardiomyopathy in young athletes. *N Engl J Med.* 1998;339:364–369

Luke A, Micheli L. Sports injuries: emergency assessment and field-side care. *Pediatr Rev.* 1999;20:291–301

Metzl JD. Strength training and nutritional supplement use in adolescent athletes. *Current Opin Pediatr.* 1999;11:292–296

Nattiv A, Agostini R, Drinkwater B, Yaeger K. The female athlete triad: the inter-relatedness of disordered eating, amenorrhea, and osteoporosis. *Clin Sports Med.* 1994;13:405–418

Rifat SF, Ruffin MT, Gorenflo DW. Disqualifying criteria in a preparticipation sports evaluation. *J Fam Prac.* 1995;41:42–50

Risser WL, Hoffman HM, Bellah GG Jr, et al. A cost-benefit analysis of preparticipation sports examinations of adolescent athletes. *J School Health.* 1985;55:270–273

Smith J, Lakowski ER. The preparticipation physical examination: Mayo clinic experience with 2,729 examinations. *Mayo Clin Proc.* 1998;73:419–429

Appendix 1 – Sample Preparticipation Examination Form

Pre-Sports Medical Screening and Health History

Name: _____

Birth Date: _____/_____/_____   Age: _____ Grade: _____

Sport(s): _____

Address: _____ City, State, Zip: _____

Telephone (H): _____ Parent/Guardian: _____

Emergency Contact: _____ Telephone: _____

Physician: _____ Telephone: _____

General Medical History (*to be completed by parent or guardian*)

Indicate if you or any member of your family have or had the following illnesses or conditions by marking (**S**) for student, (**F**) for family (sibling or parent), and (**B**) for both in the appropriate box. Please include dates where appropriate.

Asthma		Heart disorder	
Respiratory disorder		Gastrointestinal disorder	
Anemia (including sickle cell)		Kidney/Genitourinary disorder	
Hepatitis		Epilepsy or convulsive disorder	
Mononucleosis		Concussion Number: ____	
Diabetes		Frequent or severe headaches	
Thyroid disorder		History of fainting or dizziness	
Osteoporosis/ Osteopenia		Heat stroke	
High blood pressure		Absence of paired organ (eye, kidney)	

If **YES** to any of the above, please explain: _____

_____

Allergies: _____

Regular Medications: _____ Reason: _____

Do you wear protective or prescription lenses, eyeglasses, or contact lenses? _____

Have you ever been hospitalized? _____ Why? _____

Have you ever been denied athletic participation for medical reasons? _____

If yes, explain: _____

Are your menses monthly? _____

Orthopedic History (*to be completed by parent or guardian*)

Include any major musculoskeletal injury to the following areas; include sprains, dislocations, fractures, and surgery.

Area	Right	Left	Date	Injury Type/ Description
Foot				
Ankle				
Lower leg				
Thigh				
Hip				
Spine				
Shoulder				
Upper arm				
Forearm				
Wrist				
Hand				
Head				
Neck				
Other				

Do you have any other type of illness, injury, or condition that is being monitored by a doctor? (If yes, please explain)_____

I declare the above information to be accurate and a true reflection of

_____ (student's name) physical condition.

Parent or Guardian Signature: _____ Date: _____

Pre-Sports Screening (*on site portion, physician to complete*)

Blood Pressure: _____ Pulse: _____ Height: _____ Weight: _____

Eyes: PERRL _____ Other _____

Heart Rhythm: NSR _____ Arrhythmia _____

Murmur: None _____ Functional _____ Other _____

Abdomen: No OMT _____ Other _____

Visual Screening: _____

Orthopedic Screening

Knee	Rom/Stability	Normal
Ankle	Rom/Stability	Normal
Neck	Rom	Normal
Shoulder	Rom/Stability	Normal
Hamstring	Fingertip distance from the floor _____ inches.	

Scoliosis Screening Normal Other _____

Doctor Recommendations: Cleared Hold (reason) _____

Examing Doctor's Signature: _____ Date: _____

Treatment Strategies for Musculoskeletal Injuries

by Gregory L. Landry, MD, FAAP

Management of musculoskeletal injuries in primary care pediatric practice can be challenging. Most medical schools and residencies provide little training in this area. Young athletes in our practices expect the latest treatments, those that will enable the earliest possible return to sports and exercise routines.

This issue of *Adolescent Health Update* addresses general principles that guide treatment of acute and chronic injuries, and the rationale for various treatment modalities. Criteria for referral to athletic trainers, physical therapists, and orthopedic surgeons will be discussed.

Acute Injuries

Treatment of acute injuries can be divided into three phases. In the first days following injury, treatment regimens seek to minimize bleeding, edema, and pain. As these resolve, second-phase regimens address the need to restore strength and range of motion. As recovery progresses, third-phase treatment introduces sports-specific conditioning.

PHASE I

The goal of treatment in the first 48 to 72 hours after injury is to minimize bleeding, edema, and pain. This phase is easily remembered by the mnemonic RICE, which stands for Rest, Ice, Compression, and Elevation.

- *Rest* is indicated because painful use of the injured part increases bleeding and lengthens the time required for rehabilitation and return to sport. To facilitate proper rest, a sling can be prescribed for patients with arm and shoulder injuries, and crutches can be prescribed for patients with lower extremity injuries that cause a limp.
- *Ice* reduces swelling and is a great analgesic, sometimes eliminating the need for medication.
- *Compression* reduces the amount of bleeding and decreases fluid leaks from damaged capillaries. A snug elastic wrap works best in many situations, notably knee injuries and muscle contusions. A variety of compression dressings for ankles are commercially available. The air-stirrup ankle brace is comfortable and provides good compression for ankle sprains.

It is important to note that the common knee immobilizer, designed to provide comfort (especially during sleep), is neither a compression dressing nor a stabilizing brace for knee injuries. Some sports medicine specialists advise against knee immobilizers for athletes because they are often overused or used improperly. Overuse of

Learning Objectives

After reading this article, pediatricians will understand treatment modalities for musculoskeletal pain, particularly that which results from athletic injury. Pediatricians will be able to describe:

- Principles of management of both acute musculoskeletal injuries and common conditions
- Indications for referral to other health care professionals
- Treatment modalities that may be employed and their mechanisms of action
- The role of complementary or alternative therapies

Gregory L. Landry, MD, is a professor of pediatrics at the University of Wisconsin Hospitals and Clinics in Madison, Wisconsin, and the 2001 recipient of the AAP Section on Sports Medicine and Fitness Thomas E. Shaffer Award.

Case vignette: Teen with lateral ankle sprain

"Michael," a healthy 14-year-old youth who plays on his school's basketball team, presents in the office with a common lateral ankle sprain. Michael has been your patient for more than 5 years. He's an earnest kid and sports are important in his life. You know that he's already hoping to play on a college team. Initial assessment indicates that the injury is mild and the patient is motivated to cooperate in rehabilitation.

In this circumstance, the pediatrician should first describe the phase I treatment guidelines and explain why they are needed to limit bleeding and swelling. Office counseling should address functional rehabilitation, how it works, and why it can help to restore full capabilities as soon as possible. Injured athletes are likely to be frustrated; it may help to acknowledge this and then encourage the patient to channel frustrations into rehabilitation.

Since this is a mild sprain, the pediatrician can offer instruction on phase II rehabilitation in the initial visit with a handout on stretching, range of motion, and strength training for the calf and peroneal muscles. This should include demonstration of the "wall" stretch (Figure A), as well as others. (For sample stretches, please see the patient education page at the end of this article, Figures A, B, and C.) The patient should be reminded to hold each stretch for at least 10 seconds (and preferably for 30 seconds) at a time, and to avoid bouncing. Stretching should not be painful. The athlete should be instructed to do each stretch three times, and to do a set of the prescribed stretches three to four times a day.

The athlete should also be taught exercises to improve range of motion in other planes. Instruct the athlete to write the alphabet in the air with his great toe at least three times a day. Explain the effect of injury on proprioception and how this will help. For balance training, ask him to stand on the ball of the injured foot and then the uninjured foot. (Warn him that this "stork" stand will be more difficult than it looks.) If unable to do that maneuver, he may want to start by standing on the full foot before trying the ball of the foot. Many athletes are unaware of how much proprioception has been lost even with a minor injury.

Because the injury is mild and the patient is cooperative, he can be expected to follow instructions with standard supervision and intervention. The pediatrician should assure that Michael has a good picture of the plan for his care, the time required to progress to phase II and phase III rehabilitation, and how he can assure that his healing progresses optimally. Running should not occur until he can hop up and down 8 to 10 times on the injured ankle with minimal or no pain. If Michael does not have access to an athletic trainer or physical therapist, he should be seen about 7 to 10 days after the injury. It would be best to see Michael 2 to 3 days before a competition, since that is when he will be most anxious to return to sports activity.

---

knee immobilizers contributes to loss of motion and to atrophy, which are common adverse effects of an acute injury.

● *Elevation* of the injured body part above the level of the patient's heart introduces gravity as an aid to reducing hydrostatic pressure in the capillaries and, in turn, leakage of fluid into the tissues.

The RICE mnemonic does not include analgesic medication because many injuries will not require it. It may be useful to remind young athletes that RICE and rehabilitative exercises are much more important than medication. Use of anti-inflammatory medications in acute injuries is controversial; recent evidence shows that they may impair healing. The inflammatory process needs to proceed in order to allow the healing of tissues, and if that process is shortened, the restorative benefits of inflammation will be compromised. For these reasons, if analgesia is required, acetaminophen may be preferable to a nonsteroidal anti-inflammatory agent. Occasionally a mild narcotic is indicated to help the athlete sleep.

PHASE II

Phase II treatment regimens are designed to restore range of motion and strength in the injured body part. These regimens begin 48 to 72 hours after the injury, even if there is still some pain and swelling. Restoration of proprioception and balance should also be part of the program for lower extremity injuries. Loss of motion, joint effusion, and prolonged inflammation all contribute to pain with concomitant loss of muscular strength and muscular atrophy. There is a direct correlation between the length of time that muscles are not used and the likelihood that there will be a loss of strength and a delay in the return to maximum performance.

During phase II, athletes are typically depressed and frustrated by their sudden physical limitations. It is important to counsel the adolescent about what can be done to maintain fitness and what specific tasks will speed recovery.

Early mobilization is desirable whenever possible because it helps to strengthen the ligaments by encouraging proper deposition of collagen and alignment of elastin fibers. Early mobilization also improves the likelihood of successful functional rehabilitation. The duration of phase II varies with the severity of injury. The goal is improved range of motion, improved strength, and less pain. If pain persists without improvement or worsens, an orthopedic surgeon should be consulted.

Most athletes can safely begin an aerobic exercise program during phase II. The most convenient exercise is often a workout on a stationary bicycle. If the athlete has access to a pool, swimming and water exercises may be feasible. Almost any exercise with the upper extremities will be fine in the presence of a lower extremity injury. Mild pain during aerobic exercise is acceptable, provided that it does not worsen with activity and the exercise is done in a way to prevent re-injury.

The first case vignette (see box, page 786) describes principles that govern care of an athlete with a common lateral ankle sprain. Patient consultation will include discussion of stretches and devices that are useful in functional rehabilitation. The third phase of treatment, which involves working on sports-specific drills, begins when the athlete has regained strength and motion.

PHASE III

The sports-specific drills prescribed in phase III are designed to build on the functional rehabilitation that has occurred in phase II. For example,

a baseball pitcher with a shoulder injury begins throwing with short, easy throws and gradually increases the distance and the speed of throwing the ball.

The athlete with lower extremity injuries must be able to hop up and down eight to ten times on the injured leg without pain or collapse before attempting any running. This test is especially helpful for the common ankle sprain. It is also a useful office screen to assess readiness for running or competing. The running must start with jogging and progress gradually to full-speed sprints. Before returning to competition, the athlete must be able to change directions at full speed without favoring the injured ankle or limping. This provides objective functional criteria for return to play, regardless of how much the athlete, parent, or coach want the athlete to resume. When the athlete starts running, he or she should start with jogging and gradually increase speed until there is pain or limp, then stop, ice the ankle, and start over with jogging the next day. When the athlete is able to sprint full speed without pain or limp, he or she should practice changing directions (cutting) in the opposite direction of the injured ankle. This should start with half-speed cuts, then three-quarter speed, and then finally full speed. The athlete who can cut off the injured ankle at full speed with no pain or limp is ready to return to sport. Some practitioners ask athletes to run in figure-of-eight patterns of increasing speed; this approach may be less effective in building endurance.

Chronic Injuries

Chronic injuries in adolescents may not prevent the athlete from competing, but over time they can cause pain, muscle atrophy, and loss of flexibility, all of which will adversely affect performance. Chronic injuries are due to overuse. Injuries at the tissue level are due to repetitive microtrauma that exceeds the body's ability to repair tissue damage.

Every bout of exercise causes microscopic tissue damage. When there is sufficient rest between exercise bouts, the body heals the damage and actually strengthens the area under stress, which is why performance improves with training.

Case vignette: Knee pain

"Sharon," a 12-year-old who "lives to dance," presents with knee pain and a tender patellar tendon. During the evaluation, she tells you that the pain seemed to begin shortly after she was selected for an important role in her ballet class recital. When you ask her about what is involved, you learn that she is learning to do certain jumps for the performance. "Every night at home," Sharon says, "I have to practice." On exam, she is tender over the medial facet of her patella and in the patellar tendon, just below the inferior pole of the patella.

Probably the most common overuse injuries in pediatric practice produce anterior knee pain and involve the extensor mechanism of the knee, which includes the quadriceps muscles, the patella, the patellar tendon, and its attachment on the tibial apophysis. In this case, it appears that Sharon has exceeded the capacity of the patellar tendon to withstand the marked increase in load, and she has irritated her patella as well.

In this circumstance, the pediatrician should determine if the patient is engaging in any other activities that stress the anterior knee. Anterior knee pain is often seen in young athletes who are playing two or more sports. In this case, even without other activities, the nightly practices do not allow her tissues sufficient rest to heal.

The pediatrician should suggest "relative rest" by recommending that the athlete reduce the frequency or duration of practices to allow for healing. It would also be important to ask her to demonstrate the stretching routine from dance class, and to prescribe stretches for the hamstring muscles and iliotibial band if necessary. These are often more helpful than quadriceps strengthening exercises, especially in athletic individuals.

However, if the intensity and/or duration of the exercise exceed the body's ability to repair the microscopic damage, an overuse injury will result.

For example, bone takes weeks or months to remodel. If weekly running mileage increases too rapidly, a common phenomenon in adolescent distance runners who do not run year-round, a stress fracture may result. Case vignette #2 (see box, above) presents a similar problem that occurs in dancers who rapidly increase the percentage of practice time on jumps.

Care of anterior knee pain is similar regardless of whether the diagnosis is patellofemoral pain syndrome, patellar tendonitis, or Osgood-Schlatter disease. All are disorders of the extensor mechanism of the knee. As in many overuse disorders, it is important to obtain a complete history of all the activities that aggravate the pain.

Young athletes often play two or more sports. In order to prescribe "relative rest" the athlete may need to temporarily stop playing one of the sports. It is unusual for the pain to be so severe that the athlete cannot participate in any physical activities.

Overuse is one of many possible factors in the etiology of anterior knee pain. It was long thought that quadriceps weakness was an important factor, which is why quadriceps-strengthening exercises were prescribed. More recent experience suggests that quadriceps-strengthening exercises may not be necessary and may actually aggravate the pain. In many youngsters, poor flexibility, especially of the hamstring muscles and iliotibial (IT) bands, contributes to anterior knee pain.

Hamstring flexibility is best assessed with the patient supine and with the hip flexed to 90 degrees. When the knee is extended, the very flexible youngster can straighten or nearly straighten the knee to zero degrees. The inflexible adolescent may only extend the knee to 45 degrees short of full extension.

Hamstring muscles can be stretched in a variety of ways. Two of these stretches are shown in Figure B on the patient education sheet. Adolescents are more likely to do the stretches if you link them with another daily activity. The standing stretch can be performed while talking on the telephone. Either stretch can be done while watching the television.

The iliotibial band (IT band) is a thick, fibrous structure that extends from the iliac crest to Gerdy's tubercle on the proximal tibia.

It is attached to the vastus lateralis, the most lateral quadriceps muscle, and the lateral patella. IT band tightness is best assessed with the patient lying on his or her side. The hip is extended and the examiner flexes the knee. If the IT band is tight, it will hold the entire leg parallel to the examining table (Figure 1). This is commonly referred to as a positive Ober test. If the leg drifts toward the table, the IT band is flexible (a negative Ober test).

The IT band can be stretched at least two ways, as shown in Figure C on the patient education page. With the legs crossed, the trunk bends laterally toward the uninvolved side, and the IT band is stretched. With the athlete sitting and flexing the hip, the opposite elbow is placed on the outer side of the knee. The arm should pull the knee toward the opposite shoulder. This latter stretch is probably more effective. A diligent stretching program (ie, stretching several times a day) is often helpful.

Stress to the patella and extensor mechanism is more likely to occur in the child with midfoot hyperpronation (ankle valgus) seen in Figure 2. Purchasing shoes with better arch supports or using off-the-shelf arch supports will also help relieve pain. If there is any evidence of patellar instability (subluxation) on physical exam, such as tenderness over the medial retinaculum or above the adductor tubercle, or increased lateral excursion of the patella with the knee flexed to 20 degrees, then a patellar stabilizing knee sleeve might help control the pain. A knowledgeable physical therapist or athletic trainer may also try taping to prevent the patella from developing a subluxation; this will also help control the pain.

Management

Rehabilitative exercises are best taught one-on-one. Not only is it helpful to show an athlete an exercise with your own body, it is wise to watch the athlete perform the exercise to assure it is performed correctly. It is also wise to provide guidance early-on about when and how to progress the program. Some of our patients do not have access to a physical therapist (PT) or a certified athletic trainer (ATC). In these circumstances, it is entirely appropriate for a pediatrician or a

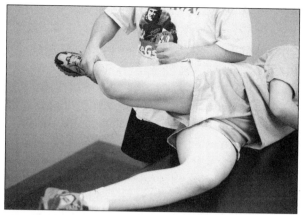

Figure 1. The Ober test for iliotibial band tightness. The hip is extended with the knee flexed to trap the IT band over the greater trochanter of the hip. If the thigh stays parallel to the table with the hip and knee flexed, the test is positive. This patient has a positive Ober test. (If the Ober test is negative, the knee drifts toward the table and the thigh is no longer parallel to the table.)

staff member to instruct the athlete on a rehabilitation program.

It is important to give the patient written instructions along with the personal demonstration. The best handouts also have an anatomic drawing to help the athlete understand the extent of the injury. There is nothing wrong with giving the athlete ideas on how to start rehabilitating an injury until he can see a PT or ATC.

REHABILITATION SPECIALISTS

Ideally, injured athletes should have an opportunity to work with an ATC or PT, professionals trained in the rehabilitation of injuries. Some

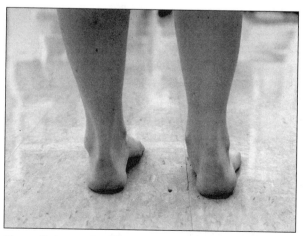

Figure 2. A neutral midfoot on the left compared to the one that is pronated on the right.

high schools have an athletic trainer available for their athletes. An ATC has completed at least an undergraduate degree and has completed core athletic training course work to achieve a list of competencies determined by the National Athletic Trainers Association (NATA). The ATC specializes in the prevention, care, and treatment of injuries in athletes.

The physical therapist has at least an undergraduate degree in physical therapy and has completed two years of course work and clinical work devoted to physical therapy. The PT specializes in the rehabilitation of injuries in all age groups from all causes. More information about these professionals may be found on Web sites for their national organizations (www.apta.org for physical therapy, and www.nata.org for athletic trainers.)

If you have choices in PT clinics, choose one that will provide feedback when rehab is not going well and whose personnel are available by telephone when you are not certain what to write on the PT consultation note.

In some states, PT referral requires a written referral from a physician. If a written referral is required, the most important part is a correct diagnosis. If uncertain about a diagnosis, it is best to consult an orthopedist or sports medicine subspecialist before consulting a PT.

When you have good working relationship with a PT, the referral can be brief. Many PT consultants want only a diagnosis (eg, lateral ankle sprain) and will then use their expertise to develop the rehabilitation program and treatment plan. For example, it is often sufficient to state, "Please instruct on a home rehab program and use modalities as indicated." If the number of visits needs to be limited, simply add, "for up to eight visits" or whatever number is desired.

PTs should give you feedback on how much history they need to help your patients. Most of our patients do not need frequent visits. For simple injuries, most of our highly motivated patients do well with a home program and a visit or two for follow-up to monitor progress.

It is also helpful to choose a PT who is familiar with "aggressive" programs designed for young athletes. Some hospital-based PTs who work with less active and more debilitated patients may have

trouble switching to the more accelerated programs for athletes. Ask team physicians for high schools and colleges what PT group serves them the best. It is important to ask about whether the group is cooperative about seeing a patient promptly when they receive a referral.

Treatment Modalities

Treatment modalities for musculoskeletal injuries involve the use of physical agents to create an environment for optimal healing while reducing pain. These include forms of heat, cold, water, electricity, and massage. The goal is a safe return to maximum capacity in a timely manner. Modalities should not be used as a substitute for rehabilitative exercises, but rather as a means to enhance the athlete's ability to perform these exercises. They are administered by PTs and ATCs, usually with a doctor's order.

COLD

Cryotherapy is the most important modality for adolescent athletes. Other modalities are used much less frequently. Cold is employed immediately after an acute injury and promptly after exercise for a chronic injury.

Cryotherapy is most useful after acute trauma because it reduces edema and controls pain. In the acute setting, cold stimulates vasoconstriction, thereby reducing bleeding. Cold therapy reduces capillary leakage in both acute and chronic injury. Athletes with a more chronic injury apply cold after a workout to minimize edema associated with microtrauma that follows a bout of exercise.

Cryotherapy can be applied with ice packs, ice buckets/baths, and ice massage. Ice packs are probably used the most in sports medicine. Crushed ice in a plastic bag is the best way to apply cold in most cases. Chemical packs are acceptable, but are expensive and quickly get warm. Commercial gel packs that are kept in the freezer are convenient, but can stay too cold for too long and are more likely to cause frostbite. It is best to have a layer of clothing or a thin towel under any cold pack. Cryotherapy achieves maximum effect after 20 minutes. After that, there is a reflex vasodilation. Ice baths are desirable when an entire joint needs to be treated, such as an ankle or elbow. They are very effective, but not well tolerated by some athletes because the initial immersion is so uncomfortable. Ice massage is most desirable for superficial injuries. Commonly done with ice that has been frozen in a paper cup, ice massage may not penetrate the tissue as deeply as ice packs. This superficial penetration is fine for tendonopathies and superficial distal extremity injuries.

SUPERFICIAL HEAT THERAPY

Heat should only be used before exercise in the subacute and chronic phases of injury and rehabilitation. Heat is almost never used immediately after exercise for any therapeutic reason. Before exercise, heat improves flexibility of the soft tissues and is associated with increased blood flow and vasodilation. This causes an increase in the permeability of vessel walls with an increase in edema. For these reasons, heat should not be used in the presence of active bleeding, inflammation, or edema.

There are several means to apply superficial heat. Hot packs, whirlpools, and paraffin baths can be applied to different body parts for various uses. Heat is often applied with hydrocollator packs, pouches of petroleum distillate or silica gel, heated in a tank of water to about 170°F. An electric heating pad is more convenient in many settings and will suffice in most cases, even though it is dry heat.

PENETRATING HEAT THERAPY

Therapeutic ultrasound is the most commonly used method to provide deep heat to muscular tissues. As the sound waves penetrate tissue, they are thought to produce oscillations of the tissue molecules that convert the sound energy to heat. Ultrasound potentially accelerates hematoma resorption, reduces pain and spasm, promotes healing, and increases extensibility of scar, all of which help regain range of motion and reduce pain. Ultrasound also can be used for phonophoresis (ultrasound with a topical medication, usually a corticosteroid). There is very little scientific evidence that phonophoresis is efficacious.

There is an increase in the extensibility of the tissues and an increase in the blood flow to the tissues for up to an hour after application of the ultrasound. Ultrasound is commonly employed in chronic injuries to progressively increase limited range of motion.

THERAPEUTIC ELECTRICAL STIMULATION

Electricity is used therapeutically to stimulate muscles or stimulate neuronal tissue, and in various forms to relieve pain, aid tissue healing, and reduce muscle spasms. Electrical muscle stimulation is used to enhance muscle contraction when there is reflex inhibition and to stimulate muscle when a limb is immobilized to minimize atrophy. It can be used to reinforce voluntary contraction during rehabilitation. It is also used to break down adhesions within muscle and to assist in relieving pain and spasm.

Transcutaneous Electrical Nerve Stimulation (TENS) is used for control of pain. It is thought to work initially via the "gate control" theory of pain reduction by stimulating large sensory nerve fiber input that suppresses the small pain nerve fibers. TENS provides pain relief beyond the time of stimulation, so it must relieve pain by other mechanisms as well. A TENS unit is typically employed for large muscle strains in the neck, trunk, or thorax, but it can be used for almost any acute or chronic injury.

Galvanic (direct) current can directly stimulate denervated muscle but is more commonly used to drive ions into tissues (iontophoresis). The theory is that a direct current will drive the molecules of the medication away from the electrode and into the skin. Corticosteroids are the most popular medications used in this procedure with anecdotal evidence of relief, especially for superficial injuries such as tendonopathies. There is some scientific evidence of the efficacy of this method but it is not conclusive. The modality has been reported to be clinically useful in treating bursitis, tendonitis, and adhesive capsulitis.

WATER

Water therapy simply means performing exercises in the presence of water. This intervention is popular because a variety of tasks can be performed safely with the buoyancy of water that would be much riskier on dry land. For example, working on balance with a sprained ankle can begin much earlier in water than on dry land. Not all athletes are comfortable working in water (especially those who can't swim), and water rehabilitation cannot be performed with an open wound. Water therapy requires access to a pool and the athlete must be supervised while working out in the pool. Water is ideal for runners with stress fractures who can "run" in the water with appropriate floatation devices.

Other modalities that may be employed are outlined in Table 1.

Summary

When an active person incurs an injury, the first task is accurate diagnosis. Following this, physician, physical therapist, athletic trainer, and athlete collaborate to generate a rehabilitation plan. First, the plan should decrease pain. This goal can be accomplished through a variety of interventions; cold and immobilization are the modalities most often employed in the acute phase.

Therapeutic exercise is the most important aspect of rehabilitation. Exercises must promote a normal range of motion through passive, active-assisted, or active exercises. Return of normal muscular flexibility and joint motion is usually necessary before working on muscle strength. Safe return to sports occurs when the athlete has completed a functional rehabilitation program with a gradual increase in intensity and duration of tasks.

Acknowledgments

The editors would like to acknowledge technical review by Reginald L. Washington, MD, FAAP, for the Committee on Sports Medicine & Fitness, and Joseph A. Congeni, MD, FAAP, for the Section on Sports Medicine and Fitness.

Table 1. Mechanical Therapies: A Glossary

Modality	Actions	Indications
—Massage therapy (examples) Friction (cross-fiber)	Pressure of massage is applied transverse to muscle fiber, tendon or ligament to break scar and adhesions in the subacute and chronic phases of injury.	Usually employed for trigger points in muscles and myofascial release. These are tender spots within the muscle thought to produce chronic pain. Anecdotally effective.
Sports massage	Rubbing and kneading of muscles especially the large muscle groups acutely and chronically.	Delayed muscle soreness after intense exercise, chronic muscle strains, particularly those of the neck and back. Anecdotally effective.
—Manual therapy	Mobilizes joints using a combination of graded oscillations and traction.	Used for a variety of chronic pain syndromes, typically by osteopathic physicians. Sometimes utilized by physical therapists.
—Manipulative therapy	Mobilizes joints using high-velocity, forceful movements at the end of joint range of motion.	Usually employed for back and neck pain by osteopaths and chiropractors. Some scientific evidence for efficacy in treatment of back pain in adults.
—Traction	Controls pain and nerve root irritation in patients with disc disease by reducing compression.	Intervertebral disc disease. Efficacious in selected adult cases.

References and Further Reading

American Academy of Pediatrics Section on Sports Medicine and Fitness. Guidelines for Parents and Athletes: Lateral Ankle Sprain and Rehabilitation. *Sports Shorts.* Issue 3, September 2000. Available at: http://www.aap.org. (Click on "You and Your Family")

Anderson B. *Stretching.* Rev ed. Bolinas, CA: Shelter Publications, Inc; 2000

Brotzman SB, ed. *Clinical Orthopaedic Rehabilitation.* St. Louis, MO: Mosby; 1996

Hergenroeder A. Acute Shoulder, Knee, and Ankle Injuries. Part 2: Rehabilitation. *Adolescent Health Update.* 1996;8:3

Mellion MB, Walsh WM, Madden C, Putukian M, eds. *The Team Physician's Handbook.* 3rd ed. Philadelphia, PA: Hanley & Belfus; 2001

Peterson L, Renstrom P. *Sports Injuries: Their Prevention and Treatment.* 3rd ed. Champaign, IL: Human Kinetics Publishers, Inc; 2001

Reid DC. *Sports Injury Assessment and Rehabilitation.* Philadelphia, PA: Churchill Livingstone; 1992 (New edition scheduled for release March 2002)

Schenck RC, ed. *Athletic Training and Sports Medicine.* 3rd ed. Rosemont, IL: American Academy of Orthopaedic Surgeons; 1999

Sullivan JA, Anderson SJ, eds. *Care of the Young Athlete.* Rosemont and Elk Grove Village, IL: American Academy of Orthopaedic Surgeons and American Academy of Pediatrics; 2000

Zachazewski JE, Magee DJ, Quillen WS, eds. *Athletic Injuries and Rehabilitation.* Philadelphia, PA: WB Saunders Company; 1996

Stretches for Functional Rehabiliation

Your recovery from injury will be quicker and more complete if you are careful to follow your doctor's instructions about what you can do from home. Please refer to these pictures and descriptions when you do the stretches your doctor has prescribed. Take care to do them exactly as instructed. Pay attention to the number of repetitions in each set and the number of times to do each set of stretches each day. Stretches should not be painful.

FIGURE A

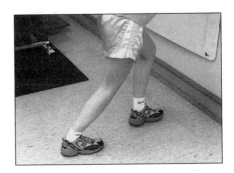

The "wall" stretch is designed to improve the flexibility of the Achilles tendon and the calf muscles. The foot must be kept flat on the floor and pointed straight toward the wall. Hold this stretch a minimum of 10 seconds (preferably 30 seconds) with no bouncing. Hold it until the muscle is tight; stretching should not be painful! Each stretch should be performed three times. Ideally, you should perform this routine three to four times daily. These are easy to do while you are on the telephone or watching television.

FIGURE B

Stretches for the hamstring muscles in the sitting and standing positions. Flexion of the back should be kept to a minimum during these maneuvers. The idea is to stretch the hamstrings, not the back. Hold each stretch a minimum of 10

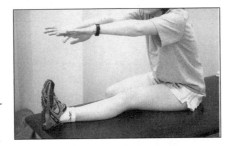
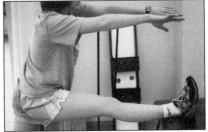

seconds (preferably 30 seconds) with no bouncing until the muscles are tight. Stretching should not be painful! Each stretch should be performed three times. Ideally, you should perform this routine three to four times daily. These are easy to do while you are on the telephone or watching television.

FIGURE C

Stretches for the iliotibial band tendon standing and sitting. While standing with the legs crossed, the trunk bends laterally toward the uninvolved side, and the IT band is stretched. While sitting and flexing the hip, use the opposite elbow over the outer side of the knee and pull the knee toward the opposite shoulder. This latter stretch is probably more effective than the standing

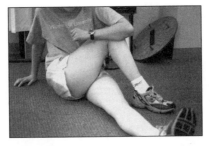
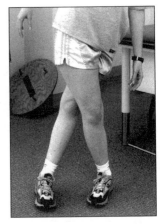

stretch. Hold each stretch a minimum of 10 seconds (preferably 30 seconds) with no bouncing until the muscles are tight; stretching should not be painful! Each stretch should be performed three times. Ideally, you should perform this routine three to four times daily. These are easy to do while you are on the telephone or watching television.

Use of Performance-Enhancing Substances

Committee on Sports Medicine and Fitness

ABSTRACT. Performance-enhancing substances include dietary supplements, prescription medications, and illicit drugs. Virtually no data are available on the efficacy and safety in children and adolescents of widely used performance-enhancing substances. This statement is intended to provide a generalized but functional definition of performance-enhancing substances. The American Academy of Pediatrics strongly condemns the use of performance-enhancing substances and vigorously endorses efforts to eliminate their use among children and adolescents. *Pediatrics* 2005;115: 1103–1106; *ergogenic, anabolic, performance enhancing, banned substance, athlete, adolescent, sport.*

Introduction

Performance-enhancing substance use in young people is a concern to pediatricians and society because of potential adverse health consequences and the effects that such practices have on moral development of the individual and on fair athletic competition for all. Health care professionals can play a valuable role in counseling the young person using or contemplating use of performance-enhancing substances by conveying factual information about the proven benefits and medical consequences of these substances and providing advice about healthful eating and training. Attempts to discourage use through scare tactics or by dismissing known performance-enhancing effects of these substances may seriously damage the credibility of the physician and do little to diminish use. Efforts to minimize use of performance-enhancing substances require the pediatrician to have an understanding of the incentives for use, a comprehensive definition of performance-enhancing substances, and familiarity with strategies for prevention.

Incentives for the Use of Performance-Enhancing Substances

The temptation for young people to use performance-enhancing substances should be easily understood by anyone who is familiar with high-level sports in our society. Success (that is, winning) is considered by many to be the most important goal of sports. At the level of professional sports, winning is the ultimate goal. This attitude permeates lower levels of sports as well, down to youth sports. Society rewards success in sports with celebrity, status, and favoritism.

For athletes of all ages, the pursuit of excellence in sports is an endeavor to be admired and encouraged. Success in sports involves obtaining an "edge" over the competition. However, sometimes the drive for success can be so engrossing and so compelling that a young person can easily lose sight of what is fair and right. Some individuals may view the use of performance-enhancing substances as a substitute for hard work. For others, performance-enhancing substances may be considered a necessary adjunct to hard work or part of the price of success. From the user's perspective, the prospects for success in sports often outweigh the prospects for serious medical complications from use of performance-enhancing substances.

For some, winning has a monetary incentive as well. The enormous salaries paid to professional athletes in the United States and elsewhere are powerful inducements for a young person with outstanding athletic talent to try anything to ensure continued athletic success.

Adolescents may be uniquely vulnerable to the lure of performance-enhancing substances. Many

doi:10.1542/peds.2005-0085

adolescents engage in risk-taking behavior and experimentation at a time when they are coping with the developmental tasks of adolescence, including defining their sexual identity, emancipating themselves from their families, achieving a sense of mastery and self-efficacy, and finding a peer group with which they can identify.[1] The adolescent, by nature, feels invincible and often shuns any suggestion that use of a substance for purposes other than legitimate therapy might pose a danger to their health or their eligibility for sports.

Adolescents are also intensely preoccupied with body image. Personal rewards perceived from enhancing size, strength, stamina, or body build can be strong motivators. A significant number of adolescents who are not involved in competitive athletics use performance-enhancing substances.[2]

The child athlete, particularly the adolescent, in today's society is caught in a struggle between ideals highly valued by society but often in direct conflict: the attitude of winning at all costs and the values of fairness and wholesomeness.

Rationale for a Broad-Based Statement on Performance-Enhancing Substances And Youth

In the last 2 decades, a considerable amount of research has been conducted with performance-enhancing substances such as creatine, amino acids, androstenedione, and dehydroepiandrosterone. Virtually no experimental research on either the ergogenic effects or adverse effects of performance-enhancing substances has been conducted in subjects younger than 18 years. The amount of scientific data from well-designed studies on the effects of these substances in adults continues to accumulate at such a rate that systematic reviews are soon made obsolete.

This statement is not intended to provide a review of currently available data on performance-enhancing substances. A list of resources for detailed information on specific performance-enhancing substances is provided at the end of this statement. Rather, this statement is intended to convey a more general policy on the basis of the following 3 points. First, the intentional use of any substance for performance enhancement is unfair and, therefore, morally and ethically indefensible. Second, use of any substance for the purpose of enhancing sports performance, including over-the-counter supplements, the composition and quality of which are not under federal regulation, may pose a significant health risk to the young person. Third, use and promotion of performance-enhancing substances tends to devalue the principles of a balanced diet, good coaching, and sound physical training.

Current Definitions of Performance-Enhancing Substances

LIMITATIONS OF CURRENT DEFINITIONS

Traditionally, sports organizations such as the International Olympic Committee and the National Collegiate Athletic Association have defined performance-enhancing substances as substances that create an unfair competitive advantage. These organizations have produced lists of banned or prohibited drugs that include substances with known performance-enhancing effects as well as substances used by athletes that have been associated with adverse health effects. Detection of illegal or banned substances by drug testing is a critical element of the enforcement and efficacy of these policies. However, current definitions of performance-enhancing substances have contextual limitations. If the substance does not have adverse medical consequences, if the substance is not detectable by drug testing, or if testing for the drug is not performed (so that a potentially dangerous substance or unfair practice may go undetected), then the substance in question would not be included in a list of banned substances.

To date, there is no definition of performance-enhancing substances that applies to all potential users. A definition of a performance-enhancing substance that is applicable to the pediatric age group should not exclude any individual who may have a substance-abuse problem or any substance that cannot be readily detected. With the prohibitive cost of testing and deficiencies associated with a detection-based banned list, widespread drug testing of children and adolescents is unlikely to be effective or practical. A definition of a performance-enhancing substance for the pediatric age group, therefore, must be independent of whether testing of the substance is conducted in that age group. Because new substances for performance enhancement as well as methods for masking the presence of these substances are continually being discovered, a definition of performance-enhancing substances must remain valid in a changing environment.

GENERAL DEFINITION OF PERFORMANCE-ENHANCING SUBSTANCES

A performance-enhancing substance is any substance taken in nonpharmacologic doses specifically for the purposes of improving sports performance. A substance should be considered performance enhancing if it benefits sports performance by increasing strength, power, speed, or endurance (ergogenic) or by altering body weight or body composition. Furthermore, substances that improve performance by causing changes in behavior, arousal level, and/or perception of pain should be considered performance enhancing.

Performance-enhancing substances include the following:

- Pharmacologic agents (prescription or nonprescription) taken in doses that exceed the recommended therapeutic dose or taken when the therapeutic indication(s) are not present (eg, using decongestants for stimulant effect, using bronchodilators when exercise-induced bronchospasm is not present, increasing baseline methylphenidate hydrochloride dose for athletic competition)
- Agents used for weight control, including stimulants, diet pills, diuretics, and laxatives, when the user is in a sport that has weight classifications or that rewards leanness
- Agents used for weight gain, including over-the-counter products advertised as promoting increased muscle mass
- Physiologic agents or other strategies used to enhance oxygen-carrying capacity, including erythropoietin and red blood cell transfusions (blood doping)
- Any substance that is used for reasons other than to treat a documented disease state or deficiency

- Any substance that is known to mask adverse effects or detectability of another performance-enhancing substance
- Nutritional supplements taken at supraphysiologic doses or at levels greater than required to replace deficits created by a disease state, training, and/or participation in sports

Strategies for Preventing Use of Performance-Enhancing Substances

The methods most widely used to prevent use of performance-enhancing substances, namely drug bans and drug testing, are primarily punitive. Drug bans imposed by organizations that regulate and oversee sports programs at various levels, from the International Olympic Committee to the National Collegiate Athletic Association and state high-school sports associations, effectively make the use of such substances "against the rules." Enforcement of drug bans has necessarily involved the use of drug testing, with positive tests carrying stiff penalties or sanctions including loss of playing privileges, removal of awards or championships from the entire team, loss of scholarships, and restrictions on future regular season and postseason play.[3] Drug testing and legal sanctions are intended to be deterrents but have little effect on most children and adolescents involved in sports.

Neither the use of drug bans nor the implementation of drug testing provides the young athlete with any framework or guidelines for resolving the conflict between the drive to win and the imperative to do the right thing.

A variety of programs educating young athletes about substance abuse in general and targeting specific performance-enhancing drugs such as anabolic steroids have been tested at the international, collegiate, and even high-school levels.[4] It is unfortunate that few evaluations of these programs have included measurement of continued drug use after the intervention, and programs appropriately studied have not been highly successful in curbing use. One program that combined drug education with training in personal skills to resist the social influences that drive the use of performance-enhancing substances was successful in decreasing the intention to use anabolic steroids among adolescent football players.[5]

Little effort has been made to target adults who are responsible for collegiate, high-school, middle-school, and youth sports programs. Permissiveness often has the same effect as active encouragement when it comes to using performance-enhancing substances. A "don't-ask" attitude should be as intolerable to parents as the provision of performance-enhancing substances to athletes by coaches would be.

Identification of the Young Person Using Performance-Enhancing Substances

Data from epidemiologic studies and case descriptions have provided information about users of performance-enhancing substances that can help pediatricians to identify them. Users of anabolic or androgenic compounds are more likely to be male; are more likely to be involved in sports that demand high levels of strength, power, size, and speed; and are likely to use other illegal substances such as tobacco and alcohol.[5-7] Young people who participate in sports that demand leanness are also more likely to use performance-enhancing substances than are those involved in sports in which leanness is not essential. Young men and women who are not competitive athletes but who are obsessed with body image and who train intensely primarily to improve their physique are also more likely to use performance-enhancing substances. Users of certain performance-enhancing substances might be identified by outward signs such as virilization in females, testicular atrophy in males, and mood changes produced by anabolic steroids. Unfortunately, most young people who use performance-enhancing substances are not readily identified by outward signs. Therefore, it is imperative that all adolescents be asked about use of performance-enhancing substances in the assessment of high-risk behaviors that should be a part of every adolescent health maintenance visit, including sports physicals, camp physicals, and all other scheduled physician-adolescent encounters.

Recommendations

To assist the pediatrician in dealing with users or potential users of performance-enhancing substances, the American Academy of Pediatrics offers the following recommendations:

1. Use of performance-enhancing substances for athletic or other purposes should be strongly discouraged.
2. Parents should take a strong stand against the use of performance-enhancing substances and, whenever possible, demand that coaches be educated about the adverse health effects of performance-enhancing substances.
3. Schools and other sports organizations should be proactive in discouraging the use of performance-enhancing substances, incorporating this message into policy and educational materials for coaches, parents, and athletes.
4. Interventions for encouraging substance-free competition should be developed that are more positive than punitive, such as programs that teach sound nutrition and training practices along with skills to resist the social pressures to use performance-enhancing substances.
5. Colleges, schools, and sports clubs should make use of educational interventions that encourage open and frank discussion of issues related to the use of performance-enhancing substances, with the aim of promoting decisions about personal drug use based on principles of fair competition and character rather than on the fear of getting caught.
6. Coaches at all levels, including youth sports, should encourage wholesome and fair competition by emphasizing healthy nutrition and training practices, taking a strong stand against cheating, and avoiding the "win-at-all-costs" philosophy.
7. Inquiries about the use of performance-enhancing substances should be made in a manner similar to inquiries about use of tobacco, alcohol, or other substances of abuse. Guidelines for patient confidentiality should be followed and explained to the patient.

8. Athletes who admit using performance-enhancing substances should be provided unbiased medical information about benefits, known adverse effects, and other risks. When appropriate, additional testing may be necessary to investigate or rule out adverse medical effects.

9. The pediatric health care professional providing care for an athlete who admits to using a performance-enhancing substance should explore the athlete's motivations for using these substances, evaluate other associated high-risk behaviors, and provide counseling on safer, more appropriate alternatives for meeting fitness or sports-performance goals.

10. Nonusers of performance-enhancing substances should have their decisions reinforced while establishing an open channel of communication if questions about performance-enhancing substances arise in the future.

11. Pediatric health care professionals should promote safe physical activity and sports participation by providing or making available sound medical information on exercise physiology, conditioning, nutrition, weight management, and injury prevention and by helping to care for sports-related medical conditions and injuries.

The November 2004 issue of "Sports Shorts" by the American Academy of Pediatrics Section on Sports Medicine and Fitness concerning performance-enhancing substances[8] is available for download and includes guidelines for pediatricians and parents.

COMMITTEE ON SPORTS MEDICINE AND FITNESS, 2002–2003

Reginald L. Washington, MD, Chairperson
David T. Bernhardt, MD
*Jorge Gomez, MD
Miriam D. Johnson, MD
Thomas J. Martin, MD
Frederick E. Reed, MD
Eric Small, MD

LIAISONS

Carl Krein, AT, PT
    National Athletic Trainers Association
Claire LeBlanc, MD
    Canadian Paediatric Society
Judith C. Young, PhD
    National Association for Sport and
    Physical Education

CONSULTANT

Oded Bar-Or, MD

STAFF

Jeanne Lindros, MPH

*Lead author

References

1. Tanner SM, Miller DW, Alongi C. Anabolic steroid use by adolescents: prevalence, motives, and knowledge of risks. *Clin J Sport Med.* 1995;5:108–115

2. Terney R, McLain LG. The use of anabolic steroids in high school students. *Am J Dis Child.* 1990;144:99–103

3. National Collegiate Athletic Association. NCAA enforcement and student-athlete reinstatement. Indianapolis, IN: National Collegiate Athletic Association. Available at: www.ncaa.org/enforcefrontF.html. Accessed January 12, 2005

4. Yesalis CE, Barhke MS. Doping among adolescent athletes. *Baillieres Best Pract Res Clin Endocrinol Metab.* 2000; 14:25–35

5. Goldberg L, Elliot D, Clarke GN, et al. Effects of a multidimensional anabolic steroid prevention intervention. The Adolescents Training and Learning to Avoid Steroids (ATLAS) Program. *JAMA.* 1996;276:1555–1562

6. Bahrke MS, Yesalis CE, Kopstein AN, Stephens JA. Risk factors associated with anabolic-androgenic steroid use among adolescents. *Sports Med.* 2000;29:397–405

7. Kindlundh AM, Isacson DG, Berglund L, Nyberg F. Factors associated with adolescent use of doping agents: anabolic-androgenic steroids. *Addiction.* 1999;94:543–553

8. American Academy of Pediatrics, Section on Sports Medicine and Fitness. Sports shorts: performance-enhancing substances. Available at: www.aap.org/family/sportsshorts12.pdf. Accessed January 12, 2005

Resources

United States Anti-Doping Agency. Available at: www.usantidoping.org. Accessed January 6, 2004

National Federation of State High School Associations. Sports medicine. Available at: www.nfhs.org/scriptcontent/va_Custom/VimDisplays/contentpagedisplay.cfm?content_id=203. Accessed January 6, 2004

National Collegiate Athletic Association. Banned drug list. Available at: http://www1.ncaa.org/membership/ed_outreach/healthsafety/drug_testing/banned_drug_classes.pdf. Accessed January 6, 2004

American Medical Society for Sports Medicine. Drugs and performance-enhancing agents in sport. *Clin J Sport Med.* 2002;12(theme issue):201–263

Gomez JE. Performance-enhancing substances in adolescent athletes. *Tex Med.* 2002;98(2):41–46

Metzl JD. Performance-enhancing drug use in the young athlete. *Pediatr Ann.* 2002;31:27–32

Ahrendt DM. Ergogenic aids: counseling the athlete. *Am Fam Physician.* 2001;63:913–922

All policy statements from the American Academy of Pediatrics automatically expire 5 years after publication unless reaffirmed, revised, or retired at or before that time.

Section VII Further Reading

Adams BB. Sports dermatology. *Adolesc Med.* 2001;12:305–322

Feinstein RA. Preparticipation physical examinations: critical controversies. *Adolesc Med.* 1997;8:149–158

Gidwani GP. Amenorrhea in the athlete. *Adolesc Med.* 1999;10:275–290

Gross RH. Foot and ankle injuries and disorders. *Adolesc Med.* 1998;9:599–609

Hurrman WW. Injuries to the hand and wrist. *Adolesc Med.* 1998;9:611–625

Kazis K, Iglesias E. The female athlete triad. *Adolesc Med.* 2003;14:87–95

Kelly AM, Pappas AM. Shoulder and elbow injuries and painful syndromes. *Adolesc Med.* 1998;9:569–587

Luckstead EF. Cardiovascular evaluation of the young athlete. *Adolesc Med.* 1998;9:441–455

Mares SC. Hip, pelvic, and thigh injuries and disorders in the adolescent athlete. *Adolesc Med.* 1998;9:551–568

Patel D, Greydanus D. Neurologic considerations for adolescent athletes. *Adolesc Med.* 2002;13:569–578

Roach JW. Knee disorders and injuries in adolescents. *Adolesc Med.* 1998;9:589–597

American Academy of Pediatrics

American Academy of Pediatrics, Committee on Sports Medicine and Fitness. Adolescents and anabolic steroids: a subject review. *Pediatrics.* 1997;99:904–908

American Academy of Pediatrics, Committee on Sports Medicine and Fitness. Cardiac dysrhythmias and sports. *Pediatrics.* 1995;95:786–788

American Academy of Pediatrics, Committee on Sports Medicine and Fitness. Climatic heat stress and the exercising child and adolescent. *Pediatrics.* 2000;106:158–159

American Academy of Pediatrics, Committee on Sports Medicine and Fitness. Medical conditions affecting sports participation. *Pediatrics.* 2001;107:1205–1209

American Academy of Pediatrics, Committee on Sports Medicine and Fitness. Medical concerns in the female athlete. *Pediatrics.* 2000;106:610–613

American Academy of Pediatrics, Committee on Sports Medicine and Fitness. Strength training by children and adolescents. *Pediatrics.* 2001;107:1470–1472

American Academy of Pediatrics, Committee on Sports Medicine and Fitness. Use of performance-enhancing substances. *Pediatrics.* 2005;115:1103–1106

Working With Families

A Consensus Statement on Health Care Transitions for Young Adults With Special Health Care Needs

American Academy of Pediatrics, American College of Family Physicians,
American College of Physicians-American Society of Internal Medicine

ABSTRACT. This policy statement represents a consensus on the critical first steps that the medical profession needs to take to realize the vision of a family-centered, continuous, comprehensive, coordinated, compassionate, and culturally competent health care system that is as developmentally appropriate as it is technically sophisticated. The goal of transition in health care for young adults with special health care needs is to maximize lifelong functioning and potential through the provision of high-quality, developmentally appropriate health care services that continue uninterrupted as the individual moves from adolescence to adulthood. This consensus document has now been approved as policy by the boards of the American Academy of Pediatrics, the American Academy of Family Physicians, and the American College of Physicians-American Society of Internal Medicine.

Introduction

Each year in the United States, nearly half a million children with special health care needs cross the threshold into adulthood.[1] One generation ago, most of those with severe disabilities died before reaching maturity; now more than 90% survive to adulthood.[2] Most young people with special health care needs are able to find their way into and negotiate through adult systems of care.[3] However, many adolescents and young adults with severe medical conditions and disabilities that limit their ability to function and result in complicating social, emotional, or behavioral sequelae experience difficulty transitioning from child to adult health care. There is a substantial number whose success depends on more deliberate guidance.[4]

Children grow up within complex living arrangements, communities, and cultures and receive medical care within an equally complex, interlocking set of relationships that includes social services, education, vocational training,

and recreation. Clearly, no single approach will work equally well for all young people, and the health care sector cannot work in isolation from the other professionals and networks that impact these young people.[5] By focusing on the health care sector in this policy statement, we do not ignore other critical relationships. Rather, we are acknowledging that physicians have an important role in facilitating transitions to adulthood and to adult health care for young people who are least likely to do it successfully on their own.

The goals of this policy statement are to ensure that by the year 2010 all physicians who provide primary or subspecialty care to young people with special health care needs 1) understand the rationale for transition from child-oriented to adult-oriented health care; 2) have the knowledge and skills to facilitate that process; and 3) know if, how, and when transfer of care is indicated.

What is Meant by "Health Care Transitions"?

Transitions are part of normal, healthy development and occur across the life span. Transition in health care for young adults with special health care needs is a dynamic, lifelong process that seeks to meet their individual needs as they move from childhood to adulthood. The goal is to maximize lifelong functioning and potential through the provision of high-quality, developmentally appropriate health care services that continue uninterrupted as the individual moves from adolescence to adulthood. It is patient centered, and its cornerstones are flexibility, responsiveness, continuity, comprehensiveness, and coordination.

Physicians are of special importance in this process because of the frequent contact with

---

PEDIATRICS (ISSN 0031 4005). Copyright © 2002 by the American Academy of Pediatrics.

many of these young people and the close relationships that often develop with them and their families.

A well-timed transition from child-oriented to adult-oriented health care allows young people to optimize their ability to assume adult roles and functioning. For many young people with special health care needs, this will mean a transfer from a child to an adult health care professional; for many others, it will involve an ongoing relationship with the same provider but with a reorientation of clinical interactions to mirror the young person's increasing maturity and emerging adulthood.

Whether the transition entails a transfer of care or not, all adults with special health care needs deserve an adult focused primary care physician. This is not to say that the child health specialist will not have an ongoing role. Rather, it is to affirm that just as children receive optimal primary care in a medical practice experienced in the care of children, so too adults benefit from receiving care from physicians who are trained and experienced in adult medicine.[5] Whether or not a transfer of care occurs, successful transition requires communication and collaboration among primary care specialists, subspecialists, young adult patients, and their families.

Why Is Planning for Transitions Important Now?

Healthy People 2010[6] established the goal that all young people with special health care needs will receive the services needed to make necessary transitions to all aspects of adult life, including health care, work, and independent living. Just as the Individuals With Disabilities Education Act of 1997[7] requires a plan for education transition, so too there should be a plan for health care transition. The challenges faced by health care professionals include ensuring age-appropriate care, advocating for improved health insurance coverage, and negotiating adequate compensation for services provided.

Optimal health care is achieved when every person at every age receives health care that is medically and developmentally appropriate. The central rationale for health care transition planning

for young people with special health care needs is to achieve this goal by ensuring that adults receive primary medical care from those trained to provide it.

Critical First Steps to Ensuring Successful Transitioning to Adult-Oriented Health Care

1. Ensure that all young people with special health care needs have an identified health care professional who attends to the unique challenges of transition and assumes responsibility for current health care, care coordination, and future health care planning. This responsibility is executed in partnership with other child and adult health care professionals, the young person, and his or her family. It is intended to ensure that as transitions occur, all young people have uninterrupted, comprehensive, and accessible care within their community.

2. Identify the core knowledge and skills required to provide developmentally appropriate health care transition services to young people with special health care needs and make them part of training and certification requirements for primary care residents and physicians in practice.

3. Prepare and maintain an up-to-date medical summary that is portable and accessible. This information is critical for successful health care transition and provides the common knowledge base for collaboration among health care professionals.

4. Create a written health care transition plan by age 14 together with the young person and family. At a minimum, this plan should include what services need to be provided, who will provide them, and how they will be financed. This plan should be reviewed and updated annually and whenever there is a transfer of care.

5. Apply the same guidelines for primary and preventive care for all adolescents and young adults, including those with special health care needs, recognizing that young people with special health care needs may require more resources and services than do other young

people to optimize their health. Examples of such guidelines include the American Medical Association's *Guidelines for Adolescent Preventive Services (GAPS),*[8] the National Center for Education in Maternal and Child Health's *Bright Futures: Guidelines for Health Supervision of Infants, Children, and Adolescents,*[9] and the US Public Health Service's *Guidelines to Clinical Preventive Services.*[10]

6. Ensure affordable, continuous health insurance coverage for all young people with special health care needs throughout adolescence and adulthood. This insurance should cover appropriate compensation for 1) health care transition planning for all young people with special health care needs, and 2) care coordination for those who have complex medical conditions.

INVITATIONAL CONFERENCE PLANNING COMMITTEE
Robert W. Blum, MD, PhD, Consultant
   University of Minnesota
David Hirsch, MD
      Past AAP Committee on Children
      With Disabilities Member
Theodore A. Kastner, MD
      AAP Committee on Children With Disabilities
Richard D. Quint, MD, MPH
      Past AAP Committee on Children
      With Disabilities Member
Adrian D. Sandler, MD, Chairperson
      AAP Committee on Children With Disabilities

CONFERENCE PARTICIPANTS
Susan Margaret Anderson, MD
      University of Virginia Children's Medical
      Center/Kluge Children's Rehabilitation Center
Maria Britto, MD, MPH
      Children's Hospital Medical Center, Division
      of Adolescent Medicine
Jan Brunstrom, MD
      St. Louis Children's Hospital
Gilbert A. Buchanan, MD
      Children's Medical Service
Robert Burke, MD, MPH
      Memorial Hospital of Rhode Island
John K. Chamberlain, MD
      University of Rochester Medical School

Barbara Cooper, Deputy Director
      Institute for Medicare Practice
Daniel Davidow, MD
      Cumberland Hospital
Theora Evans, MSV, MPH, PhD
      University of Tennessee
Thomas Gloss, Sr. Health Policy Analyst
      Health Resources and Services Administration
Patti Hackett, MEd
      Academy for Educational Development,
      Disability Studies and Services Center
Patrick Harr, MD
      American Academy of Family Physicians
William Kiernan, PhD
      The Children's Hospital
Eric Levey, MD
      Kennedy Krieger Institute
Merle McPherson, MD
      Maternal and Child Health Bureau
Kevin Murphy, MD
      Gillette Children's North Clinics
Maureen R. Nelson, MD
      Texas Children's Hospital/Baylor College
      of Medicine
Donna Gore Olson, BS
      The Indiana Parent Information Network
Gary Onady, MD, PhD
      Wright State University
Betty Presler, ARNP, PNP, PhD
      Shriners Hospital for Children
John Reiss, PhD
      Institute for Child Health Policy
Michael Rich, MD, MPH
      Children's Hospital Boston
Peggy Mann Rinehart, MD
      University of Minnesota
David Rosen, MD, MPH
      University of Michigan Health System
Peter Scal, MD
      University of Minnesota
David Siegel, MD, MPH
      University of Rochester, School of Medicine
      and Dentistry
Gail B. Slap, MD, MS
      Children's Hospital Medical Center,
      Cincinnati
Paul Clay Sorum, MD, PhD
      Albany Medical Center

Maria Veronica Svetaz, MD, MPH
    West Side Community Health Center
Patricia Thomas
    Family Voices
Margaret Turk, MD
    SUNY Health Science Center at Syracuse
Patience White, MD
    Senate Finance Committee/Children's
    National Medical Center
Philip Ziring, MD
    University of California San Francisco

Acknowledgments

This conference was funded by a supplemental grant to an existing grant for the Medical Home Initiative (No. 108100) from the Department of Health and Human Services, Health Resources and Services Administration.

References

1. Newacheck PW, Taylor WR. Childhood chronic illness: prevalence, severity, and impact. *Am J Public Health.* 1994;82:364–371

2. Blum RW. Transition to adult health care: setting the stage. *J Adolesc Health.* 1995;17:3–5

3. Gortmaker SL, Perrin JM, Weitzman M, et al. An unexpected success story: transition to adulthood in youth with chronic physical health conditions. *J Res Adolesc.* 1993;3:317–336

4. Blum RW, Garell D, Hodgman CH, et al. Transition from child-centered to adult health-care-systems for adolescents with chronic conditions. A position paper of the Society for Adolescent Medicine. *J Adolesc Health.* 1993;14:570–576

5. American Academy of Pediatrics, Committee on Children With Disabilities and Committee on Adolescence. Transition of care provided for adolescents with special health care needs. *Pediatrics.* 1996;98:1203–1206

6. Centers for Disease Control and Prevention, National Institute on Disability and Rehabilitation Research, and US Department of Education. Disability and secondary conditions. *Healthy People 2010.* Washington, DC: US Public Health Service, US Department of Health and Human Services; 2000. Available at: http://www.cdc.gov/ncbddd/dh/schp.htm. Accessed November 20, 2001

7. Individuals With Disabilities Education Act. Pub L No. 105-17 (1997)

8. American Medical Association, Department of Adolescent Health. *Guidelines for Adolescent Preventive Services (GAPS): Clinical Evaluation and Management Handbook.* Chicago, IL: American Medical Association; 2000

9. Green M, Palfrey JS, eds. *Bright Futures: Guidelines for Health Supervision of Infants, Children, and Adolescents.* 2nd ed. Arlington, VA: National Center for Education in Maternal and Child Health; 2000

10. US Preventive Services Task Force, Public Health Service. *Guidelines to Clinical Preventive Services.* 2nd ed. Washington, DC: US Public Health Service; 1996

Helping Parents Communicate With Their Teens
Part 1: Assessment and General Strategies

by Sheryl A. Ryan, MD, FAAP

Your colleague, also a pediatrician, is concerned about his eldest daughter, who recently turned 13. Once predictable, exuberant, and enthusiastic, she is now moody and sullen. Formerly a child who spent hours talking with her parents about endless topics, she is now guarded and withdrawn. The father says he feels as if his "little soul mate" has been replaced with an alien whose main function is to make him feel inadequate as a parent. The more he seeks her out, the less accessible she becomes. Her academic performance does not seem to be suffering, and there are no reports of problem behaviors from school. Still, he is anxious because lack of communication makes it difficult for him to assess her emotional status. You suggest some communication strategies. In response, he throws up his hands and says, "Teens and parents can't communicate if they're in the same room together! What's a parent to do?"

This issue of *Adolescent Health Update* begins a 2-part series on parenting and communicating with adolescents. Part 1 will present practical information to help pediatricians assess and counsel families of adolescents about effective communication and parenting. Part 2 will examine ways to apply these practical strategies in specific problem situations that challenge families.

What is Effective Parenting?

Parenting is a complex process. Adults may lack an understanding of the connection between their parenting practices and their child's development. They may be challenged by the tremendous social changes affecting the modern family. Pediatricians may be frustrated by the lack of definitive approaches to parenting issues, or they may recommend one parenting style for all types of families.

Extreme parenting styles are seldom effective. Neither the authoritarian approach ("laying down the law, no questions asked") nor the permissive approach ("don't inhibit the child's choices") is optimal. The most effective type of parenting is *authoritative*.

Authoritative parents combine sensitivity (love and nurturance) with developmentally appropriate guidance (expectations, rules, and supervision). Sensitivity includes warmth, love, acceptance, and emotional availability. Guidance includes the provision of reasonable structure, developmentally appropriate expectations, and consistent supervision. Permissive parents may be nurturing, but they communicate low expectations and offer little guidance. Authoritarian parents may have higher expectations and clearly set limits, but low levels of affection and warmth.

Waters and colleagues described an authoritative approach as one that fosters social competence, good peer relations, internalization of

---

Learning Objectives

After reading this article, pediatricians will be able to:

1. Provide families with practical knowledge about effective parenting and positive communication.
2. Discuss developmental changes in adolescents that impact parenting and communication.
3. Assess family structure, dynamics, and parenting needs.
4. Determine when parenting and communication difficulties justify outside intervention.

Sheryl A. Ryan, MD, FAAP, is an assistant professor of pediatrics, University of Rochester School of Medicine and Dentistry, Rochester, New York.

Adolescent Health Update, *Vol 11, No. 2, February 1999*

moral standards, appropriate self esteem, and compliance with rules. These attributes are less likely to be seen in adolescents whose parents are rejecting, hostile, emotionally unavailable, too permissive, or too restrictive. Table 1 describes specific guidelines for parents on how to include more authoritative elements in their everyday parenting.

Table 1*. How to Be an Authoritative Parent

Start with love and trust.
- Let your teen know that you will be there for him or her, no matter what happens.

Set clear and reasonable limits.
- Set achievable standards for behavior.
- Establish rules and expectations for this behavior.

See that both parents enforce rules consistently.
- Be firm but fair.
- Be supportive. Remember that your teen does not have your sense of experience or proportion.
- Pick your battles. Learn when to draw the line and when to be flexible.
- Be willing to reconsider a rule when it doesn't seem to apply.
- Be willing to reevaluate rules over time.

Retain your right to assert parental authority.
- Balance control with independence.
- Know how much control is too much.
- Grant freedom in stages. Avoid giving too much too soon.
- Tie increased privileges to responsible behavior.
- Teens need to experience the natural consequences of their behavior. Within reasonable limits, stand back and let that happen. (For example, while drinking and driving would not be tolerated, the teen who oversleeps should perhaps face the consequences at school.)

Work at staying close and connected with your adolescent.
- Be available.
- Spend uninterrupted time alone together.
- Get to know your teen's interests, passions, and concerns.
- Share your own concerns, interests, passions, and feelings.
- Use humor wisely.

Respect your adolescent.
- Acknowledge your teen's individuality by accepting his or her choices with respect to clothing, activities, and friends.
- Do not ridicule your teen's choices.
- Model and insist upon civil discourse.

*Adapted from Steinberg L, Levine A. *You and Your Adolescent: A Parent's Guide for Ages 10 to 20.* Chapter 1, pages 12–26.

The Impact of Adolescent Development on Parenting

Adolescence entails dramatic physical, cognitive, social, and emotional changes that alter the way parents and adolescents interact. During adolescence, most young people begin to seek advice from persons outside the home, including peers. Adolescence can be a difficult time, although most teens still accept the influence of their parents. What is it about adolescent development that challenges the ability of parents to successfully guide and nurture their teens?

Normal developmental changes that are part of the transition through adolescence prompt stress and disequilibrium in the parent-child relationship. Parents and adolescents must adapt to achieve a new balance between the parents' expectations and the adolescent's developmental needs. While this is a challenge for many families, it also creates opportunities for parents to have a positive impact on their teen's development and well being.

PSYCHOSOCIAL DEVELOPMENT

The mother of a 13-year-old boy is distraught about the dramatic changes she is seeing in her son. "He used to want to go everywhere with us," she says, "grocery shopping, to the mall, visiting relatives. Now he seems embarrassed to be around us. He doesn't even want to go on vacation with us. What are we supposed to do?"

In early adolescence (11–13 years) the physical changes of pubertal development signal dramatic and important milestones. Many young teens are concerned about whether their development is "normal" compared to their peers. With this concern about normality comes a preoccupation with one's appearance and a shift from parental and family activities to a stronger affiliation with peers. (See Table 2 for a description of developmental changes and psychosocial tasks of adolescence that may create stress within the family.)

With middle adolescence (ages 14–16), peers assume even greater importance, and the drive for separation from parents (individuation) prompts teens to test the limits of parental control and authority. Parents may misinterpret a teen's increased need to affiliate with peers and establish a better sense of personal identity as a rejection of the family. In fact, most adolescents seek to maintain strong connections with their families, and most teens' values reflect those of their parents. However, conflict over control, if it is to occur, is most likely to begin and peak during middle adolescence.

Independence can be an exciting prospect for the teen and a frightening thought for the parents. Normal behaviors may be interpreted as

Table 2. Developmental Needs and Expected Behaviors

Developmental Needs	How Teens May See It	How Parents May See It	Solutions
Independence, autonomy, and individuation	Parents are too controlling, not giving enough freedom	Teen constantly challenging the "order of command"	Negotiate rules together
	Teen doesn't have enough input into rules, household responsibilities	Teen wants to be able to "call the shots"	Link increased independence to increased responsibilities
		Teen doesn't want to follow rules, or meet responsibilities	Provide safe opportunities for exploration/freedom
		Teen wants more freedom, challenges any restriction	Maintain high expectations, allow some rebellion, but set limits and enforce rules
		Often ambivalent, erratic, moody	consistently
Peer Affiliation	Wants to spend more time with friends, less time with family	Teen rejects family to be with friend	Allow teen time to develop important friendships
		Embarrassed to be seen with family	Establish family rituals and make it clear that teen is expected to participate
			Allow teen freedom to choose friends
Identity Formation	Needs to "try on" and experiment with a lot of different identities	Egocentric, narcissistic and inconsistent	Be patient
			Keep sense of humor
			Choose your battles
	Needs privacy and space	Secretive	Respect need for privacy, but be aware that too much seclusion may be a sign of problems
Cognitive Development	Teen can think for himself	Argumentative	Provide rationale for decisions
	Can reason abstractly	Challenging	Appreciate intellectual development as positive change
		Teen "knows it all"	
		Opinionated	Remember that judgment and insight are limited

outright rejection of the family, and conflicts over parental control often result. (See Table 2) In the vignette above, a teen in early adolescence expresses his desire for individuation and greater independence. He prefers to choose his own activities, at the risk of disagreement with his parents.

Ideally, late adolescence is characterized by a relatively stable identity, important mutual friendships, and a more adult relationship with parents. Most parents, including those who have experienced conflict with their teens, will find that the older adolescent has achieved a more stable equilibrium and can more easily balance family, peer/friendship, and individual needs.

COGNITIVE DEVELOPMENT

The mother of a 15-year-old girl has asked for a few minutes to talk in private. When you are alone, she says she is becoming exasperated by her daughter's behavior. Her teen had been in the habit of saying, "Mom, you just don't get it," about certain issues, but was generally a compliant preteen. Now, her daughter is inclined to reject outright any suggestion that her mother makes. "My daughter tells me that I am so clueless about things, she can't stand to be in the same room with me," she says.

In the preteen and early adolescent years, thought and moral reasoning are concrete. The young person cannot perceive the long-term impact of decisions and behaviors. A 12-year-old girl who has been smoking cigarettes for 6 months without any appreciable limitation or health effect may conclude that she is immune to possible effects, or that those warnings were parental "scare tactics." In middle and late adolescence, however, more advanced thinking and formal operational reasoning begin to occur. Many teens in mid-adolescence can engage in abstract thinking, appreciate hypothetical situations, and apply formal logic. This may prompt some teens to test what they may have been told about risky situations, such as whether drinking really does impair their ability to drive safely. At the same time, an ability to think abstractly may also confer a new appreciation for possible effects of certain risk behaviors, such as tobacco and alcohol use.

In middle and late adolescence, previously accepted parental wisdom may be rejected or challenged. The situation described in the vignette involving the 15-year-old girl and her suddenly "clueless" mother is not atypical. While the girl's cognitive maturation is normal, her advanced reasoning skills lack judgment and perspective. Teens in mid- and late adolescence may use their abstract thinking inconsistently. They might be able to think abstractly about a philosophical point in their schoolwork, for example, but unable to apply abstract thinking to household duties or parental expectations about curfew. (See Table 2)

Pediatricians can help parents realize that abstract thought makes their adolescents more interesting people. If appropriate, the pediatrician might point out to parents that although their teen may be expressing objections to parents in what appears to be a personal manner, these challenges are normal developmental events, and not always intended to be personal.

This advice assumes that the parents have a courteous relationship with their teen, and have not personally attacked their child when giving advice. Parents who have done their best to be objective and respectful are less likely to encounter the behaviors often seen in adolescents whose parents are overly critical or harsh. Angry parents may find they have modeled behavior that is now mirrored back to them, presenting as argumentativeness that is particularly intense and negative. When the pediatrician comments on what is observed in a nonjudgmental way, parents may be better able to interpret their own or their teen's behavior, and better understand how parent/child relationships change in adolescence. Pointing out to parents that their own behavior is a potent model for their teen's behavior, perhaps by asking (gently) whether they think their teen might have reason to think this behavior is accepted among adults, may be helpful in this situation.

Role of the Pediatrician

In working with adolescents and their families, pediatricians conduct clinical assessments that take into account the contexts in which developmental events occur. The past 3 decades have featured dramatic increases in the numbers of children and adolescents who have experienced the separation or divorce of parents, the establishment of single parent or blended family households, and the phenomenon of two working parents. These demographic shifts within the population, and a reduction in the traditional supports from extended families, have altered the nature of the family unit. According to 1990 U.S. Census data, less than 10 percent of children now live in the "traditional" family of two married parents, one working, the other a homemaker.

For the pediatrician, this means that the family situations in which most adolescents are growing up are more varied than ever before. As a result, clinical assessment is more complex, and counseling may incorporate more variables. However, all healthy families share certain qualities and capabilities. They are able to ensure the physical and emotional safety of their children and teens by maintaining appropriate boundaries. They respect and value one another. They solve problems effectively. They seek help when needed.

The pediatrician who assesses family functioning in these terms can more easily formulate plans for anticipatory guidance, office counseling, or referral.

CLINICAL ASSESSMENT

The basic tools for assessment include: (1) observation; (2) a history that seeks specific information about family structure, functioning, and parenting strategies; and (3) screening for risk factors and situations, and behavior problems.

The routine health maintenance visit provides an opportunity to observe how the parents and teen interact, and the level of warmth and sensitivity between the parents and the adolescent. In adolescence, it becomes more appropriate to direct questions to the patient. Parents' reaction to this shift (and to sharing the role of information-provider with their teen) may offer clues to suggest how they are managing their adolescent's increasing maturity and independence. Parents who are comfortable allowing their teen to speak respect the teen's emerging need for privacy.

A mother is concerned about her 14-year-old son. He has recently begun leaving the house without permission and riding his bike long distances (10 miles or more), spending many hours away from home on his own. The boy is withdrawn, his eyes downcast. The mother, who is extremely anxious, provides the history exclusively, and interrupts her son whenever he attempts to answer questions directed to him. When you ask the mother to leave the room so that you and the teen can have a private chat, she hovers outside, trying to overhear your conversation and passing messages on pieces of paper under the exam room door about additional concerns that she is "afraid she might forget" to tell you later.

It is apparent that this mother is feeling threatened by her son's need for privacy, a key developmental step in attaining identify formation. (See Table 2) Her inability to respect his need for privacy was apparent from the start, and put her son's bike-riding expeditions into context.

In such a situation, the pediatrician might begin by validating the mother's concern about the long bike rides. Discussion about safety risks of these long unsupervised excursions would also offer transition to more general questions about the son's overall developmental and behavioral progress. The clinician might suggest that this mother work with her son to find less extreme ways for him to obtain the privacy and space that he needs developmentally.

If a parent's questions about problem behaviors indicate significant discord, suggest a separately-scheduled appointment with the parents alone. The American Academy of Pediatrics' guide, *The Classification of Child and Adolescent Mental Diagnoses in Primary Care: Diagnostic and Statistical Manual for Primary Care, (DSM-PC Child and Adolescent Version)* is an excellent resource for identifying specific diagnoses and codes for billing these visits.

Each family has interaction patterns that should be recognized by those who hope to help them communicate more effectively. Table 3 includes questions the pediatrician might ask to learn about these patterns. *Bright Futures: Guidelines for Health Supervision of Infants, Children, and Adolescents,* published by the National Center for Education in Maternal and Child Health with support from the Maternal and Child Health Bureau and the Medicaid Bureau of the US Department of Health and Human Services, provides a similar set of questions.

Table 3*. Questions Useful in Office Assessment of Family Function and Communication

General questions
- How are things going for you now that your son is a teenager?
- Do you have any concerns about your relationship with your daughter?

Guidance provided
- Do you have rules that your son/daughter is expected to follow?
- What happens if he/she breaks them?
- What kind of say does your teen have about household rules?
- What chores is your teen expected to do?

Sensitivity
- How do you think your son feels about being in his family?
- How close would you say you are to your daughter?

Communication style
- What do you and your teen have most difficulty talking about?
- How often do you have a conversation with your teen?
- What do you and your son/daughter argue about?
- How do you resolve the argument?
- Does one person usually win?

Family functioning/structure
- Who lives in your household?
- What other people/family members are important to your son/daughter?
- What kind of activities do you do as a whole family? How often?
- What are some of the important traditions you share with your family?

Behavior problems
- Do you have any concerns about your teen's behaviors?
- How is he/she getting along at school? In the family? With friends? At work?

Recent stressors, high risk situations
- Has any recent stress occurred in your family since we last saw your son/daughter?

*Adapted from Green M, ed. *Bright Futures: Guidelines for Health Supervision of Infants, Children, and Adolescents.*

Guidelines for Adolescent Preventive Services (GAPS), published by the American Medical Association, is also useful, and includes adolescent and parent forms.

ANTICIPATORY GUIDANCE

The pediatrician can use Table 2 as a guide when providing anticipatory guidance about developmental changes to be expected over the next year or two. Let parents know, for example, that as their 13-year-old son or daughter continues into middle adolescence, conflicts over control and time spent with peers may increase.

Certain mental health problems (eg, oppositional defiant disorder, conduct disorder, affective disorder, or other psychiatric problems), will challenge the parent independent of the parenting skills. Advise parents that although changes occur, extreme change is not normal and may reflect a serious emotional problem. For example, most teens exhibit an increased need for privacy. Parents who express concern because their adolescent has begun to spend more time alone in his or her room while maintaining a network of friends and outside interests can be told that this is normal behavior. However, an adolescent whose heightened desire for privacy is accompanied by a withdrawal from activities and friends, and who is defensive about apparent lack of interest in former activities, may have a more serious problem, such as depression, substance use, or oppositional defiant disorder. If this is the case, referral to a mental health professional may be appropriate.

The "Askable Parent"

Encourage parents to practice active listening. (Table 4) If communication is difficult, it may be helpful to point out that adolescents' increased need for privacy does not mean that they no longer need parental guidance and support. Becoming an "askable parent" consists of making oneself available when the adolescent is ready to

Table 4*. Elements of Active Listening
- Letting the adolescent finish sentences
- Paying attention to body language
- Listening with your eyes and ears
- Learning to be comfortable with silence
- Not reacting defensively even when your teenager says something critical of you
- Rephrasing the teen's comments in your own words to make sure you have understood them
- Not acting as though you have all the answers when you don't even know the questions

*Adapted from Steinberg L, Levine A. *You and Your Adolescent: A Parent's Guide for Ages 10 to 20.* Chapter 2, pages 31–32.

solicit parental advice. A brief comment, such as, "it looks like you've had a tough day," may be all the prompting a teen will need. If parents say that it is difficult to find time for private talk with their teen, suggest that they make a small change in their routine or reserve a specific time in the week, such as an early breakfast, when the teen knows that parents have set aside time to be with him or her.

In spite of the fact that most adolescents become less communicative with their parents, many parents are unaware that they themselves may communicate attitudes that exacerbate that reluctance. Table 5 offers positive and negative cues seen in parent-adolescent communication.

Information about emotional and cognitive changes in adolescence should be shared with parents and teens. Adolescents should understand that they share responsibility for positive family relationships. Talk to the teen about what is to be expected in terms of normal social and emotional development. Facts may foster insight as to

Table 5*. The Do's and Don'ts of Communication with Adolescents

Do's—Communication enhancers
- *Getting your message across clearly.*
  - ~ Be specific
  - ~ Be objective
  - ~ Be brief
  - ~ Be accurate about your feelings
  - ~ Be concrete
- *Creating times when you are available and can talk*
- *Listening actively*

Don'ts—Obstacles to communication
- Criticism and ridicule
- "Negatives"
- Giving too many orders and too much advice
- Commands, threats, sermons
- Giving unsolicited advice
- Treating adolescents' problems lightly—blanket reassurance—giving message that the adolescent's concerns are trivial
- Not speaking your mind and saying what you feel (shaming, blaming, using "you" messages rather than "I" messages)
- Imposing your own solution to a problem
- Not being specific enough about what is bothering you

*Adapted from Steinberg L, Levine A. *You and Your Adolescent: A Parent's Guide for Ages 10 to 20.* Chapter 2, pages 28–31

how their own normal development may affect interaction with their parents.

INTERVENTION FOR FAMILIES IN CONFLICT

Regalado and Halfon describe three opportunities for intervention to relieve parent-adolescent conflict. *Remediation* refers to interventions directed to the adolescent, such as diagnosing and managing behavioral, emotional, or physical problems, (eg, attention deficit disorder, conduct disorder, or a chronic medical condition) that may be the primary cause of problems in the parent-teen interaction.

In *redefinition*, the information to be shared is similar to that covered in anticipatory guidance. However, the purpose is not so much to inform parents of what might be expected, as to help them to see that their teen's behavior may be developmentally normal. Thus, the argumentativeness and challenging nature of a teen can be "redefined" not as an intentional way to reject what a parent has to say, but as a way to exercise new developmental skills around abstract reasoning. All of this can be viewed appropriately as a step in the process of testing of parental limits and achieving emancipation.

For some parents, the difficulties with their adolescent require more than redefinition. *Re-education* may be necessary to help these parents develop better skills and knowledge about parenting and communicating. (Tables 1, 4 and 5)

REFERRAL

For problems that are mild, such as those involving adolescents who are doing well academically, interacting well with peers and friends, and not involved in substance use, initial management in the office setting may obviate the need for outside referral. A message that needs to be communicated to parents is that it is crucial for them to maintain active parenting of their adolescent using suggestions such as those in Tables 2, 4, and 5. A brief office intervention may be all that is needed for them to get back on track with their teen. Referral of these families to parenting groups, support groups, or therapists who specialize in behavioral interventions may be an alternative for pediatricians who do not have the time or expertise to engage in office interventions. Some parents do well with parenting workshops or parent support groups. Follow-up within a month will determine the need to refer for further services, such as family or individual counseling.

When parents are in distress and unable to appreciate their role in their adolescent's problems, or when the adolescent is displaying behavior that compromises safety, when grades are declining, substance abuse is suspected, extracurricular activities are diminishing, or when the diagnosis is uncertain, prompt referral to a mental health professional is warranted. In these situations, follow-up by the pediatrician is needed to make sure the referral resources are meeting the needs of the teen and family.

Conclusion

Although effective parenting and communication with adolescents can be a challenge, most teens and parents are up to the task. When families encounter difficulty in growing into their new roles together, the pediatrician is in an ideal position to assess family strengths and problems, and to provide anticipatory guidance and referral. Pediatricians who give parents a realistic sense of what they might expect from their adolescent in terms of developmental challenges to the parenting process can enhance the likelihood of a smooth transition to young adulthood.

Acknowledgement

The editors would like to acknowledge technical review by William L. Coleman, MD, FAAP, for the AAP Section on Developmental and Behavioral Pediatrics.

Further Reading

Elkind D. *The Hurried Child: Growing Up Too Fast Too Soon.* Reading, MA: Addison-Wesley; 1981

Elster AB, Kuznets NJ, eds. *AMA Guidelines for Adolescent Preventive Services (GAPS).* Baltimore, MD: Williams & Wilkins; 1994

Fenwick E, Smith T. *Adolescence: The Survival Guide for Parents and Teenagers.* New York, NY: DK Publishing, Inc.; 1996

Ginott H. *Between Parent and Teenager.* New York, NY: Macmillan Publishing Company; 1996

Green M. (Ed.) *Bright Futures: Guidelines for Health Supervision of Infants, Children, and Adolescents.* Arlington, VA: National Center for Education in Maternal and Child Health; 1994

Maccoby EE, Martin JA. Socialization in the Context of the Family: Parent-Child Interaction. Mussen PH, ed. *The Handbook of Child Psychology.* 4th ed. New York, NY: John Wiley and Sons, Inc; 1983: vol 4, 1–102

Regalado M, Halfon N. Parenting: Issues for the pediatrician. *Pediatric Annals.* 1998;27:31–37

Steinberg L, Levine A. *You and Your Adolescent: A Parent's Guide for Ages 10–20.* Rev ed. New York, NY: Harper Collins Publishers, Inc; 1997

Waters E, Wippman J, Stroufe LA. Attachment, positive affect, and competence in peer groups: Two studies in contrast validation. *Child Dev.* 1979;50:821–829

Weinstein N, Bobe C, Mandell D. *Opening and Closing Pandora's Box: A Manual for Child and Adolescent Health Care Providers.* New York, NY: Children of Alcoholics Foundation (an affiliate of Phoenix House); 1998

Helping Parents Communicate With Their Teens
Part 2: Challenging Clinical Situations

by Sheryl A. Ryan, MD, FAAP and Vaughn I. Rickert, PsyD

This issue of *Adolescent Health Update* completes a two-part series on parenting of and communicating with adolescents. Part 1 (Vol 11:2) presented strategies and skills to assess families' parenting and communication styles, provide anticipatory guidance, and coordinate overall management. Part 2 presents four composite case histories representing situations commonly encountered in adolescent medicine. Considerations for the clinician, elements for anticipatory guidance, and therapeutic approaches are discussed.

Strategies to Facilitate Assessment

Adolescent patients and their parents are more likely to seek help with parenting and communication problems if the practice environment signals that they are welcome to do so. Changes in decor, including separate waiting areas for teens, can make it clear that you care for adolescents. Changes in the routine office visit, implemented as patients approach puberty, show teens and their parents that you are prepared to meet their changing psychosocial needs. (See Table 1)

As patients enter adolescence, the relationship between pediatrician and parent gradually becomes secondary to that of pediatrician and adolescent. Ideally, the clinician has fostered this shift over time, and the adolescent has already assumed the role of primary historian. Parents should be made aware of their adolescent's confidentiality rights. A clear statement made to both the adolescent and the parents at the start of the visit (for example, "It is important for me to speak directly and privately with your son/daughter about behaviors and health concerns

that are especially important during adolescence.") is one way to introduce this discussion.

Parents should understand that resolution of significant conflicts between parents and teens commonly requires more than one office visit, and pediatricians should be prepared to bill appropriately. The American Academy or Pediatrics' guide, *The Classification of Child and Adolescent Mental Diagnoses in Primary Care: Diagnostic and Statistical Manual for Primary Care (DSM-PC Child and Adolescent Version)*, commonly referred to as the *DSM-PC for Adolescents*, provides diagnoses for psychosocial

---

Learning Objectives

After reading this article, pediatricians will be able to:

1. assist adolescents and families with problems related to communication or parenting skills;
2. explain the developmental context of problematic behaviors and help parents learn to respond appropriately;
3. prepare parents for normal developmental events, such as typically increased needs for privacy and autonomy, that can be distinguished from depression;
4. discuss effective ways to deal with adolescent health risk behaviors such as drinking and driving; and
5. recognize indications for referral of adolescents with problematic behaviors to a specialist.

Sheryl A. Ryan, MD, FAAP, is an assistant professor of pediatrics, University of Rochester School of Medicine and Dentistry, Rochester, New York. Vaughn I. Rickert, PsyD, is professor and director of research, Adolescent Health Center/Pediatric Associates, Mount Sinai School of Medicine, New York, New York. At this writing, Dr. Rickert was an associate professor of obstetrics and gynecology, University of Texas Medical Branch at Galveston, Galveston, Texas.

Table 1. Creating a Suitable Environment

- Schedule additional and/or longer visits as required.
- Clarify confidentiality issues with adolescent and parents at the first visit.
- Make it clear that your primary relationship is with the adolescent.
- Recognize diversity and respect the values of each family.
- Routinely explore psychosocial status.
- Maintain a developmental perspective.

and developmental concerns related to parenting issues. The *DSM-PC* may be used to identify specific diagnoses and codes. Its use may increase recognition by insurers that pediatricians are providers of medical care for psychosocial health care concerns.

Clinical Situation 1

When a teen drinks and drives for the first time, what should parents say and do about it?

Sam, who is 17 years old, has been your patient since infancy. His father calls, distraught, on a Monday morning, and reports that, over the weekend, Sam drove to a party and returned home smelling of alcohol. Sam and the automobile were unharmed. There were no passengers. An angry confrontation had ensued. Now, both parents feel that Sam may need to be admitted to a substance abuse treatment program.

Sam, who has always been healthy, is a good student and a member of the school swim team. You have talked about substance use and reckless driving in the past, and he has denied both. You believe that Sam has been honest with you. How do you proceed?

Because it is clear from your telephone conversation with Sam's father that the parents' response to his behavior is causing significant conflict, suggest an office visit within the next few days. If possible, arrange to meet first with everyone together, then with Sam alone. This strategy allows the clinician to assess each person's perspective, the family's communication patterns, and the emotional climate.

Explain your office policy on confidentiality at the initial meeting, when all parties are present. Unless the patient may cause harm to self or others, statements made in the clinical interview

should be confidential. In the context of any evaluation for suspected substance abuse, adolescents may divulge behaviors (such as driving while intoxicated or binge drinking) that place themselves or others at risk of injury or death. In these cases, the physician may need to break confidentiality, even if the teen denies overt suicidal thoughts or behaviors.

With the parents in the room, explore for changes in Sam's school performance, involvement with friends, or extracurricular activities. Ask whether they believe Sam has driven a car while under the influence of alcohol before. Inquire about relevant parental rules, expectations, and consequences. Ask about a family history of substance use, including alcohol, and stressors in the recent past.

In this group meeting, assess family function. Parental reluctance to speak openly in front of Sam should be noted. Ask the parents if they have known Sam to experiment with other risk behaviors, and if so, how these have been handled. Ask why they feel they should admit him to a substance abuse treatment program, and whether they feel this is the only option available. Finally, invite the parents out of the room so that you can talk with Sam alone.

Ask Sam to describe the drinking and driving episode. Ask if this has occurred before, and whether there has been other substance use. Ask about his driving habits. Has he ever driven very fast, received a moving violation, or been involved in an accident? Inquire about his perception of injury risk associated with substance use. Ask about school performance and friends' use of drugs or alcohol. Ask about employment, and the specific number of hours worked per week. (Teens working more than 20 hours per week are less successful in school and are at greater risk for substance use than teens working fewer hours or not at all.) Ask about neurovegetative symptoms, such as difficulty sleeping or changes in appetite.

In this scenario, we assume that this was Sam's first episode of drinking and driving, and that he has continued to be a good student, involved in extracurricular activities and socially competent. It is clear that Sam's parents have high expectations of him. They have enjoyed a warm and open relationship. Sam has generally complied with parental rules; as a result, few consequences have been administered. Their motivation appears to be protective rather than punitive: Sam's parents are frightened about what they have heard about drunk drivers and the high rates of motor vehicle crashes among teenagers.

Your discussion with Sam and his parents would cover seven principal areas:

- The serious consequences associated with drinking and driving
- Parents as role models for responsible behavior (for example, consistent use of seat belts, not speeding, and not driving after drinking themselves)
- Normal adolescent development and common health risk behaviors
- Need for parental supervision
- Privileges tied to responsible behavior
- Limits of acceptable behavior, the consequences for going beyond these limits, and the expectation that these may need to be renegotiated as the teen gets older
- Back-up plans to ensure safety in the event that the adolescent does drink alcohol, or a friend who is driving is drinking alcohol (for example, an unconditional ride home from parents).

In talking with Sam's parents, explain that although a substance abuse treatment program may not be appropriate at this time, his actions should have consequences. These should be discussed, as should consequences for future infringements. Parental measures might include temporary suspension of his driving privileges, or conditional use of the family car. If the parents are unable to concur with the need for consequences other than a substance abuse treatment program, or are unable to develop more appropriate consequences, referral to a mental health provider for family counseling would be appropriate.

If Sam had divulged that he had consumed alcohol before driving several times in the past, it would have been necessary to discuss this with Sam's parents. Close follow-up would have been required. Referral to a substance abuse specialist would be appropriate if the pediatrician did not feel comfortable counseling Sam about cessation of this drinking behavior, or there was no improvement in the follow-up period.

Clinical Situation 2

Parental concerns about dating in early adolescence: Are these jitters justified?

You are scheduled to see 13-year-old Laura for a routine visit. The day before her appointment, Laura's mother calls to say that she and her husband have been arguing with Laura about when she may begin to date. Her husband wants to raise the issue during Laura's office visit, and asks that you support their desire to restrict dating behavior. They see this as a way to prevent their daughter from developing an early interest in sexual behaviors. How do you proceed?

Dating is one of the toughest topics for adolescents and parents because it invokes the "sex talk." Even parents who have been candid with their adolescents about physical development, sexuality, and reproduction may find this topic uncomfortable. Parents who find it difficult to communicate about or agree with their teen's requests to date, or who are uneasy about their teen's having intimate relationships, may turn to their pediatrician for help. In this situation, the pediatrician would encourage both parents to accompany Laura to her appointment, and to tell her in advance what they want to talk about.

Although, ideally, the initial meeting includes adolescent and parents, in this case Laura comes in with her mother alone. Open the clinical interview with a general inquiry as to how things are going. Next, ask the mother if there is something in particular she would like to talk about. Once the mother has spoken, you might turn to your patient and say, "Laura, what are your thoughts about what your mom just said?"

Explore Laura's definition of dating (eg, car date vs. dating in the context of group activities). Seek to establish some understanding of parental comfort about and knowledge of the boy Laura is interested in. Ask how the parents have responded in the past to these dating requests, and how Laura feels about their approach. Ask the mother about her and her husband's perspective on Laura's psychosocial development, including Laura's school performance and relationships.

Next, interview Laura privately. Ask her what dating means, how she has approached her parents, and their reaction. Explore previous dating experiences, including those her parents may not have known about. Inquire about previous intimate contact, including voluntary and involuntary sexual activity.

Ask Laura about her friends' dating experiences, and involvement in health risk behaviors such as substance use. Have she and her parents had discussions about dating and sexual activity? Is Laura informed about reproductive health issues? Determine if your patient is capable of making safe sexual decisions and able to choose dating partners who are respectful and nonviolent.

Your assessment reveals that Laura's parents:

- are worried about Laura and believe that their concerns are in her best interest;
- are uncomfortable about discussing reproductive health because they believe it will encourage sexual activity;
- believe that forbidding dating in any form will prevent Laura from becoming sexually active; and
- tend to be rigid and authoritarian and do not believe that rules should be negotiable.

Although Laura has observed the no-dating rule, she has plans to date her classmate. A goal here is to help the mother, and indirectly the father, understand that open communication with their daughter and appropriate restriction of dating behavior are not mutually exclusive. Instead, a balance of both may enhance Laura's sense of autonomy and ultimately encourage better compliance with the parents' wishes.

Laura needs the opportunity to explore her feelings about pubertal development and sexuality. Her parents would benefit from education about adolescent developmental goals, such as the need to develop a healthy body image and a sense of her sexuality, and to develop and maintain supportive relationships with her family. They also need to know that if they do not provide sexual education at home, Laura will receive it elsewhere.

The pediatrician's role is to facilitate communication without making decisions for the family.

Laura's parents have every right to say what they will permit, provided that they understand what Laura is requesting before they say no. The parents might soften their authoritarian stance so that Laura will not avoid or disregard rules completely because she hasn't had the opportunity to provide input.

Laura's parents need to appreciate that dating, per se, doesn't lead to the early onset of sexual activity. While parents can set the dating rules, they need to consider what is negotiable. They might set a curfew or restrict dating to weekends, for example, yet allow for possible exceptions for special events. Learning to communicate will help the parents respond appropriately if there are rule infractions. It will also enhance Laura's willingness to be honest.

Given the parents' discomfort with discussions about sexuality, more than one visit will be required. They should be informed that, however uncomfortable, these discussions offer a valuable opportunity to address misinformation and communicate values and behavioral expectations in a productive way. At the follow-up visit, ideally with both parents present, the pediatrician can review the progress that has been made in terms of more open communication about dating and peer activities. How has the family accommodated both Laura's desire to spend time with her friends and the parents' desire that she not begin to date just yet? If the channels of communication between Laura and her parents are better, support the family with encouragement and positive feedback. If conflict has continued or heightened, or either of the parents seems unable to recognize the need to allow Laura some autonomy (with privileges tied to responsible behavior) referral to a specialist in parenting issues and family counseling would be warranted. Table 2 presents general guidelines about dating that parents may find helpful.

Clinical Situation 3

If a teen withdraws in a time of stress, is it depression or normal behavior?

Mike, who is 12 years old, comes into your office for the first time for a routine check-up. He has no physical concerns and has always been healthy. Mike's mother explains at the outset that she is concerned

Table 2. Advice to Parents About Dating: Setting Ground Rules With Your Teen

- Admit that you grew up in a different era, but explain that your teen's safety is your first concern.
- Consider more than chronological age in setting criteria for the onset of dating. This is a case-by-case decision.
- Insist on meeting each of your teen's prospective dates before you allow unchaperoned dating. Your teen son or daughter should meet their date's parents as well.
- See that your adolescent and his or her date observe appropriate courtesies. For example, insist that the person who is driving come to the door.
- Request an itinerary for the date to determine appropriateness and safety of plans. Make it standard practice that family members let one another know where they're going, regardless of how old they are.
- Set a curfew and consequences for curfew violations and stick to them consistently.
- Keep the lines of communication open.
- Work with your teen to set up these guidelines and reassess together as needed. Adolescents who know the reason for a rule are more likely to comply with it.

about his behavior. Lately, he has become reluctant to accompany her on shopping trips or visits to his relatives, and has been spending much of his free time alone in his room. When his mother encourages him to accompany her, or openly objects to his spending

so much time alone, he argues that she has become "too nosy" and "doesn't respect his privacy."

Mike's parents have been divorced for several years and the father, a non-custodial but involved parent, has recently remarried. Mike and his mother have also recently moved to a new community. Until now, Mike's mother has tried to accommodate his increased need for privacy by leaving him alone as much as she can, but she is beginning to worry that perhaps his behavior is "unhealthy." How do you assess this young adolescent and his family?

In this case, the initial step would be to obtain a traditional history from Mike to assess for medical problems, then seek information from the mother about her specific concerns. A review of systems may reveal somatic complaints or depressive symptoms. The purpose of this interview is to assess whether Mike's withdrawal from his mother is to be attributed to normal development or depression.

A teen who is functioning well in school and reports having friends with whom he spends enjoyable time is less likely to be depressed than an adolescent whose desire for privacy includes a withdrawal from parents, friends and activities, whose academic performance has declined, and who has vague physical complaints. (See Table 3)

Table 3. Differentiating Between Depression and Normal Desire for More Time With Peers

	Depression	Developmentally Normal
Age of onset	Mean age—15 years	11–13 years
Symptoms	Vegetative signs—sleep disturbance, lethargy, appetite change, weight change	Sleeps soundly
	Irritability	Can be argumentative
	Somatic complaints	Physical symptoms usually absent
	Depressed mood	Mood swings more common but not extreme
	Subjective feelings of "boredom"	
Functioning		
Home	Impaired (social withdrawal common)	Generally normal
	May exhibit separation anxiety about leaving home, parents	May exhibit heightened conflict about family's expectations
School	May experience decrease in performance, new onset of behavioral difficulties	Generally, no change
Peers	May withdraw from peer activities, network	May express increased desire to affiliate with peers
Usual activities	May have decreased interest in prior activities, hobbies	Interested in new activities, hobbies
Associated health risk behaviors	May use substances such as tobacco, alcohol, or marijuana to self-medicate for symptoms to the extent that use interferes with normal functioning at school and home.	May experiment with tobacco, alcohol, or marijuana

Inquire about his current emotional and behavioral state, strengths and weaknesses, and whether these have changed recently. Determine when conflicts occur. Ask the mother, "Do you argue mostly when Mike is asked to spend time with the family, or has he recently become more defiant or irritable in general? Does this behavior occur at school or with his friends? Do you think the changes you have observed may be related to the family's recent move or the father's remarriage?"

Encourage Mike to speak for himself by directing questions to him, then observe the mother and son for reactions and communication patterns. Learn about Mike's behavior and functioning at home, his past and current school performance, whether he is still in touch with old friends, and whether he has established new friendships since the move.

Next, excuse Mike's mother to complete the remainder of the interview and physical exam. In your one-on-one interview, ask Mike to provide his own version of what his mother has described. Explore the changes that have occurred in his life, and acknowledge these as important transitions. Tell him that divorce, relocation, enrollment in a new school, and family structure realignments that accompany remarriage are significant stressors for all family members.

Adolescents' adaptive abilities vary tremendously. Approach this directly, perhaps by saying, "Many young people experience changes in their situation, such as divorce or remarriage of their parents, or moving to a new community and starting at a new school. These can be a real challenge to handle. How do you think you are doing managing these changes? Have you found any difficulties handling them?"

In this case, we assume that the evaluation reveals Mike to be a well-functioning adolescent. His school performance is acceptable and he has no physical complaints. Mike denies major conflicts with his mother other than her criticism about the time he spends alone. These conflicts have accelerated since their recent move, and Mike has had difficulty making friends in his new school.

Mike believes that his mother is concerned about the time he spends alone because she would like to see him spending more time with friends. He is guarded about discussing his father and his father's remarriage, or the conflict between his parents. He denies suicidal ideation and symptoms of general depression, such as irritability, boredom, feelings of sadness, difficulty sleeping, changes in appetite or weight, and decreased energy level.

Your intervention should be designed to improve the mother's understanding of normal developmental events of early adolescence. It should also support the need to maintain consistent parenting, supervision, and expectations about time spent with family members. Specifically, your intervention with this family could include:

- Reassurance that Mike is generally doing well with no specific evidence of depression. Explain to the mother that Mike's desire for privacy most likely represents a normal developmental drive to individuate. Their recent relocation and his father's remarriage may have intensified this normal developmental drive.

- Re-education if the mother has difficulty allowing Mike increased independence. Discussions about effective parenting using the authoritative parenting model and communication strategies as described in Part 1 of this series would also be helpful. Offer information about parenting programs or support groups if you feel that the mother is in need of additional assistance. She should be counseled about the signs of depression that can masquerade as a normal need for privacy. She should also understand that signs of depression or increased conflict should prompt a return visit and possible referral to a mental health professional.

- Recognition that numerous stressors are present in this family. Most notable are experiences associated with divorce, relocation, and the father's remarriage. These should be discussed as factors that may put Mike at risk for depression. They may also affect the way

Mike and his mother communicate, and can be expected to challenge the mother's ability to parent.

Close follow-up will be required to assure that Mike and his mother are negotiating this period of early adolescence successfully. Mike should be seen for follow-up in 1 month. At that time, inquire about how he and his mother have been communicating, how he is doing in school, whether he has been able to make new friends, and what activities he is involved in. A review of systems specifically related to depression should be obtained. (Table 3)

Mike's mother can provide important corroborating information about his functioning as well as her perception of his need for privacy versus withdrawal. If there are any concerns at this visit about lack of improvement, diminished functioning, or increased symptoms, immediate referral to a mental health provider would be warranted.

Clinical Situation 4

Does a sudden withdrawal from college mean that this adolescent has lost her focus?

Erica recently returned home from her first semester away at college and announced her decision to withdraw from school. Erica is unclear about what she wants, but "traveling around Europe for a while" is the current plan. Her grades in college this semester were good, but she has been unable to focus on any one area of interest and has begun to question her career plans.

Erica's parents have always described her as a perfect teenager. Now, they fear she may have "fallen in with the wrong crowd" at school and are advising her to enroll at a local college. They are afraid to confront their daughter for fear of provoking conflict, and are confused and anxious. What do you suggest to them?

Because of Erica's age, it would be appropriate in this case to begin the visit with Erica alone. Explain to the parents that the four of you will talk after you have had an opportunity to speak with her.

In the interview, explain to Erica that her parents contacted you because they were concerned about her decision to leave college for a year and you asked them to come in with her to talk about it. Tell her that while your conversation is confidential, an open discussion with all family members present will help you to respond to their concerns most effectively. Erica's response to this suggestion will give you important information about her relationship with her parents and how freely they communicate.

Ask Erica to relate her version of the current situation, the reasons for her decision to withdraw from school, how she feels about her parents' reaction, and what she hopes this year off will accomplish. Ask about her first semester and her reactions to being away from home. Explore how Erica has done academically and socially. Did she experience any academic or social difficulties making the transition from high school to college? Ask her to describe her peer relationships (close friends, intimate relationships, concerns about sexual orientation) and health risk behaviors (alcohol, tobacco or illicit substance use, and risky sexual activity). Obtain a brief medical history of recent illnesses, as well as a review of systems that includes medical and physical symptoms of depression. (See Table 3)

Finally, talk with Erica about how her family communicates about important matters, and the extent to which Erica has made her own decisions in the past. Once you have assessed Erica's functioning and current status, and the family's communication style, ask whether she would be willing to share some or all of the information she has divulged about her decision and plans for the next year.

When you are clear about what is to be considered confidential, ask her parents to join you. The family interview should be structured to give the parents an opportunity to express their concerns and their version of events. They should also be asked about stressors since Erica's last visit to your office, and her behavior (home, school, and peers). Give the parents the opportunity to reflect on their daughter's strengths and weaknesses to obtain a sense of their affection for their daughter. Ask them how they have responded to Erica's decision. Reinforce their attempts to communicate with one another.

In this scenario, we assume that both parents describe Erica as a compliant and non-challenging child and adolescent. Erica reports that she chose her college and major at her parents' suggestion. Erica feels that she has always gotten along well with her parents, but states that since she gave them "few problems" as a teenager, they rarely discussed difficult topics.

Your discussion reveals that while Erica was academically and socially successful in her first semester of college, discussions with friends had prompted questions about her career decisions and future plans. She and her parents find it hard to talk about their concerns for her future, although she feels a need for their guidance and support.

You conclude that Erica's recent decision reflects a normal developmental need to redefine her identity in terms of future aspirations and goals. You find no evidence of psychological pathology to suggest otherwise. While it might have been assumed that she had accomplished this "task" of late adolescence prior to beginning college, she allowed others to make decisions for her about college and career choice. Thus, her plans to "take time out" and reassess her future plans may reflect a high level of maturity.

This situation is well-suited to Regalado and Halfon's approach of remediation, redefinition, and re-education, as described in Part 1 of this series (Vol 11:2). The authors define *remediation* as diagnosis and management of specific behavioral or emotional problems. They describe *redefinition* as a process of framing attitudes about developmentally normal behavior that may appear to a parent to be abnormal. *Re-education* is their term for helping parents develop better parenting and communication skills.

Intervention in this family should focus primarily on redefinition, or the reframing of Erica's behavior as an important component of normal development. While Erica's parents may not agree, they need to understand that her decision is developmentally appropriate. Her behavior represents neither rebellion nor a direct challenge to their authority. In fact, it may reflect her growing competence as a young adult.

In the re-education phase, engage the parents in a discussion about how they can support Erica and how they can communicate more effectively.

Explain that as Erica begins her "year off " she is likely to need her parents' guidance and support, and that this is an opportunity for them to enhance their relationship with her.

Follow-up over the next several weeks should also be recommended, as the parents may require additional support or re-education regarding communication and parenting. This also provides an opportunity to monitor Erica's progress.

Conclusion

Adolescents and their families come to their pediatricians with a variety of psychosocial concerns. Adequate assessment and management requires an ability to respect the importance of these concerns and provide the additional time required to address them. The pediatrician who creates a comfortable context for communication with teens and their parents, and discusses parenting and communication skills in a developmental framework, will be better able to meet these needs.

Further Reading

American Academy of Pediatrics. *The Classification of Child and Adolescent Mental Diagnoses in Primary Care: Diagnostic and Statistical Manual for Primary Care (DSM-PC Child and Adolescent Version).* (Please direct inquiries to the AAP Division of Child and Adolescent Health at (800) 433-9016, ext. 7941.)

Beasley PJ, Beardslee WR. Depression in the adolescent patient. *Adolescent Medicine: State of the Art Reviews.* 1998;9:351–362

Hack S, Jellinek MS. Early identification of emotional and behavioral problems in a primary care setting. *Adolescent Medicine: State of the Art Reviews.* 1998;9:335–350

Prazar GE. A private practitioner's approach to adolescent problems. *Adolescent Medicine: State of the Art Reviews.* 1998;9:229–241

Regalado M, Halfon N. Parenting: Issues for the pediatrician. *Pediatric Annals.* 1998;27:31–37

Steinberg L, Levine A. *You and Your Adolescent: A Parent's Guide for Ages 10-20.* Rev ed. New York, NY: Harper Collins Publishers, Inc.;1997

Weitzman M, Adair R. Divorce and Children. *Ped Clin North Am.* 1988;35:1313–1323

Acknowledgment

The editors would like to acknowledge technical review by William L. Coleman, MD, FAAP, on behalf of the AAP Section on Developmental and Behavioral Pediatrics

The Teen Driver
Guidelines for Parents

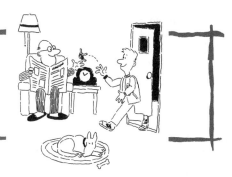

Traffic crashes are the leading cause of death for teens and young adults. More than 5,000 young people die every year in car crashes and thousands more are injured. Drivers who are 16 years old are more than 20 times as likely to have a crash as are other drivers. State and local laws, safe driving programs, and driver's education classes all help keep teens safe on the roads. Parents can also play an important role in keeping young drivers safe. This information has been developed by the American Academy of Pediatrics to inform parents about the risks that teen drivers face and how parents can help keep them safe on the roads.

Why teens are at risk

There are two main reasons why teens are at a higher risk for being in a car crash: lack of driving experience and their tendency to take risks while driving.

- **Lack of experience.** Teens drive faster and do not control the car as well as more experienced drivers. Their judgment in traffic is often insufficient to avoid a crash. In addition, teens do most of their driving at night, which can be even more difficult. Standard driver's education classes include 30 hours of classroom teaching and 6 hours of behind-the-wheel training. This is not enough time to fully train a new driver.

- **Risk taking.** Teen drivers are more likely to be influenced by peers and other stresses and distractions. This can lead to reckless driving behaviors such as speeding, driving while under the influence of drugs or alcohol, and not wearing safety belts.

Programs that help

Graduated licensing laws. Most teens get their driver's licenses in two stages: a learner's permit followed a few months later by a regular driver's license. The US Department of Transportation recommends "graduated licensing" so that learning to drive is spread over three stages. Each stage gives teens more driving privileges. Teen drivers have to meet certain restrictions for at least 6 months in each stage in order to move to the next stage. Driver's education classes would cover more and more complex decision-making and skills training during each stage. Twelve states have some form of graduated licensing laws.

Minimum drinking age and zero tolerance laws. Drunk and drugged driving are major problems for American teens. In one study, an estimated 6% to 14% of drivers younger than 21 years who were stopped at roadside sobriety checkpoints had been drinking. The misuse of alcohol and other drugs can severely hurt teenagers in many ways—especially on the road. A teen driver with a blood alcohol level (BAC) above 0.05% is more likely to be involved in a crash than is a sober teen driver.

Two types of laws exist to help lower the number of teens who drive after drinking alcohol. These are *minimum drinking* age laws and zero tolerance laws. Minimum drinking age laws prohibit the sale of alcohol to anyone under 21 years of age. These laws have helped reduce the number of alcohol-related crashes by 40%. But in some states, these laws have many loopholes and are hard to enforce. Many states have or will soon adopt zero tolerance laws that lower the allowable BAC limits for minors. Some states also require that licenses be suspended, sometimes for up to 1 year, after drivers younger than 21 years of age are arrested for driving drunk. These laws work. In Maryland, alcohol-related crashes decreased by at least 11% as a result of zero tolerance laws.

Safety belt laws. Even though all states have laws that require the use of safety belts, these laws may not apply to all passengers or all seats in a vehicle. In addition, studies show that teens do not use safety belts as often as older drivers do. Young people between 10 and 20 years old use safety belts only about 35% of the time—the lowest usage rate of any group. Strictly enforced safety belt laws, along with air bags, could greatly reduce the number of teens who are injured and killed in car crashes. In addition, teen drivers need to learn to take the responsibility of making sure all passengers are buckled up.

Curfew laws. Curfew laws ban teen driving during certain hours at night, such as midnight to 5 am. States with nighttime driving curfews for young drivers have lower crash rates than other states. The more strict the law, the fewer fatal crashes occur.

Educational efforts. Various state and national groups have programs to educate teens about unsafe driving practices, such as not wearing a safety belt and drunk driving. Pediatricians also play a role in such efforts.

There are several groups that encourage alternatives to drinking and driving by hosting social events for teens such as alcohol-free proms and parties. They also help teens and parents communicate. For example, SADD (Students Against Driving Drunk) encourages parents and teens to sign a contract in which both parties agree to avoid using alcohol or other drugs before driving and avoid riding with those who have. The contract also states that if a teen has been drinking he or she will call home for a ride. The group also encourages young people to help other teens change drinking habits and save lives on the roadways.

Safe ride programs. In some areas, "safe ride" programs help parents get involved by volunteering to drive to proms and other parties. Other programs give rides to teens who might otherwise have to drive home after drinking or ride with someone who has been drinking. A California program, for example, combines an educational program about alcohol abuse and an escort service for "stranded" teens on weekend nights. Teens can use this service in confidence. Teens volunteer to be drivers, but adults are also on-call in case questions or problems come up. Volunteer drivers stay in the car when they drop teens at home. They watch the teens enter their homes but do not talk with parents. Adults on-call handle any questions from parents.

How parents can help

Establish and discuss "house rules" about driving even before your teen gets a license. Remind your teen that these rules are in place because you care about his or her safety. If your teen complains about the rules, stand firm. You might say something like, "I don't care what other parents are doing—I care about you and don't want you to get in a crash." Remember, you control the car keys. Don't hesitate to take away driving privileges if your teen breaks any rules. Resist the urge to break the house rules yourself and let your teen drive because it is too much trouble for you to drive. Instead, try to arrange a car pool of parents and take turns driving.

You do not need to wait for graduated licensing laws to be passed in your state to adopt your own graduated driving rules. By slowly increasing driving privileges, you can help your teen get the experience needed to drive safely and responsibly. Here are some suggestions on how you can create a graduated licensing program for your teen driver. It may not be necessary to use all of the following restrictions; choose the ones that make the most sense for you and your teen.

Stage one

- teen must be at least 15½ years old or have a legal learner's permit
- teen must drive with a licensed adult driver at all times, the parent if possible
- no driving between 10 pm and 5 am or no driving after sunset
- driver and all passengers must wear safety belts
- no use of tobacco, alcohol, or other drugs
- teen must remain ticket-free and crash-free for 6 months before moving up to the next stage

Stage two

- teen must be at least 16 years old or have driven with a learner's permit for at least 6 months
- teen must drive with a licensed adult driver during nighttime hours, the parent if possible
- teen allowed to drive unsupervised during daytime hours
- passengers restricted to one nonfamily member during daytime hours

- no use of tobacco, alcohol, or other drugs
- driver and all passengers must wear safety belts
- teen must remain ticket-free and crash-free for 12 months before moving up to the next stage

Stage three

- teen must be at least 18 years old or have driven at least 2 years at the previous stage
- no restrictions on driving as long as the teen driver remains ticket-free and crash-free for 6 months
- no use of tobacco, alcohol, or other drugs
- all passengers must wear safety belts
  Other ways parents can help:
- Require that your teen maintain good grades in school before he or she can drive. Check with your auto insurance company to see if any "good student" discounts are available.
- Set a good driving example (no use of alcohol or other drugs, no speeding, always wear your safety belt, and require that safety belts be worn by all passengers).
- Remind your teen how important it is to stay focused on driving, not getting distracted by excessively loud music or talking on a cellular phone.
- Let your teen know that driving after drinking or using other drugs will not be tolerated. Tell your teen to always call you or someone else for a ride any time he or she or any other driver has been drinking or using drugs. Let your teen know that you will pick him or her up. However, if you find he or she was drinking, it may be better to wait until the next day before you discuss the incident.
- Be alert to any signs that your teen has a drinking or other substance abuse problem. If you suspect a problem, urge your teen to talk with his or her pediatrician or school counselor. Such trusted adults can refer your teen for other help, if needed.
- Support efforts to protect teens. These might include "safe ride" programs or Mothers Against Drunk Driving (MADD). Encourage alcohol-free community events.
- Encourage schools to teach about the dangers of driving after drinking or using drugs.
- Support showing safety films in schools. Also support efforts to promote safety belt use in all vehicles that take children and teens to and from school.

Driving is a privilege and a big responsibility. Teen drivers, because of their age and inexperience, are at a higher risk for car crashes. Licensing programs, rules of the road, and safe ride programs are designed to help teen drivers stay safe. Along with support and encouragement from parents, these programs are the best way to help teens learn to become responsible drivers.

American Academy of Pediatrics

DEDICATED TO THE HEALTH OF ALL CHILDREN™

The American Academy of Pediatrics is an organization of 60,000 primary care pediatricians, pediatric medical subspecialists, and pediatric surgical specialists dedicated to the health, safety, and well-being of infants, children, adolescents, and young adults.

American Academy of Pediatrics
Web site—www.aap.org

Copyright ©1996
American Academy of Pediatrics

Tips for Parents of Adolescents

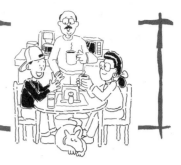

Adolescence is a time of change and challenge for your preteen or teenager. The changes that occur during adolescence are often confusing not only for your son or daughter, but for you as well. Though these years can be difficult, the reward is watching your child become an independent, caring, and responsible adult. The American Academy of Pediatrics (AAP) offers the following tips to help you face the challenges of your child's adolescence:

1. **Spend family time with your adolescent.** Although many preteens and teens may seem more interested in friends, this does not mean they are not interested in family.

2. **Spend time alone with your adolescent.** Even if your teen does not want time alone with you, take a moment here and there to remind him that your "door is always open," and you are always there if he needs to talk. Remind him often.

3. **When your adolescent talks**
   • Pay attention.
   • Watch, as well as listen.
   • Try not to interrupt.
   • Ask him to explain things further if you don't understand.
   • If you don't have time to listen when your child wants to talk, set a time that will be good for both of you.

4. **Respect your adolescent's feelings.** It's okay to disagree with your child, but disagree respectfully, not insultingly. Don't dismiss her feelings or opinions as silly or senseless. You may not always be able to help when your child is upset about something, but it is important to say, "I want to understand" or "Help me understand."

5. **When rules are needed, set and enforce them.** Don't be afraid to be unpopular for a day or two. Believe it or not, adolescents see setting limits as a form of caring.

6. **Try not to get upset if your adolescent makes mistakes.** This will help him take responsibility for his own actions. Remember to offer guidance when necessary. Direct the discussion toward solutions.

> "I get upset when I find clothes all over the floor," is much better than, "You're a slob."

Be willing to negotiate and compromise. This will teach problem solving in a healthy way. Remember to choose your battles. Some little annoying things that adolescents do may not be worth a big fight—let them go.

7. **Criticize a behavior, not an attitude.** For example, instead of saying,

> "You're late. That's so irresponsible. And I don't like your attitude,"

try saying,

> "I worry about your safety when you're late. I trust you, but when I don't hear from you and don't know where you are, I wonder whether something bad has happened to you. What can we do together to help you get home on time and make sure I know where you are or when you're going to be late?"

8. **Mix criticism with praise.** While your teen needs to know how you feel when she is not doing what you want her to do, she also needs to know that you appreciate the positive things she is doing. For example,

> "I'm proud that you are able to hold a job and get your homework done. I would like to see you use some of that energy to help do the dishes after meals."

9. **Let your child be the adolescent he wants to be, not the one you wish he was.** Also, try not to pressure your adolescent to be like you were or wish you had been at that age. Give your teen some leeway with regard to clothes, hairstyle, etc. Many teens go through a rebellious period in which they want to express themselves in ways that are different from their parents. However, be aware of the messages and ratings of the music, movies, and video games to which your child is exposed.

10. **Be a parent first, not a pal.** Your adolescent's separation from you as a parent is a normal part of development. Don't take it personally.

11. **Don't be afraid to share with your adolescent that you have made mistakes as a parent.** A few parenting mistakes are not crucial. Also, try to share with your teen mistakes you made as an adolescent.

12. **Talk to your pediatrician if you are having trouble with your adolescent.** He or she may be able to help you and your child find ways to get along.

The following is additional information you may find helpful in understanding some of the life changes and pressures your adolescent may be experiencing.

Dieting and body image

"My daughter is always trying new diets.
How can I help her lose weight safely?"

We live in a society that is focused on thinness. Adolescents see many role models in fashion magazines, on television, and in the movies that emphasize the importance of being thin. This concern about weight and body image leads many adolescents, especially girls, to resort to extreme measures to lose weight. Be aware of any diet or exercise program with which your child is involved. Be watchful of how much weight your child loses, and make sure the diet program is healthy. Eating disorders such as anorexia nervosa and bulimia nervosa can be very dangerous. If you suspect your child has an eating disorder, talk to your pediatrician right away. Ask about the brochure from the AAP called *Eating Disorders: What You Should Know About Anorexia and Bulimia.*

Many diets are unhealthy for adolescents because they do not have the nutritional value that bodies need during puberty. If your teen wants to lose weight, urge her to increase physical activity and to take weight off slowly. Let her eat according to her own appetite, but make sure she gets enough fats, carbohydrates, protein, and calcium.

Make sure your teen is not confusing a "low-fat" diet with a "no fat" diet. Teens need 30% of their calories from fat, and cutting fat out of the diet altogether is not healthy. A low-fat diet should still include 30 to 50 grams of fat daily. Many teens choose vegetarian diets. If your child decides to become a vegetarian, make certain she reads about it and becomes an educated vegetarian. She may need to see her pediatrician or a nutritionist to ensure that she is getting enough fat, calories, protein, and calcium.

Many adolescents are uncomfortable with their bodies. If your adolescent is unhappy with the way she looks, encourage her to start a physical activity program. Physical activity will stop hunger pangs, create a positive self-image, and take away the "blahs". Unfortunately, some teens may try to change their bodies by dangerous means such as unhealthy dieting (as discussed previously) or with drugs such as anabolic steroids. Encourage healthy exercise. If your child wants to train with weights, she should check with her pediatrician, as well as a trainer, coach, or physical education teacher. Help create a positive self-image by praising your child about her appearance. Set a good example by practicing what you preach. Make exercise and eating right a part of your daily routine also.

Nutrition

The growth rate during adolescence is one of the most dramatic changes the body ever goes through. It is very important for your adolescent to have a proper diet. Follow these suggestions to help keep your teen's diet a healthy one

- Limit fast food meals. Discuss the options available at fast food restaurants, and help your teen find a good balance in her diet. Fat should not come from junk food but from healthier foods such as cheese or yogurt. Vegetables and fruit are also important.
- Keep the household supply of "junk food" such as candy, cookies, and potato chips to a minimum.
- Stock up on low-fat healthy items for snacking such as fruit, raw vegetables, whole-grain crackers, and yogurt.
- Check with your pediatrician about the proper amounts of calories, fat, protein, and carbohydrates for your child.
- As a parent, model good eating habits.

Dating and sex education

"With all the sex on television, how can I teach
my son to 'wait' until he is ready?"

There are constant pressures for your adolescent to have sex. These pressures may come from the movies, television, music, friends, and peers. Teens are naturally curious about sex. This is completely normal and healthy. Talk to your adolescent to understand his feelings and views about sex. Start early and provide your teen with access to information that is accurate and appropriate. Delaying sexual involvement could be the most important decision your child can make. Talk to your teen or preteen about the following things he needs to think about before becoming sexually active:

Medical and physical risks, like unwanted pregnancy and STDs (sexually transmitted diseases) such as

- Gonorrhea
- Chlamydia
- Hepatitis B
- Syphilis
- Herpes
- HIV, the virus that causes AIDS

Emotional risks—that go along with an adolescent having sex before he is ready. The adolescent may regret the decision when he is older or feel guilty, frightened, or ashamed from the experience. Have your adolescent ask himself, "Am I ready to have sex?" "What will happen after I have sex?"

Methods of contraception—Anyone who is sexually active needs to be aware of the various methods of contraception that help prevent unintended pregnancies, as well as ways to protect against sexually transmitted diseases. Remember to tell your teen that latex condoms should always be used along with a second method of contraception to prevent pregnancy and STDs.

Setting limits—Make sure your adolescent has thought about what his limits are before dating begins.

Most importantly, let your adolescent know that he can talk to you and his pediatrician about dating and relationships. Offer your guidance throughout this important stage in your teen's life.

The following AAP brochures may help your teen in dealing with these difficult issues: *Deciding to Wait and Making the Right Choice: Facts For Teens on Preventing Pregnancy.*

If you smoke... quit

If you or someone else in the household smokes, now is a good time to quit. Watching a parent struggle through the process of quitting can be a powerful message for a teen or preteen who is thinking about starting. It also shows that you care about your health, as well as your child's.

Smoking and tobacco

"My daughter smokes behind my back. How do I convince her to quit?"

Smoking can turn into a lifelong addiction that can be extremely hard to break. Discuss with your adolescent some of the more undesirable effects of smoking, including bad breath, stained teeth, wrinkles, a long-term cough, and decreased athletic performance. Addiction can also lead to serious health problems like emphysema and cancer.

"Chew" or "snuff" can also lead to nicotine addiction and causes the same health problems as smoking cigarettes. Mouth wounds or sores also form and may not heal easily. Smokeless tobacco can also lead to cancer.

If you suspect your teen or preteen is smoking or using smokeless tobacco, talk to your pediatrician. Arrange for your child to visit the pediatrician, who will want to discuss the risks associated with smoking and the best ways to quit before it becomes a lifelong habit. Smokers young and old often are more likely to listen to advice from their doctor than from others.

Alcohol

"I know my son drinks once in a while, but it's just beer. Why should I worry?"

Alcohol is the most socially accepted drug in our society, and also one of the most abused and destructive. Even small amounts of alcohol can impair judgment, provoke risky and violent behavior, and slow down reaction time. An intoxicated teenager (or anyone else) behind the wheel of a car is a lethal weapon. Alcohol-related car crashes are the leading cause of death for young adults, aged 15 to 24 years.

Though it's illegal for people under age 21 to drink, we all know that most teenagers are no strangers to alcohol. Many of them are introduced to alcohol during childhood. If you choose to use alcohol in your home, be aware of the example you set for your teen. The following suggestions may help:

- Having a drink should never be shown as a way to cope with problems.
- Don't drink in unsafe conditions—driving the car, mowing the lawn, using the stove, etc.
- Don't encourage your child to drink or to join you in having a drink.
- Never make jokes about getting drunk; make sure that your children understand that it is neither funny nor acceptable.
- Show your children that there are many ways to have fun without alcohol. Happy occasions and special events don't have to include drinking.
- Do not allow your children to drink alcohol before they reach the legal age and teach them never, ever to drink and drive.
- Always wear your seatbelt (and ask your children to do the same.)

Drugs

"I am afraid some of my daughter's friends have offered her drugs. How can I help her make the right decision?"

Your child may be interested in using drugs other than tobacco and alcohol, including marijuana and cocaine, to fit in or as a way to deal with the pressures of adolescence. Try to help your adolescent build her self-confidence or self-esteem. This will help your child resist the pressure to use drugs. Encourage your adolescent to "vent" emotions and troubles through conversations and physical activity rather than by getting "high."

Set examples at home. Encourage your adolescent to participate in leisure and outside activities to stay away from the peer pressure of drinking and drugs. Talk with your children about healthy choices.

For more information on tobacco, alcohol, and other drugs, visit the AAP Web site at www.aap.org, or ask your pediatrician about the following AAP brochures:

Alcohol: Your Child and Drugs
Cocaine: Your Child and Drugs
Marijuana: Your Child and Drugs
Smoking: Straight Talk for Teens
Steroids: Play Safe, Play Fair
The Risks of Tobacco Use: A Message to Parents and Teens

The information contained in this publication should not be used as a substitute for the medical care and advice of your pediatrician. There may be variations in treatment that your pediatrician may recommend based on individual facts and circumstances.

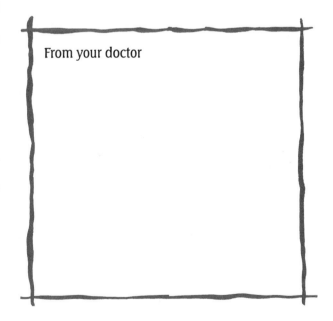

From your doctor

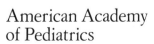

American Academy of Pediatrics

DEDICATED TO THE HEALTH OF ALL CHILDREN™

The American Academy of Pediatrics is an organization of 60,000 primary care pediatricians, pediatric medical subspecialists, and pediatric surgical specialists dedicated to the health, safety, and well-being of infants, children, adolescents, and young adults.

American Academy of Pediatrics
Web site— www.aap.org

Copyright ©1995, Updated 2/00
American Academy of Pediatrics

Section VIII Further Reading

Alderman EM. Growing up in an affluent family: unique psychosocial issues for the adolescent. *Adolesc Med.* 2001;12: 379–388

A mother's reaction to a rebellious adolescent. *Adolesc Med.* 1998;9:197–203

Austin SB, Rich M. Consumerism: its impact on the health of adolescents. *Adolesc Med.* 2001;12:389–409

Stanton B, Cuthill S, Amador C. Adolescence and poverty. *Adolesc Med.* 2001;12:525–538

Legal and Ethical Considerations

The Adolescent's Right to Confidential Care When Considering Abortion

Committee on Adolescence

ABSTRACT. In this statement, the American Academy of Pediatrics (AAP) reaffirms its position that the rights of adolescents to confidential care when considering abortion should be protected. The AAP supports the recommendations presented in the report on mandatory parental consent to abortion by the Council on Ethical and Judicial Affairs of the American Medical Association. Adolescents should be strongly encouraged to involve their parents and other trusted adults in decisions regarding pregnancy termination, and the majority of them voluntarily do so. Legislation mandating parental involvement does not achieve the intended benefit of promoting family communication, but it does increase the risk of harm to the adolescent by delaying access to appropriate medical care. The statement presents a summary of pertinent current information related to the benefits and risks of legislation requiring mandatory parental involvement in an adolescent's decision to obtain an abortion. The AAP acknowledges and respects the diversity of beliefs about abortion and affirms the value of voluntary parental involvement in decision making by adolescents.

Assuring adolescent access to health care, including reproductive health care, has been a long-standing objective of the American Academy of Pediatrics (AAP). Assured access to timely medical care is especially important for pregnant adolescents because of the significant medical, personal, and social consequences of adolescent childbearing. The AAP strongly advocates for the prevention of unintended adolescent pregnancy by supporting comprehensive health and sexuality education, abstinence, and the use of contraception by sexually active youths. For two decades the AAP has been on record as supporting the access of minors to all options regarding undesired pregnancy, including the right to obtain an abortion. Membership surveys confirm this support.[1,2]

Under current federal constitutional law, minors have the right to obtain abortions without parental consent unless otherwise specified by state law. Legislation that mandates parental involvement (parental consent or notification) as a condition of service when a minor seeks an abortion has generated considerable controversy. Recent US Supreme Court rulings, although upholding the constitutional rights of minors to choose abortion, have held that it is not unconstitutional for states to impose requirements for parental involvement as long as "adequate provision for judicial bypass" is available for minors who think that this involvement would not be in their best interest.[3,4] Subsequently, there has been renewed activity to include mandatory parental consent or notification requirements in state and federal abortion-related legislation.

The American Medical Association, the Society for Adolescent Medicine, the American Public Health Association, the American College of Obstetricians and Gynecologists, the AAP, and other health professional organizations have reached a consensus that minors should not be compelled or required to involve their parents in their decisions to obtain abortions, although they should be encouraged to discuss their pregnancies with their parents and other responsible adults. These conclusions result from objective analyses of current data, which indicate that legislation mandating parental involvement does not achieve the intended benefit of promoting family communication but does increase the risk of harm to the adolescent by delaying access to appropriate medical care.[5–9]

This statement has been approved by the Council on Child and Adolescent Health.

The recommendations in this statement do not indicate an exclusive course of treatment or serve as a standard of medical care. Variations, taking into account individual circumstances, may be appropriate.

In this statement, the AAP reaffirms its position that the rights of adolescents to confidential care when considering abortion should be protected. The AAP supports the recommendations presented in the report on mandatory parental consent to abortion by the Council on Ethical and Judicial Affairs of the American Medical Association.[5] This statement does not duplicate the extensive analysis published in that report but presents a summary of pertinent current information related to the benefits and risks of legislation requiring mandatory parental involvement in an adolescent's decision to obtain an abortion. This statement does not discuss the philosophical or religious issues related to abortion. Beliefs about abortion are deeply personal and are shaped by class, culture, religion, and personal history, as well as the current social and political climate. The AAP acknowledges and respects the diversity of beliefs about abortion. This statement affirms the value of parental involvement in decision making by adolescents and the importance of productive family communication in general. The AAP is a foremost advocate of strong family relationships and holds that parents are generally supportive and act in the best interests of their children.

Background

STATISTICAL TRENDS

One million pregnancies occur annually among American teenagers. Of these, about 400 000 occur in minors younger than 18 years of age, of which 41% are terminated by elective abortion.[10] The percentage of pregnancies terminated by induced abortion in minors increased in the 1970s, plateaued in the early 1980s, and has decreased since 1985, particularly in younger girls. Whereas 46% of pregnant adolescents 15 years of age and younger obtained abortions in 1985, only 39% did so in 1988.[10] Postulated explanations for the decline include a shift in attitudes toward abortion among adolescents, increased legal and financial barriers to abortion, particularly for low-income adolescents, and increasing social acceptance of childbearing among unmarried adolescents. Birth rates among adolescents

nationally are now the highest since the early 1970s. Approximately 80% of births to minors younger than 18 years of age are to unmarried adolescents.[11] Adoption ratios have declined during the last decade; approximately 2% to 4% of unmarried adolescents place their infants for adoption.[12]

Compared with those who choose childbirth, adolescents who choose abortion tend to come from higher socioeconomic backgrounds, have higher educational aspirations and achievements, have mothers with higher educational levels, have higher self-esteem, have greater feelings of control over life, have lower levels of anxiety, and are better able to conceptualize the future.[13-15]

STATE LAWS

The status of legislation requiring mandatory parental involvement in a minor's abortion decision is currently in flux. As of 1992, 38 states had some form of specific legislation on record, highly variable among states in both content and degree of enforcement.[9-16] However, US Supreme Court rulings in 1992 on "undue burden" standards and requirements for judicial bypass procedures raise legal questions about the validity of many existing state statutes, while allowing new or revised clauses that could be held constitutional. Groups opposed to legal abortion view parental notification requirements for minors as politically feasible; thus, adolescent rights to confidential care have become part of a larger battle regarding access to abortion in general.[17] Continuing legislative activity can be anticipated. Of 308 abortion-related bills introduced in 41 states during 1992, 61 were related to parental consent or notification, confirming the need for health professionals to be prepared to protect the best interests of adolescents with objective data on this issue.

Effect of Legislation on Family Communication

Basic principles of law and society hold that parents should be involved in and responsible for assuring medical care for their children, that parents ordinarily act in the best interests of their children, and that minors benefit from the advice and emotional support of their parents. Legislation mandating parental involvement in abortion decisions is promoted on the basis of its theoretical benefits on strengthening family responsibility and communication. Some who support reproductive choice may be ambivalent about parental notification requirements. Adults may fear that minors contemplating abortion are immature, isolated, or at risk of being coerced into decisions without adequate counseling. Many parents vote for notification clauses because they hope these laws will increase communication that otherwise might not happen.[18] The 1990 AAP membership survey showed that although 85% of members thought that mandatory parental notification for abortion would cause some adolescents to delay seeking care, 49% said there should be such laws,[2] suggesting that many AAP members assume there is benefit from such legislation. Because outcome analysis, as supported by the evidence that follows, shows a minimal benefit compared with a significant risk, there is clearly a need for current data to be better understood.

VOLUNTARY PARENTAL INVOLVEMENT

Research confirms that pregnant minors do not make abortion decisions in isolation; they actively involve adults to whom they feel close. Even when not required to, the majority of minors seeking abortions voluntarily involve at least one parent in their decisions. A survey of 1519 unmarried pregnant minors in states where parental involvement is not mandatory found that 61% told one or both parents about their intent to have abortions. The younger the minor, the more likely she was to do so (90% of those 14 years old or younger, 74% of those 16 years old).[19] Among minors who did not involve a parent, virtually all involved at least one responsible adult other than clinic staff (such as another relative, teacher, counselor, professional, or clergy). A study of inner-city, black, pregnant teenagers younger than 18 years of age confirmed that more than 91% voluntarily consulted a parent or "parent surrogate" about pregnancy decisions. The term parent surrogate refers to a close adult who is fulfilling a parental role. This person was often a grandmother,

aunt, or other relative who had "raised them" or with whom they lived, even if that adult was not the legal guardian.[20]

The importance of parent surrogates and extended families is significant when assessing the impact of attempts to legislate family communication. Most notification clauses are restricted to traditional definitions of biological parents or legal guardians and fail to address the complexity and diversity of modern family structures and adult support systems relevant to adolescents. For minors who are willing to involve parents or parent surrogates in their abortion decisions, legislation adds no benefit and actually may impede appropriate family communication channels.

INVOLUNTARY PARENTAL NOTIFICATION

Minors who choose not to inform parents about their intention to have abortions are disproportionately older (16 and 17 years old), white, and employed.[19] Very young adolescents almost always agree to voluntary parental involvement. In the unusual instance of resistance, the possibility of incest or abuse should be carefully evaluated. The most frequent reasons minors cite for not telling parents include the belief that the knowledge would damage their relationship, the fear that it would escalate conflict or coercion, and the desire to protect a vulnerable parent from stress and disappointment.[19] Adolescents who are strongly opposed to informing parents tend to predict family reactions accurately.[21] Involuntary parental notification can precipitate a family crisis characterized by severe parental anger and rejection of the minor and her partner. One third of minors who do not inform parents already have experienced family violence and fear it will recur.[19] Research on abusive and dysfunctional families shows that violence is at its worst during a family member's pregnancy and during the adolescence of the family's children.[5] Although parental involvement in minors' abortion decisions may be helpful in many cases, in others it may be punitive, coercive, or abusive.[22]

Credible reviews of available data conclude that there is no evidence that mandatory parental involvement results in the benefits to the family intended by the legislation. No studies show that forced disclosure results in improved parent-child relationships, improved communication, or improved satisfaction with the decision about pregnancy outcome.[22-24]

The current data also indicate that such legislation does not increase the likelihood that parents will be involved. The percentages of minors who inform parents about their intent to have abortions are essentially the same in states with and without notification laws.[25] In states with such laws, adolescents who are not willing to inform parents use judicial bypass mechanisms,[26] go out of state to obtain services,[27] obtain clandestine care,[28] or delay care.[29,30]

Adolescent Competency to Make Health Care Decisions

Adolescents who are willing to involve parents in their abortion decisions will likely benefit from adult experience, wisdom, and support. Legislation requiring mandatory parental consent or notification for abortion presupposes, however, that pregnant minors are not competent to make informed decisions and therefore require legal protection. The age of 18 years is a convenient legal dividing line, but it has no scientific validity as the point at which individuals become competent decision makers. Summaries of well-designed research conclude that most minors 14 to 17 years of age are as competent as adults to provide consent to abortion. They are able to understand the risks and benefits of options and to make voluntary, rational, independent decisions.[31-33] Once pregnant, an adolescent by most state laws is considered an "emancipated minor" and is held responsible and competent to consent to her own medical treatment during the pregnancy and to the medical decisions regarding her fetus or newborn (eg, amniocentesis, genetic testing, lifesaving treatment, and circumcision). No state laws require the minor's parent to consent to the minor's decision to continue the pregnancy when the parent thinks that terminating the pregnancy is in the minor's best interest or, with few exceptions, to place the infant for adoption. It is inconsistent, then, to presume that the minor is not legally competent to make decisions regarding pregnancy termination.[24,31,34]

LEGAL ISSUES

The legal issues involved in a minor's right to confidential abortion care have been well covered in other reviews.[35-38] The vast majority of court opinions and legal analyses hold that the justifications presented for mandatory parental involvement in a minor's abortion decision are not sufficiently compelling to outweigh the minor's right to privacy in deciding whether to terminate a pregnancy.[39] Teenagers perceive no difference in legal requirements for consent versus notification. Both abridge confidentiality. All analyses confirm that confidential care for adolescents is critical to improving their health. There is a "remarkable degree of consensus that adolescents should have access to confidential health services and that parental involvement, consent, or notification should not be a barrier to care."[9] There is substantial legal consensus that parental consent and notification laws, whether or not ruled constitutional, run counter to fundamental principles of family law, which ideally seek to protect the privacy of family decision making from government interference and to protect the best interests of the minor in the circumstances when the government does intervene in family affairs.[39]

Concerns About Psychological or Physical Consequences of Abortion Decisions

Some adults support mandatory parent notification, thinking that it will protect the adolescent from making a decision she might regret later. Most adolescents, however, express satisfaction with their ultimate pregnancy decisions, providing they think that the decisions were their own. No significant differences in the levels of later satisfaction with their decisions have been found between adolescents who choose abortion and those who bear children or between those who parent as opposed to those who place their infants for adoption; almost all think that they made the right choices for themselves.[40-42] The key determinant of this expressed satisfaction is the sense of "ownership" over the pregnancy decisions and the belief that their choices were not the results of coercion.[42] In other research, pregnant adolescents who chose not to communicate with parents were as satisfied with their decisions as those who did consult with parents and received support for their decisions.[20] Adolescents who communicated with nonsupportive parents were the ones more likely to express dissatisfaction with pregnancy decisions.

Extensive reviews conclude that there are no documented negative psychological or medical sequelae to elective, legal, first-trimester abortion among teenaged women.[43,44] No significant psychological sequelae have been substantiated, despite extensive searches of the scientific literature.[45-47] When facing an unwanted pregnancy, regardless of the ultimate outcome, most women experience a range of normal emotional reactions, including regret, mild depression, and anxiety. Adverse reactions after abortion are rare; most women experience relief and reduced depression and distress.[48] Some women may experience feelings of grief and guilt after termination of pregnancies, especially those who consider themselves deeply religious or who were ambivalent about their decisions, and they may benefit from appropriate therapeutic counseling.[49] The incidence of diagnosed psychiatric illness and hospitalization is considerably lower after abortion than after childbirth. Psychiatric disorders, when found, have been attributed to preexisting psychiatric illness, undergoing abortion under coercion or pressure, or concomitant highly stressful life circumstances, including abandonment.[46]

The medical risks of legal first-trimester abortion likewise are extremely low. Mortality risks seem to be five times greater for teenagers who continue their pregnancies than they are for teens who terminate them. Morbidity rates and medical complications from continuing a pregnancy are more adverse than those from abortion at all stages of gestation.[48,50] The scientific evidence indicates that legal abortion results in fewer deleterious sequelae for women compared with other possible outcomes of unwanted pregnancy. There is no rational basis for policies that put barriers in the way of an adolescent's selection of abortion because of concerns about physical or psychological consequences.

Adverse Effects of Mandatory Parental Involvement Legislation

Mandatory parental consent or notification laws do not protect the health of young women and, in fact, may do harm.

ADVERSE HEALTH IMPACT

The most damaging impact of mandatory parental notification laws is that they can delay and obstruct the access of pregnant adolescents to timely professional advice and medical care.[5,48] Teenagers are twice as likely as adults to delay the diagnosis of first-trimester pregnancy. Adolescents are often confused about their right to confidential care, and even a perceived lack of confidentiality in health care regarding sexual issues deters them from seeking services.[51] Once the minor does present for pregnancy counseling, mandatory parental involvement laws can delay medical care further. After enactment of such statutes, court proceedings in Massachusetts delayed the termination of pregnancy by as much as 6 weeks; in Minnesota, the average delay was 1 to 3 weeks, and the proportion of second-trimester abortions in teens increased by 12%.[48] In Mississippi, a parental consent requirement increased by 19% the ratio of minors to adults who underwent their procedures after 12 weeks' gestation.[52] Later-trimester procedures (after 14 weeks) increase both the medical risks and financial costs to the patient, and a prolonged delay can eliminate abortion as an accessible option.[50]

It is likely that mandatory parental consent legislation decreases access to abortion by adolescents, although confounding variables make it difficult to ascertain causal effects on abortion rates. Both abortion rates and abortion ratios have decreased nationwide in states with and without parental consent statutes. In Minnesota, after parental consent laws were enacted in 1981, at first it seemed that abortion rates decreased disproportionately in 15- to 17-year-olds, but with no increase in birth rates, leading some to hypothesize that teenagers were more motivated to avoid pregnancy.[53] However, after the Supreme Court upheld Minnesota's consent laws in 1990,[3] abortion rates in minors fell to the lowest level in 10 years, and birth rates for the same age group rose to the highest level since 1980 (*St Paul Dispatch.* June 30, 1992).

ADVERSE PSYCHOLOGICAL AND SOCIAL IMPACT

There is increasing evidence of the negative effects of delayed or denied abortion on both the emotional health of the mothers and the developmental status of the unwanted children. Later-stage abortions are associated with a greater risk of psychological sequelae for pregnant teenagers (compared with first-trimester abortions, which are without significant negative sequelae).[54] American studies have recently confirmed European research that women who are denied abortions only rarely give up their unwanted infants for adoption and may harbor resentment and anger toward their children for years. Despite strong social pressure not to acknowledge that a child is unwanted, more than one third of the women confessed to having strong negative feelings toward their children. Compared with the offspring of willing parents, the children of women who did not obtain requested abortions were much more likely to be troubled and depressed, to drop out of school, to commit crimes, and to have serious illnesses.[55,56] Compared with peers who terminate their pregnancies, adolescents who bear children are at significantly higher risk of educational deficits, economic disadvantage, and marital instability.[41,48]

ADVERSE FAMILY IMPACT

As discussed, parental involvement can have adverse effects on both minors and their families, particularly if it takes on a coercive character. The risks of violence, abuse, coercion, unresolved conflict, and rejection are significant in nonsupportive or dysfunctional families when parents are informed of a pregnancy against the adolescent's considered judgment.[1,30] In *Hodgson vs Minnesota,* the majority of the Supreme Court found that mandatory parental involvement can result in family upheaval and can be dangerous for minors in homes where physical, emotional, or sexual abuse is present.[1,39]

JUDICIAL BYPASS

The option of obtaining a judicial bypass (a court proceeding in which a judge determines whether the adolescent is mature enough to make the decision to have an abortion or whether it is in her best interest not to inform parents) is viewed by some as a reasonable compromise to protect a concerned adolescent from harm while permitting states to impose mandatory parental involvement statutes.[5] The US Supreme Court ruled in 1990 that judicial bypass mechanisms are constitutionally required if state legislation is enacted, and they are ethically essential for adolescents at risk of abuse. However, judges who preside over bypass rulings testify unequivocally that this procedure is of no benefit to minors.[57,58] It has no effect on the ultimate decision with respect to abortion or on the process by which that decision is made. Of 12 000 petitions in Massachusetts and Minnesota, only 21 were denied, and half of the denials were overturned on appeal.[24] The judicial bypass process itself poses risks of medical and psychological harm. It is detrimental to medical well-being, because it causes further delays in access to medical treatment (from 4 days to several weeks), which increase the risk of complications from delayed or second-trimester procedures.[22] It is detrimental to emotional well-being, because adolescents perceive the court proceedings as extremely burdensome, humiliating, and stressful.[24] The pregnant adolescent is required to divulge intimate details of her private life to dozens of strangers (clerks, bailiffs, court reporters, witnesses, and others) to obtain a brief (10 minute) hearing before a judge who has no firsthand knowledge of her case and typically no training in counseling adolescents or developmental issues.[39] Regardless of the Supreme Court ruling, many legal opinions hold that the judicial bypass process constitutes "undue burden" for adolescents seeking abortion care.[22,24,39]

Conclusions and Recommendations

1. Adolescents should be strongly encouraged to involve their parents and other trusted adults in decisions regarding pregnancy termination, and the majority of them voluntarily do so. A minor's decision to involve parents is determined

by the quality of the family relationship, not by laws. Family communication is inherently a family responsibility, and parents themselves create the emotional atmosphere that fosters productive dialogue. Adolescents who feel loved and supported by their parents normally will communicate with them in times of crisis. Studies show that adolescents are most likely to disclose their pregnancies if the family hasa history of warmth, rapport, and involvement of parents in past problem solving.[25,26] As emphasized in previous AAP position statements, enhancing parental skills for listening, communicating, valuing, and nurturing throughout the childhood years is the most effective means of ensuring family involvement in adolescent decisions.[1,59] The pediatrician's most valued role may be to strengthen these family communication skills and supportive behaviors.

2. Concerned professionals should make every effort to ensure that a pregnant teenager receives adult guidance and support when considering all the options available, so she can make the decision that is in her best interest. This is best achieved by adhering to existing professional ethics and standards for obtaining meaningful informed consent.[60] Physicians should ensure that the minor patient has full information and has given careful consideration to the issues involved. They should encourage minors to consult with parents, other family members, or other trusted adults if parental support is not possible. The very young adolescent is especially needy in this regard. Ultimately, the pregnant patient's right to decide should be respected regarding who should be involved and what the outcome of the pregnancy will be, which is the approach most consistent with ethical, legal, and health care principles.

3. The AAP reaffirms its position that the rights of adolescents to confidential care when considering abortion should be protected. Genuine concern for the best interests of minors argues strongly against mandatory parental consent and notification laws. Although the stated intent of mandatory parental consent laws is to enhance family communication and parental responsibility, there is no supporting evidence that the laws have these effects. No evidence exists that legislation mandating parental involvement against the adolescent's wishes has any added benefit in improving productive family communication or affecting the outcome of the decision. There is evidence that such legislation may have an adverse impact on some families and that it increases the risk of medical and psychological harm to the adolescent. Judicial bypass provisions do not ameliorate the risk.

4. The AAP reaffirms its support of measures that increase access to health care for children and youths, regardless of age or financial status, and opposes unnecessary regulations that limit or delay access to care. The documented impact of parental consent laws is to reduce minors' access to early legal abortion. Public policies should encourage sexually active adolescents to seek timely, professional health care. The threat of compelled parental notification against the adolescent's wishes, even if judicial bypass is available, is a strong disincentive to seeking care. The AAP holds that public policies can and should encourage voluntary involvement of parents or other mature adults, but specific laws mandating notification of biological parents or legal guardians as a condition of service are counterproductive.[57]

COMMITTEE ON ADOLESCENCE, 1995 to 1996
Marianne E. Felice, MD, Chair
Suzanne Boulter, MD
Edward M. Gotlieb, MD
James C. Hoyle, Jr, MD
Luis F. Olmedo, MD
I. Ronald Shenker, MD
Barbara C. Staggers, MD

LIAISON REPRESENTATIVES
Richard Sarles, MD
    American Academy of Child and
    Adolescent Psychiatry
Diane Sacks, MD
    Canadian Paediatric Society

Richard E. Smith, MD
American College of Obstetricians
and Gynecologists

SECTION LIAISON

Samuel Leavitt, MD
Section on School Health

CONSULTANTS

Roberta K. Beach, MD
Donald E. Greydanus, MD

References

1. American Academy of Pediatrics, Committee on Adolescence. Counseling the adolescent about pregnancy options. *Pediatrics.* 1989;83:135–137

2. Fleming GV, O'Conner KG. Adolescent abortion: views of the membership of the American Academy of Pediatrics. *Pediatrics.* 1993;91:561–565

3. *Hodgson v Minnesota,* 110 S 2926 (Ct 1990)

4. *Planned Parenthood of Southeastern Pennsylvania v Casey,* 112 S 2791 (Ct 1992)

5. Council on Ethical and Judicial Affairs, American Medical Association. Mandatory parental consent to abortion. *JAMA.* 1993;269:82–86

6. Society for Adolescent Medicine. Position statements on reproductive health care for adolescents. *J Adolesc Health.* 1991;12:657–661

7. American Public Health Association. Resolution 9001: adolescent access to comprehensive, confidential reproductive health care. *Am J Public Health.* 1991;81:241

8. American College of Obstetricians and Gynecologists, American Academy of Family Physicians, American Academy of Pediatrics, Organization for Obstetric, Gynecologic, and Neonatal Nurses, National Medical Association. Confidentiality in adolescent health care. *AAP News.* 1989;5:9

9. American Medical Association National Coalition on Adolescent Health, Gans JE, ed. *Policy Compendium on Confidential Health Services for Adolescents.* Chicago, IL: American Medical Association; 1993

10. Henshaw SK. Abortion trends in 1987 and 1988: age and race. *Fam Plann Perspect.* 1992;24:85–86, 96

11. National Center for Health Statistics. *Advance Report of Final Natality Statistics, 1990. Monthly Vital Statistics Report.* Hyattsville, MD: Public Health Service; 1993:41(9). US Dept of Health and Human Services publication PHS 931120

12. Bachrach CA, Stolley KS, London KA. Relinquishment of premarital births: evidence from national survey data. *Fam Plann Perspect.* 1992;24:27–32

13. Blum RW, Resnick MD. Adolescent sexual decision-making: contraception, pregnancy, abortion, and motherhood. *Pediatr Ann.* 1982;11:797–805

14. Zabin LS, Hirsch MB, Boscia JA. Differential characteristics of adolescent pregnancy test patients: abortion, childbearing, and negative test groups. *J Adolesc Health.* 1990;11:107–113

15. Plotnick RD. The effects of attitudes on teenage premarital pregnancy and its resolution. *Am Social Rev.* 1992; 57:800–811

16. Department of Government Relations, American College of Obstetricians and Gynecologists. *State Legislative Fact Sheet. State Abortion Laws 1989-1992.* Washington, DC: American College of Obstetricians and Gynecologists; 1993

17. Benshoof J. *Planned Parenthood v Casey:* the impact of the new undue burden standard on reproductive health care. *JAMA.* 1993;269:2249–2257

18. Worthington EL Jr, Larson DB, Lyons JS, et al. Mandatory parental involvement prior to adolescent abortion. *J Adolesc Health.* 1991;12:138–142

19. Henshaw SK, Kost K. Parental involvement in minors' abortion decisions. *Fam Plann Perspect.* 1992;24: 196–207,213

20. Zabin LS, Hirsch MB, Emerson MR, Raymond E. To whom do inner-city minors talk about their pregnancies? Adolescents' communication with parents and parent surrogates. *Fam Plann Perspect.* 1992;24:148–154,173

21. Benshoof J, Pine RN, Paltrow LW, et al. *Brief for petitioners in Hodgson v Minnesota and Minnesota v Hodgson,* US Supreme Court, Ott 1989 term, cases 88–1125 and 88–1309:13–16

22. Donovan P. Judging teenagers: how minors fare when they seek court-authorized abortions. *Fam Plann Perspect.* 1983;15:259–267

23. Donovan PA. *Our Daughters' Decisions: The Conflict in State Law on Abortion and Other Issues.* New York, NY: Alan Guttmacher Institute; 1992

24. Crosby MC, English A. Mandatory parental involvement/judicial bypass laws: do they promote adolescents' health? *J Adolesc Health.* 1991;12:143–147

25. Blum RW, Resnick MD, Stark TA. The impact of parental notification law on adolescent abortion decision-making. *Am J Public Health.* 1987;77:619–620

26. Blum RW, Renick MD, Stark TA. Factors associated with the use of court bypass by minors to obtain abortions. *Fam Plann Perspect.* 1990;22:158–160

27. Cartoof VG, Klerman LV. Parental consent for abortion: impact of the Massachusetts law. *Am J Public Health.* 1986;76:397–400

28. Binkin N, Gold J, Gates W Jr. Illegal-abortion deaths in the United States: why are they still occurring? *Fam Plann Perspect.* 1982;14:163–167

29. *Missouri Monthly Vital Statistics.* Jefferson City, MO: Missouri Department of Health; 1990:23

30. Declaration of Lenore E. Walker, PhD, *American Academy of Pediatrics v VandeKamp,* 214 App 3d831 (Cal 1989), filed Nov 23, 1987

31. Moreno JD. Treating the adolescent patient: an ethical analysis. *J Adolesc Health Care.* 1989;10:454–459

32. Ambuel B, Rappaport J. Developmental trends in adolescents' psychological and legal competence to consent to abortion. *Law Hum Behav.* 1992;16:129–154

33. Weithorn LA, Campbell SB. The competency of children and adolescents to make informed treatment decisions. *Child Dev.* 1982;53:1589–1598

34. American College of Obstetricians and Gynecologists, Moore KG, ed. *Public Health Policy Implications of Abortion.* Washington, DC: American College of Obstetricians and Gynecologists; 1990

35. English A. Treating adolescents: legal and ethical considerations. *Med Clin North Am.* 1990;74:1097–1112

36. Holder AR. *Legal Issues in Pediatrics and Adolescent Medicine.* 2nd ed. New Haven, CT: Yale University Press; 1985

37. Holder AR. Minors' rights to consent to medical care. *JAMA.* 1987;257:3400–3402

38. Council on Scientific Affairs, American Medical Association. Confidential health services for adolescents. *JAMA.* 1993;269:1420–1424

39. Greenberger MD, Conner K. Parental notice and consent for abortion: out of step with family law principles and policies. *Fam Plann Perspect.* 1991;23:31–35

40. Resnick MD. Adolescent pregnancy options. *J Sch Health.* 1992;62:298–303

41. Zabin LS, Hirsch MB, Emerson MR. When urban adolescents choose abortion: effects on education, psychological status, and subsequent pregnancy. *Fam Plann Perspect.* 1989;21:248–255

42. Resnick MD, Blum RW, Bose J, Smith M, Toogood R. Characteristics of unmarried adolescent mothers: determinants of child rearing versus adoption. *Am J Orthopsychiatry.* 1990;60:577–584

43. Zabin LS, Sedivy V. Abortion among adolescents: research findings and the current debate. *J Sch Health.* 1992;62:319–324

44. Hardy JB, Zabin LS. *Adolescent Pregnancy in an Urban Environment: Issues, Programs, and Evaluation.* Washington, DC: Urban Institute Press; 1991

45. American Psychological Association. *Psychological Sequelae of Abortion.* Washington, DC: American Psychological Association; 1987

46. Stotland NL. The myth of the abortion trauma syndrome. *JAMA.* 1992;268:2078–2079

47. Blumenthal SJ. An overview of research findings. In: Stotland NL, ed. *Psychiatric Aspects of Abortion.* Washington, DC: American Psychiatric Press; 1991

48. Council on Scientific Affairs, American Medical Association. Induced terminations of pregnancy before and after *Roe v Wade:* trends in mortality and morbidity of women. *JAMA.* 1992;268:3231–3239

49. Tentoni SC. A therapeutic approach to reduce postabortion grief in university women. *J Am Coll Health.* 1995; 44:35–37

50. Gates W Jr, Grimes DA. Morbidity and mortality of abortion in the United States. In: Hodgson JE, ed. *Abortion and Sterilization: Medical and Social Aspects.* New York, NY: Academic Press, Inc; 1981:155–180

51. Cheng TL, Savageau JA, Sattler AL, Dewitt TG. Confidentiality in health care: a survey of knowledge, perceptions, and attitudes among high school students. *JAMA.* 1993;269:1404–1407

52. Henshaw SK. The impact of requirements for parental consent on minors' abortions in Mississippi. *Fam Plann Perspect.* 1995;27:120–122

53. Rogers JL, Boruch RF, Stems GB, DeMoya D. Impact of the Minnesota parental notification law on abortion and birth. *Am J Public Health.* 1991;81:294–298

54. Cates W Jr. Adolescent abortions in the United States. *J Adolesc Health.* 1980;1:18–25

55. Dagg PK. The psychological sequelae of therapeutic abortion—denied and completed. *Am J Psychiatry.* 1991; 148:578–585

56. David HP, Dytrych Z, Matejek Z, Schuller V, eds. *Born Unwanted: Developmental Effects of Denied Abortion.* New York, NY: Springer Publishing Co; 1988

57. *American Academy of Pediatrics v Lungren,* San Francisco 884–574 (Cal 1992)

58. Teare C. California affirms minors' right to abortion. *Youth Law News.* 1994;15(4):1–3

59. American Academy of Pediatrics, Committee on School Health and Committee on Adolescence. Education of the family. *AAP News.* 1986;11:14

60. American Academy of Pediatrics, Committee on Bioethics. Informed consent, parental permission, and assent in pediatric practice. *Pediatrics.* 1995;95:314–317

HIPAA and Adolescent Privacy in a Nutshell

Edward M. Gotlieb M.D., F.A.A.P., F.S.A.M.

The Final Privacy Rule of the Health Insurance Portability and Accountability Act of 1996 went into effect in the United States on April 14, 2003. Although HIPAA privacy rules apply generally to all, there are specific areas of HIPAA which are different, or differently applied to adolescent patients, and specifically those considered to be "emancipated minors."

The Personal Representative has the right to limit access to protected health information under HIPAA.

A minor's parent or guardian, or the adolescent himself or herself, if specified by state law, is considered to be the minor's "personal representative," and has control over protected health information.

> "Where the parent, guardian, or other person acting in loco parentis, is not the personal representative...and where there is no applicable access provision under State or other law, including case law, a covered entity may provide or deny access...to a parent, guardian, or other person acting in loco parentis, if such action is consistent with State or other applicable law, provided that such decision must be made by a licensed health care professional, in the exercise of professional judgment."
>
> under paragraphs (g)(3)(i)(A), (B), or (C) of this section under Sec. 164.524

Generally, State Law governs adolescent privacy. A licensed health care provider may use professional discretion in certain cases.

- The privacy rule contained in HIPAA states "[S]tate law governs disclosures to parents. In cases where state law is silent or unclear, the revisions would preserve state law and professional practice by permitting a health care provider to use discretion to provide or deny a parent access to such records as long as that decision is consistent with state or other law."

- HIPAA "allows a covered health care provider to choose not to treat a parent as a personal representative of the minor when the provider is concerned about abuse or harm to the child." (Sec. 164.502(g)(5).)

- "...a covered provider may disclose health information about a minor to a parent in the most critical situations, even if one of the limited exceptions discussed above apply. Disclosure of such information is always permitted as necessary to avert a serious and imminent threat to the health or safety of the minor." (Sec. 164.512(j).)

An adolescent's parent may cede confidentiality to the adolescent.

- HIPAA "allows the minor to exercise control of protected health information when the parent has agreed to the minor obtaining confidential treatment" Sec. 164.502 (g)(3)(i)(C)

The Use of Chaperones During the Physical Examination of the Pediatric Patient

Committee on Practice and Ambulatory Medicine

ABSTRACT. The intent of this statement is to inform practitioners about the purpose and scope of an appropriate physical examination for children, adolescents, and young adults, and the need to communicate this information to the parents and the patient. Issues of patient comfort, confidentiality, and the use of a chaperone are addressed. An appropriate physical examination should result in efficient, sensitive, and effective health care.

An appropriate physical examination is often a critical component of a visit to the pediatrician by a child, adolescent, or young adult. There are multiple goals of the physical examination, including detection of developmental delays and/or physical abnormalities, which may be congenital or acquired, and detection of clues to the cause of a current illness. The extent of the examination is determined by both the reason for the visit and by diagnostic considerations raised during the history taking. Some physical examinations will be highly focused and the child, adolescent, or young adult will be fully clothed. At other times, during a physical examination, the patient may be partially or completely unclothed. In these cases an appropriate gown should be provided.

The purpose and scope of the physical examination should be made clear to the parents. It should also be made clear to the patient if he or she is old enough to understand. If any part of the examination will be physically or psychologically uncomfortable, the parents and patient should be so informed in advance of the examination. Similarly, the pediatrician must be sensitive to the patient's and parent's feelings about an examination, particularly if the breasts, ano-rectal area, and/or genitalia require inspection or palpation. In some cases, either the patient, the parent,

the pediatrician, or some combination of these persons may wish to have a chaperone present. In those cases, the chaperone protects the interest of the patient and the pediatrician. However, there are a variety of circumstances, including those in which the patient requests confidentiality, that would render the presence of a chaperone problematic. Physician judgment and discretion must be paramount in evaluating the needs for a chaperone; however, the highest priority should be given to the requests of the patient and the parent. If a patient is offered and declines the use of a chaperone, the pediatrician should document this fact in the chart. Communication in advance regarding the components of the physical examination being performed is of critical importance in any event.

Attention to these principles should result in more efficient, sensitive, and effective health care for children, adolescents, and young adults while preventing misunderstandings about the reasons for and conduct of the examination.

COMMITTEE ON PRACTICE AND AMBULATORY MEDICINE, 1995 TO 1996

Peter D. Rappo, MD, Chairperson
Edward O. Cox, MD
John L. Green, MD
James W. Herbert, MD
E. Susan Hodgson, MD
James Lustig, MD
Thomas C. Olsen, MD
Jack T. Swanson, MD

AAP SECTION LIAISONS
A. D. Jacobson, MD, Section on Administration and Practice Management

---

PEDIATRICS (ISSN 0031 4005). Copyright © 1996 by the American Academy of Pediatrics.

Robert Sayers, MD, Section on Uniformed Services
Julia Richerson Atkins, MD, Resident Section

Lɪᴀɪsᴏɴ Rᴇᴘʀᴇsᴇɴᴛᴀᴛɪᴠᴇs
Todd Davis, MD, Ambulatory Pediatric Association
Michael O'Neill, MD, Canadian Paediatric Society

Section IX Further Reading

The **National Center for Youth Law** is a private, nonprofit law office serving the legal needs of children and their families.
www.youthlaw.org

The **Center for Adolescent Health & the Law** supports laws and policies that promote the health of adolescents and their access to comprehensive health care.
www.cahl.org

Index

A